D1601816

Atlas of **CLINICAL GASTROENTEROLOGY**

Third Edition

ELSEVIER CD-ROM LICENCE AGREEMENT

PLEASE READ THE FOLLOWING AGREEMENT CAREFULLY BEFORE USING THIS PRODUCT. THIS PRODUCT IS LICENSED UNDER THE TERMS CONTAINED IN THIS LICENCE AGREEMENT ('Agreement'). BY USING THIS PRODUCT, YOU, AN INDIVIDUAL OR ENTITY INCLUDING EMPLOYEES, AGENTS AND REPRESENTATIVES ('You' or 'Your'), ACKNOWLEDGE THAT YOU HAVE READ THIS AGREEMENT, THAT YOU UNDERSTAND IT, AND THAT YOU AGREE TO BE BOUND BY THE TERMS AND CONDITIONS OF THIS AGREEMENT. ELSEVIER LIMITED ('Elsevier') EXPRESSLY DOES NOT AGREE TO LICENSE THIS PRODUCT TO YOU UNLESS YOU ASSENT TO THIS AGREEMENT. IF YOU DO NOT AGREE WITH ANY OF THE FOLLOWING TERMS, YOU MAY, WITHIN THIRTY (30) DAYS AFTER YOUR RECEIPT OF THIS PRODUCT RETURN THE UNUSED PRODUCT AND ALL ACCOMPANYING DOCUMENTATION TO ELSEVIER FOR A FULL REFUND.

DEFINITIONS As used in this Agreement, these terms shall have the following meanings:

'Proprietary Material' means the valuable and proprietary information content of this Product including without limitation all indexes and graphic materials and software used to access, index, search and retrieve the information content from this Product developed or licensed by Elsevier and/or its affiliates, suppliers and licensors.

'Product' means the copy of the Proprietary Material and any other material delivered on CD-ROM and any other human-readable or machine-readable materials enclosed with this Agreement, including without limitation documentation relating to the same.

OWNERSHIP This Product has been supplied by and is proprietary to Elsevier and/or its affiliates, suppliers and licensors. The copyright in the Product belongs to Elsevier and/or its affiliates, suppliers and licensors and is protected by the copyright, trademark, trade secret and other intellectual property laws of the United Kingdom and international treaty provisions, including without limitation the Universal Copyright Convention and the Berne Copyright Convention. You have no ownership rights in this Product. Except as expressly set forth herein, no part of this Product, including without limitation the Proprietary Material, may be modified, copied or distributed in hardcopy or machine-readable form without prior written consent from Elsevier. All rights not expressly granted to You herein are expressly reserved. Any other use of this Product by any person or entity is strictly prohibited and a violation of this Agreement.

SCOPE OF RIGHTS LICENSED (PERMITTED USES) Elsevier is granting to You a limited, non-exclusive, non-transferable licence to use this Product in accordance with the terms of this Agreement. You may use or provide access to this Product on a single computer or terminal physically located at Your premises and in a secure network or move this Product to and use it on another single computer or terminal at the same location for personal use only, but under no circumstances may You use or provide access to any part or parts of this Product on more than one computer or terminal simultaneously.

You shall not (a) copy, download, or otherwise reproduce the Product or any part(s) thereof in any medium, including, without limitation, online transmissions, local area networks, wide area networks, intranets, extranets and the Internet, or in any way, in whole or in part, except for printing out or downloading nonsubstantial portions of the text and images in the Product for Your own personal use; (b) alter, modify, or adapt the Product or any part(s) thereof, including but not limited to decompiling, disassembling, reverse engineering, or creating derivative works, without the prior written approval of Elsevier; (c) sell, license or otherwise distribute to third parties the Product or any part(s) thereof; or (d) alter, remove, obscure or obstruct the display of any copyright, trademark or other proprietary notice on or in the Product or on any printout or download of portions of the Proprietary Materials.

RESTRICTIONS ON TRANSFER This Licence is personal to You, and neither Your rights hereunder nor the tangible embodiments of this Product, including without limitation the Proprietary Material, may be sold, assigned, transferred or sublicensed to any other person, including without limitation by operation of law, without the prior written consent of Elsevier. Any purported sale, assignment, transfer or sublicense without the prior written consent of Elsevier will be void and will automatically terminate the Licence granted hereunder.

TERM This Agreement will remain in effect until terminated pursuant to the terms of this Agreement. You may terminate this Agreement at any time by removing from Your system and destroying the Product and any copies of the Proprietary Material. Unauthorized copying of the Product, including without limitation, the Proprietary Material and documentation, or otherwise failing to comply with the terms and conditions of this Agreement shall result in automatic termination of this licence and will make available to Elsevier legal remedies. Upon termination of this Agreement, the licence granted herein will terminate and You must immediately destroy the Product and all copies of the Product and of the Proprietary Material, together with any and all accompanying documentation. All provisions relating to proprietary rights shall survive termination of this Agreement.

LIMITED WARRANTY AND LIMITATION OF LIABILITY Elsevier warrants that the software embodied in this Product will perform in substantial compliance with the documentation supplied in this Product, unless the performance problems are the result of hardware failure or improper use. If You report a significant defect in performance in writing to Elsevier within ninety (90) calendar days of your having purchased the Product, and Elsevier is not able to correct same within sixty (60) days after its receipt of Your notification, You may return this Product, including all copies and documentation, to Elsevier and Elsevier will refund Your money. In order to apply for a refund on your purchased Product, please contact the return address on the invoice to obtain the refund request form ('Refund Request Form'), and either fax or mail your signed request and your proof of purchase to the address indicated on the Refund Request Form. Incomplete forms will not be processed. Defined terms in the Refund Request Form shall have the same meaning as in this Agreement.

YOU UNDERSTAND THAT, EXCEPT FOR THE LIMITED WARRANTY RECITED ABOVE, ELSEVIER, ITS AFFILIATES, LICENSORS, THIRD PARTY SUPPLIERS AND AGENTS (TOGETHER 'THE SUPPLIERS') MAKE NO REPRESENTATIONS OR WARRANTIES, WITH RESPECT TO THE PRODUCT, INCLUDING, WITHOUT LIMITATION THE PROPRIETARY MATERIAL. ALL OTHER REPRESENTATIONS, WARRANTIES, CONDITIONS OR OTHER TERMS, WHETHER EXPRESS OR IMPLIED BY STATUTE OR COMMON LAW, ARE HEREBY EXCLUDED TO THE FULLEST EXTENT PERMITTED BY LAW.

IN PARTICULAR BUT WITHOUT LIMITATION TO THE FOREGOING NONE OF THE SUPPLIERS MAKE ANY REPRESENTIONS OR WARRANTIES (WHETHER EXPRESS OR IMPLIED) REGARDING THE PERFORMANCE OF YOUR PAD, NETWORK OR COMPUTER SYSTEM WHEN USED IN CONJUNCTION WITH THE PRODUCT, NOR THAT THE PRODUCT WILL MEET YOUR REQUIREMENTS OR THAT ITS OPERATION WILL BE UNINTERRUPTED OR ERROR-FREE.

EXCEPT IN RESPECT OF DEATH OR PERSONAL INJURY CAUSED BY THE SUPPLIERS' NEGLIGENCE AND TO THE FULLEST EXTENT PERMITTED BY LAW, IN NO EVENT (AND REGARDLESS OF WHETHER SUCH DAMAGES ARE FORESEEABLE AND OF WHETHER SUCH LIABILITY IS BASED IN TORT, CONTRACT OR OTHERWISE) WILL ANY OF THE SUPPLIERS BE LIABLE TO YOU FOR ANY DAMAGES (INCLUDING, WITHOUT LIMITATION, ANY LOST PROFITS, LOST SAVINGS OR OTHER SPECIAL, INDIRECT, INCIDENTAL OR CONSEQUENTIAL DAMAGES ARISING OUT OF OR RESULTING FROM: (I) YOUR USE OF, OR INABILITY TO USE, THE PRODUCT; (II) DATA LOSS OR CORRUPTION; AND/OR (III) ERRORS OR OMISSIONS IN THE PROPRIETARY MATERIAL.

IF THE FOREGOING LIMITATION IS HELD TO BE UNENFORCEABLE, OUR MAXIMUM LIABILITY TO YOU IN RESPECT THEREOF SHALL NOT EXCEED THE AMOUNT OF THE LICENCE FEE PAID BY YOU FOR THE PRODUCT. THE REMEDIES AVAILABLE TO YOU AGAINST ELSEVIER AND THE LICENSORS OF MATERIALS INCLUDED IN THE PRODUCT ARE EXCLUSIVE.

If the information provided in the Product contains medical or health sciences information, it is intended for professional use within the medical field. Information about medical treatment or drug dosages is intended strictly for professional use, and because of rapid advances in the medical sciences, independent verification of diagnosis and drug dosages should be made.

The provisions of this Agreement shall be severable, and in the event that any provision of this Agreement is found to be legally unenforceable, such unenforceability shall not prevent the enforcement or any other provision of this Agreement.

GOVERNING LAW This Agreement shall be governed by the laws of England and Wales. In any dispute arising out of this Agreement, you and Elsevier each consent to the exclusive personal jurisdiction and venue in the courts of England and Wales.

Atlas of CLINICAL GASTROENTEROLOGY

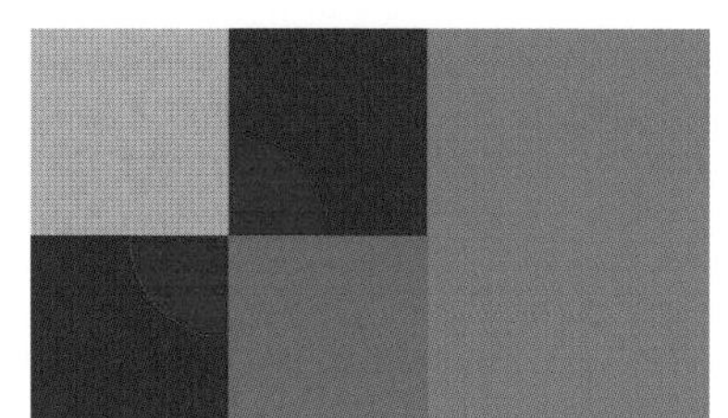

Third Edition

Alastair Forbes BSc MD FRCP ILTM
Consultant Gastroenterologist and Reader in Gastroenterology
Department of Medicine, St Mark's Academic Institute
St Mark's Hospital
London, UK

J J Misiewicz BSc MBBS FRCP
Consultant Physician
Department of Gastroenterology & Nutrition
Central Middlesex Hospital
London, UK

Carolyn C Compton MD PhD
Professor and Chair of Pathology
Department of Pathology
McGill University
Montreal, Canada

Marc S Levine MD
Professor of Radiology
Department of Radiology, University of Pennsylvania School of Medicine
Hospital of the University of Pennsylvania
Philadelphia, PA, USA

M Shafi Quraishy MBBS FRCP FRCP(Edin) FRCP&S(Glasg)
Gastroenterologist and Honorary Consultant in Teaching and Training
Department of Medicine, St Mark's Academic Institute
St Mark's Hospital
London, UK

Stephen E Rubesin MD
Professor of Radiology
Department of Radiology, University of Pennsylvania School of Medicine
Hospital of the University of Pennsylvania
Philadelphia, PA, USA

Paul J Thuluvath MD FRCP
Associate Professor of Medicine and Director of Liver Transplantation
Division of Gastroenterology
Johns Hopkins University
Baltimore, MA, USA

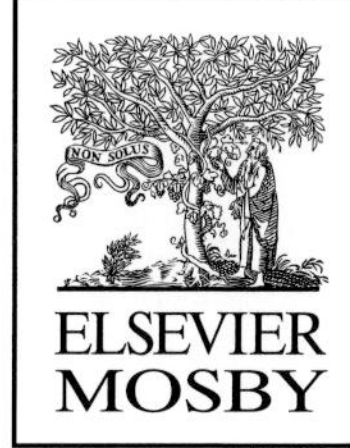

Edinburgh London New York Oxford Philadelphia St Louis Sydney Toronto 2005

ELSEVIER
MOSBY

An imprint of Elsevier Ltd

Second edition 1994
Third edition 2005

ISBN 07234283X

British Library Cataloguing in Publication Data
A catalogue record for this book is available from the British Library

Library of Congress Cataloging in Publication Data
A catalog record for this book is available from the Library of Congress

Notice
Medical knowledge is constantly changing. Standard safety precautions must be followed, but as new research and clinical experience broaden our knowledge, changes in treatment and drug therapy may become necessary or appropriate. Readers are advised to check the most current product information provided by the manufacturer of each drug to be administered to verify the recommended dose, the method and duration of administration, and contraindications. It is the responsibility of the practitioner, relying on experience and knowledge of the patient, to determine dosages and the best treatment for each individual patient. Neither the Publisher nor the authors assumes any liability for any injury and/or damage to persons or property arising from this publication.
The Publisher

Printed in Spain

Commissioning Editor: Rolla Couchman
Project Development Manager: Belinda Kuhn
Project Manager: Rory MacDonald
Illustration Manager: Mick Ruddy
Design Manager: Andy Chapman

The Publisher's policy is to use **paper manufactured from sustainable forests**

CONTENTS

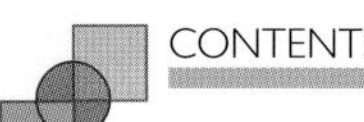

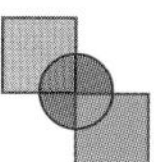

PREFACE

The third edition of the Atlas of Clinical Gastroenterology constitutes an extensive revision of the previous edition. The opportunity has been taken to bring the text and images up-to-date, and to incorporate advances – especially those in gastrointestinal imaging - made over the past 10 years.

The illustrations continue to provide extensive visual documentation of normal and abnormal anatomy, histology, endoscopy, and radiology of the alimentary tract, supported by relevant text. As before we do not intend the atlas to be a textbook of gastrointestinal or hepatobiliary disease, and it should not be used, or judged, as such. However, we anticipate that the notes and illustrations will form a useful and convenient source of information on the various aspects of the normal and abnormal alimentary tract. We are confident that the atlas and its electronic partner will again find an important place in gastrointestinal teaching at all levels.

Gastroenterology and hepatology are progressing rapidly, and technological advances in imaging techniques are key to the development of these specialities. Diagnostic procedures and methods are described, and histopathological, radiological, and endoscopic appearances are presented in some detail, reflecting their importance in practice. We would emphasise however that we have deliberately minimised the therapeutic aspects of the discipline. Pharmacology is not especially pictorial, and we did not feel that we could do justice to the potentially hazardous nature of many gastrointestinal interventions safely within the space available. Nonetheless we have shown some of the results of interventions, such as the endoscopic appearances of the post-operative stomach, since these may be a source of confusion to the inexperienced diagnostician.

The editors hope that readers will find the atlas useful and stimulating. We would like to thank the many colleagues who generously helped with the material included in this publication, and who are acknowledged in the text.

AF, CC, ML, SR, PT, SQ and JJM

ACKNOWLEDGEMENTS

The editors gratefully acknowledge all those who helped in the extensive revision of this atlas. Particular thanks are due to our colleagues at Elsevier for their graphic skills, for their close attention to the compilation of the comprehensive index, and for their support and encouragement throughout. It has proved a good partnership.

THE ESOPHAGUS

1

NORMAL ESOPHAGUS

The esophagus is a muscular tube connecting the oropharynx to the stomach. It begins at the lower margin of the cricopharyngeus muscle and is approximately 25 cm long. It is composed of striated muscle in the upper third, smooth muscle in the lower two thirds, and is lined throughout by squamous epithelium.

In the mediastinum, the esophagus is closely related to the two trunks of the vagus nerve, the trachea, the aorta, and the heart (Figs 1.1–1.4). Both aortic and left bronchial impressions can be visualized during a barium swallow examination (Fig. 1.5). In addition to demonstrating the normal mucosal pattern of the esophagus, a barium swallow may show a slight constriction approximately 2 cm above the diaphragm, below which is an area of dilatation known as the vestibule, or phrenic ampulla (Fig. 1.6). This area of dilatation should not be confused with the radiological appearances of hiatus hernia (see below). The esophagus enters the stomach at an angle, just below the diaphragmatic crura and approximately 40 cm from the incisor teeth.

Food is transported from the pharynx to the stomach by coordinated contraction of the muscular layers of the body of the esophagus. This peristaltic contraction wave is relatively slow and moves down the esophagus at a rate of 2–6 cm per second. When initiated by swallowing, it is known as primary peristalsis, as distinct from secondary peristalsis, which originates below the hypopharynx with no antecedent swallowing movement. The barrier functions of the esophagus depend on the upper cricopharyngeal sphincter and the lower esophageal sphincter (LES). The LES is a zone of high pressure (normally between 15 and 35 mmHg) extending over the lowest 3–4 cm of the esophagus; it has no definite anatomical

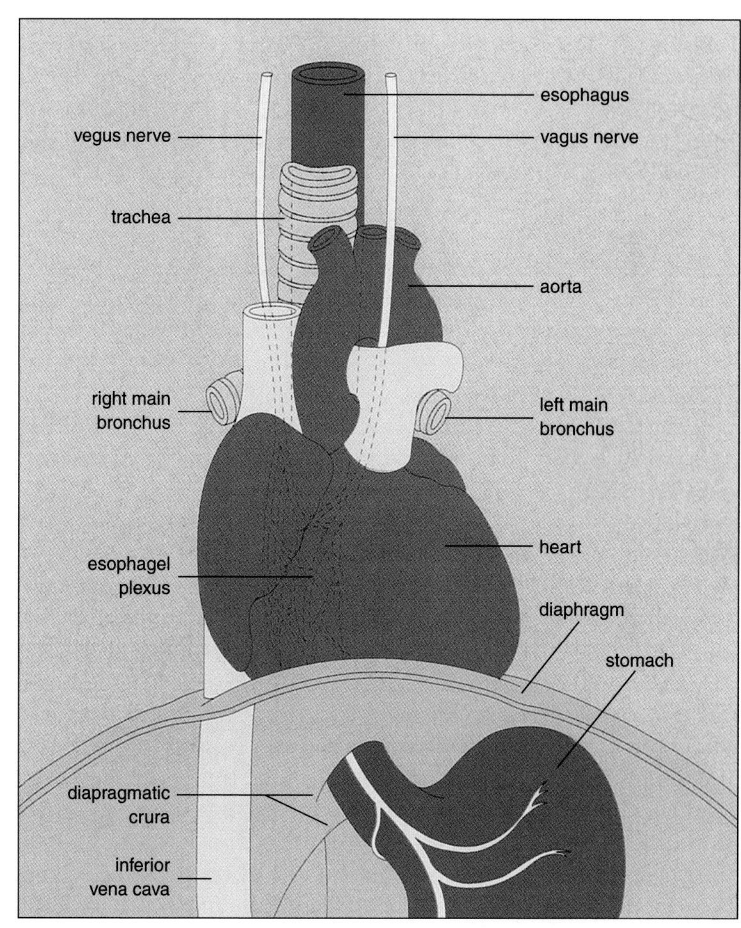

Fig. 1.1 Diagram showing the anatomical relations of the esophagus.

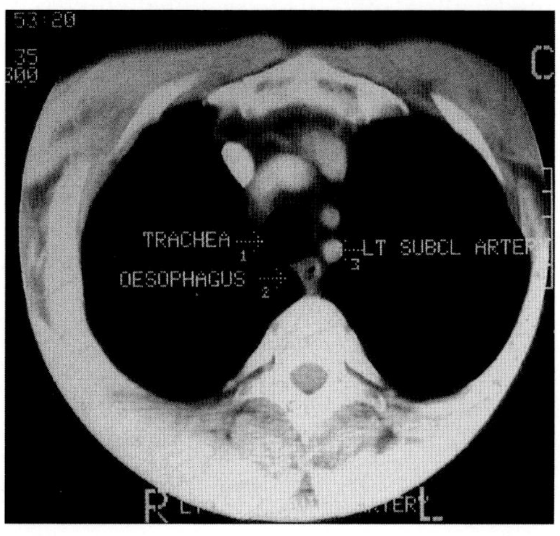

Fig. 1.2 Transverse CT scan of the thorax above the level of the tracheal bifurcation showing the relationship of the esophagus to the trachea and major vessels.

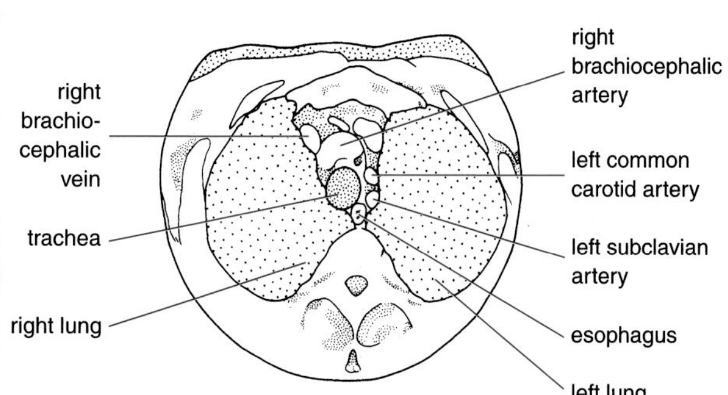

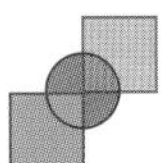

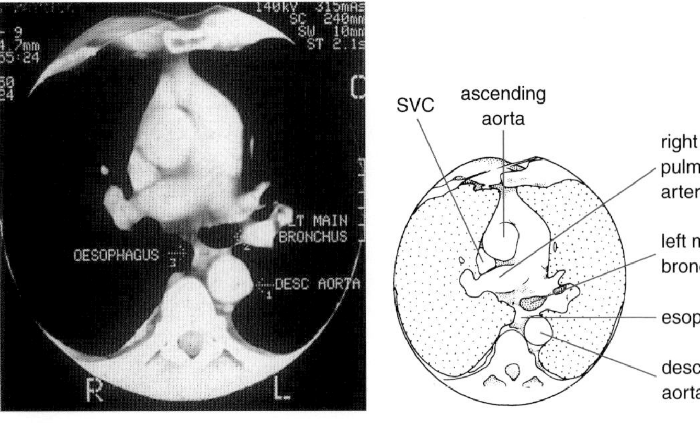

Fig. 1.3 Thoracic CT scan at the level of the aortic arch showing the relationship of its posterior part and of the left main bronchus to the esophagus.

counterpart. Manometric studies of esophageal motility are usually accomplished using a transnasal catheter (Fig. 1.7). On swallowing, the normal cricopharyngeus relaxes before passage of the bolus, and then contracts; this is followed by a peristaltic contraction along the body of the esophagus, and the LES relaxes just prior to the contraction wave reaching it, thus allowing passage of the bolus into the stomach (Fig. 1.8). The LES alone is not, however, sufficient to prevent gastro-esophageal reflux, and is aided by compression of the subdiaphragmatic portion of the esophagus as a result of a rise in intragastric or intra-abdominal pressure. The angled entry of the esophagus into the stomach is an additional protective factor.

The pH within the esophagus is usually 5–7, and prolonged periods with a pH of less than 4 are generally considered abnormal; assessment is best made by continuous 24 hour pH monitoring (Figs 1.9, 1.10).

Endoscopically, the body of the esophagus appears as a smooth featureless tube with visible submucosal blood vessels (Fig. 1.11). At the gastro-esophageal junction, the transition from esophageal to gastric mucosa is easily seen as an irregular circumferential line known as the Z-line (or the ora serrata, or gastric rosette) (Figs 1.12, 1.13). Peristaltic waves will often be seen during the examination.

The luminal surface of the esophagus is lined by non-keratinized squamous epithelium. Papillae, which are extensions of the lamina propria, penetrate for a short distance into the epithelium. The lamina propria is separated from the underlying submucosa by a thin layer of smooth muscle, the muscularis mucosae. The circular muscle layer is deep to the submucosa, the myenteric plexus lying between this and the outermost longitudinal muscle (Figs 1.14, 1.15).

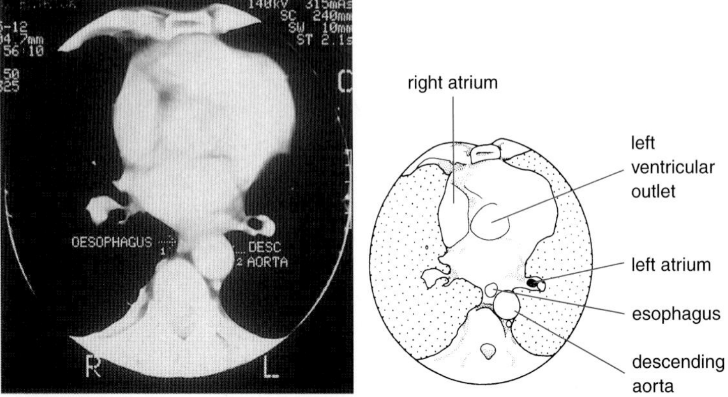

Fig. 1.4 Thoracic CT scan at the level of the left atrium showing the relationship of the esophagus to the aorta and the cardiac structures.

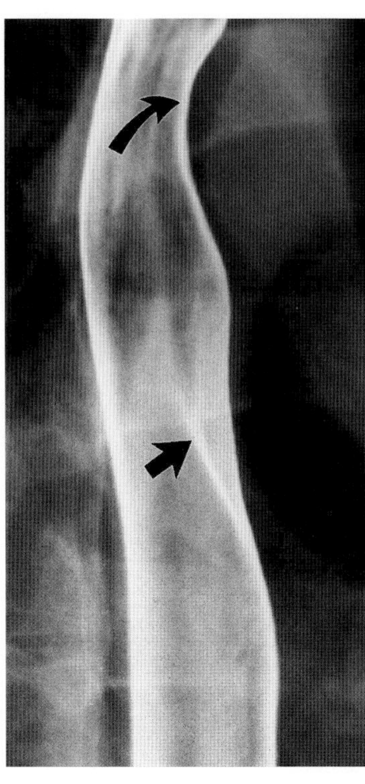

Fig. 1.5 Double-contrast esophagram showing normal indentations on the esophagus from the aortic arch (curved arrow) and the left main bronchus (straight arrow). (Reproduced with permission from reference 1).

DIVERTICULA

Gastrointestinal diverticula are pouches lined by one or more layers of the gut wall. They occur immediately above the upper esophageal sphincter (Zenker's diverticulum, or pharyngeal pouch), near the midpoint of the esophagus, and immediately above the lower esophageal sphincter (epiphrenic diverticulum). Their etiology is not clear, but the impression that abnormal motility and lack of co-ordination of sphincter relaxation are responsible for diverticula at the upper and lower ends of the esophagus has led to their designation as pulsion diverticula. Mid-esophageal diverticula, however, are thought to be due to traction from inflammatory adhesions within the mediastinum, quite commonly following tuberculosis.

The pharyngeal pouch (Zenker's diverticulum) has walls consisting only of esophageal mucosa prolapsing above or through the cricopharyngeus muscle (Figs 1.16, 1.17). It may become large enough to obstruct the esophageal lumen and thereby produce dysphagia (Fig. 1.18); aspiration of its contents can lead to serious respiratory complications. By contrast, mid-esophageal diverticula are frequently asymptomatic (Figs 1.19, 1.20). Symptoms from an epiphrenic diverticulum (Figs 1.21, 1.22) are thought to be related to the associated motor abnormalities, rather than to the presence of the diverticulum itself. Asymptomatic diverticula may be perforated at endoscopy if unrecognized, and the false lumen entered in error. Intramural diverticulosis is unlikely to be recognized endoscopically or to cause problems, but has characteristic appearances on barium swallow (Figs 1.23, 1.24). Post-infective pseudodiverticula are also seen (Fig. 1.24).

GASTRO-ESOPHAGEAL REFLUX

The reflux of gastric or intestinal contents into the esophagus may cause the symptoms of heartburn (pyrosis), and may be complicated by esophagitis, including Barrett's syndrome (see below), ulceration, and later strictures. Pathological gastro-esophageal reflux can occur with or without a hiatus hernia, and in a number of other conditions including pregnancy and scleroderma. Certain pharmacological agents and smoking are also strongly implicated. In all of

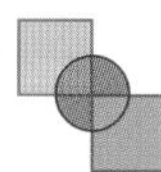

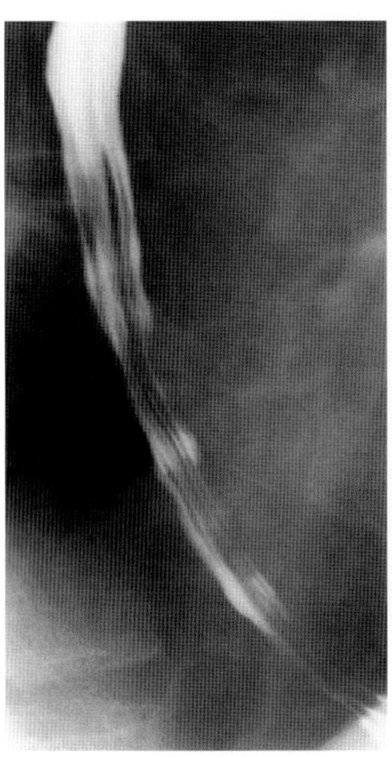

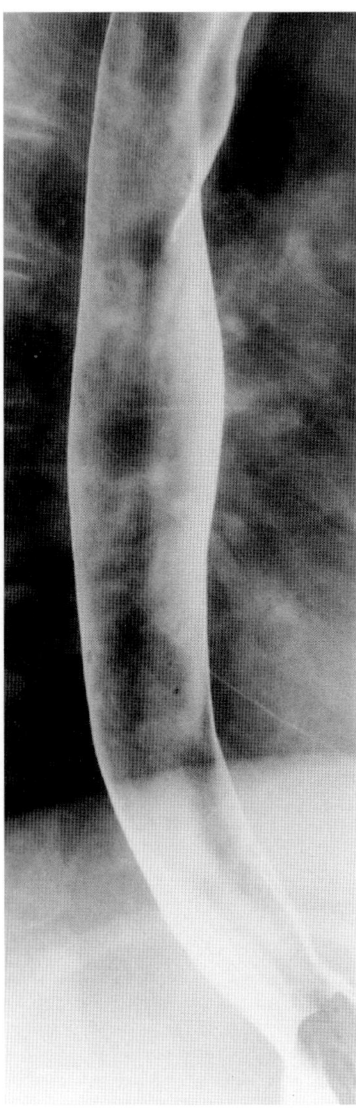

■ **Fig. 1.6** Double-contrast esophagram showing the normal appearance of the esophagus in the distended and contracted states. Note how the mucosa has a smooth, featureless appearance when the esophagus is distended (right) and how the folds are thin and straight when the esophagus is collapsed (left).

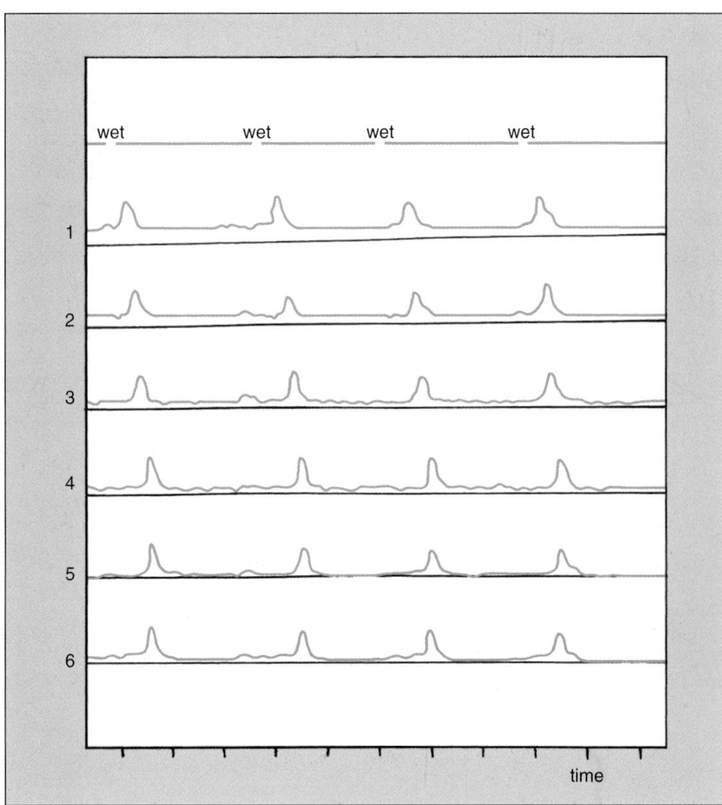

■ **Fig. 1.8** Manometry showing normal distal esophageal peristalsis. Channels 1–4 are at 5 cm intervals; channels 4–6 at 5 cm above lower esophageal sphincter. Marks on the horizontal axis represent 5-second intervals; intervals between grid lines on vertical axis represent 200 mmHg. Wet = swallows of 5 ml water. Courtesy of Dr J de Caestecker.

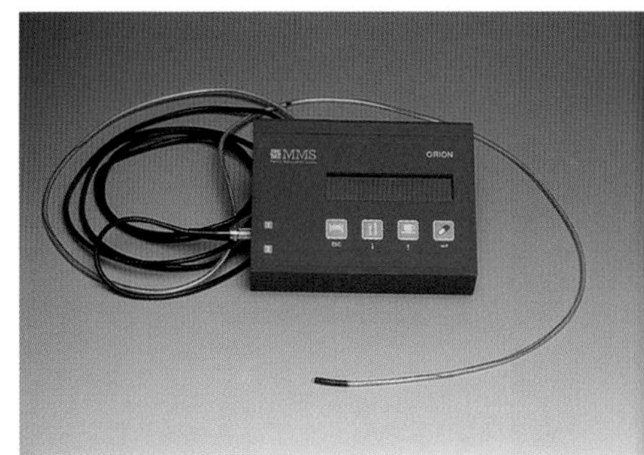

■ **Fig. 1.9** Equipment for 24-hour ambulatory esophageal pH measurement. The electrode shown in the foreground is passed transnasally. The blue recording device – which measures 11 x 8 cm – is carried on the patient's waistband during the study. Courtesy of Dr T Nicholls.

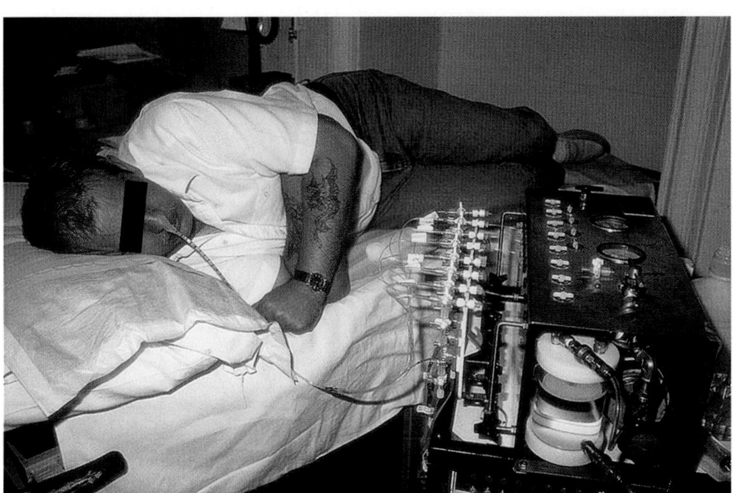

■ **Fig. 1.7** Patient undergoing esophageal manometry. The multiple pressure transducers are to the right (the computer and monitor screen are out of frame). Courtesy of Dr T Nicholls.

these situations there is decreased resting lower esophageal sphincter pressure. In patients with reflux, the pressure is typically 10 mmHg or less (compared with at least 15 mmHg in the normal individual). Reflux is readily demonstrated by pH studies (Fig. 1.25) and prolonged periods with a pH of less than 4 are clinically important (Fig. 1.26). The presence of reflux on barium swallow (Fig. 1.27) is not always associated with symptoms, but the 'herring-bone' or 'feline' pattern of multiple transverse folds (Fig. 1.28) correlates well with pathological reflux. Gastro-esophageal reflux may also be demonstrated by isotope techniques.

HIATUS HERNIA

A hiatus hernia is present when part of the stomach lies within the thoracic cavity above the diaphragm. Most herniae are of the sliding type, in which a variable portion of the stomach slides up through the diaphragmatic opening, so that the gastro-esophageal junction lies above the level of the diaphragm (Figs 1.29–1.31). This

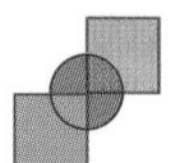

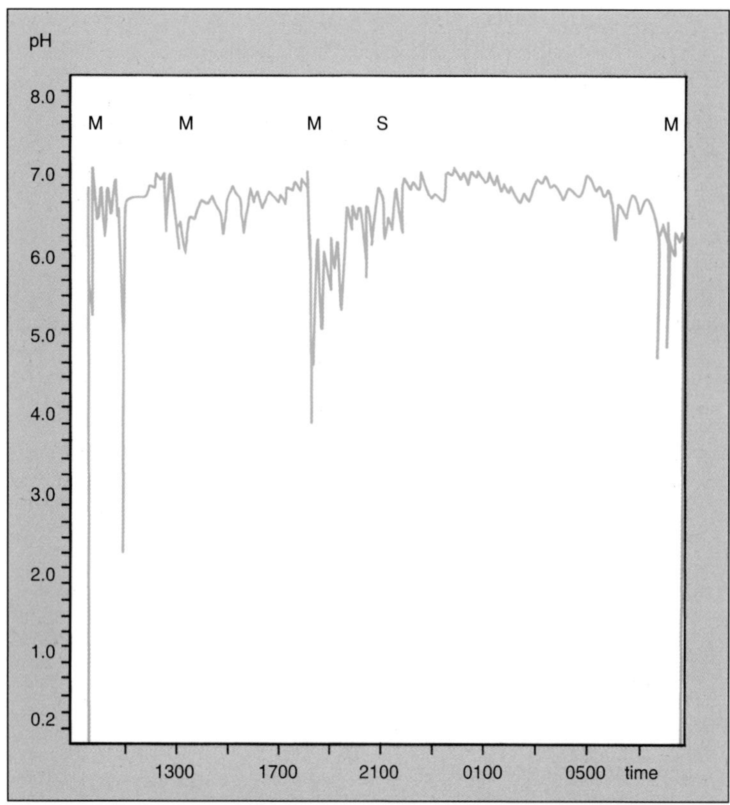

■ **Fig. 1.10** Normal 24-hour tracing. Time on horizontal axis; pH on vertical axis. M = meal; S = supine/sleep. Note some brief reflux events after meals. Courtesy of Dr J de Caestecker.

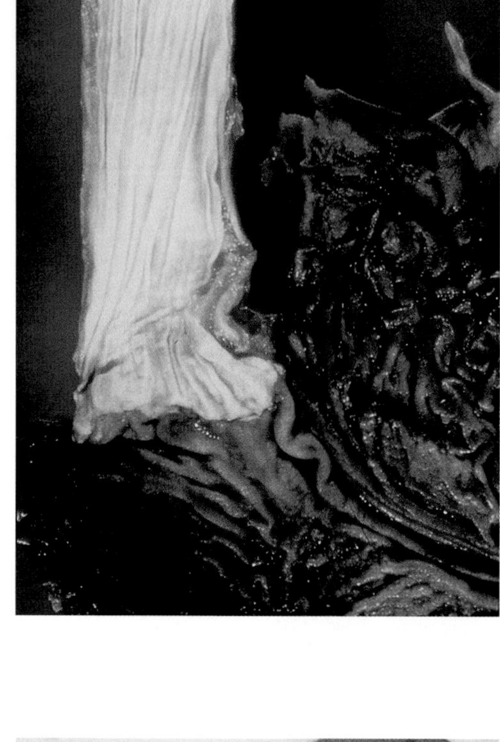

■ **Fig. 1.13** Normal esophagus. Macroscopic image of the normal esophagus showing smooth white-pink squamous mucosa and a sharply demarcated gastro-esophageal junction with a regular contour.

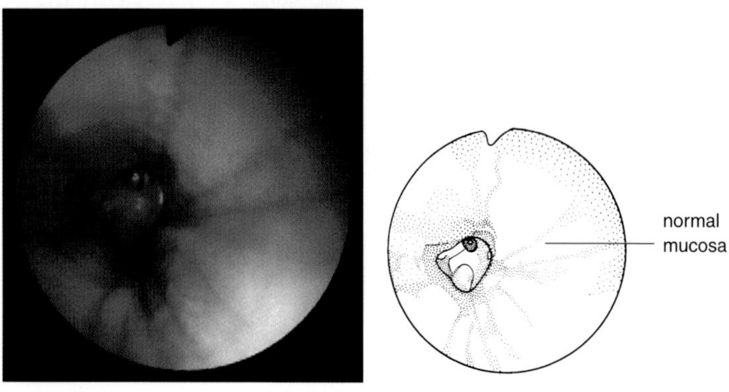

■ **Fig. 1.11** Endoscopic view of the normal body of the esophagus with pale pink mucosa.

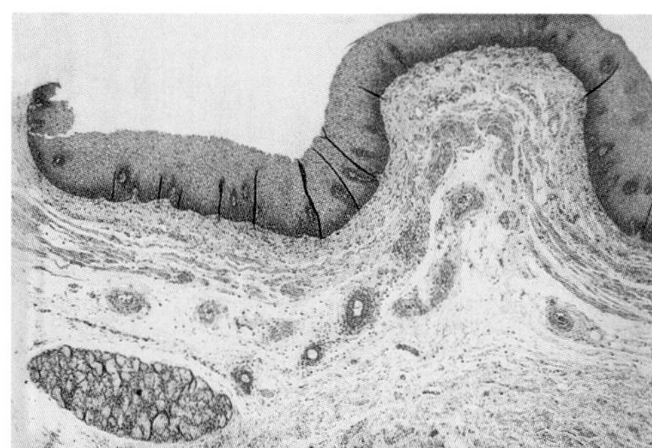

■ **Fig. 1.14** Histology of the normal distal esophagus showing non-keratinizing squamous mucosa and a mucin-producing submucosal gland with its excretory duct cuffed by small collections of lymphocytes.

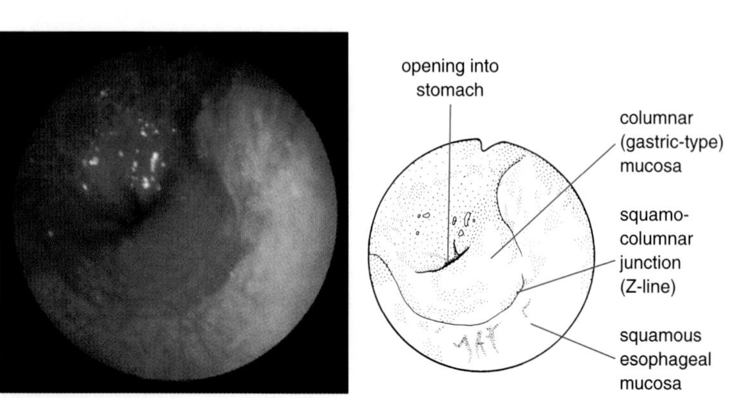

■ **Fig. 1.12** Normal squamo-columnar mucosal transition or Z-line.

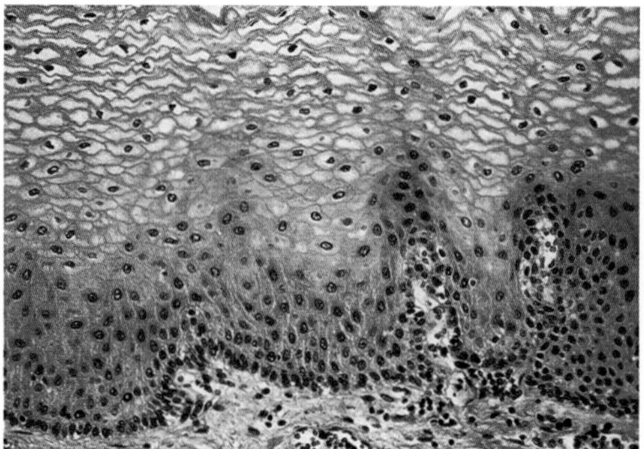

■ **Fig. 1.15** Normal esophageal epithelium, the basal aspect of which shows small immature squamous cells that acquire abundant, glycogen-rich (clear) cytoplasm as they mature towards the surface.

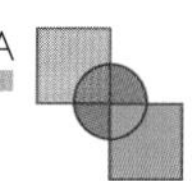

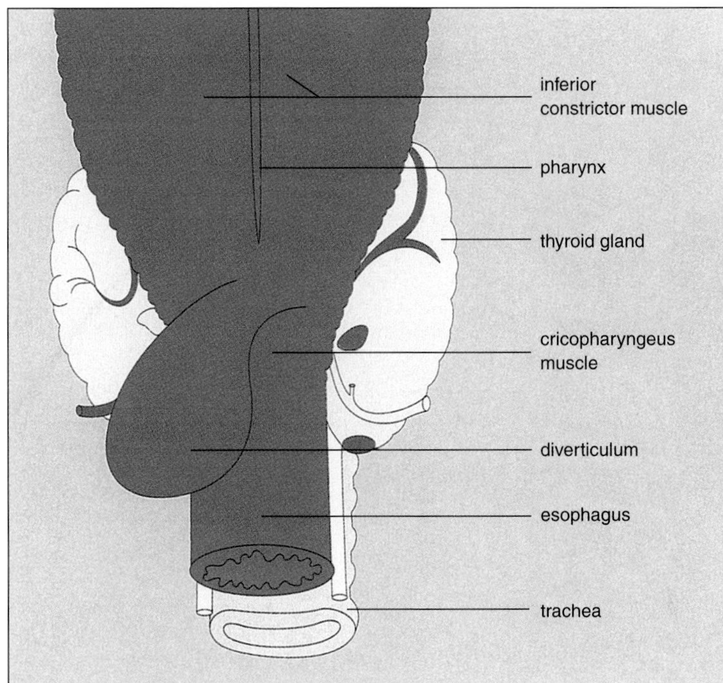

■ **Fig. 1.16** Diagram of a pharyngeal pouch protruding (typically to the left) between the oblique fibers of the inferior pharyngeal constrictor and the transverse cricopharyngeus muscle.

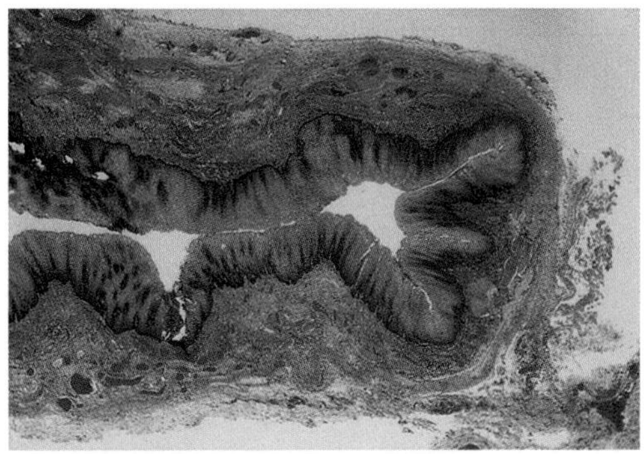

■ **Fig. 1.17** Histological appearance of a Zenker's diverticulum lined by mildly hyperplastic squamous mucosa with a mildly inflamed lamina propria and an attenuated muscularis mucosae.

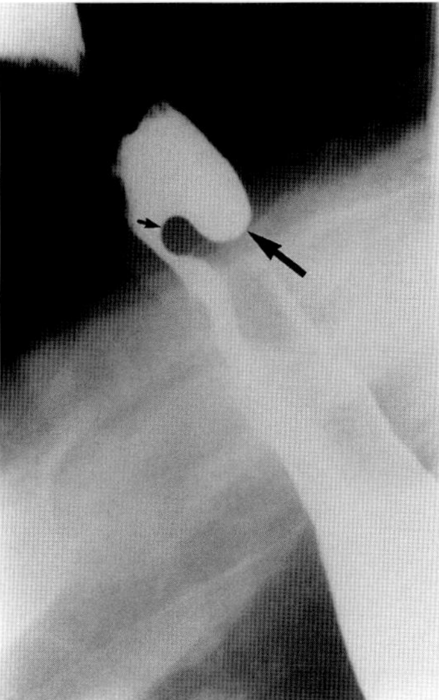

■ **Fig. 1.18** Barium swallow showing a Zenker's diverticulum as a focal out-pouching (large arrow) from the posterior aspect of the pharyngo-esophageal junction just above a prominent cricopharyngeus (small arrow) which fails to relax normally during swallowing.

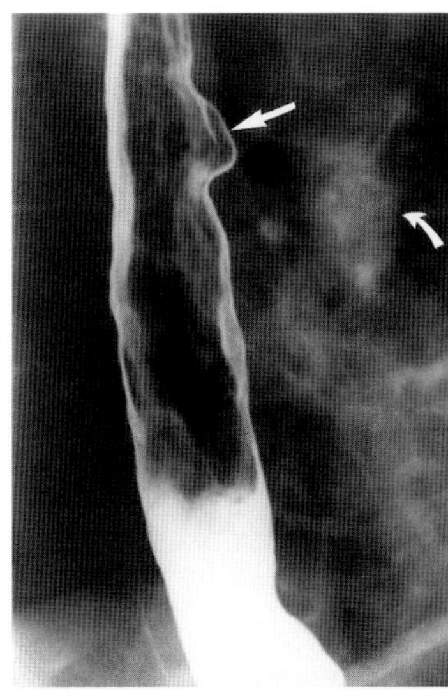

■ **Fig. 1.19** Double-contrast esophagram showing a traction diverticulum as a triangular out-pouching (straight arrow) from the left lateral wall of the mid esophagus due to scarring from old granulomatous disease. Note calcified lymph nodes (curved arrow) in the left hilum.

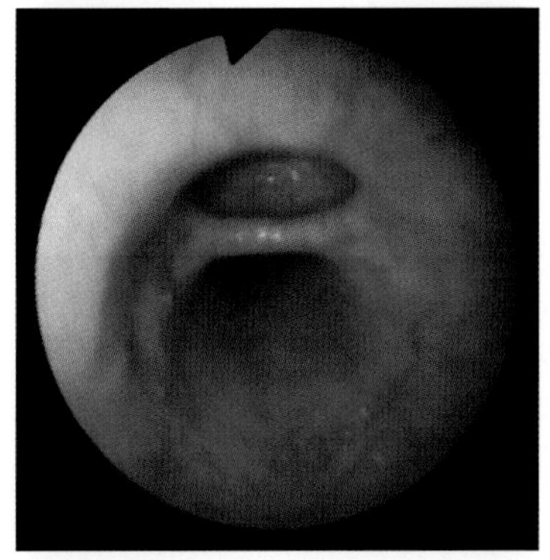

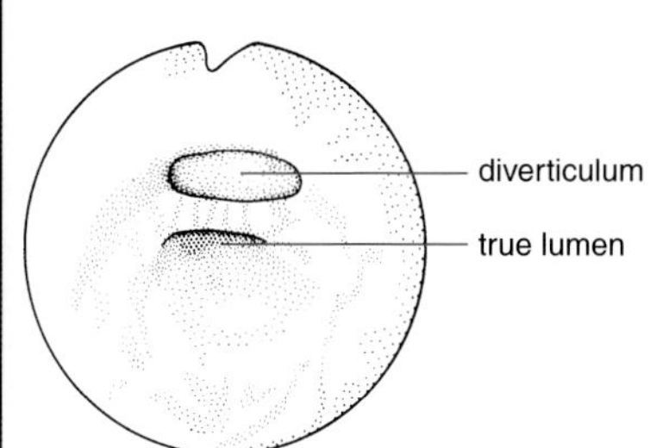

■ **Fig. 1.20** Endoscopic view of a mid-esophageal diverticulum.

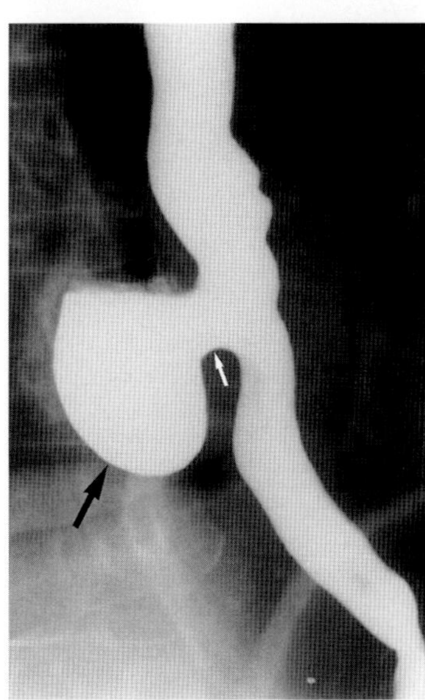

■ **Fig. 1.21** Double-contrast esophagram showing an epiphrenic diverticulum as a large out-pouching (black arrow) with a discrete neck (white arrow) on the right lateral wall of the distal esophagus.

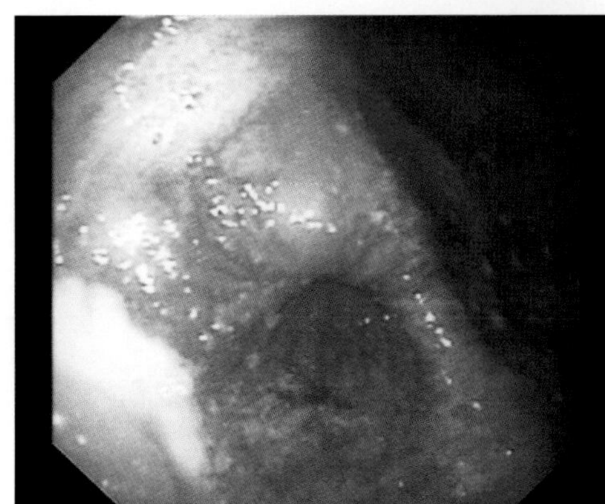

■ **Fig. 1.22** Endoscopic view of epiphrenic diverticulum with stagnant food debris.

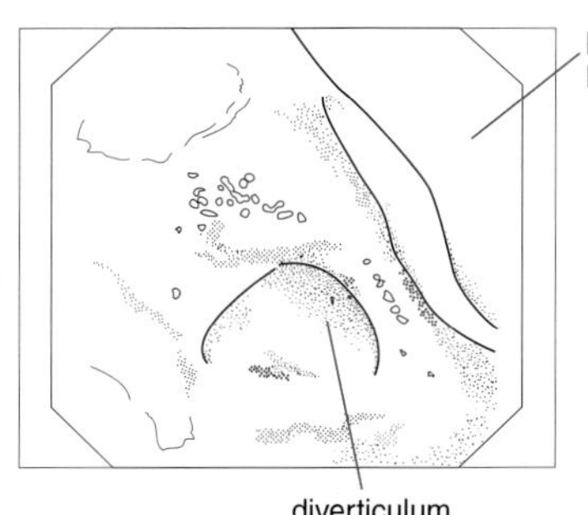

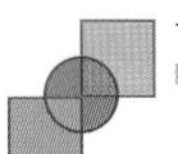

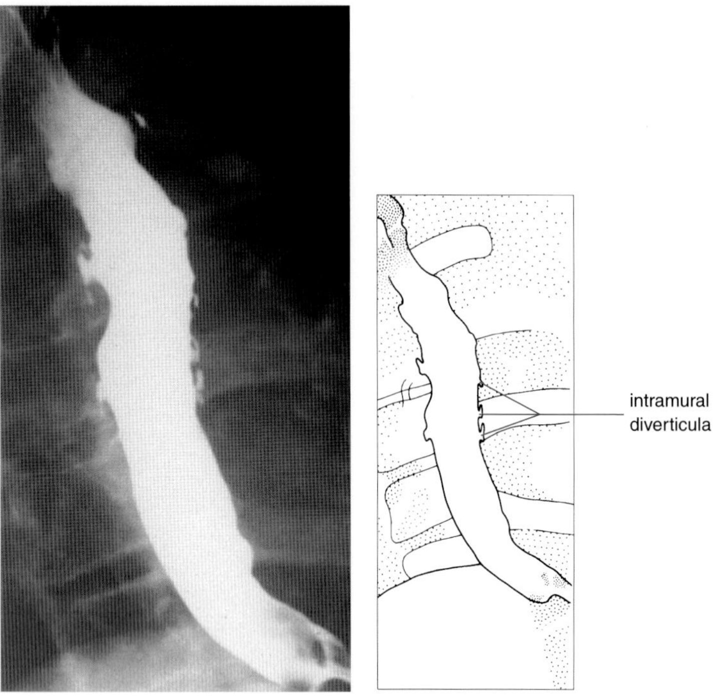

Fig. 1.23 Barium swallow demonstrating multiple intramural diverticula.

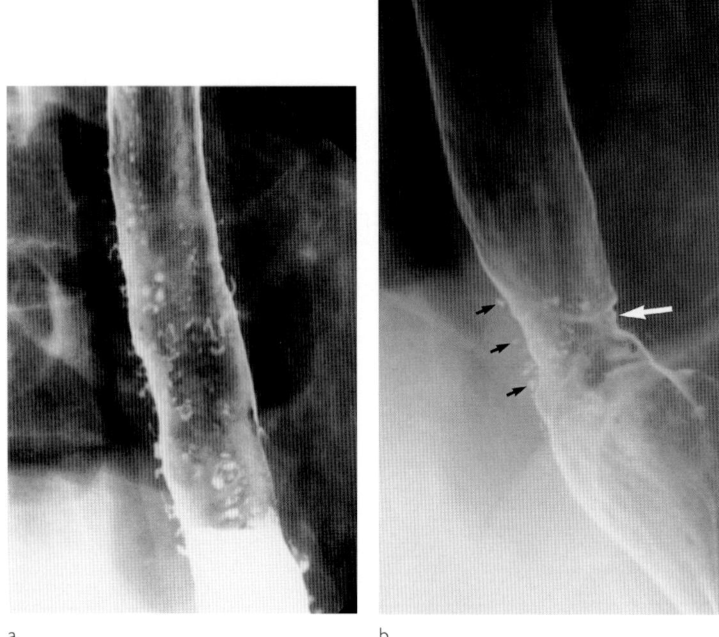

Fig. 1.24 Double-contrast esophagrams in two patients with esophageal intramural pseudodiverticulosis. (a) The first patient has innumerable pseudodiverticula seen both en face and in profile in the mid and distal esophagus. (b) In contrast, the second patient has a mild peptic stricture (white arrow) in the distal esophagus with a focal cluster of pseudodiverticula in the region of the stricture. Note how the pseudodiverticula seen in profile (black arrows) appear to be floating outside the wall of the esophagus, a feature that is characteristic of these structures. (Fig. 1.24b reproduced with permission from reference 1.)

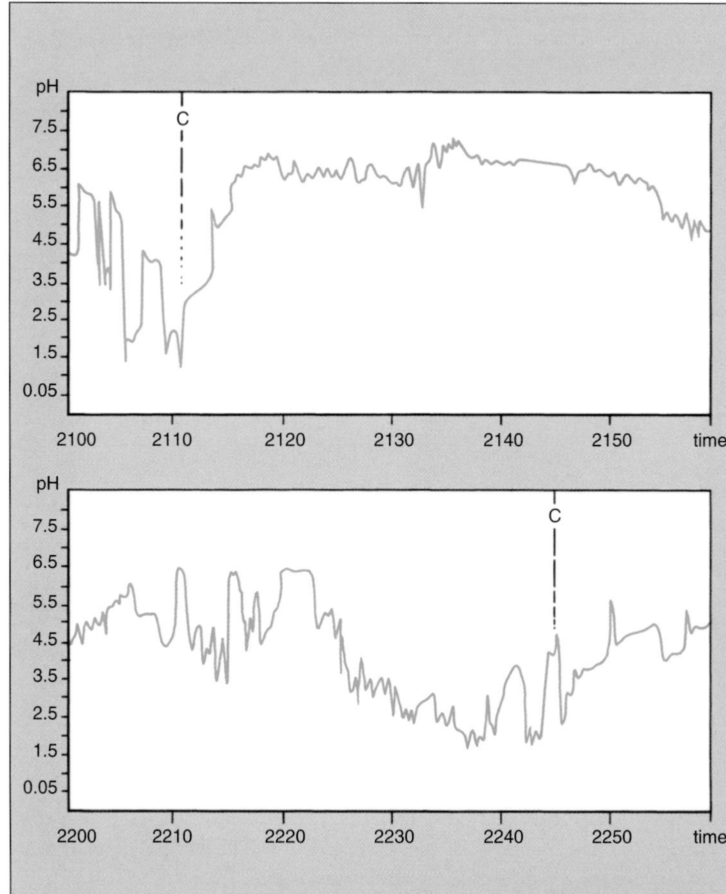

Fig. 1.25 Abnormal esophageal pH tracing showing correlation with chest pain (C indicates pain as recorded by patient) with episodes of acid reflux. Courtesy of Dr J de Caestecker.

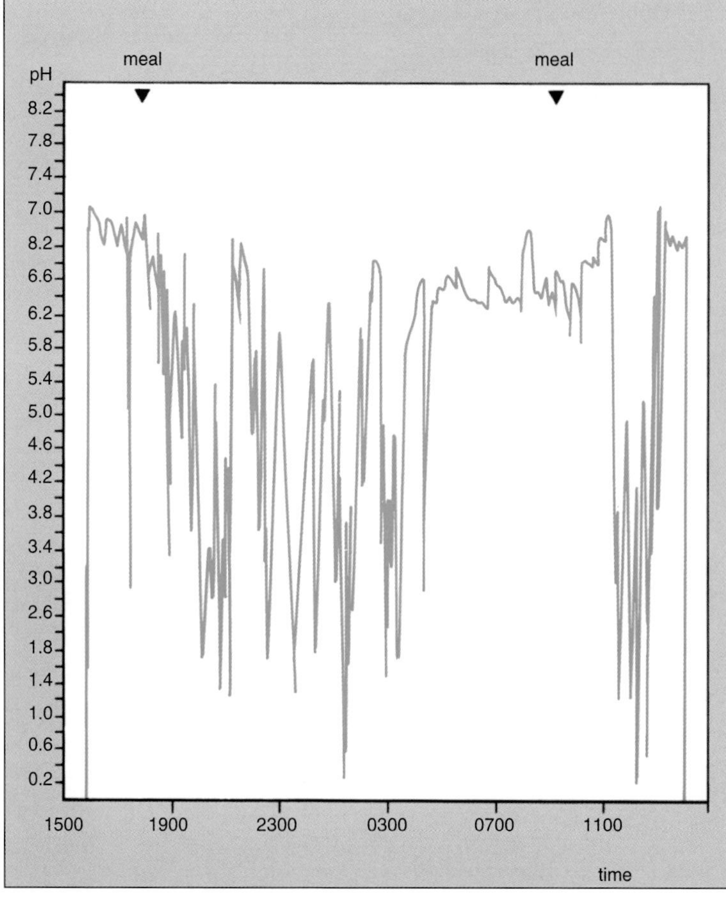

Fig. 1.26 Abnormal 24-hour pH tracing. Note increased frequency and duration of reflux after meals, but also long-duration reflux episodes overnight. Courtesy of Dr J de Caestecker.

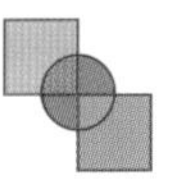

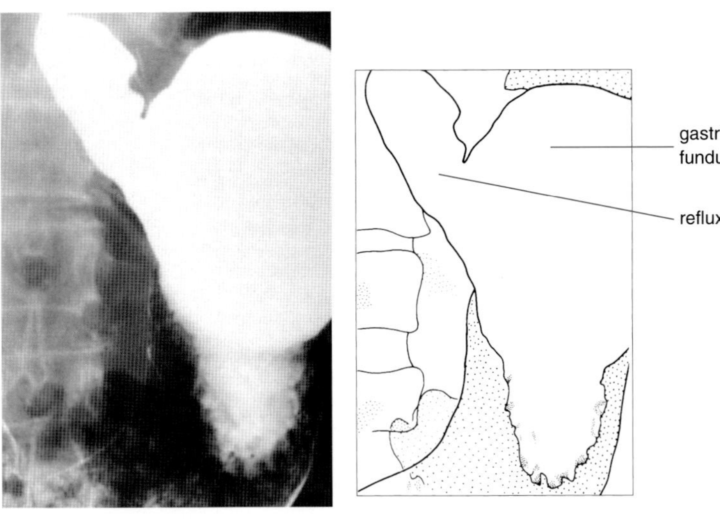

Fig. 1.27 Barium swallow (supine view) showing spontaneous gastro-esophageal reflux.

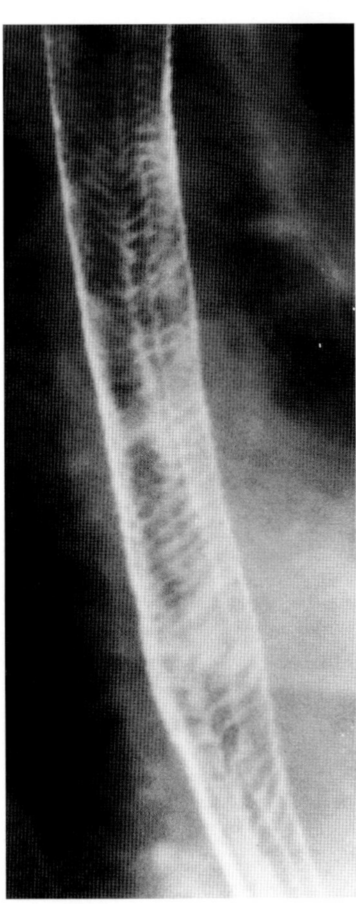

Fig. 1.28 Double-contrast esophagram showing the feline esophagus as multiple thin transverse folds in the esophagus. These folds are usually seen as a transient finding and are often associated with gastro-esophageal reflux.

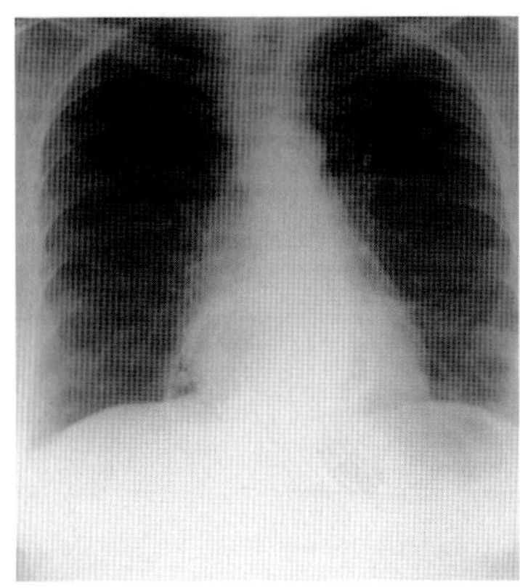

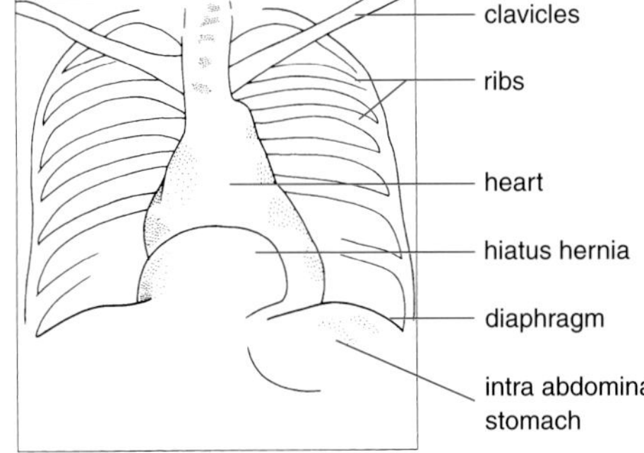

Fig. 1.29 Chest radiograph showing a hiatus hernia in a patient with retrosternal discomfort.

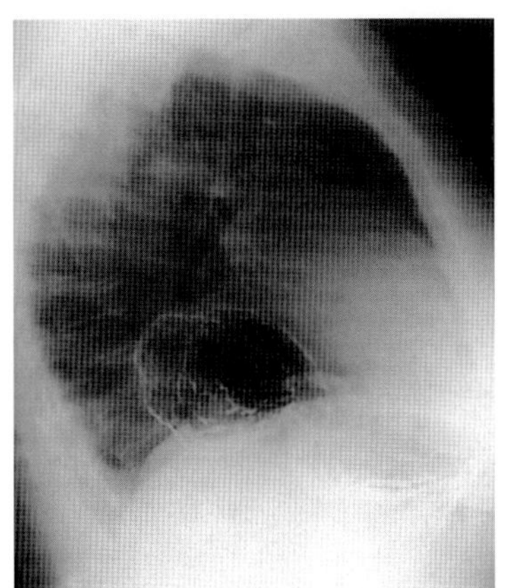

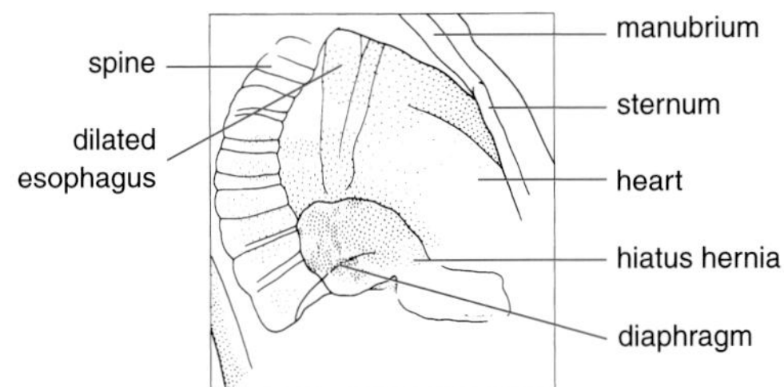

Fig. 1.30 Lateral chest radiograph of the same patient as in Fig. 1.29 confirming the position of a large hiatus hernia after ingestion of barium.

is often, but not necessarily, accompanied by weakening of the lower esophageal sphincter and by gastro-esophageal reflux. At endoscopy, the gastro-esophageal junction is seen lying above the indentation of the diaphragmatic crura, and the hernia may also be readily recognized from the stomach with the endoscope retroverted, when a wide and lax gastro-esophageal junction can be seen around the instrument (Fig. 1.32). Surgical intervention to tighten the hiatal orifice can prevent further reflux with concurrent alteration in the endoscopic appearance (Fig. 1.33).

Rolling or para-esophageal herniae are much less common. The gastro-esophageal junction is then normally situated, below the level of the diaphragm, but a part of the stomach herniates anteriorly through the diaphragm to lie within the thoracic cavity (Fig. 1.34). Reflux is less likely, but patients experience a feeling of fullness and discomfort after meals. Strangulation and infarction are much more likely complications than in sliding herniae. A small proportion of hiatus herniae has rolling and sliding components. Ulceration of the herniated stomach may occur with either type.

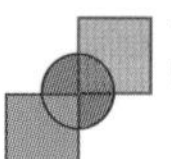

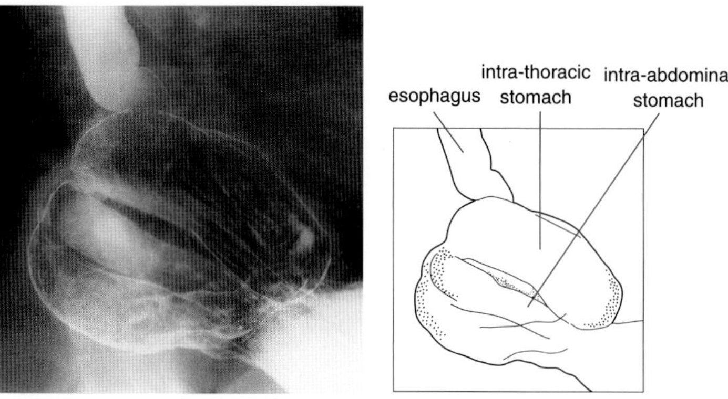

■ **Fig. 1.31** Upper gastrointestinal barium study showing a large sliding hiatus hernia above the diaphragm. (Reproduced with permission from reference 1.)

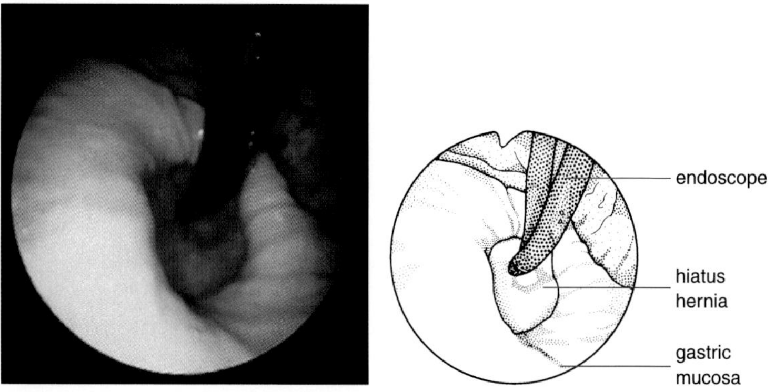

■ **Fig. 1.32** Retroflexed endoscopic view of hiatus hernia from the stomach. The mucosal constriction around the shaft of the instrument is due to diaphragmatic hiatus.

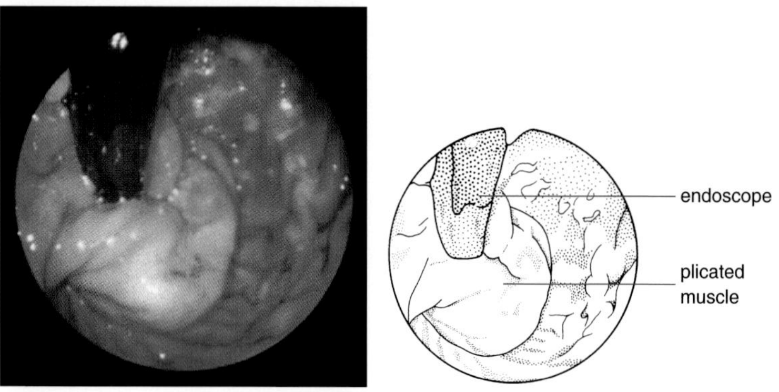

■ **Fig. 1.33** Endoscopic view from the stomach following successful Nissen fundoplication.

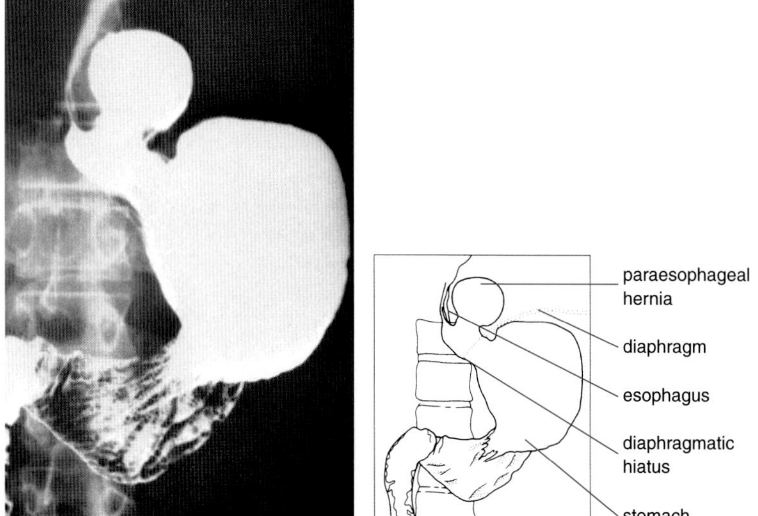

■ **Fig. 1.34** Barium meal showing a rolling hiatus hernia.

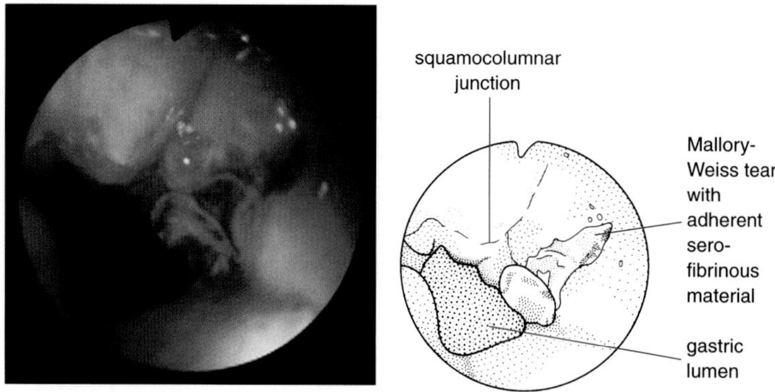

■ **Fig. 1.35** Endoscopic view of Mallory–Weiss tear at gastro-esophageal junction.

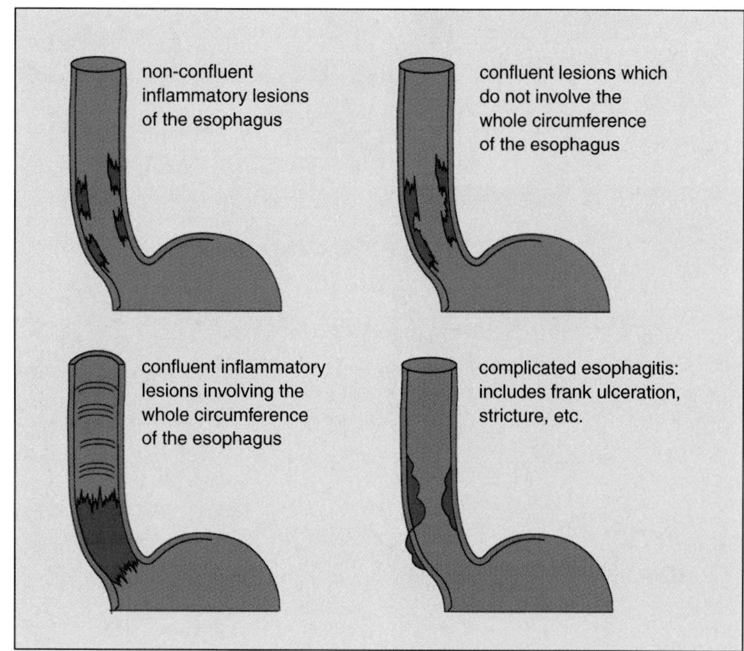

■ **Fig. 1.36** The Los Angeles scale for classification of esophagitis and its diagrammatic representation. (a) Mucosal breaks confined to the mucosal fold, each no longer than 5 mm. (b) At least one mucosal break longer than 5 mm confined to the mucosal fold but not continuous between two folds. (c) Mucosal breaks that are continuous between the tops of mucosal folds but not circumferential. (d) Extensive mucosal breaks engaging at least 75% of the esophageal circumference.

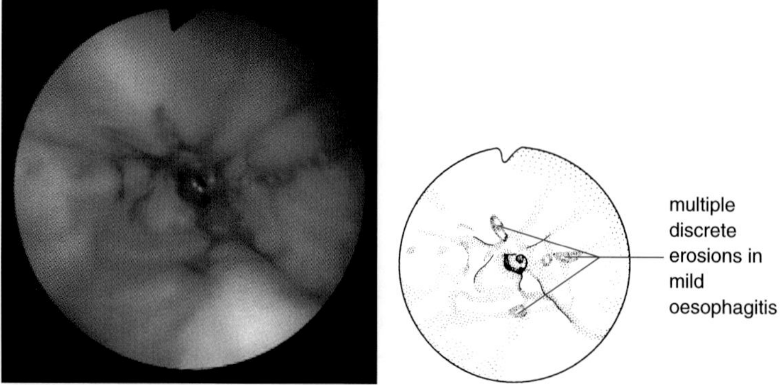

■ **Fig. 1.37** Endoscopic view of grade A esophagitis with solitary erosions.

MALLORY–WEISS TEARS

Repeated strenuous retching or vomiting may be responsible for tears in the proximal cardiac mucosa – Mallory–Weiss tears (Fig. 1.35) – which frequently extend across the esophagogastric junction. It is probable that the tears result from the transient but

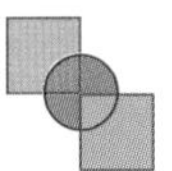

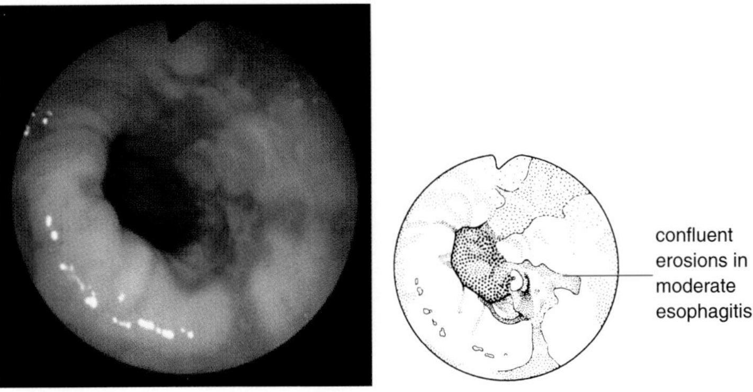

Fig. 1.38 Grade C esophagitis: erosions crossing mucosal folds but not involving the whole circumference.

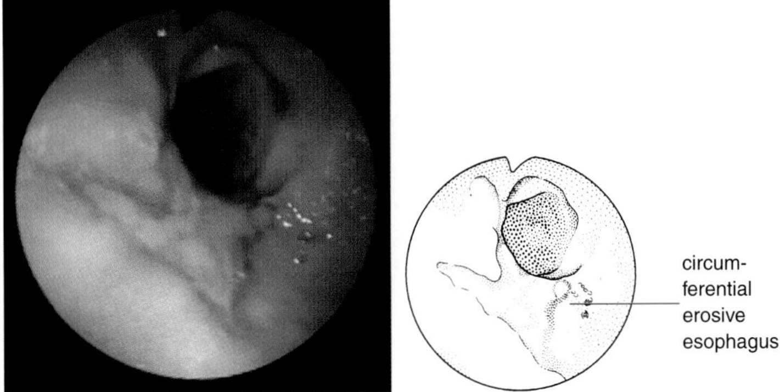

Fig. 1.39 Grade D esophagitis with circumferential erosions.

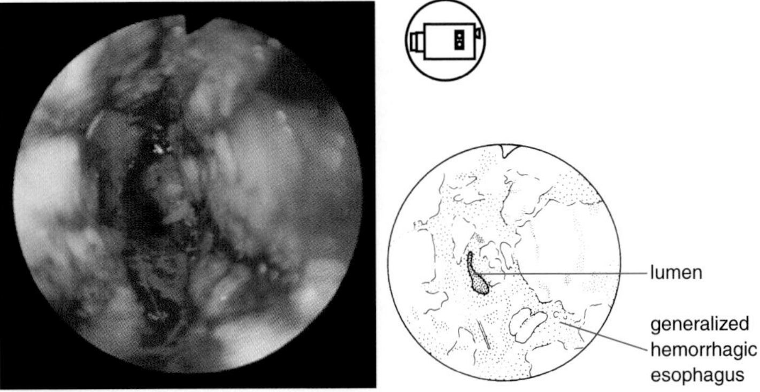

Fig. 1.40 Endoscopic view of severe grade D esophagitis complicated by stricture and hemorrhage.

forceful herniation that occurs in this situation. Significant hemorrhage may result.

ESOPHAGITIS

Esophagitis is now usually graded according to an endoscopically defined four-point scale (Figs 1.36–1.40). It is usually associated with acid reflux (peptic esophagitis), with a variable contribution from other gastric secretions and from biliary reflux. The correlation of symptoms with endoscopic and radiological appearances (Figs 1.41, 1.42) is not always good, and histological changes may be diagnostic in the presence of normal imaging (Figs 1.43, 1.44). Reflux shown on pH studies may be responsible for symptoms in the absence of endoscopic or even histological evidence of esophagitis.

Esophagitis may be associated with swallowed medications (Fig. 1.45), particularly in the elderly where posture and mild

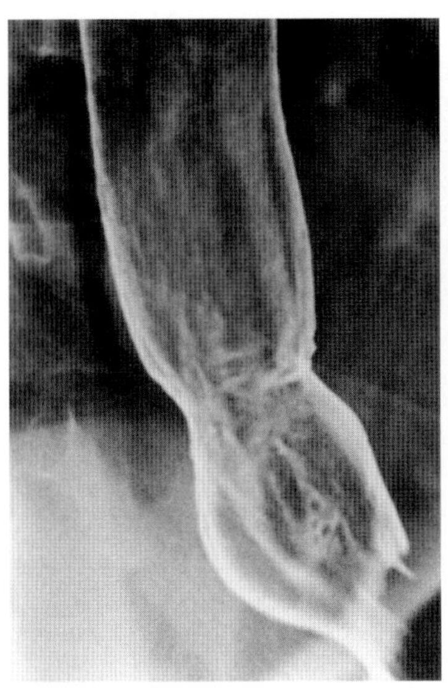
a

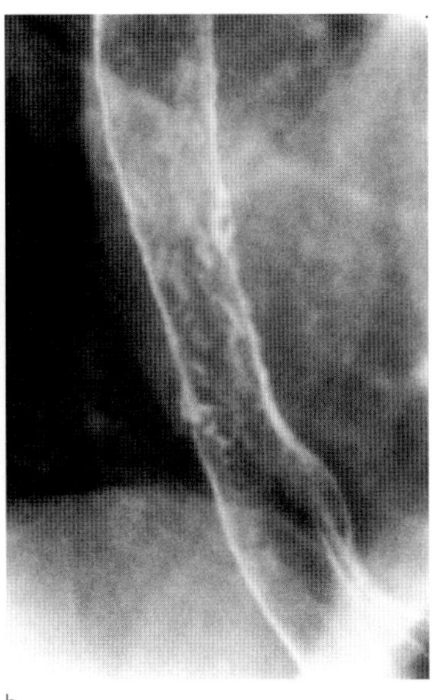
b

Fig. 1.41 (a,b) Double-contrast esophagrams showing multiple tiny ulcers in the distal esophagus in two patients with reflux esophagitis. The ulcers are clustered together above the gastro-esophageal junction in one patient but involve a longer segment of the distal esophagus in the other. (Fig. 1.41a reproduced with permission from reference 2; Fig. 1.41b reproduced with permission from reference 1.)

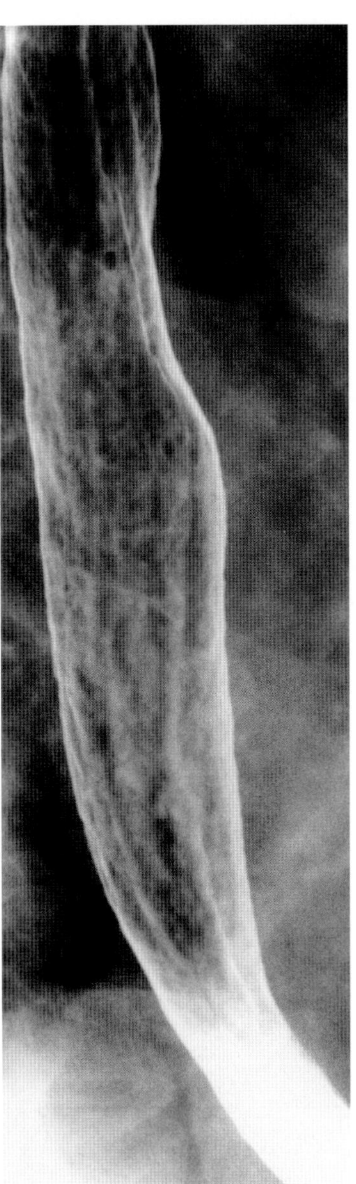

Fig. 1.42 Double-contrast esophagram showing reflux esophagitis with a granular mucosa. Note the poorly defined radiolucencies that fade peripherally due to edema and inflammation of the mucosa.

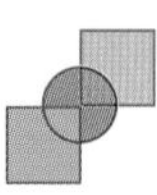

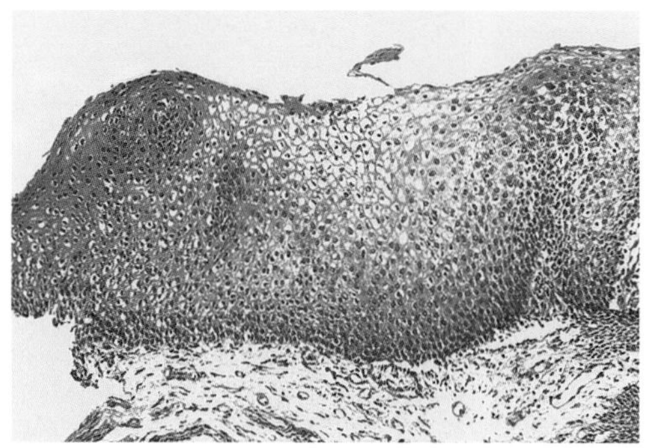

Fig. 1.43 Eosinophilic esophagitis caused by gastro-esophageal reflux. Microscopic view of reflux esophagitis showing a thickened, mildly spongitic esophageal mucosa with patchy mild glycogen depletion of the superficial aspect causing a parakeratotic appearance.

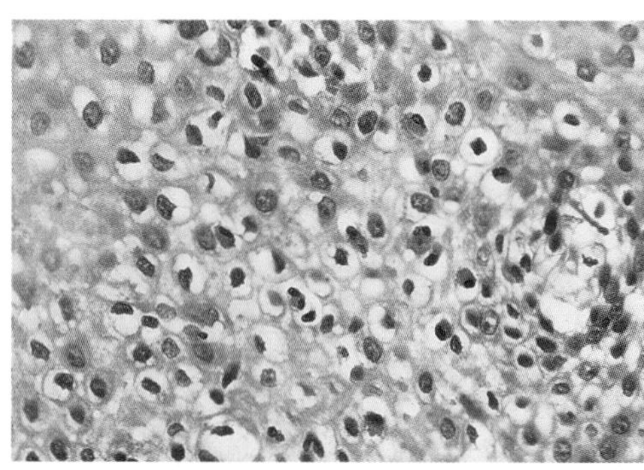

Fig. 1.44 High magnification appearance of reflux esophagitis characterized by intraepithelial infiltration by eosinophils.

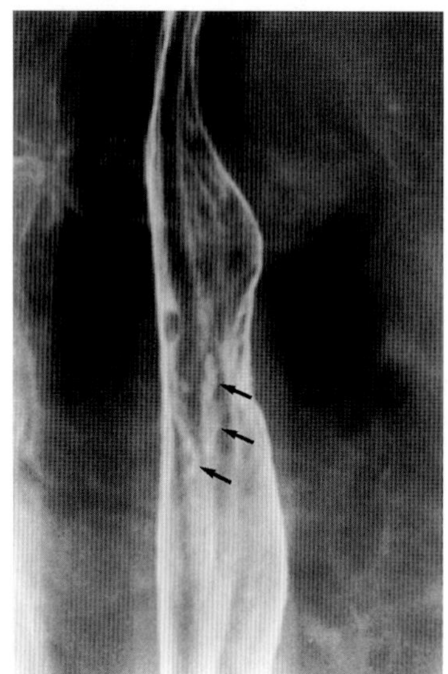

Fig. 1.45 Double-contrast esophagram showing several small, serpiginous ulcers (arrows) in the mid esophagus due to recent tetracycline ingestion in a patient with drug-induced esophagitis.

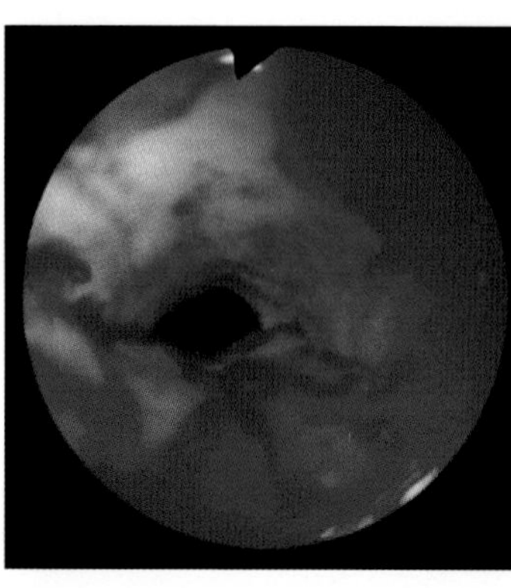

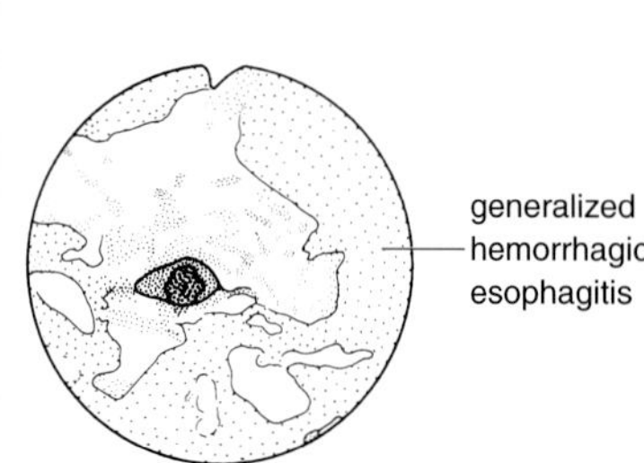

Fig. 1.46 Endoscopic view of acute phase of caustic esophageal damage.

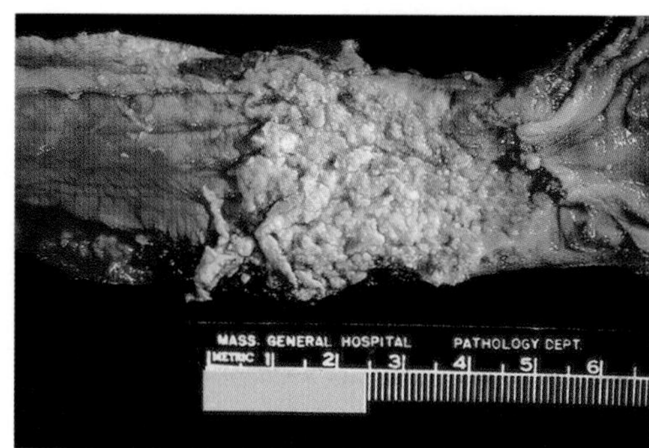

Fig. 1.47 Macroscopic post-mortem view of severe corrosive esophagitis showing deep ulceration and pseudomembrane formation over the distal third of the esophagus secondary to lye ingestion.

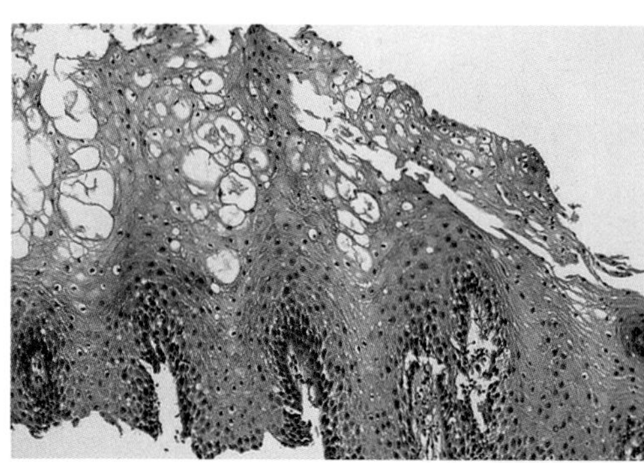

Fig. 1.48 Microscopic appearance of chemical esophagitis showing direct, moderate to severe injury and marked spongiosis of the luminal aspect of the mucosa.

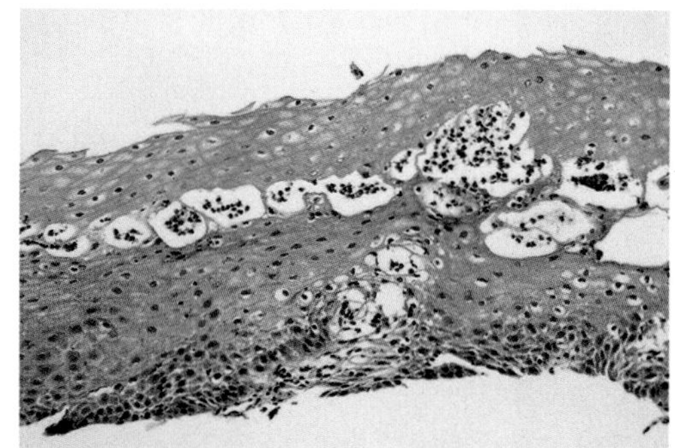

Fig. 1.49 Microscopic appearance of severe chemical injury with necrosis of the superficial half of the mucosa and collections of neutrophils forming microabscesses within the mucosal papillae and at interface between the necrotic and viable squamous epithelium.

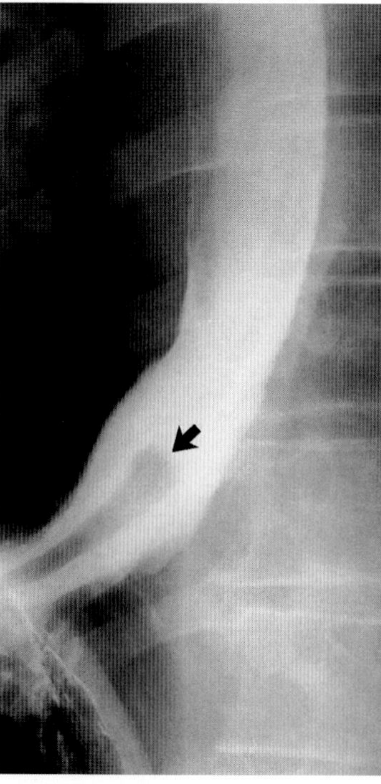

Fig. 1.50 Prone single-contrast esophagram showing an inflammatory esophagogastric polyp as a prominent fold that arises at the gastric cardia and extends into the distal esophagus as a smooth polypoid protuberance (arrow). Endoscopy is not warranted when a typical inflammatory polyp is seen on barium studies.

impairment of motility contribute, and is a serious complication of acci-dental or suicidal ingestion of strong alkali (Figs 1.46–1.49). Severe esophagitis may also follow otherwise successful radiotherapy for esophageal carcinoma (see below). The so-called sentinel polyp may remain after healing of esophagitis of whatever cause (Fig. 1.50).

Esophageal ulcer

Most patients with reflux esophagitis have superficial mucosal ulceration (e.g. Fig. 1.39), but only a minority will develop deeper ulceration involving the muscle layers of the esophagus (Fig. 1.40). Frank ulcers also occur with a number of infective causes (see below). Hematemesis may occur but is rarely severe, except when from ulceration overlying varices; this is a recognized complication of injection sclerotherapy (Fig. 1.51), and less of a risk after banding. Perforation of esophageal ulcers is unusual.

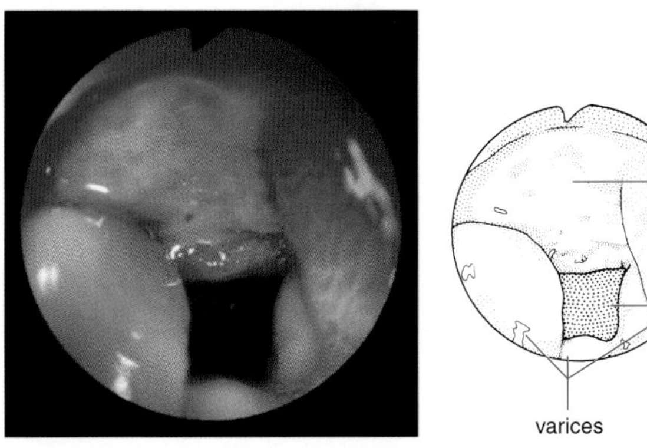

Fig. 1.51 Endoscopic view of a giant ulcer complicating sclerotherapy to distal esophageal varices.

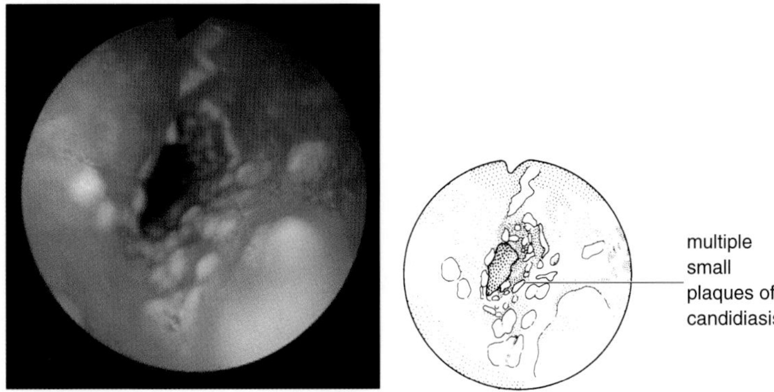

Fig. 1.52 Endoscopic view of mild, patchy esophageal candidiasis.

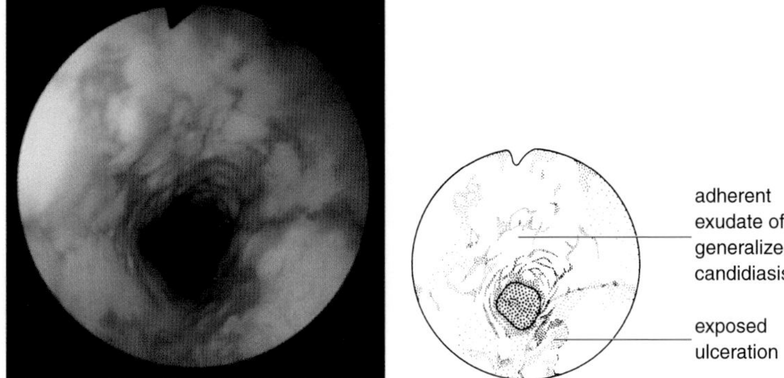

Fig. 1.53 Endoscopic view of severe esophageal candidiasis in which the mucosa is completely covered with a thick layer of adherent exudates.

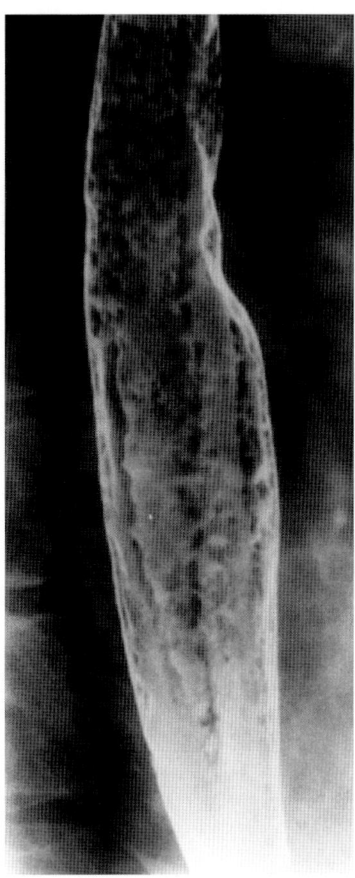

Fig. 1.54 Double-contrast esophagram showing Candidal esophagitis with multiple discrete plaque-like lesions separated by segments of normal intervening mucosa. Note how the plaques have a linear configuration and are oriented along the long axis of the esophagus. These findings are characteristic of candidiasis. (Reproduced with permission from reference 3.)

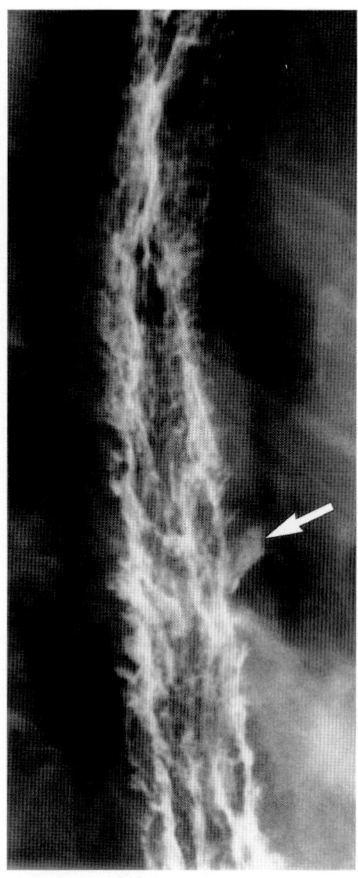

Fig. 1.55 Double-contrast esophagram showing advanced *Candidal* esophagitis with a grossly irregular or 'shaggy' esophagus due to innumerable coalescent plaques and pseudomembranes with trapping of barium between these lesions. Some of the plaques may eventually slough, producing one or more deep ulcers (arrow) superimposed on a background of diffuse plaque formation. As in this case, many patients with fulminant *Candidal* esophagitis are found to have AIDS.

Infective esophagitis

Infective esophagitis other than of candidal origin remains relatively rare other than in the markedly immunosuppressed. Candidal esophagitis (Fig. 1.52) typically occurs in patients on repeated courses of antibiotics especially in those with malignant disease, diabetes, or on immunosuppressant drugs. It may be so mild as to be an incidental finding on endoscopy, but is occasionally part of a systemic infection severe enough to cause death. The characteristic symptom is odynophagia (pain on swallowing), true dysphagia being less frequent. Unlike reflux esophagitis, which tends to be maximal distally, candidiasis may affect the proximal esophagus and often involves multiple sites. The white adherent patches seen endoscopically represent clumps of yeast hyphae, superimposed on a background of hyperemic and, in severe cases, ulcerated esophageal mucosa (Fig. 1.53). The radiological changes are subtle except in advanced disease when the esophageal wall takes on an irregular plaque-like or 'shaggy' appearance (Figs 1.54, 1.55). Exfoliative cytology, direct smears of esophageal material, and mucosal biopsy may all show yeast forms (Figs 1.56–1.58). The endoscopic appearances should be distinguished from those of esophageal keratosis (Fig. 1.59).

Herpes simplex esophagitis is unusual other than in human immunodeficiency virus (HIV) infection. It can be identified radiologically (Fig. 1.60), but is easier to diagnose endoscopically and

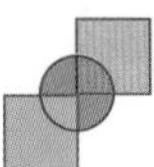

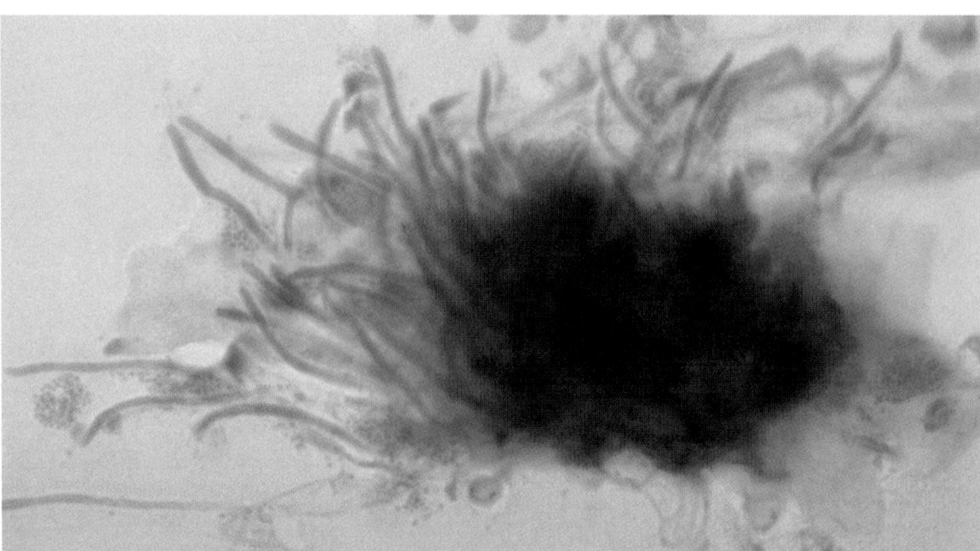

Fig. 1.56 A cytological preparation showing candidal hyphae growing outwards from a central fungal ball. Papanicolau stain (x 900). Courtesy of Dr E Hudson.

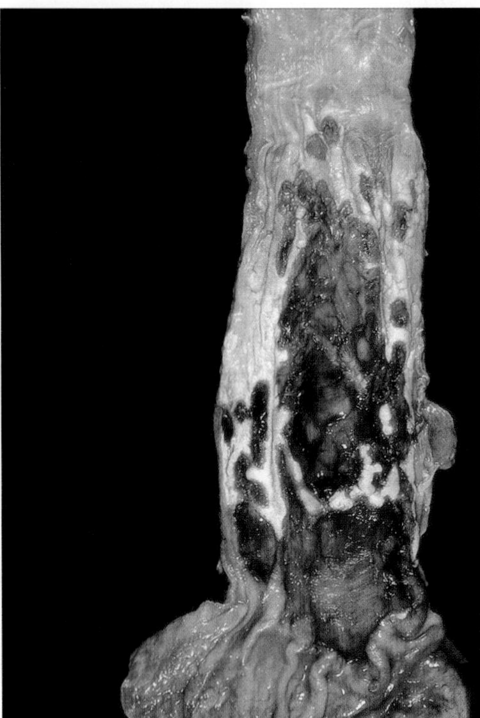

Fig. 1.57 Macroscopic view of severe fungal esophagitis in which the ulcers are characteristically irregular in contour and filled with necrotic debris, giving them a shaggy appearance.

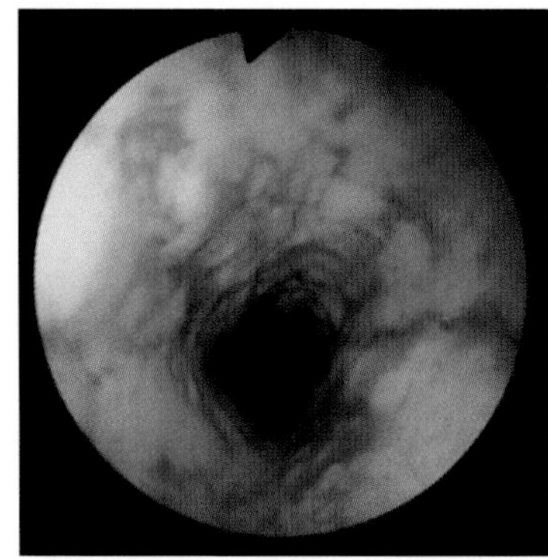

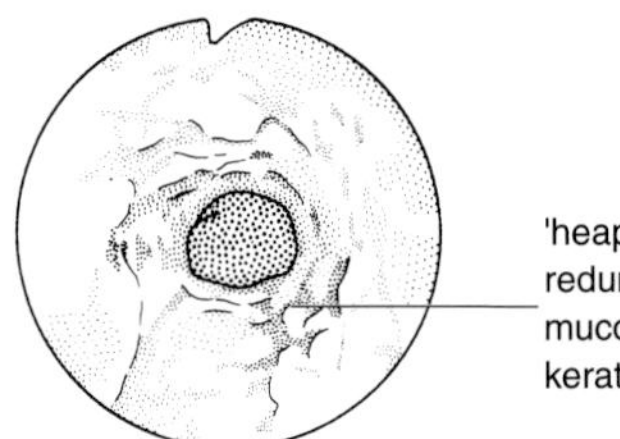

Fig. 1.59 Endoscopic appearance of esophageal keratosis.

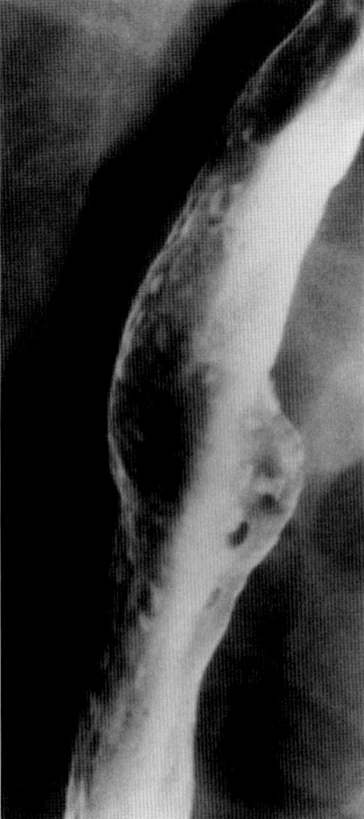

Fig. 1.60 Double-contrast esophagram showing multiple small, discrete ulcers in the upper and mid esophagus due to herpes esophagitis. Note how the ulcers are surrounded by radiolucent mounds of edematous mucosa. In the appropriate clinical setting, these findings are characteristic of herpes esophagitis. (Reproduced with permission from reference 4.)

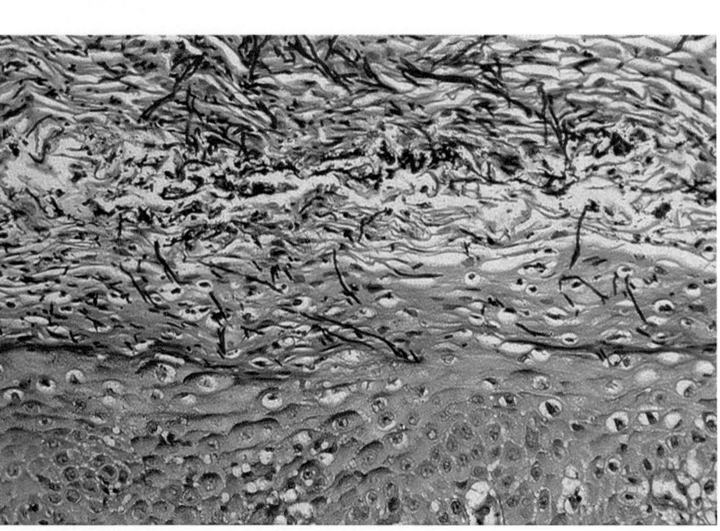

Fig. 1.58 High-magnification histological appearance of the esophageal mucosa in candidal esophagitis showing yeast forms and invasive pseudohyphae stained by PAS.

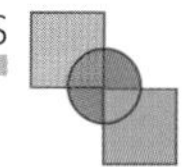

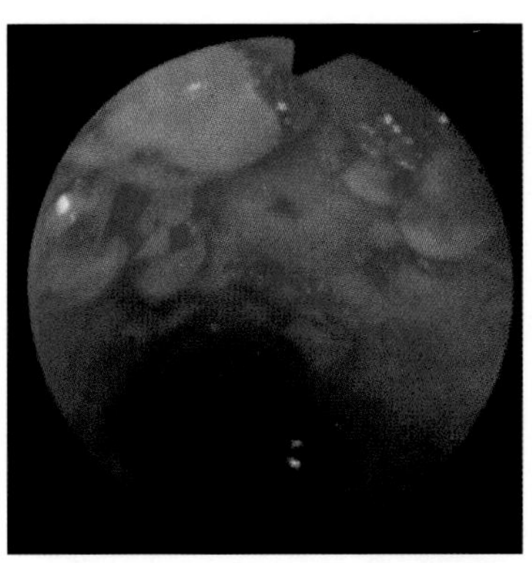

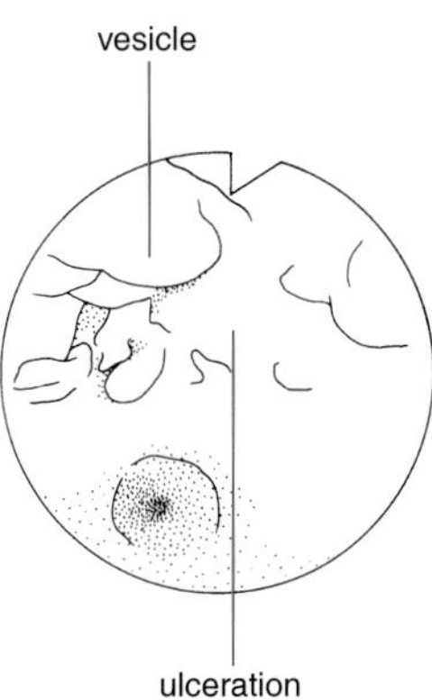

■ **Fig. 1.61** Endoscopic view of esophagitis due to herpes simplex virus showing diagnostic herpetic vesicles and multiple ulcers.

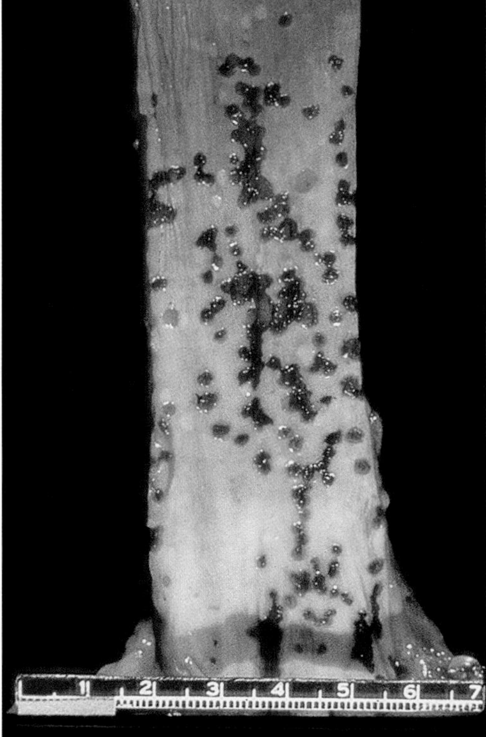

■ **Fig. 1.62** Macroscopic appearance of viral esophagitis showing characteristic 'punched-out' ulcers studding the distal esophagus.

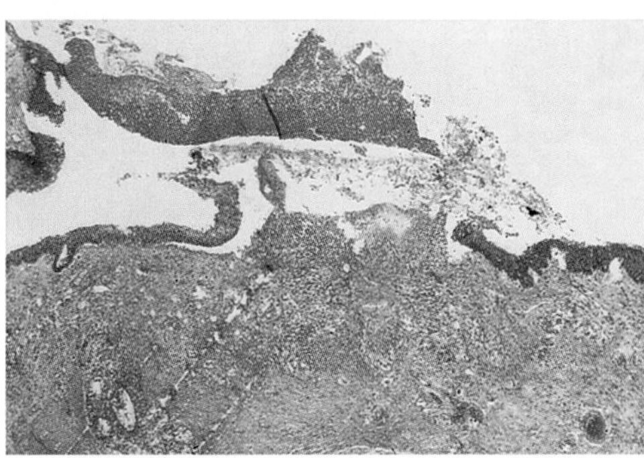

■ **Fig. 1.63** Microscopic view of a discrete aphthous ulcer overlain by fibrinous exudate typical of herpes simplex esophagitis.

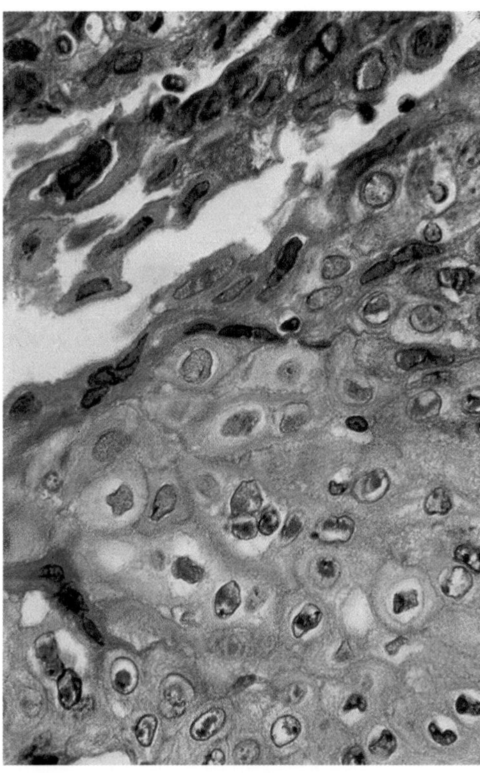

■ **Fig. 1.64** High-magnification view of squamous cells at the edge of an aphthous ulcer showing the intranuclear inclusions, nuclear irregularities, and multiple nuclei characteristic of herpes simplex infection.

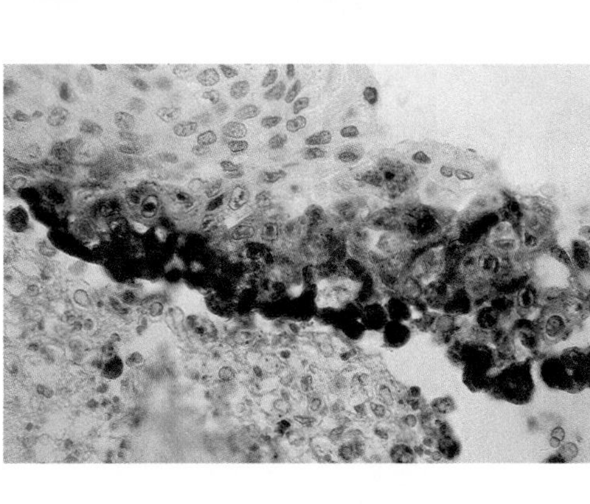

■ **Fig. 1.65** Immunohistochemical stain for herpes simplex type I demonstrates the presence of viral infection of desquamated esophageal mucosal cells within exudates overlying an ulcerated area.

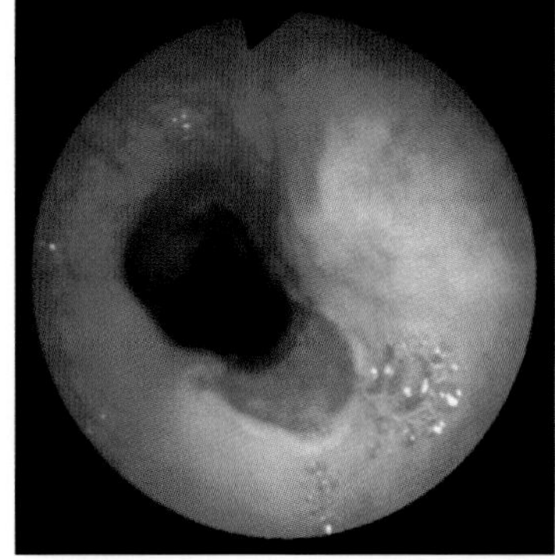

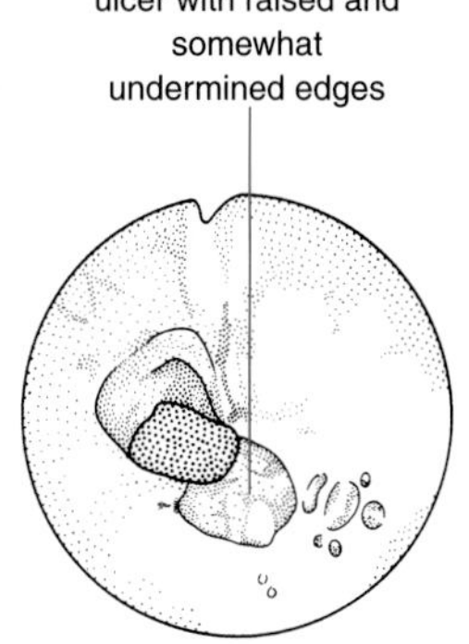

■ **Fig. 1.66** Endoscopic view of ulceration from cytomegalovirus infection. Note the raised edges and the potential, in more advanced cases, for confusion with neoplastic disease.

especially so if unruptured vesicles are present (Fig. 1.61). Otherwise it produces a non-specific erosive esophagitis. In the absence of vesicles, histological examination of biopsies should confirm the diagnosis (Figs 1.62–1.65).

Esophagitis from cytomegalovirus infection can be responsible for large punched-out ulcers that may be thought malignant (Fig. 1.66). The radiological features can be strongly suggestive (Fig. 1.67), but histology (with or without immunohistochemistry) showing the viral inclusions and an associated inflammatory response is required for confirmation of the diagnosis (Figs 1.68–1.70).

Oral hairy leukoplakia (seen mainly in AIDS patients) has a counterpart in the esophagus where it may be responsible for odynophagia or dysphagia (Figs 1.71, 1.72). It is attributed to Epstein–Barr virus infection. HIV esophagitis is also recognized in the absence of secondary infection (Fig. 1.73).

Although the premalignant potential of papillomas at other sites in the body appears lacking, the development of papilloma virus-related lesions in the esophagus is of more than passing interest.

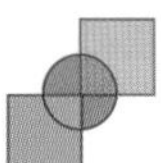

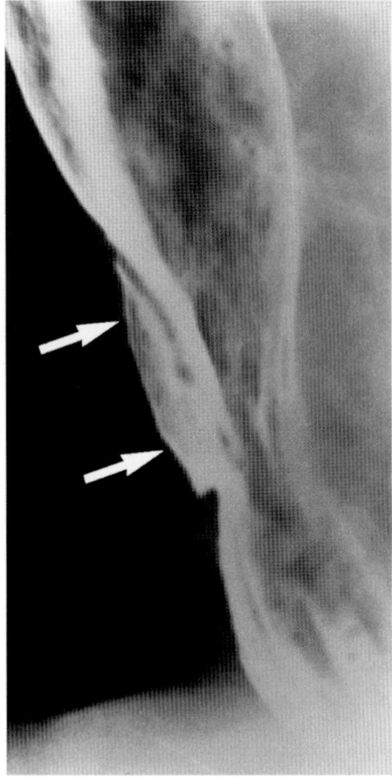

a

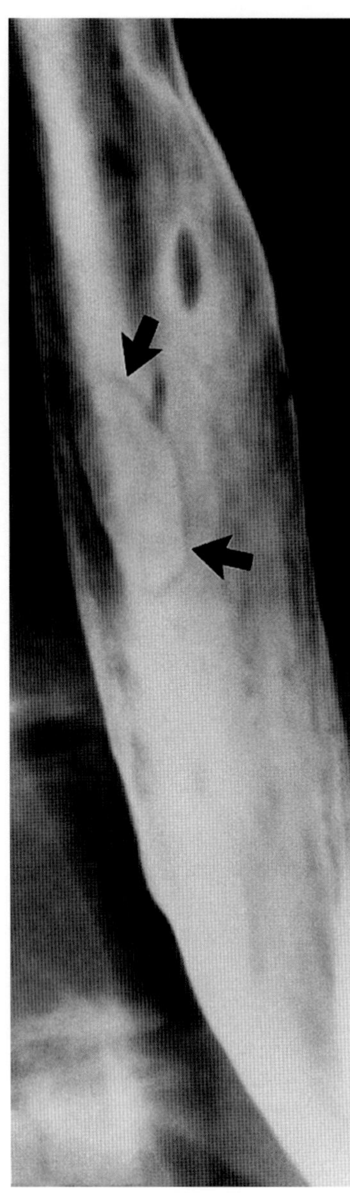

b

■ **Fig. 1.67** Double-contrast esophagrams showing giant ulcers in two patients with cytomegalovirus (CMV) esophagitis. One patient (a) has a long, flat ulcer seen in profile (white arrows) in the distal esophagus, whereas the other (b) has a large ovoid ulcer seen en face (black arrows) in the mid esophagus with a thin rim of edema surrounding the ulcer. Because herpetic ulcers rarely become this large, the presence of one or more giant ulcers should suggest the possibility of CMV esophagitis in patients with AIDS. (Fig. 1.67a courtesy of Sidney W Nelson, M.D.; Seattle, WA; Fig. 1.67b courtesy of Kyunghee C Cho, M.D.; Newark, NJ; both figs reproduced with permission from reference 2.)

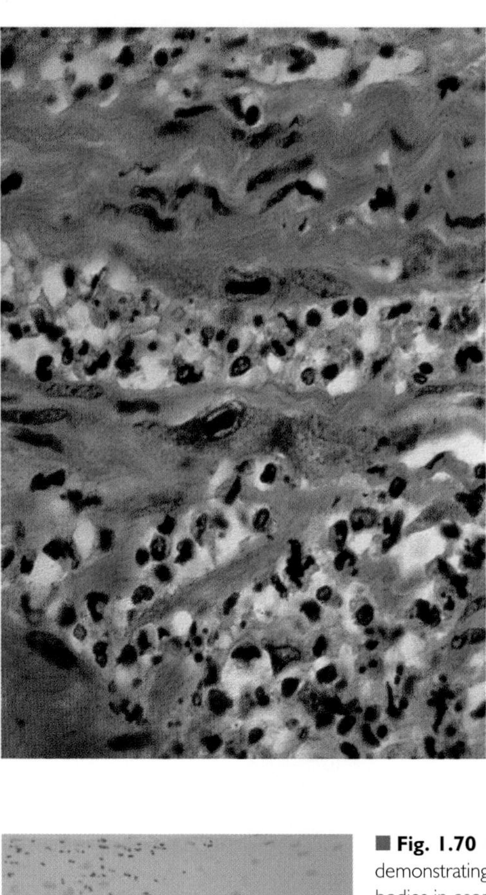

■ **Fig. 1.69** High magnification of virally infected stromal cells at the base of an aphthous ulcer in cytomegalovirus esophagitis showing enlarged nuclei with prominent amphophilic intranuclear inclusions surrounded by a clear halo and irregular condensation of the nucleoplasm against the nuclear membrane.

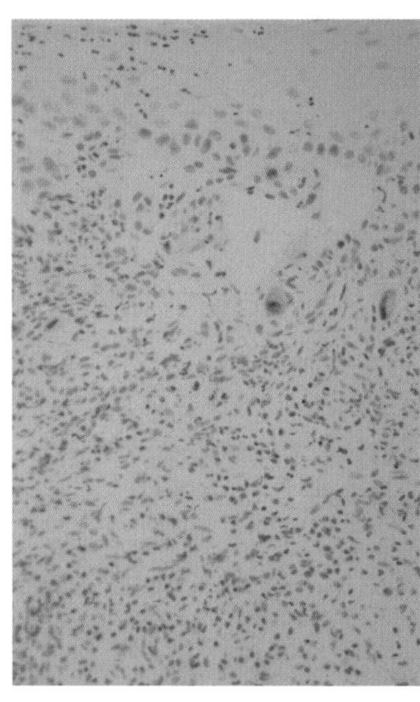

■ **Fig. 1.70** Immunohistochemical staining demonstrating cytomegalovirus inclusion bodies in esophagitis (staining brown).

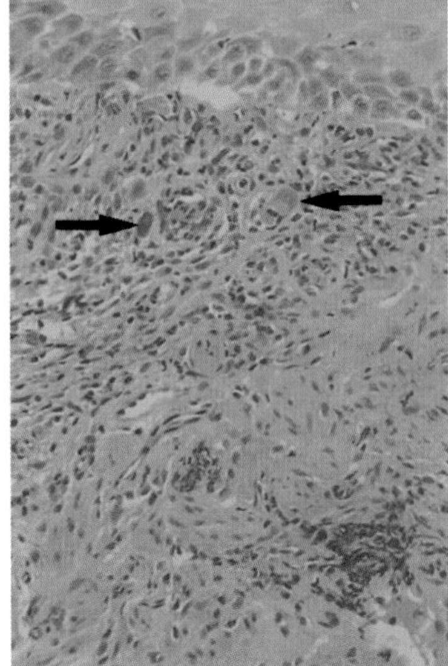

■ **Fig. 1.68** Histological appearance of cytomegalovirus esophagitis (arrows indicate inclusions).

■ **Fig. 1.71** Appearance of hairy leukoplakia in a patient with AIDS. Courtesy of Dr SA Morse.

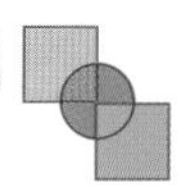

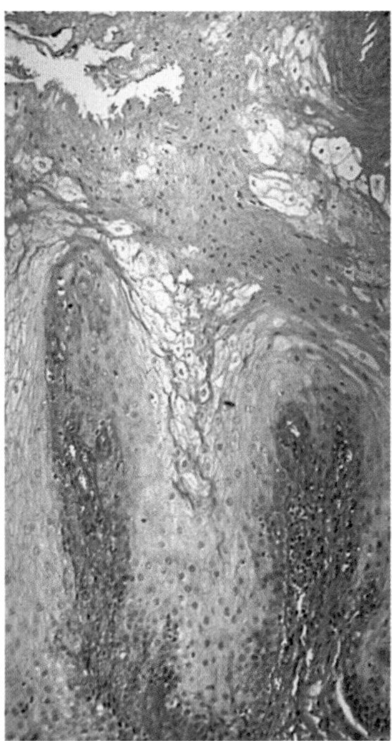

■ **Fig. 1.72** Hugely thickened squamous epithelium of hairy leukoplakia. Courtesy of Dr N Francis.

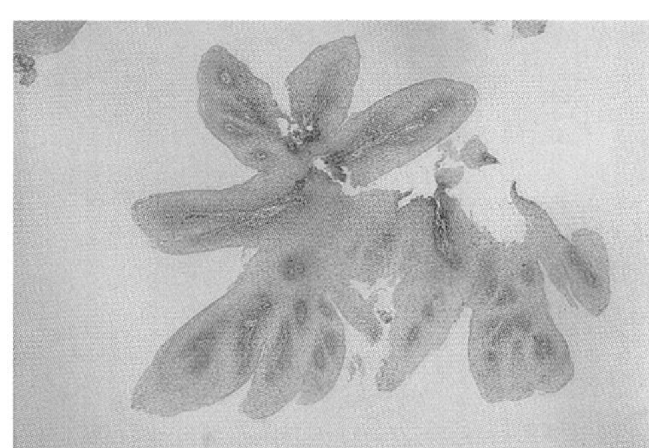

■ **Fig. 1.74** Microscopic appearance of an esophageal papilloma showing the characteristic 'church-spire' spiking growth pattern of the squamous epithelium.

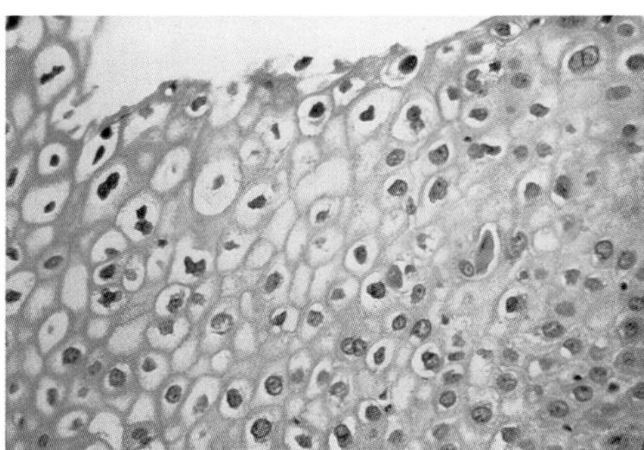

■ **Fig. 1.75** High-magnification microscopic appearance of the squamous epithelium of an esophageal papilloma showing the vacuolization and pleomorphism (koilocytosis) of the cells that is characteristic of human papilloma virus infection.

■ **Fig. 1.76** Immunohistochemical stain for human papilloma virus in an esophageal papilloma. Immunostaining for human papilloma virus demonstrates infection of the koilocytotic squamous cells.

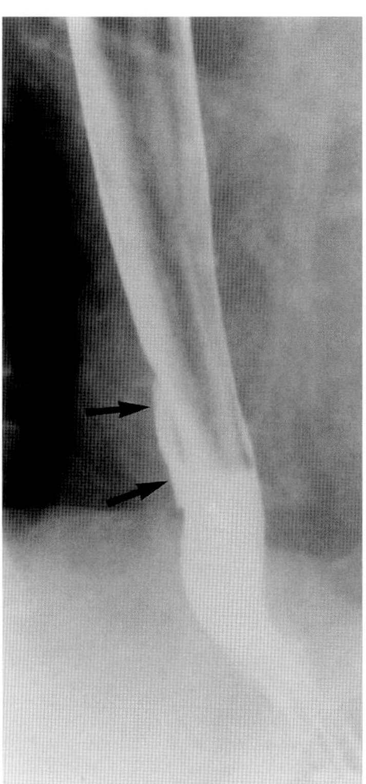

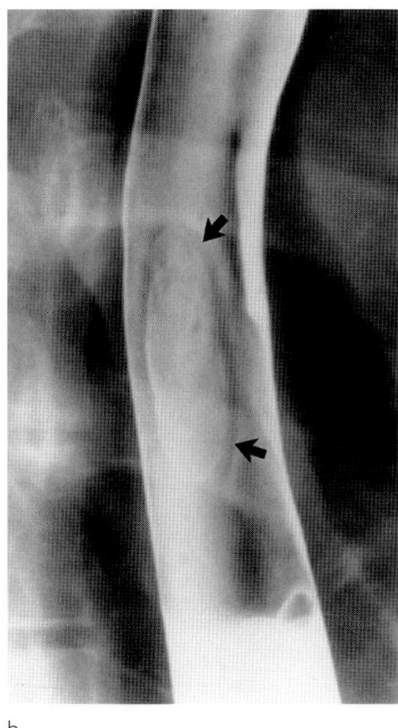

a b

■ **Fig. 1.73** Double-contrast esophagrams showing giant ulcers in two patients with human immunodeficiency virus (HIV) esophagitis. One patient (a) has a large, flat ulcer seen in profile (long arrows) in the distal esophagus, whereas the other (b) has a giant, ovoid ulcer seen en face (short arrows) in the mid esophagus. Note the resemblance to the ulcers in Fig. 1.67. Endoscopic brushings, biopsies, and cultures are required to differentiate HIV from CMV, so that appropriate therapy can be initiated in these patients. (Fig. 1.73b reproduced with permission from reference 5.)

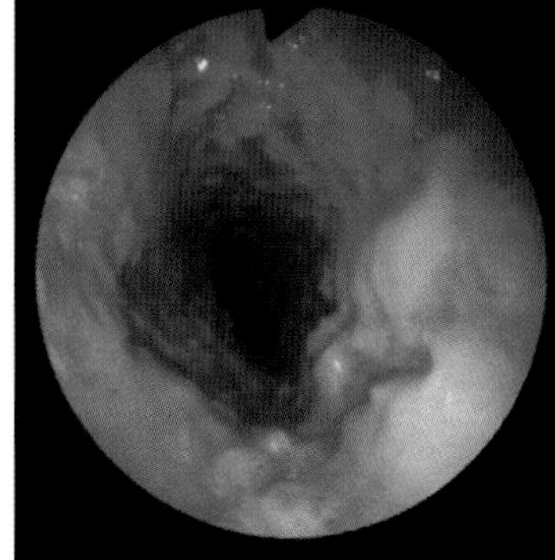

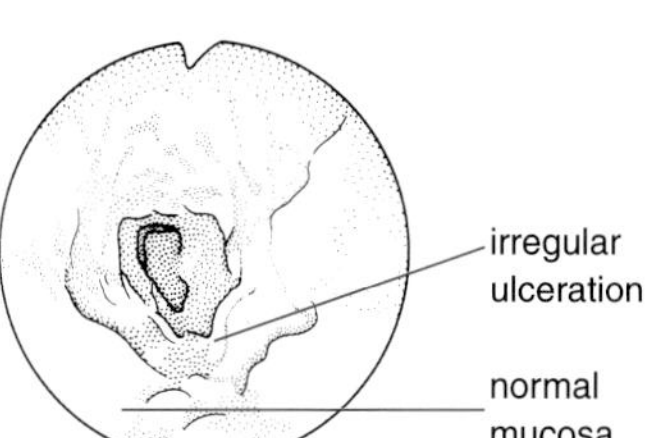

■ **Fig. 1.77** Endoscopic appearance of the esophageal ulceration as occasionally seen in Crohn's disease.

Endoscopically they are indistinguishable from other benign polyps, but the histological changes are distinctive (Figs 1.74–1.76).

Esophageal symptoms and endoscopic appearances similar to those of infective esophagitis may occur in Crohn's disease (Fig. 1.77); the correct diagnosis is likely to be apparent from the knowledge of Crohn's disease at other sites and/or from granulomata seen histologically.

ESOPHAGEAL STRICTURE

Prolonged and/or severe reflux may lead to fibrosis and stricture formation (peptic stricture) accompanied by progressive dysphagia, initially for solids and later for liquids. Although the radiological diagnosis of a benign stricture is usually correct, particularly when it occurs above a hiatus hernia (Fig. 1.78), endoscopy with multiple

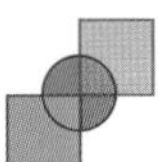

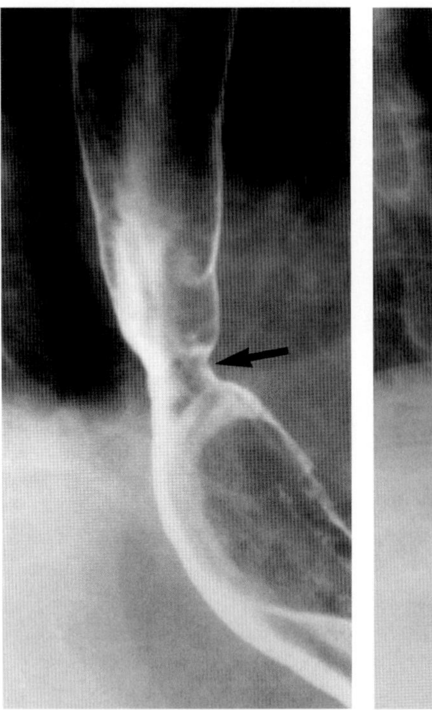

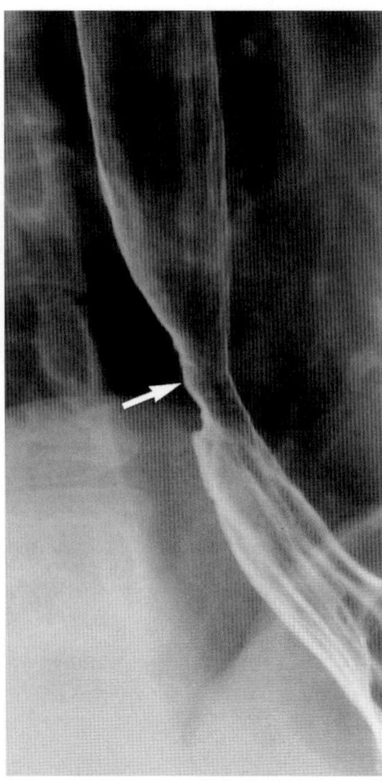

■ **Fig. 1.78** Double-contrast esophagram in two patients with peptic strictures. One patient has a short area of narrowing (black arrow) in the distal esophagus above a hiatal hernia, whereas the other has a longer area of asymmetric narrowing (white arrow). These strictures can have a variable length, depending on the degree of scarring.

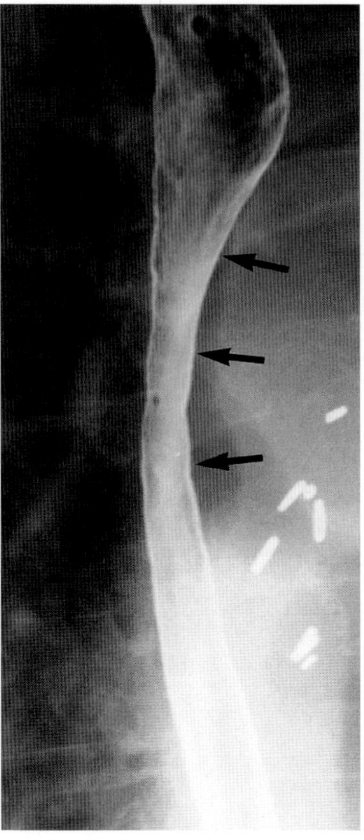

■ **Fig. 1.80** Double-contrast esophagram showing a radiation stricture as a smooth, tapered area of concentric narrowing (arrows) in the mid esophagus. This patient had undergone radiation therapy and surgery (note surgical clips) for carcinoma of the lung.

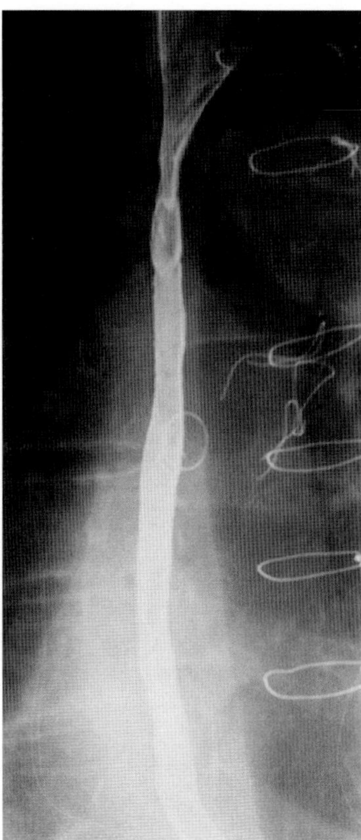

■ **Fig. 1.81** Double-contrast esophagram showing a caustic stricture as an unusually long segment of narrowing involving the lower two-thirds of the thoracic esophagus. This patient had ingested lye many years earlier, and coincidentally had required cardiac surgery and hence thoracotomy.

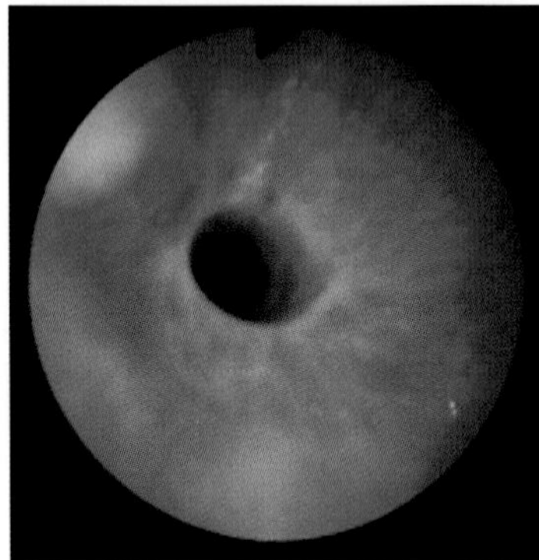

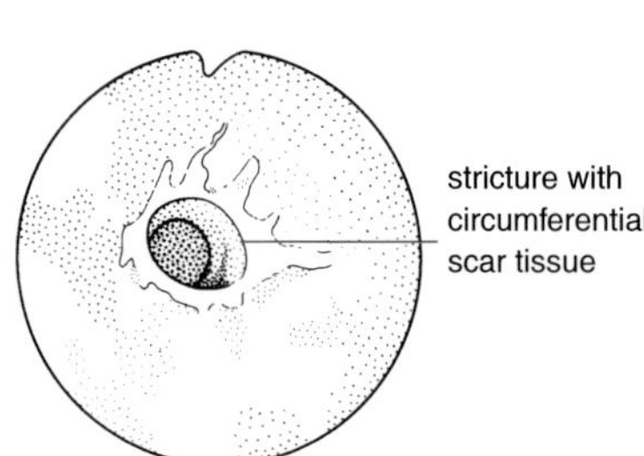

■ **Fig. 1.79** Endoscopic view of benign esophageal stricture (in this case the late result of circumferential damage caused by long-term ingestion of NSAIDs).

biopsies and/or brush cytology to exclude malignancy is always advisable (Fig. 1.79). Benign esophageal strictures may follow otherwise successful radiotherapy (Fig. 1.80), and tend to be especially severe after ingestion of caustic soda or other corrosive agents (Fig. 1.81).

Esophageal strictures may be successfully managed by endoscopic or radiological dilatation using semirigid dilators or balloons (Fig. 1.82). No technique is without the risk of complications including bleeding and perforation (Fig. 1.83).

Dysphagia may also result from the extrinsic compression of the esophagus. Non-neoplastic conditions such as left atrial enlargement or aortic aneurysm may be to blame, as well as compression or involvement of the esophagus by (for example) bronchial carcinoma or malignant mediastinal nodes (Fig. 1.84).

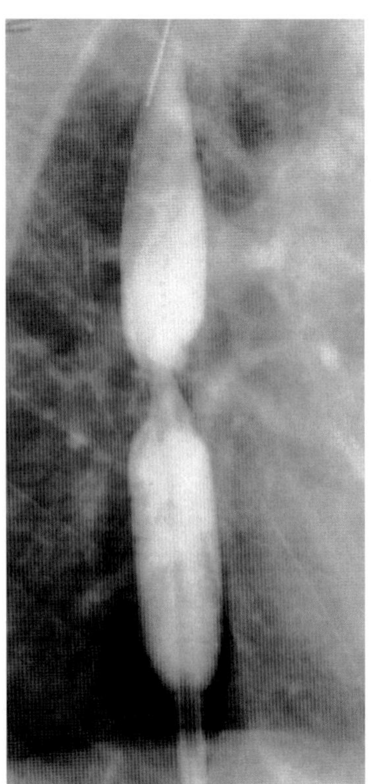

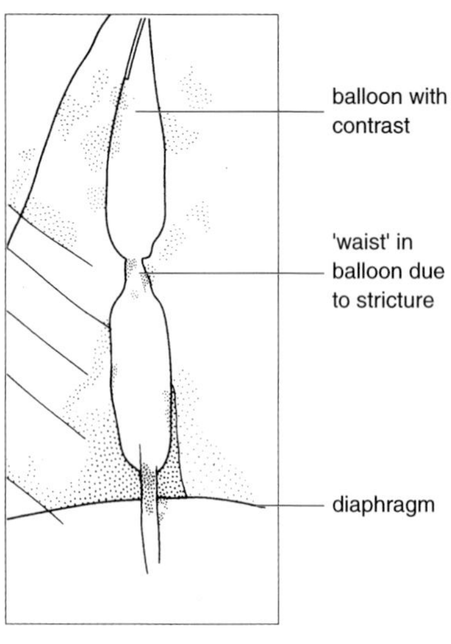

■ **Fig. 1.82** Endoscopic view of eccentric benign esophageal stricture with associated esophagitis. A guide wire is in place through the stricture in preparation for dilation.

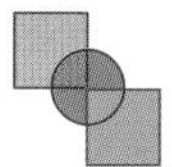

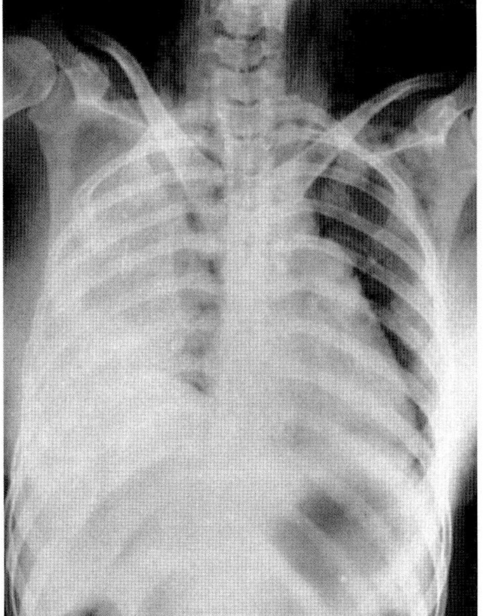

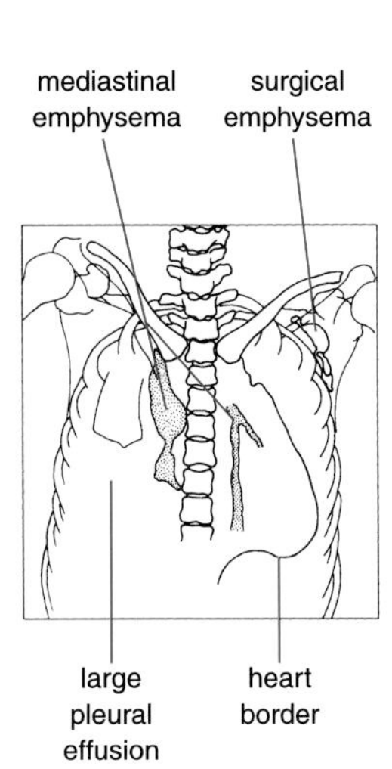

■ **Fig. 1.83** Chest radiograph showing consequences of esophageal perforation following dilation of a stricture. There is a right pleural effusion, mediastinal emphysema and gross surgical emphysema in the neck and upper chest wall.

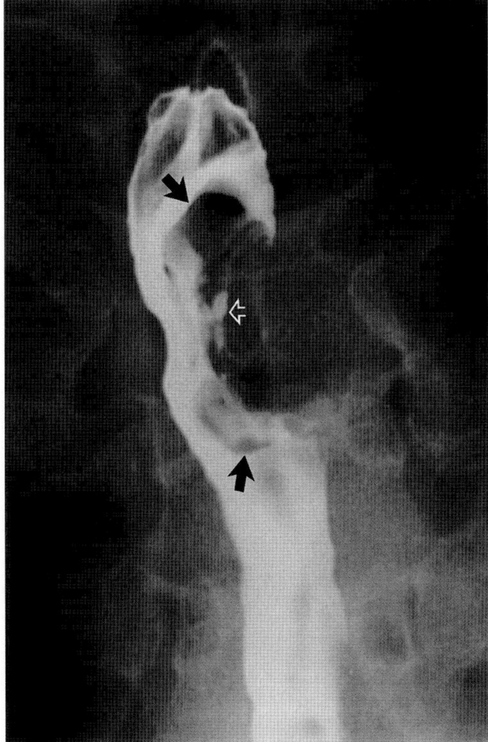

■ **Fig. 1.84** Double-contrast esophagram showing esophageal involvement by mediastinal adenopathy from carcinoma of the lung. Note the large area of lobulated mass effect (black arrows) with central ulceration (white arrow) due to invasion of the esophagus by tumor in the mediastinum.

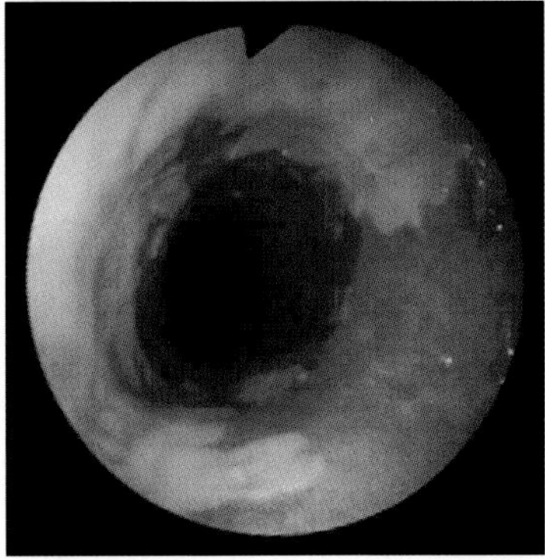

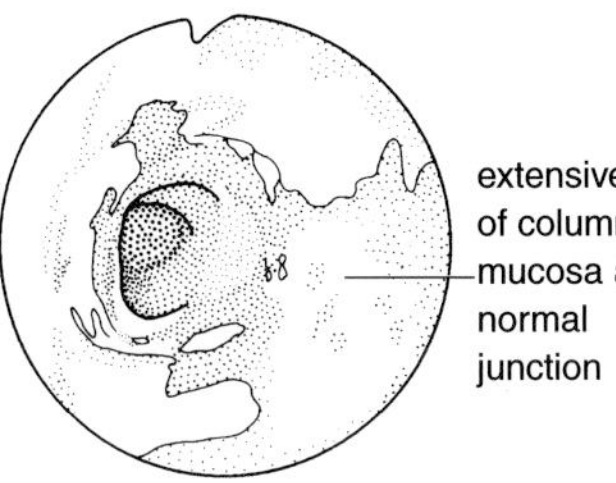

■ **Fig. 1.85** Endoscopic view of Barrett's syndrome. Areas of deeper pink, metaplastic, columnar epithelium alongside the normal pale pink, squamous esophageal mucosa. The columnar epithelium extends at least 3 cm above the gastro-esophageal junction.

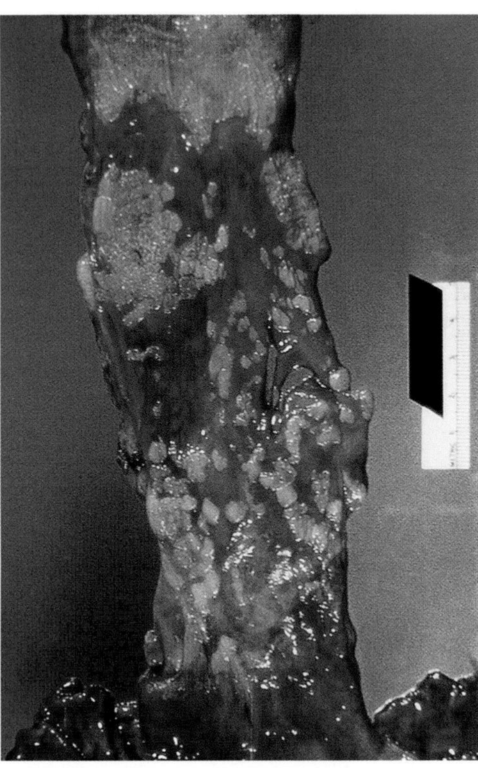

■ **Fig. 1.86** Macroscopic appearance of the distal esophagus in Barrett's syndrome showing irregular pale islands of residual squamous mucosa amid broad areas of metaplastic mucosa having the same red-pink color as the mucosa of the gastric fundus, the proximal aspect of which is seen at the bottom of the photograph.

BARRETT'S SYNDROME

It is highly probable that the partial replacement of the normal squamous epithelium of the esophageal mucosa by areas of columnar epithelium (Barrett's syndrome) is a direct complication of gastro-esophageal reflux. At endoscopy, the normal mucosa of the distal esophagus is replaced by areas of redder mucosa that look more like the gastric lining. These may be in continuity with the stomach or appear as discrete islands in the lower esophagus (Figs 1.85, 1.86). Given the irregularity of the normal Z-line (see Fig. 1.12), Barrett's is usually diagnosed endoscopically only when at least 3 cm of the esophagus is affected or there are discrete islands. There is considerable debate around the significance of short-segment (visible endoscopically but less than 3 cm) Barrett's, and indeed of ultra-short-segment disease in which identification is purely from the histological features of biopsies taken from the esophago-gastric junction zone. Radiological diagnosis may also be possible (Fig. 1.87).

The histological hallmark is the presence of columnar epithelium of intestinal type – intestinal metaplasia – but other cell types may also be present (Figs 1.88–1.89).

The clinical importance of Barrett's syndrome lies in its premalignant potential (see below). Most authorities now advocate regular endoscopic surveillance in those potentially fit for esophagectomy. Confirmed severe dysplasia at multiple sites in Barrett's epithelium is increasingly accepted as an indication for esophageal resection.

ESOPHAGEAL CARCINOMA

Historically, most esophageal carcinomas were of squamous cell type and occurred approximately equally at all sites in the esophagus. However, this predominance has been almost overturned by the rapid increase in incidence (up by around 15% per year in the USA) of adenocarcinoma (accounting for less than 5% of all esophageal tumors until recently). Adenocarcinoma of the esophagus is no longer rare in Western countries, and while it accounts for perhaps

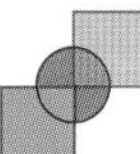

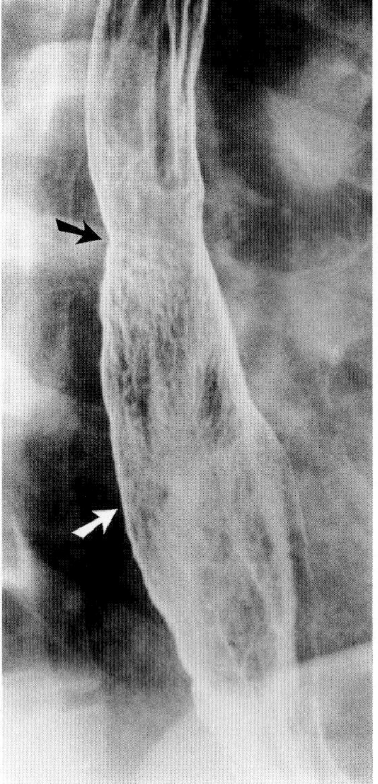

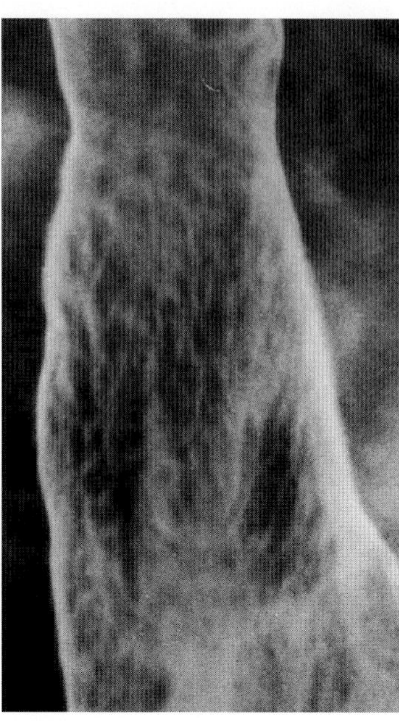

■ **Fig. 1.87** Double-contrast esophagram showing Barrett's esophagus with a reticular mucosal pattern. Note the mild stricture (black arrow) in the mid esophagus with a distinctive reticular pattern seen extending a considerable distance distally from the stricture (to the level of the white arrow). The reticular pattern is better seen on a close-up view of this region. (Both figures reproduced with permission from reference 6.)

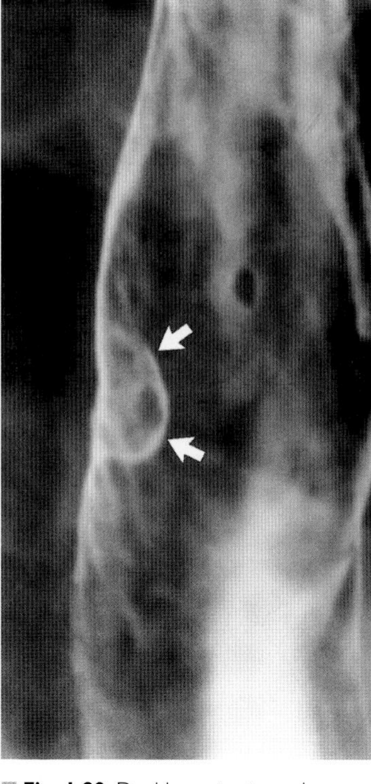

■ **Fig. 1.90** Double-contrast esophagram showing an early esophageal cancer as a small, sessile polyp (arrows) in the mid esophagus. (Courtesy of Seth N. Glick, M.D.; Philadelphia, PA; reproduced with permission from reference 1.)

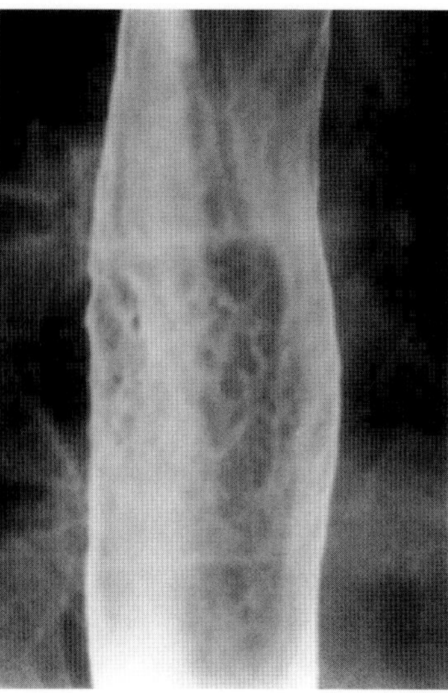

■ **Fig. 1.91** Double-contrast esophagram showing a superficial spreading carcinoma as a focal area of mucosal nodularity in the mid esophagus. Note how the nodules are poorly defined, producing a confluent area of disease. This appearance should be differentiated from the discrete plaque-like lesions of *Candida* esophagitis in Fig. 1.54. (Reproduced with permission from reference 1.)

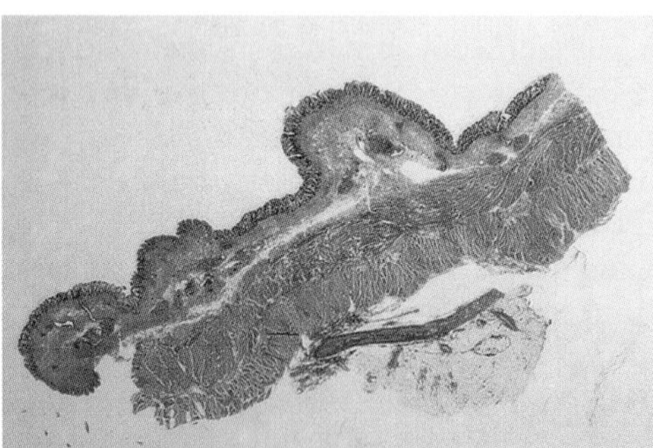

■ **Fig. 1.88** Whole-mount longitudinal section through the distal esophagus involved by Barrett's esophagus shows metaplastic glandular mucosa covering a submucosa that contains submucosal glands, which identify the section topographically as originating from the esophagus rather than the stomach.

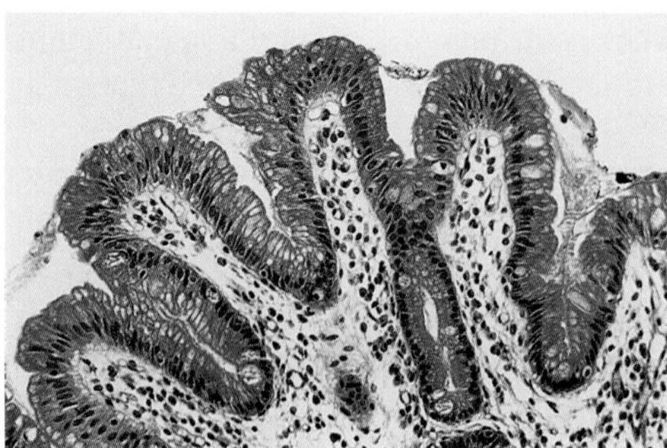

■ **Fig. 1.89** High-magnification micrograph showing metaplastic glandular mucosa characteristic of Barrett's esophagus and termed 'specialized Barrett's epithelium' composed of goblet cells and columnar mucus-producing cells resembling gastric surface epithelium.

only 5% of proximal esophageal malignancies, it is now the commonest histological type in the distal third of the esophagus, most of which probably arise from prior Barrett's syndrome, with 0.5% of Barrett's-affected patients developing cancer each year. It canbe difficult to make a clear distinction from upwards extension of adenocarcinoma of the gastric cardia but there is evidence to suggest that the etiology may be similar.

Patients present with dysphagia, initially for solids and later for liquids as the tumor progresses. Weight loss, anorexia and occasionally pain or hematemesis are accompanying symptoms. Radiologically, tumors may produce only subtle changes (Fig. 1.90): asymmetrical, diffuse thickening of the esophageal wall (Figs 1.91, 1.92); polypoid intrusions into the esophageal lumen (Fig. 1.93); or strictures with characteristically 'shouldered' appearances (Fig. 1.92), unlike the smoother tapering of benign strictures (e.g. Fig. 1.81). Endoscopy reflects the radiological findings (Figs 1.94, 1.95) and allows biopsy and cytological sampling to confirm the diagnosis. CT scanning and endoscopic ultrasound examination (Figs 1.96, 1.97) can be particularly helpful in assessing the operability of esophageal malignancies, since surgical resection remains the only hope of cure. The distinction between predominantly exophytic and constricting tumors is important if endoscopic palliation is to be employed, since the exophytic tumors can be expected to do well with endoluminal ablative therapies (e.g. laser or alcohol) (Fig. 1.98). Good results for constricting tumors are more likely to follow the placement of an esophageal prosthesis (Fig. 1.99), and with the slimmer introducer sets of self-expanding metal stents the need for prior balloon dilatation to facilitate their passage is increasingly questioned as an unnecessary addition to the risks of the procedure.

The macroscopic appearances of esophageal tumors correspond to the imaging and can be classified as fungating, ulcerative, or infiltrative (Fig. 1.100). Only rarely, in patients with mild symptoms and those identified from surveillance of Barrett's syndrome, is early carcinoma diagnosed.

The histology of squamous tumors encompasses a spectrum from essentially *in situ* tumors (Fig. 1.101), through early (Fig. 1.102) and deep invasion (Fig. 1.103) to the deeply invading poorly differentiated tumor. Both the degree of differentiation and the extent

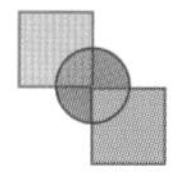

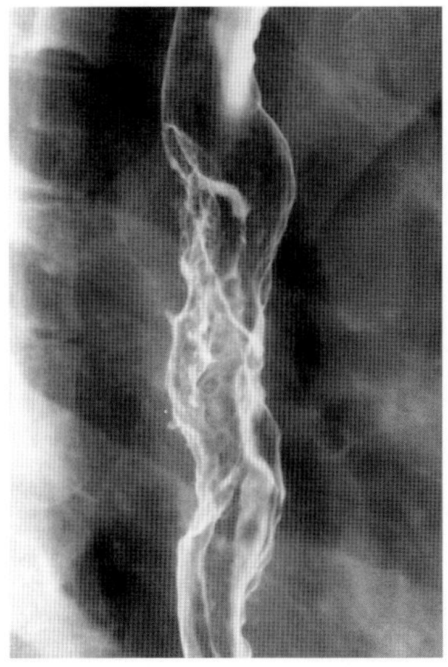

■ **Fig. 1.92** Double-contrast esophagram showing an infiltrating esophageal carcinoma as an irregular area of narrowing in the mid esophagus with ulceration, nodularity, and abrupt proximal and distal borders. (Reproduced with permission from reference 1)

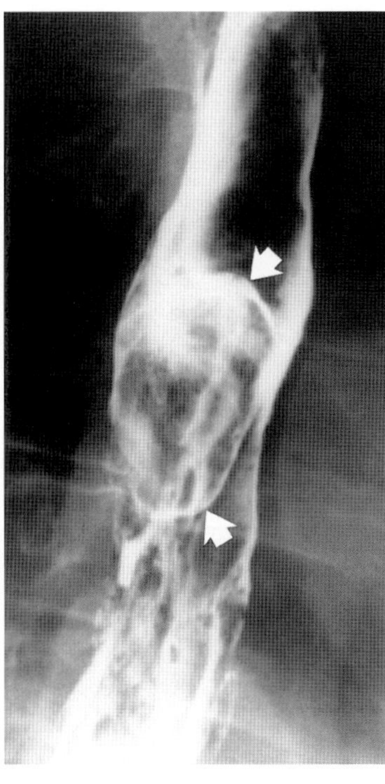

■ **Fig. 1.93** Double-contrast esophagram showing a polypoid esophageal carcinoma as a large protruded lesion (arrows) in the mid esophagus. (Reproduced with permission from reference 1.)

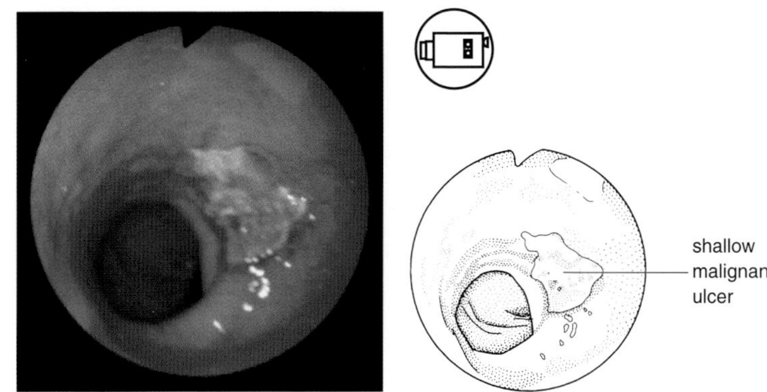

■ **Fig. 1.94** Endoscopic appearance of early ulcerative malignancy (adenocarcinoma) of the distal esophagus. The importance of biopsy in distinction from benign esophagitis is demonstrated.

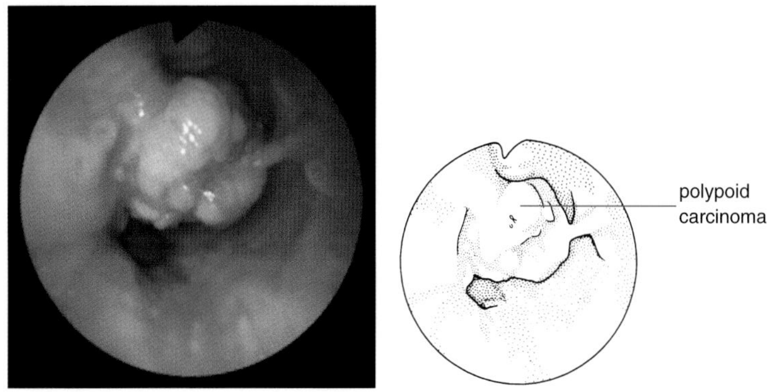

■ **Fig. 1.95** Endoscopic appearance of an exophytic carcinoma in the distal esophagus.

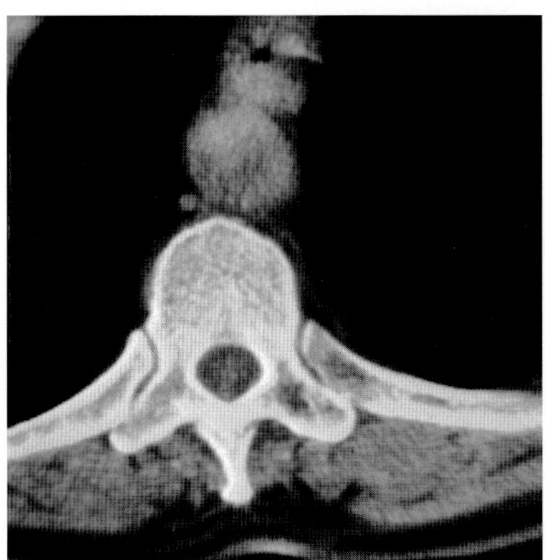

■ **Fig. 1.96** CT appearance of esophageal carcinoma; the abnormally thick-walled esophagus lies anterior to the aorta.

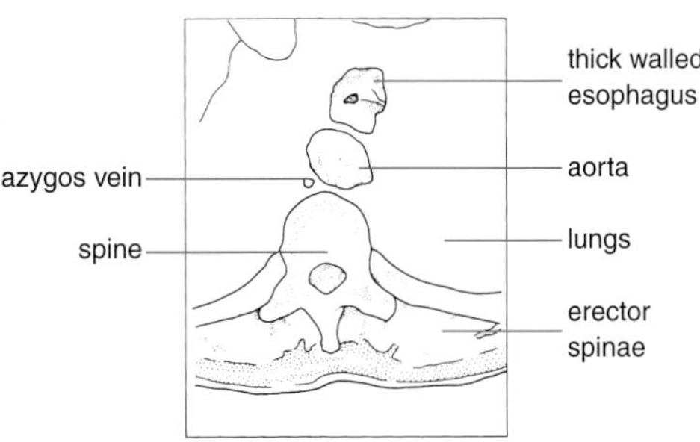

■ **Fig. 1.97** Endoscopic ultrasound study in esophageal carcinoma. Depth of invasion through esophageal muscle is clearly demonstrated.

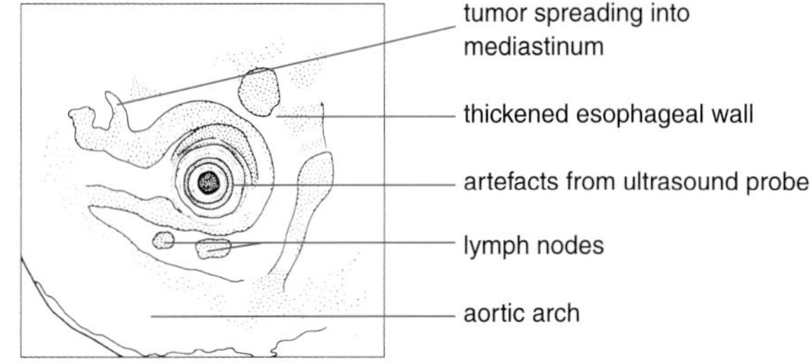

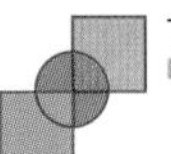

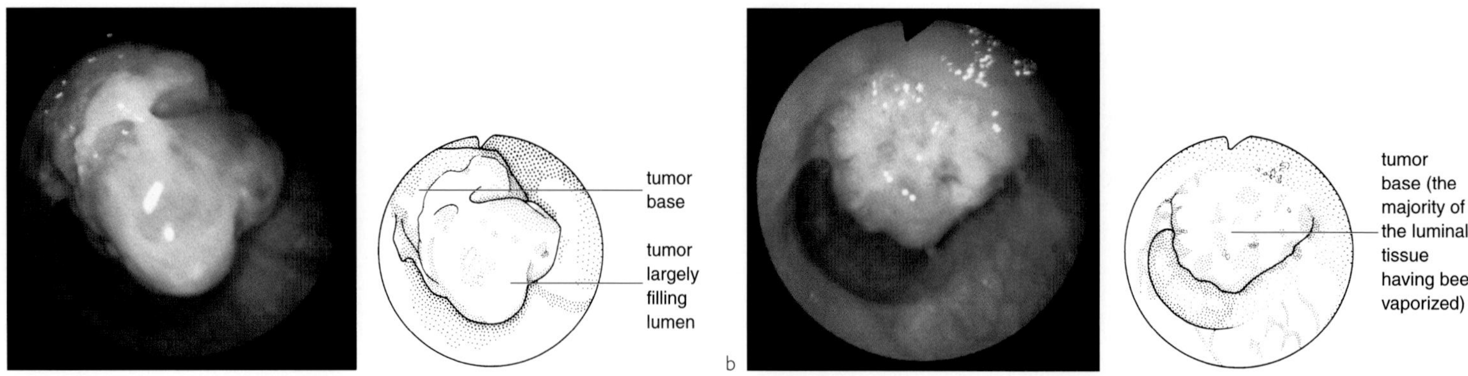

■ **Fig. 1.98** Endoscopic appearance of exophytic esophageal carcinoma before and after a single treatment with Nd-YAG laser.

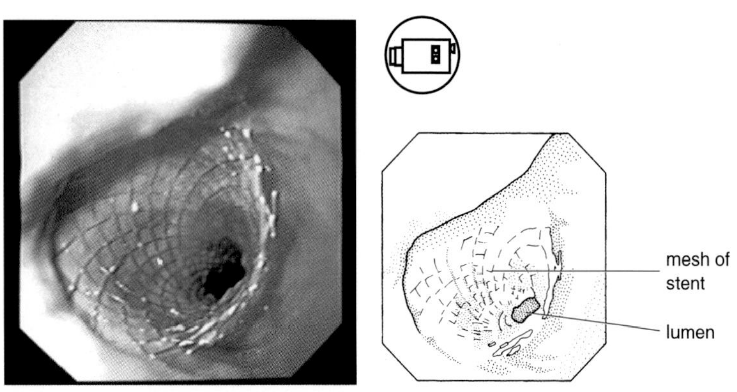

■ **Fig. 1.99** Endoscopic appearance of the esophagus at the upper end of an expandable metal stent used for an inoperable esophageal carcinoma. The partial epithelialization of the stent is apparent.

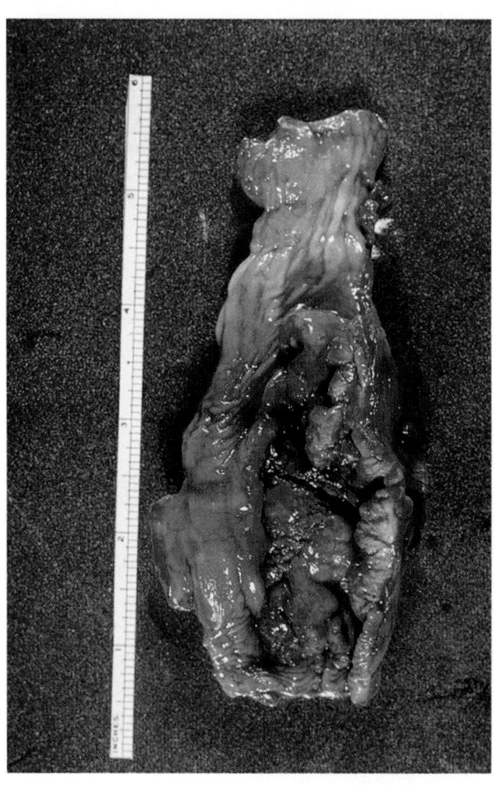

■ **Fig. 1.100** Macroscopic appearance of a large, exophytic but centrally ulcerated squamous cell carcinoma of the mid esophagus.

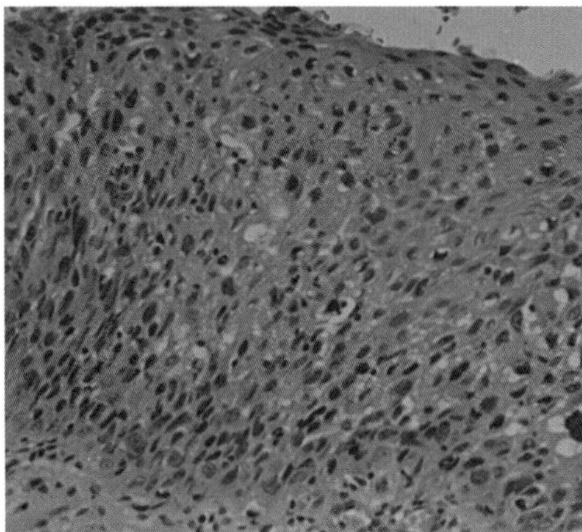

■ **Fig. 1.101** Histological appearance of esophageal carcinoma. In *in situ* carcinoma there is nuclear pleomorphism throughout the mucosa but no invasion. H&E stain (x420).

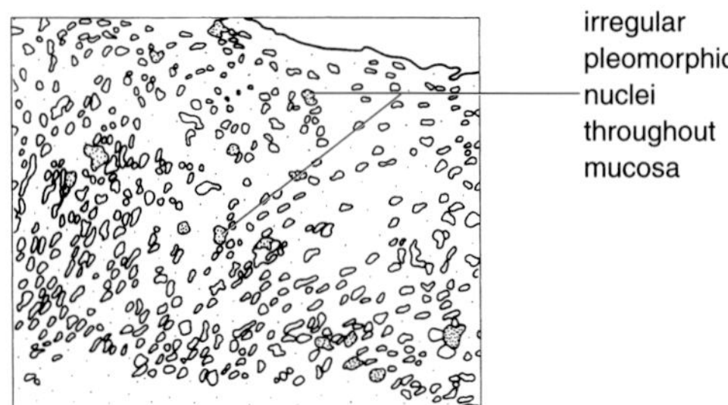

of infiltration through the esophageal wall have prognostic significance.

The upward extension of a gastric adenocarcinoma masquerading as an esophageal tumor is demonstrated histologically (Fig. 1.104); a comparable macroscopic specimen illustrates the difficulty of distinction between a true junctional carcinoma and an extending tumor of the cardia or fundus (Fig. 1.105). The microscopic appearances of Barrett's cancers may be seen helpfully alongside the originating non-neoplastic epithelium (Figs 1.106, 1.107) and these origins can be discerned even in the more advanced tumor (Fig. 1.108).

Late progression of esophageal carcinoma may lead to the development of broncho-esophageal fistula (Fig. 1.109), or to the overgrowth

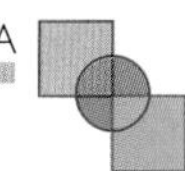

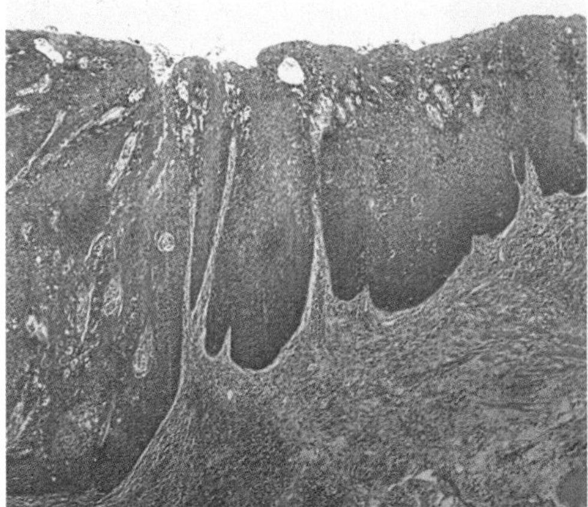

■ **Fig. 1.102** Histological appearance of early invasive squamous carcinoma with downgrowth of malignant epithelium into the submucosa. H&E stain (x100).

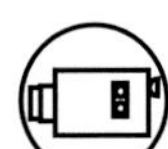

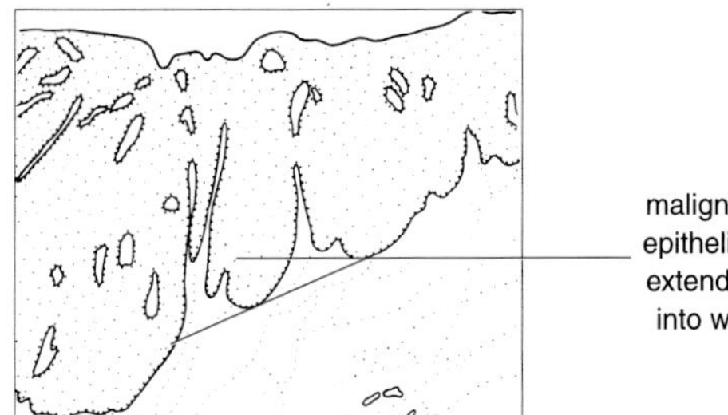

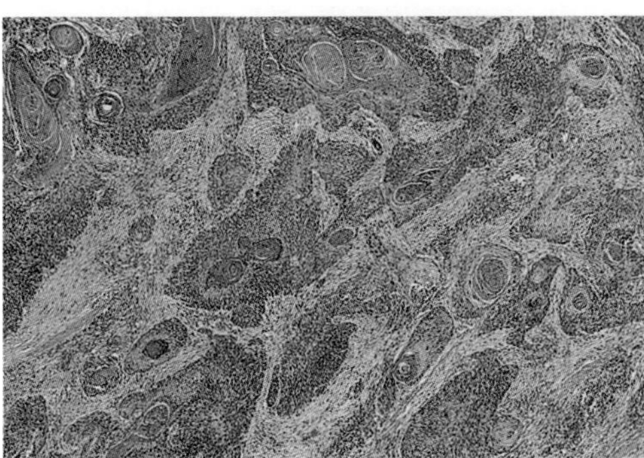

■ **Fig. 1.103** Microscopic appearance of tongues of well-differentiated squamous cell carcinoma showing central keratinization ('keratin pearl' formation) invading the esophageal wall.

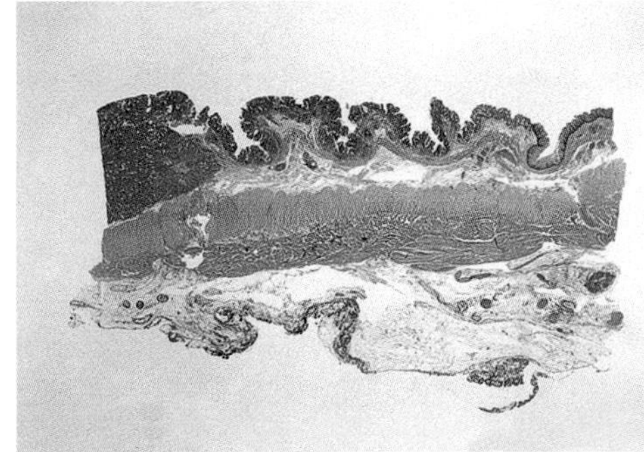

■ **Fig. 1.105** Adenocarcinoma of the esophagus arising from Barrett's esophagus. Whole-mount longitudinal section through the distal esophagus shows an infiltrating adenocarcinoma (far left) flanked by dysplastic Barrett's mucosa (right).

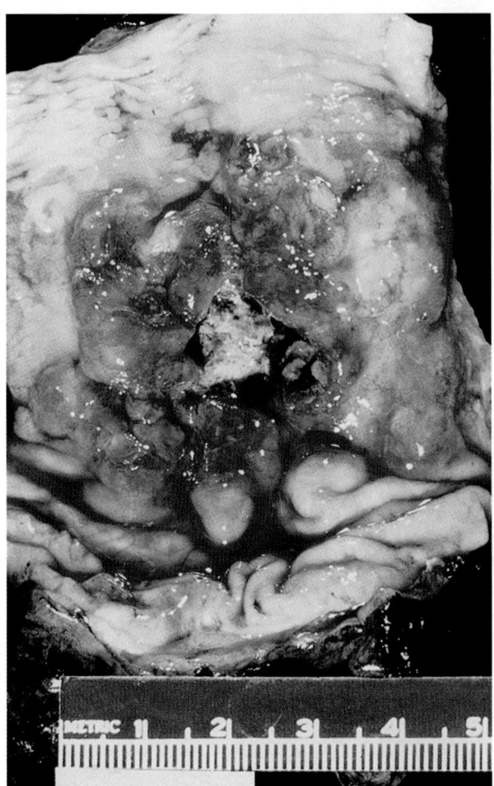

■ **Fig. 1.104** Macroscopic appearance of an ulcerating adenocarcinoma of the distal esophagus arising in a background of Barrett's esophagus.

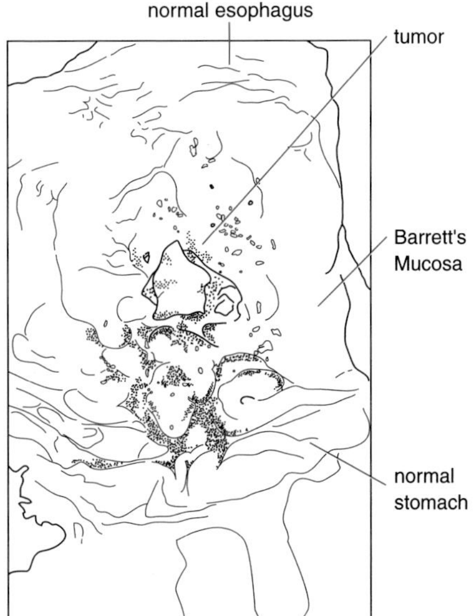

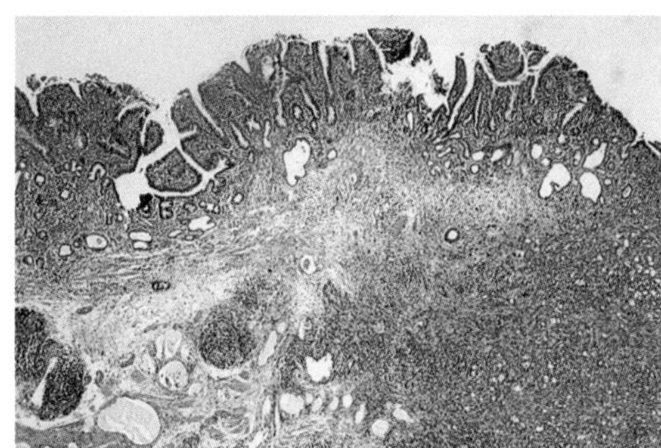

■ **Fig. 1.106** Adenocarcinoma of the esophagus arising from Barrett's esophagus. Microscopic appearance of invasive esophageal adenocarcinoma (right) and the dysplastic Barrett's mucosa (left) from which it arose.

■ **Fig. 1.107** High-magnification appearance of Barrett's epithelium with high-grade dysplasia, adjacent to the invasive carcinoma, characterized by irregular glands and mucosal contours and hyperchromatic, pleomorphic epithelial cells showing nuclear disarray and loss of polarity.

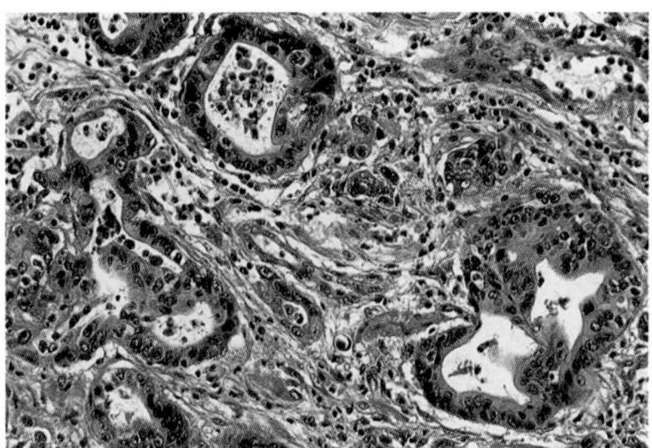

■ **Fig. 1.108** High-magnification appearance of the irregular small glands of invasive, moderately differentiated adenocarcinoma arising from Barrett's esophagus.

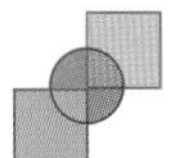

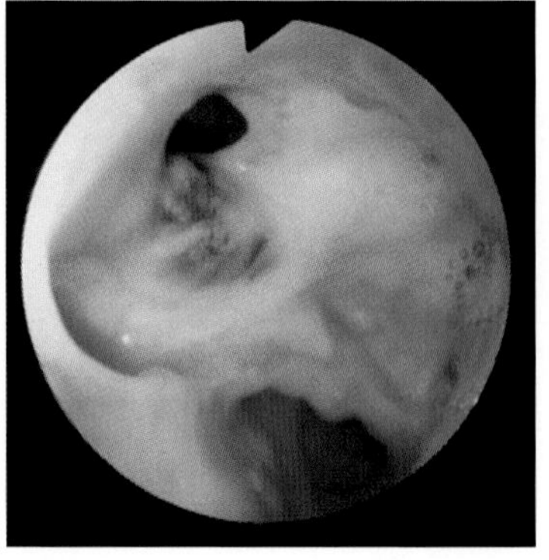

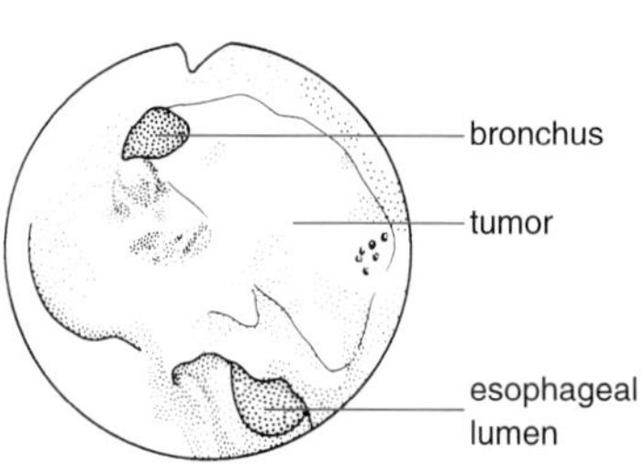

■ **Fig. 1.109** Endoscopic view of a malignant broncho-esophageal fistula. The esophageal lumen is the lower of the two openings.

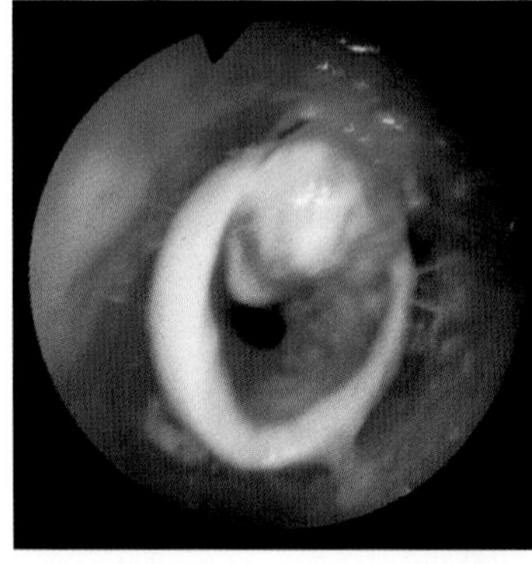

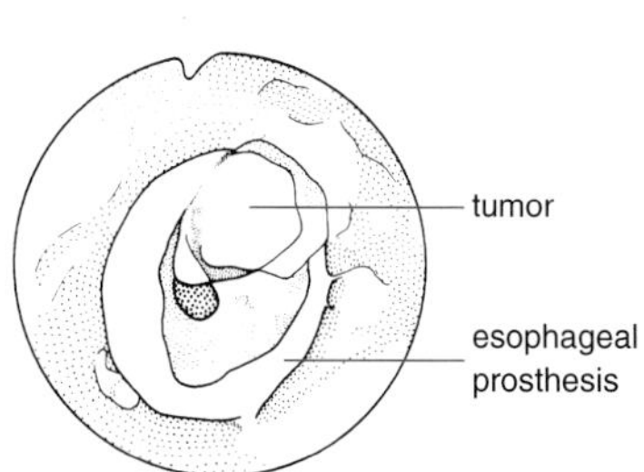

■ **Fig. 1.110** Late overgrowth of prosthesis by tumor progression.

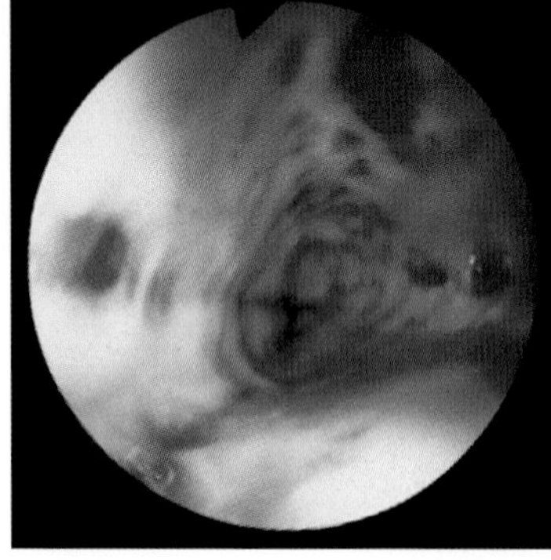

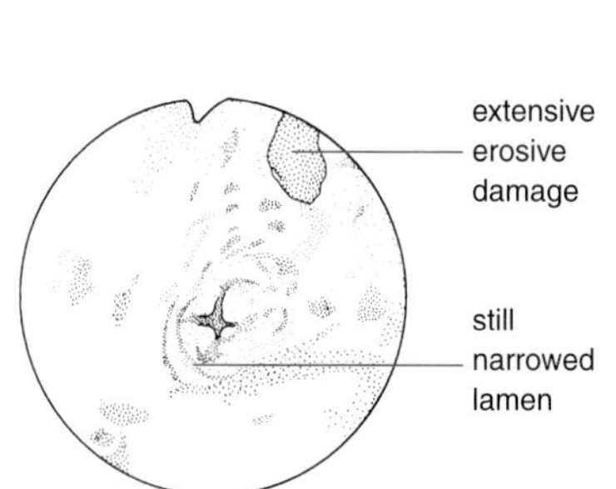

■ **Fig. 1.111** Endoscopic appearance of the extensive necrosis produced by intraluminal irradiation of an esophageal tumor.

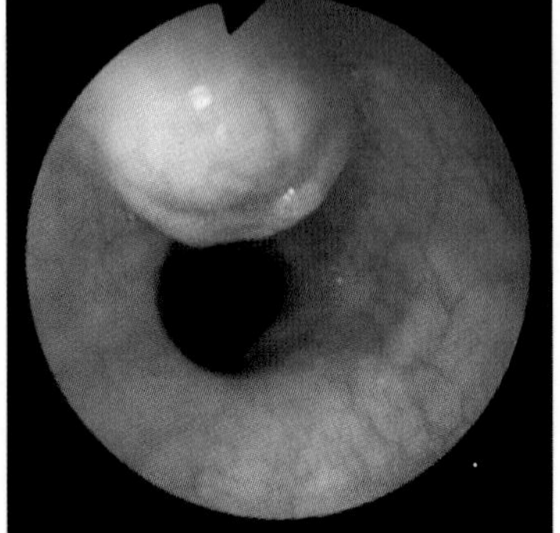

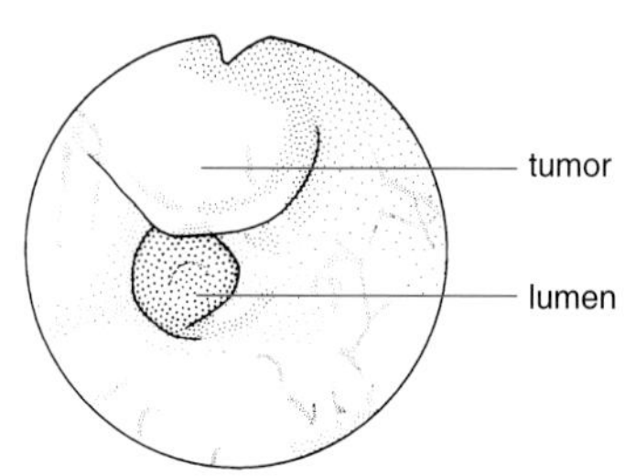

■ **Fig. 1.112** Endoscopic appearance of adenoid cystic carcinoma of the esophagus.

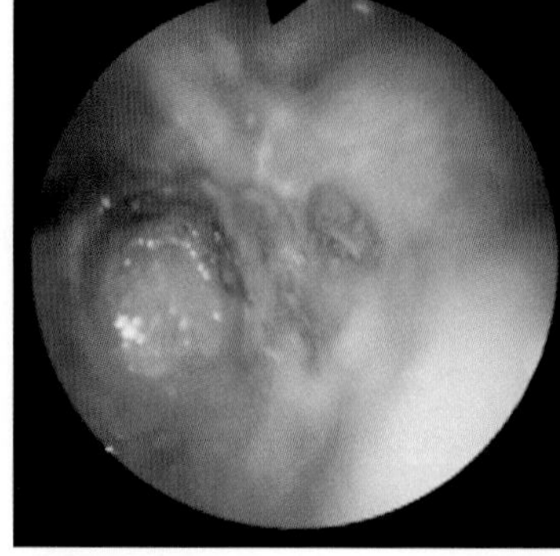

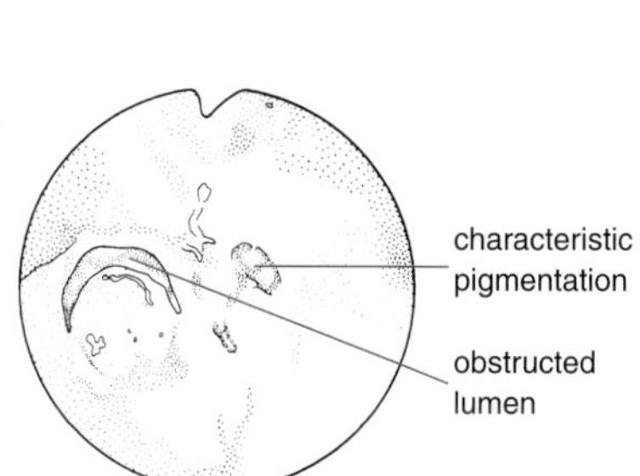

■ **Fig. 1.113** Endoscopic appearance of esophageal melanoma.

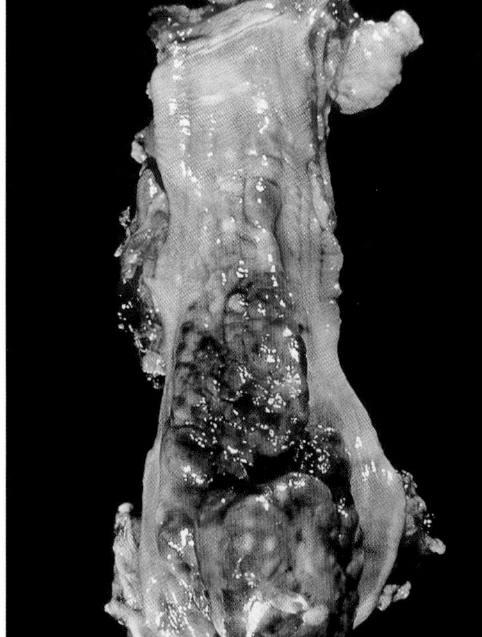

■ **Fig. 1.114** Macroscopic appearance of melanoma of the esophagus showing the blue-black pigmentation that is characteristic of this rare tumor type.

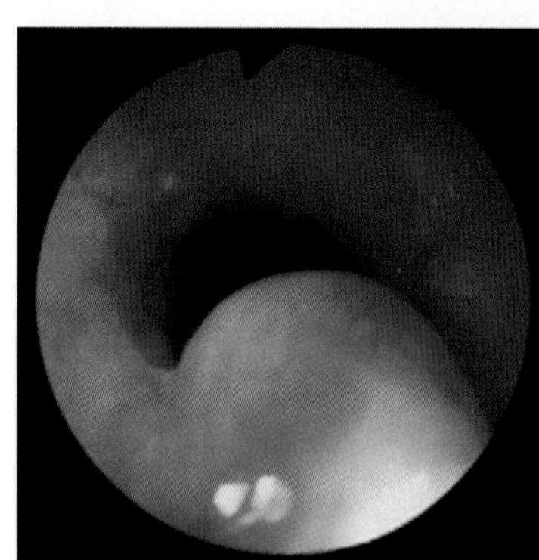

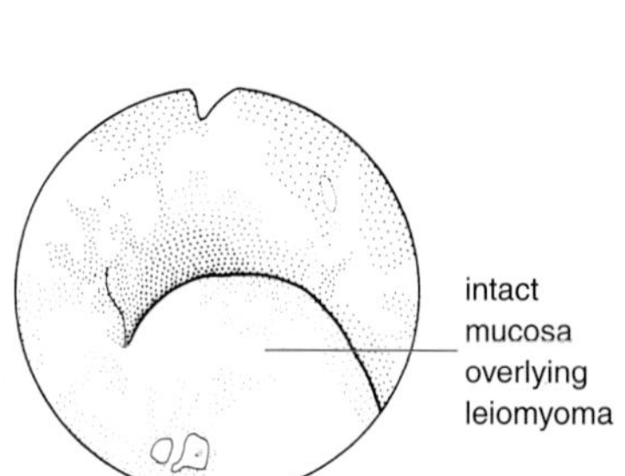

■ **Fig. 1.115** Endoscopic appearance of esophageal stromal tumor (of leiomyoma type).

of a palliative prosthesis (Fig. 1.110). Radiotherapy may be associated with a severe necrotic esophagitis (Fig. 1.111), and although this may be transient, late stricturing is also seen (see Fig. 1.81).

Other neoplasms and polyps

A variety of benign and less common malignant tumors of the esophagus are also recognized (Figs 1.112–1.117), including the

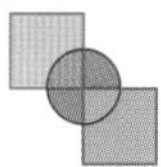

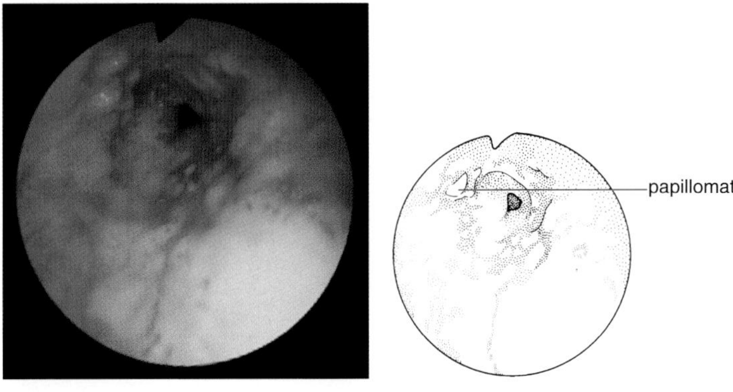

■ **Fig. 1.116** Endoscopic appearance of distal esophageal papillomatosis.

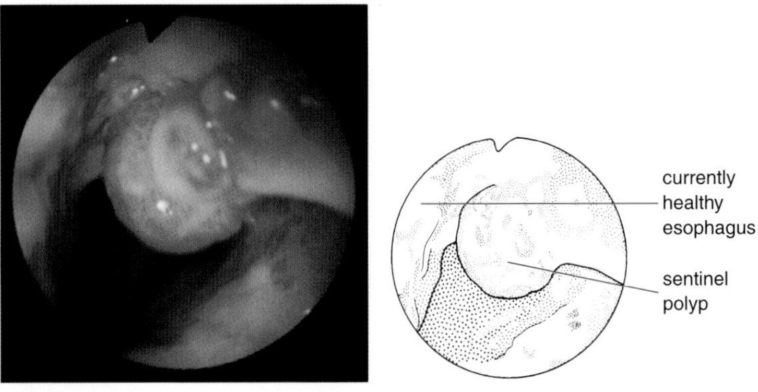

■ **Fig. 1.117** Endoscopic view of esophageal sentinel polyp associated with previous esophagitis.

benign sentinel polyp that marks the site of previous inflammation (Fig. 1.117). Rare, but important because it is so easily missed endoscopically and yet is readily curable once found, is the pedunculated submucosal tumor. The bizarre complaint of a fleshy lump being regurgitated into the mouth and then repeatedly swallowed may occur (Fig. 1.118).

RINGS AND WEBS

Esophageal webs are thin membranes of connective tissue covered by normal squamous epithelium. Although they may occur anywhere along the esophagus, they are usually situated in the upper third and are frequently asymmetrical (Fig. 1.119). The association of a very proximal esophageal web and iron-deficiency anemia is known as the Paterson–Brown–Kelly (or Plummer–Vinson) syndrome and occurs most often in middle-aged women. Such patients may also have leukoplakia of the oropharynx (Fig. 1.120) and koilonychia. These webs regress spontaneously with treatment of the anemia and, although there are no aberrant epithelial changes in the web (Fig. 1.121), the syndrome is associated with an increased incidence of post-cricoid carcinoma.

Two types of esophageal rings have been described. The Schatzki ring is a symmetrical, submucosal, fibrous thickening that occurs at the squamo-columnar junction at the lower end of the esophagus. It measures 1–3 mm in thickness (Fig. 1.122). The ring can be seen endoscopically above the diaphragmatic indentation (Fig. 1.123). The other type of ring occurs just proximal to the site of the Schatzki ring, at the junction of the distal esophagus and the uppermost part of the lower esophageal sphincter and is thought to be muscular. Manometrically, this corresponds to a high-pressure zone, and is frequently associated with esophageal motor disorders and diffuse esophageal spasm (see below). Both webs and rings cause intermittent dysphagia for solids, and occasional bolus impaction. The disruption of webs and rings caused by diagnostic endoscopy may be therapeutic.

ACHALASIA OF THE CARDIA

Achalasia is a disorder of esophageal motility of unknown etiology, which usually affects the middle-aged. The clinical and pathophysiological features are also produced by esophageal involvement with *Trypanosoma cruzi* infection (Chagas' disease; see Chapter 6), and rarely, but crucially, as a consequence of metastatic carcinoma (see below). Patients generally present with dysphagia for both liquids and

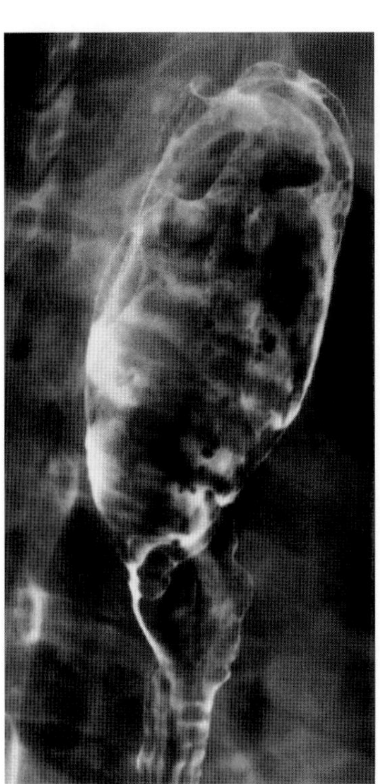

a

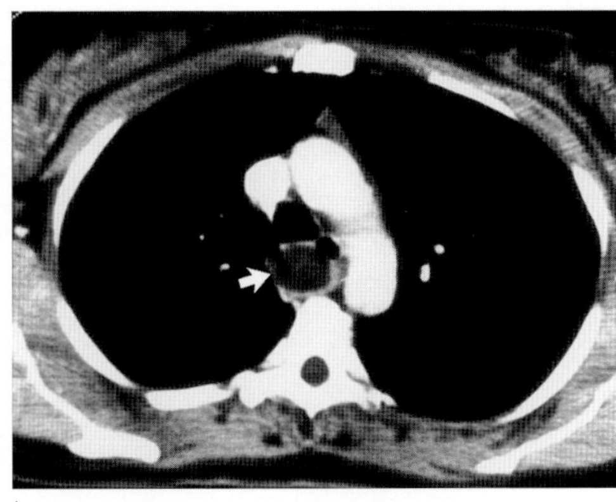

b

■ **Fig. 1.118** (a) Double-contrast esophagram showing a giant fibrovascular polyp as a smooth, expansile, sausage-shaped mass expanding the lumen of the upper thoracic esophagus. (b) A CT scan in the same patient shows a fat-density mass (arrow) expanding the esophagus with a thin rim of contrast surrounding the lesion, confirming its intraluminal location. Fibrovascular polyps often contain areas of fat-density on CT because of their high adipose content. (Reproduced with permission from reference 7.)

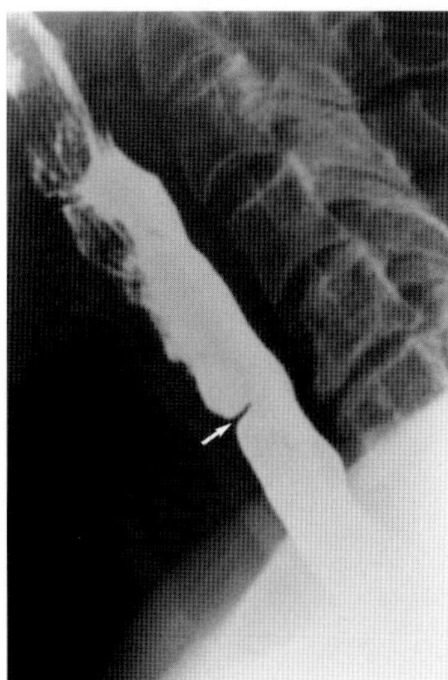

■ **Fig. 1.119** Double-contrast esophagram showing a cervical esophageal web as a thin indentation (arrow) on the anterior aspect of the cervical esophagus. This is the typical appearance of a cervical web.

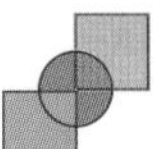

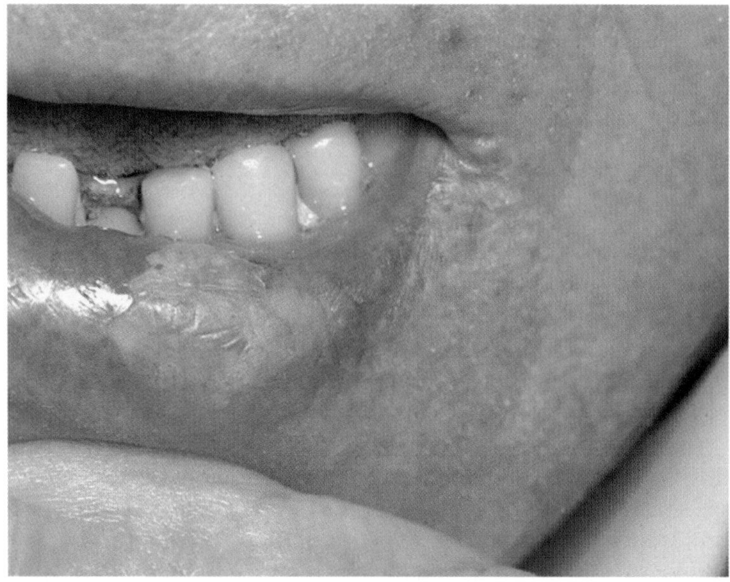

■ **Fig. 1.120** White thickened plaque of leukoplakia on the labial mucosa. Courtesy of Dr S Goolamali.

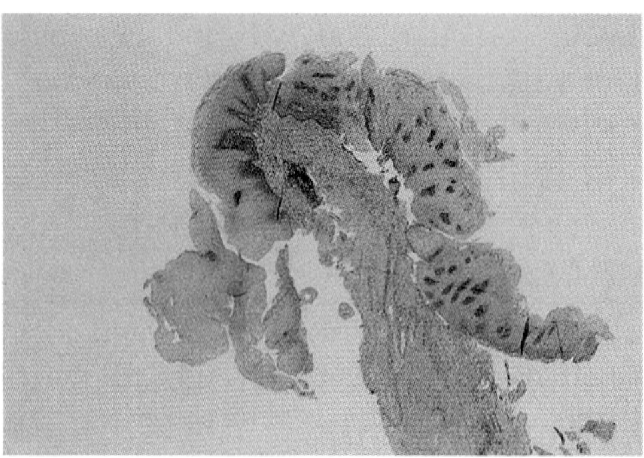

■ **Fig. 1.121** Microscopic appearance of a resected esophageal web showing the characteristic redundancy (pleat) of the otherwise normal squamous mucosa.

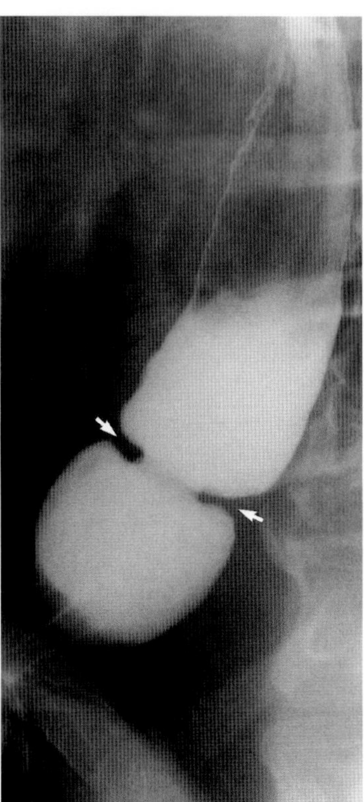

■ **Fig. 1.122** Prone single-contrast esophagram showing a Schatzki ring as a smooth, symmetric ring-like constriction (arrows) at the gastro-esophageal junction above a hiatal hernia. Note how the ring has a vertical height of only several millimeters. Such rings are best seen when the esophagus is optimally distended during continuous drinking of low-density barium in the prone position.

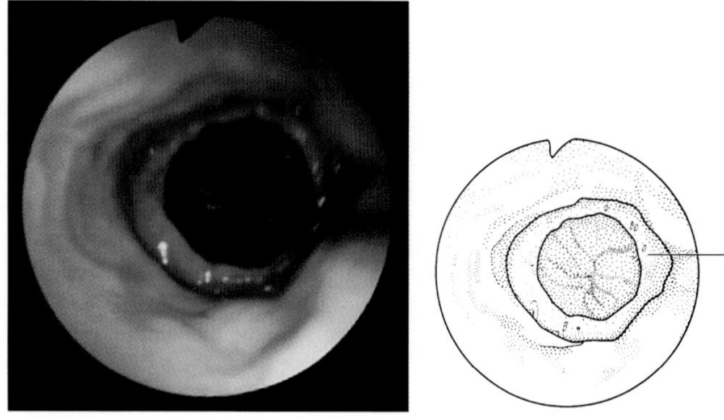

■ **Fig. 1.123** Endoscopic view of a Schatzki ring situated at the junction of the pale pink esophageal and deeper pink gastric mucosa.

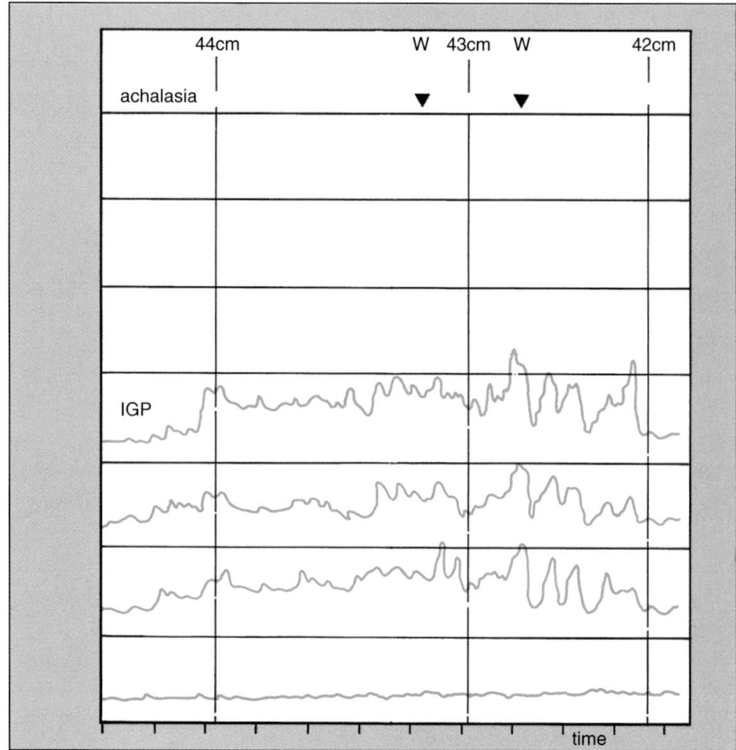

■ **Fig. 1.124** Manometry of achalasia. Station pull-through of lower esophageal sphincter: the three recorded channels are at the same level but at 120 degrees to each other. Marks on the horizontal axis represent 10-second intervals. Vertical axis: scale between major intervals = 100 mmHg. IGP = intragastric pressure. Rise in pressure at 44 cm indicates LES; note j = high resting pressure (around 50 mmHg). W = wet swallows – note lack of sphincter relaxation to intragastric pressure. Courtesy of Dr J de Caestecker.

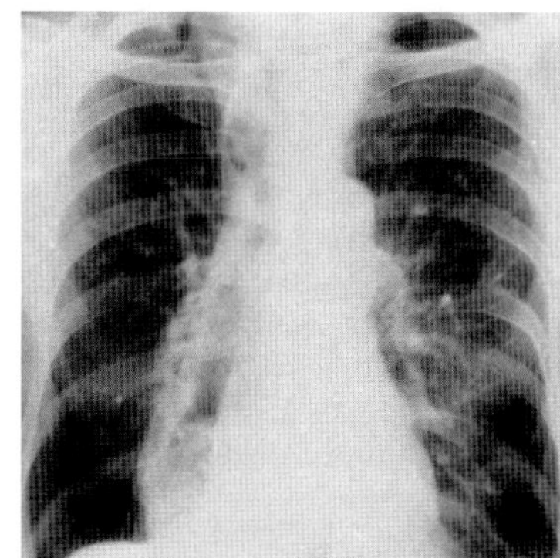

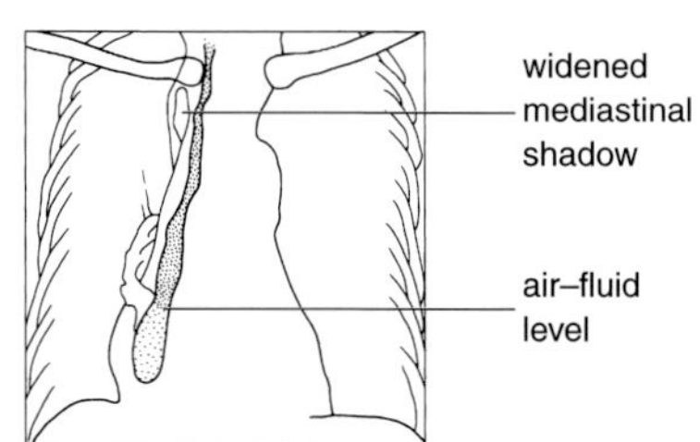

■ **Fig. 1.125** Chest radiograph showing a widened mediastinum due to the dilated esophagus of achalasia. An air–fluid level is visible.

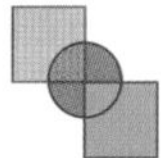

solids, although some, particularly in the early stages of the disease, may have chest pain. Regurgitation of esophageal contents may lead to aspiration pneumonia, or other respiratory complications.

The impaired motility is associated with a lack of peristalsis in the distal two thirds of the esophagus, and incomplete or absent relaxation of the lower esophageal sphincter in response to voluntary swallowing. Manometry usually demonstrates a high resting pressure, and confirms the lack of full sphincter relaxation (down to intragastric pressure) (Fig. 1.124). These abnormalities lead to progressive dilatation of the esophagus above the lower esophageal sphincter. In severe cases, a plain chest radiograph will show the dilated esophagus with an air–fluid level behind the heart, secondary to the accumulation of food and secretions (Figs 1.125, 1.126). Barium studies (Fig. 1.127) help to emphasize the distinction from a large hiatus hernia (see Figs 1.29–1.30). The endoscopic appearances are those of a normal but very dilated esophagus

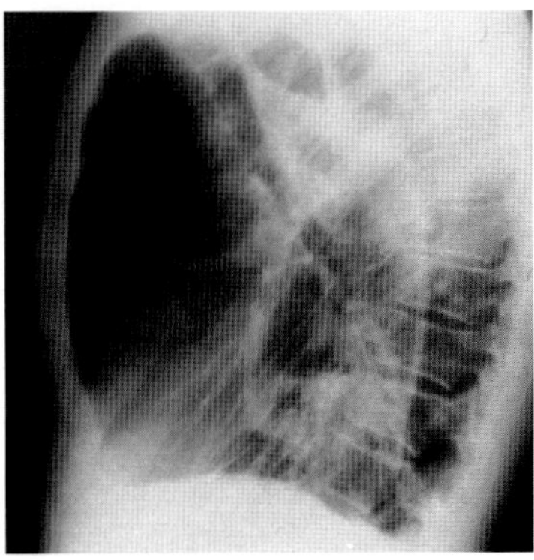

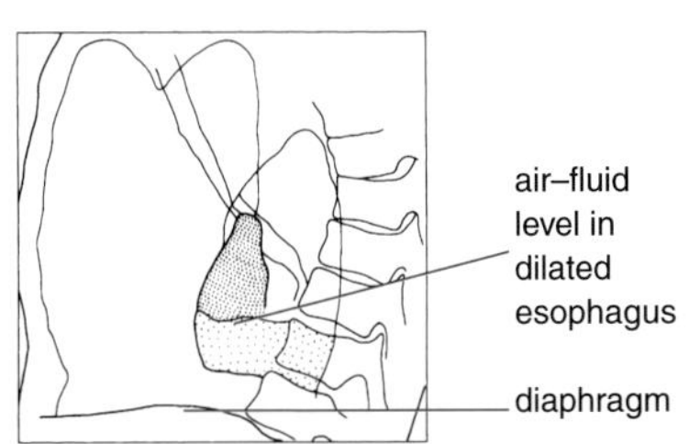

Fig. 1.126 A lateral film also shows the air–fluid level in the dilated esophagus.

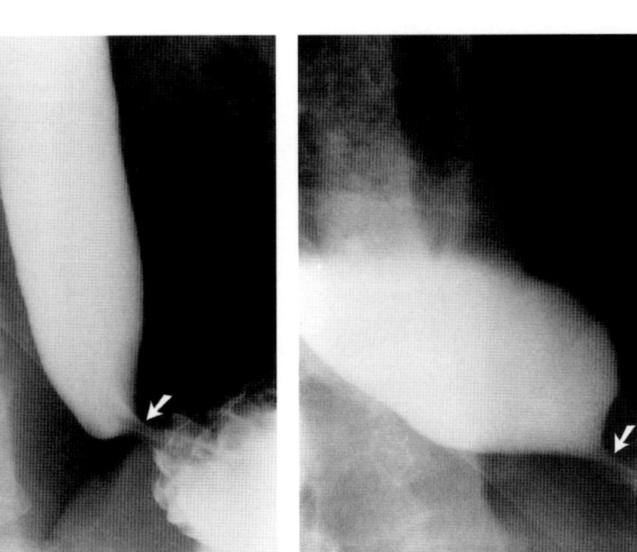

Fig. 1.127 Single-contrast esophagrams in two patients with primary achalasia. Both patients had absent primary peristalsis at fluoroscopy and beak-like narrowing (arrows) of the distal esophagus near the gastro-esophageal junction due to failure of relaxation of the lower esophageal sphincter. In the patient with more advanced achalasia, note how the esophagus is more dilated and filled with debris.

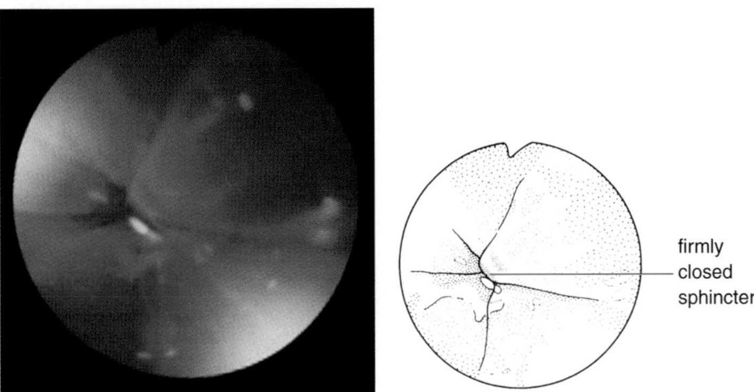

Fig. 1.128 Endoscopic view of achalasia after thorough lavage, showing firmly closed sphincter zone.

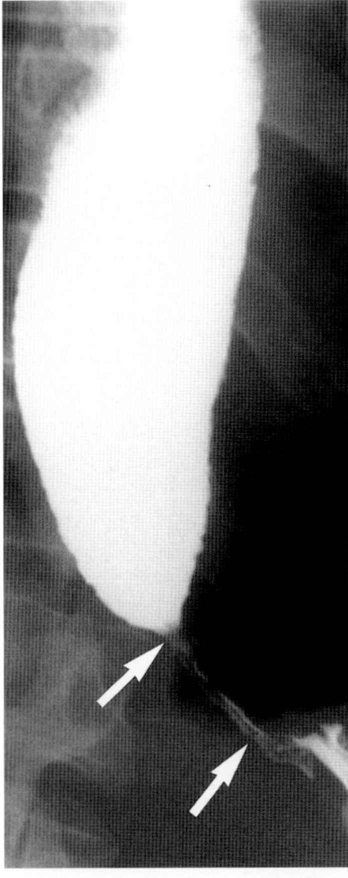

Fig. 1.129 Single-contrast esophagram showing secondary achalasia with tapered narrowing (arrows) of the distal esophagus and proximal dilatation. In this case, however, note how the narrowed segment extends several centimeters above the gastro-esophageal junction, an unusual finding in patients with primary achalasia. This was an elderly patient with dysphagia who had metastatic carcinoma of the lung causing secondary achalasia. (Reproduced with permission from reference 8.)

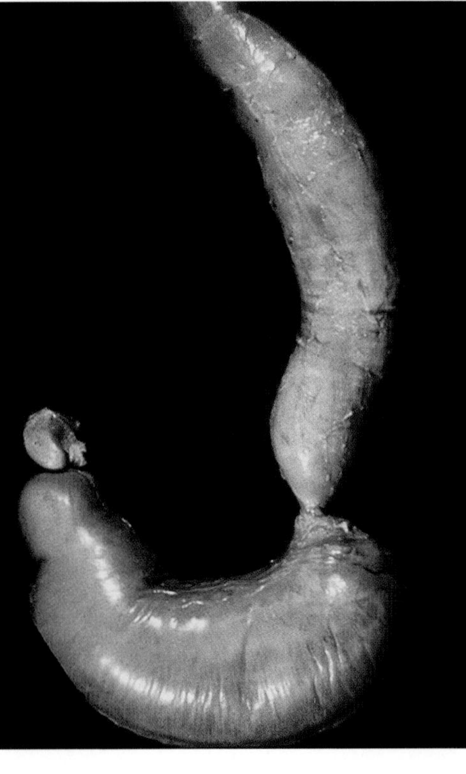

Fig. 1.130 Achalasia in Chagas' disease. Macroscopic appearance at autopsy of a grossly dilated esophagus above a constricted gastro-esophageal sphincter. (Courtesy of Dr. James Maguire.)

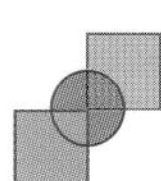

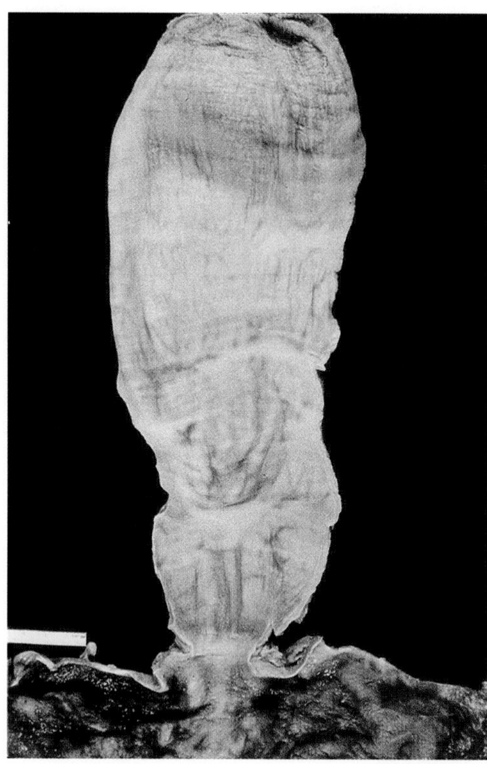

■ **Fig. 1.131** Achalasia in Chagas' disease. Macroscopic appearance of the massively dilated esophagus, opened longitudinally, in achalasia secondary to Chagas' disease. (Courtesy of Dr. James Maguire.)

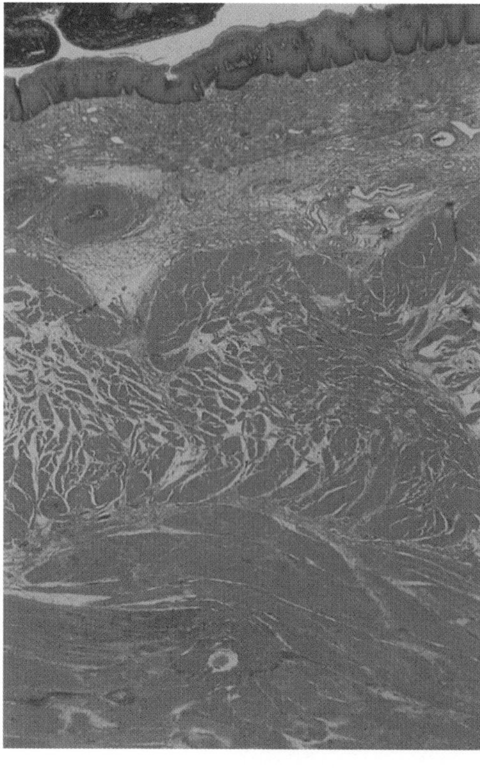

■ **Fig. 1.132** Histology of achalasia, Striking muscular hypertrophy has primarily affected the circular layer and, in part, may reflect denervation. H&E stain (x 4). Courtesy of Dr FA Mitros.

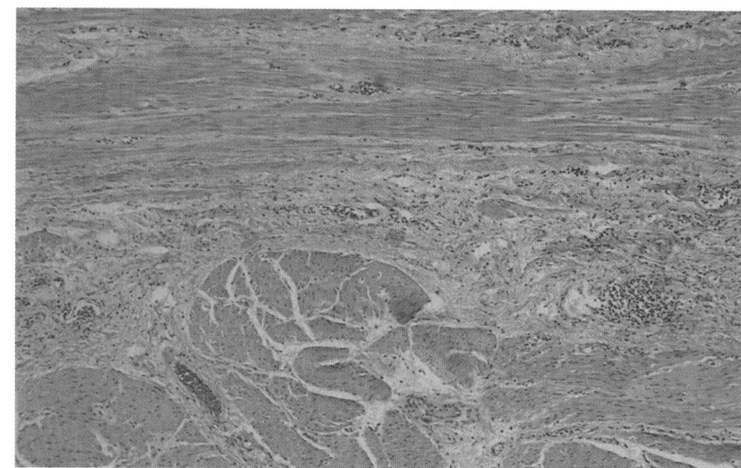

■ **Fig. 1.133** Histology of achalasia showing a segment of myenteric plexus near the gastro-esophageal junction that is devoid of ganglion cells. H&E stain (x 16). Courtesy of Dr FA Mitros.

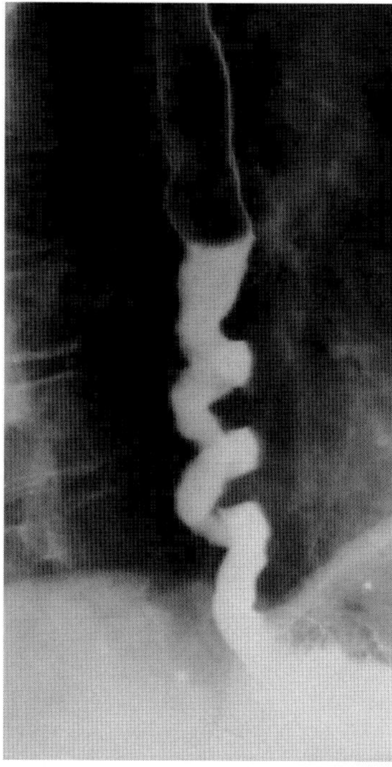

■ **Fig. 1.134** Barium swallow showing diffuse esophageal spasm with a typical 'corkscrew' deformity.

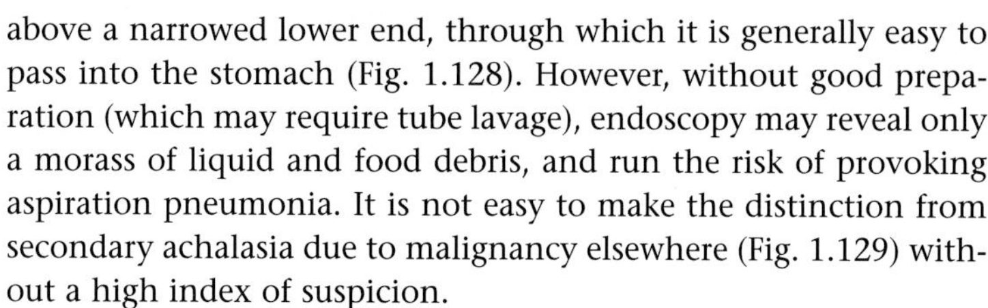

above a narrowed lower end, through which it is generally easy to pass into the stomach (Fig. 1.128). However, without good preparation (which may require tube lavage), endoscopy may reveal only a morass of liquid and food debris, and run the risk of provoking aspiration pneumonia. It is not easy to make the distinction from secondary achalasia due to malignancy elsewhere (Fig. 1.129) without a high index of suspicion.

Macroscopically, the achalasic esophagus is grossly dilated above a narrow distal segment (Figs 1.130, 1.131). Special staining techniques on full-thickness biopsies demonstrate the loss of ganglion cells in the myenteric plexus. The normal non-argyrophilic ganglion cells are decreased in number, especially in the dilated portion of the esophagus; argyrophilic ganglion cells are not affected (Figs 1.132, 1.133).

Surgical myectomy probably offers only modest advantages over balloon dilatation, and initial promise of pharmacological methods has not been sustained. Newer endoscopic approaches using radiofrequency ablation are under active scrutiny. On a lifetime basis there is a small increased risk of squamous carcinoma within the dilated segment; if the achalasia was previously unrecognized this may then be confused with a simple obstructing tumor with upstream dilatation.

ESOPHAGEAL SPASM

Esophageal spasm is a disorder of esophageal motility characterized clinically by episodic dysphagia and chest pain resembling angina. Although the symptoms may occur without warning, they are frequently provoked by swallowing or by the ingestion of hot or very cold liquids, and they are associated with objective evidence of gastro-esophageal reflux in approximately 50% of cases. Diffuse esophageal spasm may produce a characteristic 'corkscrew'

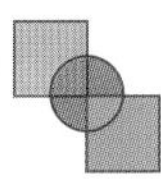

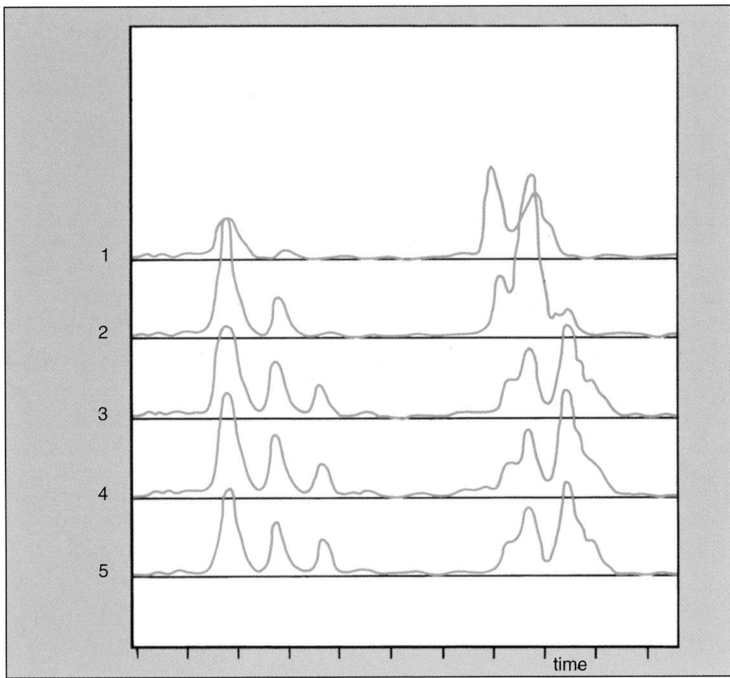

■ **Fig. 1.135** Manometry of diffuse esophageal spasm. Most of the classic features are shown. The first pressure wave is simultaneous (i.e. non-peristaltic) and multi-peaked. The second wave-front is peristaltic but also multi-peaked; the amplitude is increased (>200 mmHg). Marks on the horizontal axis represent 5-second intervals.

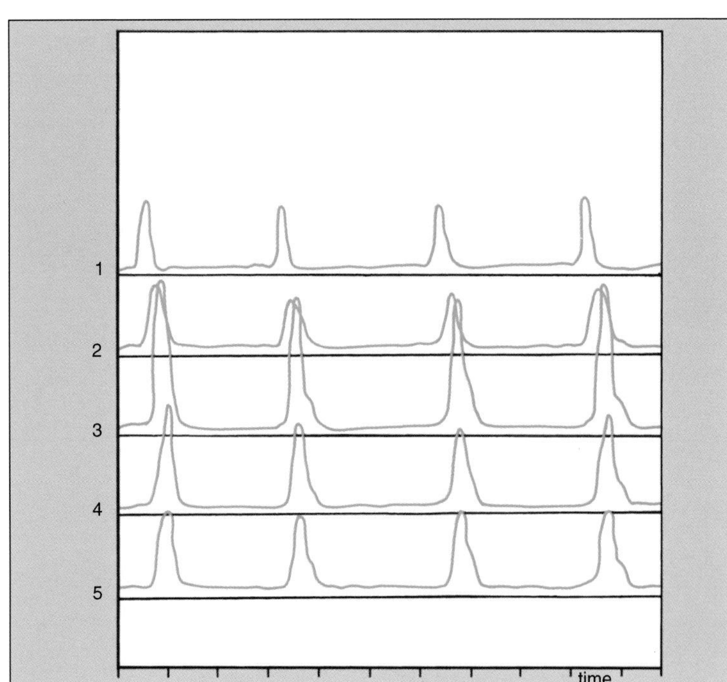

■ **Fig. 1.137** Manometry of 'nutcracker' esophagus: normally propagated peristalsis of increased amplitude (>200 mmHg) in distal channels. Marks in the horizontal axis represent 5-second intervals. Courtesy of Dr J de Caestecker.

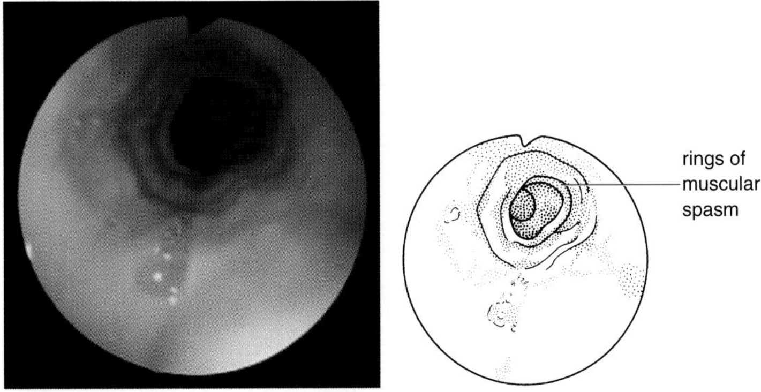

■ **Fig. 1.136** Endoscopic view of esophagus showing multiple 'rings' of diffuse spasm.

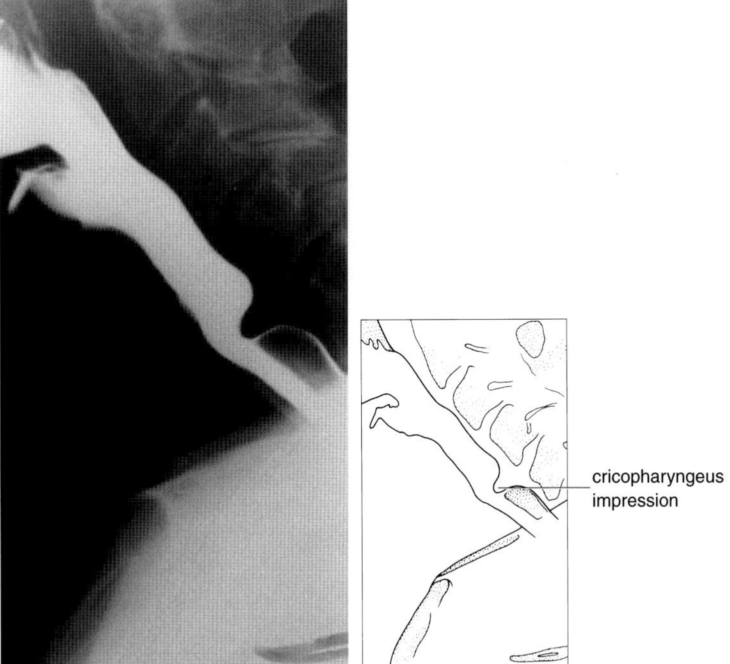

■ **Fig. 1.138** Delayed relaxation of the cricopharyngeus as shown on a lateral view at barium swallow.

appearance of the esophagus on barium swallow (Fig. 1.134), but less severe cases will be recognized usually only from manometric studies (Fig. 1.135). Endoscopy is not usually helpful, although multiple simultaneous 'ring' contractions may be seen (Fig. 1.136). The so-called 'nutcracker' esophagus is associated with severe pain and with muscular contraction of markedly increased amplitude and duration but of normal propagation (Fig. 1.137). The resting pressure within the body of the esophagus may be increased, as may lower esophageal sphincter pressure; however, relaxation on swallowing is normal. Secondary diffuse spasm may occasionally occur in association with distal obstruction, and it is wise to precede manometric studies by endoscopic assessment of the upper gastrointestinal tract. Occasionally, globus hystericus may be suggested erroneously by localized delay in relaxation of the cricopharyngeus (Fig. 1.138).

SCLERODERMA (SYSTEMIC SCLEROSIS)

Pronounced esophageal motor dysfunction as a result of smooth muscle dysfunction is common in scleroderma and in the mixed connective tissue disease overlap syndromes (Fig. 1.139). Manometry shows low-pressure peristalsis (Fig. 1.140) and this may precede other systemic (non-gastroenterological) manifestations of the disease: the clear distinction from achalasia is then helpful. Radiologically, there is absent peristalsis and dilatation of the esophagus with free gastro-esophageal reflux – hence the frequent association with esophagitis and late stricture formation. Symptoms of dysphagia predominate in most patients, but those of reflux esophagitis may also be troublesome.

The histology of the esophagus in scleroderma shows progressive atrophy of the smooth muscle coat; replacement with fibrous tissue

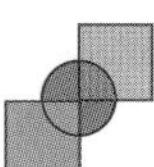

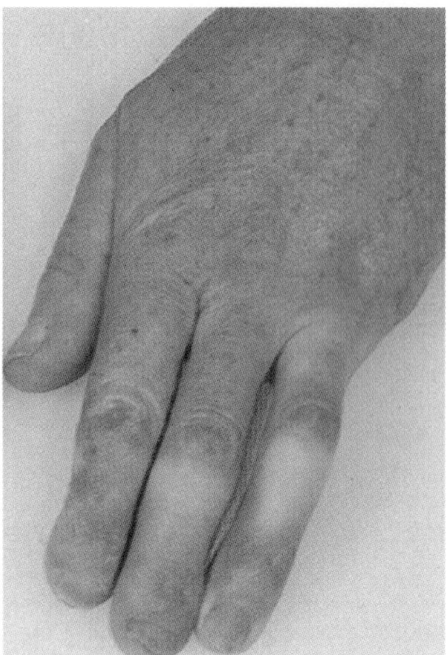

■ **Fig. 1.139** The hand in scleroderma showing shiny tethered skin, pulp atrophy, pitting scars, digital ulceration and early flexion contractures. There is active Raynaud's phenomenon. The fifth digit was amputated for gangrene. Courtesy of Prof C Black.

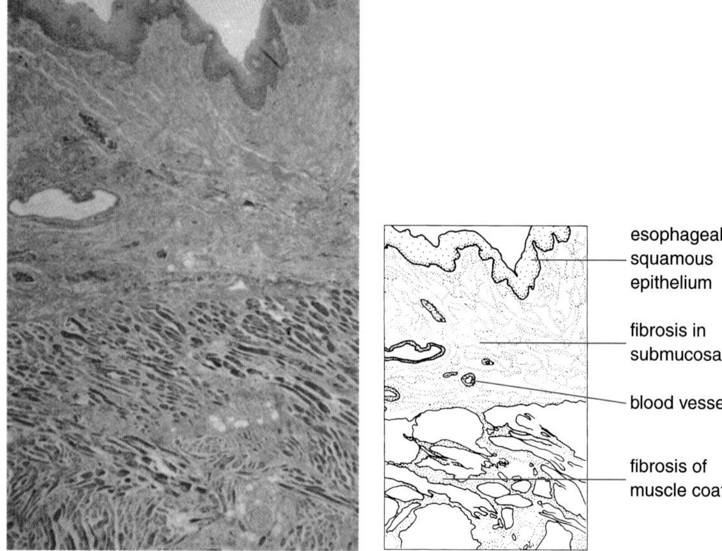

■ **Fig. 1.141** Histological appearance of scleroderma showing increased fibrosis of the submucosa (blue), fragmenting the muscularis and beginning to disrupt the main muscle coat. Martius Scarlet Blue stain (x20).

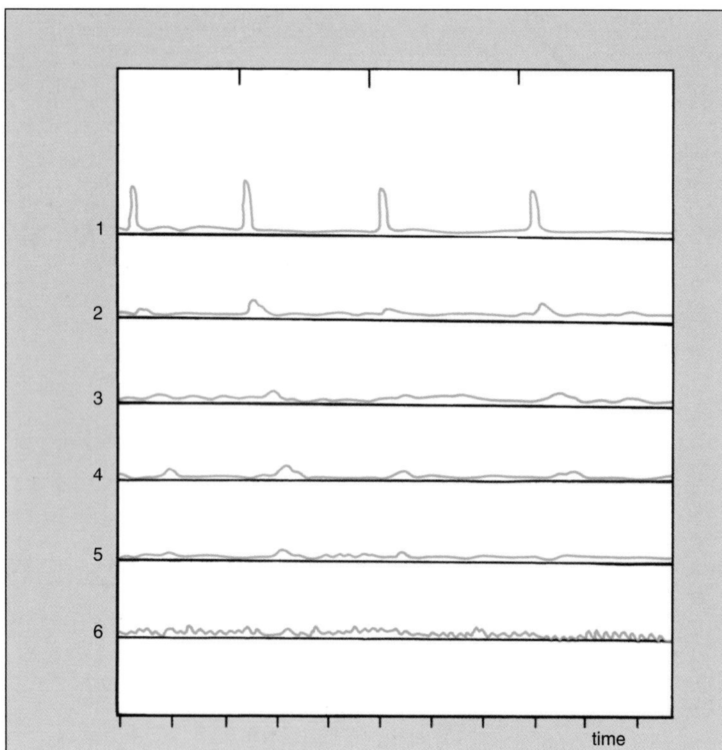

■ **Fig. 1.140** Manometry of scleroderma – in this case associated with severe esophagitis. Marks on the horizontal axis represent 5-second intervals. Low-pressure peristalsis is shown in the distal five channels with normal pressure waves in the proximal channel. This type of motility disorder is usually associated with poor clearance of refluxed gastric acid. Courtesy of Dr J de Caestecker.

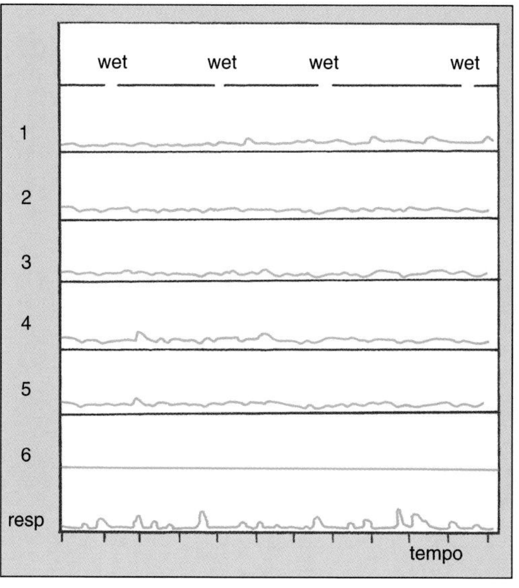

■ **Fig. 1.142** Aperistalsis shown on manometry in a patient with dystrophia myotonica. Marks on the horizontal axis represent 5-second intervals. Wet = swallows of 5 ml water; rep = respiratory tracing. Courtesy of Dr J de Caestecker.

may also involve the submucosa (Fig. 1.141). However, there is considerable variation between patients, and either muscular or submucosal changes may predominate. Involved arteries and arterioles show characteristically mucoid intimal thickening.

Similar abnormalities of motility and sphincter function occur in other collagen vascular disorders, and in patients with Raynaud's syndrome who have no other cutaneous manifestations of scleroderma. Complete aperistalsis may be seen in dystrophia myotonica (Fig. 1.142).

ESOPHAGEAL VARICES

Esophageal varices are submucosal esophageal veins dilated by increased pressure within the portal venous system. They provide a major channel for portal–systemic collateral circulation. Hepatic cirrhosis or thrombosis of the splenic, portal or hepatic veins are the usual causes (see Chapter 12). Varices are most prominent in the distal esophagus but extend for a variable degree proximally. They are an important cause of severe upper gastrointestinal bleeding. Barium swallow will show large varices but (whether single or double contrast) it is not a sensitive investigation (Fig. 1.143). As well as demonstrating smaller varices, endoscopy permits the immediate therapeutic option of variceal banding or injection sclerotherapy (Fig. 1.144). Visceral angiography is less used, but also has therapeutic potential if selective embolization can be achieved (Fig. 1.145). The histological appearances are normally available only after death, but confirm the transmural nature of the varices (Figs 1.146, 1.147).

ESOPHAGEAL ATRESIA

Embryologically the lung bud, a median ventral outgrowth of the foregut, is carried caudally and divides into two, becoming the trachea ventrally and the esophagus dorsally. Any alteration in this

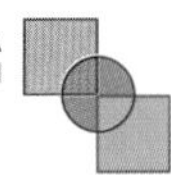

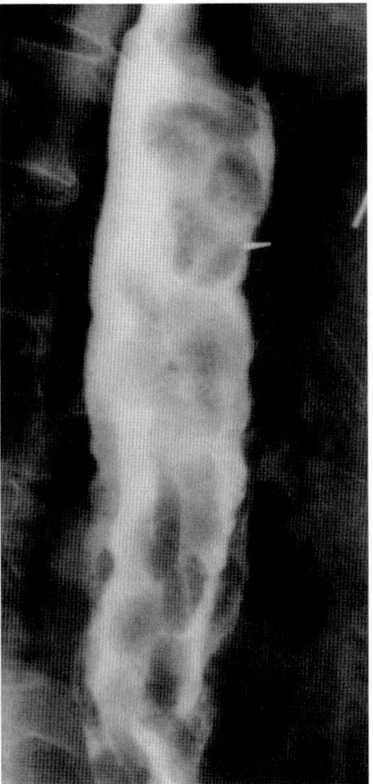

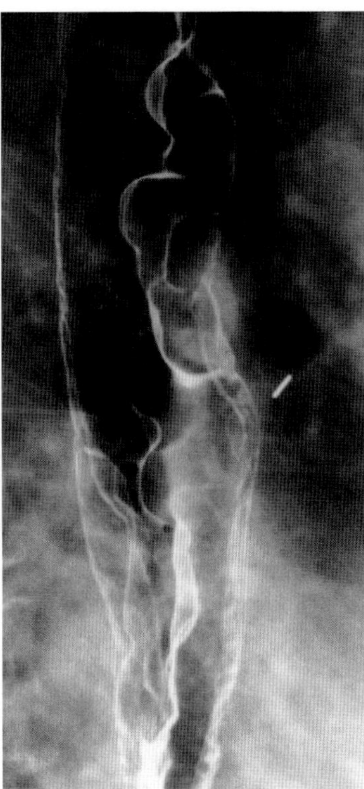

■ Fig. 1.143 Single-contrast and double-contrast esophagrams showing esophageal varices as considerably thickened, serpiginous defects in the mid and distal esophagus in a patient with portal hypertension.

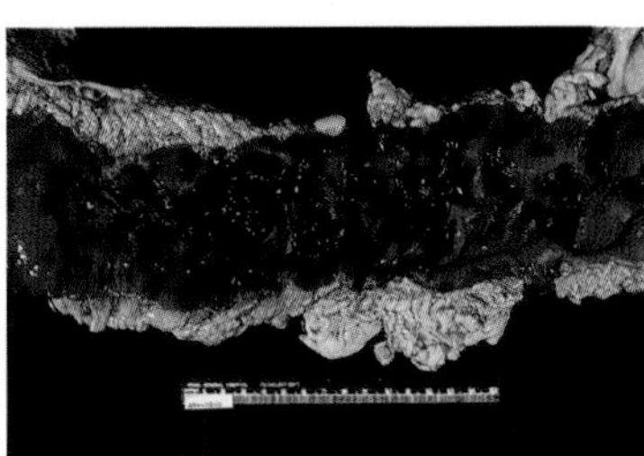

■ Fig. 1.146 Macroscopic appearance of distal esophagus involved by extensive varices with hemorrhage.

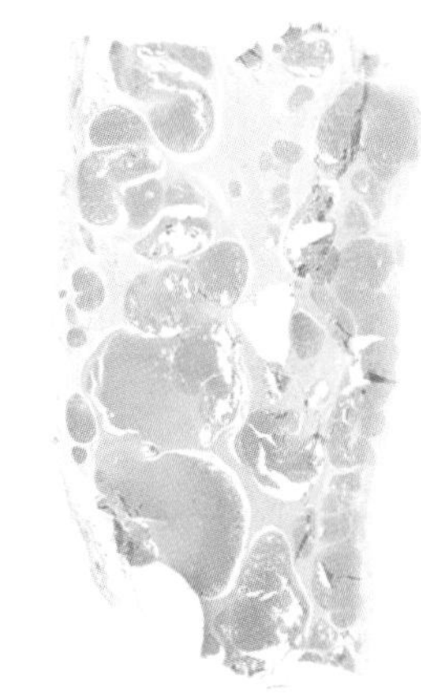

■ Fig. 1.147 Whole-mount section through the distal esophagus showing transmural involvement by congested varices.

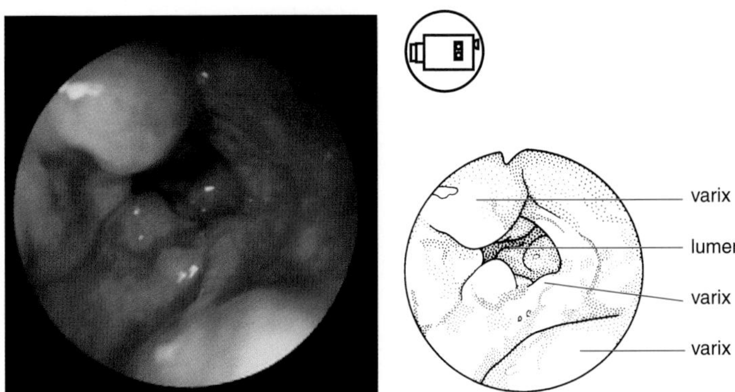

■ Fig. 1.144 Endoscopic view of large esophageal varices protruding into the lumen.

process leads to anomalies in the development of the esophagus, trachea, or both, frequently with an accompanying esophageal fistula. In the commonest anomaly, the upper esophagus ends in a blind pouch, and the lower portion is connected to the trachea near to its bifurcation (Figs 1.148, 1.149). There may be associated cardiovascular abnormalities such as coarctation of the aorta or a patent ductus arteriosus. Polyhydramnios in the third trimester of pregnancy may be the first clue. After birth, the presence of copious saliva around the infant's mouth, with a triad of choking, coughing and cyanosis with the first feed, should alert the physician to the possibility of esophageal atresia. The degree of feeding difficulty and the risk of aspiration pneumonia depend on the anatomical extent of the anomaly (Fig. 1.150).

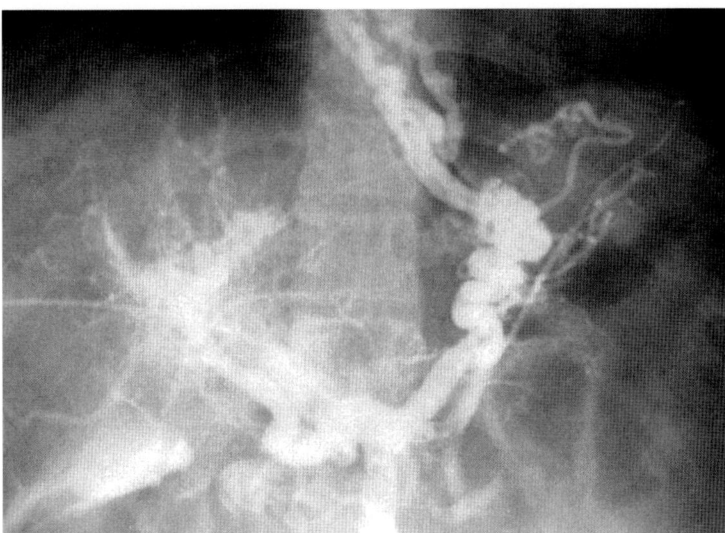

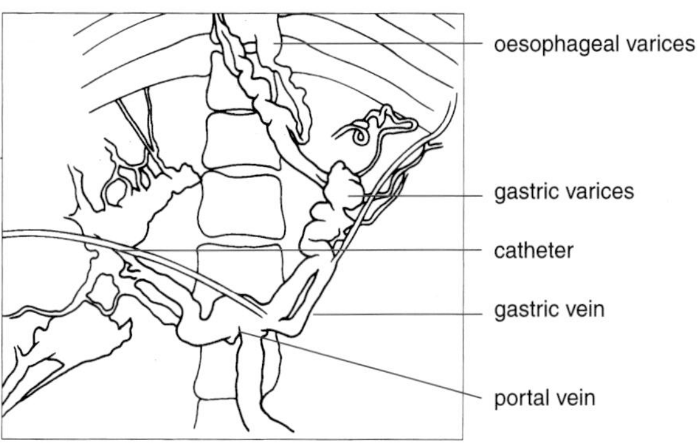

■ Fig. 1.145 Transhepatic portogram in a patient with a thrombosed portal vein following childhood umbilical sepsis. Note the large collateral gastric vein feeding gastric and esophageal varices. Courtesy of Dr R Dick.

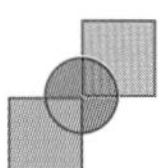

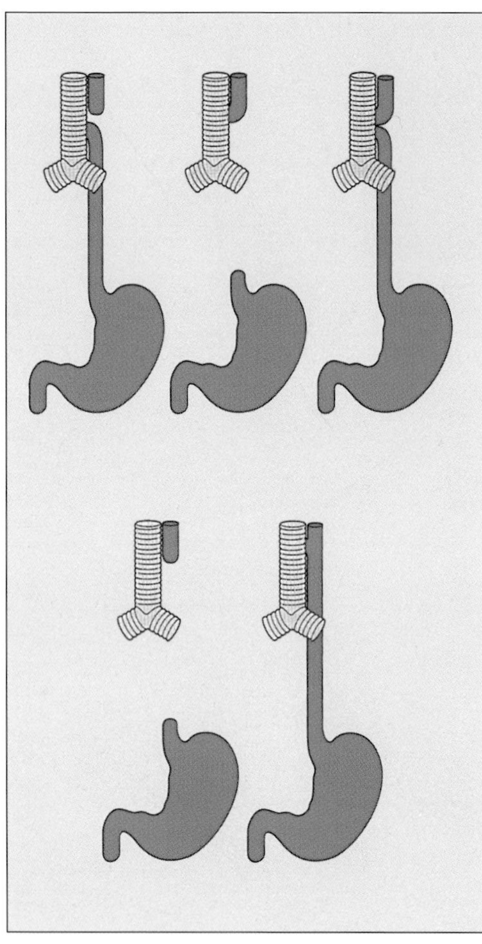

■ **Fig. 1.148** Diagram illustrating various types of tracheo-esophageal fistula.

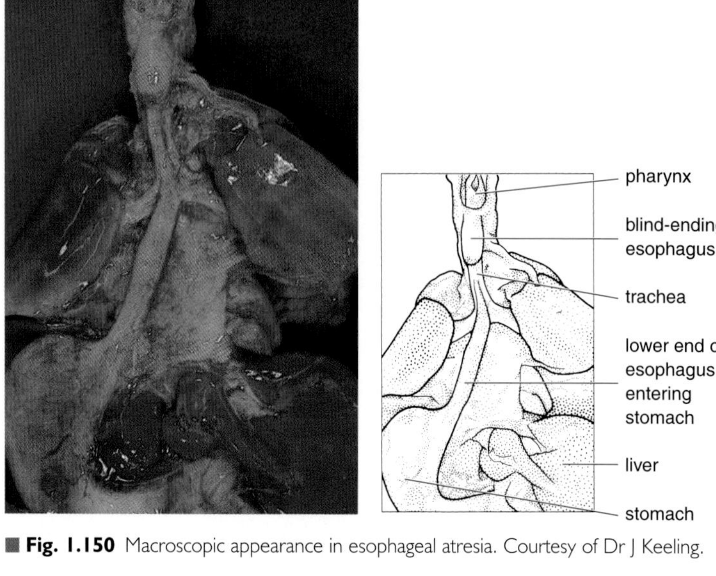

■ **Fig. 1.150** Macroscopic appearance in esophageal atresia. Courtesy of Dr J Keeling.

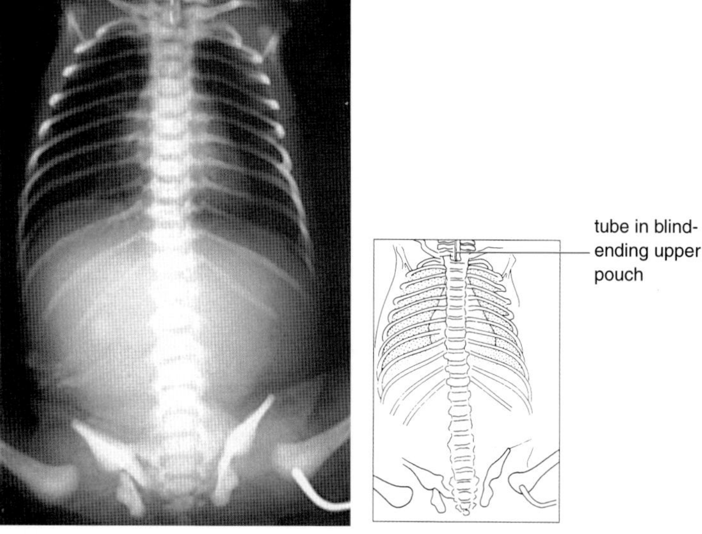

■ **Fig. 1.151** Plain radiograph of a neonate with esophageal atresia. A tube can be seen in the blind-ending upper pouch. There is no gas in the abdomen. Courtesy of Ms V Wright.

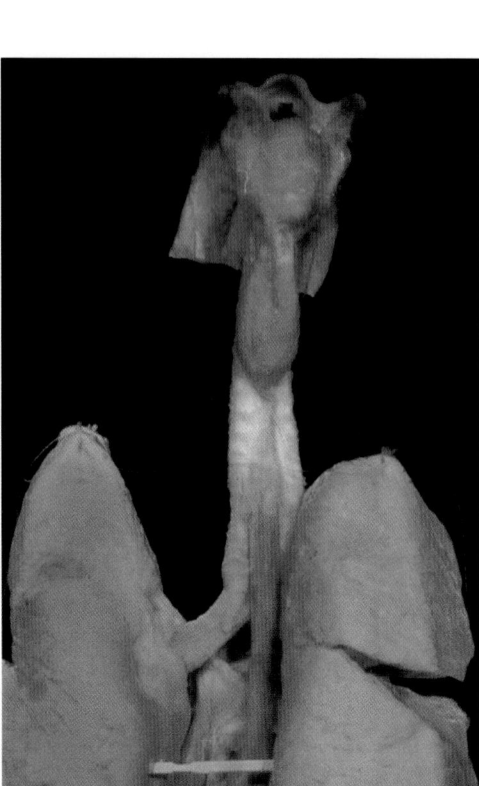

■ **Fig. 1.149** Macroscopic appearance of tracheo-esophageal fistula. This shows the most common variety in which the upper part of the esophagus ends blindly, and the lower end enters the trachea above its bifurcation. The example shown was an incidental finding in a still-born infant. Courtesy of the Royal College of Surgeons.

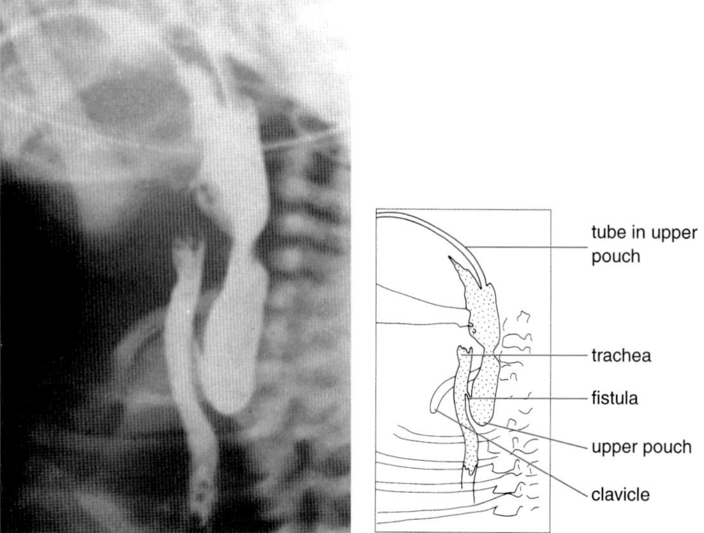

■ **Fig. 1.152** Lateral view of a non-ionic contrast study in esophageal atresia demonstrating a fistula to the trachea. Courtesy of Dr C Hall.

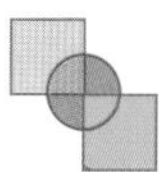

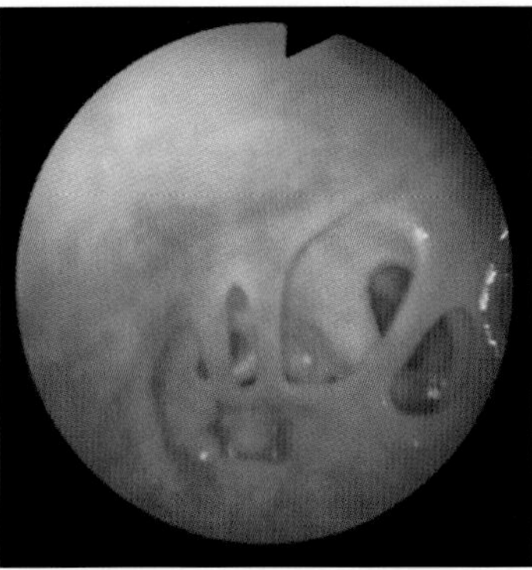

■ **Fig. 1.153** Endoscopic appearance of a congenital malformation of the distal esophagus.

Plain radiographs may show a gasless abdomen in infants with atresia if there is no tracheo-esophageal fistula (Fig. 1.151), or reveal a blind esophageal pouch on a lateral view (Fig. 1.152). If the diagnosis is suspected, passage of a fine tube and testing the pH of the aspirate is also helpful. Cautious barium radiology is diagnostic (this being less damaging to the airways in the event that aspiration is provoked with water-soluble contrast media).

Congenital anomalies of the esophagus of less physiological consequence may also be found incidentally at endoscopy in adults (Fig. 1.153).

FOREIGN BODIES

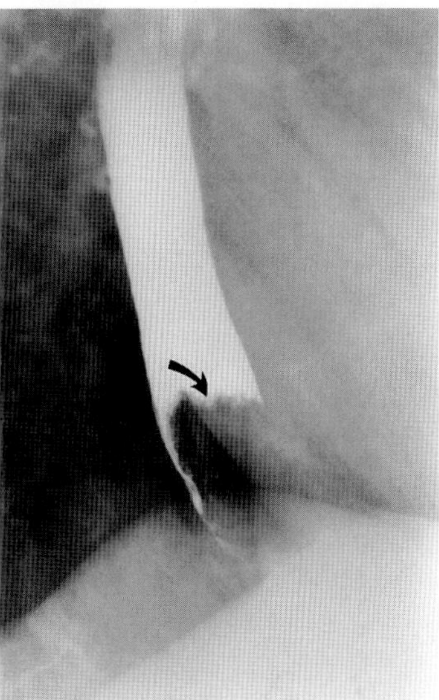

■ **Fig. 1.154** Single-contrast esophagram showing an impacted piece of meat in the distal esophagus as a polypoid defect (arrow) with associated obstruction. Such patients often have underlying rings or strictures as the cause of impaction, so a follow-up barium study should be performed to re-evaluate the esophagus after the impaction has been relieved. (Reproduced with permission from reference 1.)

Swallowed foreign bodies may become impacted in the esophagus. Obstruction by food bolus usually occurs only in the edentulous or in those with an esophageal stricture (Figs 1.154, 1.155), but fish bones are a potentially troublesome exception. Young children may swallow a variety of objects, and this can also happen in the psychiatrically disturbed, and prisoners. Foreign bodies tend to lodge at the cricopharyngeus or at the esophago-gastric junction. The former presents the risk of asphyxiation, the latter that of esophageal perforation, particularly with mercury batteries, which should always be removed. Once objects enter the stomach, most will pass through the remainder of the gastrointestinal tract uneventfully (but see Chapter 2).

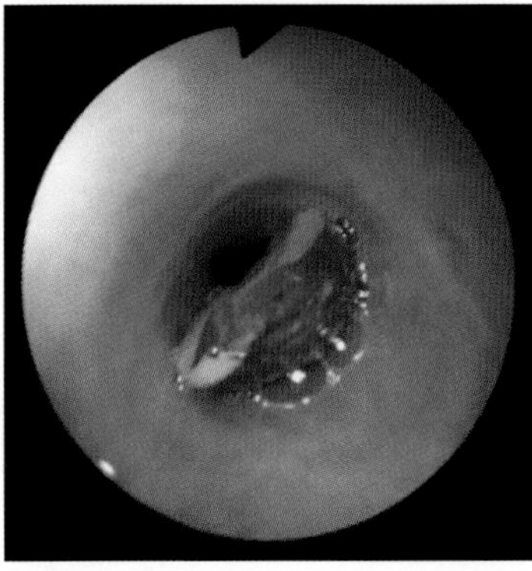

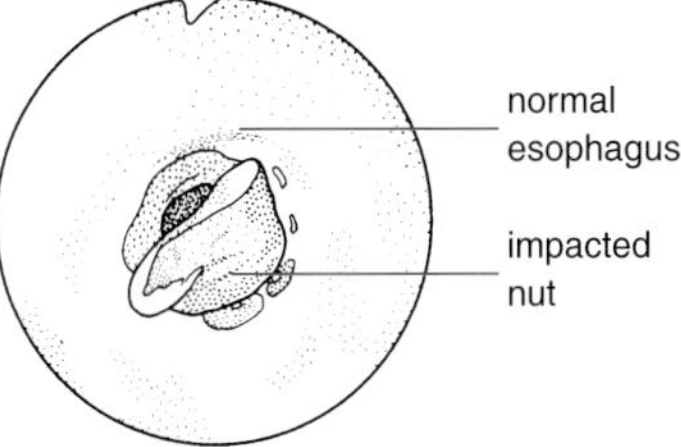

■ **Fig. 1.155** Endoscopic view of a fragment of walnut impacted into a benign esophageal stricture.

REFERENCES

1. Levine MS (ed.) Radiology of the esophagus. Philadelphia: WB Saunders, 1989, Figs 1.9A, 2.4, 5.25B, 7.2, 7.4A, 7.7A, 7.10A, 10.13, and 12.13.
2. Gore RM, Levine MS (eds) Textbook of gastrointestinal radiology. Philadelphia: WB Saunders, 2000, Figs 21.3B, 22.14A, and 22.14B.
3. Levine MS, Macones, AJ, Laufer I. Candida esophagitis: accuracy of radiographic diagnosis. Radiology 1985; 154: 581–587, Fig. 1C.
4. Levine MS, Rubesin SE, Laufer I. Double contrast gastrointestinal radiology. Philadelphia: WB Saunders, 2000, Fig. 5.49A.
5. Levine MS, Goercher G, Katzka DA, Herlinger H, Rubesin SE, Laufer I. Giant, human immunodeficiency virus-related ulcers in the esophagus. Radiology 1991; 180: 323–326, Fig. 2.
6. Levine MS, Kressel HY, Caroline DF, Laufer I, Herlinger H, Thompson JJ. Barrett esophagus: reticular pattern of the mucosa. Radiology 1983; 147: 663–667, Figs 1A and 1B.
7. Levine MS, Buck JL, Pantongrag-Brown L, Buetow PC, Hallman JR, Sobin LH. Fibrovascular polyps of the esophagus: clinical, radiographic, and pathologic findings in 16 patients. AJR 1996; 166: 781–787, Figs 3A and 3C.
8. Woodfield CA, Levine MS, Rubesin SE, Langlotz CP, Laufer I. Diagnosis of primary versus secondary achalasia: reassessment of clinical and radiographic criteria. AJR 2000; 175: 727–731, Fig. 3.

THE STOMACH

2

NORMAL STOMACH

The stomach lies between the esophagus and the duodenum, and acts primarily as an initial mixing chamber for digestion of ingested food. It comprises several distinct zones (Fig. 2.1). The cardia is situated just below the esophageal opening (Figs 2.2, 2.3), and the fundus constitutes the part that lies cephalad to the esophago-gastric junction. The main part of the stomach is the body, which has a shorter, lesser curve and a longer, dependent greater curve (Figs 2.4, 2.5). The mucosa of the body and fundus is thrown into folds, or rugae. The distal third of the stomach, the antrum, is smooth with no rugae, and is demarcated proximally by the incisura angularis (Fig. 2.6) and distally by the pylorus (Figs 2.7, 2.8). The pyloric

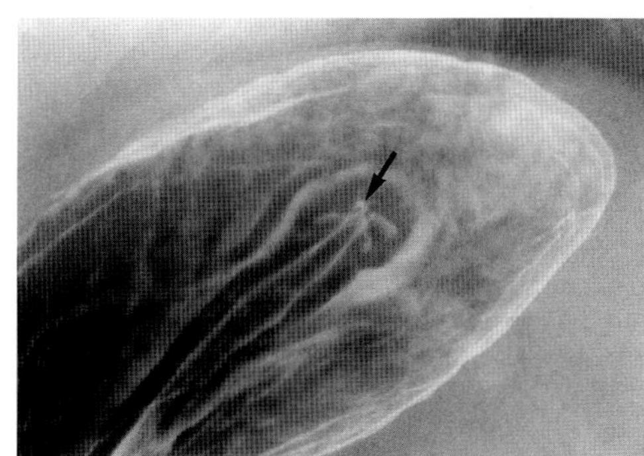

Fig. 2.3 Recumbent right lateral view of the gastric fundus showing the cardiac rosette as three or four stellate folds radiating to a central point at the gastro-esophageal junction (arrow).

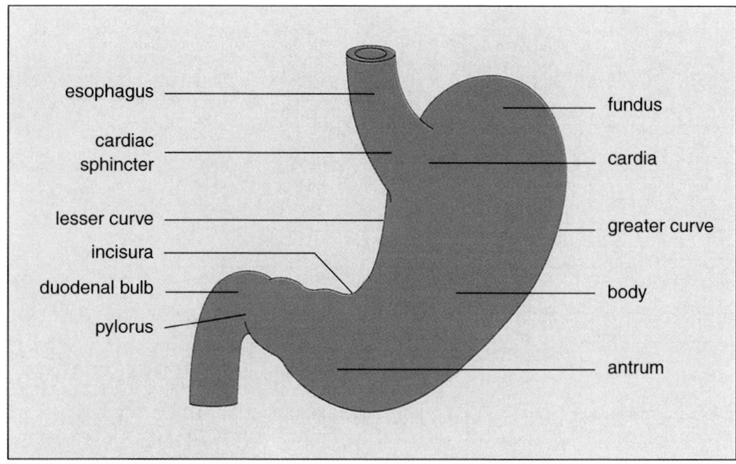

Fig. 2.1 Diagram showing the normal anatomy of the stomach.

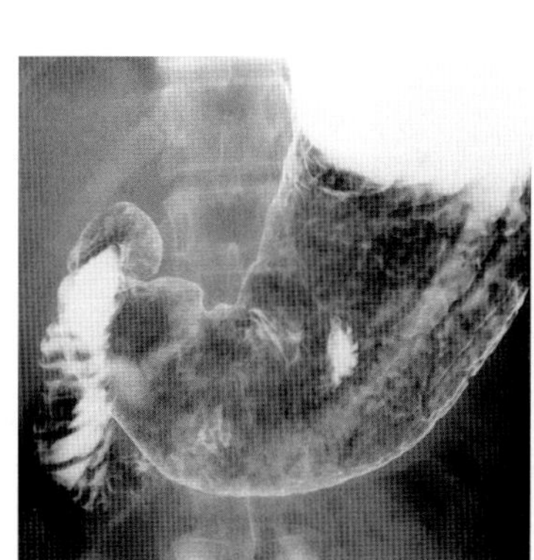

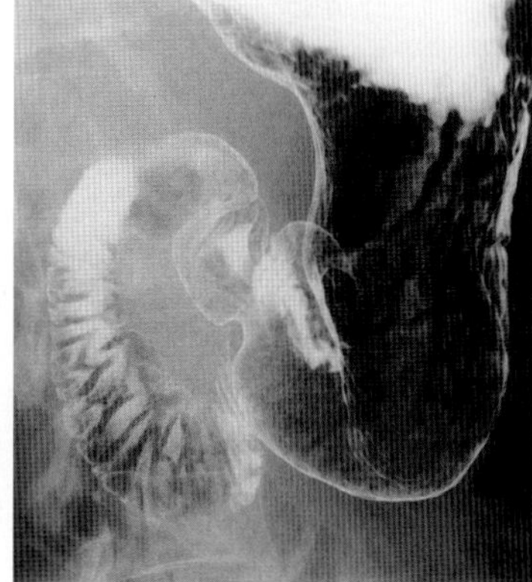

Fig. 2.4 Frontal and left posterior oblique views from a double-contrast upper gastrointestinal study showing the normal appearance of the stomach and duodenum.

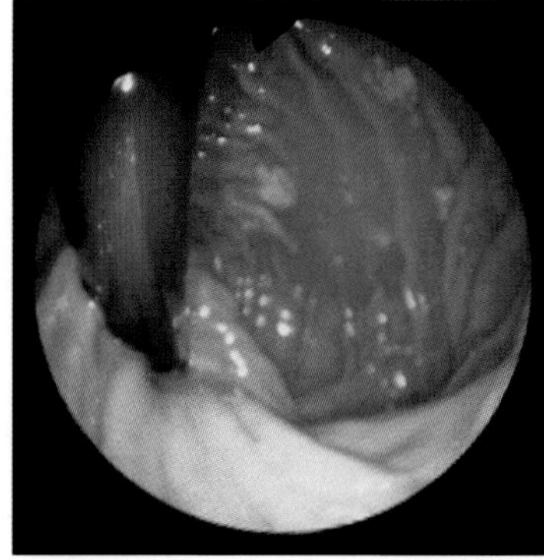

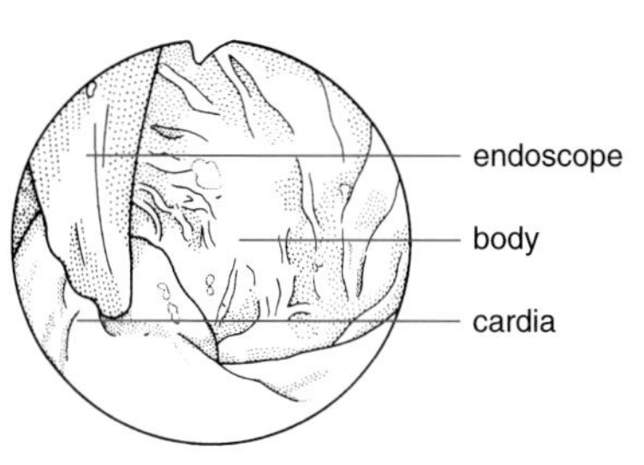

Fig. 2.2 Endoscopic view of the cardia; the instrument is retroflexed and its entry through the cardia into the body of the stomach is seen from below.

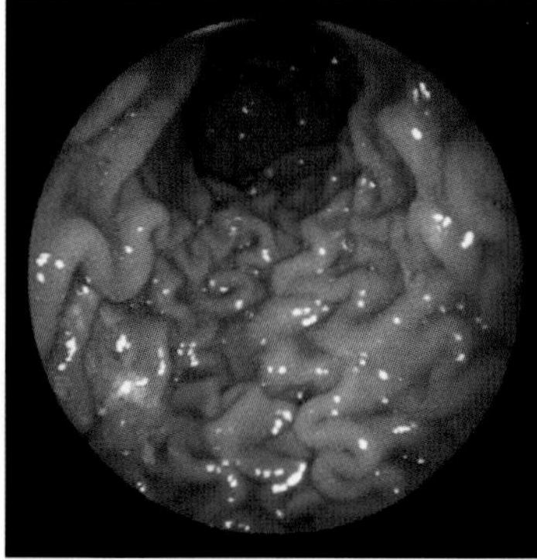

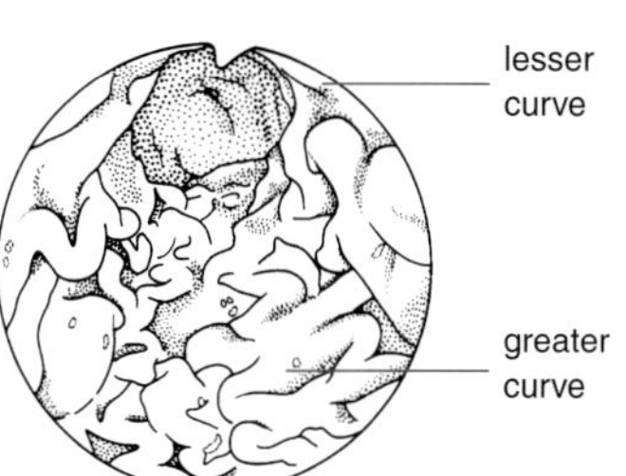

Fig. 2.5 Endoscopic view mainly of the greater curve of the stomach.

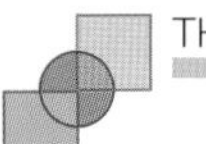

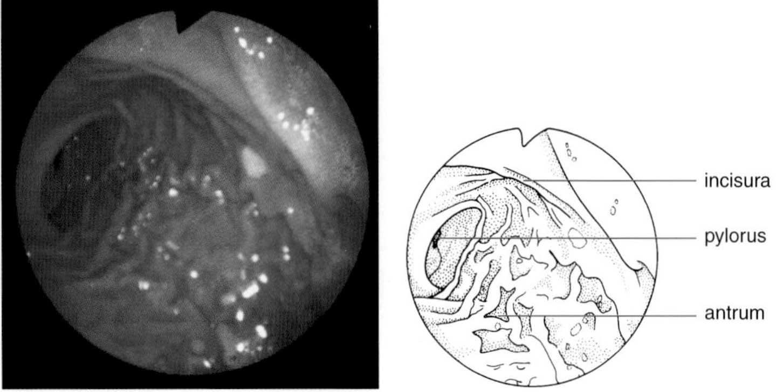

■ **Fig. 2.6** Endoscopic view of the distal stomach showing the incisura, antrum, and pylorus.

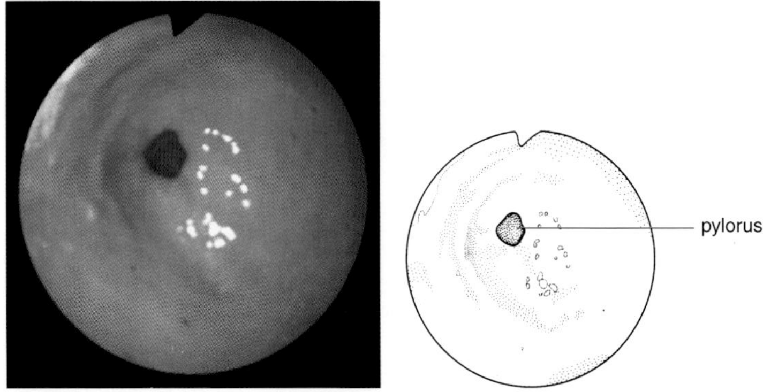

■ **Fig. 2.7** Normal antrum and pylorus.

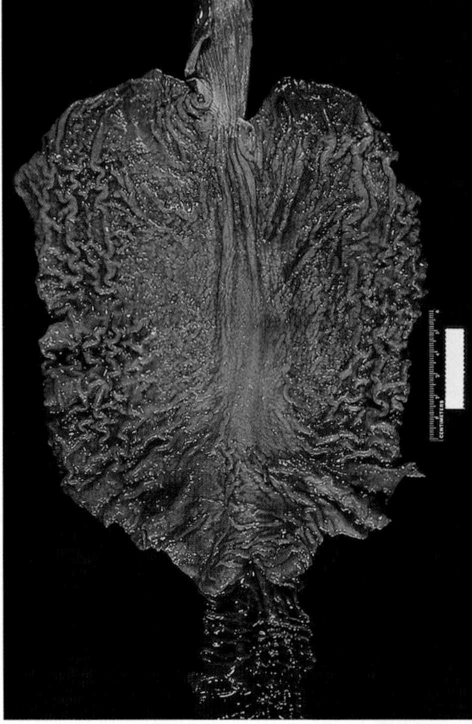

■ **Fig. 2.8** Macroscopic image of the normal stomach opened along the greater curvature showing longitudinal folds of the body and fundus and transverse folds of the antrum.

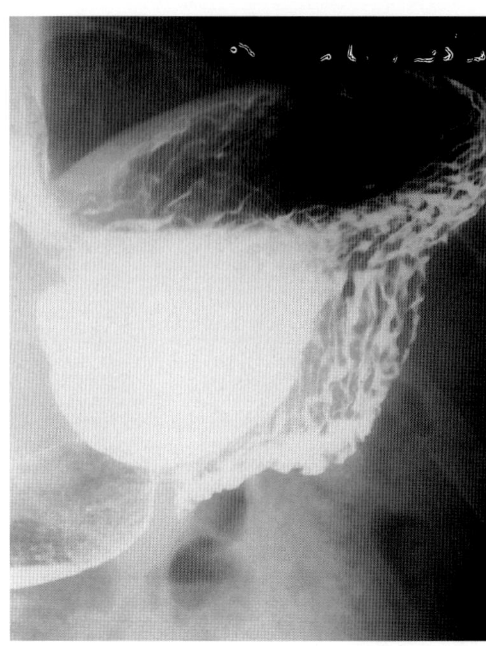

■ **Fig. 2.9** Barium study showing the 'cup and spill' normal variant.

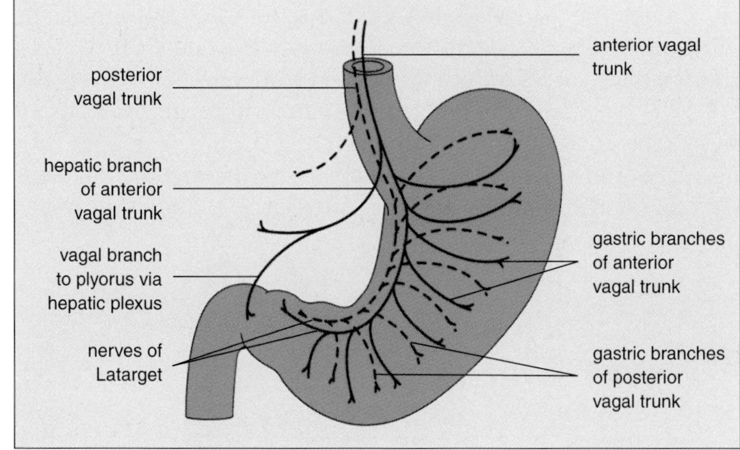

■ **Fig. 2.10** Diagram showing the anatomical arrangement of the vagus nerve and its branches.

sphincter itself is formed from a concentration of circular muscle. Occasionally the fundus will hang down across the body of the stomach; this normal variant is known, from its radiological appearance, as the 'cup and spill' deformity (Fig. 2.9).

The stomach is innervated by vagal parasympathetic nerves, and by sympathetic nerves from the celiac plexus. The vagus divides into anterior and posterior trunks (Fig. 2.10); the anterior trunk is further divided into an anterior gastric division that supplies the anterior wall of the stomach, and a hepatic division that supplies the proximal duodenum. The posterior gastric wall is supplied by the posterior gastric division of the posterior vagal trunk. In addition to afferent fibers, the vagus contains three types of efferent fiber – cholinergic stimulatory, adrenergic inhibitory, and non-adrenergic inhibitory – which help in the control of secretion and motility.

The mucosa of the fundus and body of the stomach are covered by regular columnar epithelia which extend for a short distance into the gastric pits. The gastric glands open into the base of these pits (Fig. 2.11). The glands of the body incorporate two types of specialized secretory cells (Fig. 2.12): the parietal (or oxyntic) cells, which produce hydrochloric acid and vitamin B_{12}-binding intrinsic factor (Fig. 2.13); and pepsin-producing chief cells (Fig. 2.14). Antral (pyloric) glands do not contain acid- or pepsin-producing cells, but are mucus secreting (Figs 2.15, 2.16). The majority of gastrin-producing ('G') cells are found in the antrum, interspersed between the mucus cells (Figs 2.17–2.20).

The stomach is lined by a layer of mucus, a gelatinous material composed predominantly of glycoproteins and mucopolysaccharides secreted by the surface epithelium (Figs 2.21, 2.22). The mucus protects the gastric mucosa from surface injury by physical irritants,

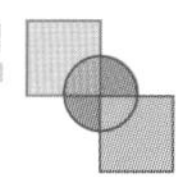

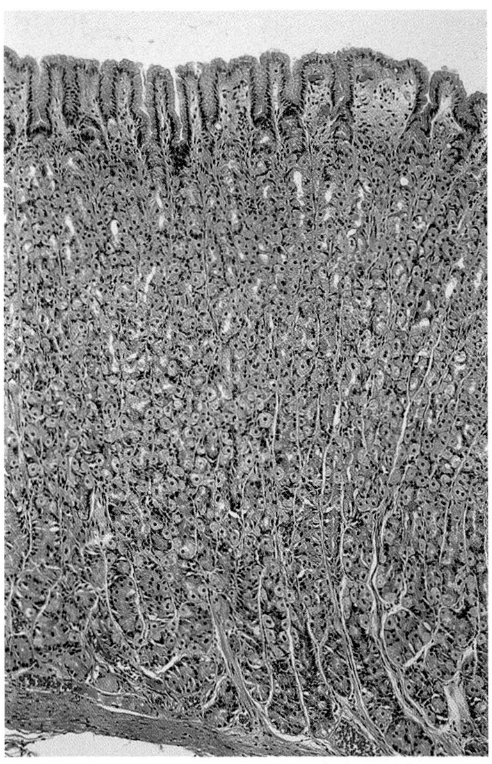

■ **Fig. 2.11** Microscopic appearance of the normal oxyntic mucosa of the body and fundus showing short pits, long straight glands with little intervening stroma, and no inflammatory cells in the lamina propria.

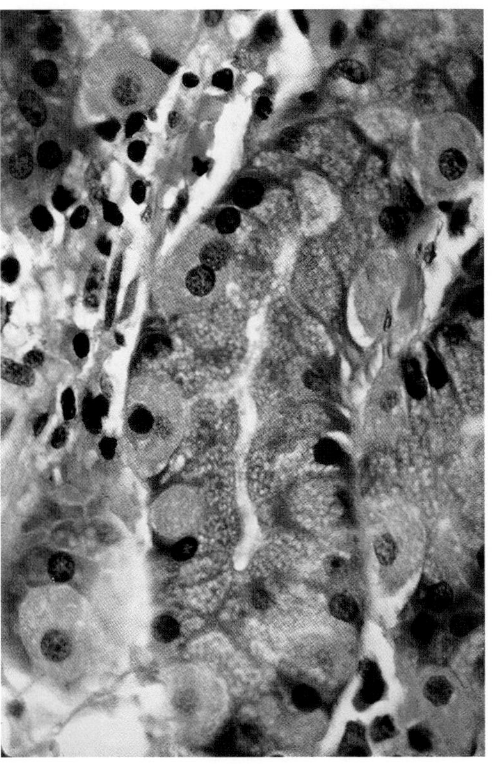

■ **Fig. 2.12** High magnification of normal oxyntic glands showing HCl- and intrinsic factor-producing parietal cells with eosinophilic (pink) cytoplasm and pepsin-producing chief cells with basophilic (purple) cytoplasm.

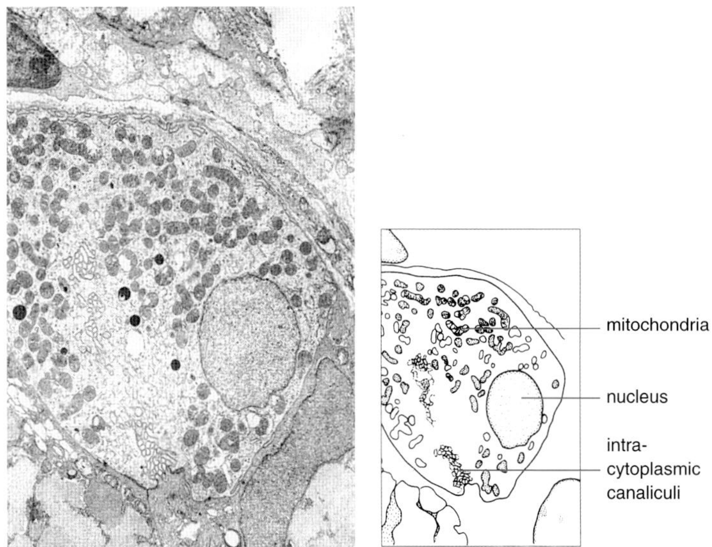

■ **Fig. 2.13** Electron micrograph of a parietal cell showing abundant mitochondria and the intracytoplasmic canalicular system of the cell (x 3000). Courtesy of Dr D. Day.

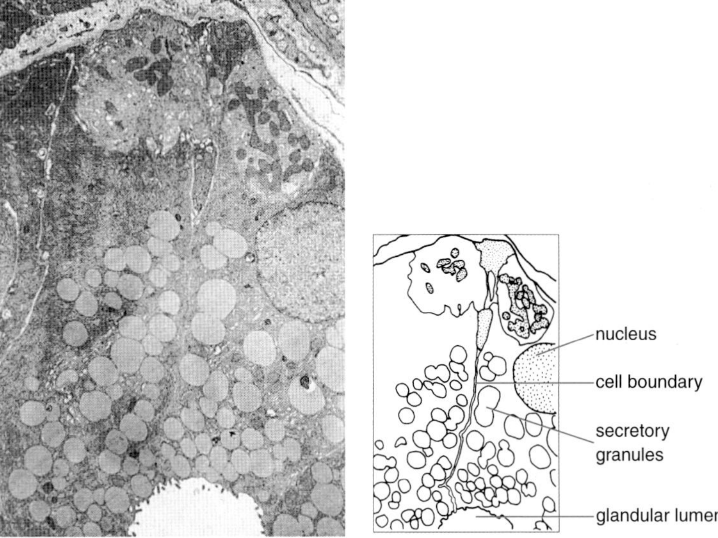

■ **Fig. 2.14** Electron micrograph showing the typical granules of a chief, or pepsin-producing, cell from the body of the stomach (x 3000). Courtesy of Dr D. Day.

and buffers gastric acid under basal conditions, although its effect in buffering stimulated acid secretion is negligible. The mucus layer is also important in allowing colonization by *Helicobacter pylori* (see below).

The vagus acts on parietal cells to stimulate acid production, and on G cells to stimulate gastrin release, in both cases via the action of acetylcholine. In addition, acetylcholine potentiates the parietal cell response to other secretagogs. Gastrin is also released directly by exposure to peptides and amino acids, and by antral distension. Although stimulation of H_2 receptors on the parietal cells by histamine also stimulates acid production, the final common pathway for gastric acid secretion is now known to be via the hydrogen-potassium ATPase system. Both histamine and the gastrin analog, pentagastrin, can, however, provoke maximal acid production (the basis of the augmented histamine-pentagastrin test for assessment of acid secretory capacity).

Although the volume of the resting stomach is 50 ml or less, receptive relaxation of the body of the stomach occurs as food and liquid are ingested, partly mediated by ghrelin, so that there is little rise in intragastric pressure. Peristaltic waves are initiated by the gastric pacemaker in the fundus of the stomach, and then occur at a rate of about three per minute. These gradually propel the viscous gastric contents into the distal antrum. Unlike the cardia, in the resting state the pylorus is always open, and it closes only during peristalsis (Fig. 2.23). The rate at which contents pass into the duodenum depends on physical and chemical composition: solids, hypertonic fluids and especially lipids, all empty at a slower rate than isotonic fluids. Scintigraphy using separate labels for the solid and liquid phase readily demonstrates this (Figs 2.24–2.27). As pressure rises in the antrum, a proportion of the antral contents passes through the open pylorus into the duodenum. Duodenal receptors then

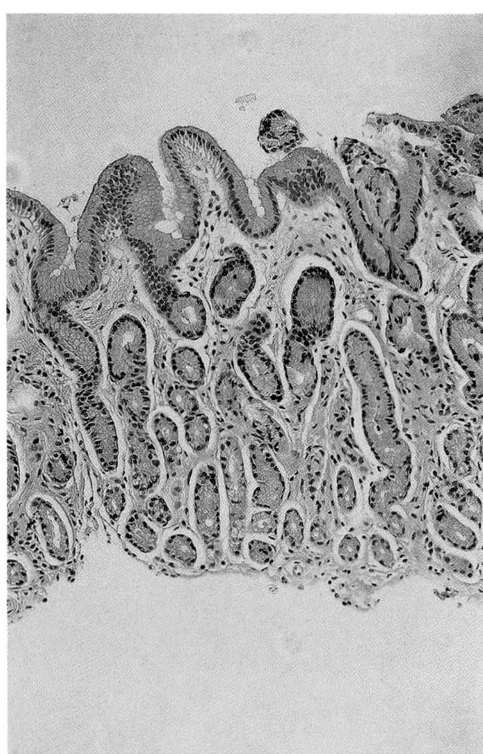

■ **Fig. 2.15** Microscopic appearance of the normal antral mucosa showing pits that are identical to those of the body/fundus but glands that are short, more widely spaced, and composed of mucus cells.

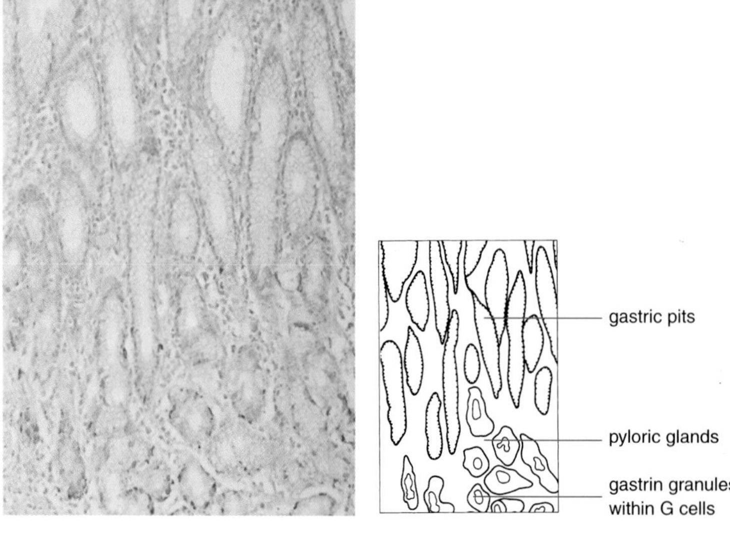

■ **Fig. 2.17** Photomicrograph of the gastric antrum, showing G cells (part of the APUD system) within the pyloric glands. Grimelius, silver impregnation (x 120).

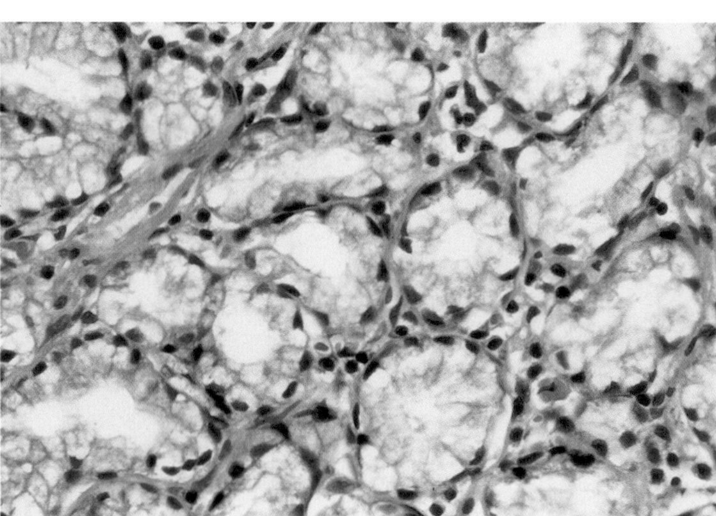

■ **Fig. 2.16** Microscopic appearance of the normal antral mucosal glands lined by simple cuboidal, mucin-producing epithelium.

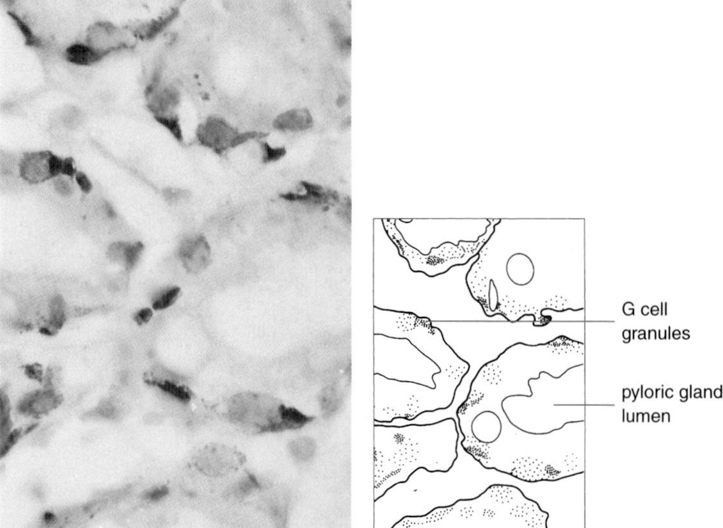

■ **Fig. 2.18** High power view of Fig. 2.16 showing brown-staining G cell granules (x 800).

contribute negative feedback leading the pylorus to contract abruptly, causing antral pressure to increase and thus propel contents back into the body of the stomach. This antral 'pump' or 'mill' therefore ensures the thorough mixing of gastric contents and digestive juices, and a controlled emptying of the stomach.

BENIGN GASTRIC ULCER

The classical presentation of benign gastric ulcer with weight loss and indigestion made worse by eating is not often seen; patients more often describe symptoms that would fit equally well for duodenal ulcer. Investigation with barium meal or (preferably) endoscopy is appropriate for either. Benign ulcers may occur at any site in the stomach, but are commonest on the lesser curve away from acid-secreting epithelium. Barium meal examination showing an ulcer crater with radiating mucosal folds reaching to its rim (Figs 2.28–2.30) strongly suggests that the ulcer is benign, but all gastric ulcers should be examined endoscopically (Fig. 2.31) and histologically, with a later endoscopy to check healing (Fig. 2.32). It is important to take multiple biopsies even from apparently benign ulcers (see Figs 2.99 and 2.100 – both are from the same ulcer but only one shows adenocarcinoma).

The macroscopic appearances of a benign ulcer are consistent with the endoscopic appearances (Figs 2.33, 2.34) and the presence of radiating mucosal folds is again typical. Histologically, the intact gastric mucosa extends to the margins of the ulcer crater (Fig. 2.35), the base of the ulcer consisting mainly of granulation tissue. With chronicity, fibrosis may completely replace the gastric muscle, seen then only at the margins of the lesion (Fig. 2.36).

Ulcers on the greater curve are more often malignant than ulcers elsewhere in the stomach, but a common benign variant is the 'sump' ulcer, which occurs in the most dependent part of the stomach and is often associated with ingestion of anti-inflammatory drugs (Figs 2.37, 2.38, 2.39). Juxta-pyloric ulcers are invariably benign and can be considered with duodenal ulcers, which they resemble in clinical behavior.

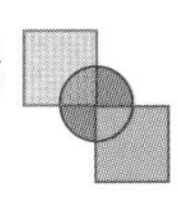

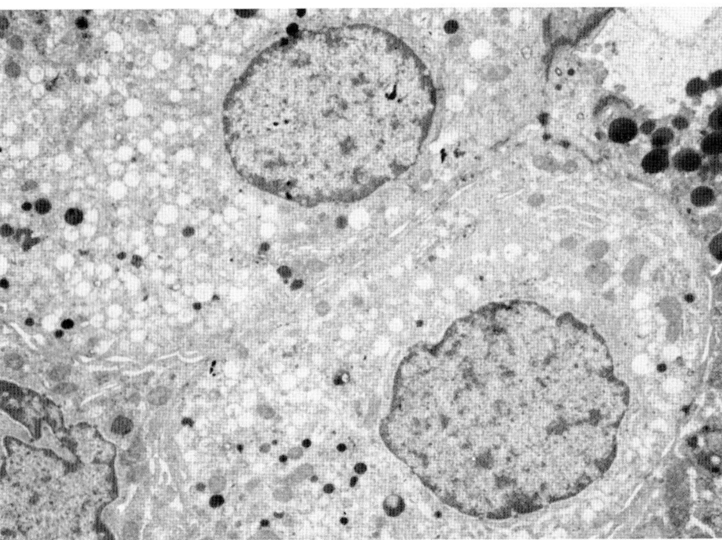

■ **Fig. 2.19** Electron micrograph of G cells demonstrating the two patterns (dense and clear) of gastrin neurosecretory granules (x 7500). Courtesy of Professor J. Polak.

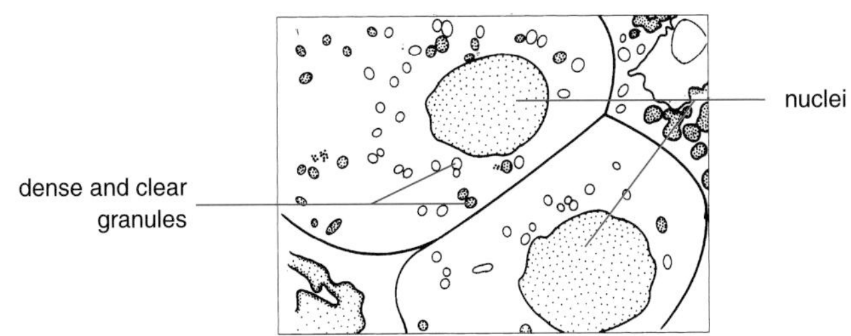

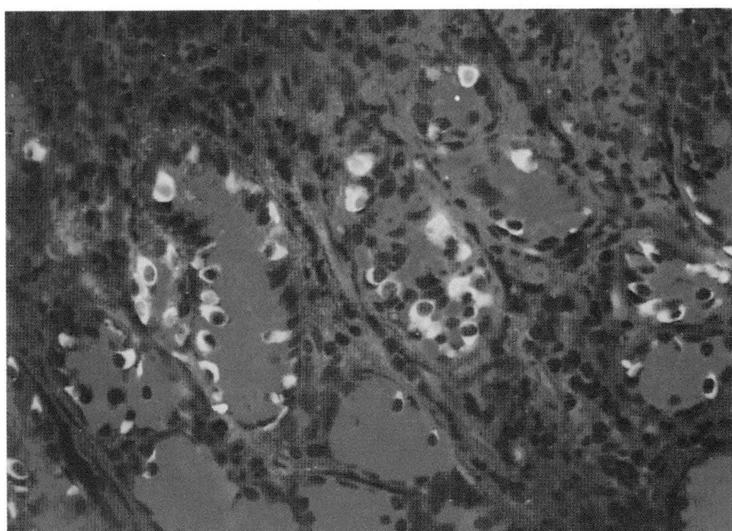

■ **Fig. 2.20** Green-fluorescing G cells in the pyloric glands, demonstrated by fluorescein-labeled anti-gastrin. The pyloric glands appear brown from mucin which has taken up the PAS (periodic acid Schiff) counterstain. Courtesy of Prof J. Polak.

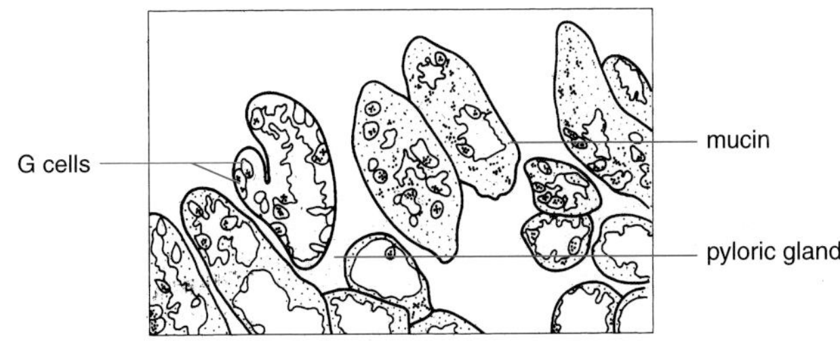

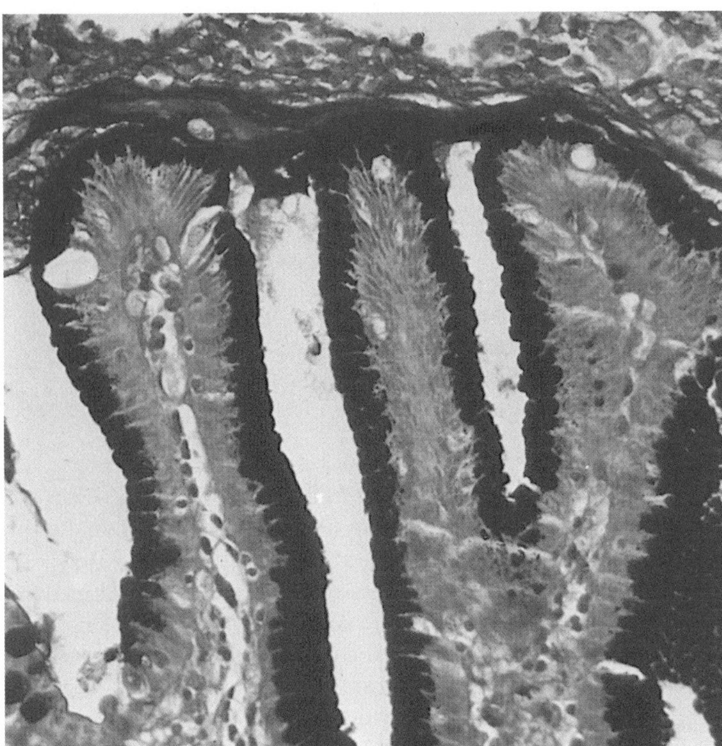

■ **Fig. 2.21** Histology of the surface gastric mucosa showing the covering layer of mucin. H&E stain (x 320).

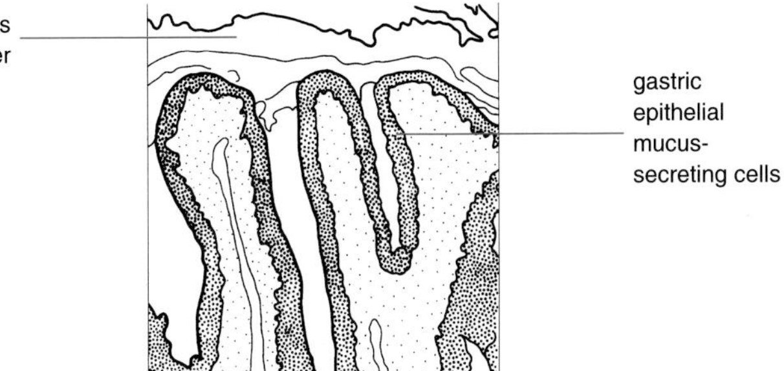

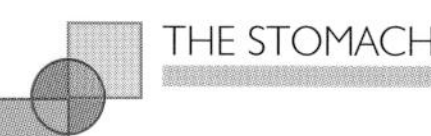

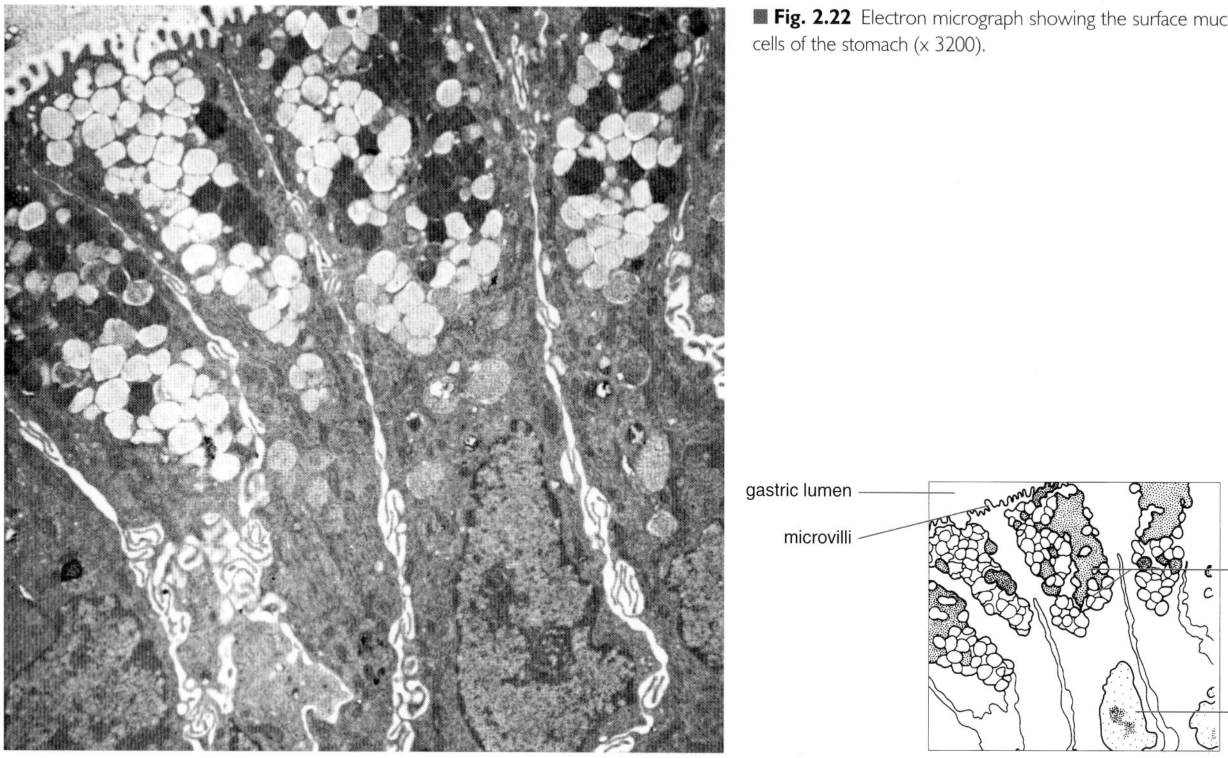

■ **Fig. 2.22** Electron micrograph showing the surface mucus-secreting epithelial cells of the stomach (x 3200).

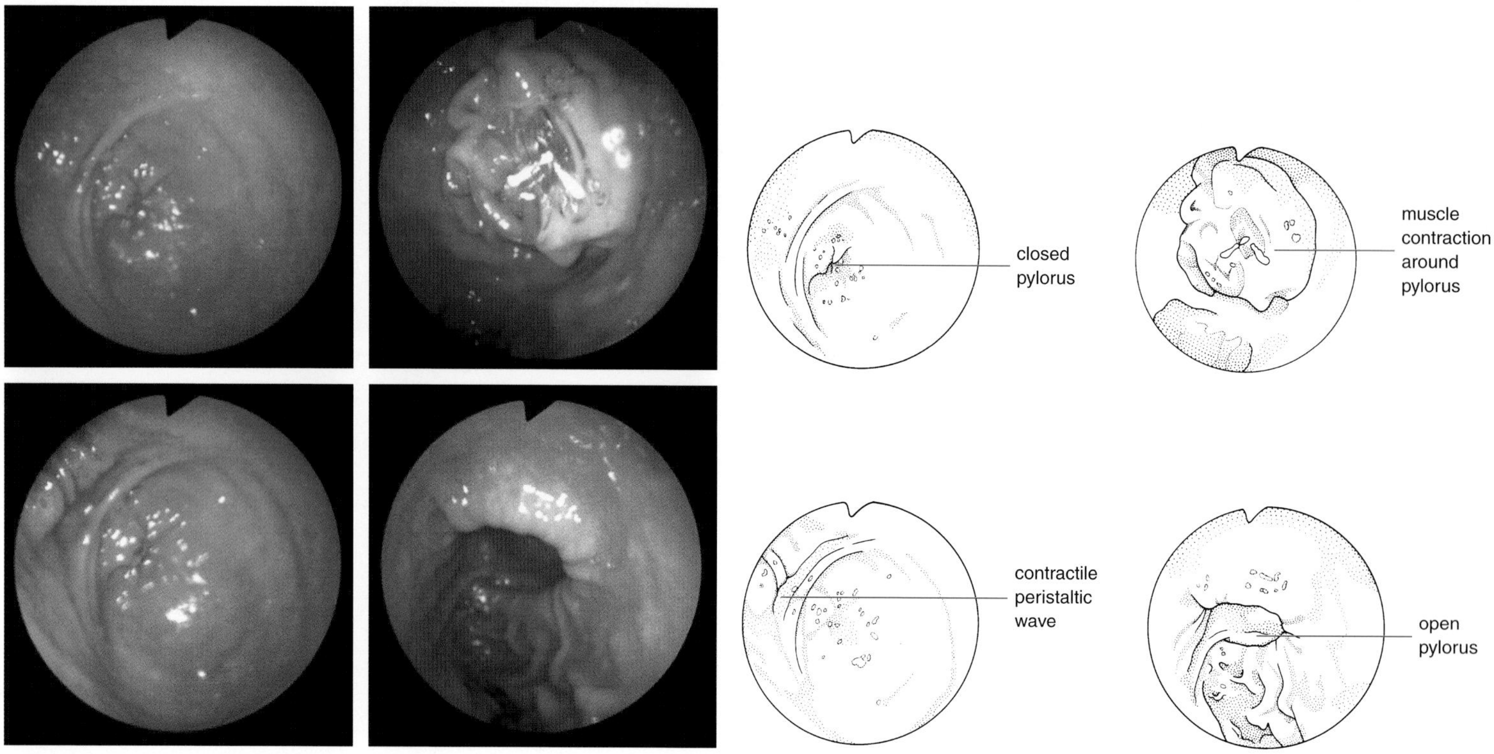

■ **Fig. 2.23** Sequential endoscopic views (clockwise from bottom left) showing a peristaltic contraction wave advancing along the body of the stomach to the antrum and closing the pylorus, which finally reopens to the resting state (bottom right).

Complications of gastric ulcers

The major complications of gastric ulceration are bleeding and perforation; either may be the first manifestation of the ulcer. Erosion of a vessel in the base of an ulcer is a common cause of significant hemorrhage (Fig. 2.40), and the endoscopic observation of a visible vessel indicates a significantly higher risk of rebleeding (Fig. 2.41). This, and the increasing recognition that endoscopic intervention by thermal therapy (laser, diathermy, or argon plasma coagulation) perhaps preceded by injection of dilute adrenaline (epinephrine) solutions, can reduce the risk of rebleeding and death, has led to an increased use of early endoscopy in hematemesis. Occasionally the endoscopist will see an actively bleeding vessel; this poses the worst prognosis for rebleeding and is a strong indication for immediate endoscopic intervention and surgery if not rapidly successful (Fig. 2.42). More rarely, a bleeding vessel will be found in the proximal stomach with no apparent ulcer: the so-called Dieulafoy lesion (Figs 2.43, 2.44).

Perforation of a peptic ulcer usually presents as an abdominal catastrophe with peritonitis and characteristic subphrenic gas (see

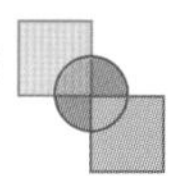

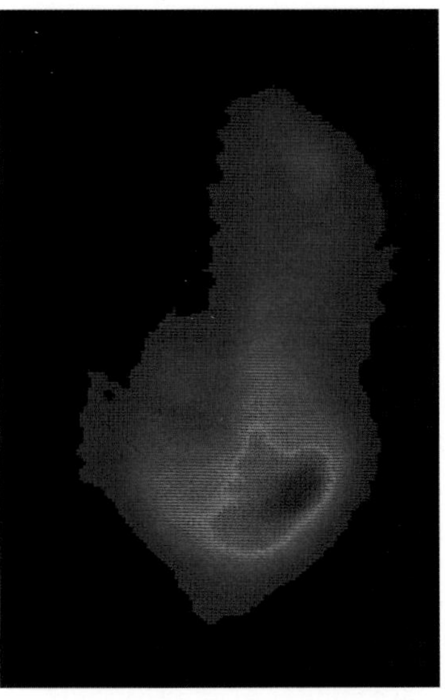

Fig. 2.24 Scintigraphic study of gastric emptying: normal distribution of liquid at 5 minutes after ingestion. Courtesy of Mr G.P. Morris and Cancer Research UK.

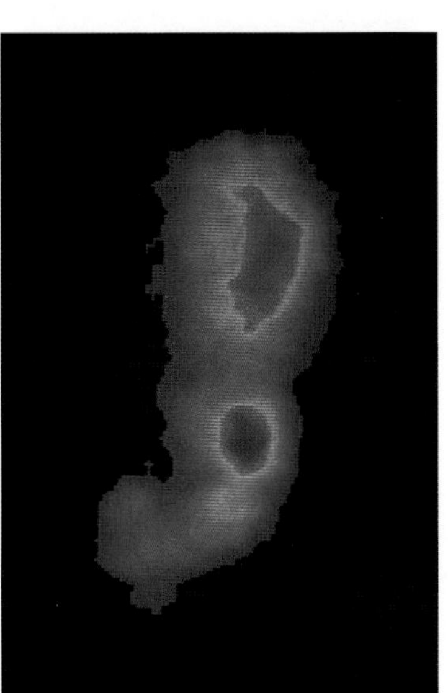

Fig. 2.25 Scintigraphic study of gastric emptying: normal distribution of solid at 5 minutes after ingestion. Courtesy of Mr G.P. Morris and Cancer Research UK.

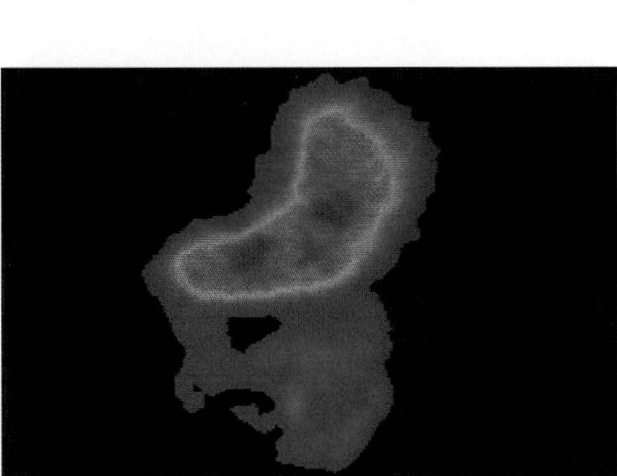

Fig. 2.26 Scintigraphic study of gastric emptying: normal passage of liquid to the small bowel at 1 hour after ingestion. Courtesy of Mr G.P. Morris and Cancer Research UK.

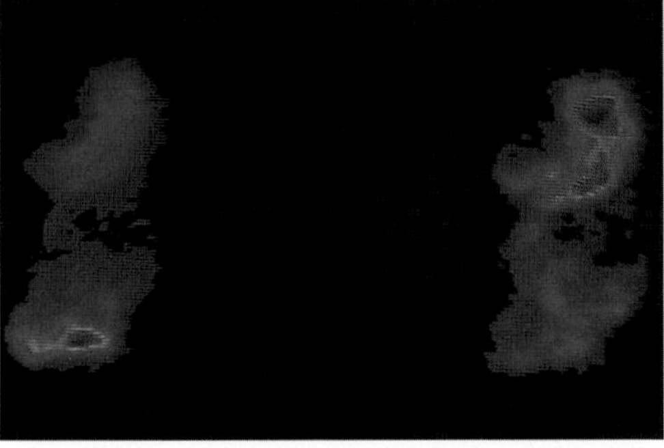

Fig. 2.27 Scintigraphic study of gastric emptying: comparison of normal transit of liquid (to the terminal ileum) (left), to that of solids (right) at 2 hours after ingestion. Courtesy of Mr G.P. Morris and Cancer Research UK.

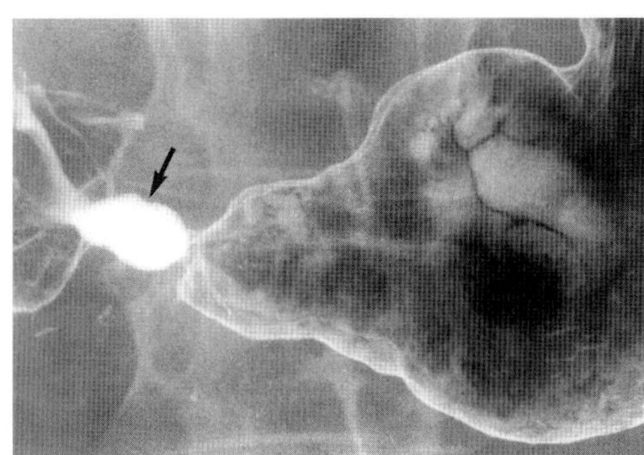

Fig. 2.28 Double-contrast barium study showing a large ulcer crater filled with barium (arrow) in the pyloric channel.

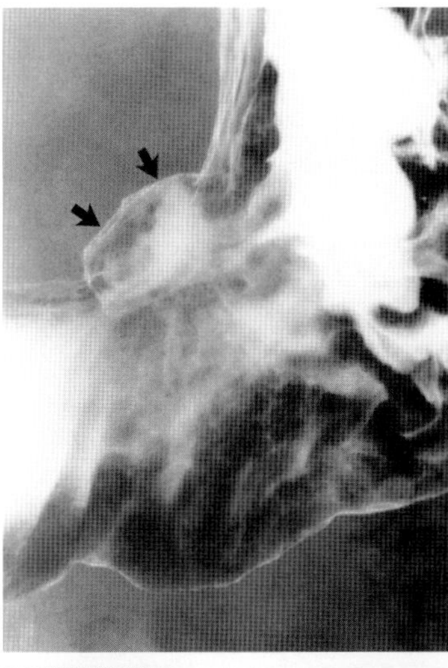

Fig. 2.29 Double-contrast barium studies showing benign ulcers (arrows) on the lesser curvature of the gastric body in two patients.

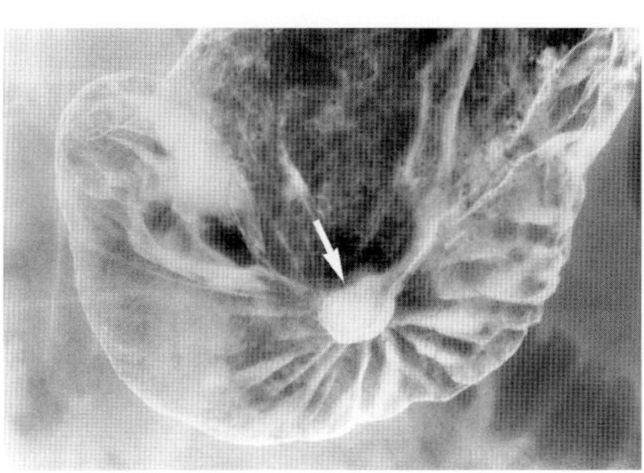

Fig 2.30 Double-contrast barium study showing barium collecting in a benign ulcer (arrow) on the posterior wall of the proximal antrum. Note the gastric folds seen radiating toward the edge of the ulcer crater. (Reproduced with permission from reference 1.)

Chapter 3), but a chronic ulcer may erode into adjacent structures thereby forming fistulae (Fig. 2.45).

Chronic benign prepyloric and antral ulcers may also be responsible for gastric outlet obstruction (Fig 2.46) although this is less often seen since the advent of more effective medical therapies.

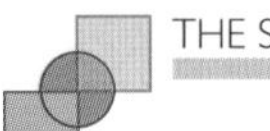

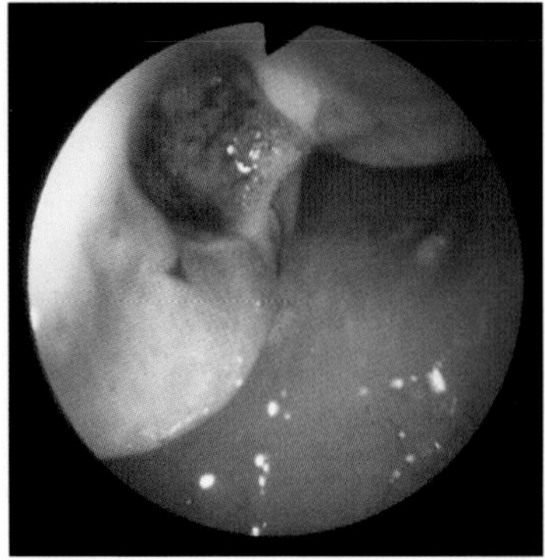

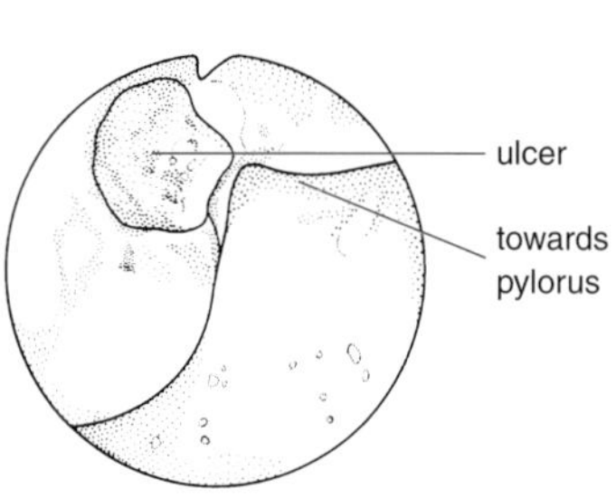

■ **Fig. 2.31** Endoscopic appearance of a chronic antral gastric ulcer showing its well-demarcated edge and flat base.

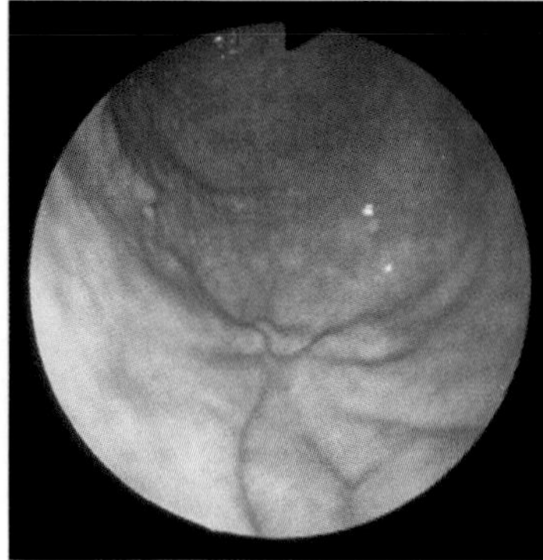

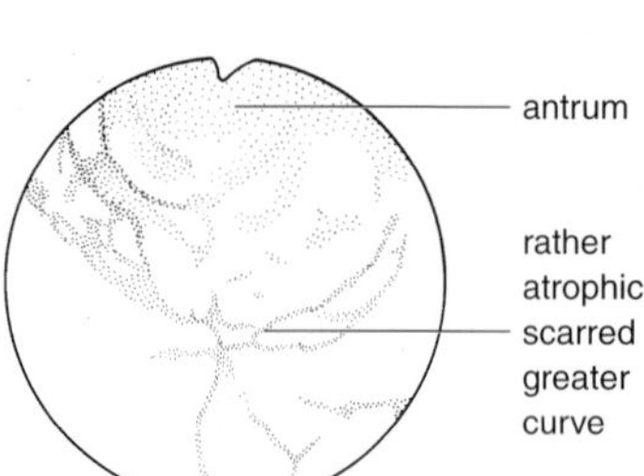

■ **Fig. 2.32** Scarring of the greater curve seen after the healing of a benign ulcer (associated with the ingestion of non-steroidal anti-inflammatory drugs).

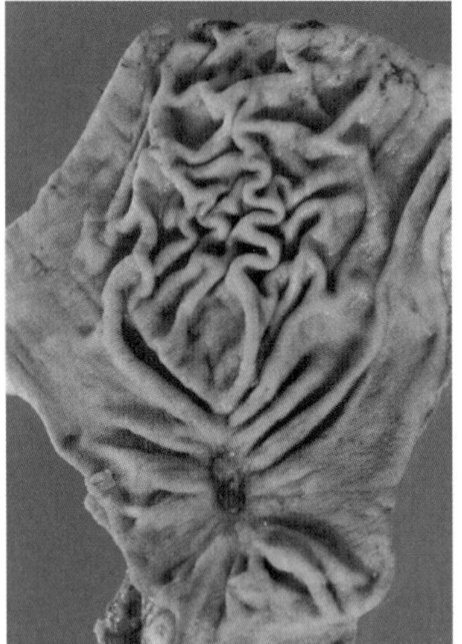

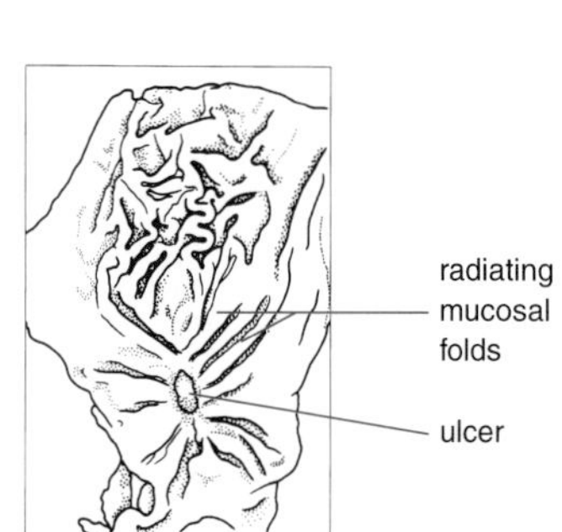

■ **Fig. 2.33** Partial gastrectomy specimen showing a benign ulcer on the lesser curve in the proximal antrum.

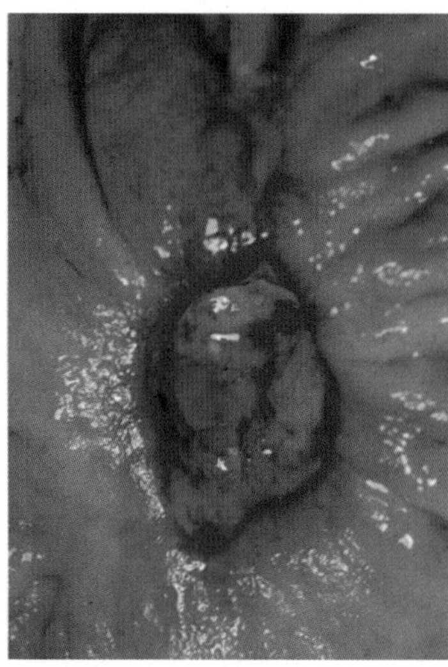

■ **Fig. 2.34** Partial gastrectomy specimen showing a chronic ulcer with recent hemorrhage.

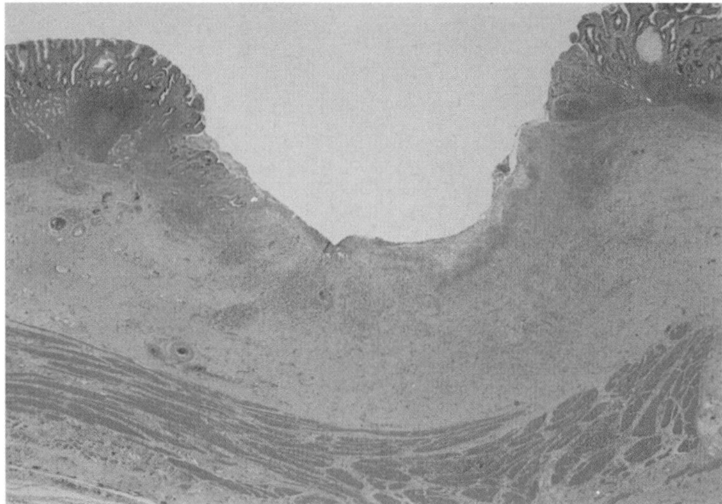

■ **Fig. 2.35** The histological appearance of a benign gastric ulcer. Limited fibrosis is present but the muscle coat in the floor of the ulcer is intact. H&E stain (x 12).

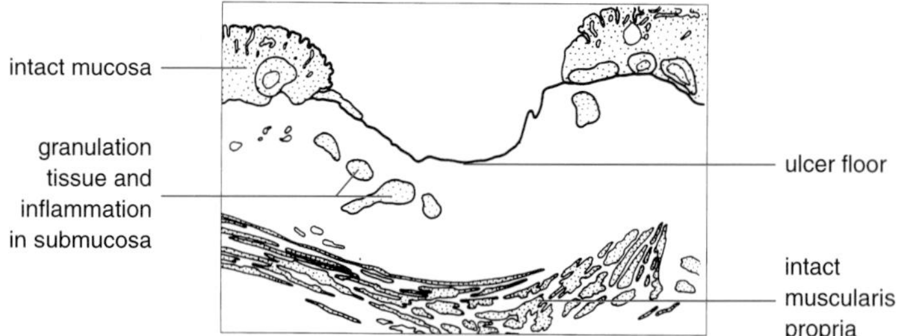

GASTRITIS

Gastritis – inflammation of the gastric mucosa – took on new significance with the recognition that antral gastritis (the erstwhile type B gastritis) is the result of infection with *Helicobacter pylori* (as is most duodenal ulceration). Several earlier classifications were combined into the Sydney system which incorporates topography, etiology (when known), and morphology. It limits gastritis to three basic patterns – acute, chronic, and 'special' – and allows reporting with an etiological prefix and/or a morphological suffix (Fig. 2.47). It is questionable whether uncomplicated gastritis itself is responsible for symptoms.

Acute gastritis

Acute gastritis is often the result of injury by drugs such as non-steroidal anti-inflammatory agents or alcohol, and is frequently seen in the seriously ill patient in the intensive care unit. The most important

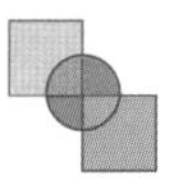

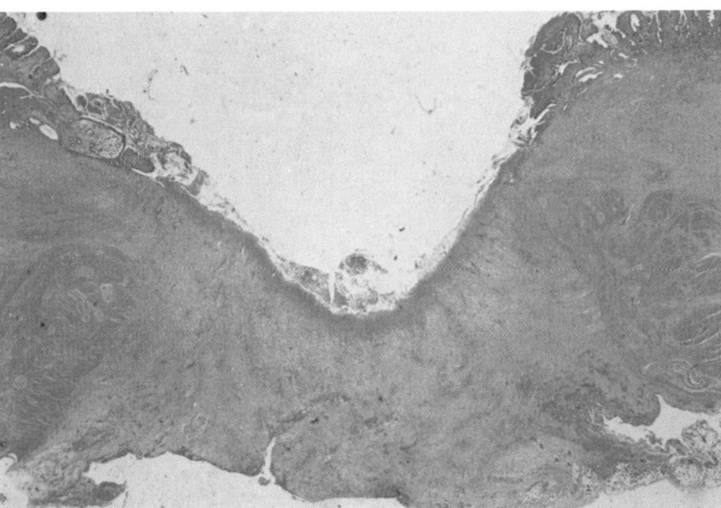

■ **Fig. 2.36** The histological appearance of a chronic benign gastric ulcer. In contrast to Fig. 2.33, there is complete fibrous replacement of the muscle coat of the stomach wall. Surviving muscle is seen at both edges. H&E stain (x 12).

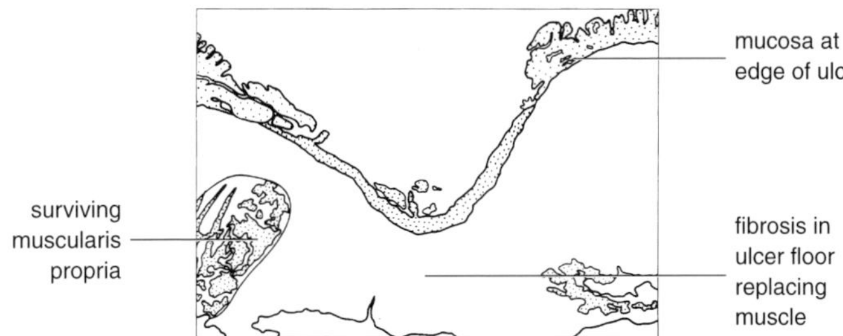

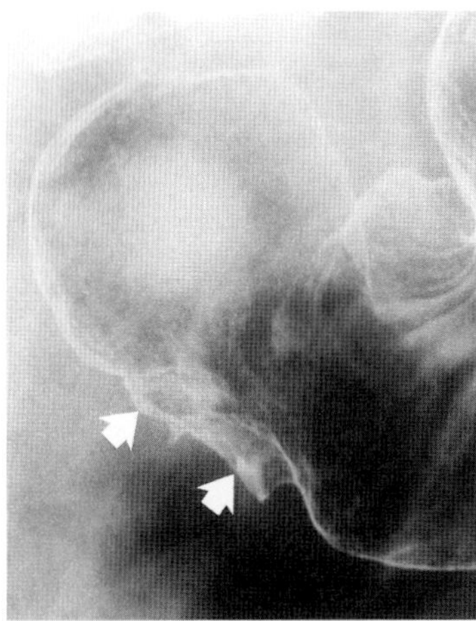

■ **Fig. 2.37** Double-contrast barium study showing a flat ulcer (arrows) on the greater curvature of the gastric antrum due to chronic aspirin therapy. (Reproduced with permission from reference 1.)

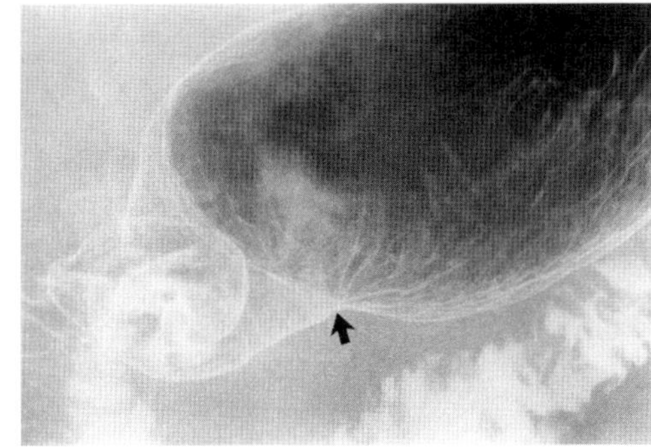

■ **Fig. 2.38** Double-contrast barium study showing radiating folds and focal retraction of the greater curvature of the proximal antrum (arrow) as a result of scarring from chronic aspirin gastropathy.

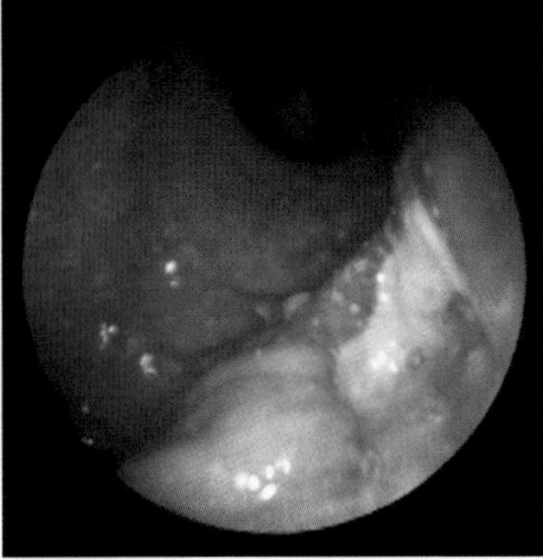

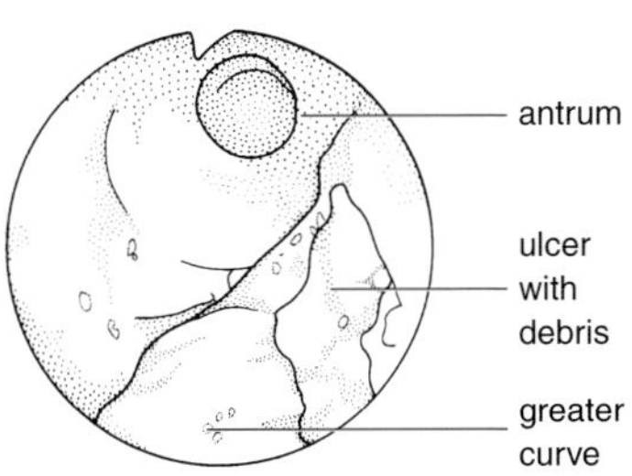

■ **Fig. 2.39** Endoscopic view of a greater curve ulcer caused by ingestion of non-steroidal anti-inflammatory tablets.

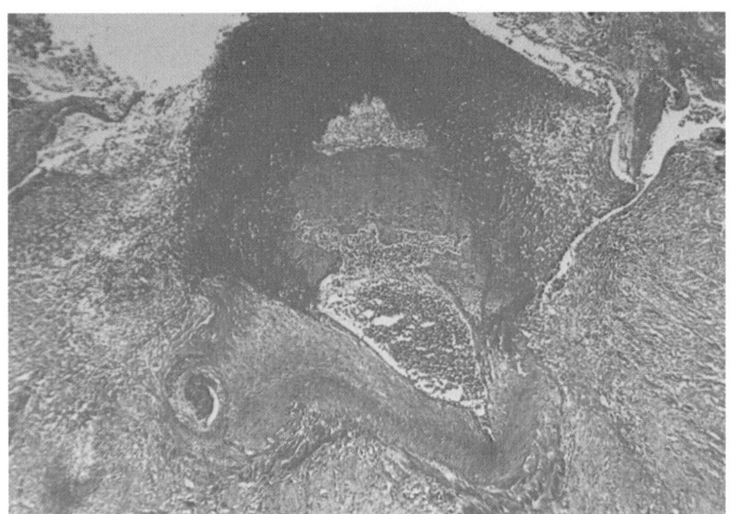

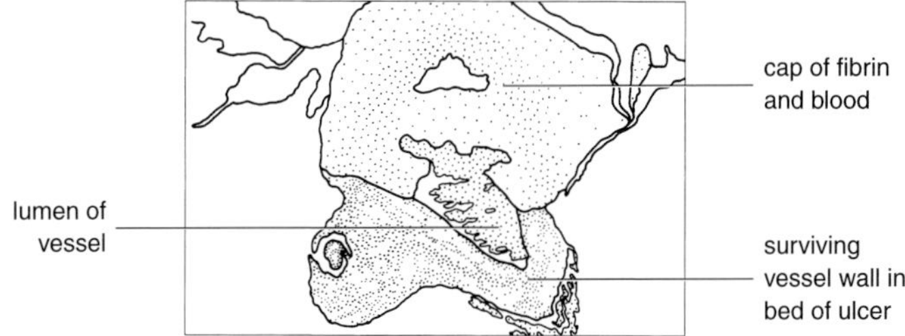

■ **Fig. 2.40** Histological appearance of a benign gastric ulcer, with an artery involved by erosion of the ulcer. A cap of fibrin and blood replaces the luminal aspect of the arterial wall. H&E stain (x 30).

clinical feature is gastrointestinal hemorrhage, which may be both generalized and profuse. Radiology is helpful only if a double-contrast technique is used; it may then show small, shallow erosions in which a central pit of barium is surrounded by a lucent halo or more linear defects (Figs 2.48. 2.49). Endoscopically and macroscopically, lesions appear as multiple hemorrhagic spots with small superficial erosions against a background of hyperemia (Figs 2.50–2.52). Biopsy is not usually appropriate, as additional bleeding may result, and the histology shows only non-specific necrosis of the superficial mucosa and focal loss of the surface epithelium (Figs 2.53–2.55). In more severe cases the mucosa can become severely disrupted to the extent of perforation (Figs 2.56, 2.57).

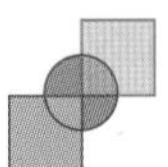

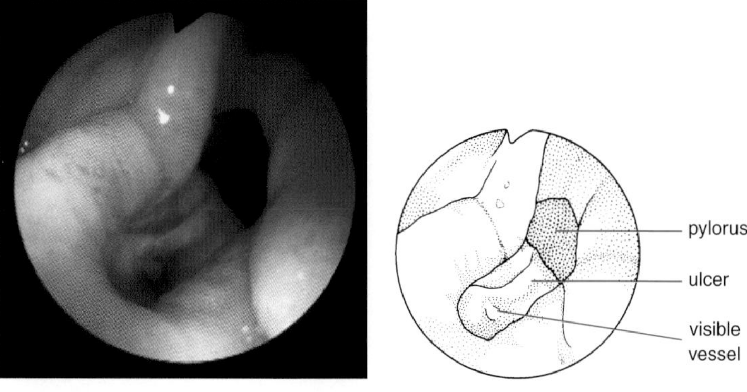

■ **Fig. 2.41** Endoscopic appearance of pyloric channel ulcer with a visible vessel in its base.

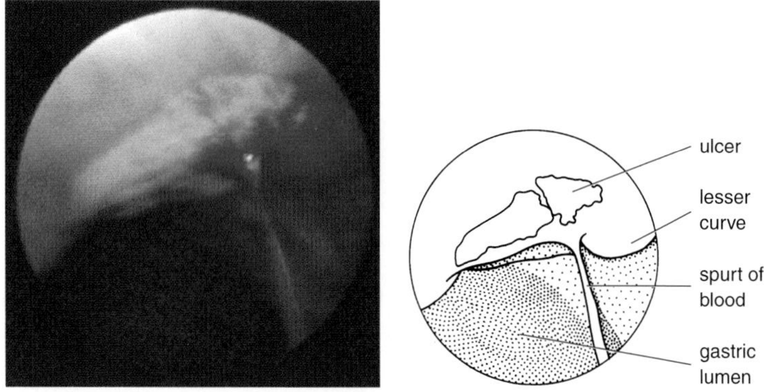

■ **Fig. 2.42** Endoscopic view of a benign ulcer with a spurting vessel in its base.

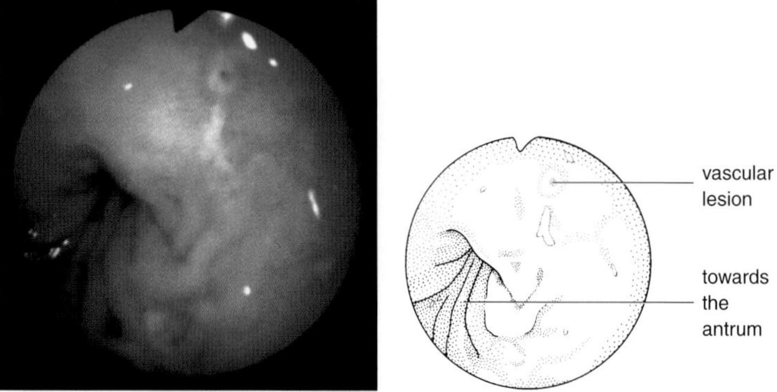

■ **Fig. 2.43** Endoscopic appearance of Dieulafoy lesion in which a vessel is seen in the absence of definite associated ulceration.

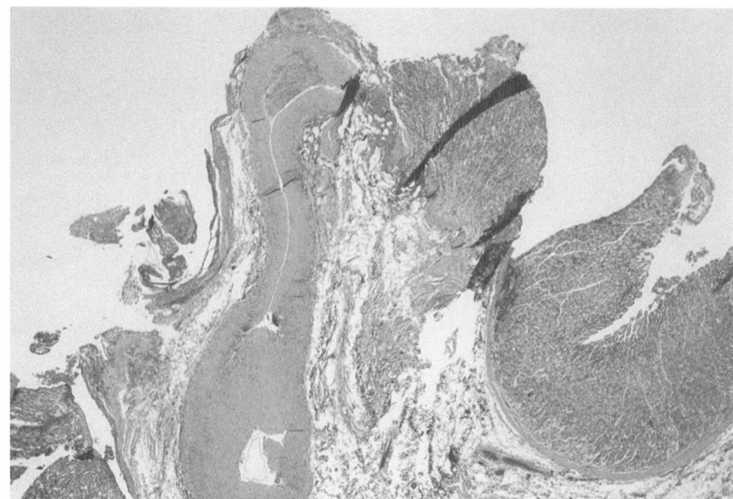

■ **Fig. 2.44** Dieulafoy's ulcer. Microscopic appearance of a large-bore ('caliber-persistent') muscular artery in an abnormally superficial location within the gastric mucosa from a partial gastrectomy performed on an emergent basis for massive hemorrhage from this site.

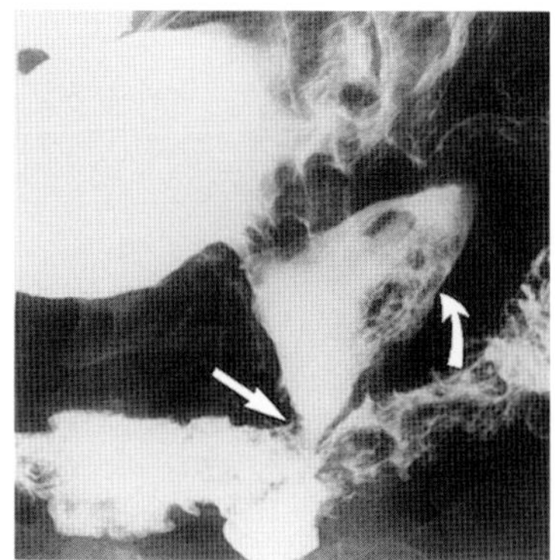

■ **Fig. 2.45** Double-contrast barium study showing a giant ulcer (curved arrow) on the greater curvature of the gastric body with barium entering the transverse colon via a gastrocolic fistula (straight arrow). This patient was on high doses of aspirin. (Reproduced with permission from reference 2.)

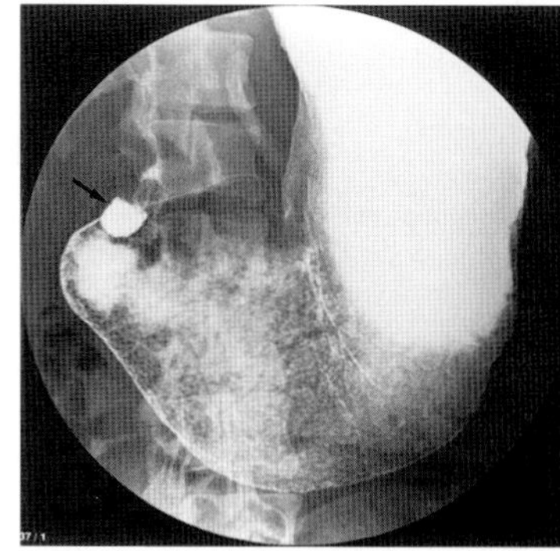

■ **Fig. 2.46** Single-contrast barium study showing a prepyloric ulcer (arrow). Also note dilatation of the stomach and dilution of barium by fluid in this patient with associated gastric outlet obstruction.

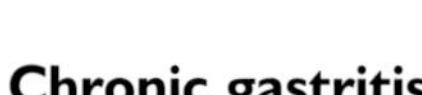

Chronic gastritis

Chronic atrophic gastritis, which usually spares the antrum, is associated with parietal cell antibodies, reduced secretion of acid and intrinsic factor, and hence with pernicious anemia and other autoimmune disorders (Figs 2.58–2.62). By contrast, in the early stages of chronic gastritis associated with *Helicobacter pylori* infection, activity is maximal in the antrum, acid secretion is not much affected, and B_{12} malabsorption is not found (Figs 2.63–2.71). Later in its evolution one sees atrophy (Fig 2.72) and in all situations of atrophic gastritis there is an increased risk of gastric carcinoma. The presence of *H. pylori* may be detected by culture of antral biopsies, on histology, or by one of a number of techniques dependent on the organism's high urease activity. Placement of antral biopsies in a urea-containing medium allows simple detection from the pH change that occurs as ammonia is produced by the organism: commercial test kits are available (Fig. 2.73). False-negative results probably reflect sampling error, which may be overcome by sampling (in effect) from the whole of the stomach by breath testing. Labeled urea is taken orally and the quantity of isotope in exhaled carbon dioxide subsequently measured. Most centers now use the non-radioactive ^{13}C isotope with its detection by mass spectrometry, which has become substantially cheaper than was once the case (Fig. 2.74). Serological tests are also available; an elevated IgM antibody is indicative of current activity, but IgG antibody is probably a better guide overall.

Opportunistic gastritis

It is not only *H. pylori* that can cause an infective gastritis, but it is unusual for problems to arise other than in the immunocompromised or those on potent acid suppression in the context of intensive care. Cytomegalovirus and cryptosporidial infections are responsible for characteristic forms of gastritis (Figs 2.75, 2.76).

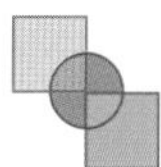

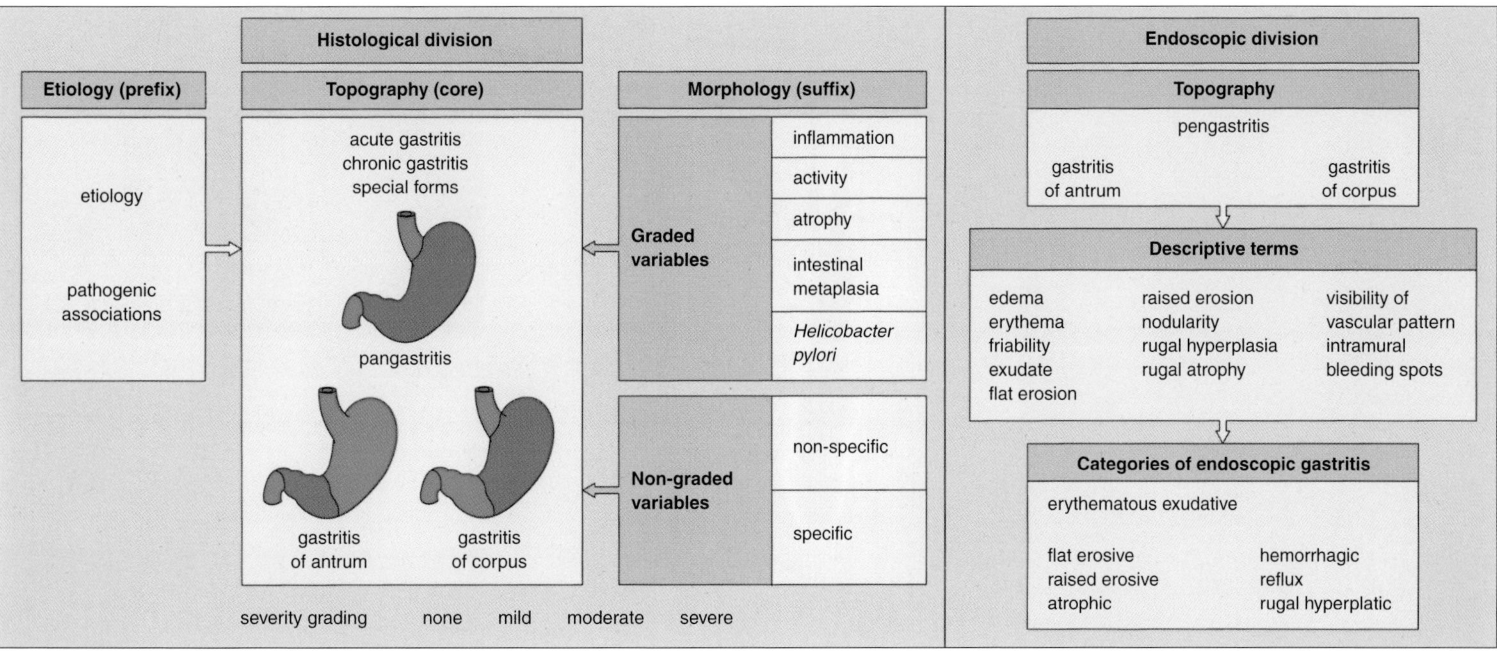

Fig. 2.47 The Sydney system for classification of gastritis.

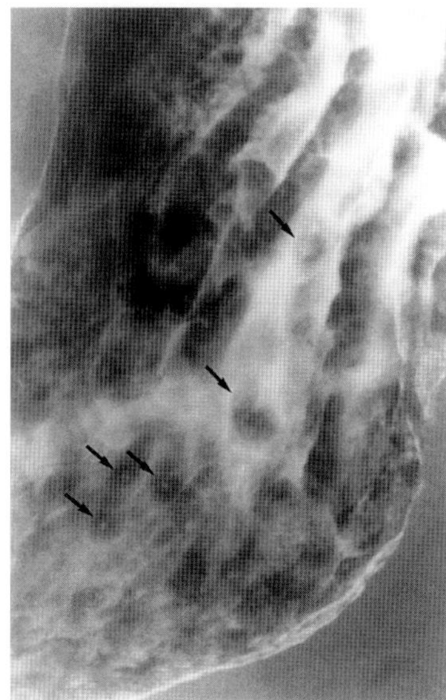

Fig. 2.48 Double-contrast barium study showing multiple varioliform erosions as punctate collections of barium surrounded by radiolucent mounds of edema (arrows) in the gastric body.

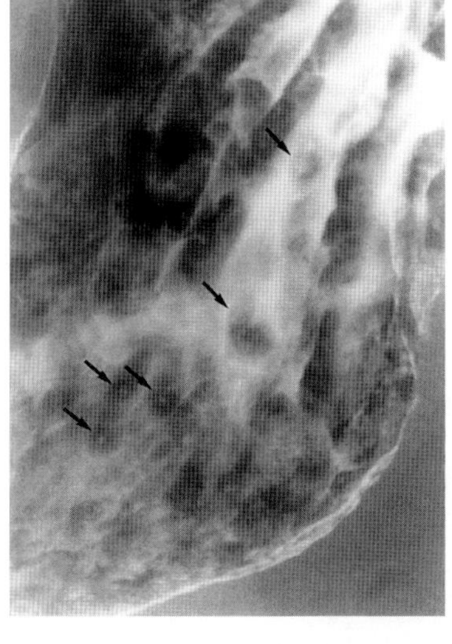

Fig. 2.49 Double-contrast barium study showing linear and serpiginous erosions (arrowheads) clustered together near the greater curvature of the gastric antrum. This patient was taking a non-steroidal anti-inflammatory drug.

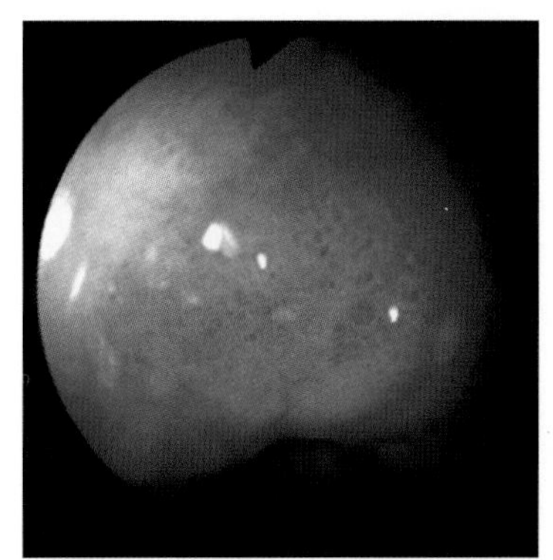

Fig. 2.50 Endoscopic view of gastric erosions in association with punctate hemorrhages.

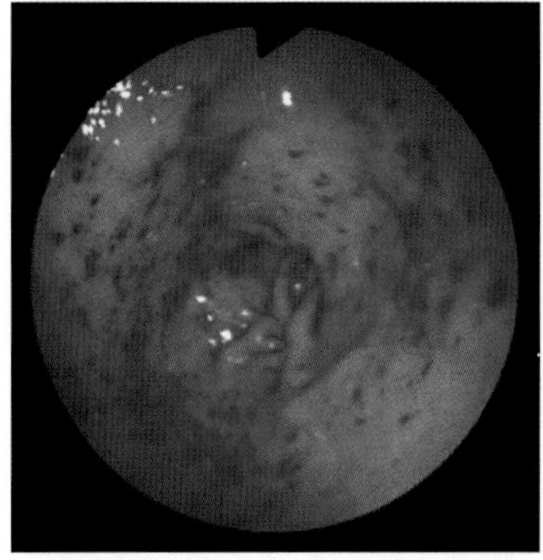

Fig. 2.51 Hemorrhagic gastritis associated with purpuric lesions in a patient with severe thrombocytopenia.

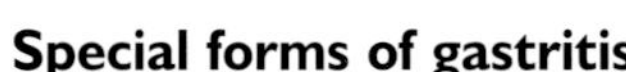

Special forms of gastritis

Eosinophilic gastritis affects the distal stomach. Dyspepsia is common, and thickened antral folds may cause pyloric obstruction. Bleeding, protein-losing enteropathy, and eosinophilic ascites are also described. Other sites in the gastrointestinal tract may also be affected, but peripheral eosinophilia is rarely prominent. The diagnosis is generally made from gastric histology; the changes are most marked in the antrum, where there is submucosal edema and a variable eosinophilic infiltrate, which may include occasional giant cells, and which may extend through to the serosal surface (Fig. 2.77).

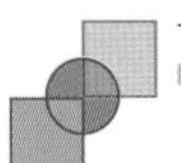

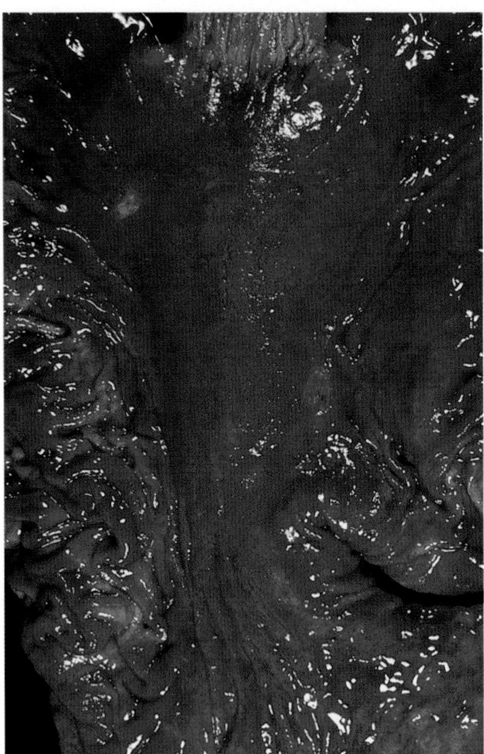

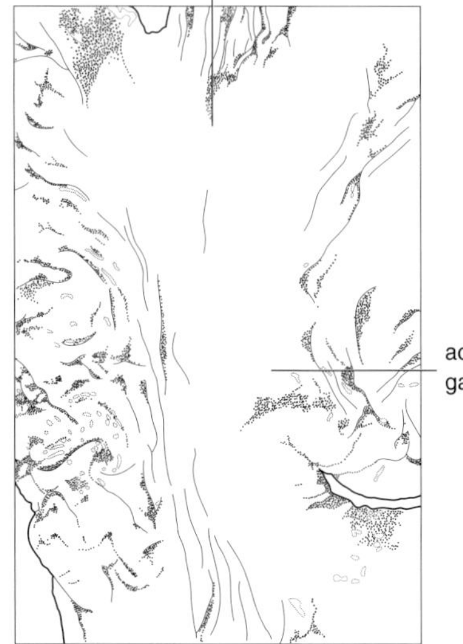

■ **Fig. 2.52** Acute erosive gastritis. Macroscopic appearance of severe acute hemorrhagic gastritis with discrete erosions on the lesser curvature.

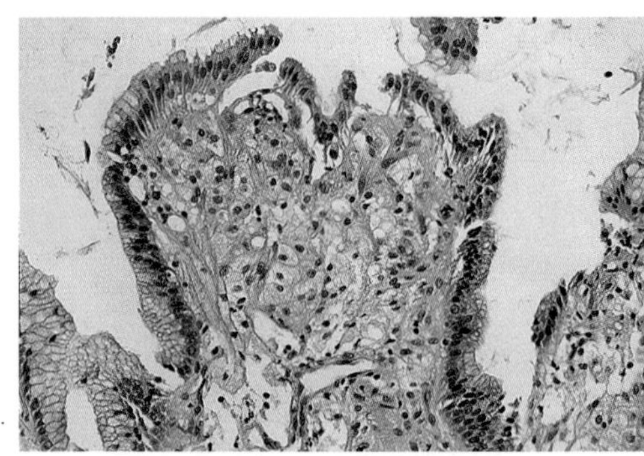

■ **Fig. 2.54** High magnification of healing erosive gastritis showing collections of foamy macrophages characteristic of mucosal xanthoma formation at the site of previous stromal hemorrhage.

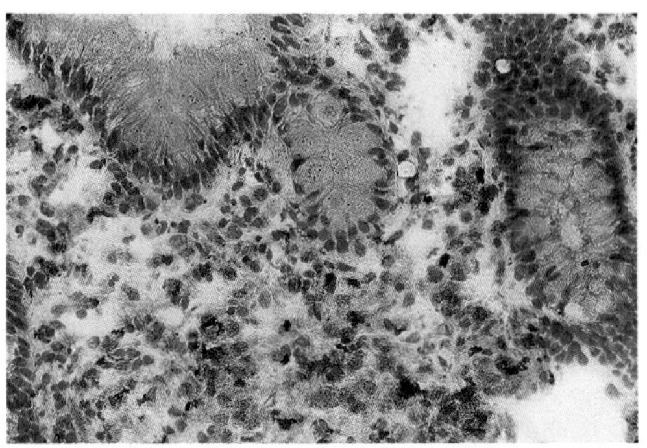

■ **Fig. 2.55** Healing erosive gastritis with xanthoma formation. An oil red O stain identifies the cytoplasmic content of the foamy macrophages as neutral lipid, a breakdown product of red cell membranes.

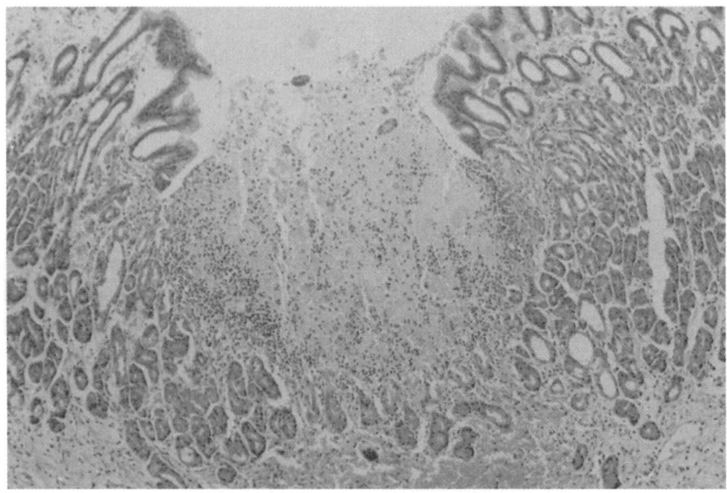

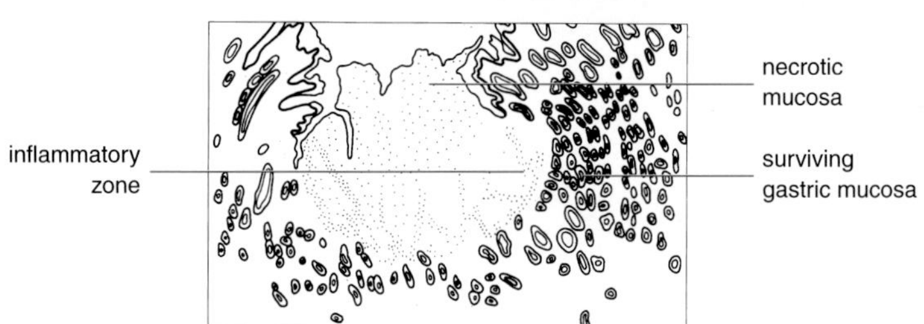

■ **Fig. 2.53** Microscopic appearance of acute erosive gastritis showing a discrete focus of partial-thickness necrosis of the mucosa without evidence of chronicity such as fibrosis or widespread inflammatory cell infiltration. Inflammation is limited to the interface between the viable and necrotic mucosa.

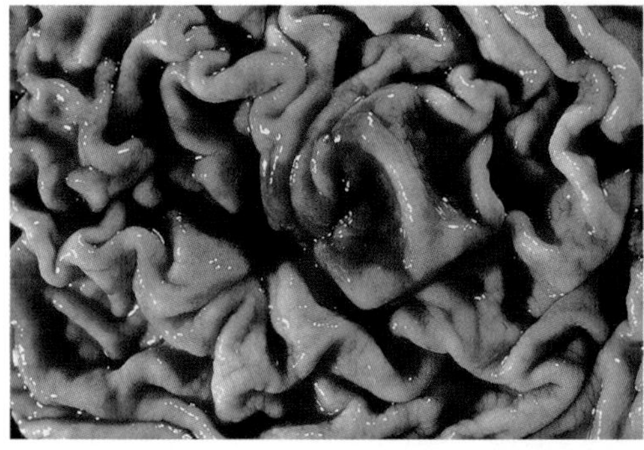

■ **Fig. 2.56** Macroscopic appearance of a partial gastrectomy with severe focal chemical gastritis and perforation due to non-steroidal anti-inflammatory drugs.

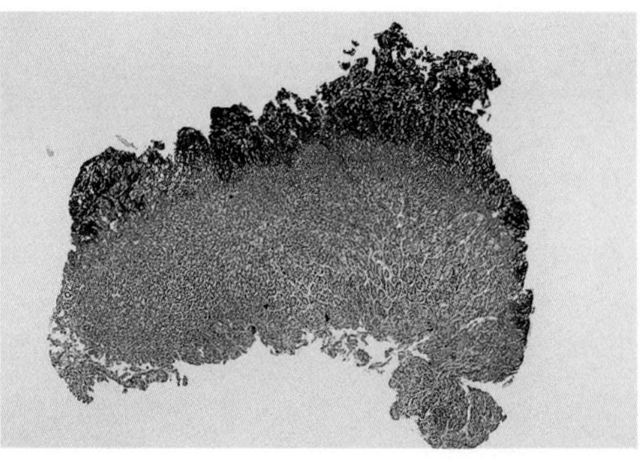

■ **Fig. 2.57** Severe focal chemical gastritis. Microscopic appearance of superficial mucosal necrosis ('chemical burn') of the gastric mucosa secondary to direct chemical injury from aspirin.

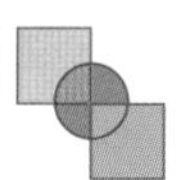

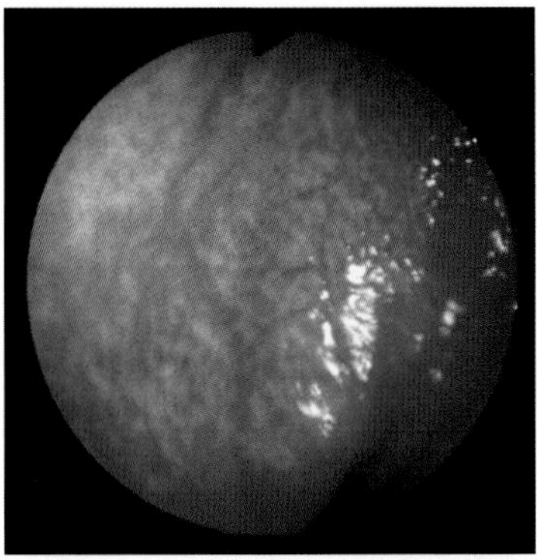

Fig. 2.58 Endoscopic appearance of chronic gastritis associated with pernicious anemia.

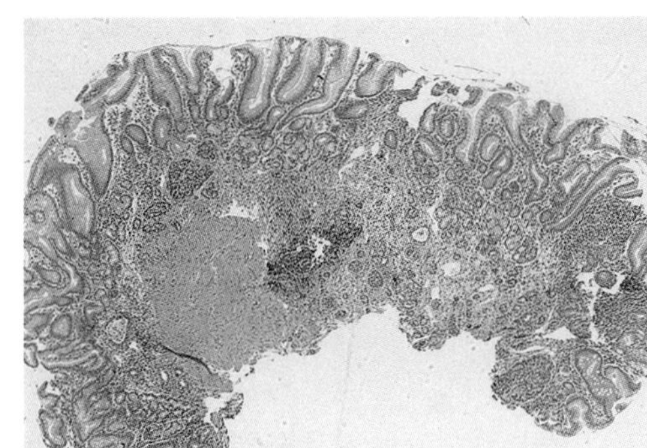

Fig. 2.62 The microscopic appearance of the oxyntic mucosa in autoimmune gastritis showing neuroendocrine cell hyperplasia with micro-carcinoid formation secondary to long-standing gastrin stimulation resulting from parietal cell destruction and achlorhydria.

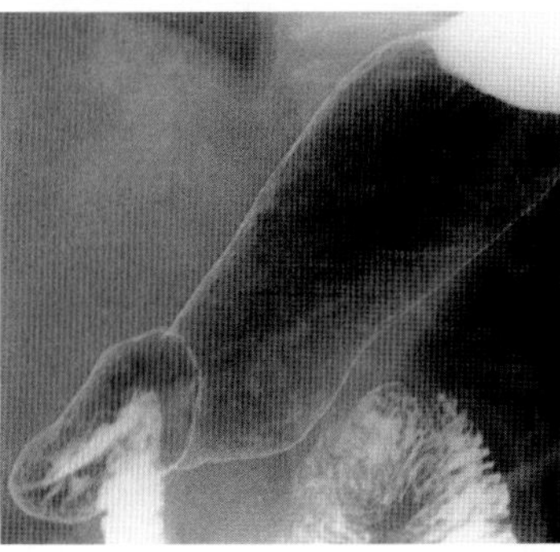

Fig. 2.59 Double-contrast barium study showing decreased distensibility of the stomach and a paucity of folds, producing a 'bald' appearance that is characteristic of atrophic gastritis.

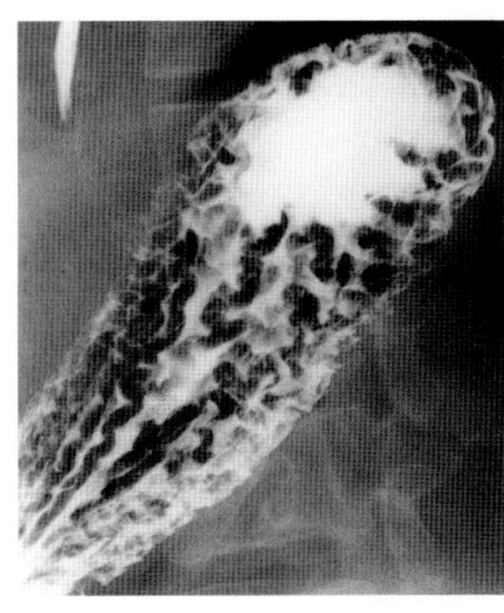

Fig. 2.63 Double-contrast barium study showing moderately thickened, irregular folds in the gastric fundus and body due to infection by *Helicobacter pylori*.

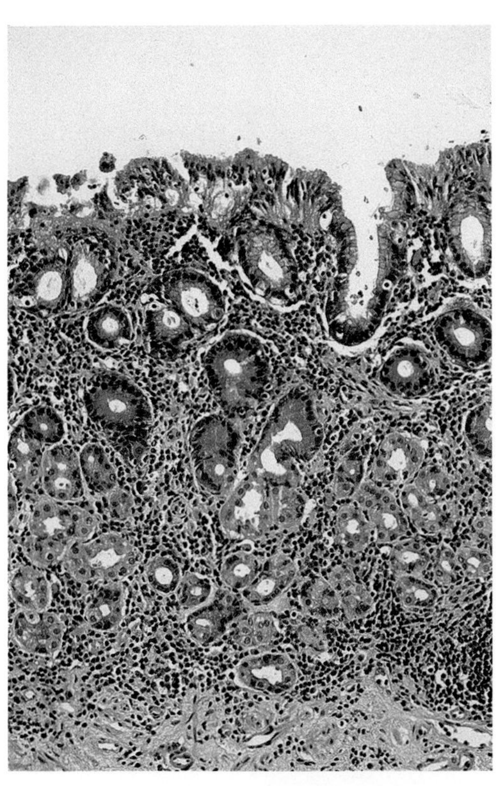

Fig. 2.60 Autoimmune gastritis with atrophy of the gastric corpus. Microscopic appearance of autoimmune gastritis with marked lymphocytic infiltration of the stroma diffusely and glands focally and dramatic reduction in oxyntic gland length and number.

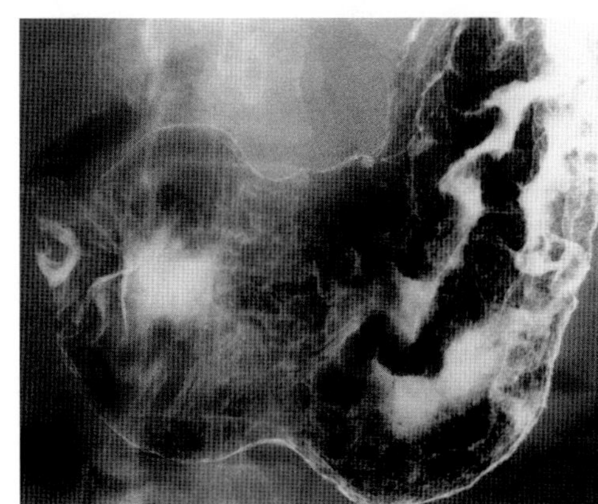

Fig. 2.64 Double-contrast view showing markedly thickened, lobulated folds in the gastric body (also known as polypoid gastritis) in a patient with marked *H. pylori* gastritis. Ménétrier's disease and lymphoma (see Fig. 2.82) could produce similar findings. (Reproduced with permission from reference 3.)

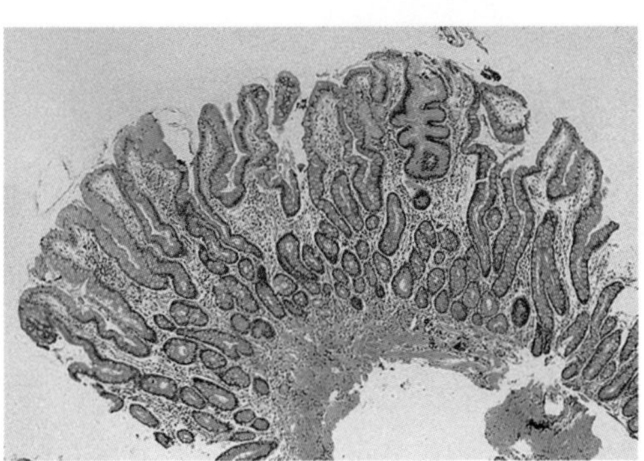

Fig. 2.61 Microscopic appearance of long-standing autoimmune gastritis with complete atrophy of the oxyntic mucosa and diffuse intestinal metaplasia.

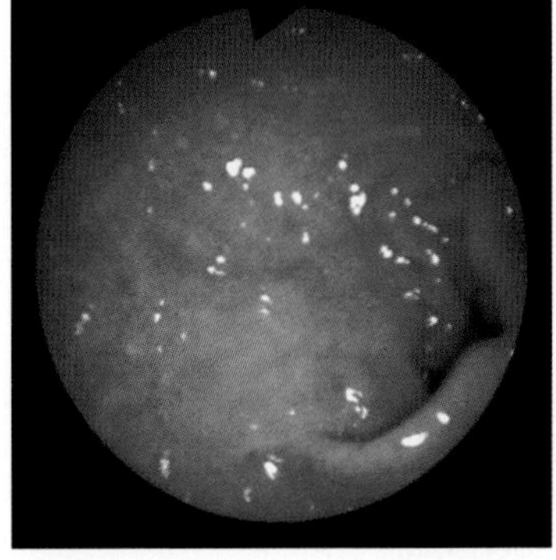

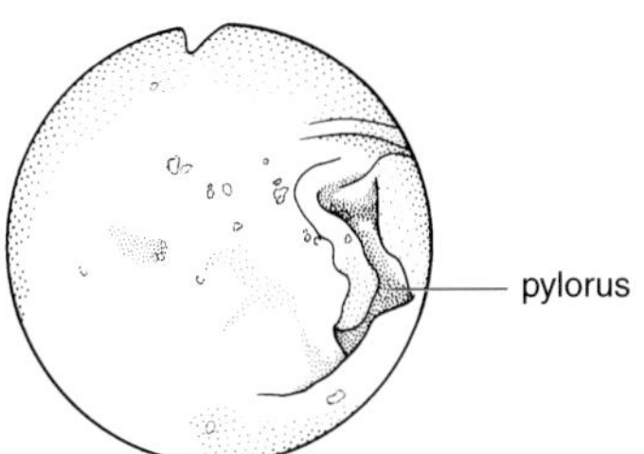

Fig. 2.65 Endoscopic appearance of antral gastritis associated with *Helicobacter pylori*.

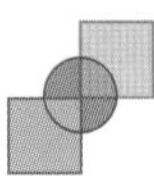

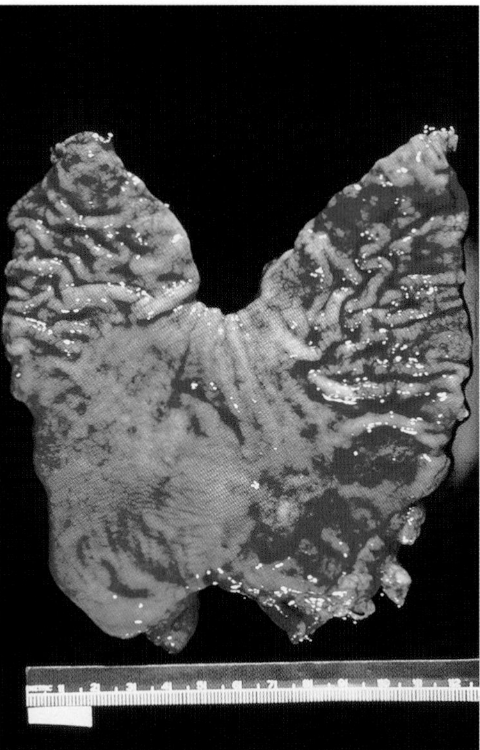

■ **Fig. 2.66** Partial gastrectomy specimen showing chronic antral gastritis caused by *Helicobacter pylori* with flattening of the antral mucosa and loss of the characteristic mucosal folds.

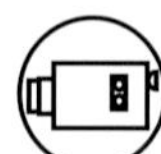

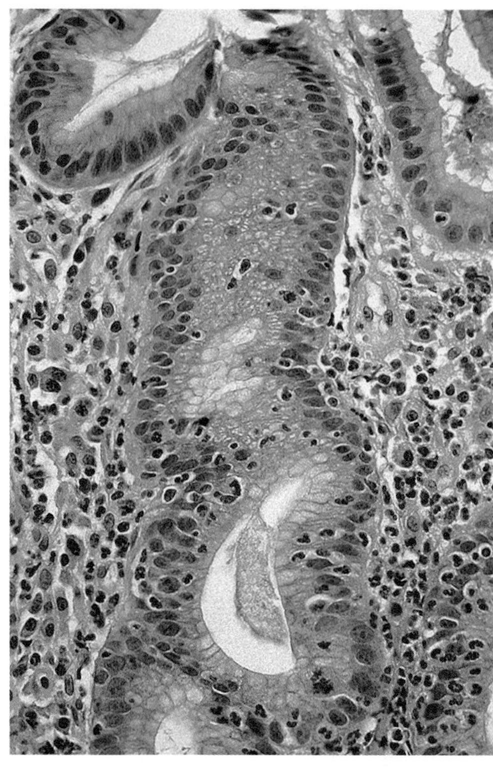

■ **Fig. 2.69** High-magnification microscopic appearance of *Helicobacter pylori* gastritis showing a hyperplastic gastric pit surrounded by stromal plasma cells but infiltrated by neutrophils ('pititis').

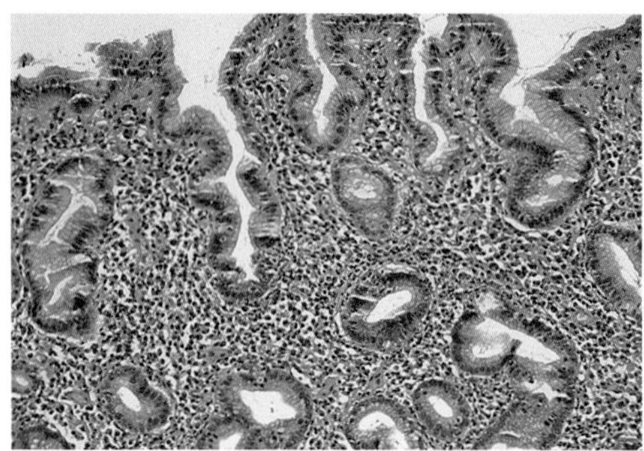

■ **Fig. 2.67** Microscopic appearance of the antrum in *Helicobacter pylori* gastritis showing a characteristically dense lymphoplasmacytic stromal infiltrate.

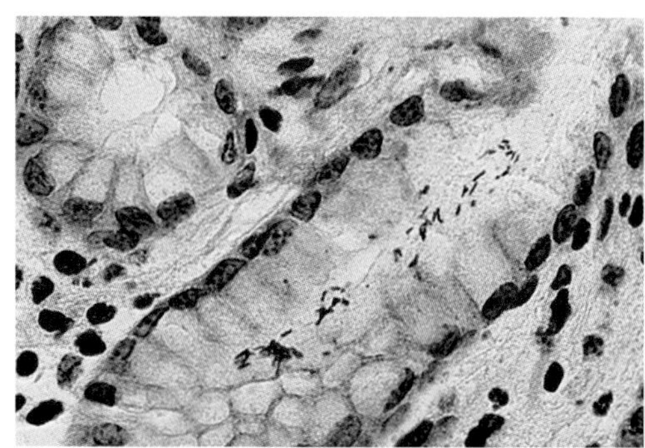

■ **Fig. 2.70** Warthin–Starry silver stain in *Helicobacter pylori* gastritis demonstrating the short, plump spiral bacilli in the pits of the antral mucosa.

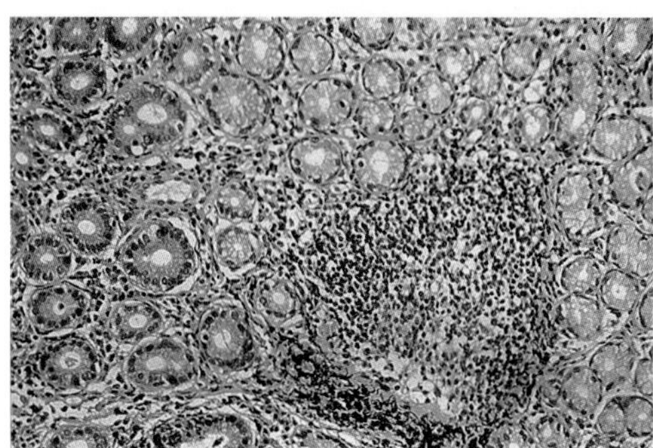

■ **Fig. 2.68** Microscopic appearance of *Helicobacter pylori* gastritis showing lymphoid follicle formation in the antral lamina propria, a feature that is strongly associated with *Helicobacter pylori* infection.

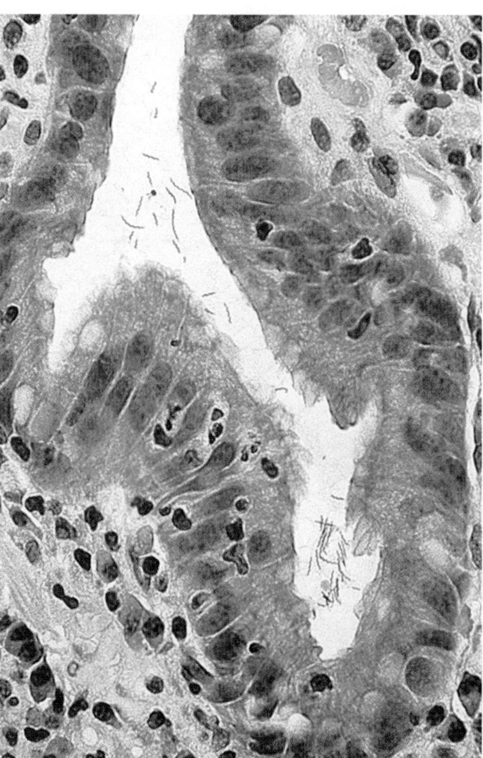

■ **Fig. 2.71** High-magnification microscopic appearance of *Helicobacter heilmanni* showing infecting organisms that are characteristically very long and tightly spiraled with a 'zig-zag' appearance.

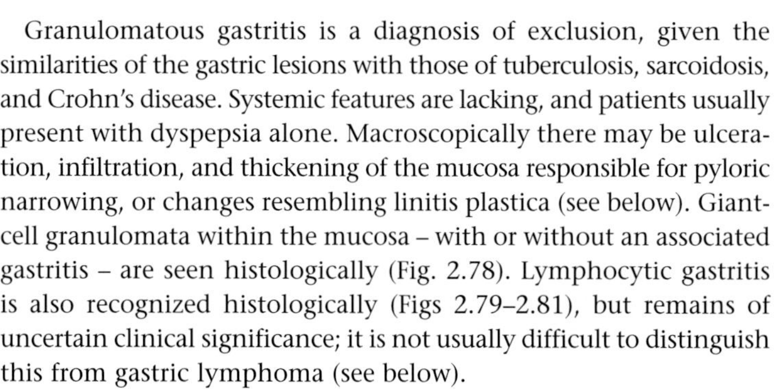

Granulomatous gastritis is a diagnosis of exclusion, given the similarities of the gastric lesions with those of tuberculosis, sarcoidosis, and Crohn's disease. Systemic features are lacking, and patients usually present with dyspepsia alone. Macroscopically there may be ulceration, infiltration, and thickening of the mucosa responsible for pyloric narrowing, or changes resembling linitis plastica (see below). Giant-cell granulomata within the mucosa – with or without an associated gastritis – are seen histologically (Fig. 2.78). Lymphocytic gastritis is also recognized histologically (Figs 2.79–2.81), but remains of uncertain clinical significance; it is not usually difficult to distinguish this from gastric lymphoma (see below).

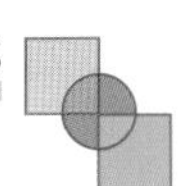

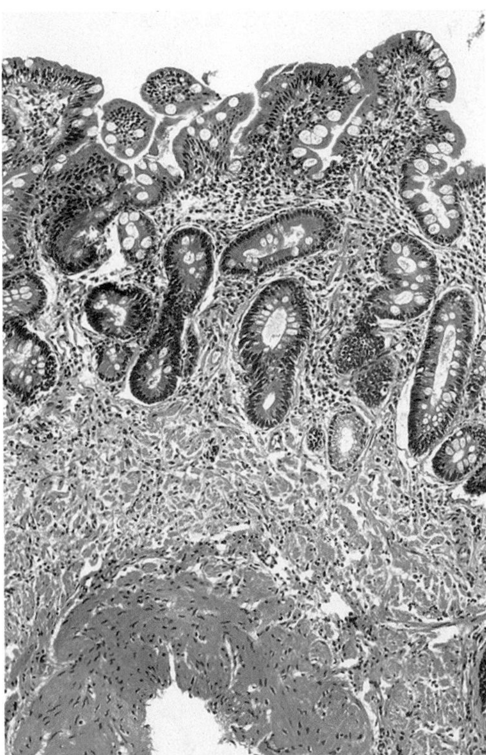

■ **Fig. 2.72** Microscopic appearance of the gastric antrum in chronic inactive *Helicobacter pylori* gastritis showing short sparse antral glands with subjacent fibrosis and widespread intestinal metaplasia.

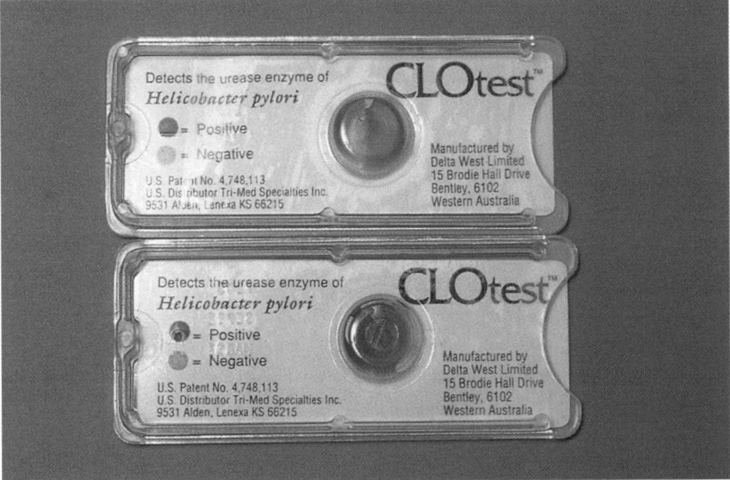

■ **Fig. 2.73** Detection of *H. pylori* by urease activity in antral biopsies. The upper slide shows a negative biopsy which has not changed the pH nor the color of the indicator. The lower, positive biopsy has produced large quantities of urease with associated color change.

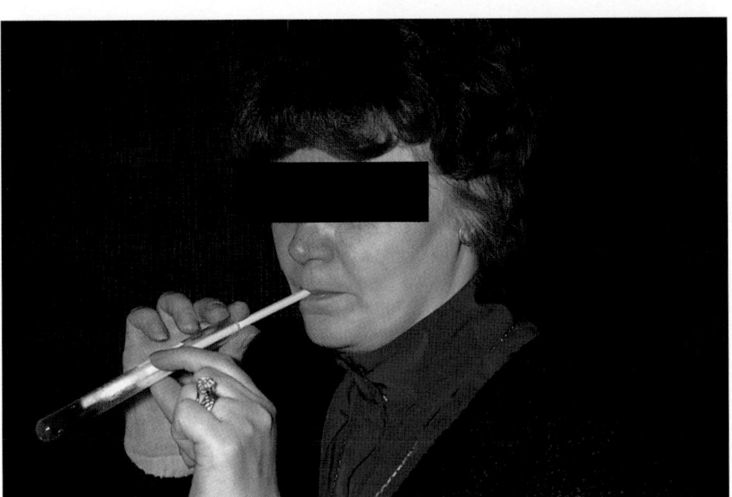

■ **Fig. 2.74** The non-radioactive carbon 13 urea breath test can be done safely in fertile women and in children; expired breath samples are obtained very simply by blowing through a straw into a sealable test tube. Courtesy of Dr R. Logan.

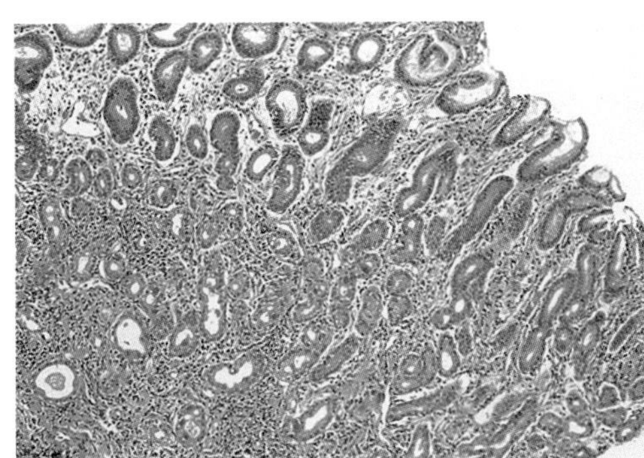

■ **Fig. 2.75** Microscopic appearance of CMV gastritis showing a patchy, dense mixed inflammatory infiltrate associated with virally infected glands, the lining cells of which contain large eosinophilic intranuclear inclusions.

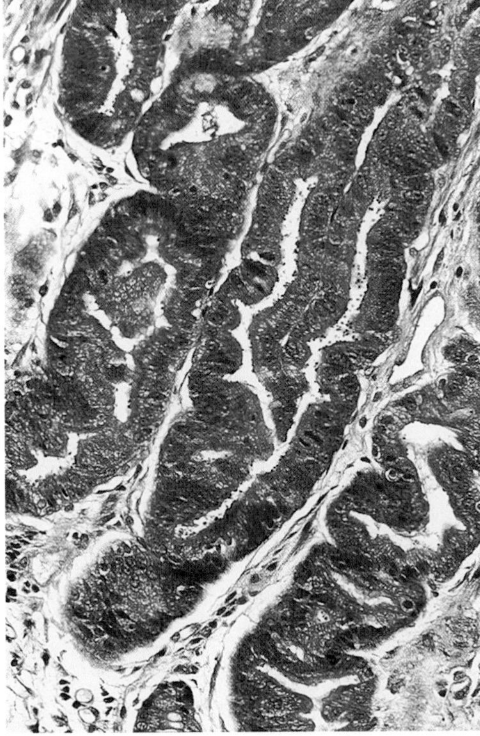

■ **Fig. 2.76** Microscopic appearance of the antral pits in opportunistic upper gastrointestinal infection by cryptosporidia showing numerous small round non-invasive organisms studding the surfaces of the foveolar cells.

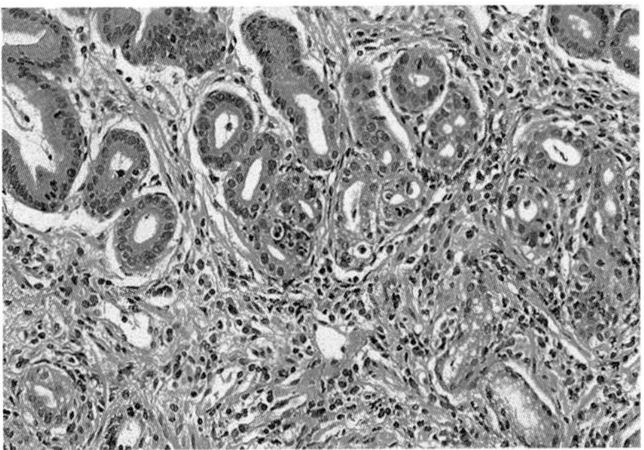

■ **Fig. 2.77** Microscopic appearance of eosinophilic gastritis showing infiltration of both stroma and glands by eosinophils, focal-forming eosinophilic microabscesses.

Ménétrier's disease – giant hypertrophic gastritis – causes generalized (or less commonly localized) enlargement of the folds of the gastric body (Fig. 2.82). Gastric polyposis, carcinoma, and giant rugal hypertrophy comprise the radiological differential diagnosis. Endoscopically, the giant folds are readily seen and may have a nodular or polypoid appearance (Fig. 2.83). The surface is frequently congested or even ulcerated, but protein loss and hypoproteinemia, which is characteristic of the condition, also occur without frank ulceration (Fig 2.84). Superficial biopsies are often normal, and deep biopsies, which reveal elongation and dilatation of the gastric pits, may be necessary for confident histological diagnosis. Some replacement of

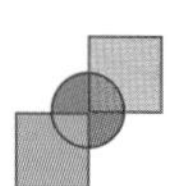

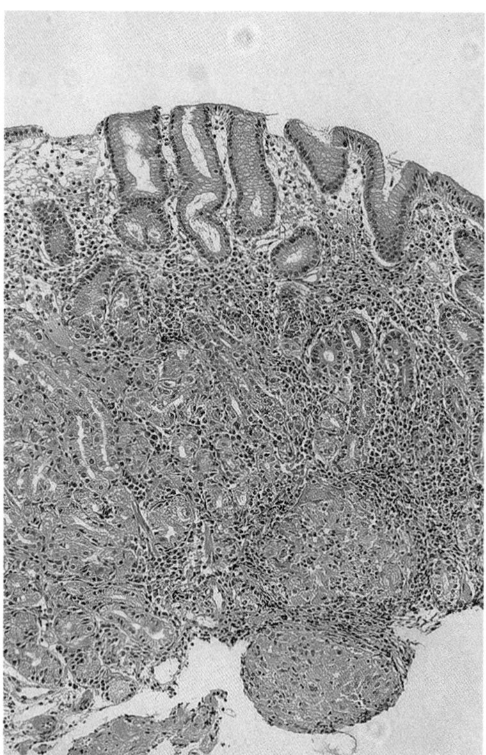

■ **Fig. 2.78** Microscopic appearance of granulomatous gastritis showing well-formed non-caseating granulomata surrounded by chronic inflammation in the deep lamina propria of the gastric antrum in a patient with Crohn's disease of the upper gastrointestinal tract.

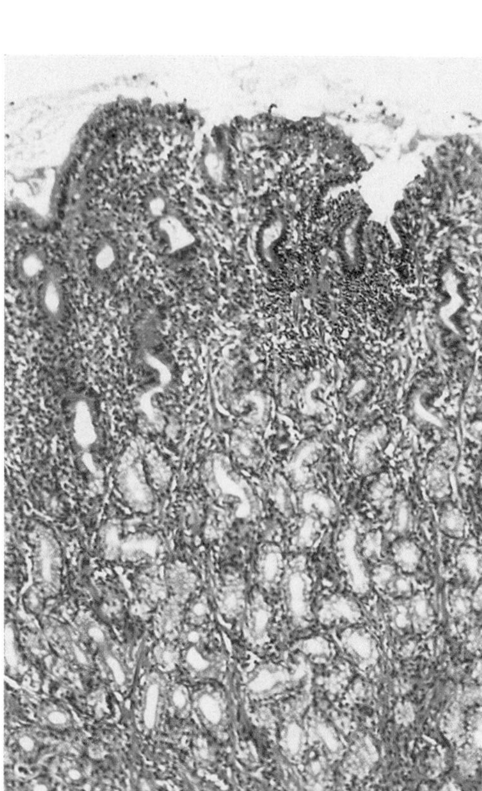

■ **Fig. 2.79** Low-magnification microscopic appearance of the antrum in lymphocytic gastritis with a moderately dense inflammatory infiltrate of the superficial lamina propria.

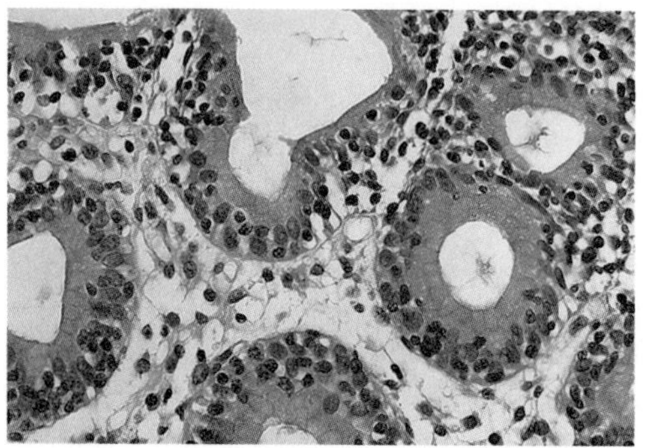

■ **Fig. 2.80** High-magnification microscopic appearance of lymphocytic gastritis showing markedly increased numbers of intraepithelial lymphocytes within the glandular and surface epithelium.

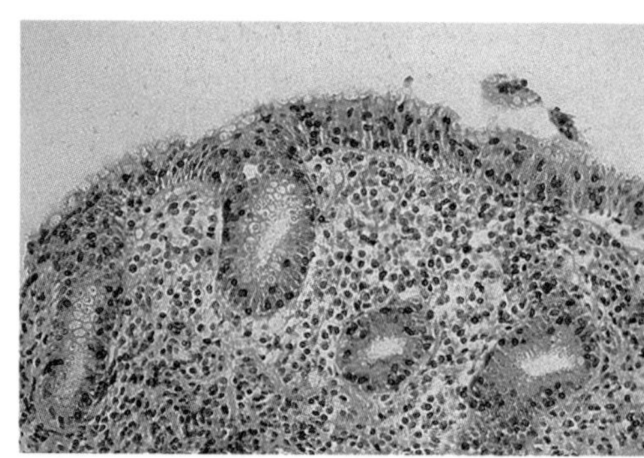

■ **Fig. 2.81** An immunohistochemical stain demonstrates that the lymphocytes infiltrating the epithelium in lymphocytic gastritis are CD4-positive T cells.

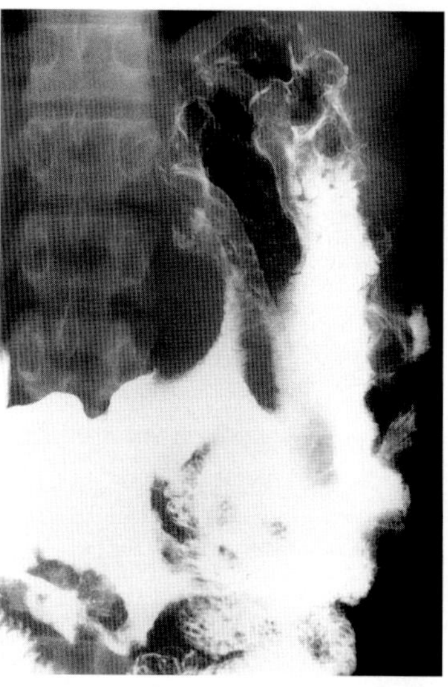

■ **Fig. 2.82** Ménétrier's disease. Characteristic macroscopic appearance of Ménétrier's disease showing extreme enlargement of the rugal folds in the gastric body and fundus without involvement of the antrum.

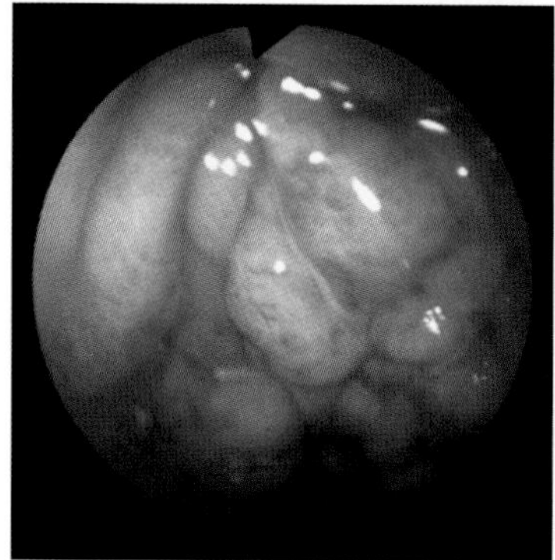

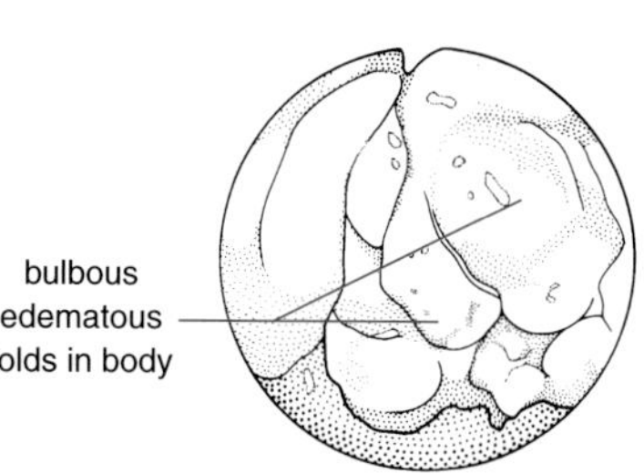

■ **Fig. 2.83** Endoscopic appearance of Ménétrier's disease showing apparently polypoid protrusions and generally edematous gastric mucosa.

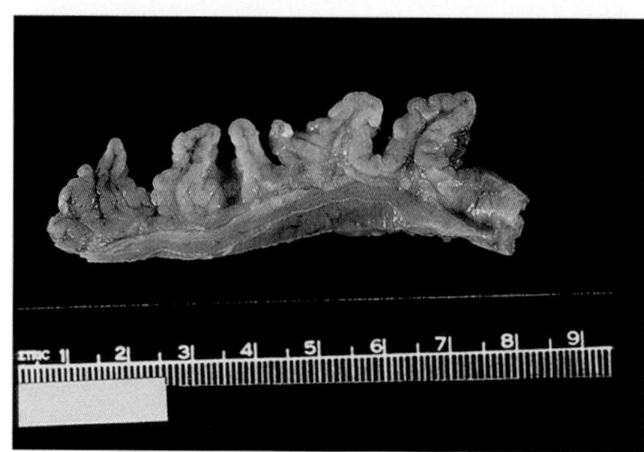

■ **Fig. 2.84** Ménétrier's disease. Macroscopic appearance of a transverse section through the gastric wall showing the markedly thickened and elongated rugal folds of the body.

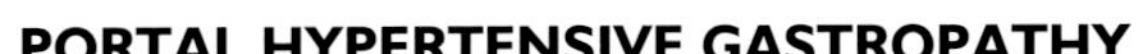

the acid-secreting glands by simple (and sometimes cystic) mucous glands is typical (Figs 2.85, 2.86). A distinction should be drawn here from the rugal hypertrophy of Zollinger–Ellison syndrome (see Chapter 3) in which the abnormality derives from oxyntic gland hypertrophy (Fig 2.87).

Gastritis, or even frank infarction, may result from ischemic damage in patients with prolonged hypotension or with misplaced arterial chemotherapy for hepatic tumors (Fig. 2.88); similar changes are associated with irradiation.

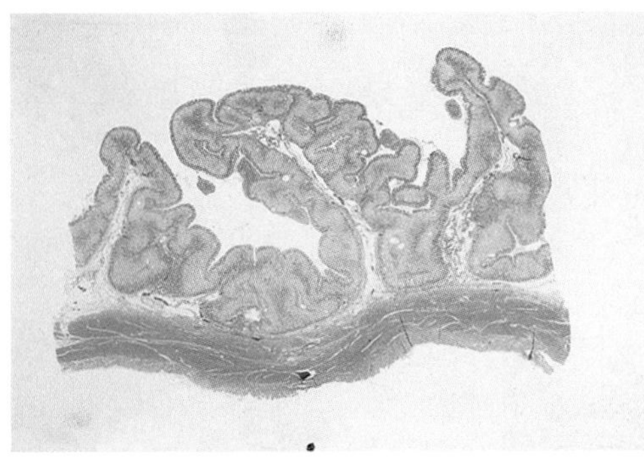

Fig. 2.85 Whole-mount microscopic appearance of Ménétrier's disease showing enlarged rugal folds and thickened mucosa.

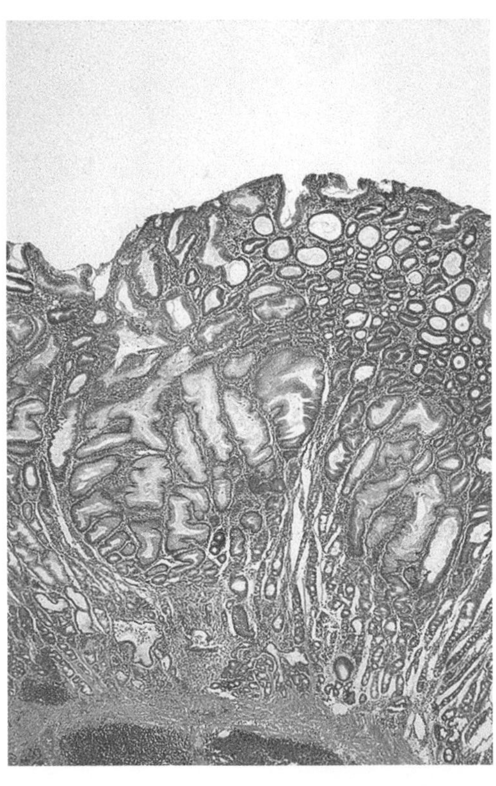

Fig. 2.86 Microscopic appearance of Ménétrier's disease showing markedly elongated, tortuous pits. The hyperplastic pits comprise most of the thickness of the mucosa; the underlying glands are atrophic.

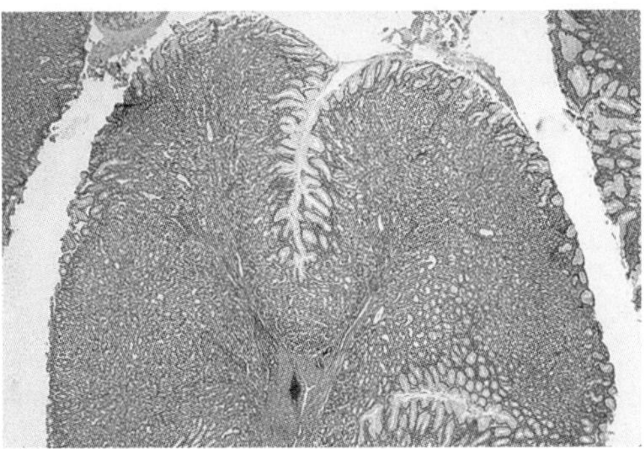

Fig. 2.87 Microscopic appearance of the gastric body in the Zollinger–Ellison syndrome characterized by rugal fold enlargement and mucosal thickening that is caused by hypertrophy of the oxyntic glands rather than the pits as seen in Ménétrier's disease.

PORTAL HYPERTENSIVE GASTROPATHY

Portal hypertension is considered more fully in Chapter 12, but is responsible for characteristic changes, such as congestive gastropathy and watermelon stomach (Figs 2.89, 2.90), which may otherwise be confused with simple gastritis. The histology also is characteristic with prominent vascular ectasia (Fig 2.91). Gastric fundal varices also occur (Figs 2.92–2.94).

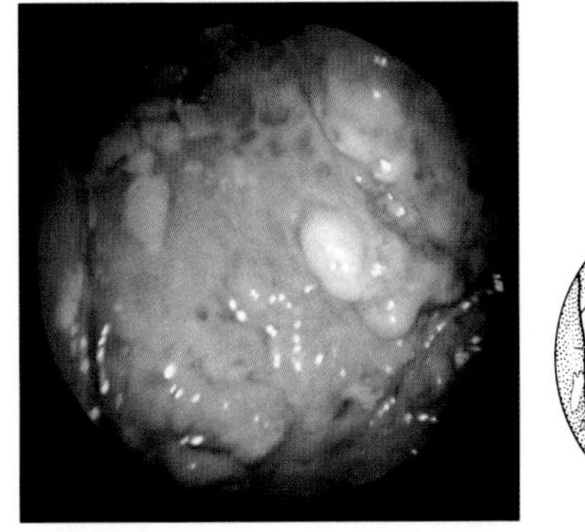

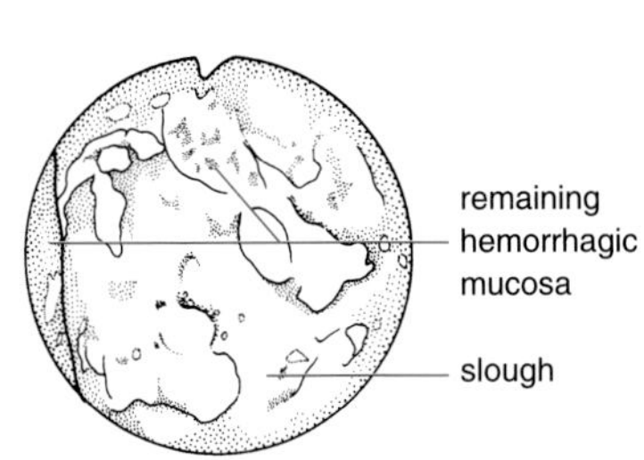

Fig. 2.88 Endoscopic appearance of the severe mucosal sloughing seen in ischemic gastritis.

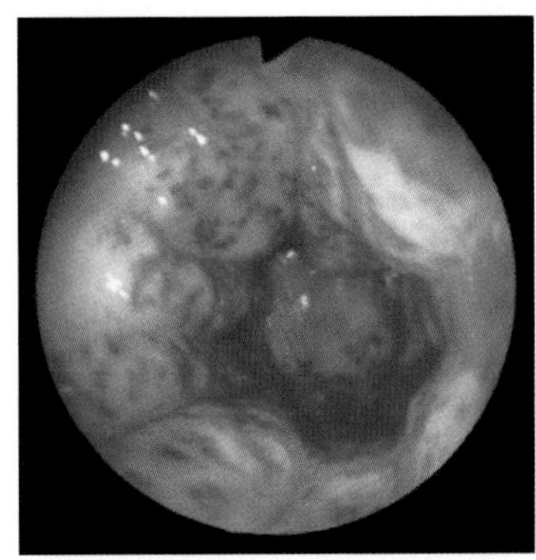

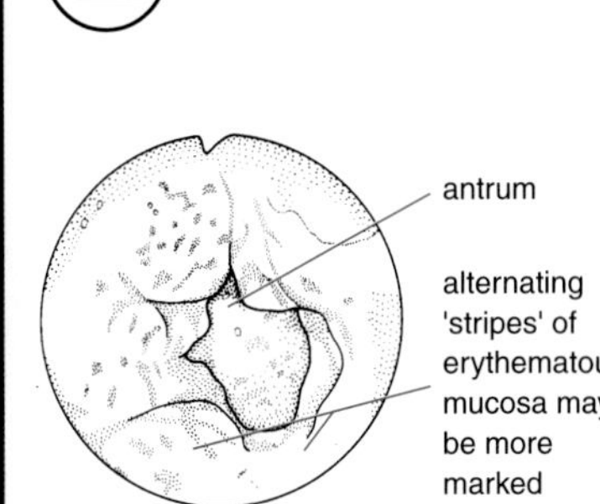

Fig. 2.89 Water-melon stomach.

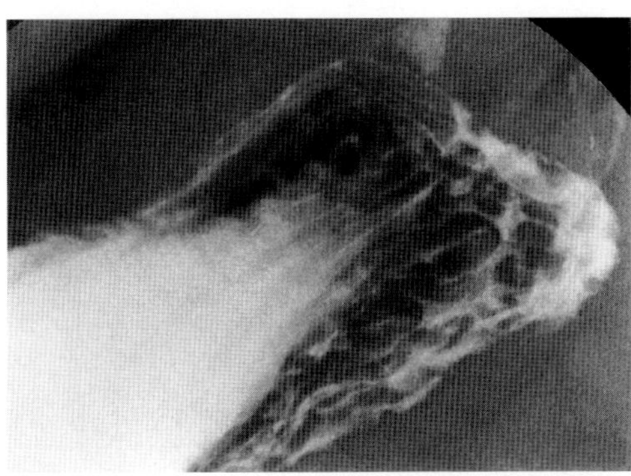

Fig. 2.90 Double-contrast view showing slightly thickened, nodular folds in the gastric fundus in a patient with non-alcoholic hepatic steatosis and hepatitis. This appearance was caused by portal hypertensive gastropathy. (Reproduced with permission from reference 4.)

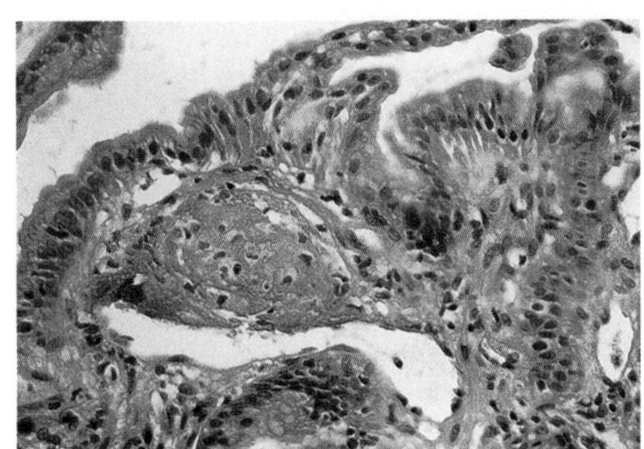

Fig. 2.91 Microscopic appearance of gastric antral vascular ectasia showing markedly ectatic thin-walled vessels below the mucosal surface, the largest of which contains an adherent fibrin thrombus.

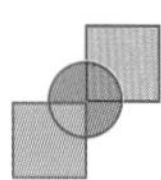

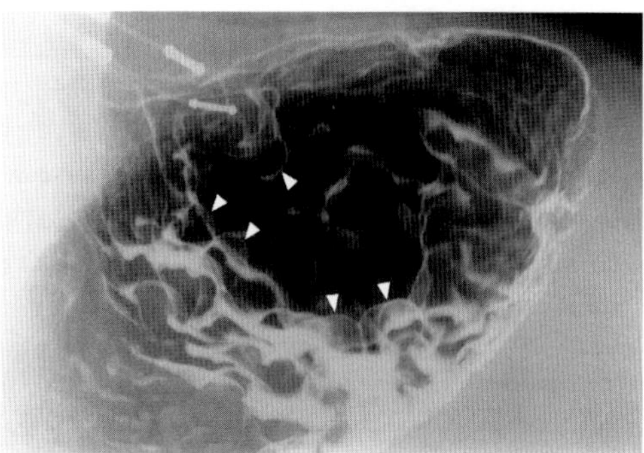

Fig. 2.92 Double-contrast barium study showing gastric varices as multiple submucosal nodules (arrowheads) and serpentine folds in the gastric fundus. These findings are typical of varices in the stomach.

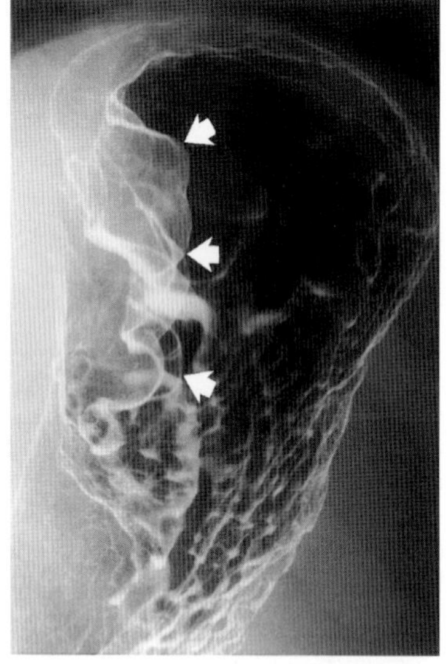

Fig. 2.93 Double-contrast barium study showing a conglomerate mass of varices (arrows) in the gastric fundus in a patient with portal hypertension. Lymphoma or a malignant gastrointestinal stromal tumor could produce similar findings. (Reproduced with permission from reference 5.)

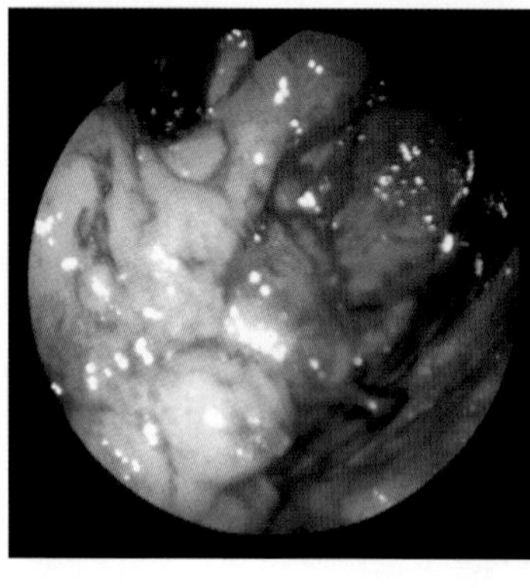

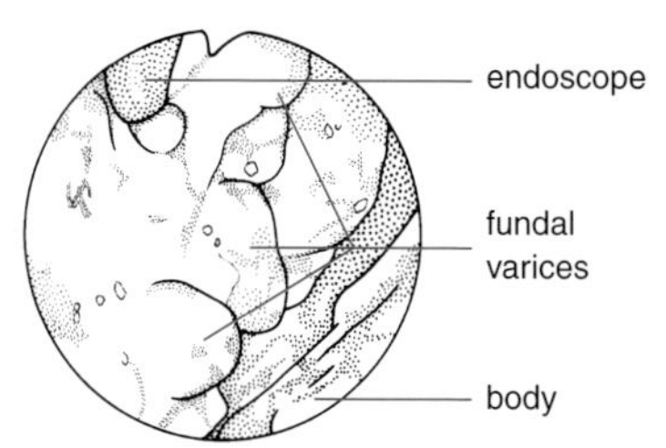

Fig. 2.94 Gastric fundal varices responsible for recent bleeding, in a patient with portal hypertension.

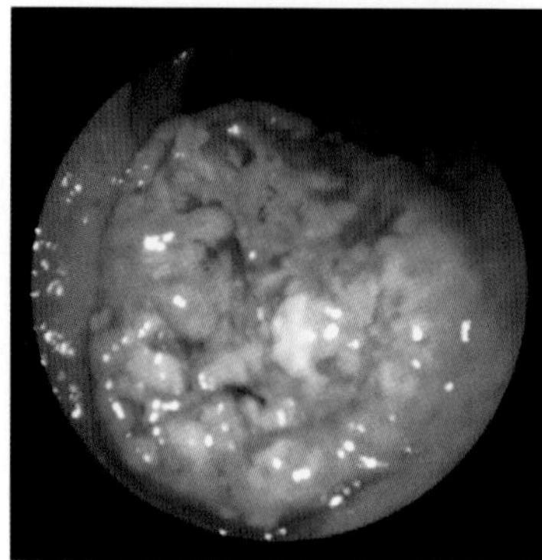

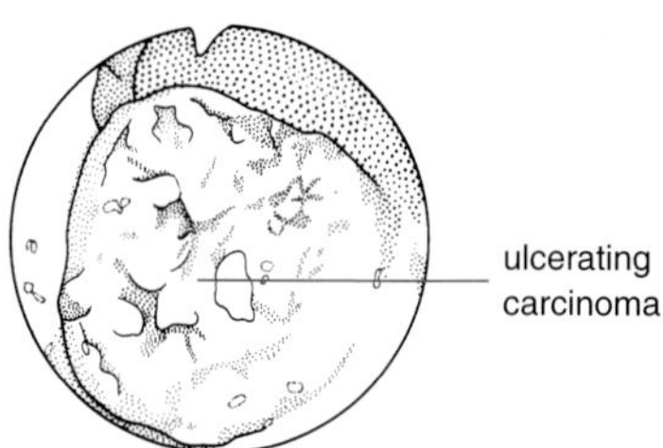

Fig. 2.95 Endoscopic appearance of an obvious, ulcerating carcinoma.

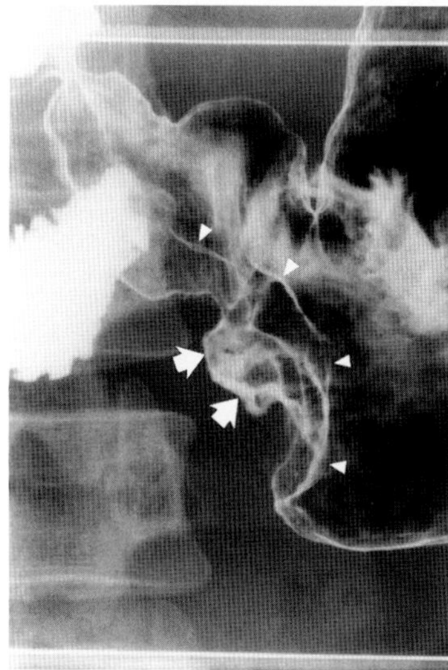

Fig. 2.96 Double-contrast barium study showing a polypoid carcinoma etched in white (arrowheads) with central ulceration (arrows) on the greater curvature of the gastric antrum. (Reproduced with permission from reference 6.)

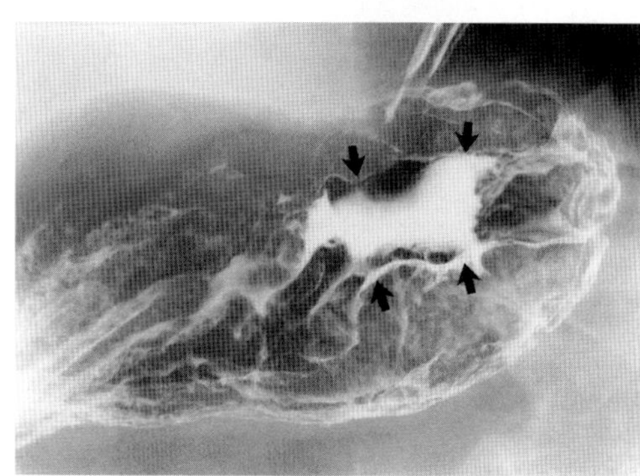

Fig. 2.97 Double-contrast barium study showing a carcinoma of the cardia as an irregular ulcer crater (arrows) with thickened, lobulated folds abutting the ulcer. Note how this lesion has obliterated the normal cardiac rosette.

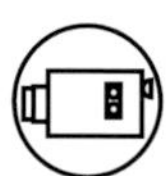

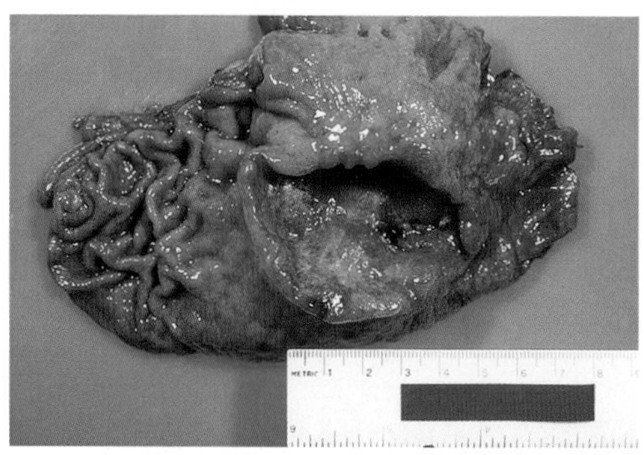

Fig. 2.98 Ulcerating gastric carcinoma (Borrmann type 3 gross morphology). Partial gastrectomy specimen showing a large, irregular raised mass with central ulceration and irregular contours characteristic of a malignant neoplasm.

GASTRIC CARCINOMA

Gastric carcinoma remains, worldwide, one of the more common gastrointestinal malignancies, responsible for 12% of all cancer deaths. Although early gastric cancer, with its much better prospect for cure, is being recognized more often (especially in Japan), the majority of Western patients present late and therefore have a poor prognosis. The antrum and the lesser curve of the stomach are the most commonly involved sites (Fig. 2.95) but these cancers may develop anywhere in the stomach (Fig. 2. 96) and as many as 40% involve the cardia (Fig. 2.97). The macroscopic appearances include the overtly neoplastic ulcer with rolled edges (Fig. 2.98), the apparently benign ulcer (Figs 2.99, 2.100), and fungating, nodular tumors (Figs 2.101–2.102). Less common is the scirrhous, infiltrating type known as linitis plastica, in which the malignancy spreads widely throughout all layers of the stomach wall (Figs 2.103, 2.104); ulceration may be minimal or absent and the endoscopic abnormality trivial, apart from an easily missed reduction in distensibility of the stomach (Fig. 2.105), but there is rarely any doubt at laparotomy (Figs 2.106, 2.107).

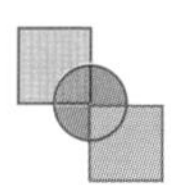

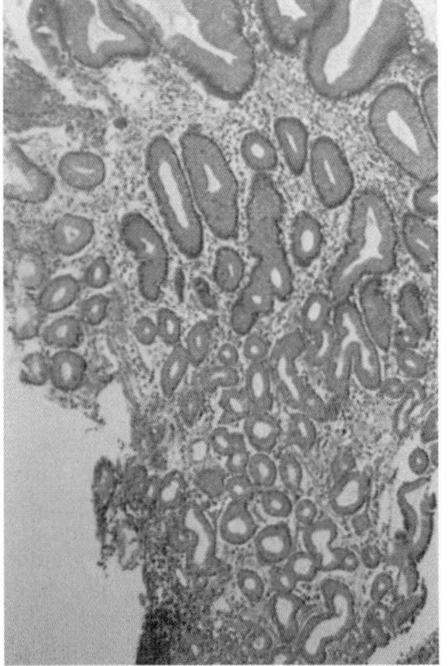

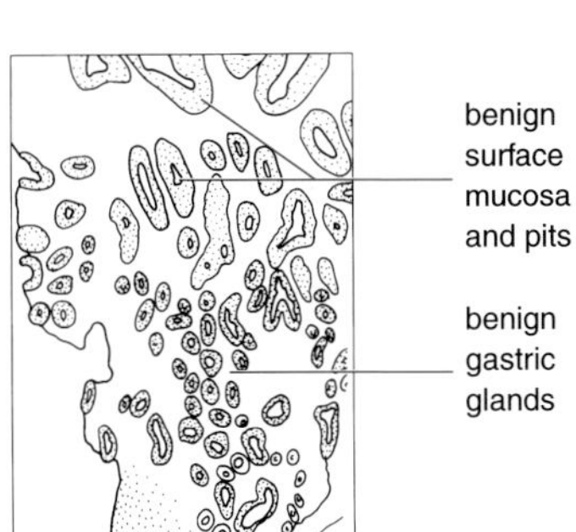

■ **Fig. 2.99** One of ten biopsy pieces from an apparently benign gastric ulcer showing appearances of chronic inflammation only. H&E stain (x 25).

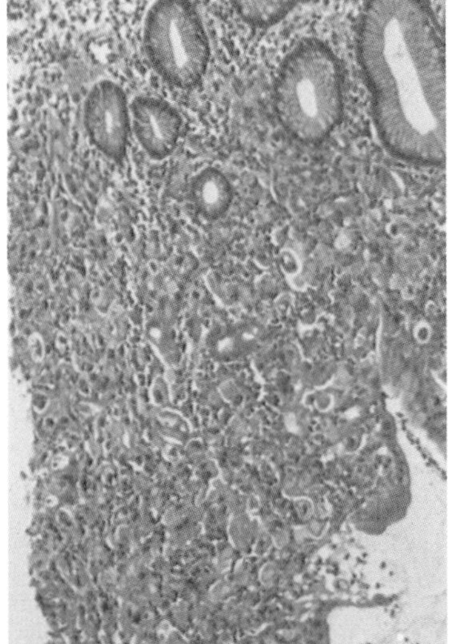

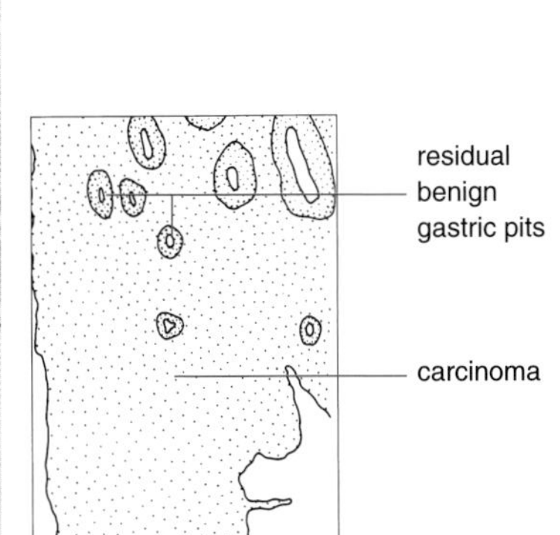

■ **Fig. 2.100** The single malignant biopsy from amongst ten pieces from the same case as in Fig. 2.99 illustrating the potential hazard of inadequate sampling. H&E stain (x 75).

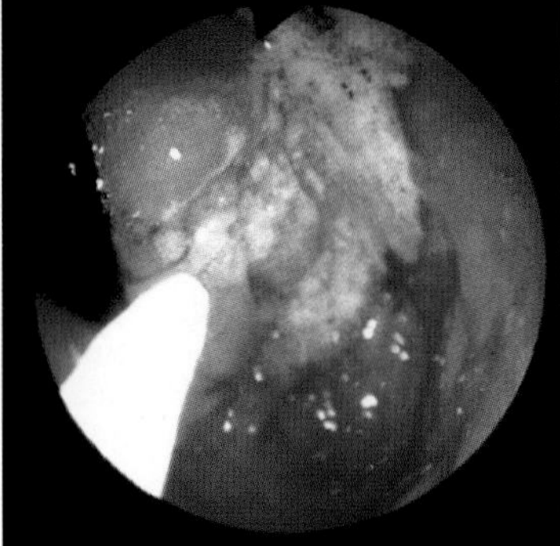

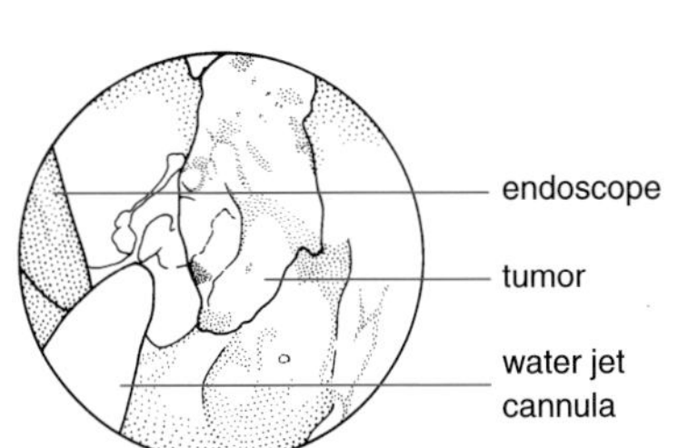

■ **Fig. 2.101** Adenocarcinoma at the cardia causing esophageal obstruction, seen here with the endoscope retroflexed. The lesion is being washed, prior to biopsy, with a water jet.

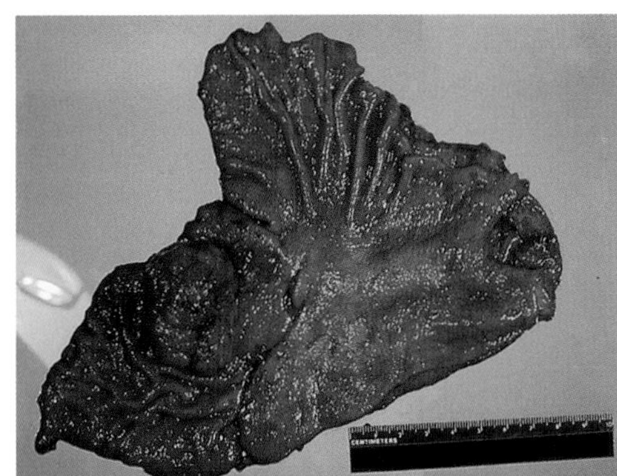

■ **Fig. 2.102** Fungating gastric carcinoma (Borrmann type 2 gross morphology). Partial gastrectomy specimen showing a fungating carcinoma in the transitional zone between the body and antrum.

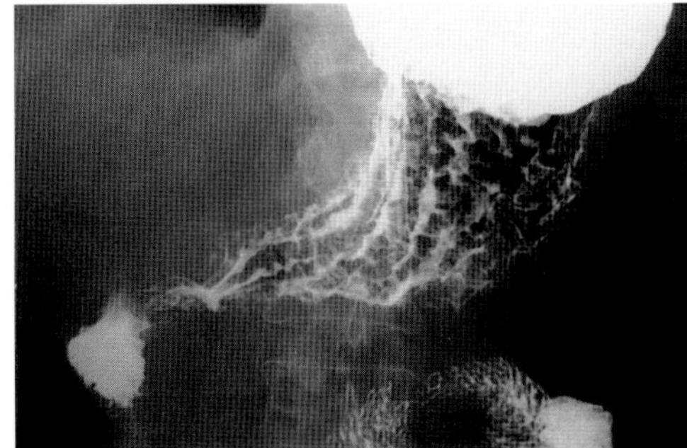

■ **Fig. 2.103** Double-contrast barium study showing marked narrowing of the gastric antrum with an irregular contour and thickened, nodular folds (i.e., a linitis plastica appearance) due to a primary scirrhous carcinoma of the stomach. At one time, these tumors were mainly thought to arise in the gastric antrum, extending proximally into the body and fundus.

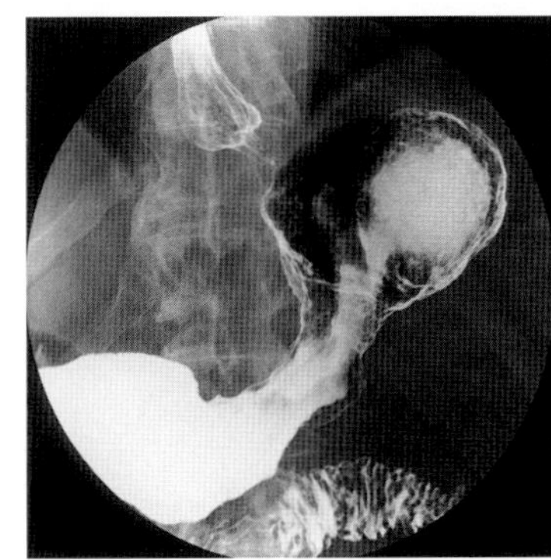

■ **Fig 2.104** Double-contrast barium study showing irregular narrowing of the gastric body due to a scirrhous carcinoma. As many as 40% of these tumors are now thought to be confined to the fundus or body of the stomach with sparing of the antrum.

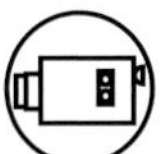

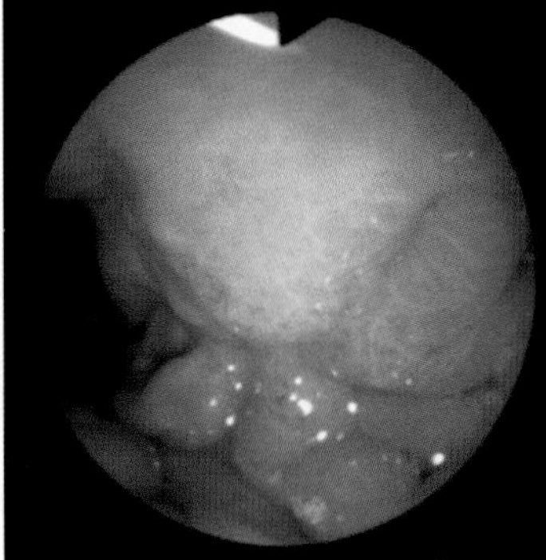

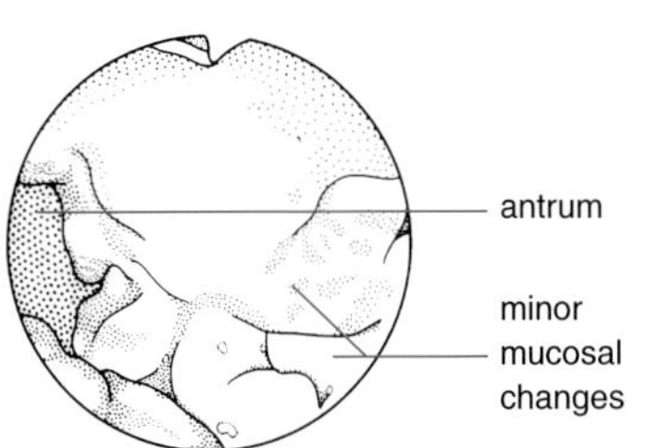

■ **Fig. 2.105** Endoscopic appearance of linitis plastica. The absence of marked mucosal changes is demonstrated.

Gastric cancer may be classified histologically as intestinal or diffuse. In the intestinal form, the tumors are more likely to be exophytic masses and a glandular pattern is more obvious (Figs 2.108, 2.109). Diffuse and signet-ring tumors are less well defined, are associated with a linitus presentation, and contain solitary or small clusters of malignant cells (Figs 2.110, 2.111); gland formation is rare. The cytological appearances of brushings from a benign ulcer can also be readily distinguished from those from a malignant ulcer (Figs 2.112, 2.113).

The TNM classification is now preferred in order to refine staging and prognosis (Fig. 2.114). Early gastric carcinoma is defined as that confined to the mucosa or to the mucosa and submucosa, and falls

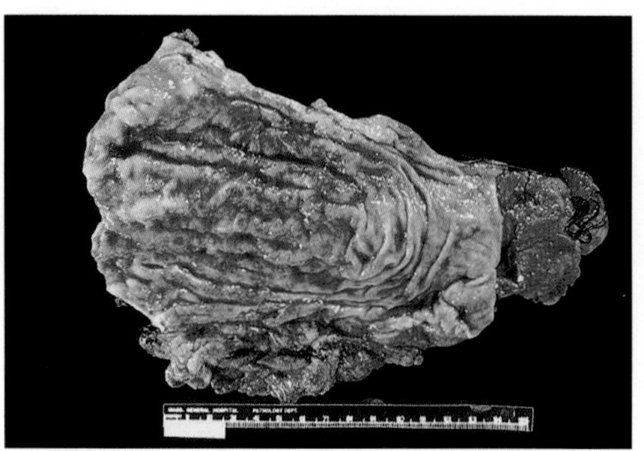

■ **Fig. 2.106** Linitis plastica/diffusely infiltrative carcinoma (Borrmann type 4 gross morphology). A partial gastrectomy specimen in linitis plastica showing a pattern mimicking hypertrophic gastropathy with massive expansion of the gastric folds.

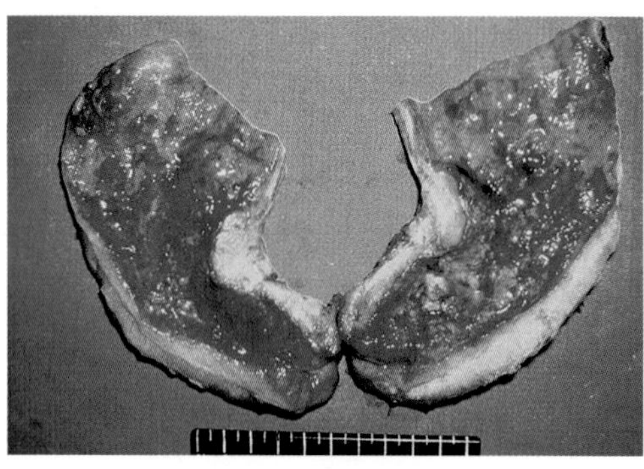

■ **Fig. 2.107** Linitis plastica/diffusely infiltrative carcinoma (Borrmann type 4 gross morphology). The cut surface of the gastric wall in linitis plastica showing the characteristic marked thickening with stenosis of the lumen. In this case, the normal pattern of mucosal folds is obliterated by the infiltrating tumor.

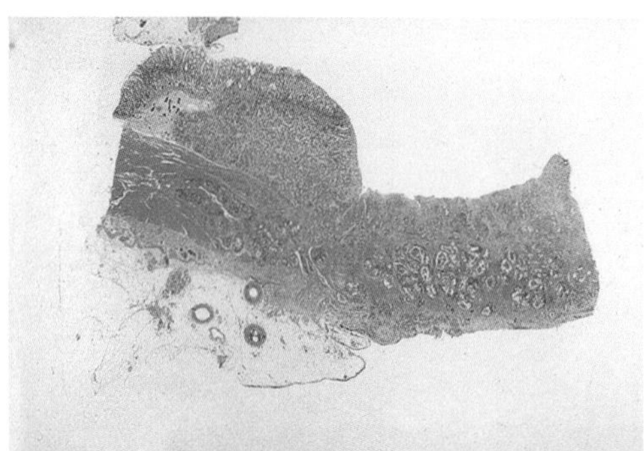

■ **Fig. 2.108** Whole-mount microscopic section through an ulcerating gastric adenocarcinoma showing a carcinomatous mass at the ulcer edge and malignant glands extending through the gastric wall at the base of the ulcer.

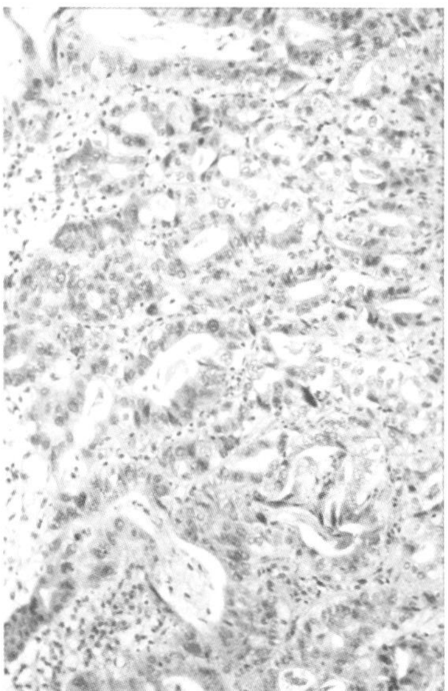

■ **Fig. 2.109** Gastric adenocarcinoma. High-magnification microscopic appearance of moderately differentiated invasive adenocarcinoma showing malignant glands of varying sizes and shapes with small amounts of mucin in their lumens.

into three main types on endoscopic and histological criteria (Fig. 2.115). With appropriate attention to detail, barium studies and endoscopy will permit recognition of early gastric cancer (Figs 2.116, 2.117). Although CT scanning is of help in staging gastric carcinoma (Fig. 2.118), it is not of comparable sensitivity for local extension to that achievable with endoscopic ultrasound (Fig. 2.119).

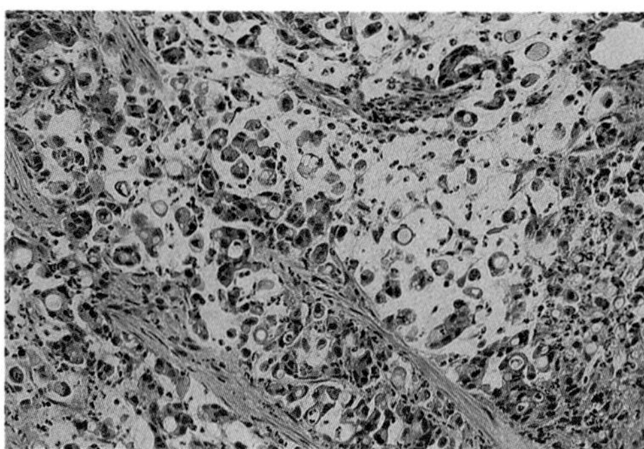

■ **Fig. 2.110** Signet-ring cell carcinoma in linitis plastica. Characteristic microscopic appearance of signet-ring cell carcinoma showing a diffusely infiltrating growth pattern. Gland formation is minimal to absent.

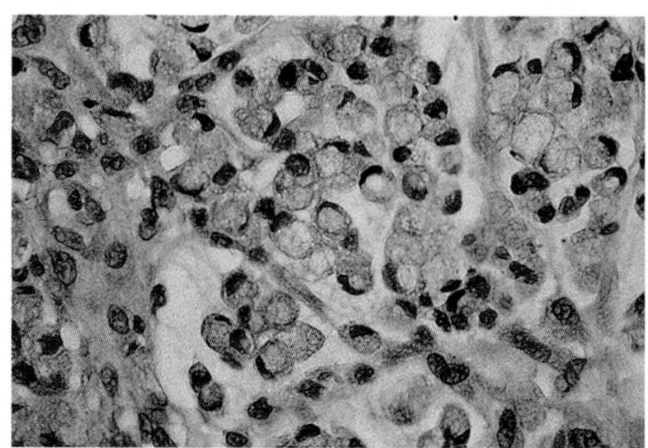

■ **Fig. 2.111** High-magnification microscopic appearance of signet-ring cell adenocarcinoma showing the characteristic non-cohesive malignant cells with large cytoplasmic mucin vacuoles that displace the nucleus to the side.

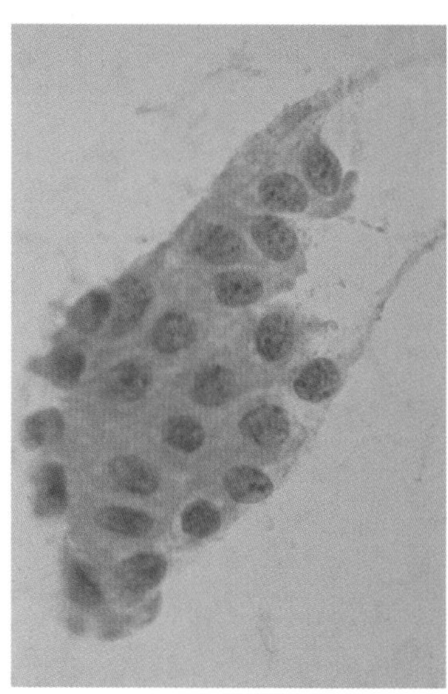

■ **Fig. 2.112** Cytological preparation showing benign gastric epithelial cells. Papanicolaou stain (x 500). Courtesy of Dr E.A. Hudson.

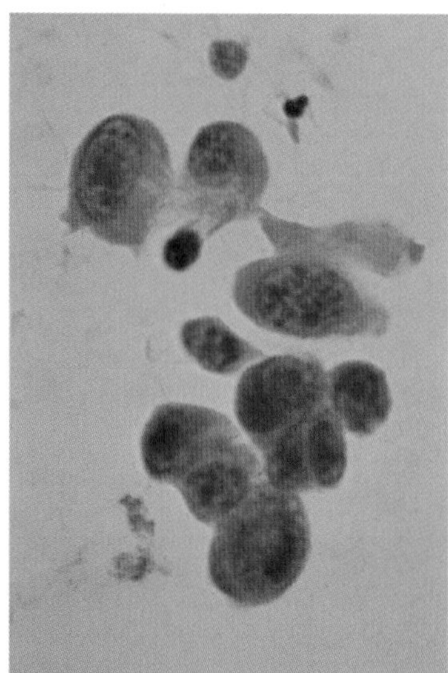

■ **Fig. 2.113** Cytological preparation of malignant gastric epithelial cells, in which the nuclear–cytoplasmic ratio is increased, and there are hyperchromatic nuclei with coarsely clumped chromatin. Papanicolaou stain (x 500). Courtesy of Dr E.A. Hudson.

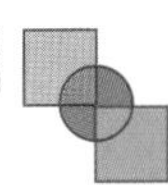

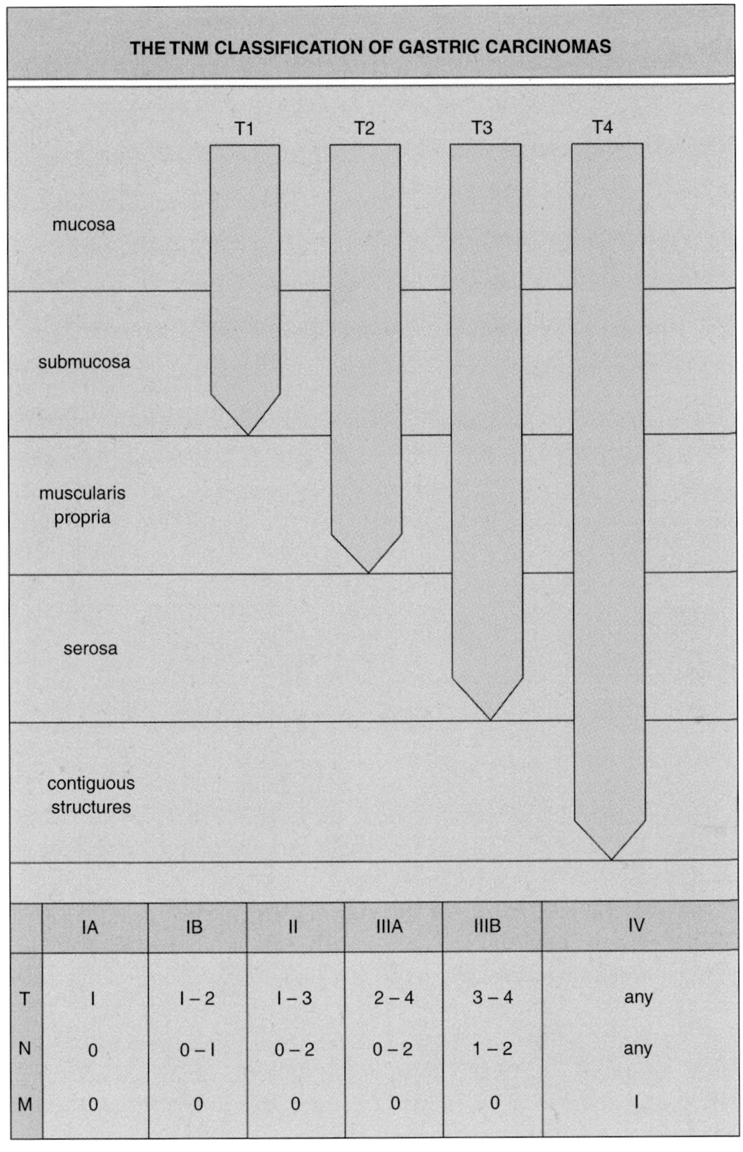

	IA	IB	II	IIIA	IIIB	IV
T	I	I – 2	I – 3	2 – 4	3 – 4	any
N	0	0 – I	0 – 2	0 – 2	1 – 2	any
M	0	0	0	0	0	I

■ **Fig. 2.114** TNM classification of gastric carcinoma.

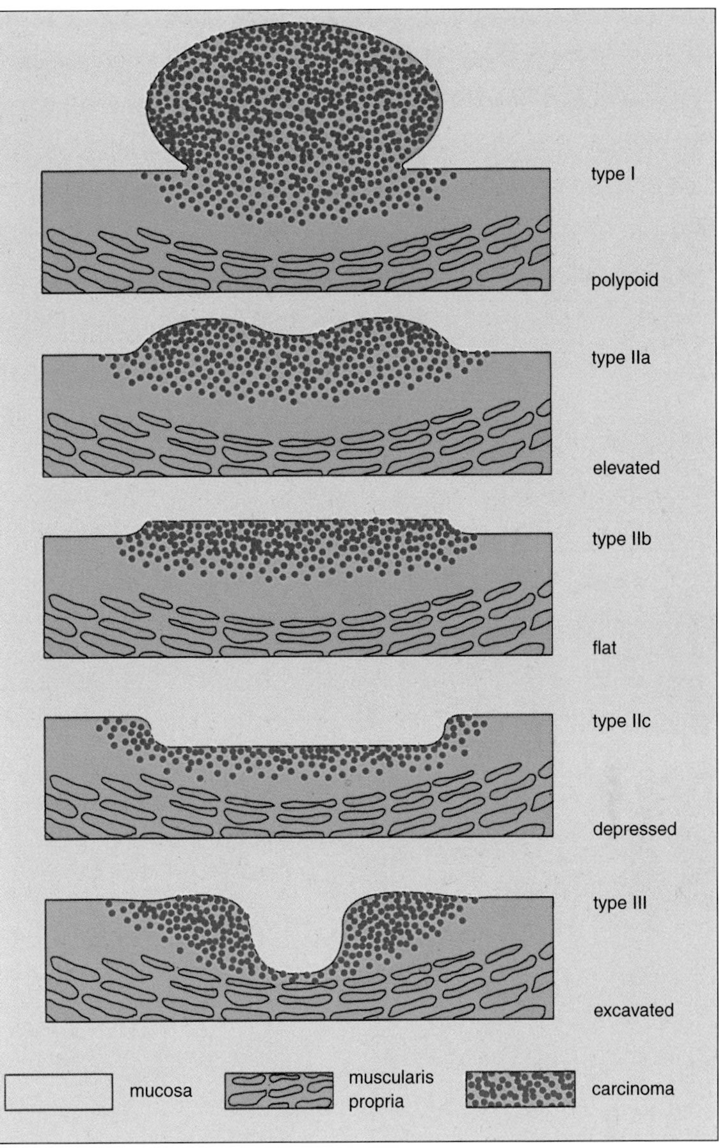

■ **Fig. 2.115** Macroscopic classification of early gastric cancer based on endoscopic appearances.

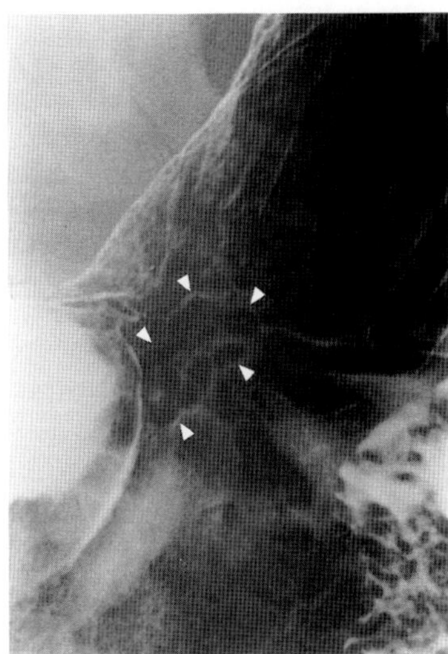

■ **Fig. 2.116** Double-contrast barium study showing an early gastric cancer as a small polypoid lesion (arrows) near the lesser curvature of the gastric body. The abnormal folds are an important radiological sign of early cancer.

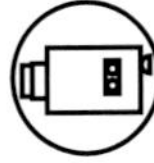

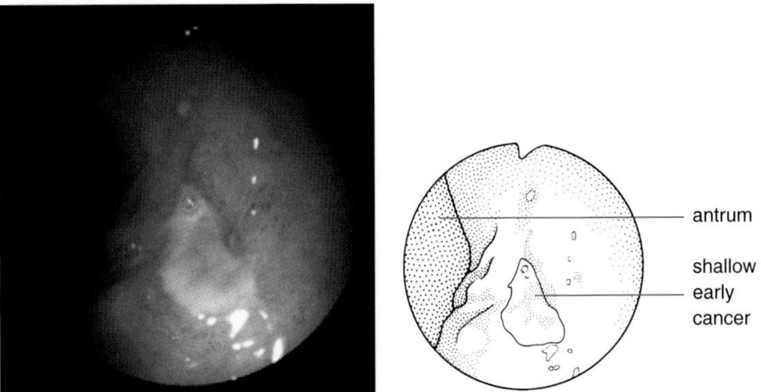

■ **Fig. 2.117** Endoscopic view of early gastric cancer.

Protuberant early gastric cancer is usually well-differentiated with obvious glandular formation (Figs 2.120, 2.121), while less well-differentiated histology and signet-ring cells are commoner in flat, excavated lesions (Figs 2.122, 2.123).

PREMALIGNANT AND OTHER HIGH-RISK STATES

Certain conditions are associated with an increased risk of developing gastric carcinoma. These include pernicious anemia, adenomatous polyps, intestinal metaplasia (Fig. 2.124), and previous gastric surgery, but chronic gastritis associated with *H. pylori* is probably numerically most important. The importance of Barrett's syndrome in the pathogenesis of adenocarcinoma in the esophago-gastric junctional zone is considered in Chapter 1.

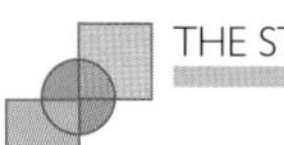

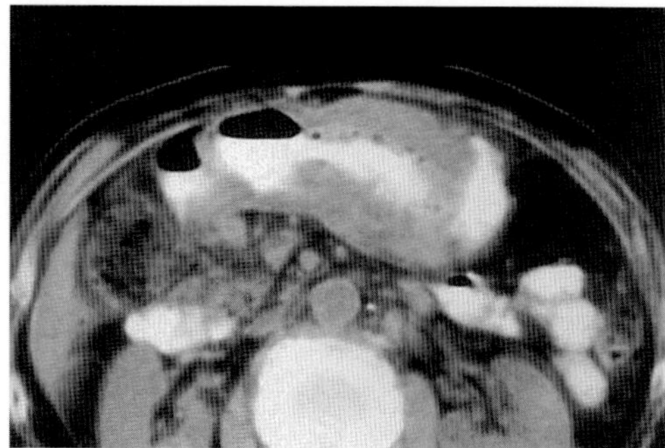

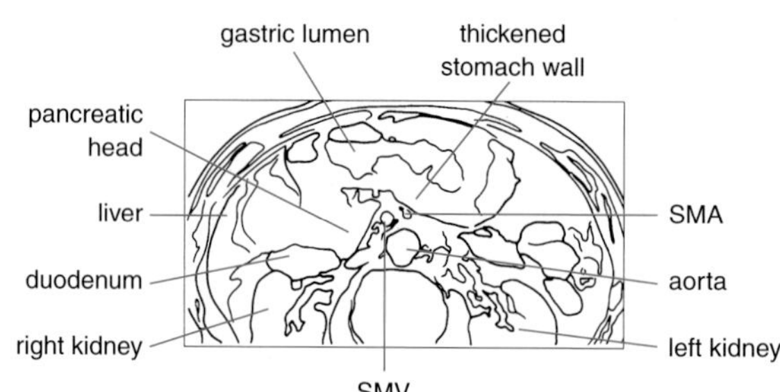

Fig. 2.118 CT appearance of gastric carcinoma.

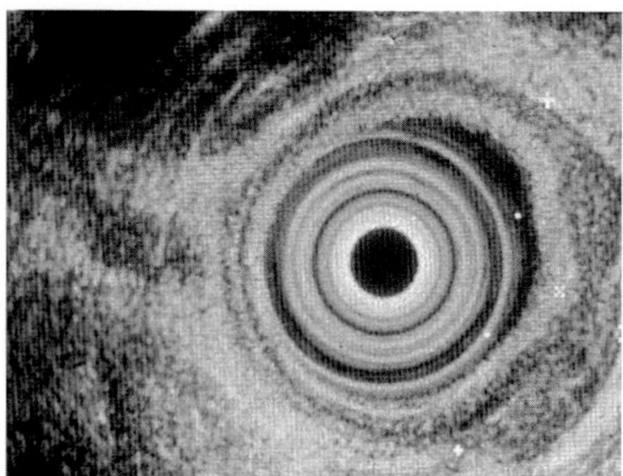

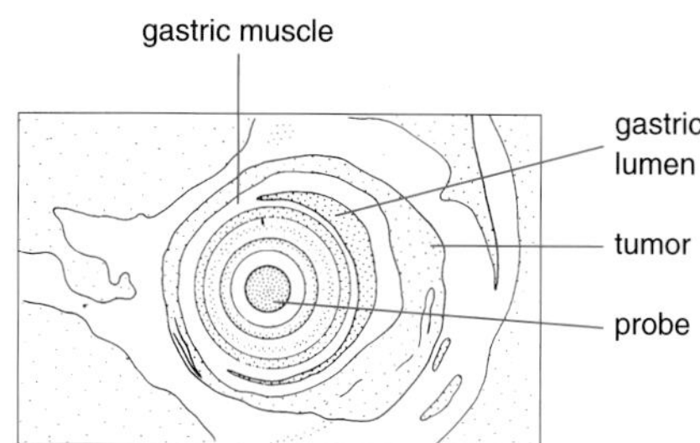

Fig. 2.119 Endoscopic ultrasound scan of early gastric carcinoma, from which it was concluded that the tumor did not infiltrate beyond the muscularis propria. Histological examination of the resection specimen confirmed this.

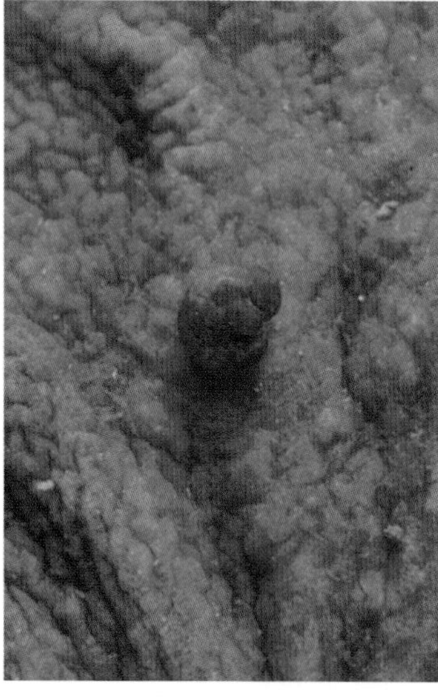

Fig. 2.120 Macroscopic appearance of early gastric cancer of protruding or polypoid type.

The place of surveillance gastroscopy (Fig. 2.125) is not yet firmly established, partly because of the small proportion of positive results amongst screened patients, and partly because the presence of dysplasia or metaplasia has not always been found to be a good predictor of subsequent malignancy. The specific variety of intestinal metaplasia characterized by incomplete cell differentiation and sulfomucin secretion, known as type III intestinal metaplasia (Fig. 2.126) has a much stronger association with carcinoma, but the stain is toxic, and limiting screening to this group will not be readily feasible until an alternative histochemical or immunological test is available.

Gastric polyps

Gastric polyps may be hamartomatous (Figs 2.127, 2.128), regenerative or hyperplastic (Figs 2.129–2.134), as well as true neoplasms. Although hyperplastic polyps can grow to a huge size (Fig. 2.130) they do not undergo malignant transformation.

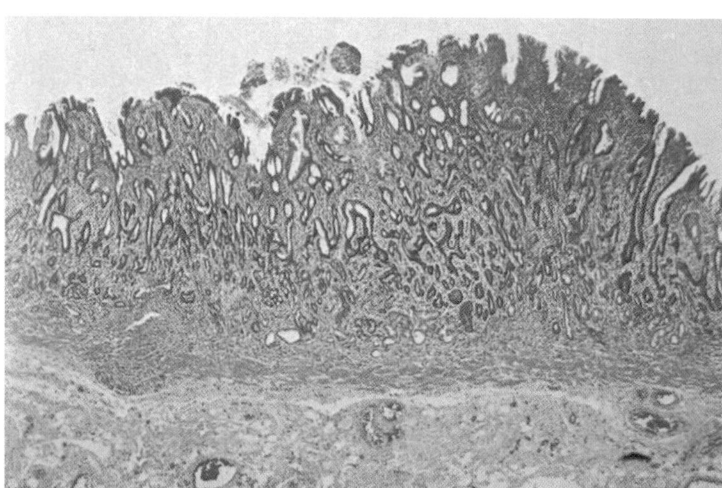

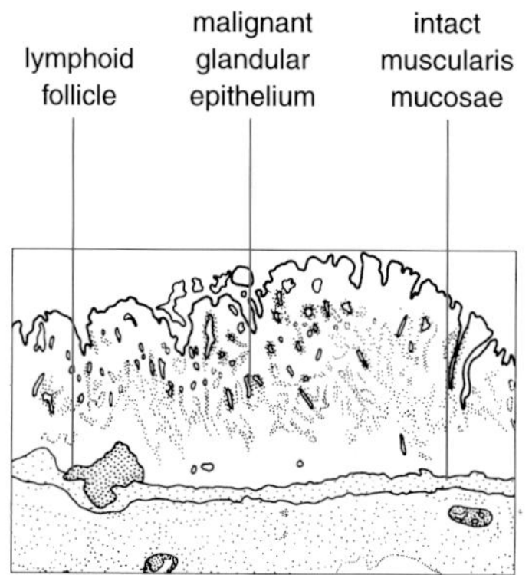

Fig. 2.121 The histological appearance of early gastric carcinoma in which there is invasion of the mucosa that does not extend into the muscularis (intestinal type). H&E stain (x 30).

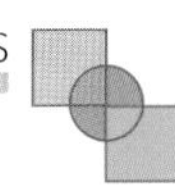

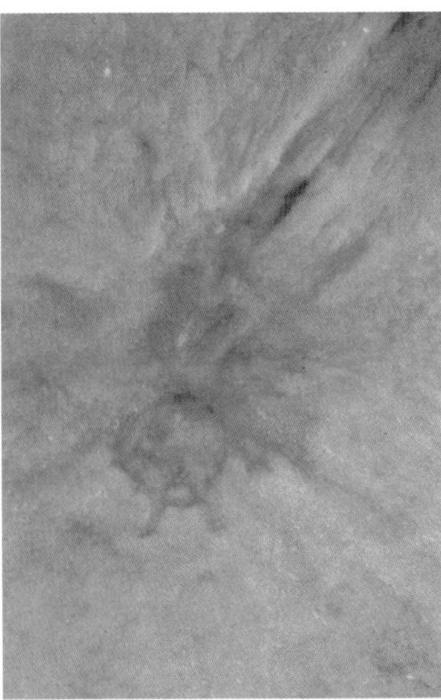

■ **Fig. 2.122** Macroscopic appearance of early cancer of the depressed type.

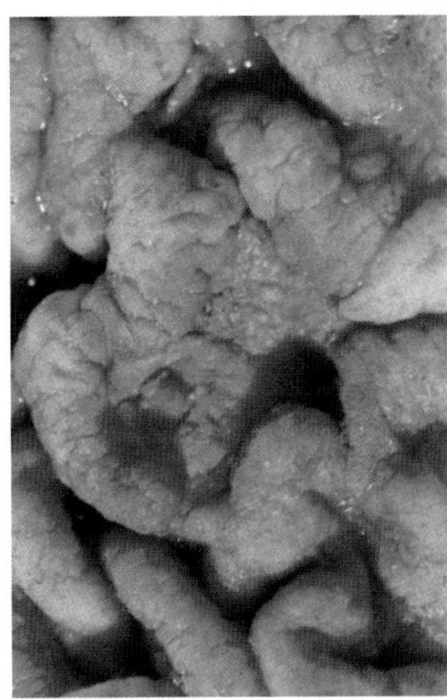

■ **Fig. 2.123** Macroscopic appearance of early cancer of the excavated type.

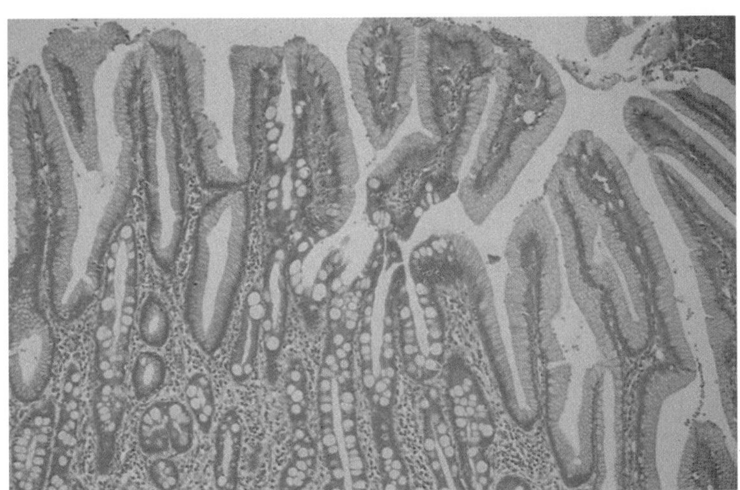

■ **Fig. 2.124** Histological appearance of intestinal metaplasia. The uniform columnar cells of the normal gastric epithelium clearly contrast with the apparently vacuolated goblet cells of the metaplastic epithelium. H&E stain (x 75).

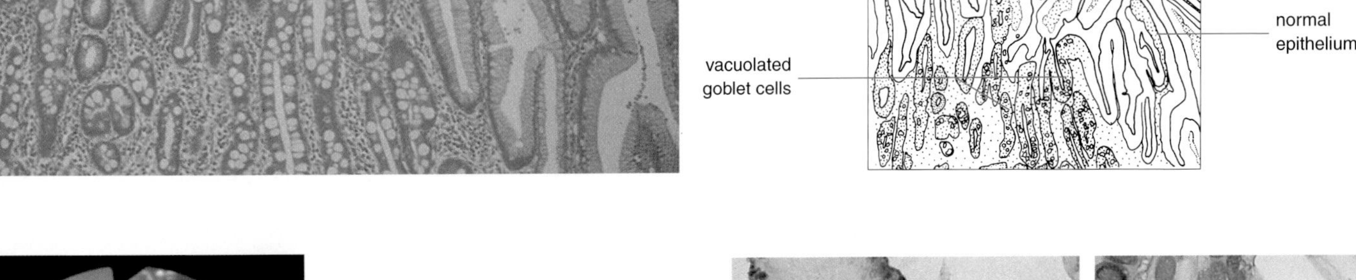

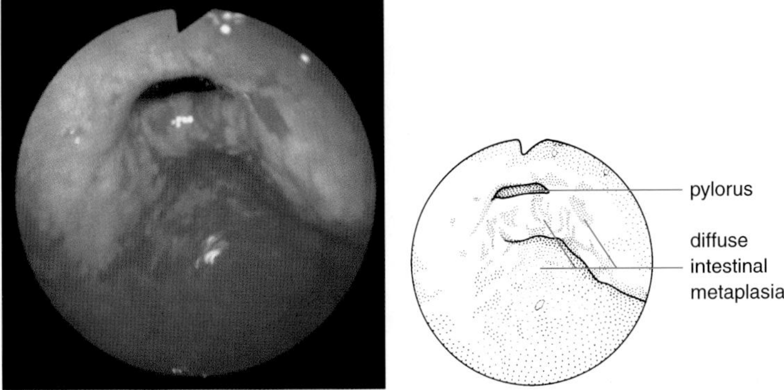

■ **Fig. 2.125** Endoscopic appearance of marked intestinal metaplasia affecting the antrum.

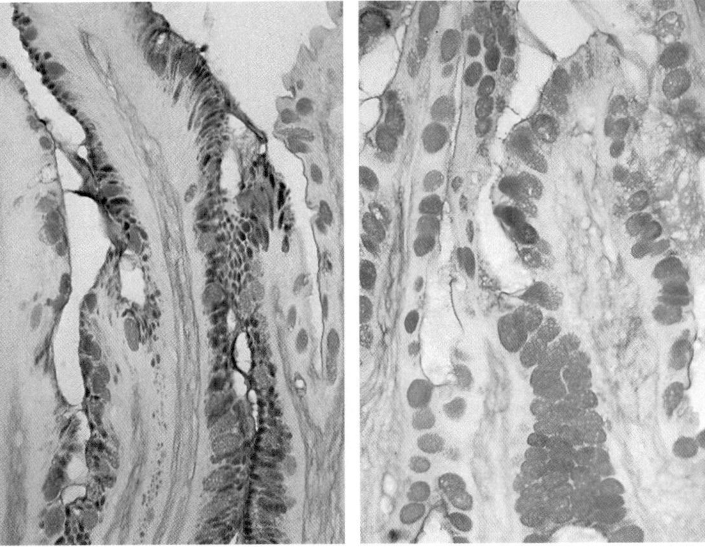

■ **Fig. 2.126** (Left) Histology of incomplete (type III) intestinal metaplasia in which the columnar cells contain sulfomucin and are stained brown. Sialomucin-containing goblet cells stain blue. (Right). In complete intestinal metaplasia (type I), goblet cells secreting sialomucin are stained blue, and the columnar cells are unstained, with the brush border delineated (high iron diamine/Alcian blue stain). Courtesy of Dr B. Morson and Prof J. Jass.

It is probably only adenomatous polyps (Fig. 2.135) that have malignant potential, with a higher risk when multiple (Fig. 2.136) or when the diameter exceeds 2 cm. Barium studies demonstrate apparently translucent filling defects (Fig. 2.137), and at endoscopy, adenomatous polyps are more obviously distinct from surrounding mucosa than the commoner regenerative/hyperplastic type (contrast with Fig. 2.131). The histology is typical of adenomas (Fig. 2.138).

Adenomatous polyps in the duodenum are common in familial adenomatous polyposis (FAP) (see Chapters 3 and 7), but unusual

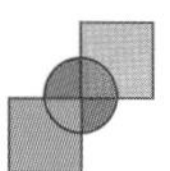

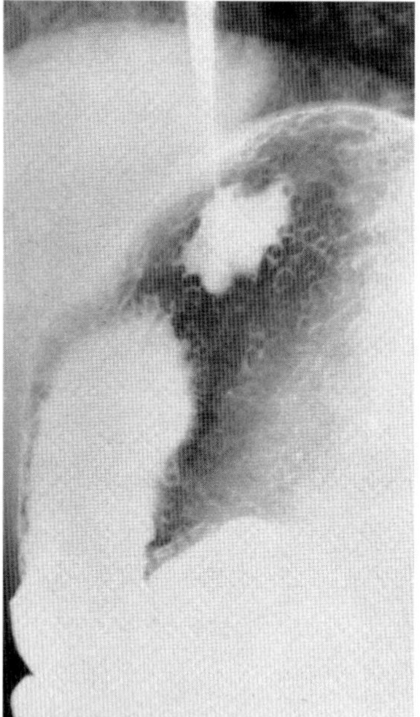

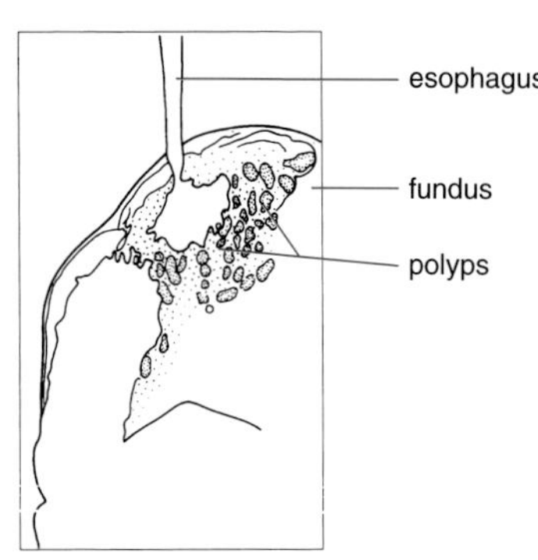

Fig. 2.127 Barium meal showing numerous filling defects caused by small hamartomatous polyps.

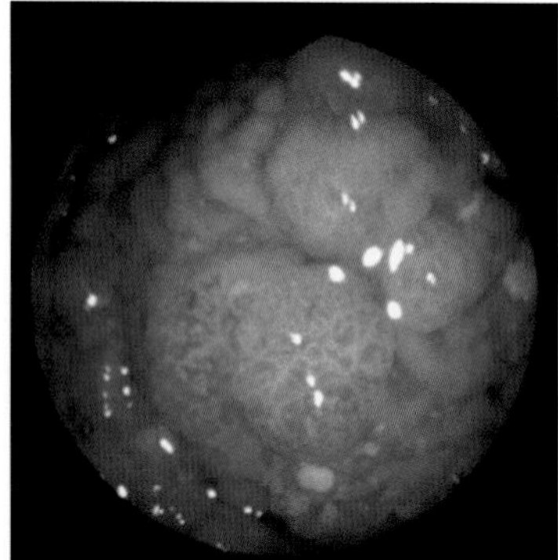

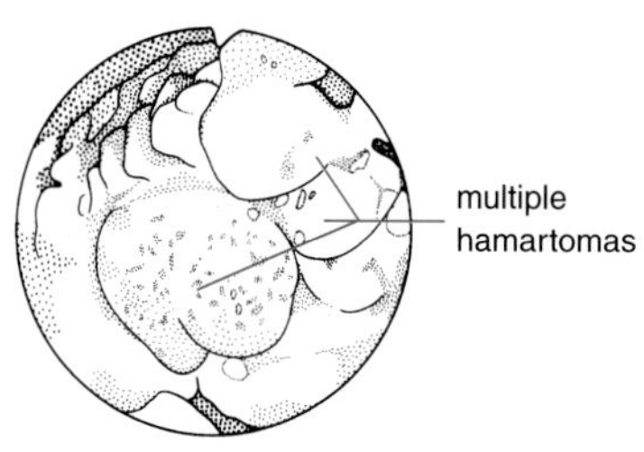

Fig. 2.128 Endoscopic appearance of multiple hamartomas in Peutz–Jegher's syndrome.

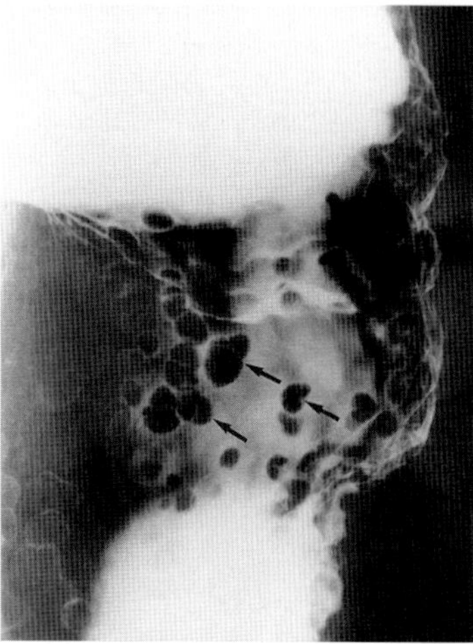

Fig. 2.129 Double-contrast barium study showing multiple small, rounded hyperplastic polyps (arrows) in the gastric body.

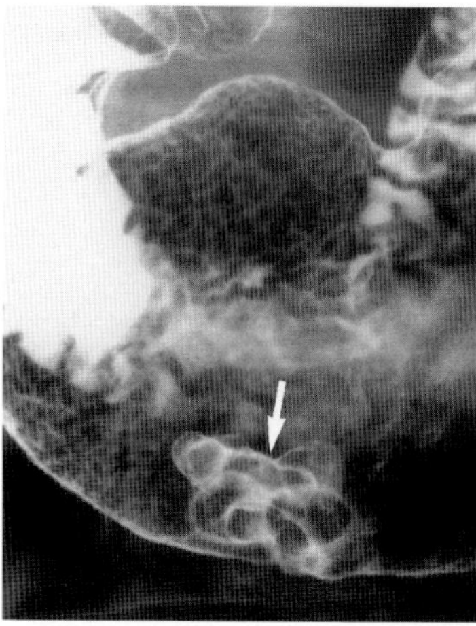

Fig. 2.130 Double-contrast barium study showing a giant hyperplastic polyp as a multilobulated mass (arrow) on the greater curvature of the gastric antrum. (Reproduced with permission from reference 6.)

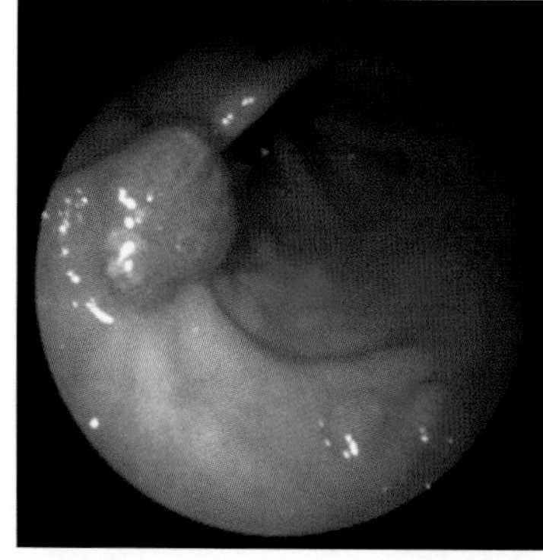

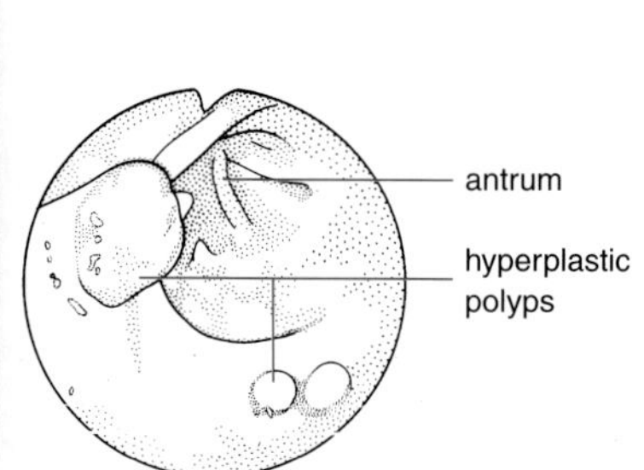

Fig. 2.131 Endoscopic appearance of hyperplastic polyps.

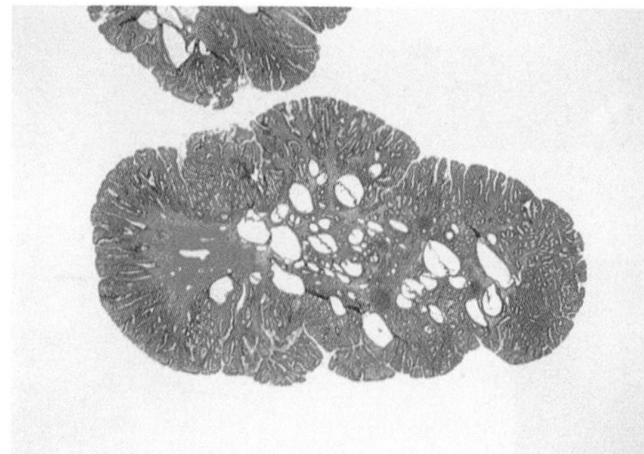

Fig. 2.132 Whole-mount microscopic appearance of a hyperplastic polyp showing dilatation of the pits and residual glands entrapped within the splayed smooth muscle of the polyp head.

proximal to the ampulla of Vater. However at least 50% of FAP patients who have reached their fourth decade have large numbers of fundic gland polyps in the proximal stomach (Figs 2.139–2.141), and occasional adenomas do occur – probably only when there is bile reflux.

OTHER TUMORS

Gastrointestinal stromal tumors

A considerable range of different histological subtypes is now grouped within the general umbrella of gastrointestinal stromal tumors. Since they have relatively characteristic endoscopic appearances it is probably still worth identifying leiomyomas specifically. They are the commonest benign tumors of the stomach, and in some autopsy series have proved the commonest gastrointestinal tumors. Leiomyomas arise from the gastric smooth muscle, and, because they are submucosal and rarely impinge on the lumen, are frequently asymptomatic; endoscopic ultrasound is then the ideal investigation (Fig. 2.142). Large tumors typically produce smooth filling defects, and, less often, are pedunculated (Fig. 2.143). The classical appearance of a polypoid, submucosal tumor with hemorrhage from its ulcerated tip is readily diagnosed endoscopically (Fig. 2.144) with similar features at resection (Fig. 2.145). Endoscopic biopsies may reveal only normal epithelium, but if tissue deep enough is obtained

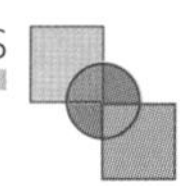

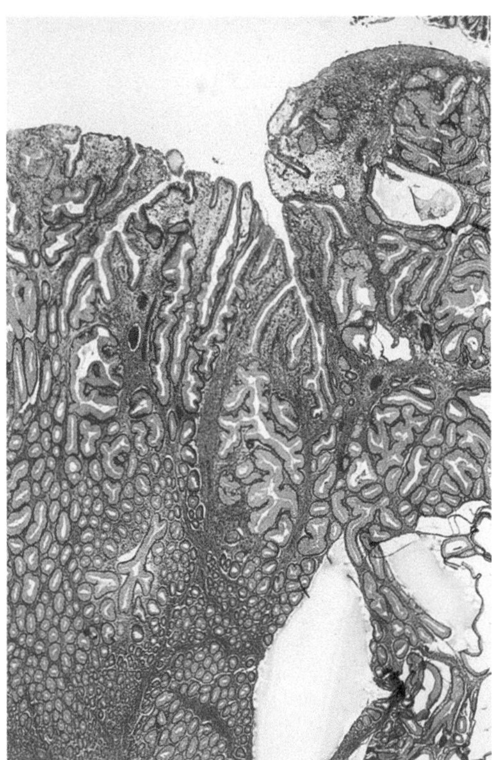

Fig. 2.133 Microscopic appearance of a hyperplastic polyp showing the characteristic elongation and tortuousness of the gastric pits that comprise most of the mass of the polyp head.

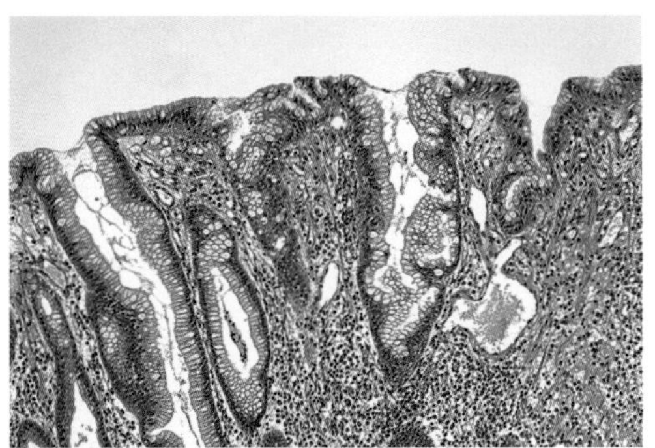

Fig. 2.134 High-magnification appearance of the surface of a hyperplastic polyp showing the crowding and tufting of the hyperplastic foveolar epithelium and the chronic inflammation of the stroma.

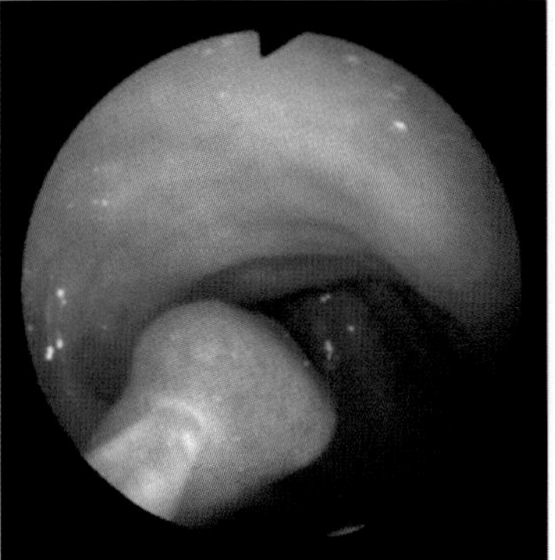

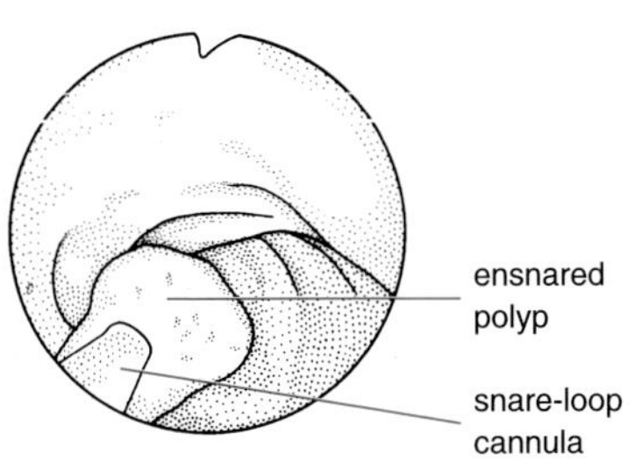

Fig. 2.135 Endoscopic appearance of a benign adenomatous gastric polyp. A diathermy snare has been passed around the polyp, which is about to be removed by electrocautery.

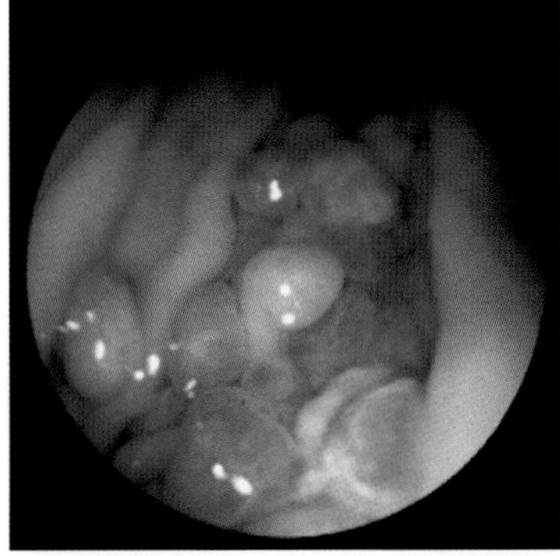

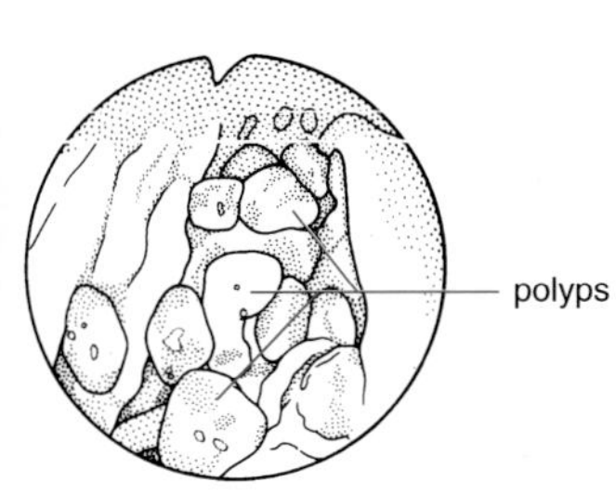

Fig. 2.136 Multiple benign adenomatous polyps.

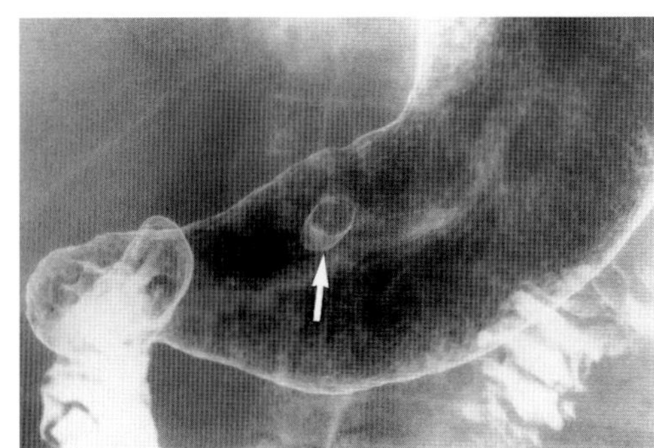

Fig. 2.137 Double-contrast barium study showing a solitary, slightly lobulated adenomatous polyp (arrow) in the antrum. (Reproduced with permission from reference 6.)

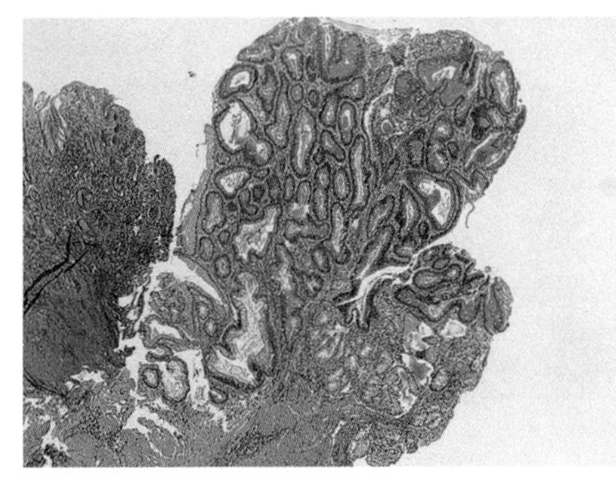

Fig. 2.138 Microscopic appearance of a gastric tubular adenoma showing the dysplastic glands that comprise the entire polyp head.

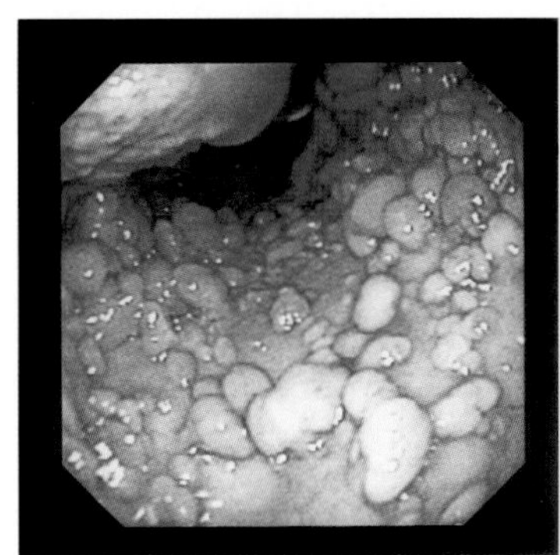

Fig. 2.139 Endoscopic appearance of fundic gland gastric polyposis affecting body and fundus in a patient with familial adenomatous polyposis.

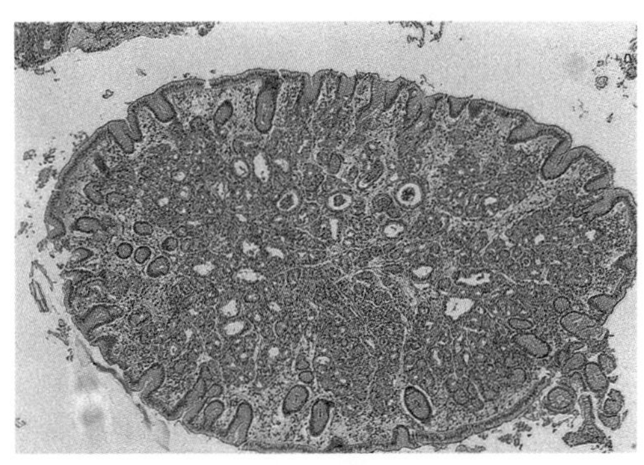

Fig. 2.140 Microscopic appearance of a fundic gland polyp showing the characteristic cystic dilatation of the oxyntic glands that comprise most of the polyp mass.

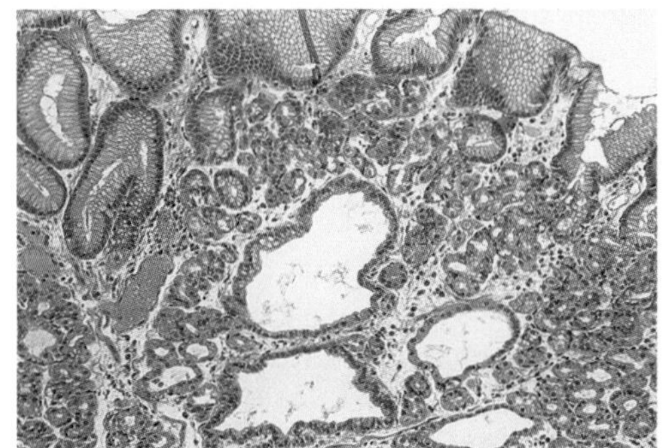

Fig. 2.141 High-magnification microscopic appearance of a fundic gland polyp showing the cytologically normal but histologically disorganized oxyntic glands in the polyp head and the short, normal pits. Dysplasia may very rarely occur in the surface epithelium of these polyps when associated with a familial adenomatous polyposis syndrome.

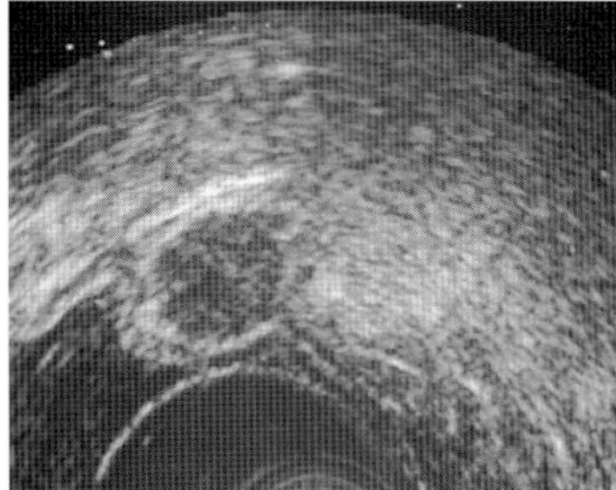

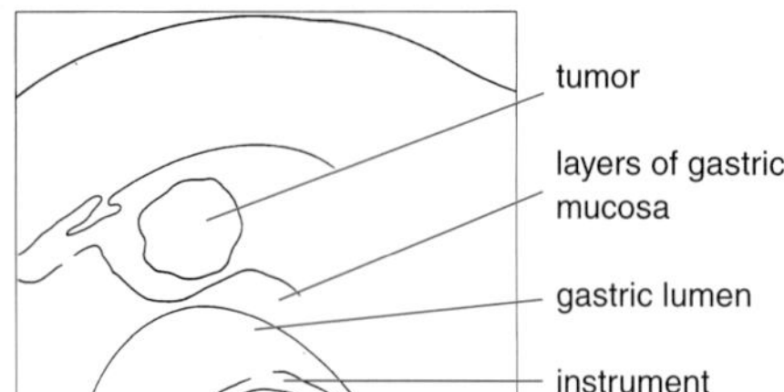

Fig. 2.142 Endoscopic ultrasound appearance of gastric stromal tumor of the leiomyoma type. The tumor lies deep to the submucosa in the muscle layer.

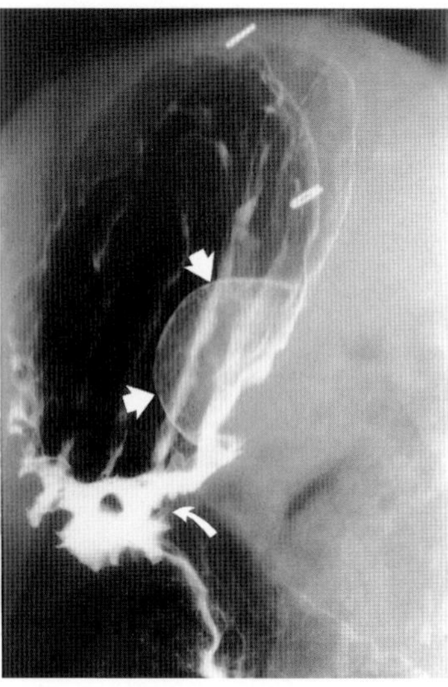

Fig. 2.143 Double-contrast barium study showing a gastric leiomyoma as a smooth, submucosal mass (straight arrows) in the gastric fundus. (Note gastrojejunal anastomosis (curved arrow) in this patient with a Billroth II partial gastrectomy.)

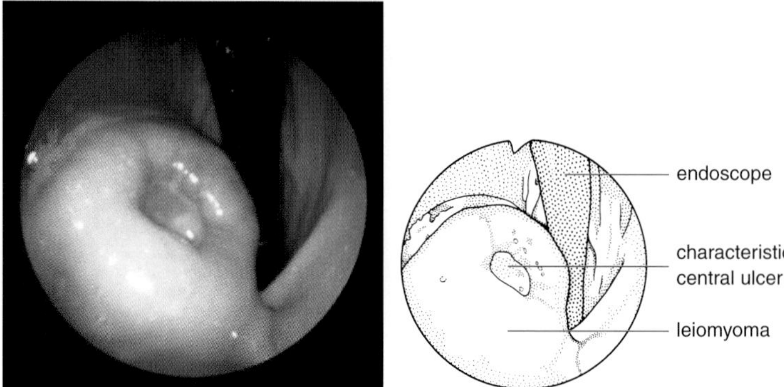

Fig. 2.144 Endoscopic appearance of gastric leiomyoma with central ulceration. The lesion protrudes obviously into the gastric lumen and was responsible for presentation with hematemesis.

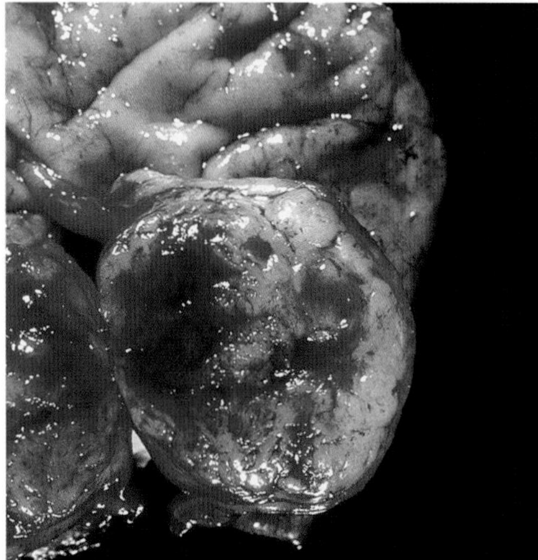

Fig. 2.145 Partial gastrectomy specimen containing a low-grade gastrointestinal stromal tumor (GIST) of the stomach showing the bulging, pale tan cut surface and well-demarcated borders.

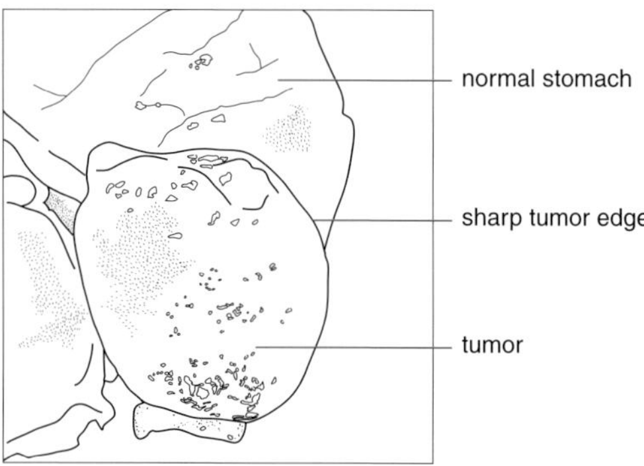

it will show interlacing bundles and whorls of smooth muscle (Figs 2.146, 2.147). The problem with all of the gastrointestinal stromal tumors is the great difficulty in determining malignant potential: although size and mitotic activity are valuable indicators, malignancy can in some respects be confirmed only by the presence of metastases, or obviously aggressive features on imaging (Figs 2.148, 2.149).

Lymphoma

Gastric lymphoma may be an isolated lesion or part of a disseminated process; it is, for example, more common in AIDS. The radiology tends predominantly to depict thickened folds (Fig. 2.150), and the lesion which crosses the gastro-duodenal junction is usually

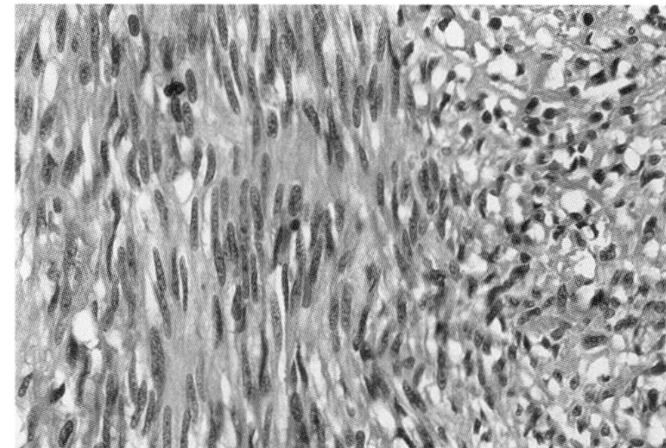

Fig. 2.146 Microscopic appearance of a low-grade GIST showing interlacing fascicles of plump, uniform spindle cells with a low mitotic index.

lymphomatous (Fig. 2.151). The endoscopic appearances range from the barely visible to gross lesions (Fig. 2.152); as for early carcinoma, biopsy is essential.

Many gastric lymphomas are of origin in mucosa-associated lymphoid tissue (MALTomas); they may exhibit characteristic radiological features with poorly defined confluent nodules (Fig. 2.153) to be distinguished from simple lymphoid hyperplasia (Fig. 2.154).

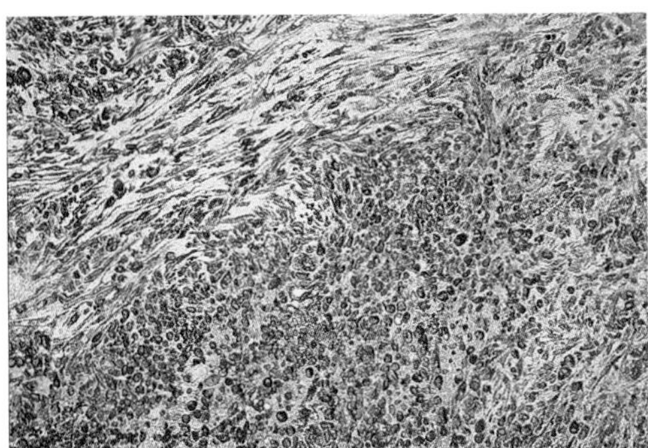

Fig. 2.147 Immunohistochemical stain for cKIT (CD117) in a low-grade GIST showing marked diffuse expression of this marker for interstitial cells of Cajal (intestinal pacemaker cells).

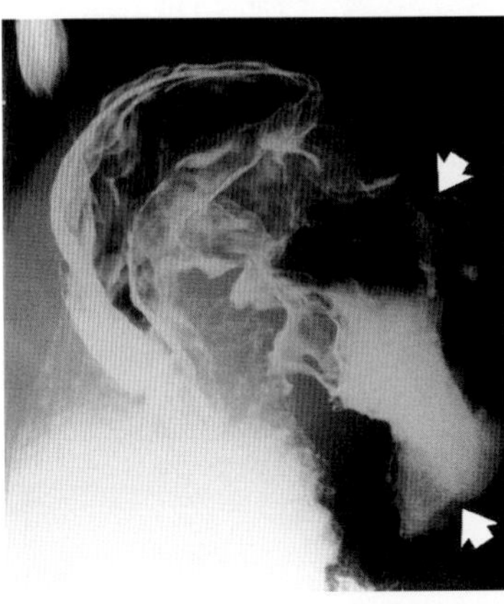

Fig. 2.148 Malignant gastrointestinal stromal tumor with cavitation. Double-contrast barium study shows a cavitated lesion containing a giant extraluminal collection of barium (arrows).

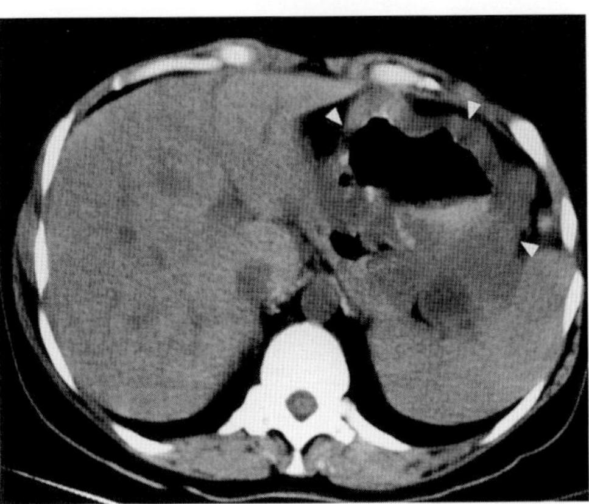

Fig. 2.149 A CT scan in the same patient as Fig 2.148 shows a heterogeneous mass (arrowheads) containing a large central gas collection due to necrosis and cavitation of the tumor. Lymphoma and hematogenous metastases (especially from malignant melanoma) could produce identical findings.

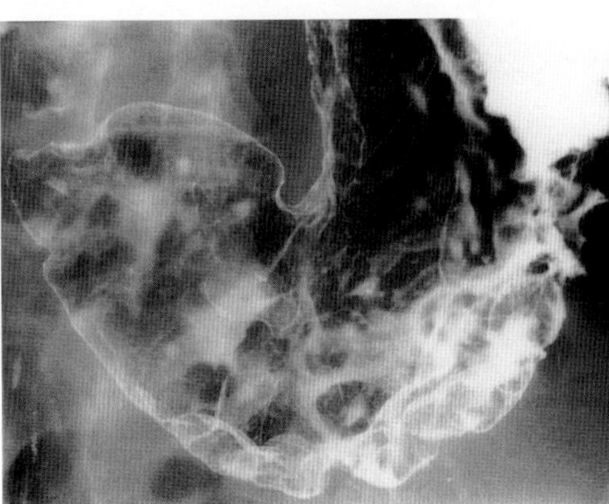

Fig. 2.150 Double-contrast barium study showing thickened, lobulated folds in the gastric body due to non-Hodgkin's lymphoma.

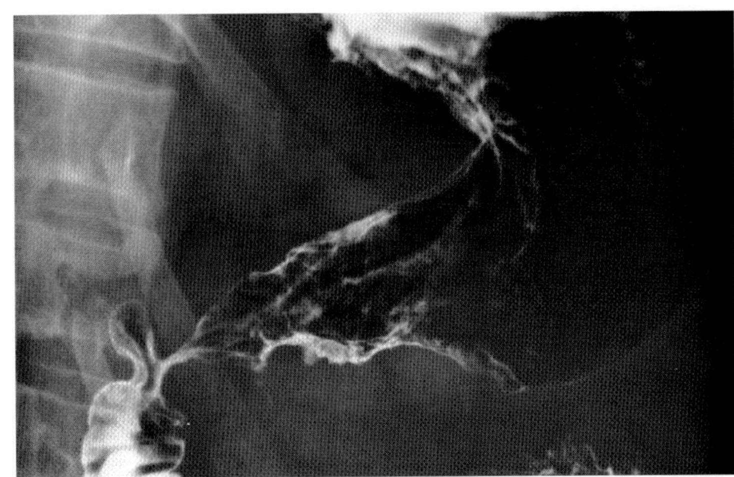

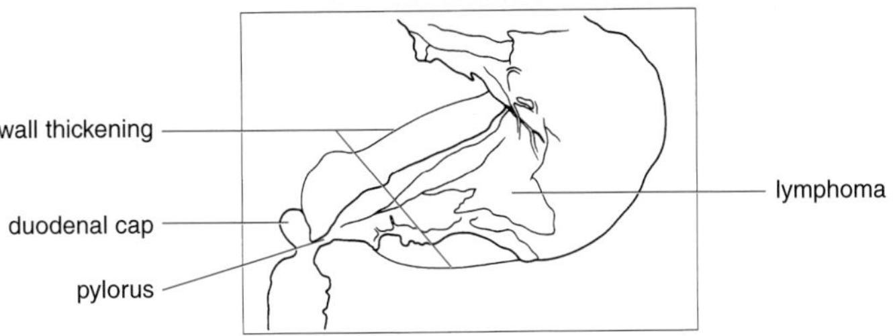

Fig. 2.151 Barium meal showing a large irregular annular mass in the distal stomach which extends across the gastroduodenal junction. The substantial thickening of the wall that is demonstrated, and, more particularly, the characteristic involvement of the duodenum, supported the correct interpretation that this was lymphomatous.

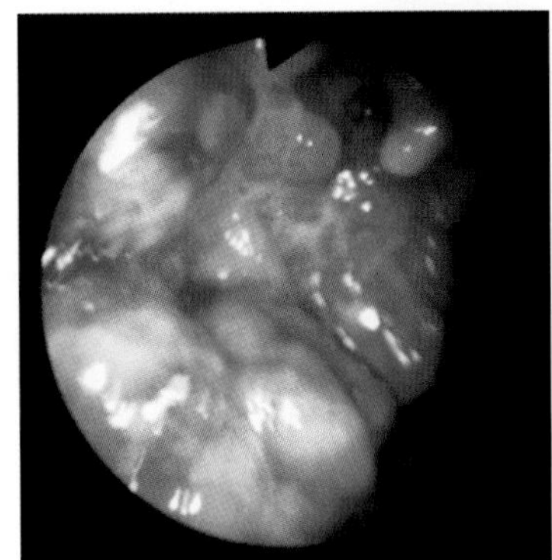

Fig. 2.152 Endoscopic appearance of gastric lymphoma.

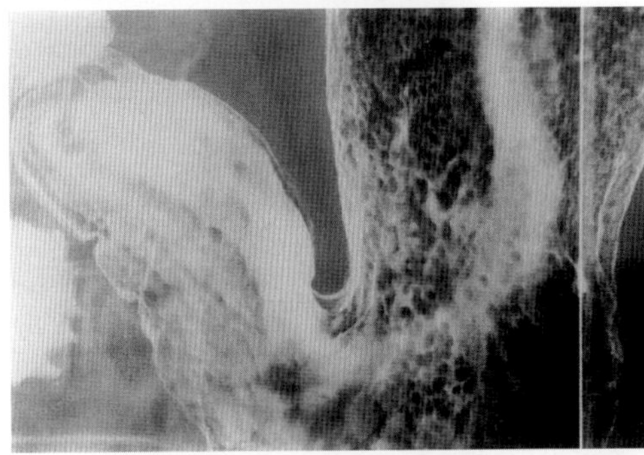

Fig. 2.153 Double-contrast barium study showing confluent, poorly defined nodules of varying sizes in the gastric body due to a low-grade gastric MALT lymphoma. Note how the appearance differs from that of the uniform, well-defined nodules of lymphoid hyperplasia in Fig. 2.154. (Reproduced with permission from reference 8.)

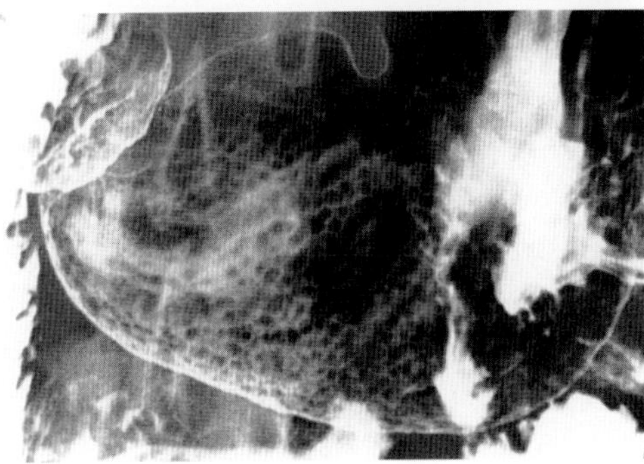

Fig. 2.154 Double-contrast barium study showing innumerable tiny, round nodules in the gastric antrum in a patient with lymphoid hyperplasia secondary to chronic *H. pylori* gastritis. (Reproduced with permission from reference 7.)

The MALToma is now known to be another manifestation of chronic *H. pylori* infection, moreover one that is responsive to eradication therapy if tackled early in its evolution. However, surgical resection is still needed for more advanced lesions (Fig. 2.155) and permits a more detailed histological examination (Figs 2.156, 2.157).

Other types of gastric lymphoma may also occur, including Hodgkin's disease. The previously termed benign, follicular, lymphoid hyperplasia, or pseudolymphoma, is also now known to be a true monoclonal lymphoma.

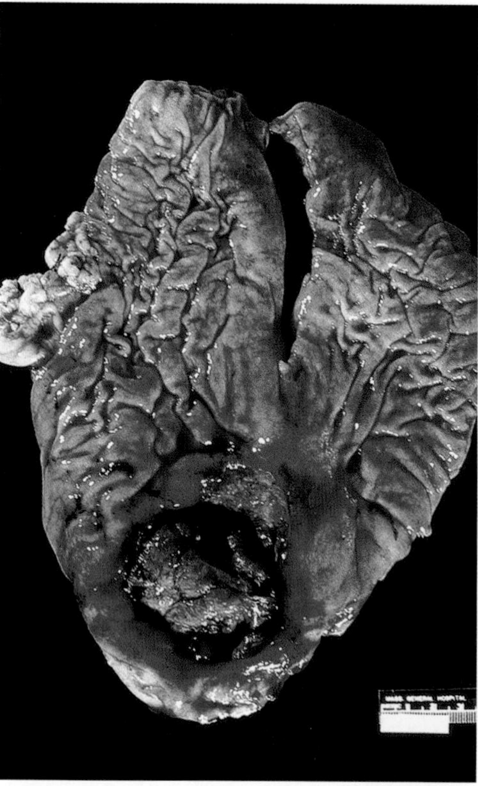

Fig 2.155 Partial gastrectomy specimen with diffuse involvement by an extra-nodal marginal zone B-cell lymphoma of mucosa-associated lymphoid tissue (MALT lymphoma) showing both diffuse infiltration and expansion of gastric folds of the body and a raised, ulcerated mass in the antrum.

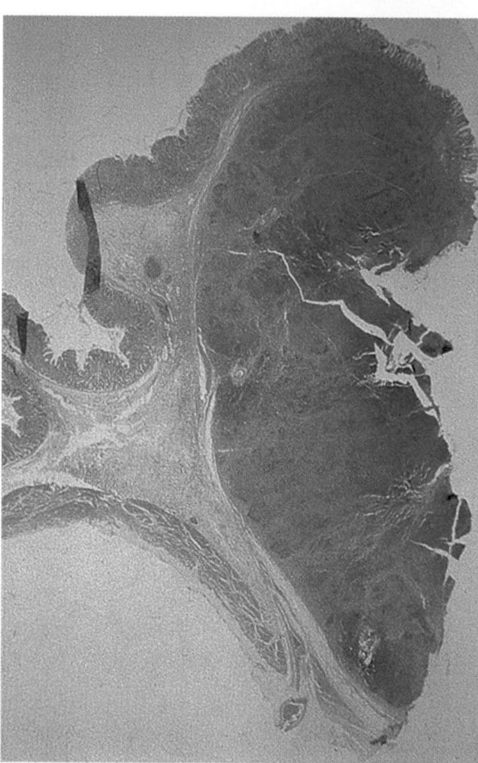

Fig. 2.156 Whole-mount microscopic view of a gastric MALT lymphoma showing diffuse confluent infiltration of the submucosa and ulceration of the mucosa.

Other gastric neoplasms and lesions which may mimic them

The stomach is an occasional site for metastatic spread, usually from an adenocarcinoma of origin in the pancreas, ovary or breast (Figs 2.158, 2.159). Other non-epithelial tumors such as gastric carcinoids are also seen (Fig. 2.160). Gastric involvement with Kaposi's

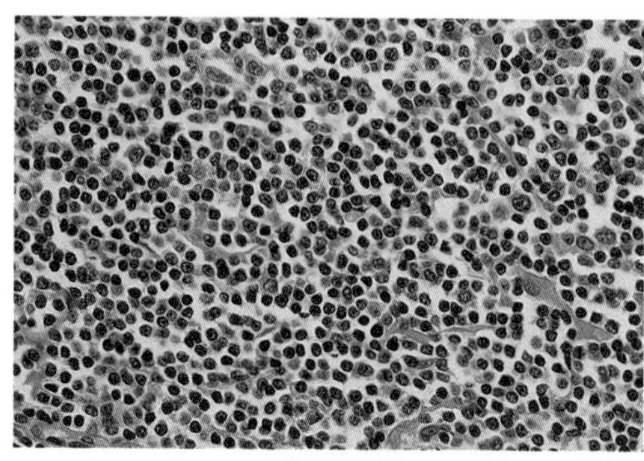

Fig. 2.157 High-magnification microscopic appearance of a low-grade gastric MALT lymphoma showing the characteristic centrocyte-like cells and small numbers of larger, nucleolated blast cells.

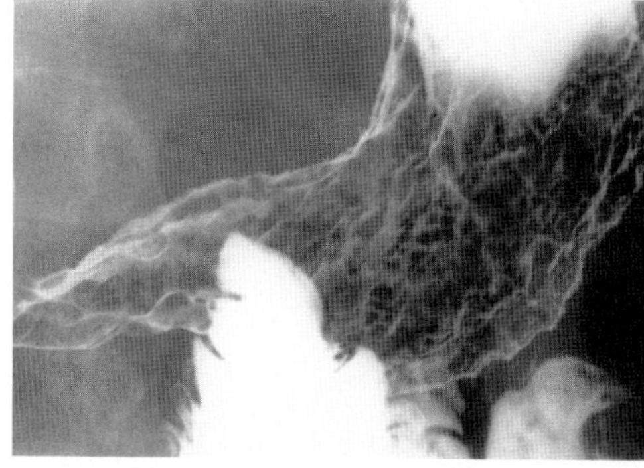

Fig. 2.158 Double-contrast barium study showing decreased distensibility of the gastric antrum with nodularity of the mucosa as a result of metastatic breast cancer encasing the stomach. The findings can be indistinguishable from those of a primary scirrhous carcinoma (see Fig. 2.103). (Reproduced with permission from reference 9.)

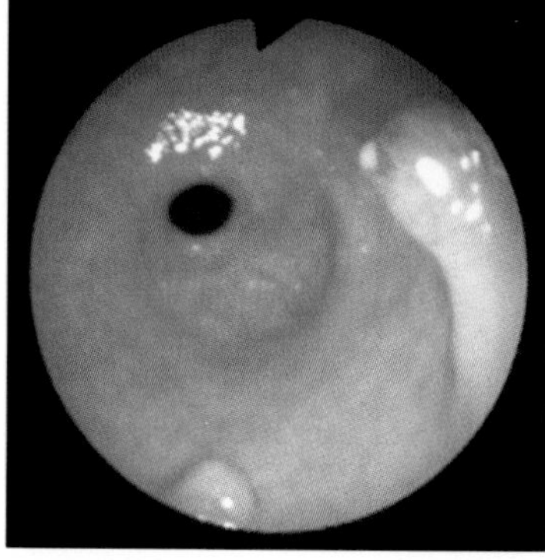

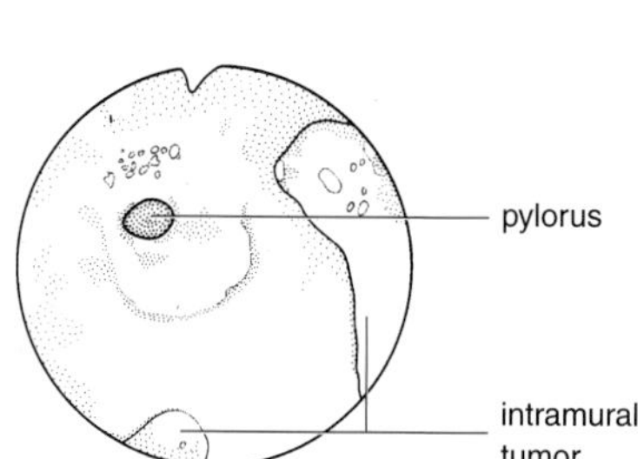

Fig. 2.159 Intramural gastric carcinoma seen endoscopically – in this case the result of secondary deposits from disseminated breast cancer.

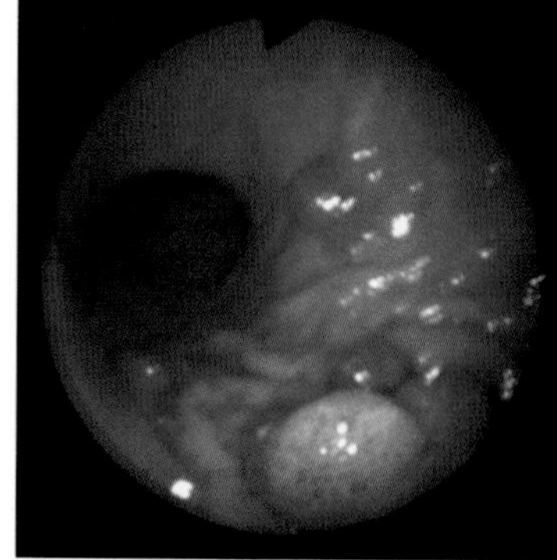

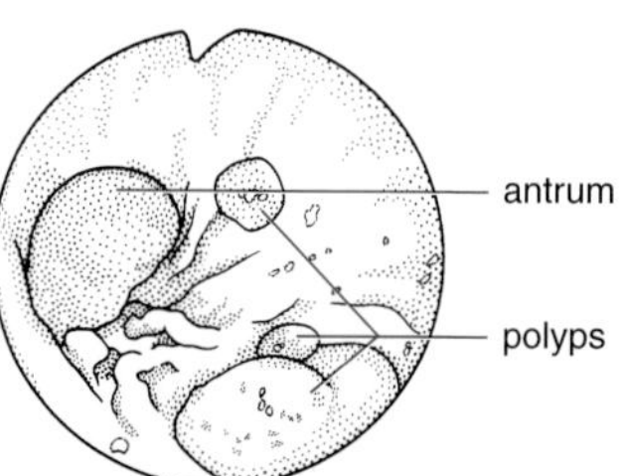

Fig. 2.160 Endoscopic appearance of the multiple polyps sometimes seen in gastric carcinoid – here on a background of severe atrophic gastritis.

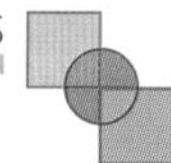

sarcoma is not infrequently seen in AIDS patients (Figs 2.161, 2.162). The histological appearance of deep endoscopic biopsies is similar to that of Kaposi's at other gastrointestinal sites.

Ectopic islands of pancreatic tissue may be recognized endoscopically (Fig. 2.163) – confusion with neoplasia is readily overcome by biopsy, which reveals normal pancreatic histology (see Chapter 9). Gastric xanthoma is less likely to be confused with more sinister pathology (Fig. 2.164).

DIVERTICULA

Gastric diverticula are uncommon chance findings on radiology or endoscopy. The majority are congenital and occur high on the posterior wall just below the gastro-esophageal junction (Fig. 2.165). A smaller number are prepyloric and follow previous peptic ulceration. Endoscopically, they appear as small, round, sharp-edged openings, which alter with peristalsis (Fig. 2.166). Dyspeptic symptoms occasionally result.

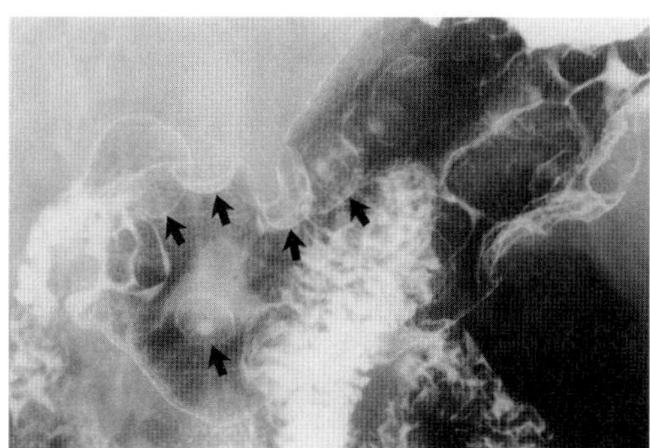

Fig. 2.161 Double-contrast barium study showing multiple submucosal masses (arrows) in the stomach due to Kaposi's sarcoma.

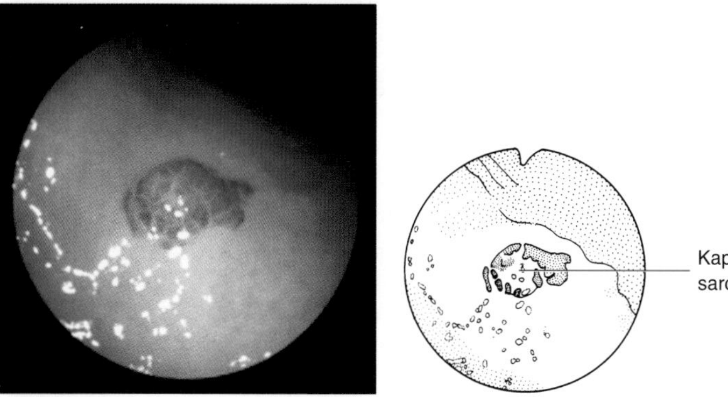

Fig. 2.162 Endoscopic appearance of gastric Kaposi's sarcoma in an AIDS patient with multiple cutaneous lesions.

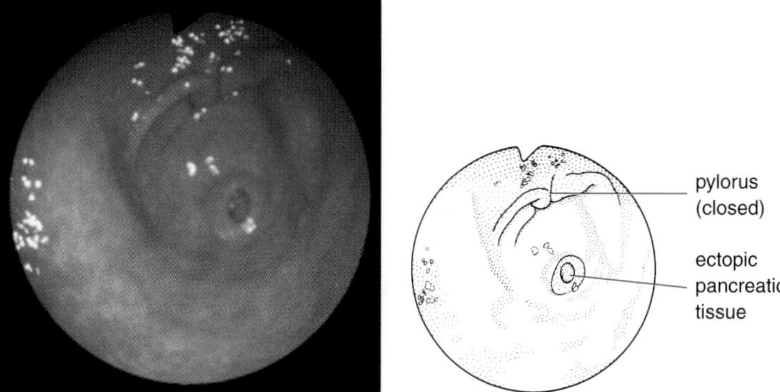

Fig. 2.163 Typical endoscopic appearance of ectopic pancreatic tissue – seen here in the antrum.

CONGENITAL HYPERTROPHIC PYLORIC STENOSIS

This condition is second only to inguinal hernia as a reason for surgical intervention during the first year of life. It is not truly congenital, as the pyloric muscle hypertrophies, causing progressive narrowing of the pyloric canal during the first few weeks of life ultimately leading to pyloric obstruction. Males are affected more commonly than females and there is often a family history. Non-bilious vomiting of increasing frequency and severity, associated with weight loss, and dehydration, are typical. The upper abdomen may be distended (Fig. 2.167) with visible gastric peristalsis and a palpable lump representing the hypertrophied pylorus. The differential diagnosis is not usually a problem and contrast radiology is now obsolete, given the ready confirmation of the diagnosis by ultrasound scanning (Figs 2.168, 2.169). At laparotomy, the hypertrophied pylorus is visible, and pyloromyotomy (Ramstedt's operation) is the usual procedure (Figs 2.170, 2.171).

Adult pyloric stenosis

Pyloric stenosis in later life is usually the result of scarring, with or without concurrent edema, in association with pyloric-channel and duodenal ulcer (see above and Chapter 3). Occasionally antral

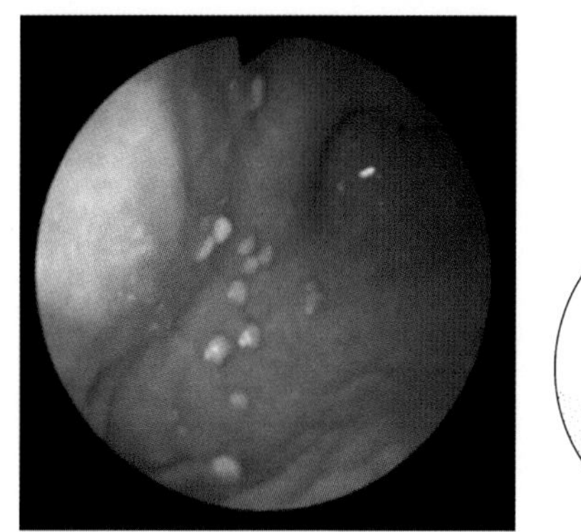

Fig. 2.164 Gastric xanthomata.

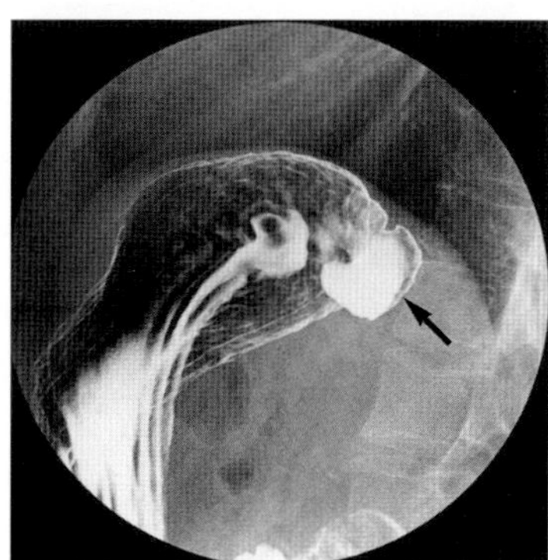

Fig. 2.165 Double-contrast barium study showing a gastric diverticulum as a discrete out-pouching (arrow) from the posterior wall of the fundus.

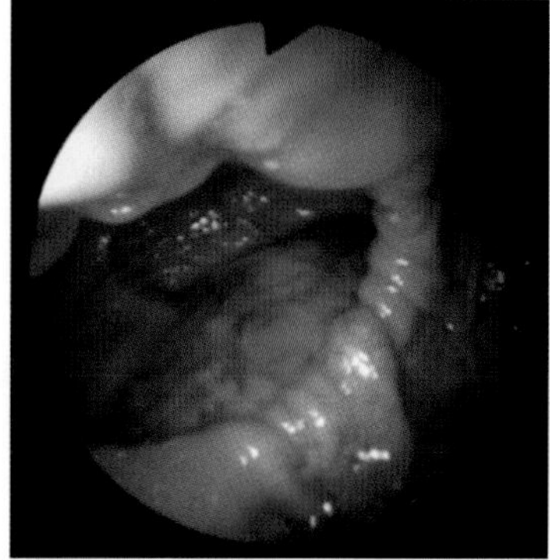

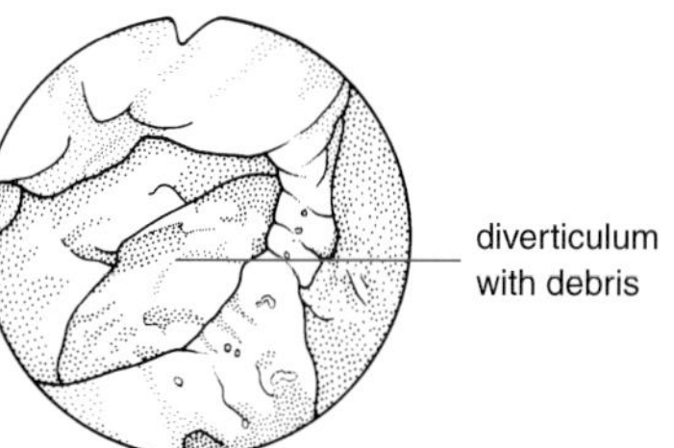

Fig. 2.166 Endoscopic appearance of a gastric diverticulum

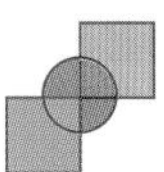

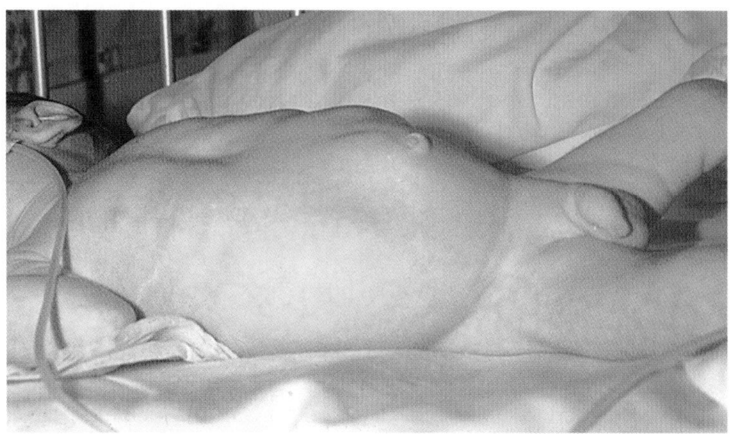

■ **Fig. 2.167** A neonate with hypertrophic pyloric stenosis showing the distended stomach. Courtesy of Dr V. Wright.

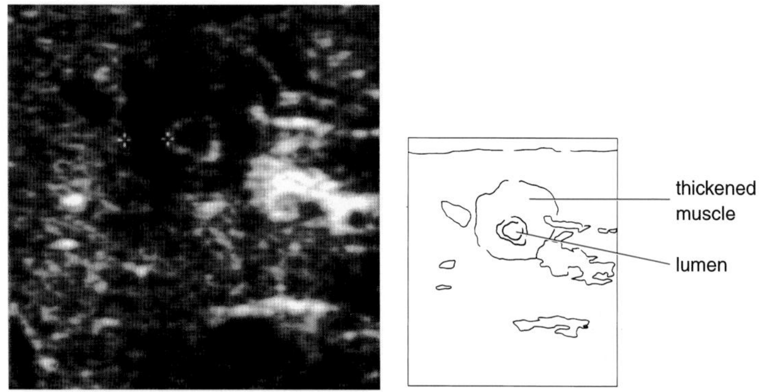

■ **Fig. 2.168** Transverse ultrasound scan illustrating the typical appearance of the thickened muscle in pyloric stenosis.

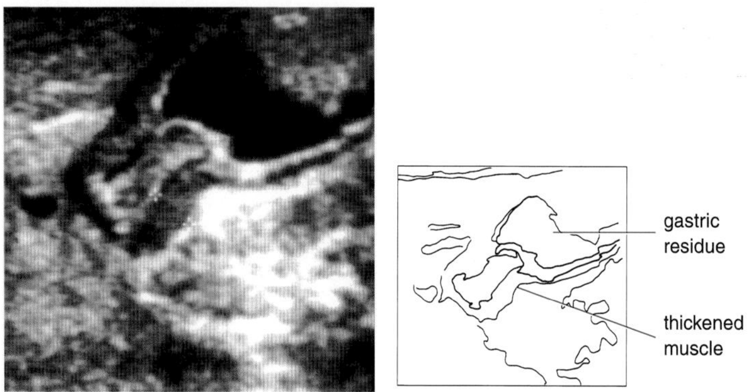

■ **Fig. 2.169** Longitudinal ultrasound scan of the same patient, showing also significant gastric residue.

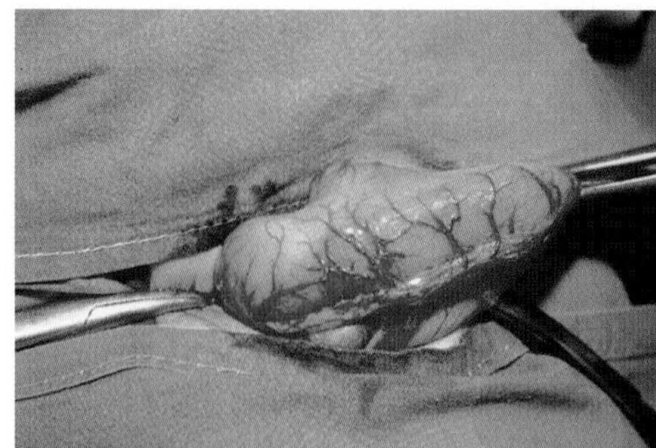

■ **Fig. 2.170** Appearance of hypertrophic pyloric stenosis at laparotomy. Courtesy of Mr H.H. Nixon.

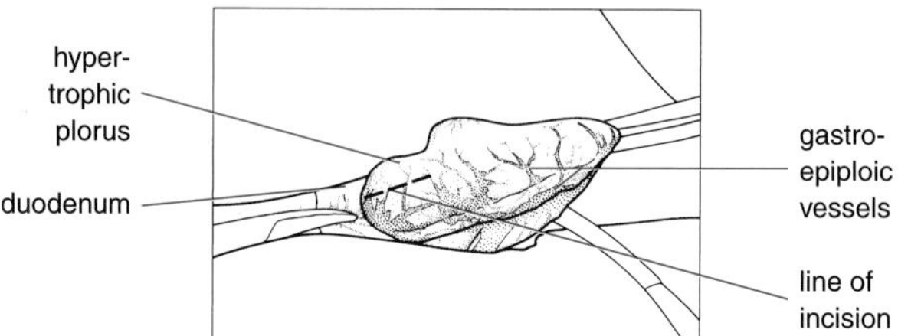

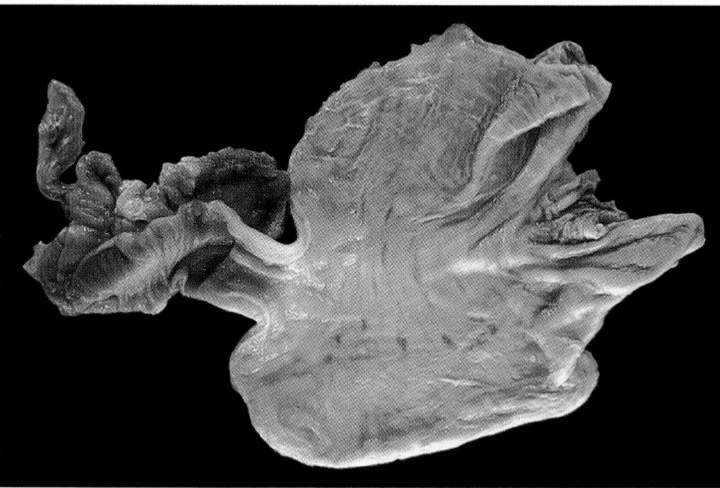

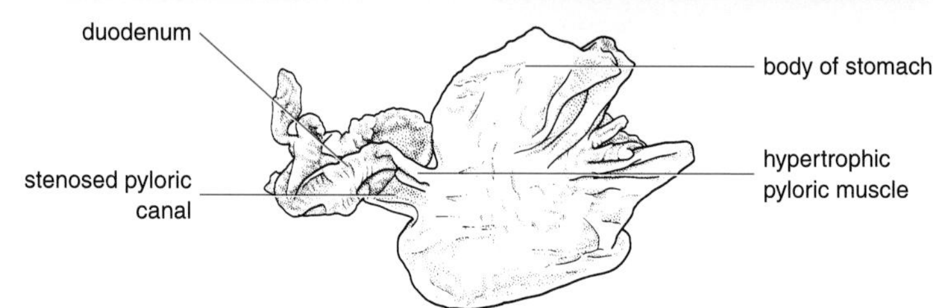

■ **Fig. 2.171** Post-mortem specimen from a patient with congenital hypertrophic pyloric stenosis. Courtesy of Dr J.S. Wigglesworth.

carcinomas or duodenal tumors are responsible. Much more rarely, adults present with unexplained pyloric stenosis, and it is thought that these patients have a mild, late-presenting form of the infantile condition. The occurrence of infantile and adult forms in different members of the same family and the concordant histological changes favor this hypothesis. An antral web or diaphragm may cause similar troubles (Fig. 2.172).

Functional gastric outlet obstruction

Symptomatic gastric outlet obstruction, with a persistent sensation of satiety relieved by vomiting, may exist in the absence of an anatomical or mechanical cause. Although it is sometimes a non-specific feature of non-ulcer dyspepsia or irritable bowel syndrome, delayed gastric emptying also results from diabetic neuropathy and visceral myopathy (see Chapter 7). It can be best documented by isotopic emptying studies (Fig. 2.173); delay may principally affect solids, liquids, or both equally.

Gastric volvulus

Gastric volvulus may be asymptomatic, responsible for mild dyspepsia, or for severe, even intractable, vomiting. The stomach may rotate on one of three basic axes (Fig. 2.174), an oblique angle being the most common. At contrast radiology it may be difficult to determine the axis of rotation (Fig. 2.175), and the endoscopist may be completely disorientated and sometimes unable to find the pylorus (Fig. 2.176). Symptomatic cases require surgical fixation. Distinction should be made from the radiological appearance of the normal (asymptomatic) 'cup and spill' variant (see Fig. 2.9).

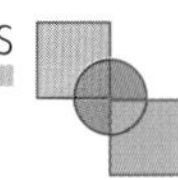

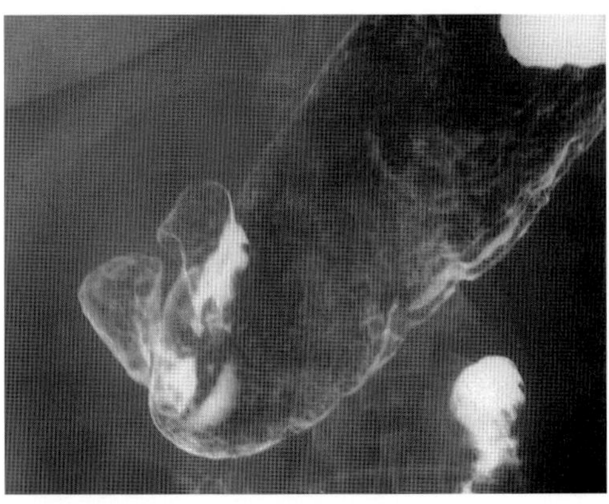

■ **Fig. 2.172** Barium meal showing an antral web responsible for gastric outlet obstruction.

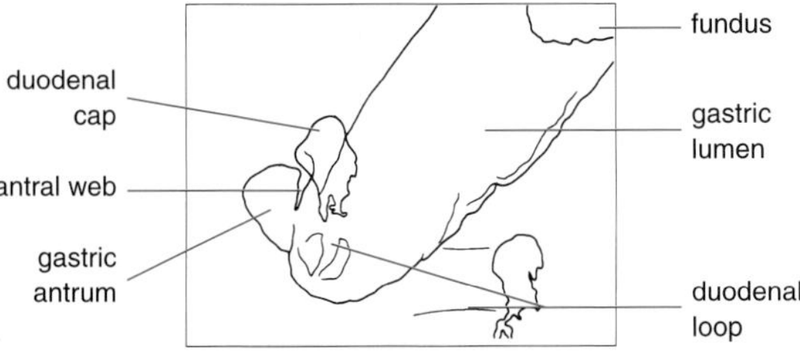

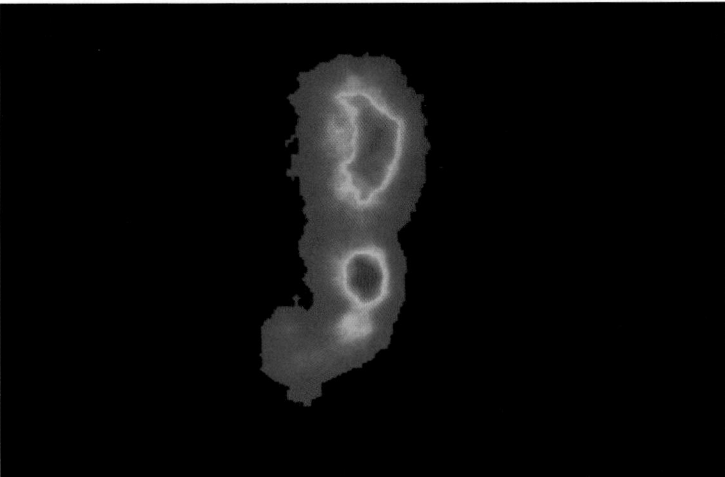

■ **Fig. 2.173** The impaired emptying of diabetic gastroparesis demonstrated by delayed transit of a test meal: the isotopically labeled solid component has not left the stomach at 1 hour (compare with Figs 2.25 and 2.27). Courtesy of Mr G.P. Morris and Cancer Research UK.

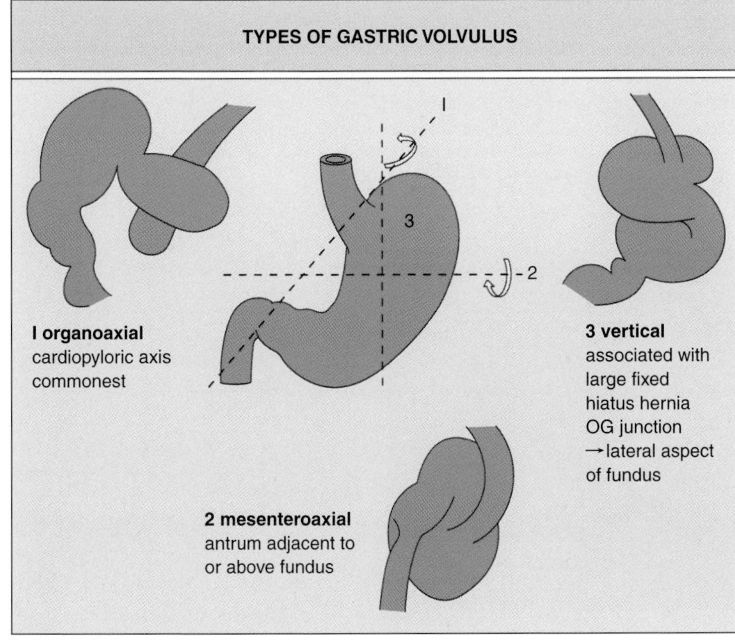

■ **Fig. 2.174** Diagram illustrating the three potential axes for gastric volvulus.

FOREIGN BODIES AND BEZOARS

Swallowed foreign bodies are rarely responsible for gastric damage (see also Chapter 1) and, having traversed the esophago-gastric junction, rarely impact more distally unless huge (Fig. 2.177). However, serious complications, including intestinal perforation, or, very rarely, penetration of major vessels with subsequent hemorrhage, are described: sharp objects should therefore be removed, endoscopically if possible. A particular hazard is presented by mercury batteries, which leak rapidly and then cause severe mucosal damage: they too should be removed.

More peculiar to the stomach is the formation of bezoars, which are concretions of foreign material built up gradually, usually over many months. Typically, they are composed largely of swallowed hair (trichobezoar) (Fig. 2.178) or fibrous residues of foodstuffs (phytobezoar), accumulated secondary to gastric stasis or partial gastric outlet obstruction (particularly in the post-operative stomach).

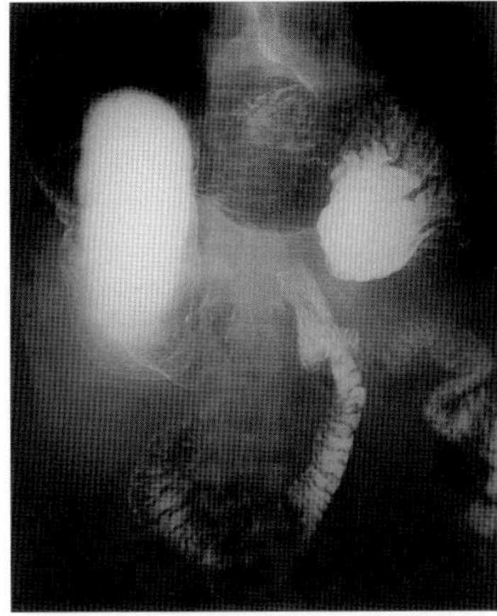

■ **Fig. 2.175** Single-contrast barium study showing an upside-down intrathoracic stomach due to an organoaxial gastric volvulus with flipping of the stomach into the chest via a large diaphragmatic rent.

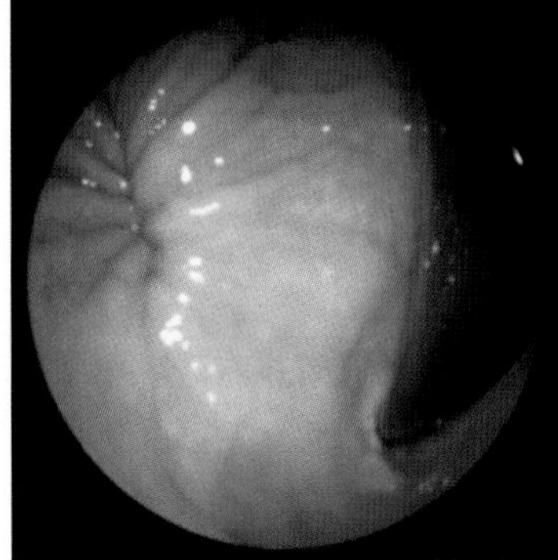

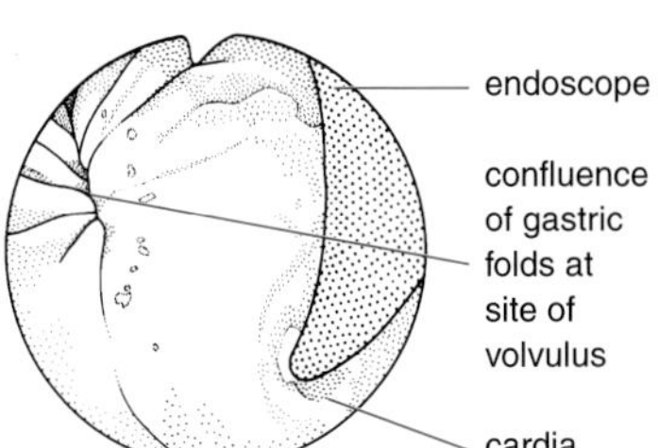

■ **Fig. 2.176** Endoscopic appearance of gastric volvulus.

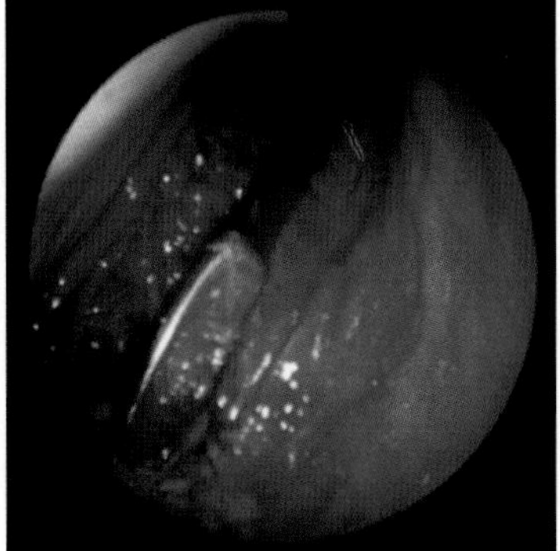

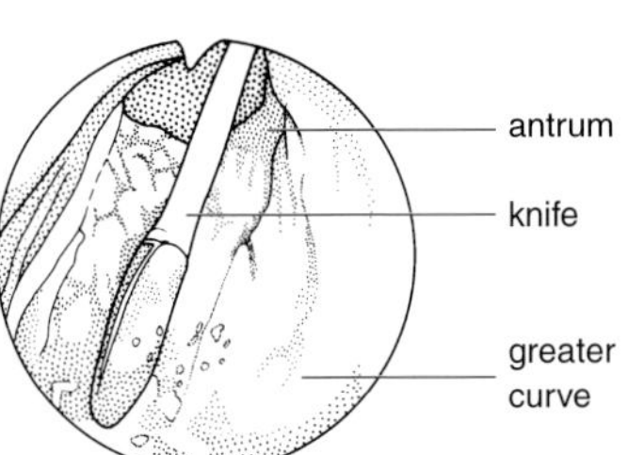

■ **Fig. 2.177** Swallowed foreign bodies may be seen in, and retrieved from, the stomach: in this case a table knife.

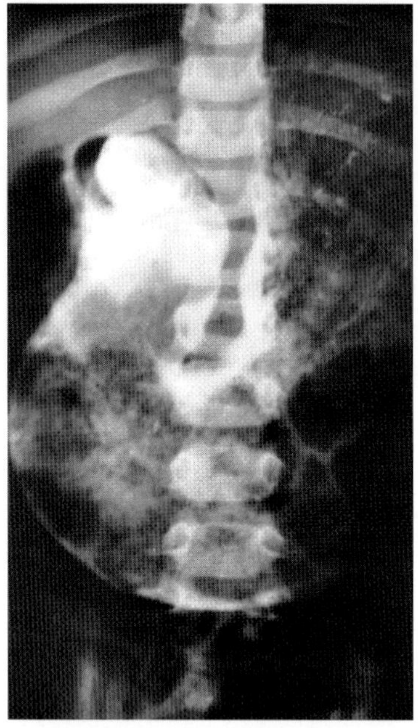

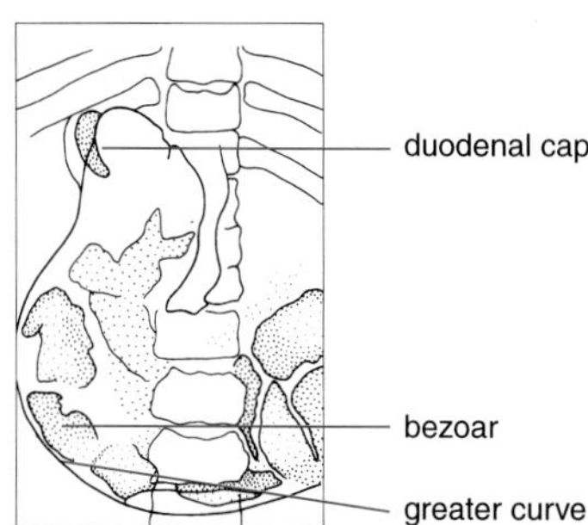

Fig. 2.178 Barium meal showing a trichobezoar as a large, irregular filling defect within the lumen extending from the fundus to the antrum. This was the result of a mixture of cotton wool and hair swallowed by a 5-year-old.

Bezoars eventually become symptomatic, and may be complicated by ulceration or perforation.

THE POST-OPERATIVE STOMACH

The availability of potent antisecretory drugs and regimes that permit the eradication of *H. pylori* has markedly reduced the need for traditional peptic ulcer surgery. Increased skills with laparoscopic intervention may, however, lead to a revival of vagotomy for ulcer disease. Truncal vagotomy (Fig. 2.179; see also Fig. 2.10) generally causes major impairment of gastric motility and is usually combined with pyloroplasty (Fig. 2.180) and/or gastroenterostomy (Fig. 2.181), unnecessary with more selective vagotomy which preserves the enervation of the antrum (nerves of Laterjet) (see Figs 2.10, 2.179). Uncontrolled bleeding from peptic ulcers necessitates a Billroth II type gastrectomy, which would also often be used for acquired pyloric obstruction (Figs 2.182, 2.183). The Billroth I partial gastrectomy is not now often performed. Total gastrectomy for gastric carcinoma leaving an esophago-jejunal anastomosis is readily appreciated endoscopically (Fig. 2.184).

There are a number of post-operative complications (not least the increased frequency of malignancy in the partially resected stomach), and post-operative radiological and endoscopic assessment may be required. The appearances can be confusing and stomal ulcers are easily missed. It is usually possible endoscopically to identify and enter the afferent and efferent loops of a Billroth II gastrectomy (see Fig. 2.183), but when difficulty is experienced, the endoscope tends to follow the efferent loop more readily. Careful examination of both sides of the stoma is essential to avoid missing small ulcers (Fig. 2.185). The non-specific gastritis of the operated stomach is almost to be considered a normal phenomenon (Figs 2.186, 2.187), but the threshold for biopsies should be low if early malignancy or premonitory dysplasia are not to be missed (Figs 2.188, 2.189). CT scanning is not routine in the follow-up of patients with previous gastric carcinoma, but will occasionally show dramatic evidence of recurrence (Fig. 2.190). Retained sutures may be seen and are usually innocent, only rarely acting as a nidus for ulceration (Fig. 2.191).

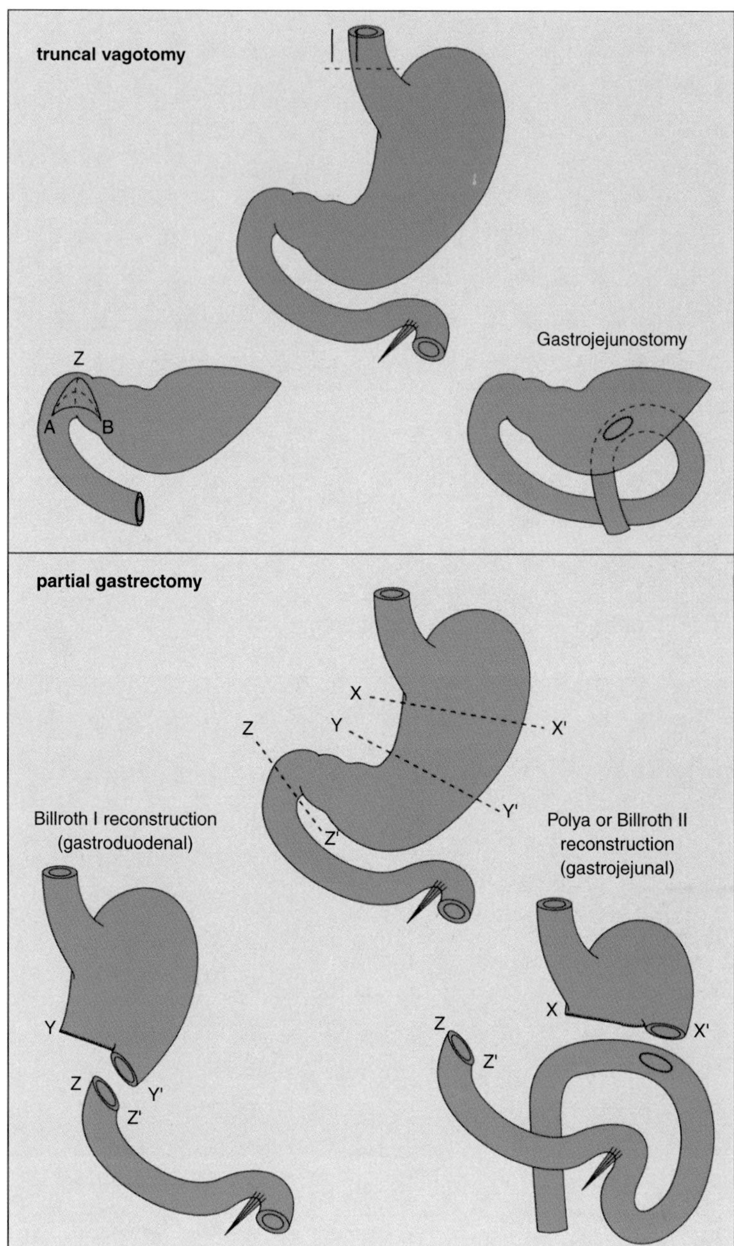

Fig. 2.179 Diagram illustrating some of the commoner gastric operations. In truncal vagotomy the whole stomach is denervated. The pyloroplasty incision is made from A to B across the pylorus, which is then sutured from X to Z, so widening the lumen of the pyloric channel. In partial gastrectomy, the stomach is usually resected between X–X' and Z–Z', the more localized antrectomy limiting resection to Y–Y' and Z–Z'. The reconstruction follows the general pattern of the Billroth I or Billroth II technique. Courtesy of Professor M. Hobsley.

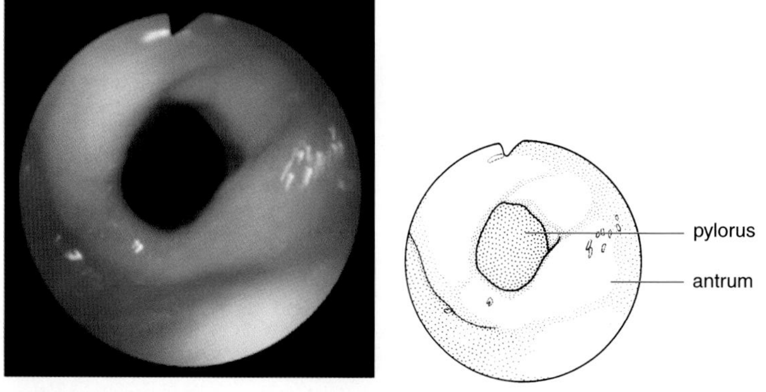

Fig. 2.180 Endoscopic appearance of pyloroplasty showing a widely and continually patent pylorus.

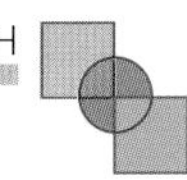

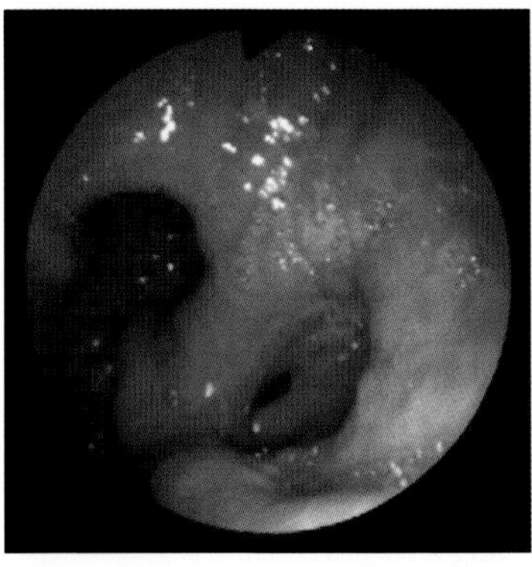

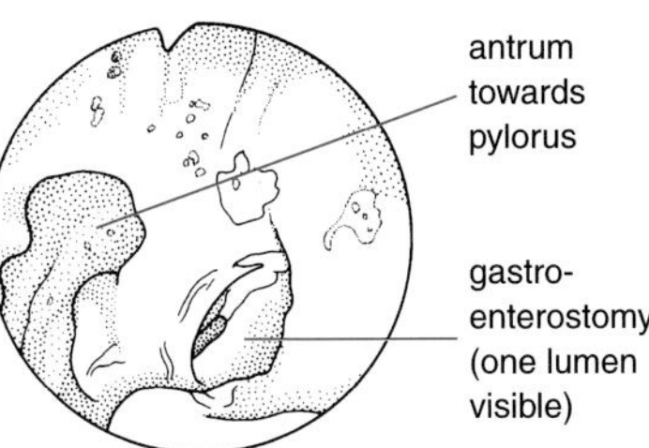

■ **Fig. 2.181** Endoscopic appearance of the intact stomach with a gastroenterostomy, which illustrates how confusion can arise when the operative details have not been clear prior to the examination.

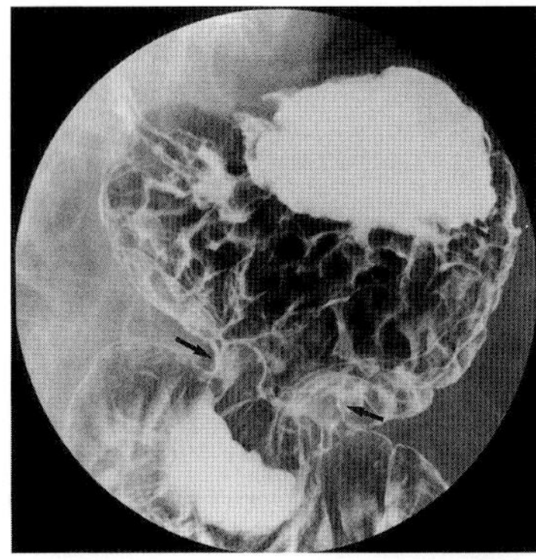

■ **Fig. 2.182** Double-contrast barium study showing a Billroth II partial gastrectomy with a widely patent gastro-jejunal anastomosis (arrows). Also note thickened folds in the gastric remnant due to bile reflux gastritis.

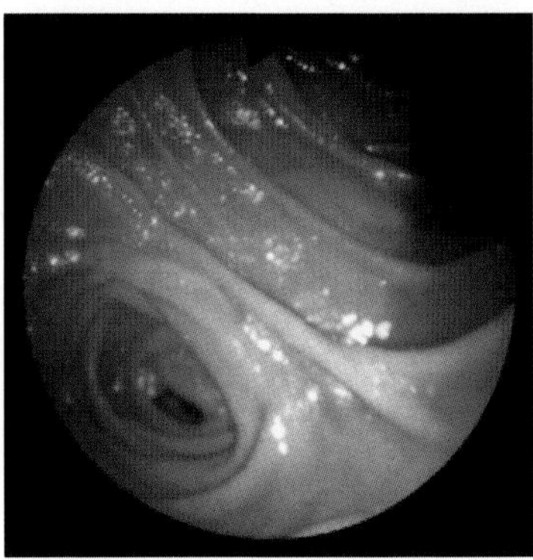

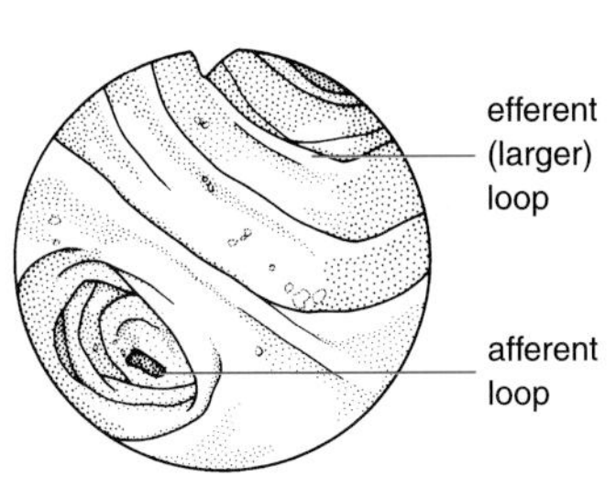

■ **Fig. 2.183** Endoscopic appearance of Billroth II gastrectomy showing afferent and efferent loops.

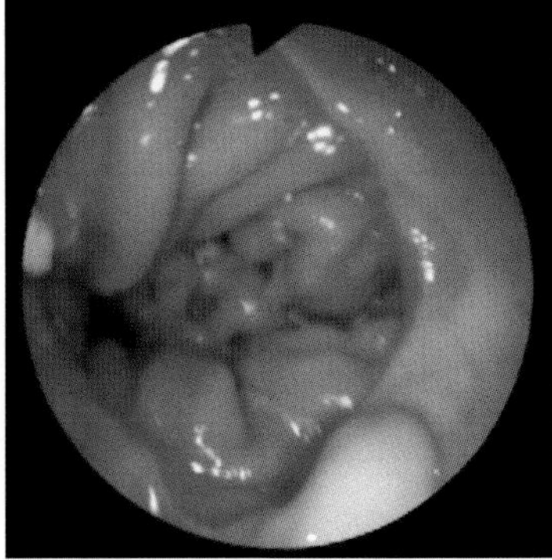

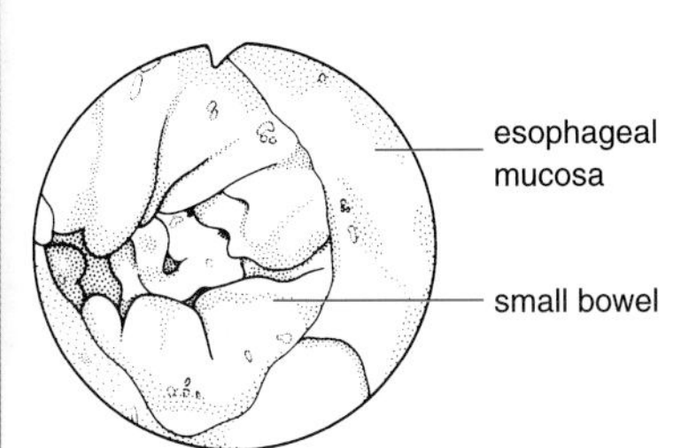

■ **Fig. 2.184** Endoscopic appearance of the esophago-jejunal anastomosis following total gastrectomy.

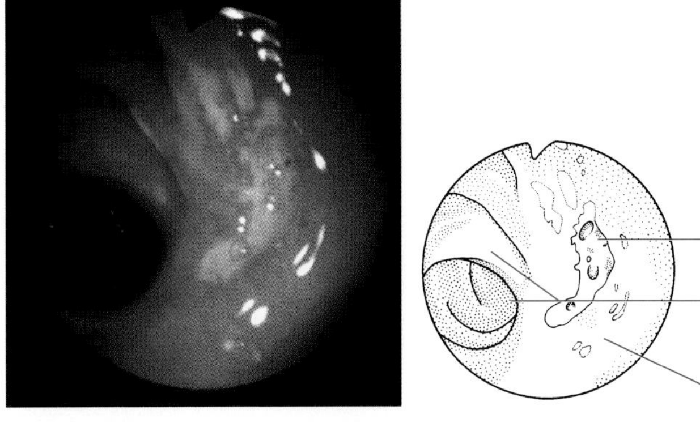

■ **Fig. 2.185** Endoscopic appearance of stomal ulcer within the stomal ring in a patient with a previous Billroth II gastrectomy.

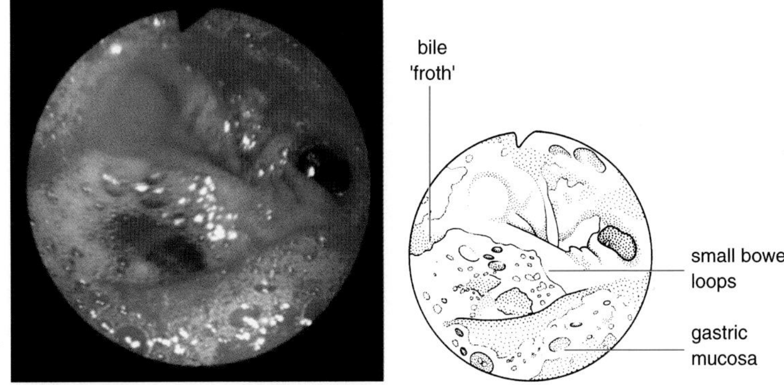

■ **Fig. 2.186** Marked erythema and edema seen in association with biliary reflux following Billroth II gastrectomy.

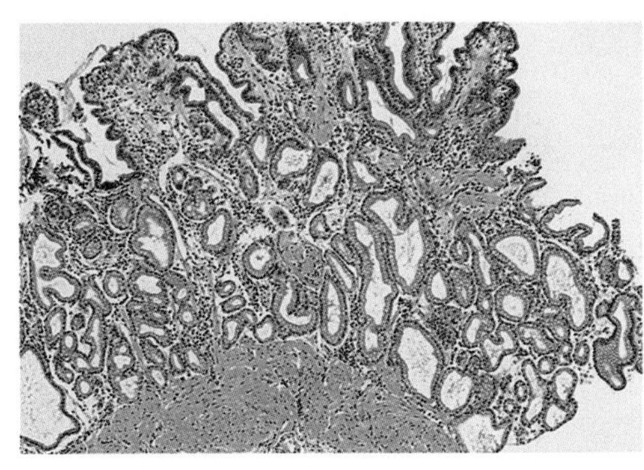

■ **Fig. 2.187** Histological appearance of chronic chemical gastritis secondary to reflux of small intestinal contents into the gastric body remnant of a Billroth II anastomosis showing cystic dilatation of glands that have undergone pseudopyloric metaplasia (chronic gastritis cystica).

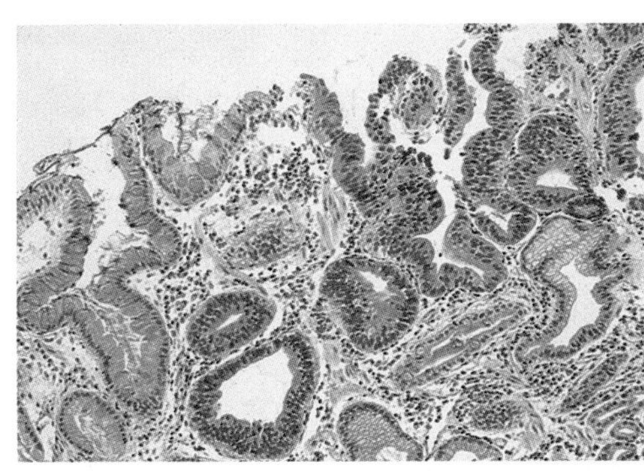

■ **Fig. 2.188** Microscopic appearance of epithelial dysplasia of the gastric remnant, a late complication of chronic chemical gastritis in Billroth II procedure.

Morbid obesity is again being managed surgically, but with much less destructive operations than have had currency in the past; the band gastroplasty appears safe and effective, but renders subsequent visualization of the duodenum problematic (Fig. 2.192). The endoscopic placement of a fluid-filled balloon designed to be left in the stomach for some months has not proved a great long-term success.

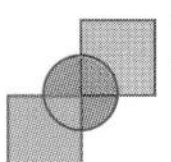

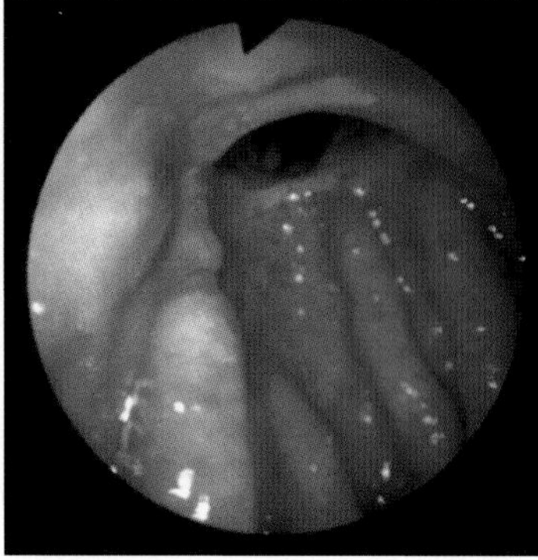

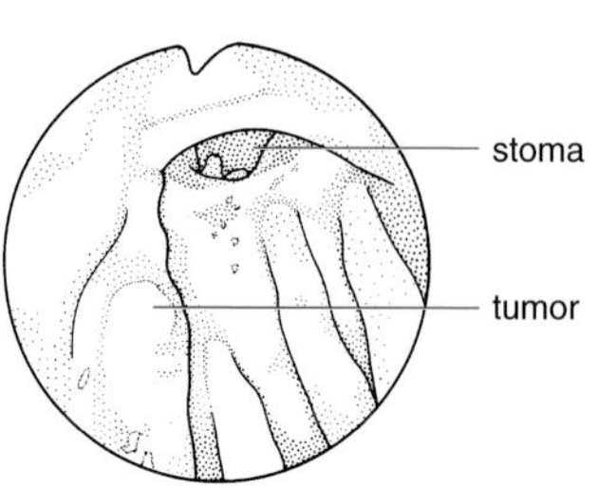

■ **Fig. 2.189** Endoscopic appearances of early carcinoma complicating a Billroth II partial gastrectomy. Neoplastic change is indicated by subtle color change and minor distortion of a prestomal fold.

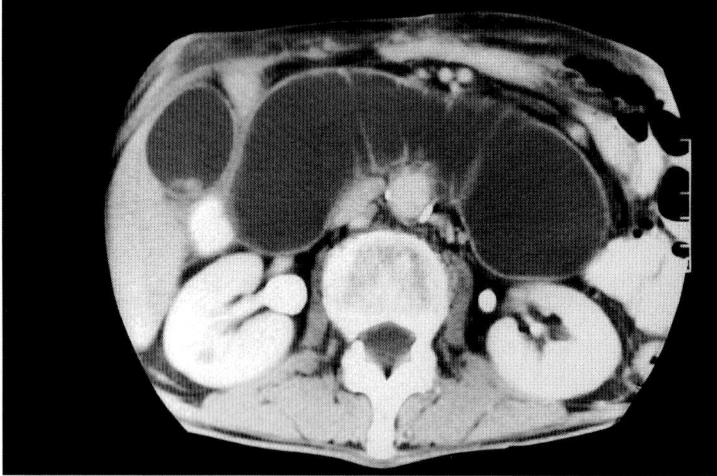

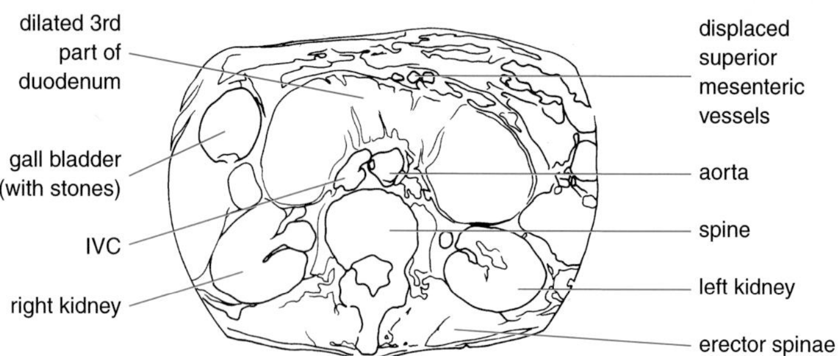

■ **Fig. 2.190** CT scan showing obstruction of the afferent loop in a patient with a previous resection for gastric carcinoma. In addition to the intestinal obstruction, the pressure within the afferent loop was also responsible for biliary and pancreatic duct dilatation.

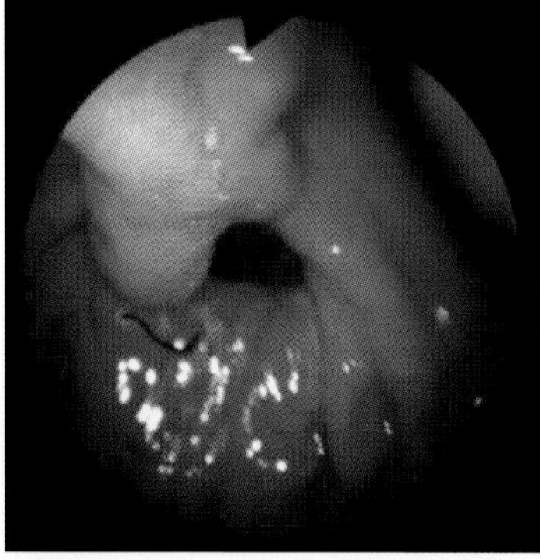

■ **Fig. 2.191** Endoscopic appearance of a retained suture with associated mild ulceration.

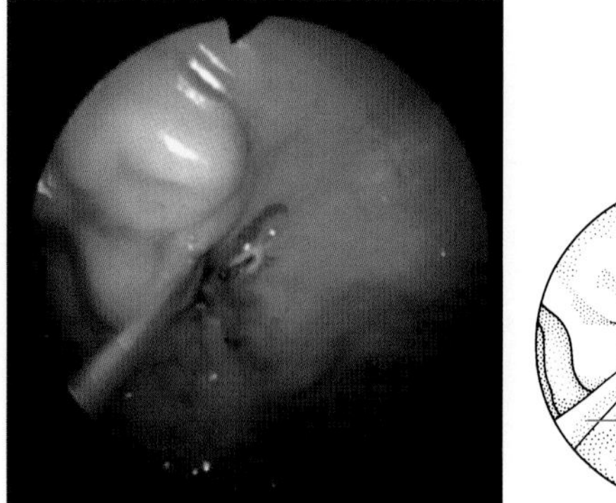

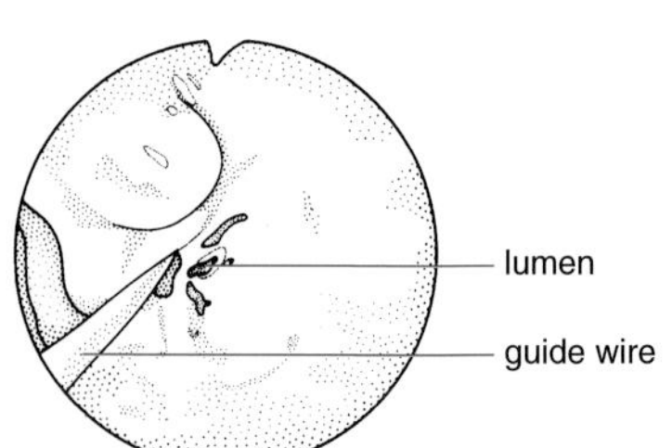

■ **Fig. 2.192** Endoscopic appearance of stomach following gastroplasty for morbid obesity. A guide wire is inserted through the small remaining lumen.

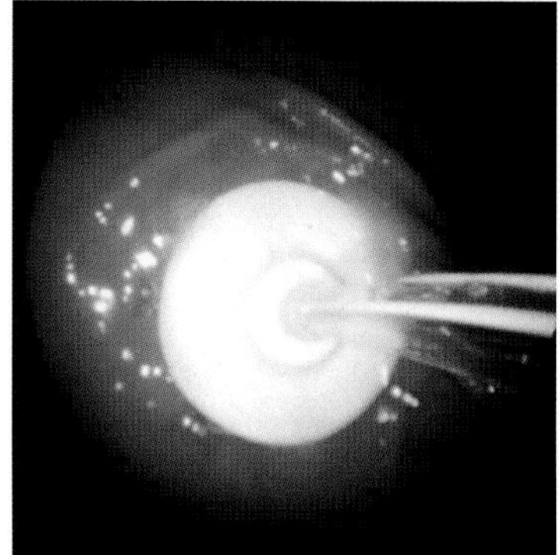

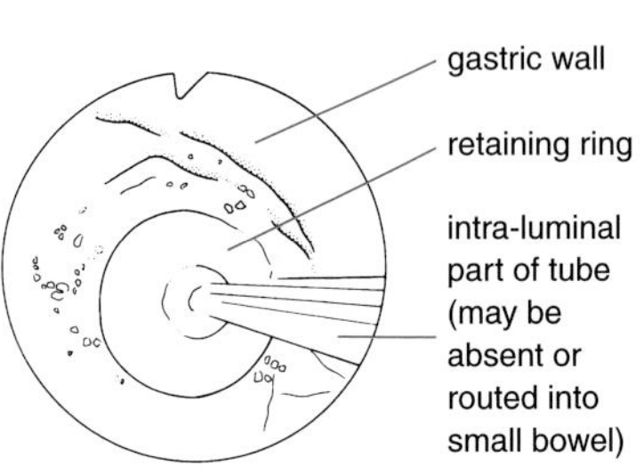

■ **Fig. 2.193** Endoscopic appearance of a satisfactorily placed gastrostomy tube in a patient unable to swallow following a stroke.

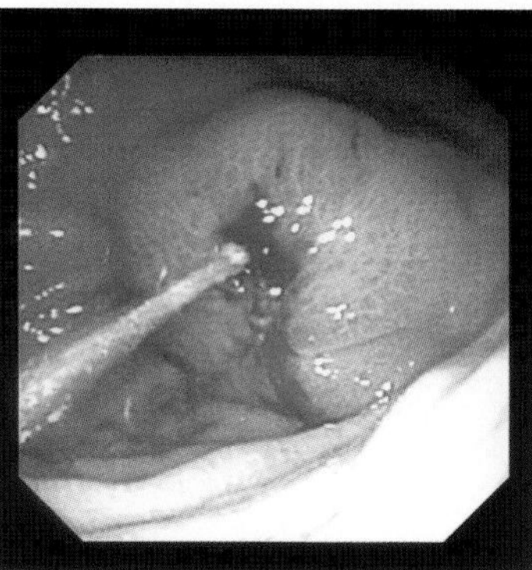

■ **Fig. 2.194** Endoscopy in a patient with buried bumper syndrome. The gastrostomy tube had ceased to function and only a mucosal mound was visible until the tube was vigorously flushed, at which point a jet of water emerged from its center. Surgical removal was necessary.

By contrast, nutritional support is increasingly provided by the enteral route, and a percutaneous endoscopic gastrostomy tube is generally better tolerated than long-term nasogastric intubation (Fig. 2.193). Although usually remarkably well-tolerated for long periods, there is a danger of the so-called buried bumper syndrome if the tube is not regularly manipulated. In this condition there is mucosal overgrowth, which can lead to the complete disappearance of the internal retaining collar (Fig 2.194).

REFERENCES

1. Levine MS, Rubesin SE, Laufer I. Double contrast gastrointestinal radiology. Philadelphia: WB Saunders, 2000, Figs 7.45 and 7.65B.
2. Levine MS, Kelly MR, Laufer I, Rubesin SE, Herlinger H. Gastrocolic fistulas: the increasing role of aspirin. Radiology 1993; 187: 359–361, Fig. 1B.

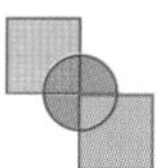

3. Sohn J, Levine MS, Furth EE, Laufer I, Rubesin SE, Herlinger H, Lichtenstein GR. *Helicobacter pylori* gastritis: radiographic findings. Radiology 1995; 195: 763–767, Fig. 5A.
4. Chang D, Levine MS, Ginsberg GG, Rubesin SE, Laufer I. Portal hypertensive gastropathy: radiographic findings in eight patients. AJR 2000; 175: 1609–1612, Fig. 1.
5. Levine MS, Kieu K, Rubesin SE, Herlinger H, Laufer I. Isolated gastric varices: splenic vein obstruction or portal hypertension? Gastrointest Radiol 1990; 15: 188–192, Fig. 2A.
6. Gore RM, Levine MS (eds). Textbook of gastrointestinal radiology. Philadelphia: WB Saunders, 2000, Figs 34.2B, 34.6A, and 35.8C.
7. Torigian DA, Levine MS, Navdeep SG, Rubesin SE, Fogt F, Schultz CF, Furth EE, Laufer I. Lymphoid hyperplasia of the stomach: radiographic findings in five adult patients. AJR 2001; 177: 71–75, Fig. 1A.
8. Yoo CC, Levine MS, Furth EE, Salhany KE, Rubesin SE, Laufer I, Herlinger H. Gastric mucosa-associated lymphoid tissue lymphoma: radiographic findings in six patients. Radiology 1998; 208: 239–243, Fig. 4A.
9. Levine MS, Kong V, Rubesin SE, Laufer I, Herlinger H. Scirrhous carcinoma of the stomach: radiologic and endoscopic diagnosis. Radiology 1990; 175: 151–154, Fig. 4A.

THE DUODENUM

3

NORMAL DUODENUM

The duodenum, which is the most proximal and fixed part of the small intestine, joins the stomach to the jejunum. It is approximately 25 cm long, and its configuration divides it into four parts: the duodenal bulb, and then the descending, horizontal, and ascending portions (Fig. 3.1). On barium meal the duodenal bulb appears triangular (Fig. 3.2) with shallow longitudinal folds that become obliterated when the cap is distended (Fig. 3.3). Endoscopically the cap is smooth-lined and takes the form of a short bulbous cylinder (Fig. 3.4). The second part of the duodenum descends retroperitoneally to the right of the midline, adjacent to the head of the pancreas, at the level of the first and second lumbar vertebrae (L1 and L2). The ampulla of Vater (papilla) opens at its approximate midpoint and is most easily recognized endoscopically (Fig. 3.5) by its relationship to the longitudinal fold. The ampulla is also readily identified by the novel endoscopy capsule, which is considered in more detail in Chapters 4 and 5 (Fig. 3.6). The pancreatic and biliary ducts, which enter the duodenum at this point, are considered in Chapter 9 and Chapters 10 and 14, respectively. The third part of the duodenum is also retroperitoneal, crosses the midline at L3, continues close to the head of the pancreas, and is itself crossed anteriorly by the

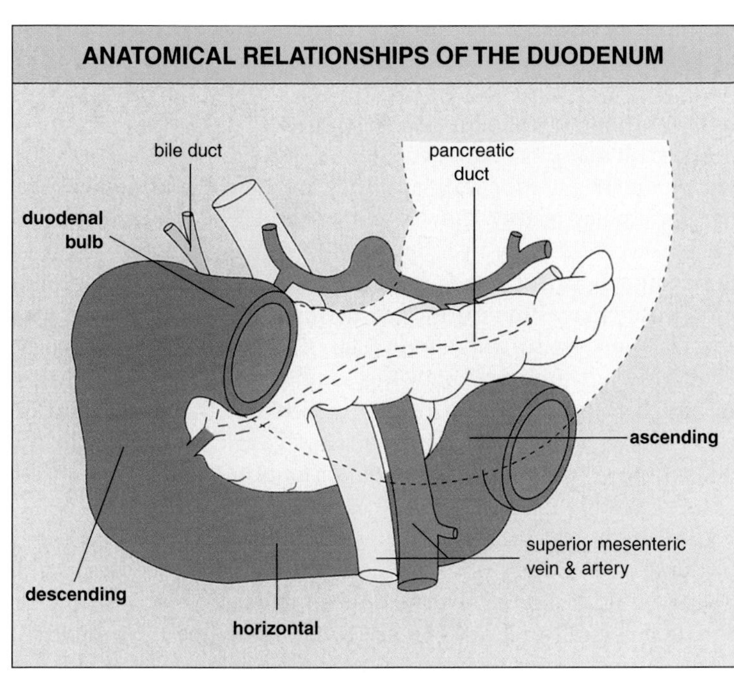

■ **Fig. 3.1** The anatomical relationships of the duodenum.

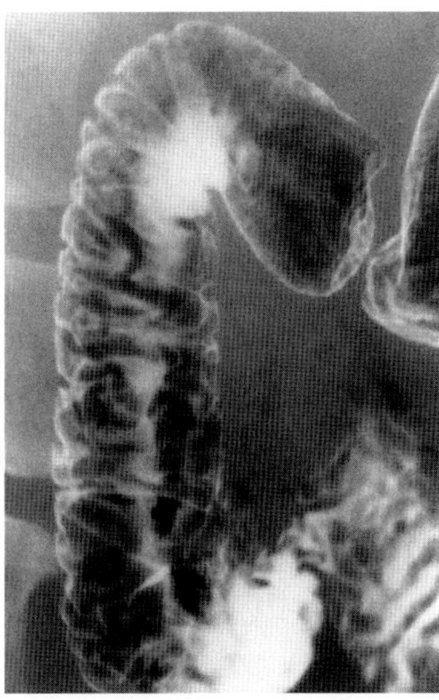

■ **Fig. 3.2** Left posterior oblique view from double-contrast barium study showing the normal appearance of the duodenal bulb and sweep.

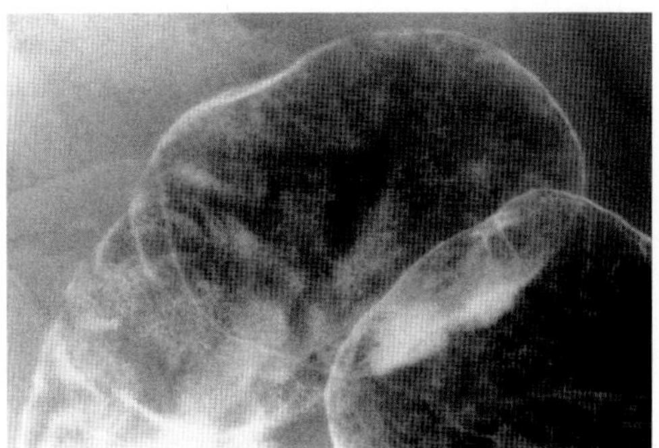

■ **Fig. 3.3** Close-up double-contrast view showing a fine reticular surface pattern in the duodenal bulb as a normal finding.

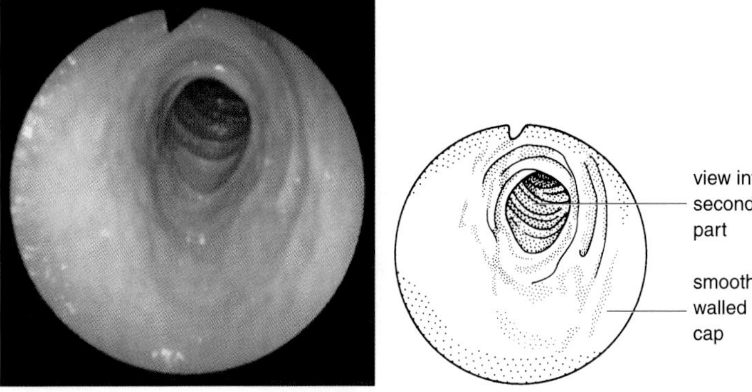

■ **Fig. 3.4** Endoscopic appearance of the normal duodenal cap.

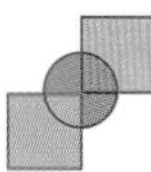

superior mesenteric artery and vein (see Fig. 3.1). The fourth part of the duodenum ascends obliquely below the body of the pancreas, before turning abruptly downwards and anteriorly, where its junction with the jejunum is anchored by a fibromuscular structure, the ligament of Treitz. The smooth internal appearance of the duodenal bulb is quite different from that in the more distal parts, all of which have the circular folds characteristic of the small intestine, the valvulae conniventes (Fig. 3.7). With conventional endoscopy it is difficult to get beyond the third part of the duodenum and usually impossible to get past the ligament of Treitz, but the use of a longer, specifically designed enteroscope (or a pediatric colonoscope) permits more distal examination if necessary.

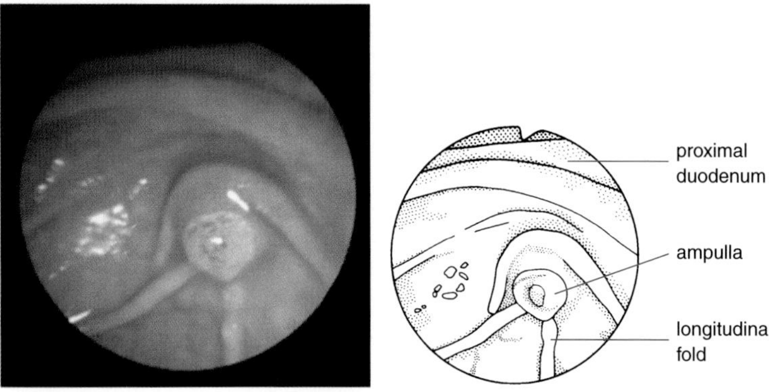

■ **Fig. 3.5** Endoscopic appearance of the normal second part of the duodenum showing the ampulla of Vater and its relationship to the longitudinal fold.

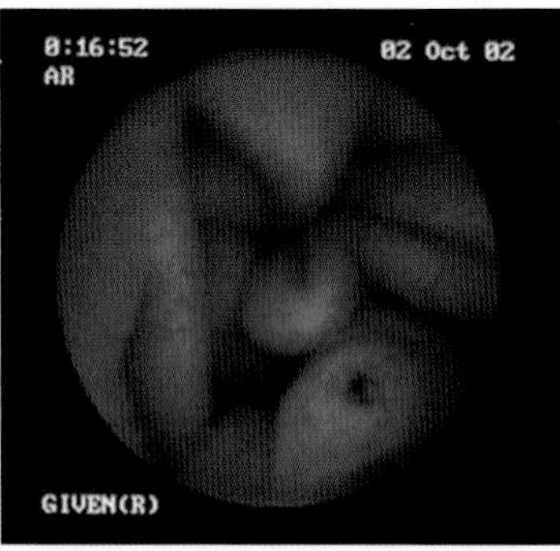

■ **Fig. 3.6** The inferior image quality of the Given capsule is notable, but the ampulla is still readily identifiable in the lower part of the image. Courtesy of Dr N Kalantzis.

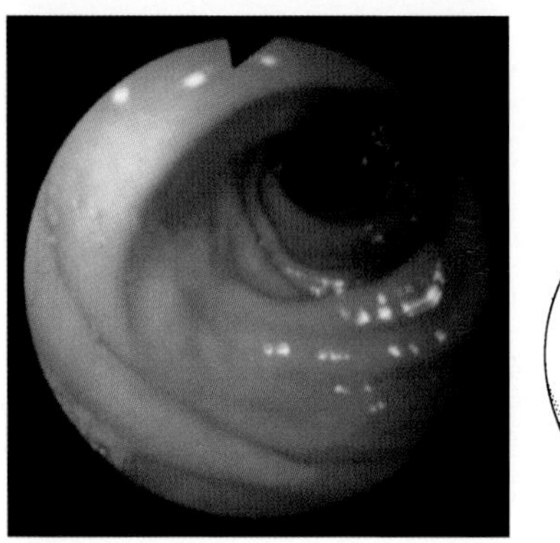

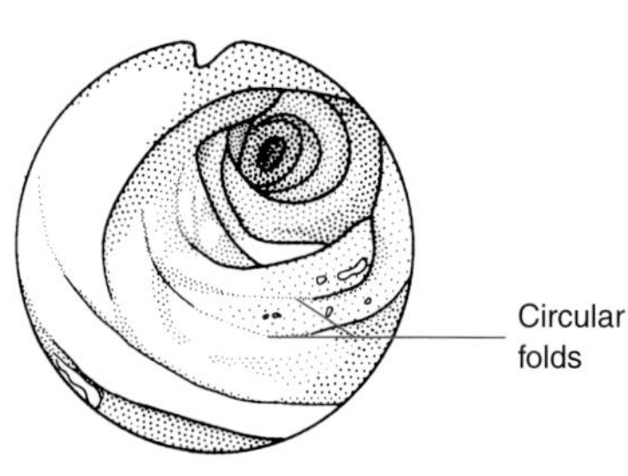

■ **Fig. 3.7** Endoscopic appearance of the second part of the duodenum: the beginning of the third part is seen in the distance.

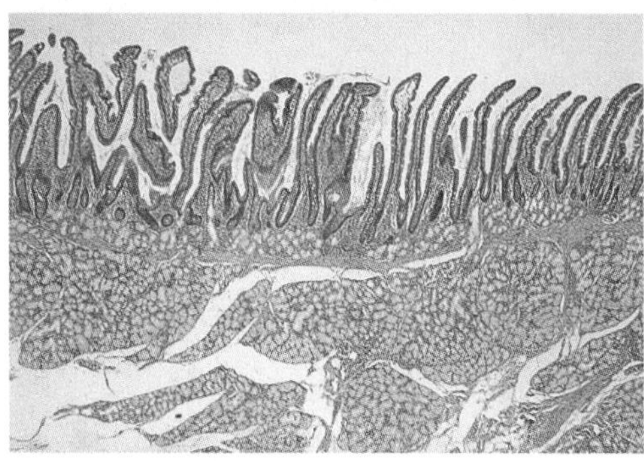

■ **Fig. 3.8** Microscopic appearance of the normal duodenum showing tall villi and mucin-producing Brunner's glands filling the submucosal and deep lamina propria.

The duodenal wall comprises mucosa, muscularis mucosae, and submucosa, within circular and longitudinal muscle coats (Fig. 3.8). The mucosa, in common with the rest of the small bowel, has tall villi, although, in general, duodenal villi are broader than those in the jejunum. Between the villi are the crypts of Lieberkühn, which dip down into the muscularis mucosae. There is a gradual maturation of cells from the crypt base to the tip of the villus. The surface epithelium of the villi and crypts bears a mixture of absorptive and goblet cells; the former have prominent microvilli on their luminal border. In the submucosa, and peculiar to the duodenum, are Brunner's glands. These mucus- and bicarbonate-secreting glands open into the crypts and are most numerous in the first part of the duodenum. Paneth cells and cells of the APUD system are also found within the crypts, and it is common for the muscularis mucosae to be somewhat disorganized around the glandular elements.

DUODENAL ULCER

The lesion most commonly affecting the duodenum is ulceration, and it is now known that both antral infection with *Helicobacter pylori* and the presence of gastric acid are virtual prerequisites. However, these two factors are not 'sufficient cause,' since the frequency of duodenal ulcer is less than would be predicted given the high prevalence of *H. pylori* (historically in the West and currently in the developing world) and the relative rarity of achlorhydria. Certain *H. pylori* strains (such as those expressing cagA) are more likely to cause disease, but this is not the full explanation. In the UK, males, who have a lifetime risk of duodenal ulcer of at least 10%, are more commonly affected than females. There is also a higher incidence in patients of blood group O, in non-secretors of blood group antigens and in individuals with high pepsinogen I levels. Smoking and drugs are important cofactors in the etiology, and drugs such as the non-steroidal anti-inflammatories are the commonest cause of duodenal ulcer in the absence of *H. pylori* infection. Many ulcer patients have exaggerated acid secretion in response to pentagastrin stimulation, and patients with the Zollinger–Ellison syndrome (the result of gastrin-producing neoplasia), who have gross acid hypersecretion, usually have multiple problematic duodenal ulcers.

The great majority of duodenal ulcers occur in the bulb, most commonly on the anterior wall, and they are almost never malignant. Barium studies readily show acute ulcers (Figs 3.9 and 3.10), but there can be difficulty in interpretation when a previously scarred duodenum is investigated (see Fig 3.26 for example). Endoscopy more easily makes the distinction between current ulceration with scarring, and old scarring alone (Figs 3.11–3.13), and presents the additional advantage of allowing sampling for *H. pylori* antritis. Although *H. pylori* is most readily detected in the gastric antrum (see Chapter 2), it is found in areas of gastric metaplasia in the duodenum when there is duodenal ulceration (Figs 3.14, 3.15; see also Fig. 3.38).

Ulcers at, or just distal to, the junction of the first and second parts of the duodenum are often termed post-bulbar ulcers. Because of their location such ulcers can be difficult to diagnose endoscopically and radiologically (Figs 3.16, 3.17), but recognition is important since they are less likely to be *H. pylori*-related. A variety of infections, and Crohn's disease (Fig. 3.18), may be responsible for

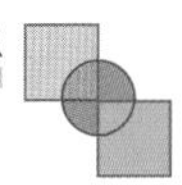

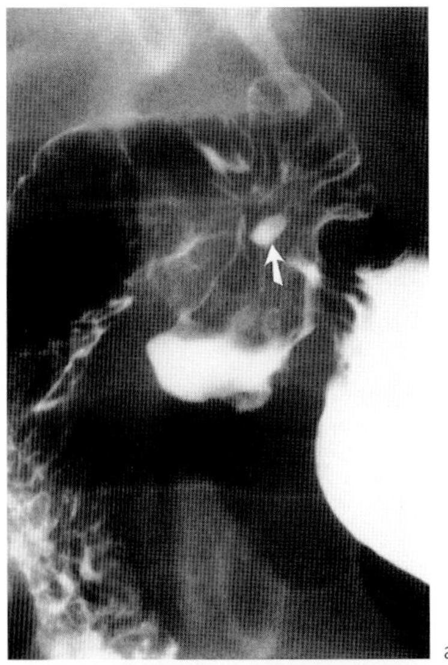

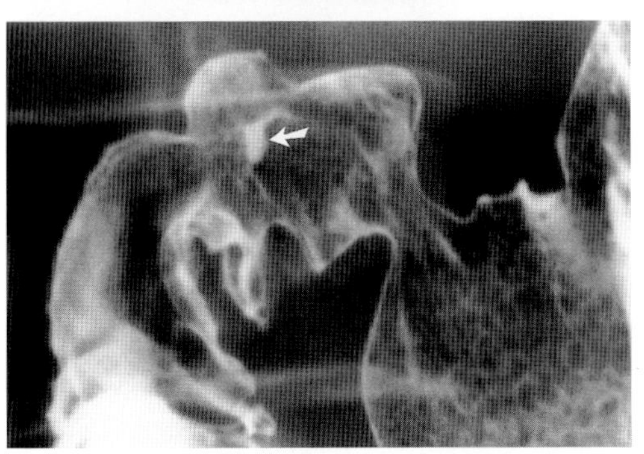

Fig. 3.9a, b Double-contrast barium studies showing duodenal ulcers (arrows) in two patients. Note radiating folds and deformity of adjacent bulb due to edema and spasm accompanying these ulcers. (Fig. 3.5a reproduced with permission from reference 1; Fig. 3.5b reproduced with permission from reference 2.)

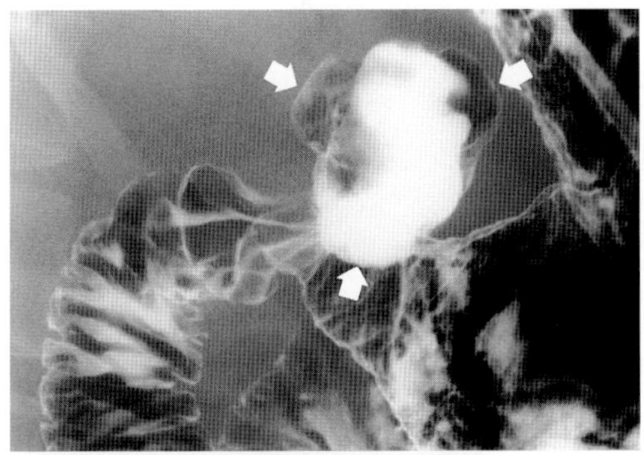

Fig. 3.10 Double-contrast barium study showing a giant duodenal ulcer as a large collection of barium (arrows) replacing the duodenal bulb. (Reproduced with permission from reference 1.)

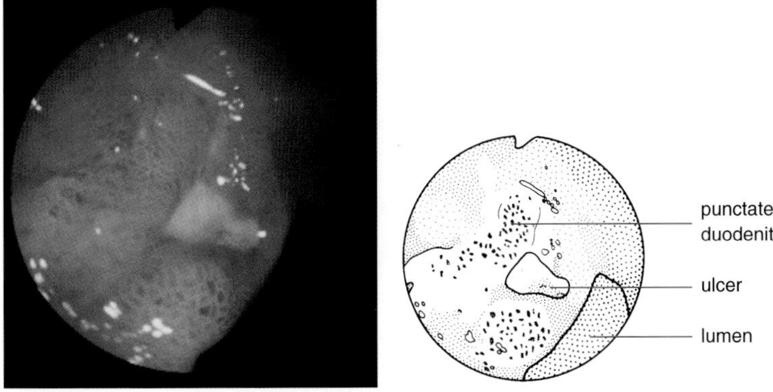

Fig. 3.11 Endoscopic appearance of acute duodenal ulcer with some associated duodenitis.

these ulcers, and consideration should again be given also to a diagnosis of Zollinger–Ellison syndrome. Endoscopic assessment and biopsy are always appropriate in these, in the non-healing bulbar ulcer and, to a lesser extent, when multiple bulbar ulcers are found (Figs 3.19, 3.20).

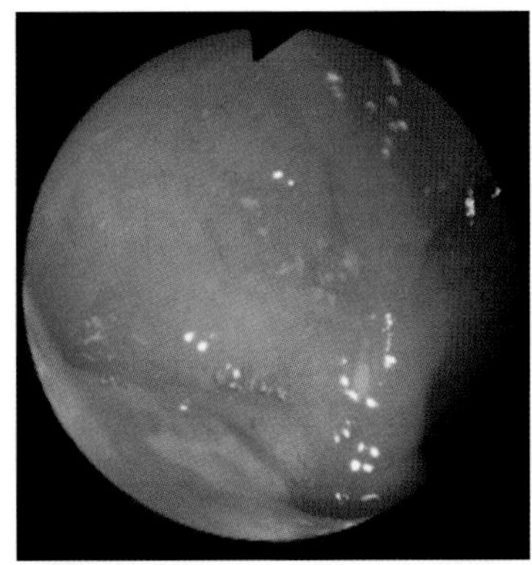

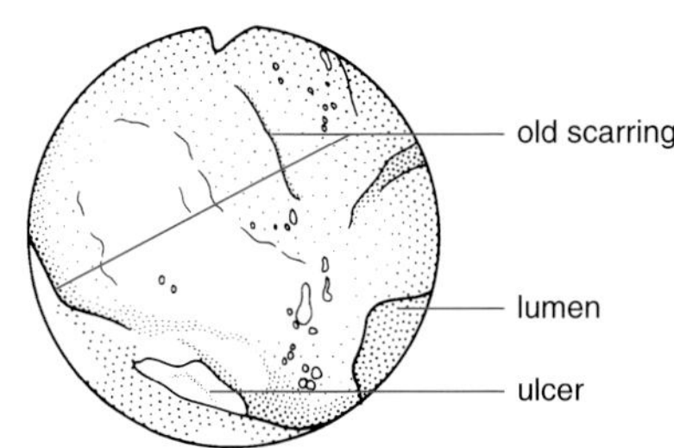

Fig. 3.12 Endoscopic view of a duodenal ulcer in a badly scarred duodenal bulb; a prior barium examination had shown the deformity but was inconclusive as to current ulceration.

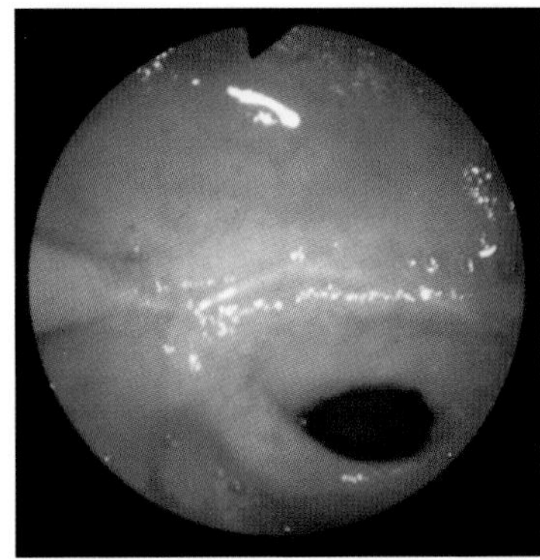

Fig. 3.13 Endoscopic view showing scarring and retraction after the healing of a duodenal ulcer; there is no current ulceration.

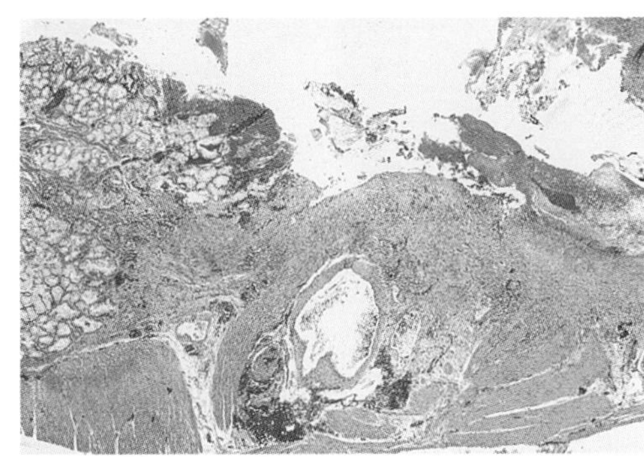

Fig. 3.14 Microscopic appearance of a duodenal ulcer extending deep into the submucosa. Fibrosis and hemorrhage are seen around a large muscular vein in the ulcer base (center).

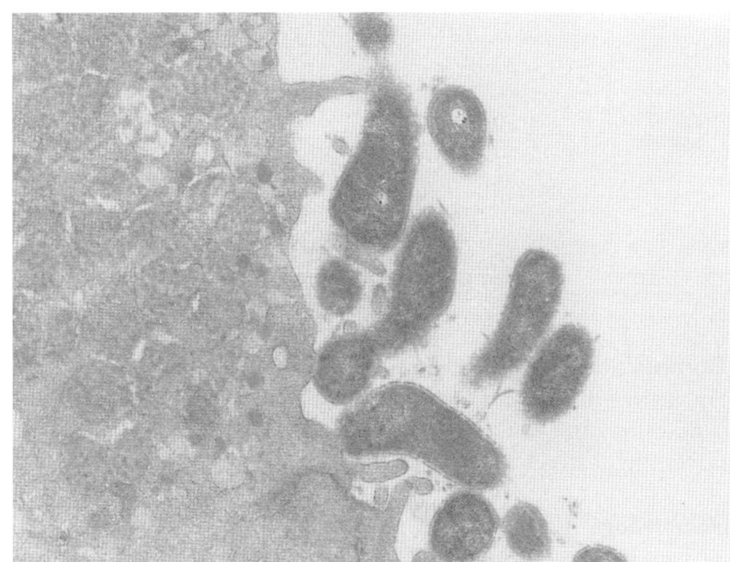

Fig. 3.15 Transmission electron micrograph showing duodenal gastric metaplasia. *H. pylori* are adhering to the mucosa via attachment pedestals (x 15 000). Courtesy of Dr M.M. Walker and Dr R. Logan.

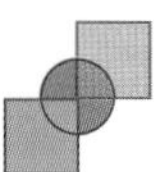

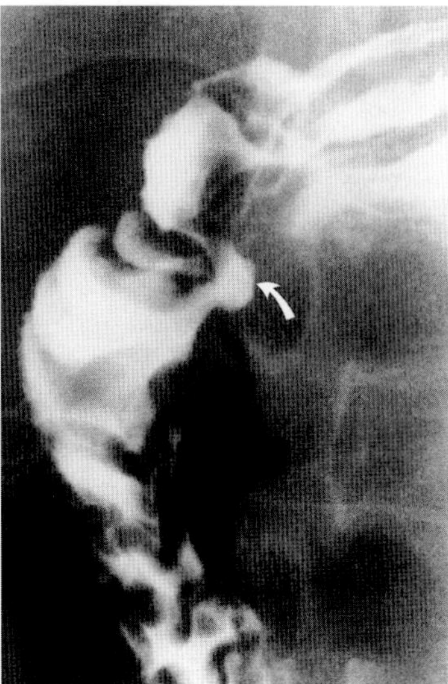

Fig. 3.16 Double-contrast barium study showing a post-bulbar duodenal ulcer (arrow) on the medial wall of the proximal descending duodenum just above the level of the papilla. Note radiating folds and an associated indentation of the lateral wall.

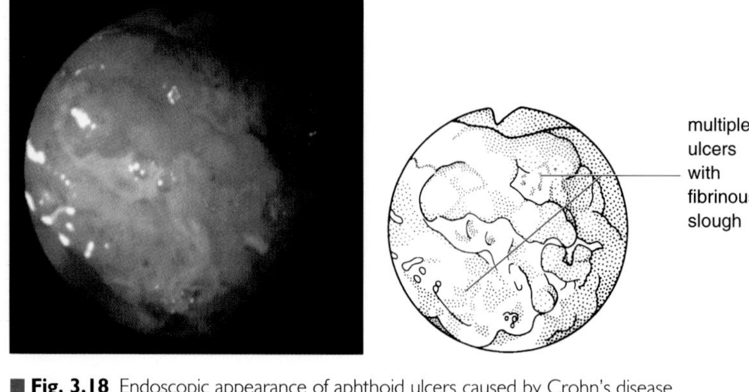

Fig. 3.18 Endoscopic appearance of aphthoid ulcers caused by Crohn's disease (confirmed histologically).

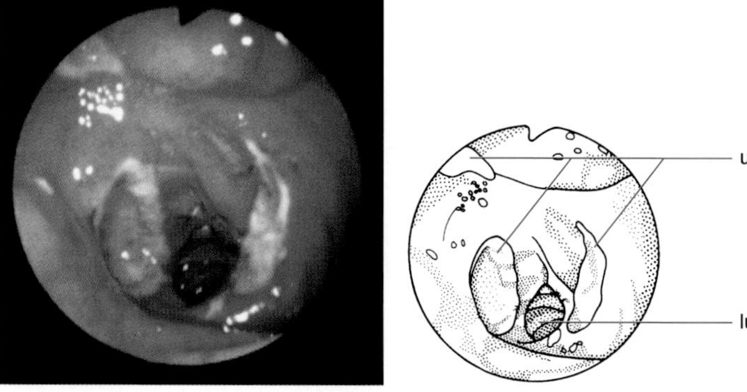

Fig. 3.19 Endoscopic appearance of multiple duodenal ulcers. The 'kissing' ulcers seen here were not in fact from Zollinger–Ellison syndrome but correctly prompted an estimation of the fasting gastrin.

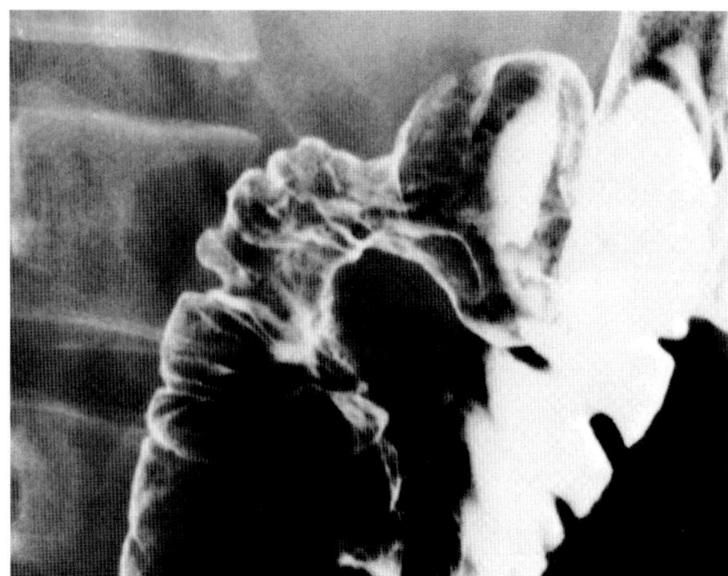

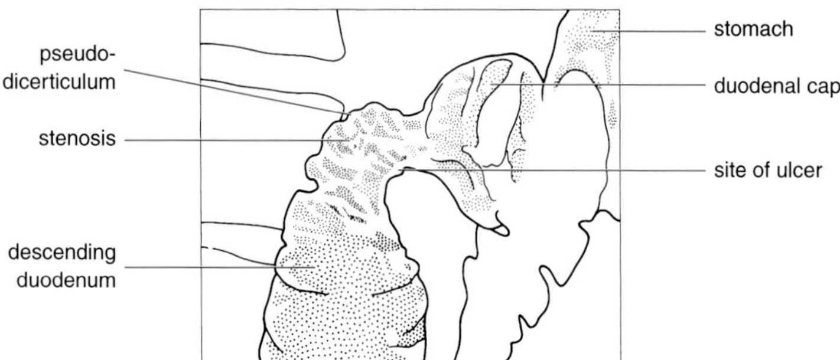

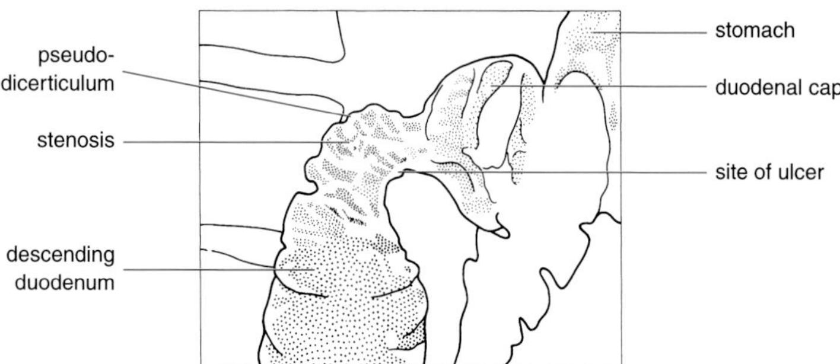

Fig. 3.17 Hypotonic duodenogram of a post-bulbar ulcer. The ulcer itself is difficult to see, although the deformity, with stenosis and some pseudo-diverticular change, is evident.

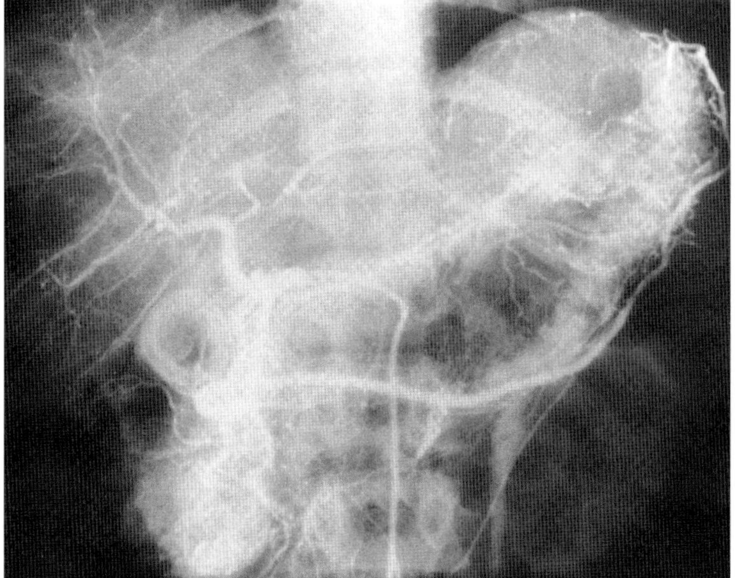

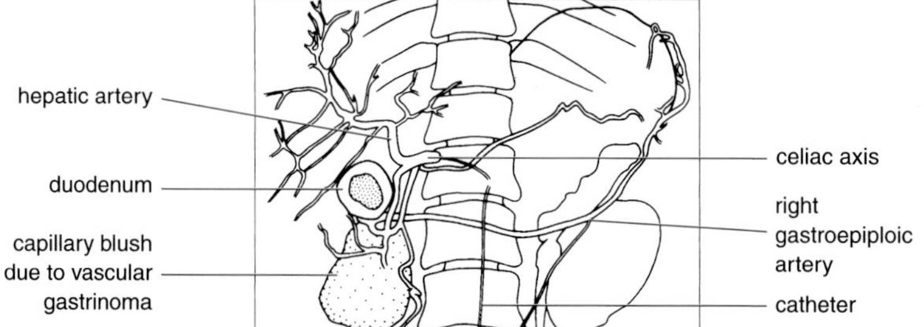

Fig. 3.20 Celiac axis angiography in a patient with Zollinger–Ellison syndrome; the gastrinoma is demonstrated, appearing as a capillary blush.

Complications of duodenal ulcer

The main complications of duodenal ulcer disease are hemorrhage, perforation, and stenotic gastric outlet obstruction; each may be a presenting feature.

Hemorrhage

Bleeding occurs at some time in up to a fifth of duodenal ulcer patients. It is most commonly a dramatic event with sudden onset of hematemesis and melena, although insidious bleeding may present with iron-deficiency anemia. Endoscopy is the preferred means of diagnosis but

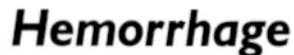

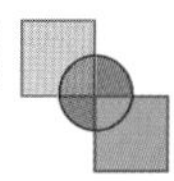

may be difficult because of intraluminal blood. The use of a washing jet is then particularly helpful. Stigmata of recent hemorrhage, such as adherent clot (Figs 3.21, 3.22) or a visible vessel in the base of the ulcer (Figs 3.23, 3.24), indicate an increased risk of continuing or recurrent bleeding. The importance of obtaining an early and accurate diagnosis is emphasized by the increasing recognition that, in patients with stigmatic ulcers, endoscopic intervention (using thermal therapies such as heater probes, diathermy, laser or argon plasma coagulation, or metal clips or simple infiltration with adrenaline/epinephrine) has a beneficial effect on prognosis.

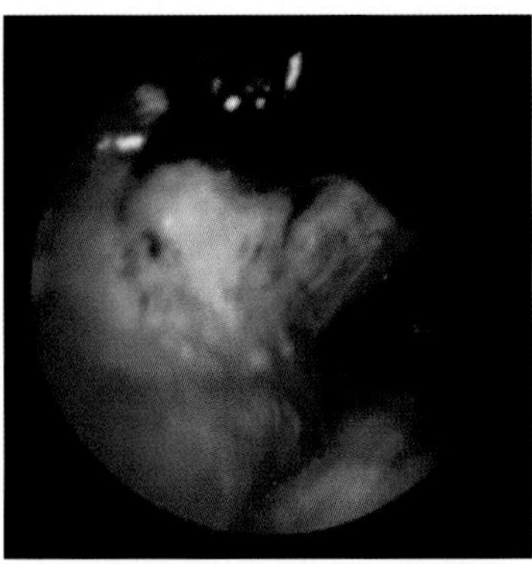

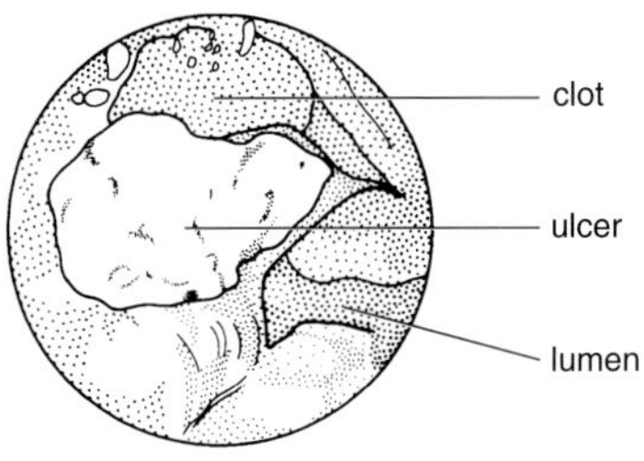

Fig. 3.21 Endoscopic view of a duodenal ulcer which has clot adherent to the base, one of the stigmata of recent bleeding which indicates a high risk of recurrent hemorrhage.

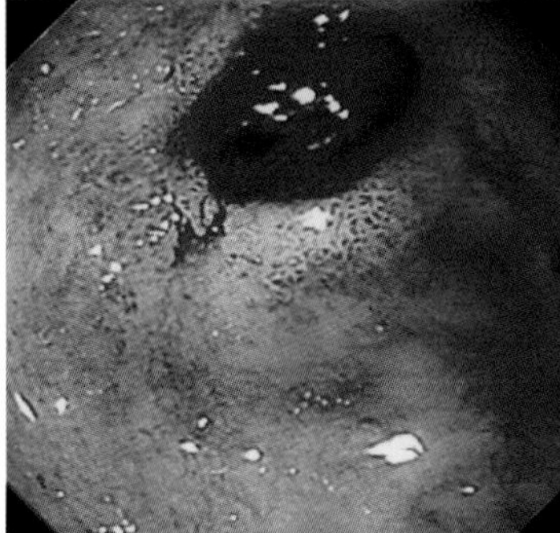

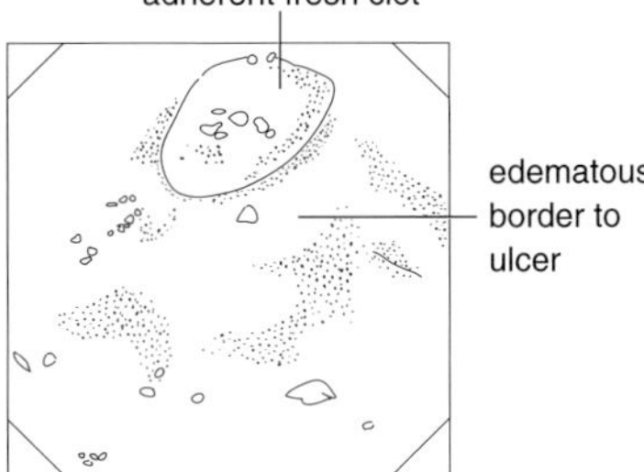

Fig. 3.22 Another example of adherent clot, in this case almost obscuring the underlying ulcer.

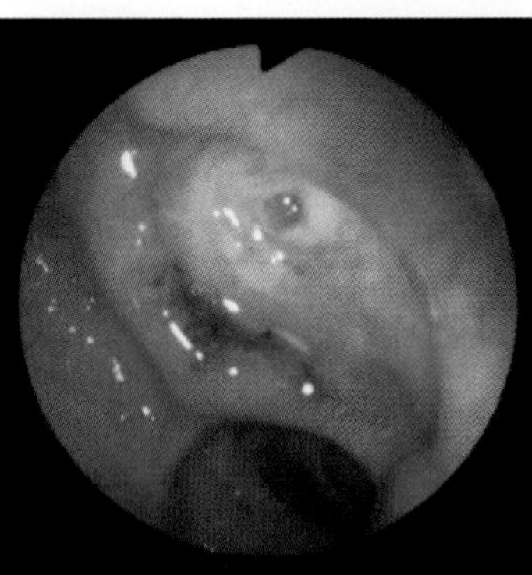

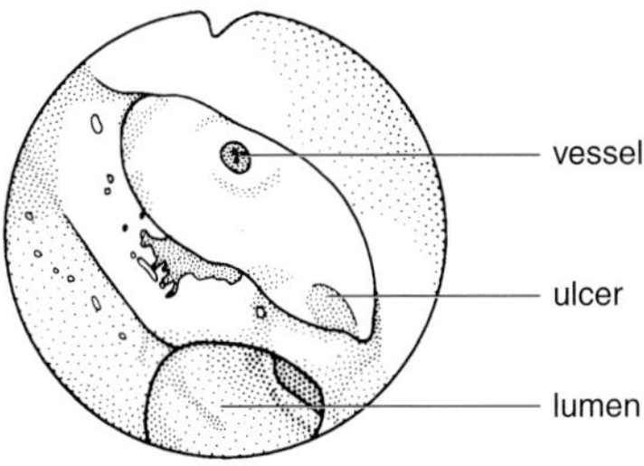

Fig. 3.23 Duodenal ulcer with a protruding vessel – again stigmatic for high risk of re-bleeding.

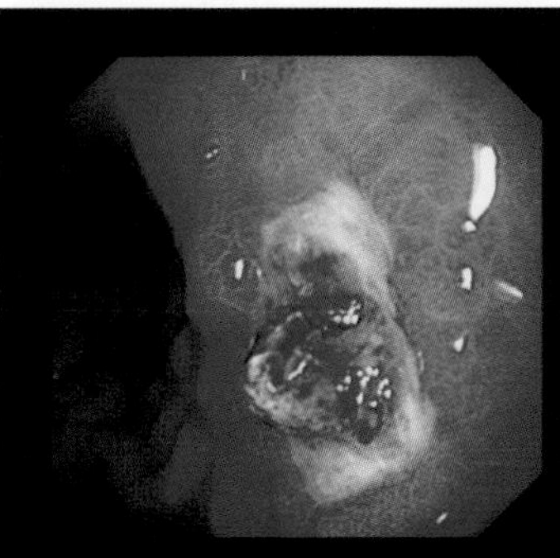

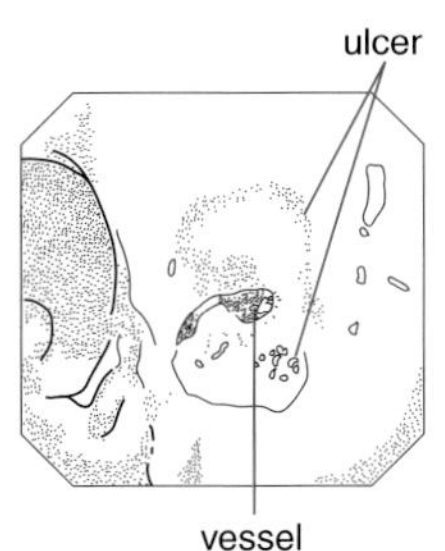

Fig. 3.24 Large visible vessel in the center of a posterior wall duodenal ulcer.

Perforation

Ulceration extending through the duodenal wall results in free perforation or, less often, in the penetration of an adjacent viscus. Anterior perforation usually leads to sudden onset of severe abdominal pain followed by signs of peritonitis. An erect plain radiograph helpfully confirms subphrenic air (Fig. 3.25). Penetration more usually follows a long history of symptoms, with a more or less dramatic deterioration at the time of penetration. The pancreas is most often affected and, depending upon the site and extent of the penetration, pancreatitis or obstructive jaundice may result.

Gastric outlet obstruction (pyloric stenosis)

Gastric outlet obstruction is a less common complication of duodenal ulceration, and most patients have a long prior history. Scarring and narrowing of the pyloric canal and/or duodenal cap (Figs 3.26, 3.27) may eventually progress to complete obstruction with vomiting, which may be projectile and often contains stale food. Mild features of pyloric stenosis are not infrequently encountered when an acute ulcer causes marked inflammatory edema. In severe cases, metabolic alkalosis, an audible succussion splash more than 4 hours after eating, and visible gastric peristalsis are seen. The diagnosis may be strongly suggested on the plain radiograph (Fig. 3.28). Contrast examination

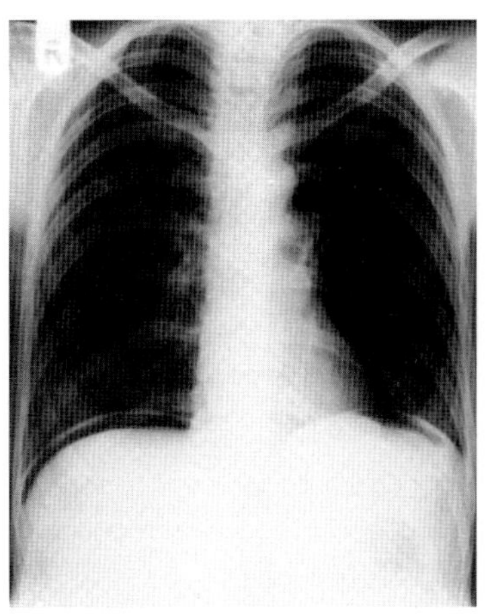

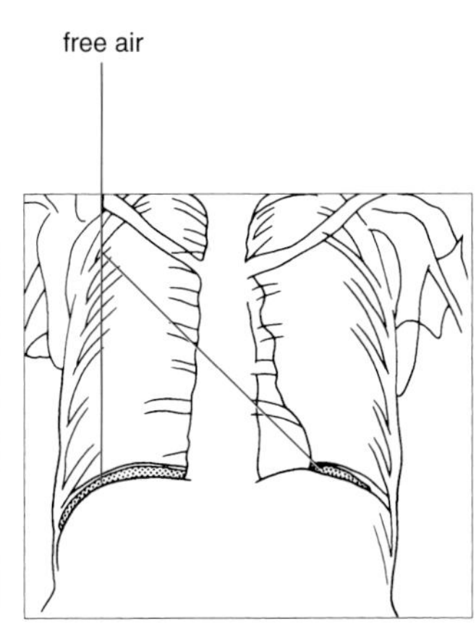

Fig. 3.25 Erect radiograph showing free gas under both hemi-diaphragms as a result of a perforated duodenal ulcer. (Similar features may of course be seen with a perforated gastric ulcer.)

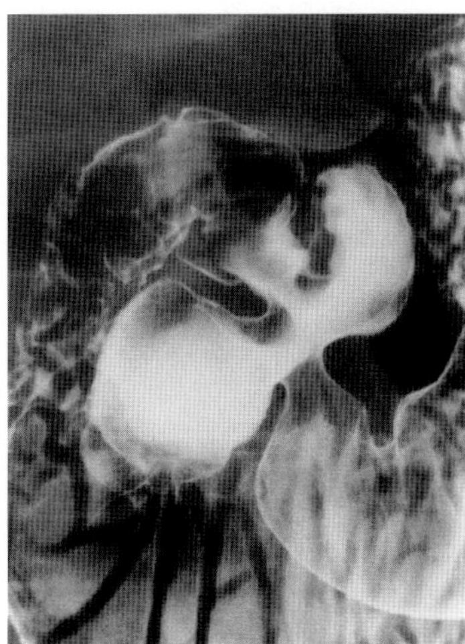

Fig. 3.26 Double-contrast barium study showing marked narrowing and deformity of the duodenal bulb due to scarring from previous peptic ulcer disease.

(Fig. 3.29) documents the site of obstruction but not necessarily the cause. Endoscopy carries a greater risk of pulmonary aspiration, but, following careful washout, may not only confirm the diagnosis (Fig. 3.30), but also allow therapeutic intervention using dilating balloons. Antral or proximal duodenal neoplasia (see Chapter 2, and below) or, more rarely, adult hypertrophic pyloric stenosis (see Chapter 2), are rarely responsible.

DUODENITIS

Duodenitis may be associated with duodenal ulcer disease (see Fig. 3.11), but its pathological significance remains uncertain; mild cases are often found incidentally (Fig. 3.31). Endoscopically, the appearances are those of hyperemia and congestion (Fig. 3.32), progressing in more severe cases to irregularity with superficial erosions (Fig. 3.33). Characteristic focal erosions, which really represent aphthous ulcers, may sometimes be seen in the duodenum in Crohn's disease (Fig. 3.34).

The histology of duodenitis, likewise, encompasses a spectrum of disease severity based on the inflammatory cell infiltrate and the degree of villous abnormality (Figs 3.35–3.37). The association of *H. pylori* infection and duodenal ulcer may depend on the prior development of gastric metaplasia within the duodenal cap (see Figs 3.14, 3.15, 3.38).

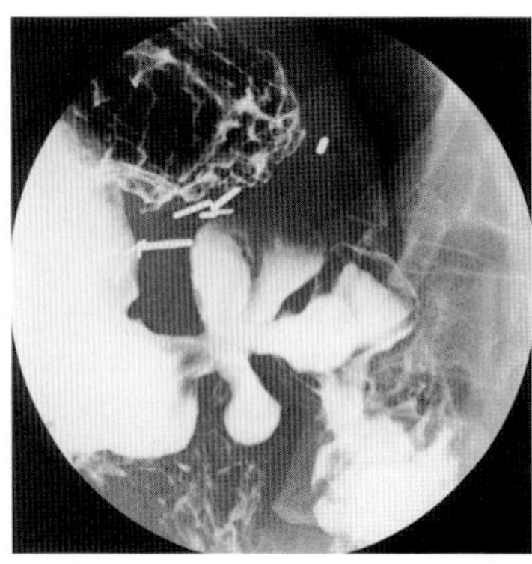

Fig. 3.27 Double-contrast barium study showing a clover leaf deformity of the duodenal bulb with multiple out-pouchings or pseudo-diverticula due to severe scarring from previous peptic ulcer disease. (Reproduced with permission from reference 1.)

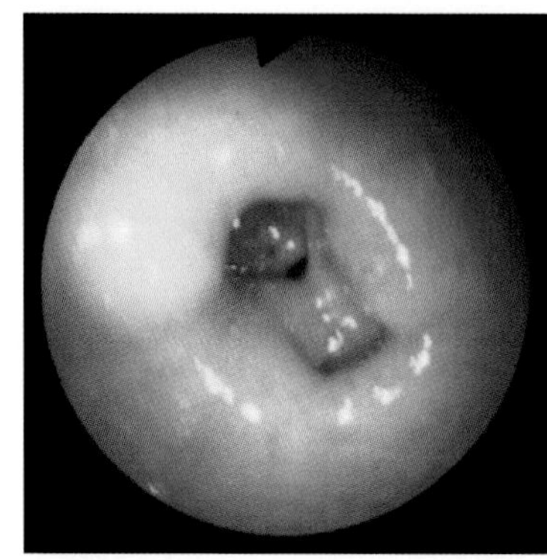

Fig. 3.30 A virtually pinhole stricture beyond the pylorus – the result of previous duodenal ulceration.

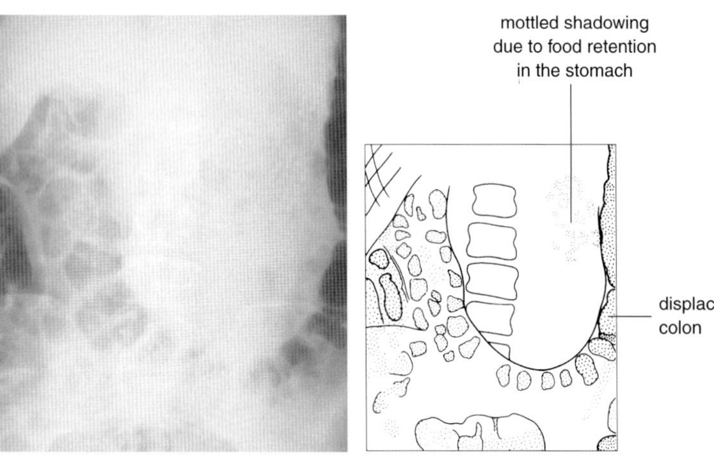

Fig. 3.28 Plain abdominal radiograph showing gross enlargement of the stomach secondary to a stenotic chronic duodenal ulcer causing gastric outlet obstruction. Note how the transverse colon is displaced anteriorly by the distended stomach.

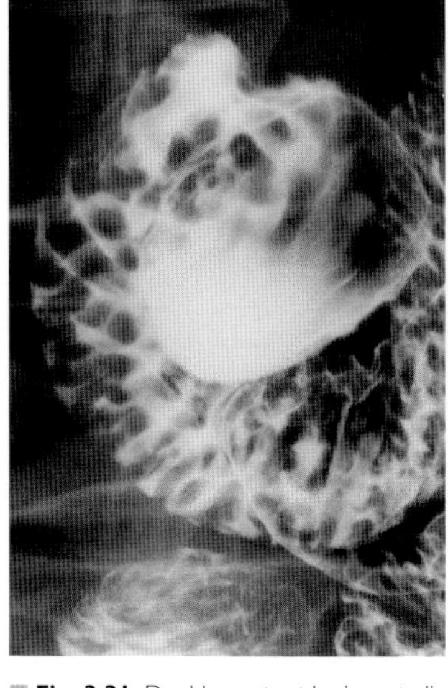

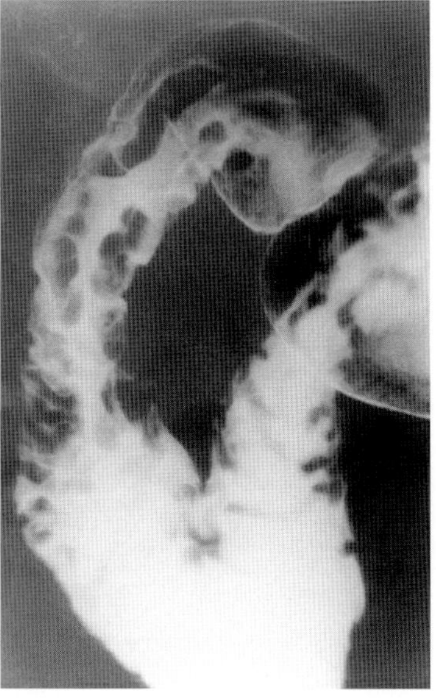

Fig. 3.31 Double-contrast barium studies showing thickened, nodular folds in the proximal duodenum in two patients with duodenitis.

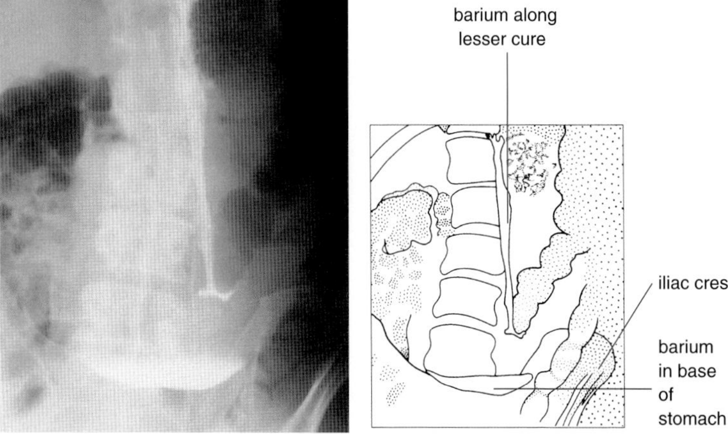

Fig. 3.29 The appearance after a mouthful of barium was given to the patient shown in Fig. 3.28. Note the pool of barium at the base of the stomach, and its proximity to the iliac crest.

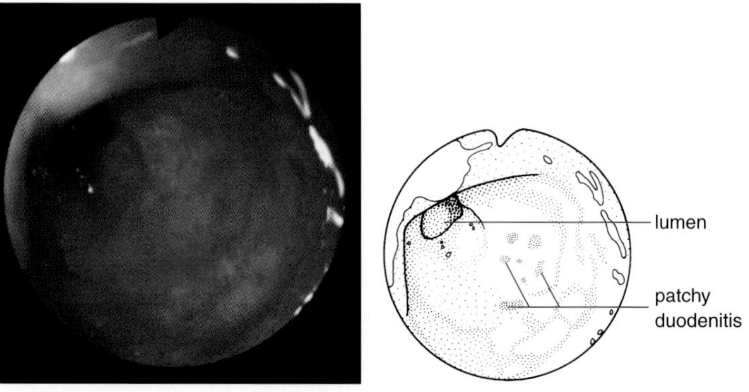

Fig. 3.32 Endoscopic appearance of patchy mild duodenitis.

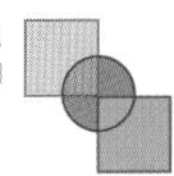

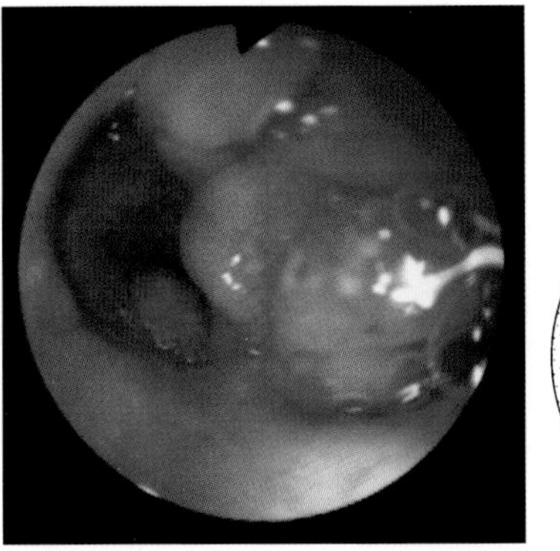

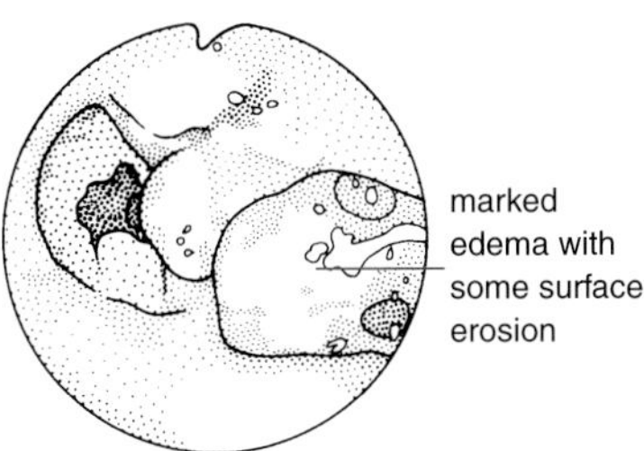

■ **Fig. 3.33** Endoscopic appearance of severe erosive duodenitis.

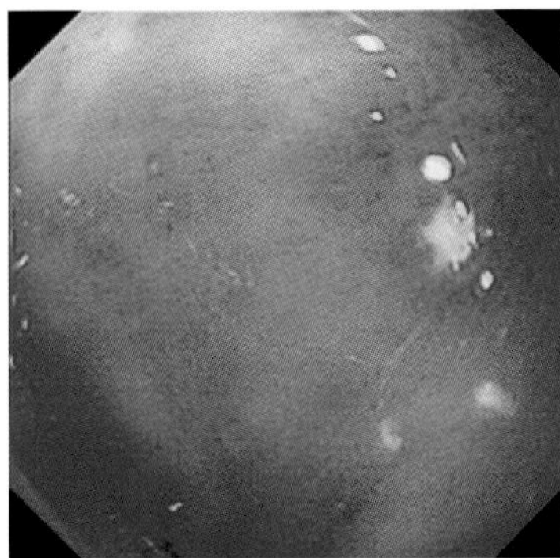

■ **Fig. 3.34** Focal erosion in the duodenal cap in Crohn's disease (aphthous ulceration).

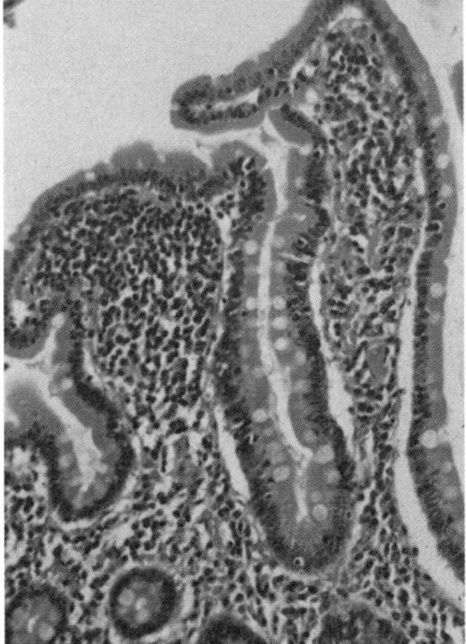

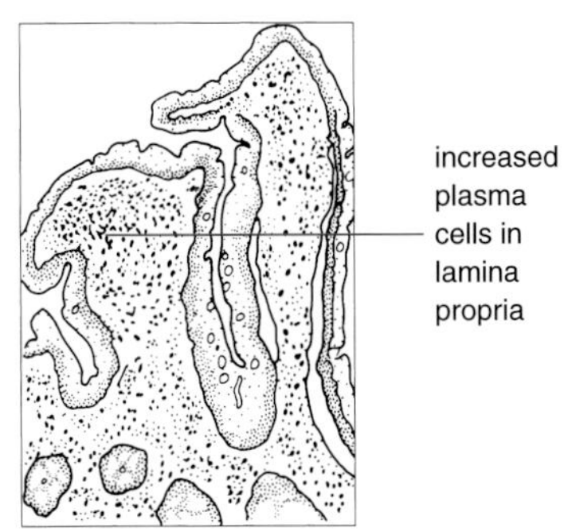

■ **Fig. 3.35** Histological appearance of mild duodenitis showing increased numbers of plasma cells in the lamina propria. H&E stain (x 125).

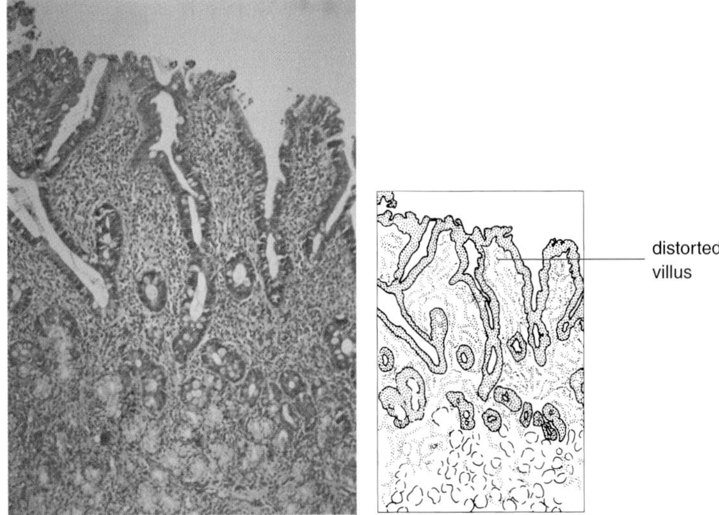

■ **Fig. 3.36** Histological appearance of moderate duodenitis in which there is some villous distortion. H&E stain (x 50).

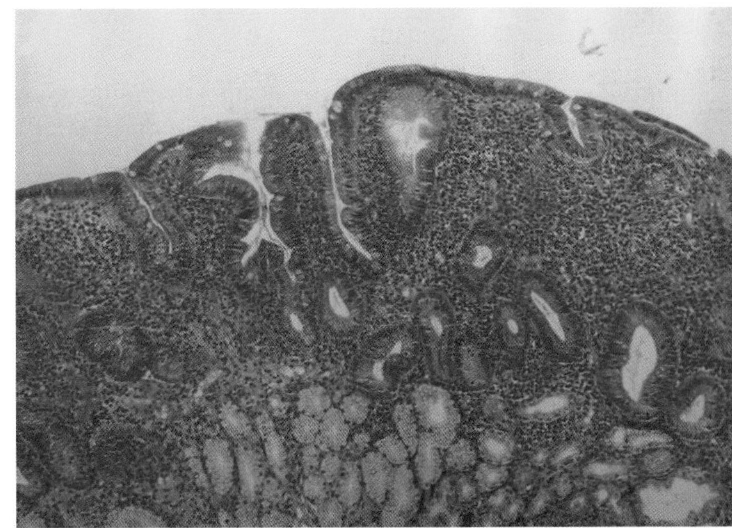

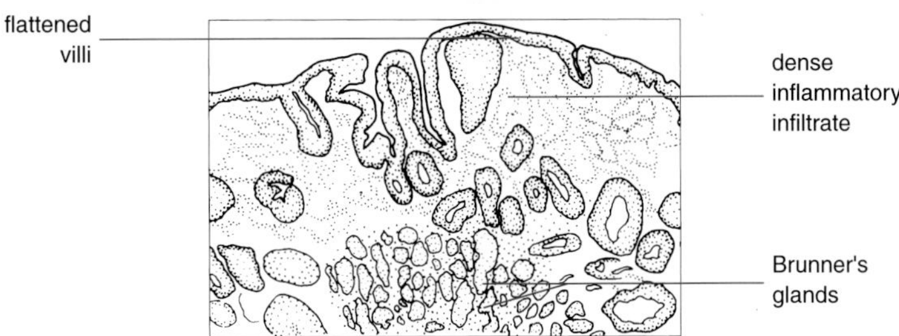

■ **Fig. 3.37** Histological appearance of more severe duodenitis in which the villous pattern is lost; subtotal villous atrophy is associated with a heavy inflammatory cell infiltrate in the lamina propria. H&E stain (x 70).

DUODENAL DIVERTICULA

Duodenal diverticula may be acquired or congenital. Acquired diverticula in the proximal duodenum are usually the result of scarring and adhesions from peptic ulcer disease (Fig. 3.39). Congenital examples typically arise from the second part of the duodenum (Fig. 3.40); the ampulla of Vater is usually closely adjacent, and may lie within the diverticulum (Fig. 3.41). There is a definite but unexplained association between common bile duct stones and duodenal diverticula. Stasis within large and/or multiple diverticula of the duodenum or more distal small intestine can result in bacterial overgrowth (see Chapter 4).

DUODENAL POLYPS AND TUMORS

A variety of polyps and polypoid tumors arise in the duodenum; all are uncommon. Polyps occur very much more frequently in two familial conditions considered in more detail elsewhere: familial adenomatous polyposis (FAP) (Figs 3.42, 3.43), and Peutz–Jeghers syndrome (see Chapters 4 and 7). In the case of FAP, and with better management of the colonic cancer risk, duodenal neoplasia has become a major cause of morbidity and death. Most FAP patients have duodenal adenomas by the age of 35, and these may progress to carcinoma (see below).

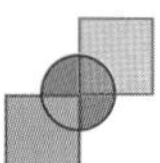

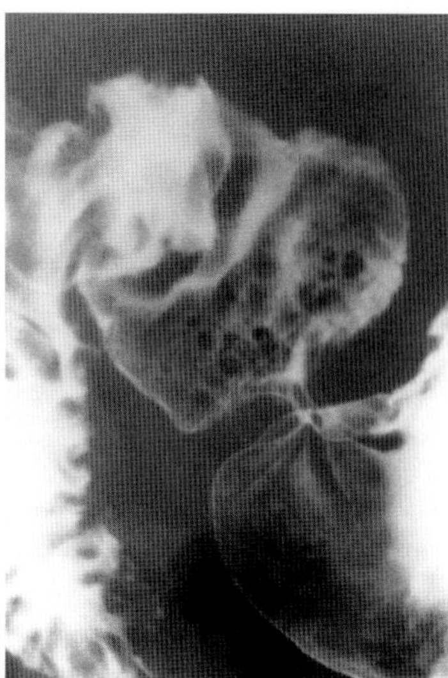

■ **Fig. 3.38** Double-contrast barium study showing heterotopic gastric mucosa as discrete, angulated filling defects near the base of the duodenal bulb.

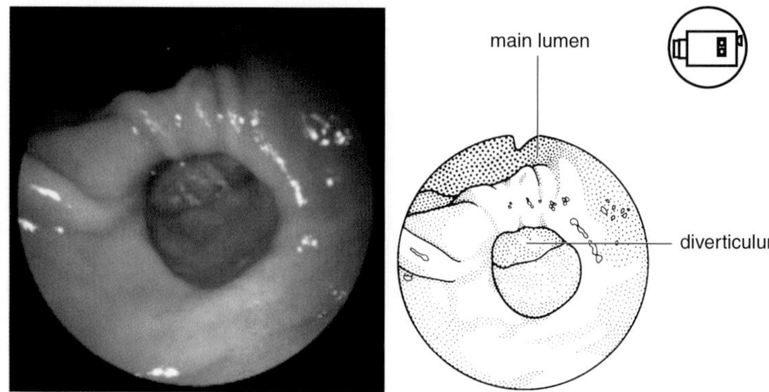

■ **Fig. 3.41** Endoscopic appearance of a peri-ampullary diverticulum. The ampulla in this case opens just inside the diverticulum.

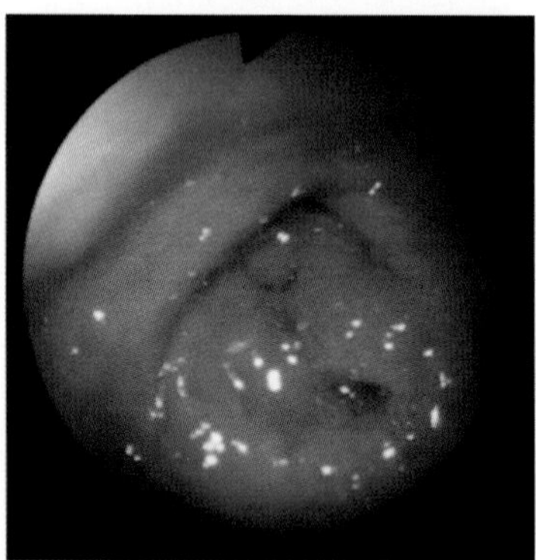

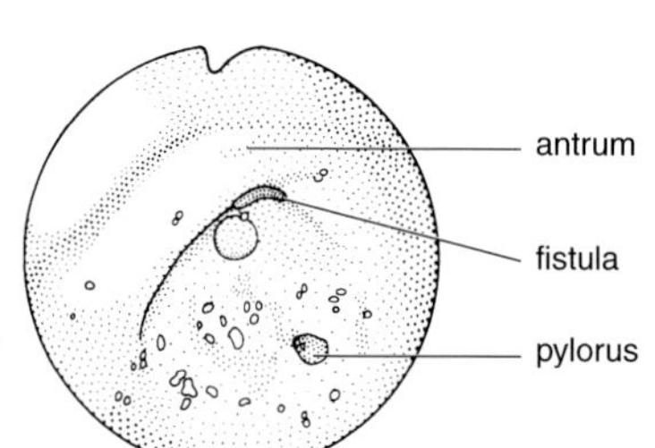

■ **Fig. 3.39** Endoscopic appearance of a gastro-duodenal fistula and diverticulum resulting from a previous penetrating antral ulcer. This appearance is sometimes described as the 'double pylorus'.

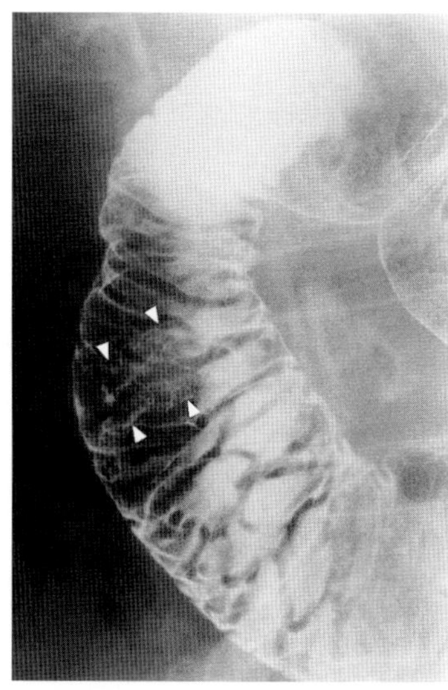

■ **Fig. 3.42** Double-contrast barium study showing a subtle villous tumor as a discrete polypoid mass (arrowheads) with a reticulo-nodular surface due to trapping of barium in the interstices of the lesion. (Reproduced with permission from reference 2.)

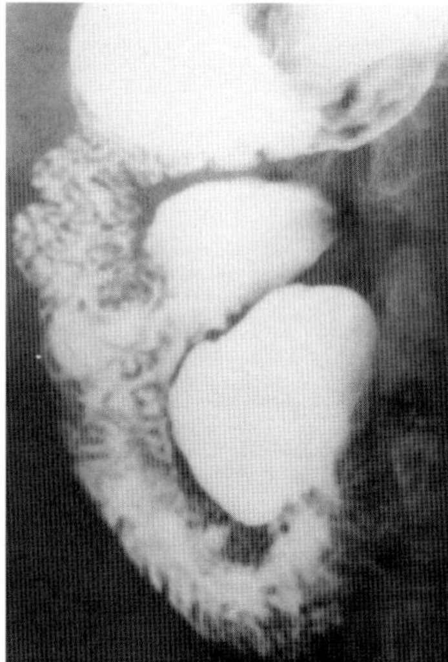

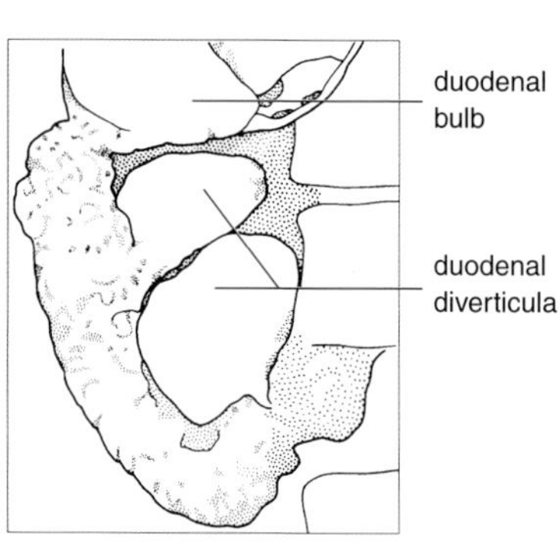

■ **Fig. 3.40** Barium meal showing two large duodenal diverticulae arising from the medial border of the second part of the duodenum.

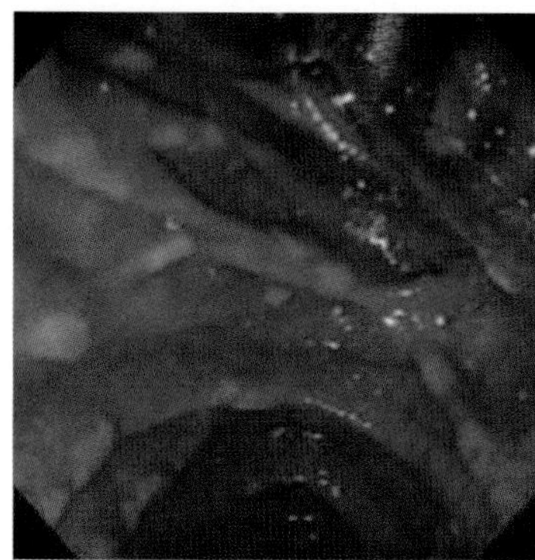

■ **Fig. 3.43** Endoscopic appearances of the flat mucosal lesions of early adenomas in the duodenum of FAP.

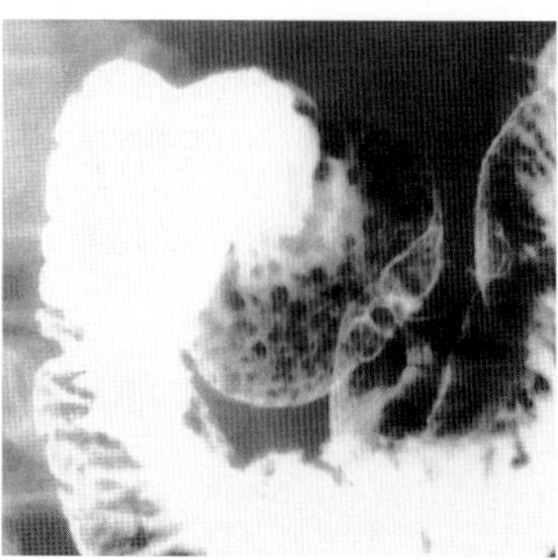

■ **Fig. 3.44** Double-contrast barium study showing tiny, round nodules in the duodenal bulb due to Brunner's gland hyperplasia. Lymphoid hyperplasia of the duodenum could produce identical findings (see Fig. 3.45). (Reproduced with permission from reference 2.)

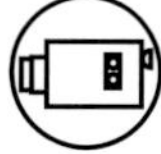

Brunner's gland hyperplasia may be responsible for an apparently polypoidal proximal duodenum on barium meal or at endoscopy (Fig. 3.44). Lymphoid hyperplasia has some similar features but generally exhibits smaller smooth nodules of very even size (Fig. 3.45). Correct recognition is valuable, both conditions being of a harmless nature.

Gastrointestinal stromal tumors (including lipomata and leiomyomas), and non-familial adenomas may also present as polyps, which occasionally bleed or cause obstruction of the duodenum or bile duct. Although barium meal readily demonstrates them, endoscopy is preferred as it allows both histological assessment and removal (Figs 3.46, 3.47). Formal resection will still sometimes be necessary in the larger and more sessile lesion that is beyond the limits for safe endoscopic mucosal resection (Figs 3.48, 3.49).

The frequency of duodenal carcinoma is low, but is greatly overrepresented in FAP (see Chapter 7) in which patients have a lifetime risk of no less than 25% of developing duodenal carcinoma. Surveillance upper gastrointestinal endoscopy is warranted.

Lymphoma rarely affects the duodenum in isolation (see Chapter 4) but produces a characteristic lobulated pattern on barium meal (Fig. 3.50). Extrinsic 'bulging' into the duodenum from an impacted common bile duct stone (Fig. 3.51) can usually be correctly interpreted from the clinical context, but confusion with a submucosal tumor may only be resolved by additional imaging (CT, MRI or endoscopic retrograde cholangiopancreatography (ERCP)) (see Chapter 13). Ampullary carcinoma is considered in Chapter 9.

VASCULAR DISEASE AFFECTING THE DUODENUM

By far the most common cause of duodenal bleeding is hemorrhage from peptic ulceration, but the multiple telangiectasiae of Osler–Weber–Rendu syndrome (Fig. 3.52; see also Chapter 4), and frank hemangiomata (Fig. 3.53) may also be responsible. Although duodenal varices may be seen in patients with portal hypertension (Fig. 3.54), it is unusual for significant hemorrhage to result.

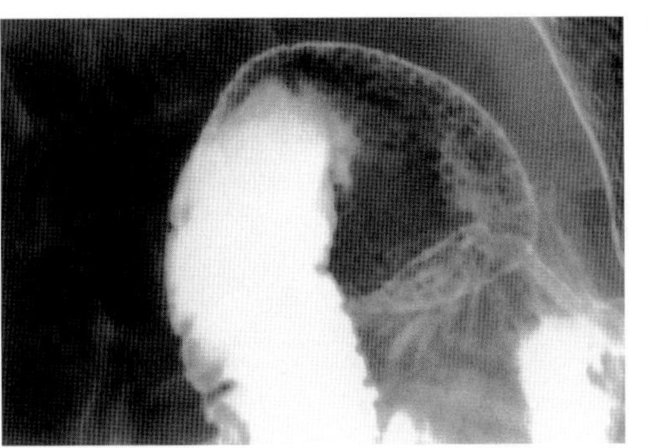

Fig. 3.45 Double-contrast barium study showing innumerable, tiny, round nodules in the duodenal bulb due to lymphoid hyperplasia. Brunner's gland hyperplasia could produce identical findings (see Fig. 3.44). (Reproduced with permission from reference 2.)

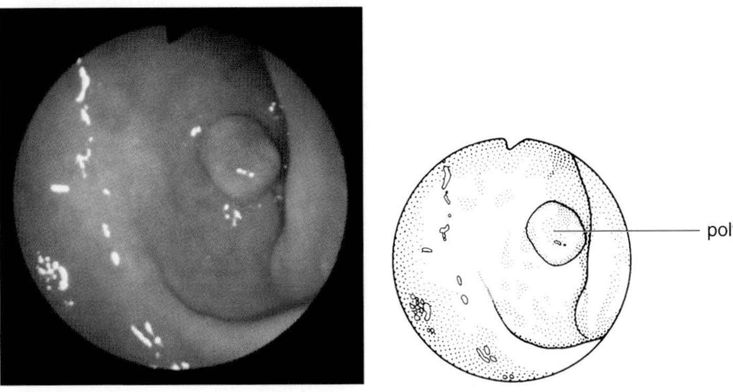

Fig. 3.46 Endoscopic appearance of a duodenal hyperplastic polyp.

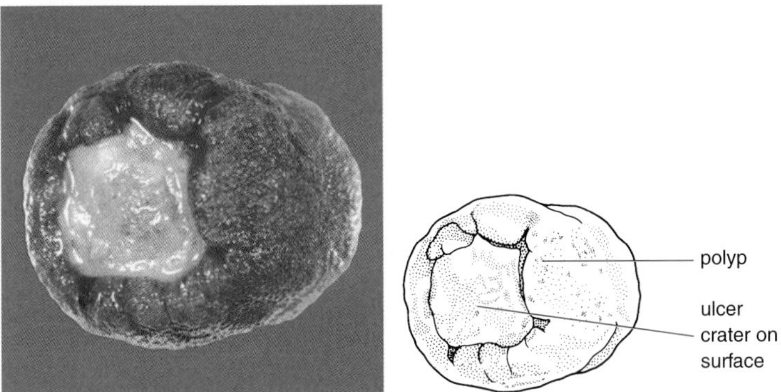

Fig. 3.47 Macroscopic appearance of a polyp removed from the duodenum by snare electrocautery. The ulcerated surface of the polyp which had previously been responsible for significant hemorrhage is demonstrated (the stalk is on the opposite aspect and is not seen).

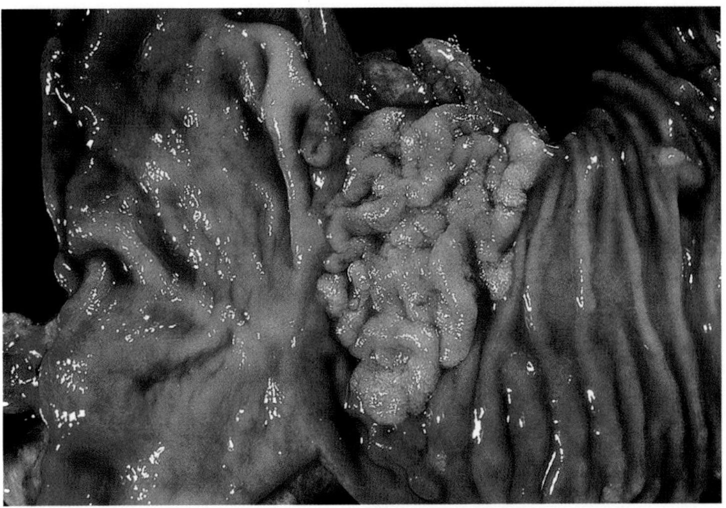

Fig. 3.48 Macroscopic view of a villous adenoma of the proximal duodenum showing a pale, raised cerebriform gross appearance.

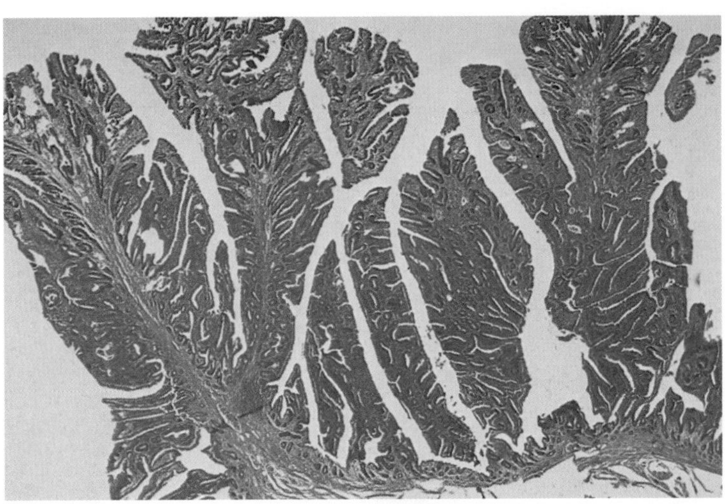

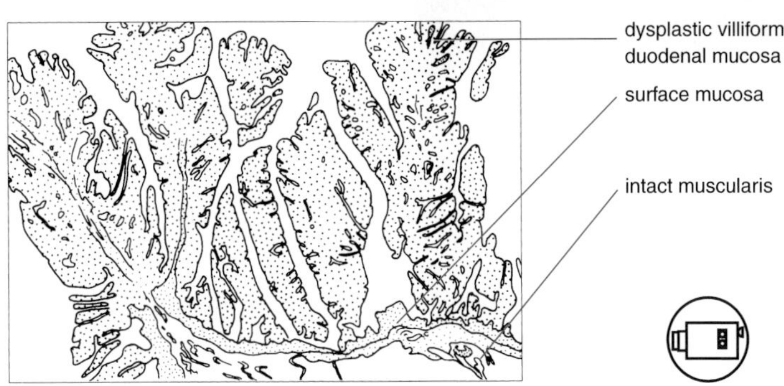

Fig. 3.49 Histological appearance of a villous adenoma in the duodenum showing fronds of dysplastic mucosa but no invasion. H&E stain (x 30).

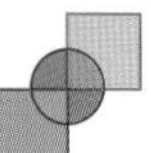

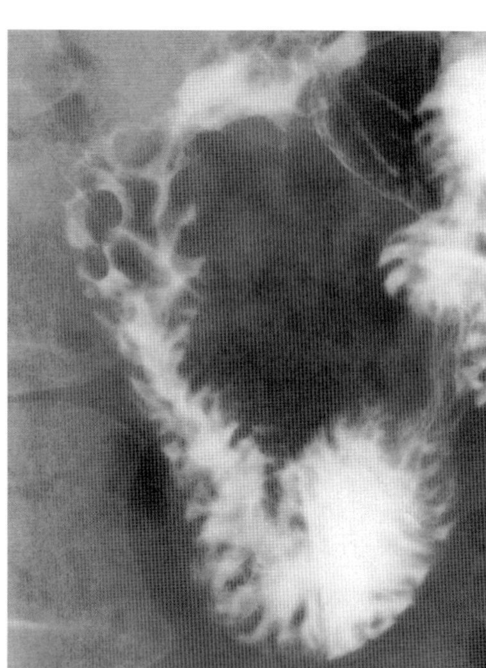

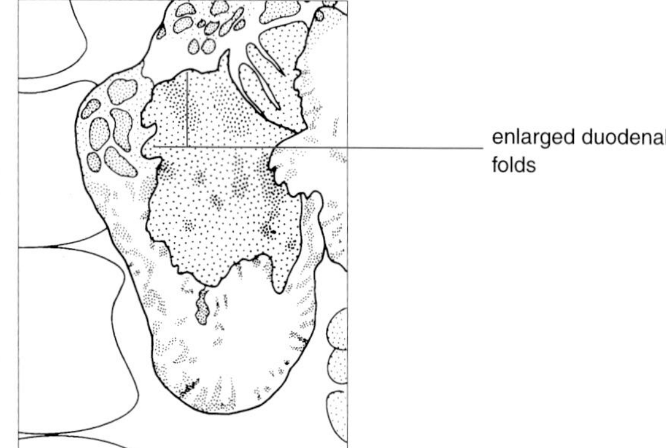

■ **Fig. 3.50** Characteristic appearance of duodenal lymphoma on barium contrast study.

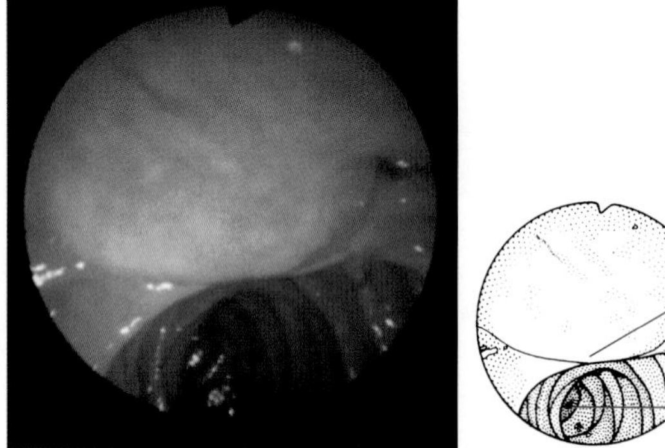

■ **Fig. 3.51** The endoscopic appearance when a dilated common bile duct bulges into the duodenum: in this case the result of a large common bile duct stone.

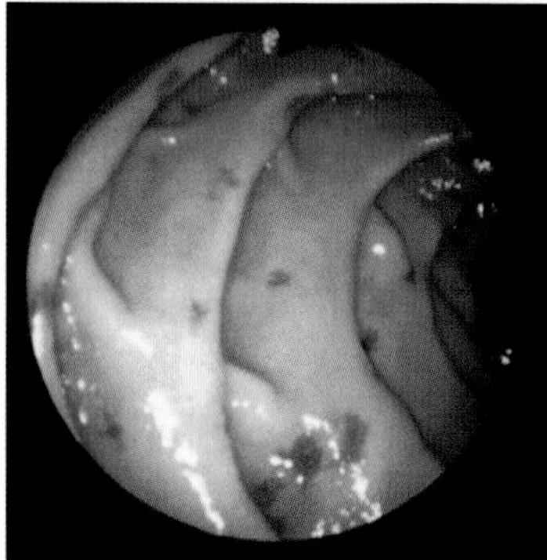

■ **Fig. 3.52** The endoscopic appearances of multiple telangiectasiae in a patient with Osler–Weber–Rendu syndrome involving the duodenum.

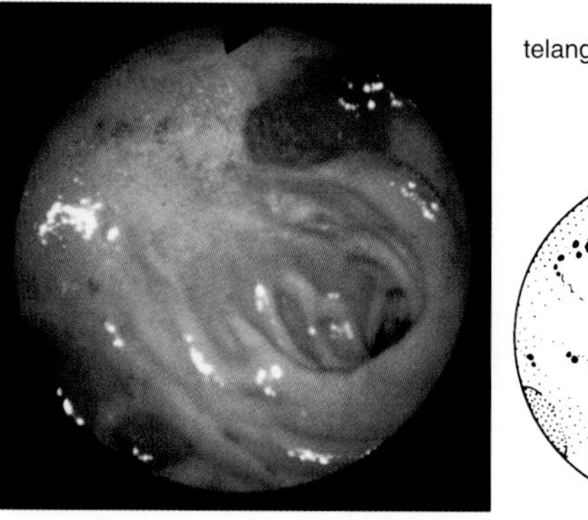

■ **Fig. 3.53** Endoscopic appearance of hemorrhagic duodenal hemangiomata.

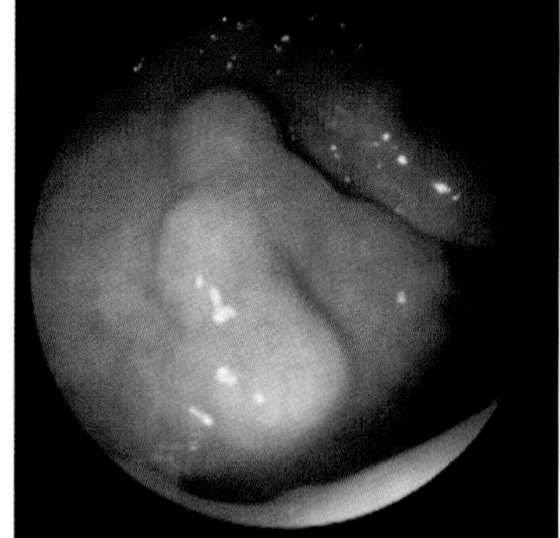

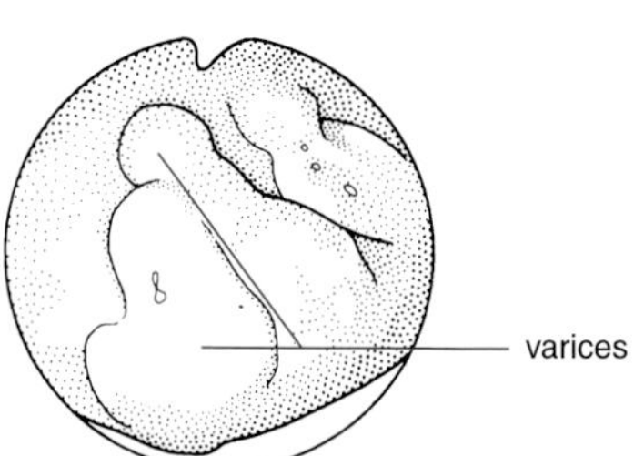

■ **Fig. 3.54** The characteristic appearance of duodenal varices seen at endoscopy.

Compression of the celiac axis by the median arcuate ligament of the diaphragm or by neurofibrous tissue of the celiac ganglion is thought to be responsible for the so-called celiac axis compression syndrome, in which recurrent episodes of upper abdominal pain occur after meals and are sometimes associated with nausea and vomiting. Whether the symptoms are related to intestinal ischemia (in the absence of narrowing of the mesenteric vessels) remains controversial since the pancreatico-duodenal arcades should provide an adequate collateral circulation. Narrowing of the celiac axis is certainly not uncommon at autopsy in patients who have had no suggestive symptoms in life. A neurogenic origin for the pain, from compression of the celiac ganglion and contributory vasospasm, has not been excluded. On examination an epigastric bruit may be heard. Celiac axis angiography demonstrates narrowing of the celiac artery at its origin (Fig. 3.55), which may be amenable to surgical release or reconstruction.

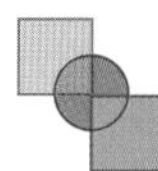

CONGENITAL DUODENAL OBSTRUCTION

Congenital obstruction of the duodenum varies in extent, from a simple stenosis or diaphragm partially obstructing the lumen (Fig. 3.56), to a complete block with a gap between the two ends of bowel (duodenal atresia). The site of obstruction is distal to the ampulla of Vater in about 80% of cases. Vomiting, which occurs within a few hours of birth, is usually, therefore, of bile-stained fluid. Associated congenital anomalies, including Down's syndrome, are common. Examination is often otherwise unrewarding apart from the presence of upper abdominal distention. The typical 'double bubble' sign with absence of distal abdominal gas may be seen on abdominal radiograph (Fig. 3.57), but in incomplete obstruction, contrast studies may be necessary (Fig. 3.58). Occasionally, even with complete atresia, some gas may be seen beyond the obstructing segment and is thought to reach there by passing through the minor papilla into the major papilla. It is occasionally possible to make the diagnosis before birth if obstetric ultrasound has shown polyhydramnios (Fig. 3.59).

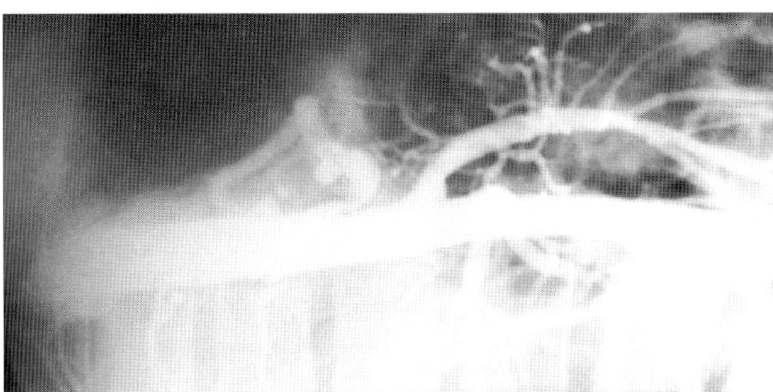

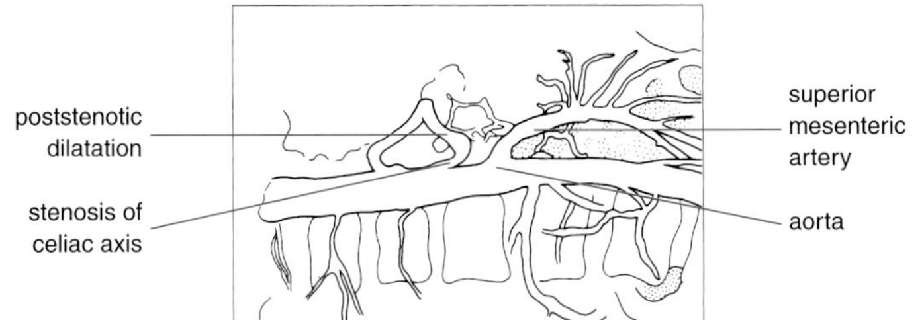

Fig. 3.55 Lateral aortogram showing stenosis at the origin of the coeliac axis. Courtesy of Mr A. Marston.

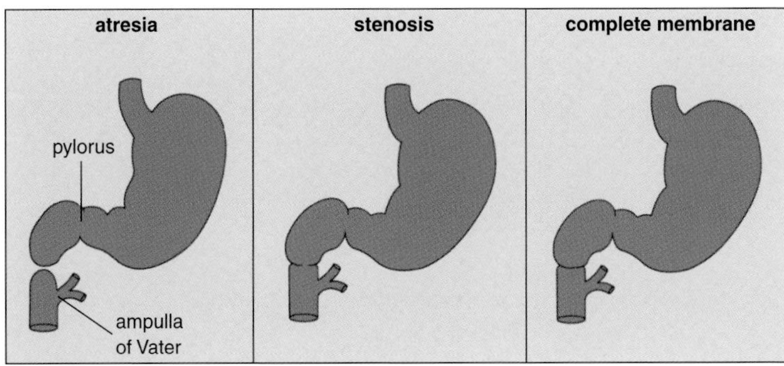

Fig. 3.56 The different types of duodenal atresia. All the examples shown are above the ampulla of Vater.

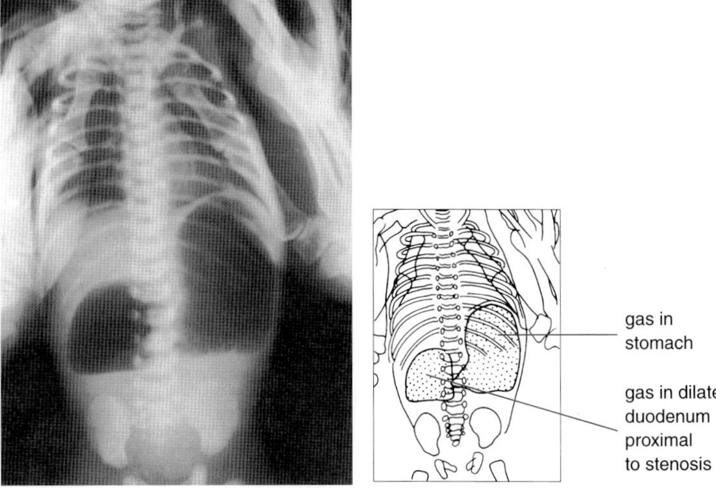

Fig. 3.57 Plain radiograph showing the 'double bubble' sign in duodenal atresia. Courtesy of Dr G.M. Steiner.

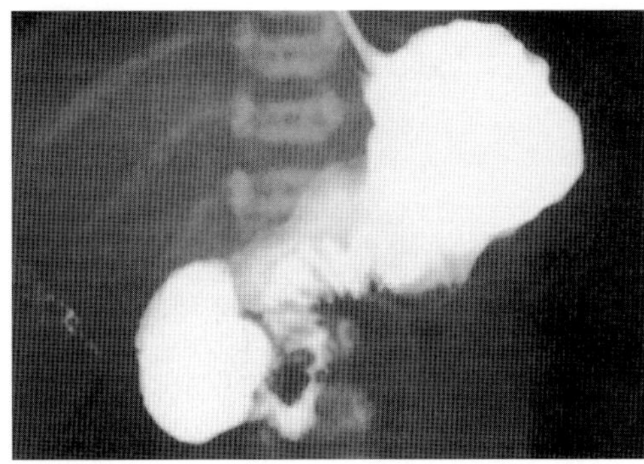

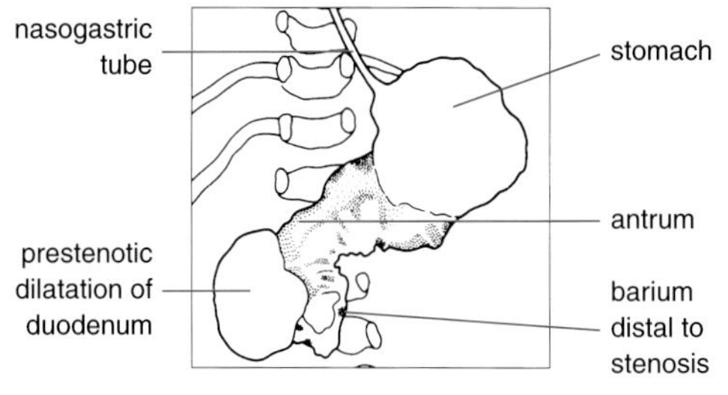

Fig. 3.58 Typical barium meal appearance in a patient with projectile vomiting. Partial occlusion of the second part of the duodenum with prestenotic dilatation is demonstrated. Courtesy of Dr K.J. Shah.

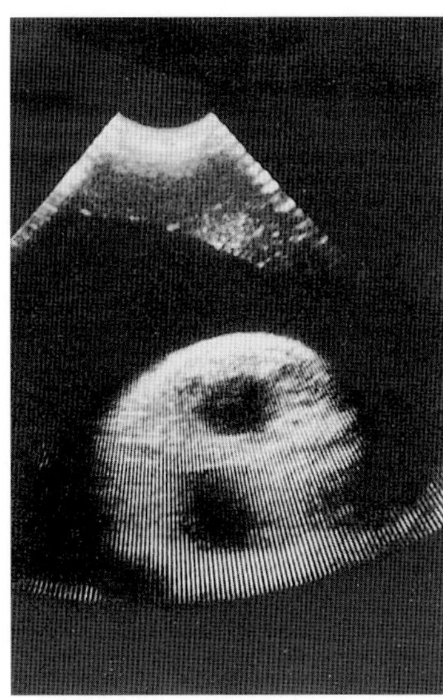

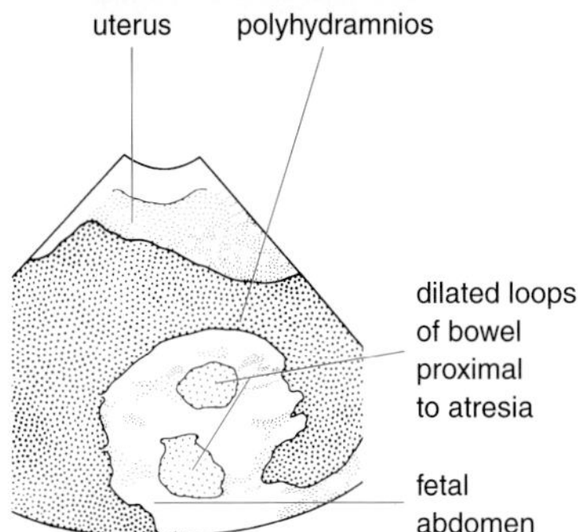

Fig. 3.59 Obstetric ultrasound scan showing polyhydramnios in a fetus subsequently shown to have duodenal atresia. Courtesy of Dr H. Carty.

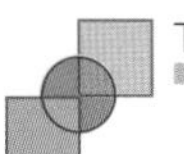

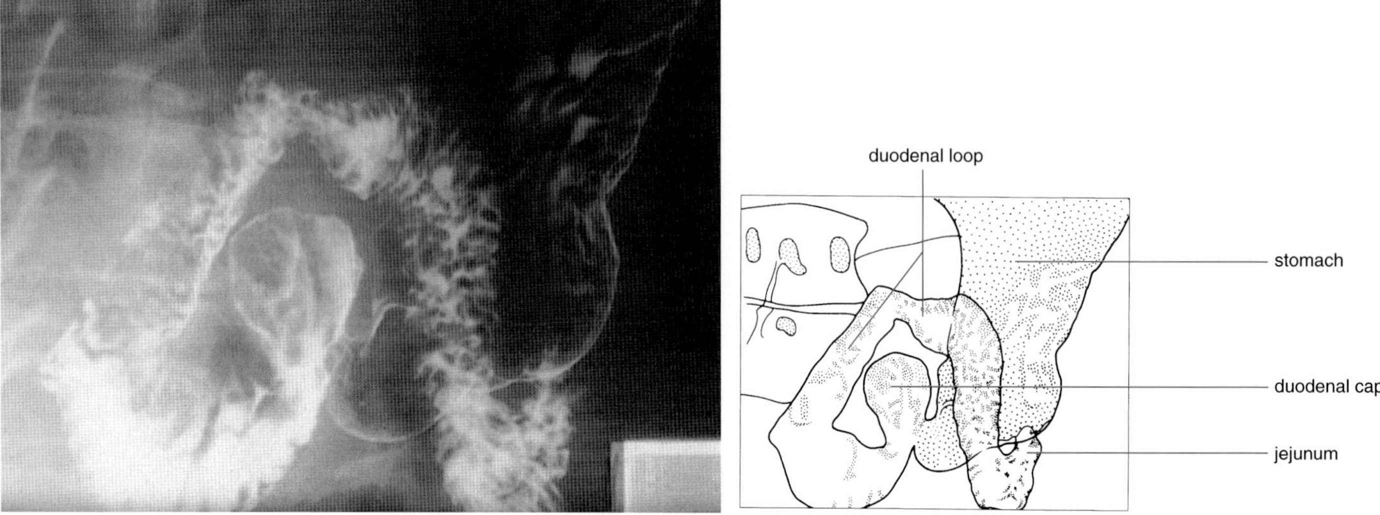

Fig. 3.60 Barium meal in a patient with a congenital reversal of the duodenal loop, showing the bizarre position of the duodenal cap, with the duodenal loop lying above it.

Congenital reversal of the duodenal loop presents a curious pattern on barium meal (Fig. 3.60), which is of little clinical significance but may be associated with, or be part of, other congenital abnormalities (see Chapter 4).

REFERENCES

1. Gore RM, Levine MS (eds) Textbook of gastrointestinal radiology. Philadelphia: WB Saunders, 2000, Figs 32.24B, 32.30, and 32.32B.
2. Levine MS, Rubesin SE, Laufer I. Double contrast gastrointestinal radiology. Philadelphia: WB Saunders, 2000, Figs 9.22, 9.38, 9.39A, and 9.41.

SMALL INTESTINE I

4

NORMAL SMALL INTESTINE

The jejunum forms the proximal small intestine, and the ileum the distal: there is no sharp demarcation between the two. As one passes distally, the bowel wall becomes progressively thinner and the lumen narrower; the mesentery of the ileum contains more fat and has a more complex pattern of arterial arcades (Fig. 4.1). The small bowel is anchored proximally by the retroperitoneal fixation of the duodenum at the ligament of Treitz, and is relatively immobile distally because of the fixation of the cecum to the posterior abdominal wall. Between these two points there is considerable mobility about the extensive mesentery. The normal small bowel is at least 2 m in length (mean around 3.5 m), but elongation of the intestinal smooth muscle occurs after death, resulting in a typical autopsy length of at least 6 m.

In the proximal jejunum (and in the post-bulbar duodenum) circular folds, or valvulae conniventes, are well developed and numerous (Fig. 4.2). They are usually absent in the distal ileum, and their degree of prominence largely accounts for the radiological features distinguishing between the different areas of the small bowel (Figs 4.3–4.6).

The small intestinal mucosa is arranged into multiple finger-like villi, the surfaces of which are composed of enterocytes and scattered goblet cells. The crypts of Lieberkühn open between the bases of the villi. In the duodenum, the villi are broad, and of leaf- or spade-like format (see Chapter 3). In the jejunum, they are most finger-like,

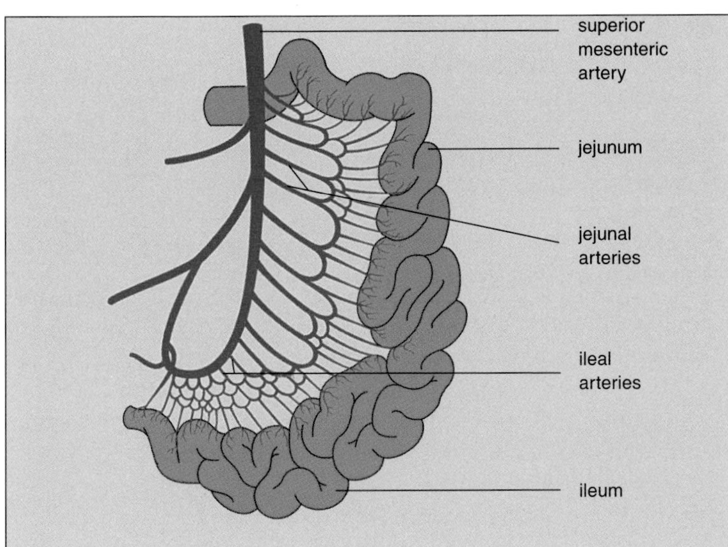

■ **Fig. 4.1** Diagram showing the patterns of arterial arcades to the jejunum and the ileum.

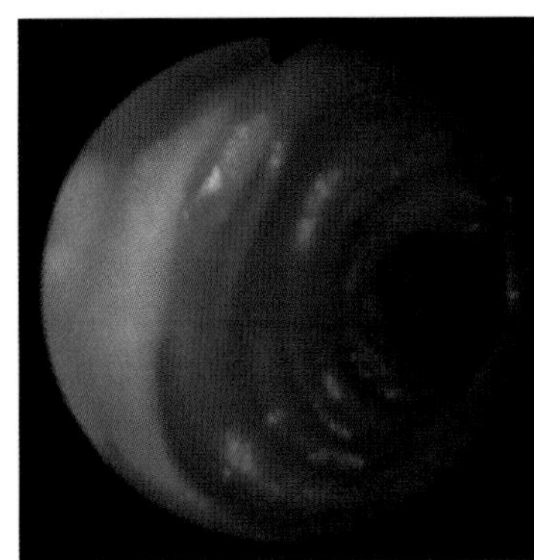

■ **Fig. 4.2** Normal jejunum seen through a flexible enteroscope of the 'push' type. Courtesy of Dr A. Van Gossum.

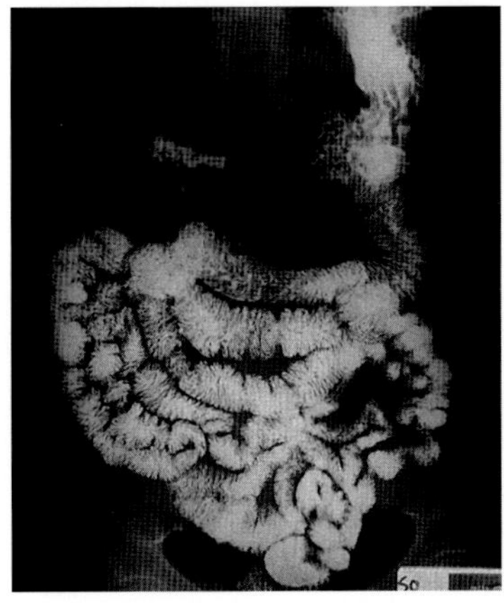

■ **Fig. 4.3** Normal barium follow-through showing the overall pattern of the small bowel.

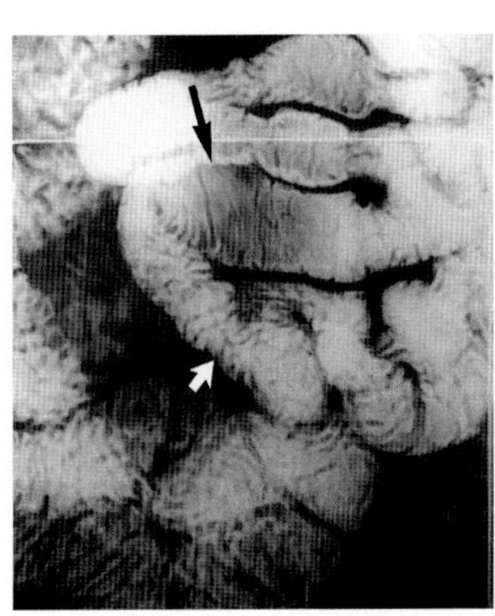

■ **Fig 4.4** Spot radiograph from normal small bowel follow-through. When the small intestine is distended and the loops do not overlap (black arrow), the jejunal valvulae conniventes are well seen. When the small bowel loops overlap each other or the loops are not distended (white arrow), the valvulae conniventes are only demonstrated as a 'feathery' pattern.

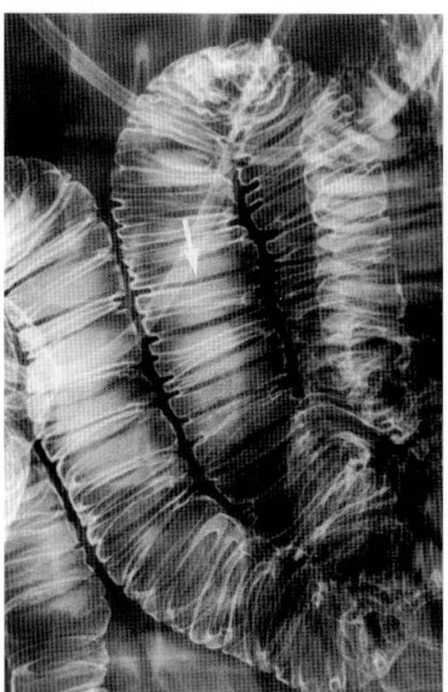

■ **Fig. 4.5** Spot radiograph of the jejunum from a normal enteroclysis (small bowel enema). The valvulae conniventes (representative folds identified by arrow) are smooth, 1–2 mm in width, and lie perpendicular to the longitudinal axis of the small bowel. There are about 2 folds per centimeter in the jejunum. (Reproduced with permission from Rubesin, reference 4, Fig. 2.). The differences in the display of the small bowel structures from those of the normal follow-through can be appreciated.

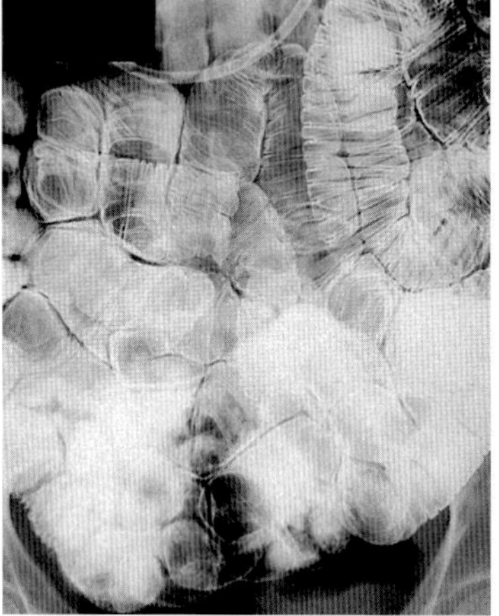

■ **Fig. 4.6** By following the barium with methylcellulose suspension a double-contrast enteroclysis view is later obtained of virtually the whole ileum. Courtesy of Dr N.G. Reading.

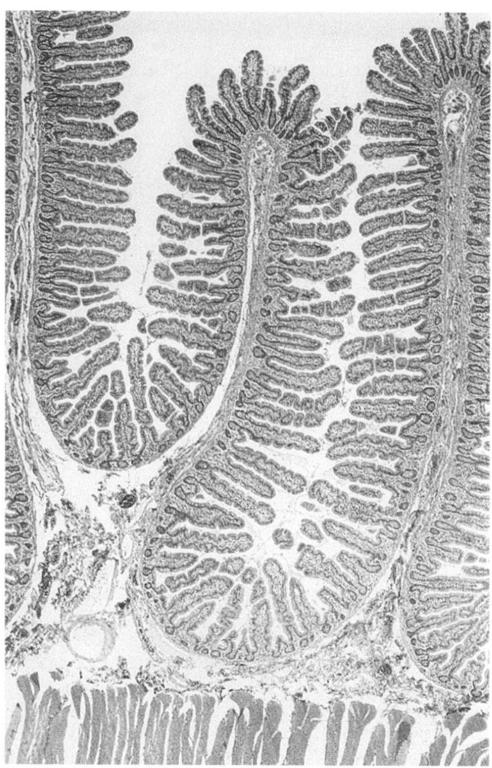

■ **Fig. 4.7** Normal jejunal mucosa. Microscopic view of plicae circulares showing villi of uniform height projecting from the surface.

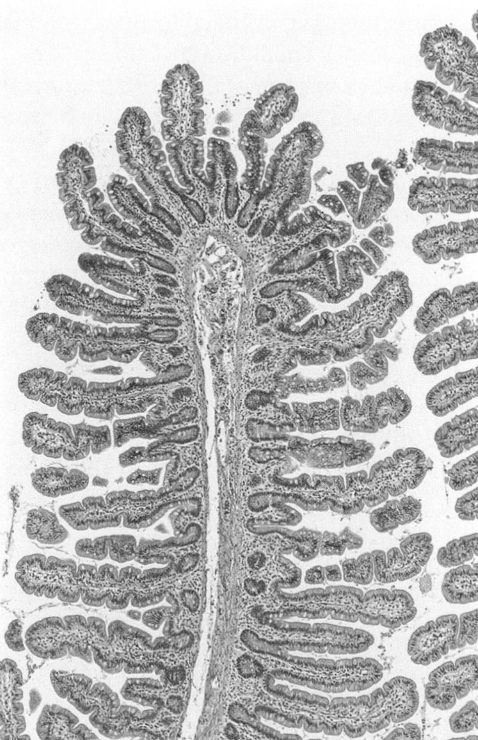

■ **Fig. 4.8** Higher magnification of the tip of a single mucosal fold of the normal jejunum showing a villus: crypt height ratio of about 4–5:1.

becoming taller and more slender still in the ileum (Figs 4.7–4.9). These features are easily appreciated through the dissecting microscope (Fig. 4.10). It is notable that the proportion of leaf forms in the proximal small bowel is normally higher in people living in the tropics, even to the extent of suggesting mild partial villous atrophy; the villus height:crypt depth ratio remains within the normal range of 3:1 to 4:1 nonetheless.

Enterocytes are relatively homogeneous columnar epithelial cells, with key roles in secretion and absorption accomplished in part through their brush border of microvilli (Figs 4.11–4.13). The cell turnover is amongst the most rapid of all cells with a typical lifespan of just 2–3 days. Continual renewal occurs from intestinal stem cells (enteroblasts) in the base of the crypt with migration upwards onto the villi as differentiation occurs. Goblet cells, more abundant in the ileum, 'M' cells, and tuft cells are also found on the villi. M cells, which have no microvilli, are usually found over Peyer's patches (Figs 4.14, 4.15) and form an integral part of the luminal sampling processes of the gut-associated lymphoid tissue. Tuft cells have prominent microvilli but their function is still unknown. Epithelial lymphocytes are normally present, but in health there are rarely more than 40 for each 100 enterocytes. Paneth cells and endocrine cells of the APUD system including 'L' cells which secrete gut hormones such as the glucagon-like peptides are found in the crypts. A small number of lymphoid cells, eosinophils, and histiocytes is usually to be seen in the lamina propria, which provides the villus with a core of supporting connective tissue that encloses blood and lymphatic vessels.

INTESTINAL OBSTRUCTION

Intestinal obstruction occurs when the passage of intestinal contents is impeded. Mechanical obstruction may be within the lumen, within the bowel wall, or extrinsic (as in the case of adhesions and herniae), and it requires differentiation from functional causes or pseudo-obstruction (see below and Chapter 7), and from the 'paralytic ileus' that follows intra-abdominal surgery.

The clinical features associated with obstruction vary according to its site. When the obstruction is proximal pain and bilious vomiting with little distention will predominate; lower small bowel obstruc-

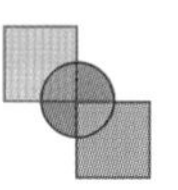

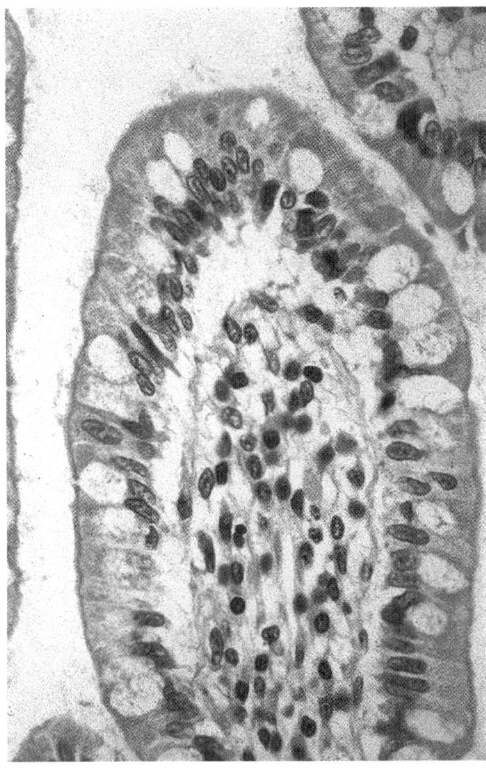

■ **Fig. 4.9** Normal jejunal mucosa. High-magnification appearance of a single villus showing the bright pink brush border (microvillus brush border) of the enterocytes and the clear cytoplasmic mucin vacuoles of the goblet cells.

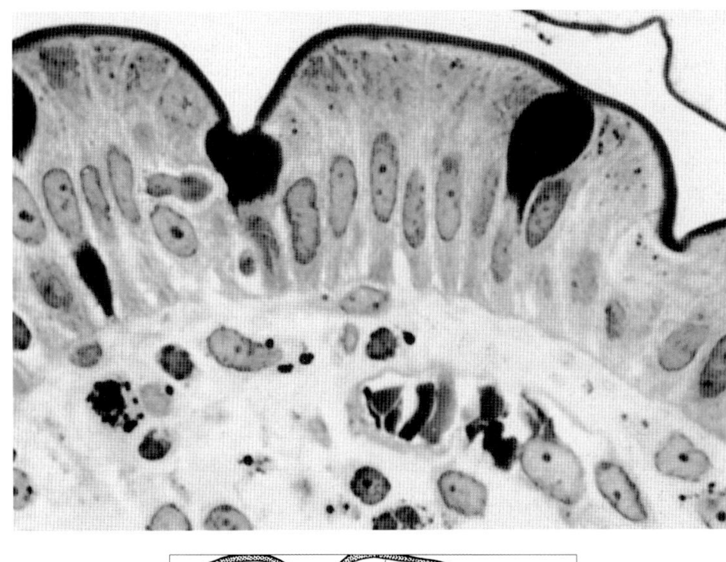

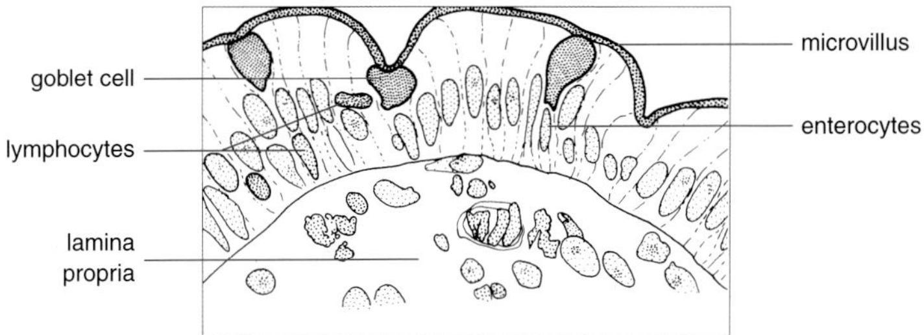

■ **Fig. 4.11** Electron micrograph of normal jejunal mucosa: Epon section (x 70 000). Courtesy of Dr M.N. Marsh.

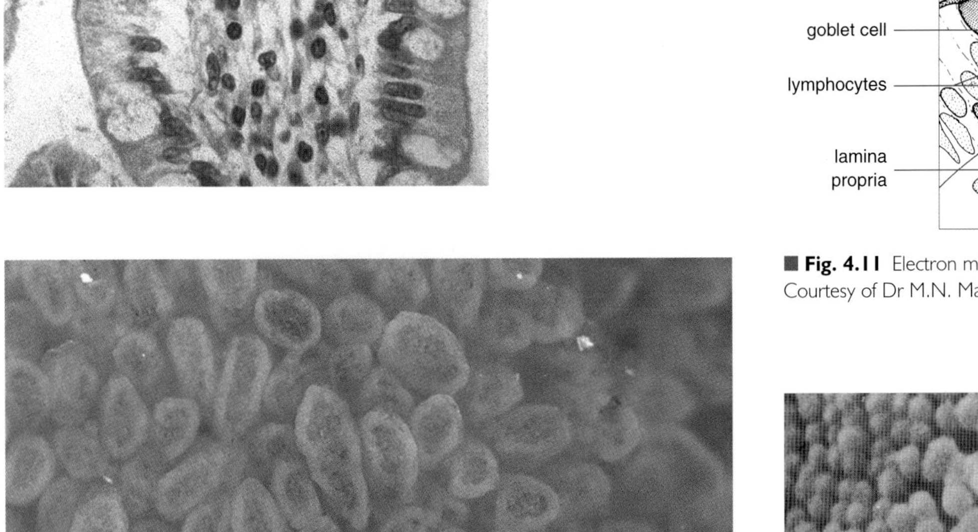

■ **Fig. 4.10** Dissecting microscope appearance of jejunal mucosa showing normal finger-like villi.

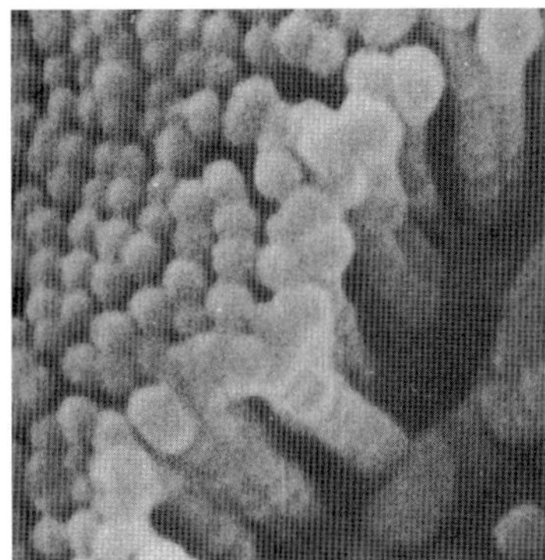

■ **Fig. 4.12** Electron micrograph of the microvillous border showing individual enterocytes (x 160). Courtesy of Dr M.N. Marsh.

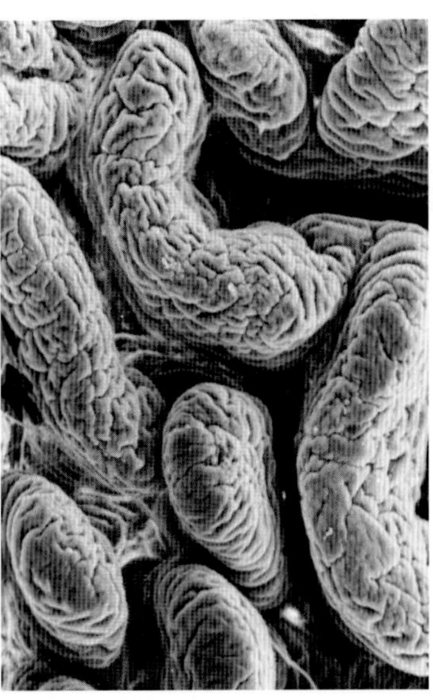

■ **Fig. 4.13** Scanning electron micrograph showing normal mucosa with leaf-like forms (x 140).

tion is more often associated with distention and feculent vomiting secondary to bacterial overgrowth within the obstructed segment. Peristalsis may be visible in thin patients (Fig. 4.16) until motility becomes impaired, and examination may demonstrate the cause of the obstruction if (for example) a strangulated hernia is present (see below).

The plain radiograph is usually confirmatory (Figs 4.17, 4.18). Small bowel distention is differentiated radiologically from colonic distention by the outlining of the valvulae conniventes by intestinal gas, and by the distribution of distended loops, which mainly occupy the center of the abdomen (Fig. 4.17); in small bowel obstruction of mechanical cause there is usually little or no colonic gas. Excessive gas and fluid in the small bowel is readily apparent on the erect film as a series of air–fluid levels (see Fig. 4.18). Only rarely will the plain radiograph show a clinically unsuspected reason for obstruction, such

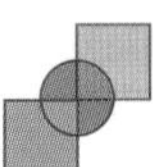

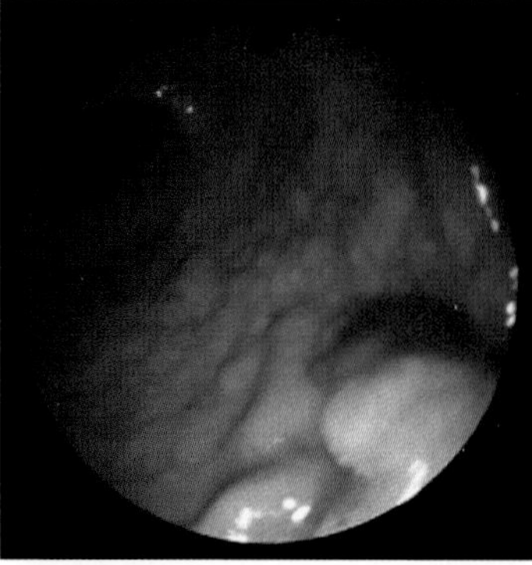

■ **Fig. 4.14** Endoscopic appearance of normal Peyer's patches in the terminal ileum.

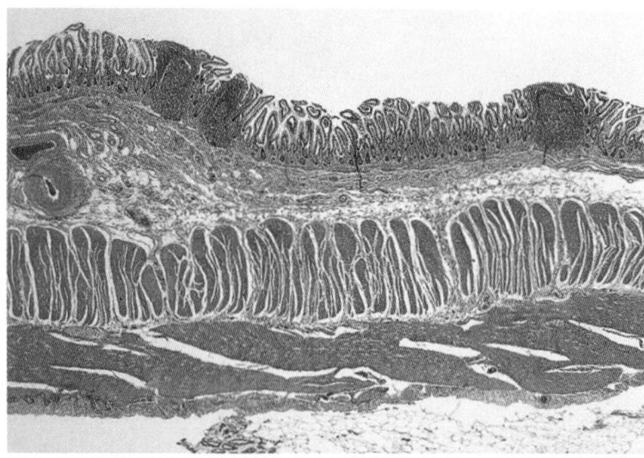

■ **Fig. 4.15** Low-magnification microscopic view of normal ileal mucosa showing the mucosal lymphoid follicles (germinal centers) known as Peyer's patches.

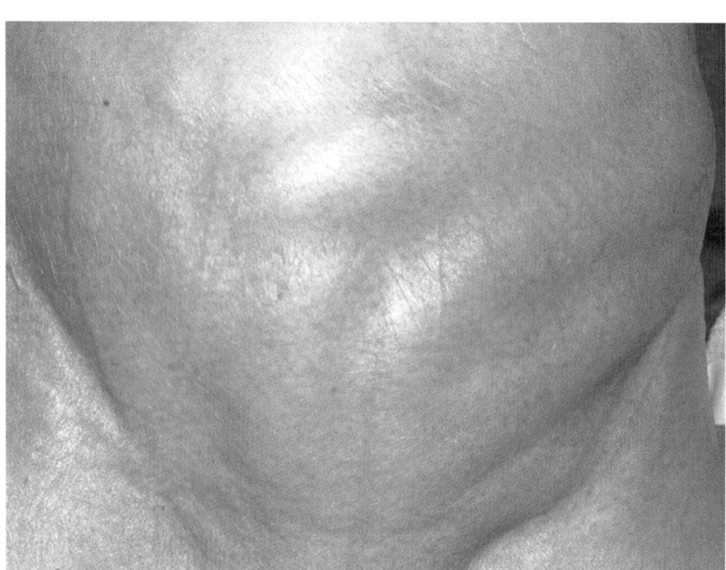

■ **Fig. 4.16** A patient with intestinal obstruction showing loops of distended small bowel. Peristalsis was visible. Courtesy of Mr D.N.L. Ralphs.

as a large gallstone within the intestinal lumen (gallstone ileus) (Fig. 4.19); an air cholangiogram secondary to the spontaneous biliary-enteric fistula is then usual (Fig. 4.20). CT scanning is now firmly established as an investigation of choice in intestinal obstruction since, in many cases, this reveals both the anatomical site of obstruction and its etiology (Figs 4.21–4.23). CT is also helpful in avoiding surgery when a functional cause of obstruction is present and laparotomy inappropriate. CT scanning can readily distinguish band adhesions from internal herniation or indeed from intussusception from a mass lesion, but conventional contrast imaging may be more accessible to the non-radiologist (Figs 4.24–4.28). Large bowel obstruction is considered further in Chapter 7.

GLUTEN-SENSITIVE ENTEROPATHY – CELIAC DISEASE

Celiac disease is a disorder of the small bowel mucosa in which villous atrophy is responsible for generalized malabsorption. It usually responds rapidly to the withdrawal of gluten-containing cereals

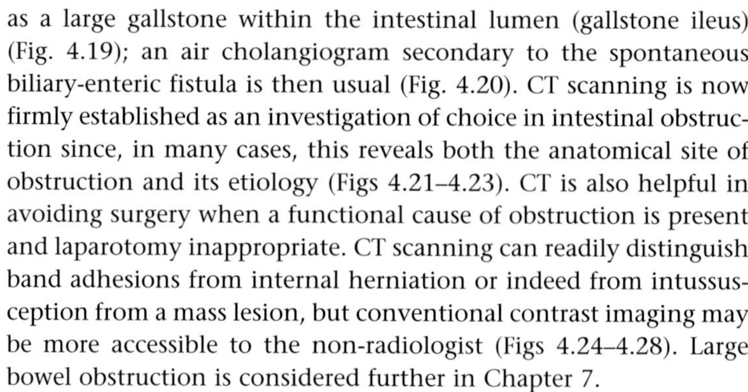

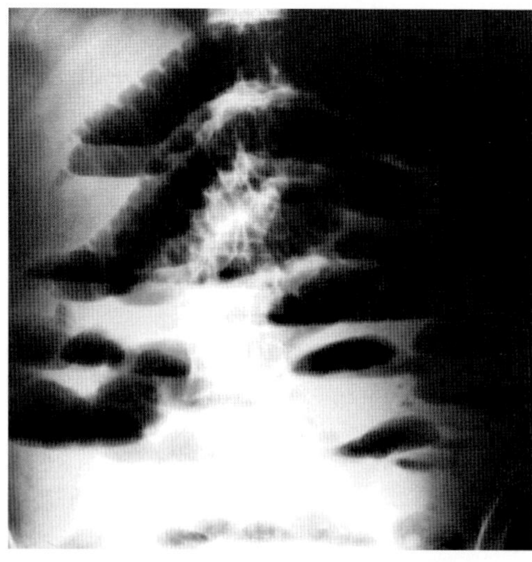

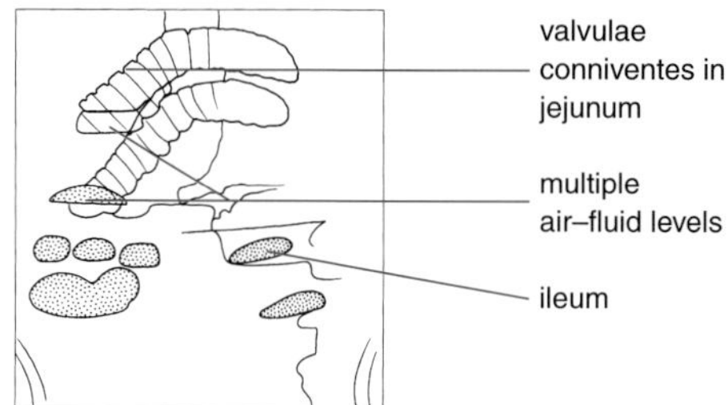

■ **Fig. 4.18** Abdominal radiograph (erect view), showing multiple air–fluid levels in the small bowel due to obstruction.

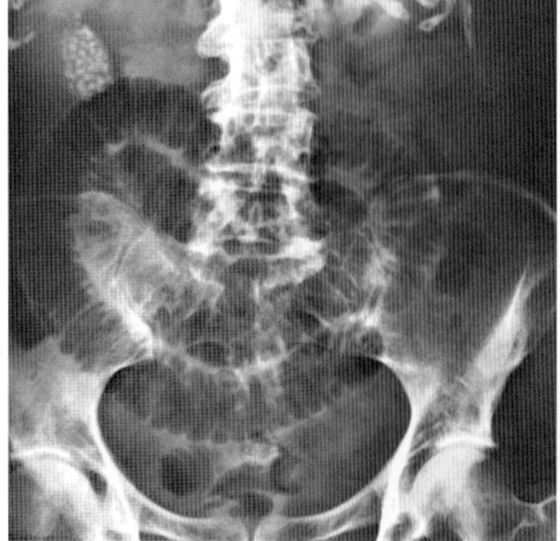

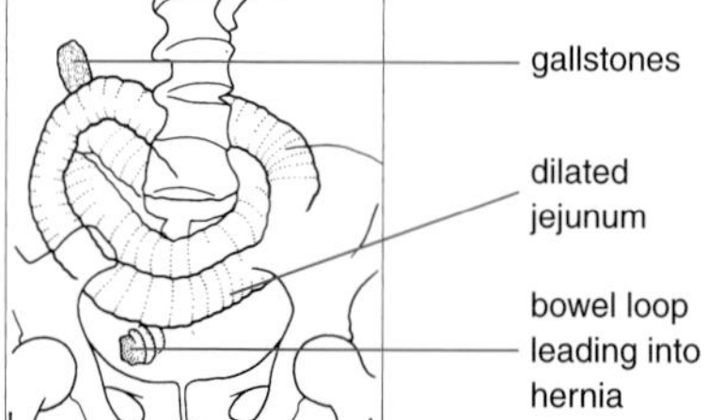

■ **Fig. 4.17** Supine abdominal radiograph of a patient with an obstructed femoral hernia. Distended loops of jejunum lie centrally, and the valvulae conniventes are clearly outlined by intraluminal gas. A bowel loop is trapped in the hernia in the right side of the pelvis. Note also the gallstones.

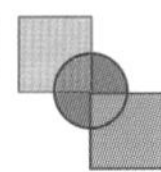

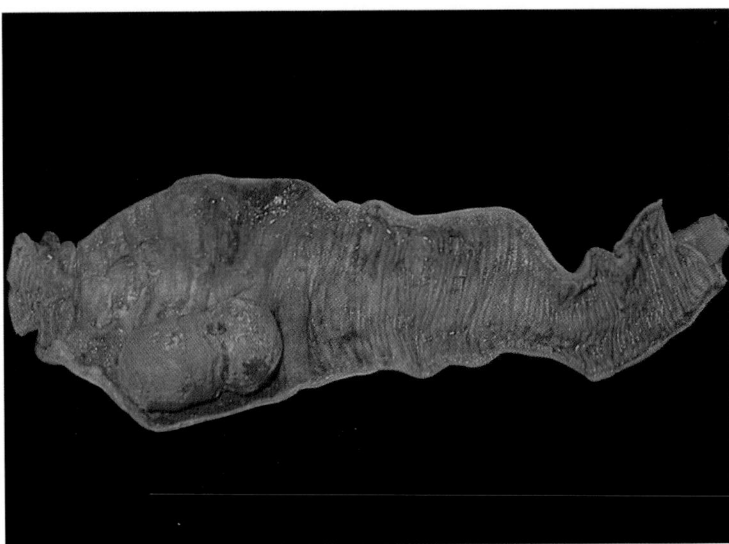

■ **Fig. 4.19** Resection specimen of small intestine with a calcified gallstone within a dilated loop of bowel.

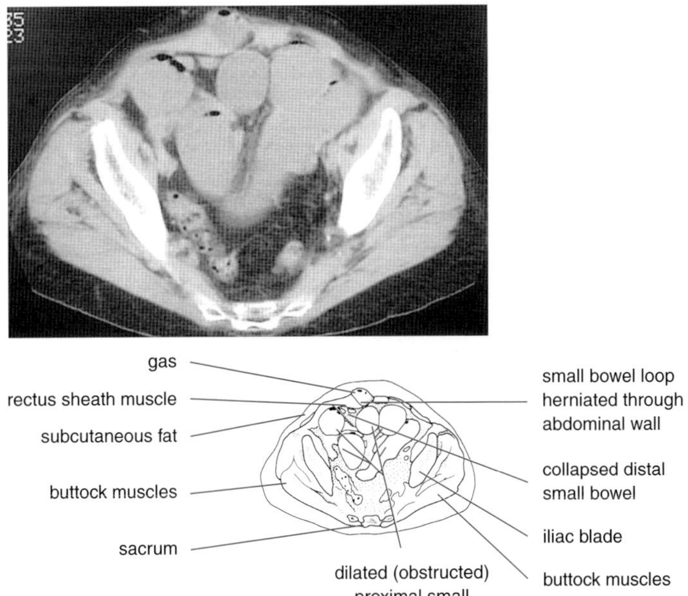

■ **Fig. 4.21** CT scan of a patient with small bowel obstruction in whom the cause of the obstruction was not evident clinically. The scan shows clear evidence of an abdominal wall hernia causing the obstruction, which was confirmed at surgery

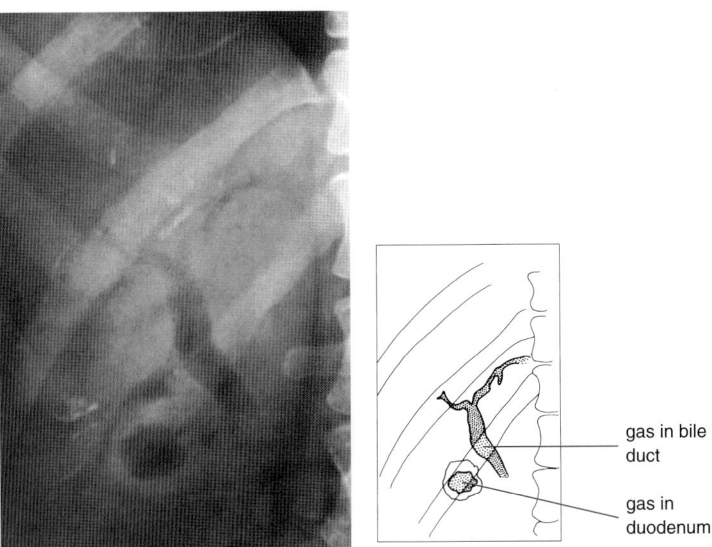

■ **Fig. 4.20** Radiograph showing air cholangiogram secondary to a cholecystoenteric fistula in a patient with intestinal obstruction from gallstones.

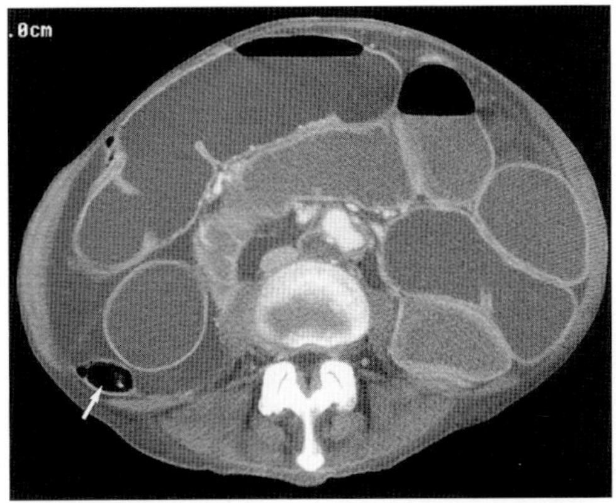

■ **Fig. 4.22** CT through the mid abdomen shows many dilated, fluid-filled small bowel loops. The ascending colon (arrow) is compressed. Ascites is present in the right paracolic gutter.

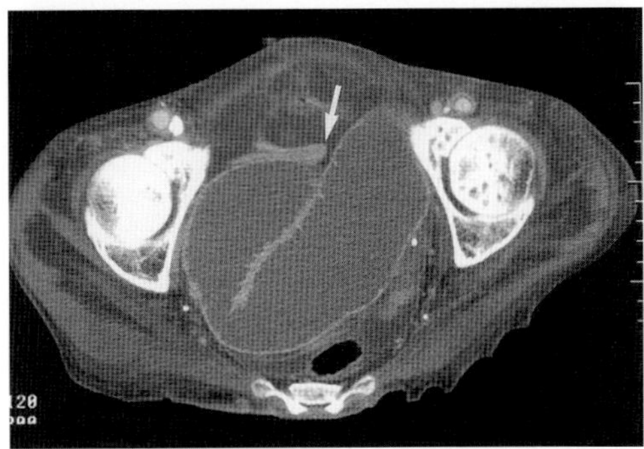

■ **Fig 4.23** CT through the pelvis shows an abrupt transition (arrow) from a markedly dilated small bowel loop to collapsed loop. No mass is seen at this transition, only an abrupt angulation caused by adhesions.

(wheat, barley, rye). Presentation is typically in early childhood when cereals are first introduced into the diet, with weight loss, weakness, and diarrhea with dramatic steatorrhea (Fig. 4.29); however, presentation later in childhood (Figs 4.30, 4.31) or as an adult with more subtle symptoms, is well recognized. Clues such as a history of poor overall growth and delayed menarche may help to initiate appropriate investigation. Clubbing, pathological bruising from malabsorption of vitamin K, iron- and/or folic acid-deficient anemia, osteomalacia, proximal myopathy, and hypocalcemia are all rarely seen. Hematological investigations typically show a dimorphic anemia with a raised red-cell-distribution-width (even if the net MCV is normal), and Howell–Jolly bodies, which are a result of the splenic atrophy typical of long-standing disease (Fig. 4.32).

The most specific widely available marker for the diagnosis is the presence of circulating endomysial antibody (>95% sensitivity and specificity); its target antigen – tissue transglutaminase (TTGA) – has now been identified, and assays for TTGA now exist for routine diagnostic use. Contrast studies are rarely appropriate in the diagnostic process but when performed show a malabsorption pattern, with dilatation of the lumen; coarsely thickened folds, nodular mucosa, and flocculation and clumping of the barium, may also be seen (Figs 4.33, 4.34) on follow-through examinations. CT scanning may demonstrate mild lymphadenopathy (Fig. 4.35). Radiological signs of osteomalacia, such as Looser's zones, are now rarely seen (Fig. 4.36), but abnormalities of bone densitometry (and biopsy, when performed) are common (Fig. 4.37).

Full diagnosis of celiac disease is still considered to require histological assessment of the small bowel mucosa, and the subsequent reversal of the abnormalities on a gluten-free diet. Pinch biopsies taken from the distal duodenum at endoscopy usually provide adequate material for diagnosis, but duodenitis may also cause villous atrophy,

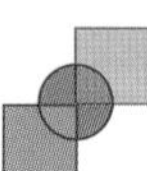

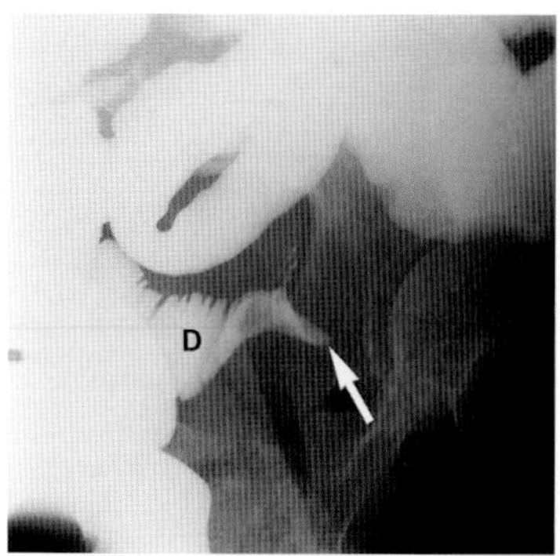

Fig 4.24 Barium enema with retrograde flow into the distal ileum shows non-distended distal small bowel (D) and a smooth beak-like narrowing (arrow) at the site of the obstructing adhesion.

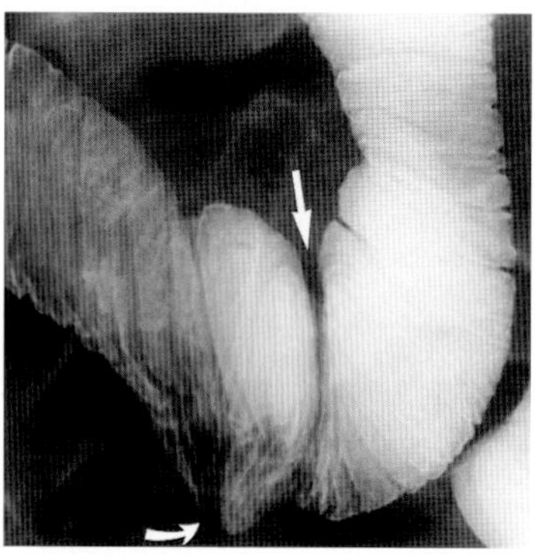

Fig. 4.25 Enteroclysis demonstrating partially obstructing adhesion. An adhesive band (straight arrow) crosses the lumen of the mid small bowel. Adhesions cause angulation of the bowel wall and tethering of folds (curved arrow).

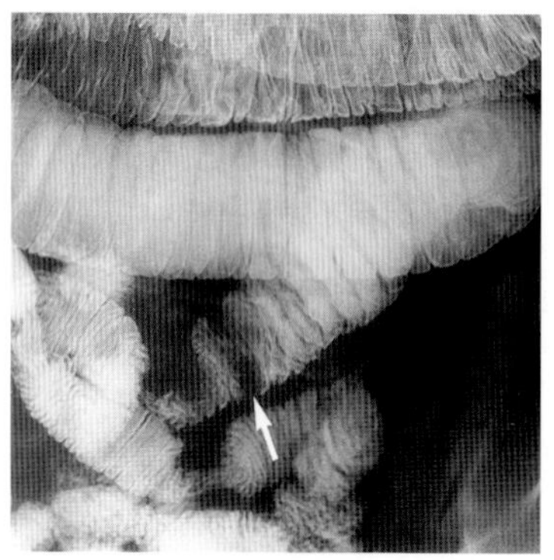

Fig. 4.26 Enteroclysis demonstrating adhesion mid small intestine causing partial obstruction. An adhesive band is seen as a smooth ring-like band (arrow) crossing the bowel. The small bowel folds are preserved. The bowel proximal to the band is moderately dilated. (Reproduced with permission from reference 1, Fig. 23.23.)

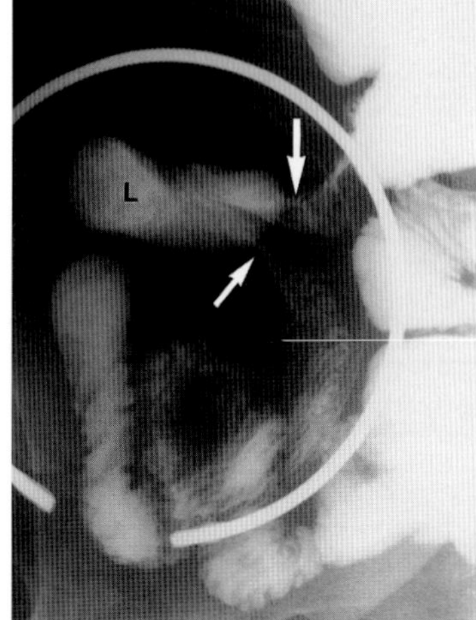

Fig. 4.27 Enteroclysis demonstrating internal hernia. A loop of mid small bowel (L) is within an internal hernia. The intestines entering (long arrow) and exiting (short arrow) the hernia are identified. (Reproduced with permission from reference 8, Fig. 52.32A.)

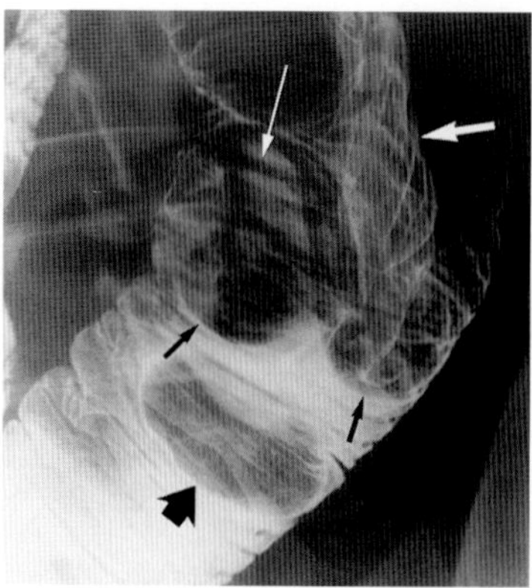

Fig. 4.28 Enteroclysis demonstrating partial small bowel obstruction due to intussusception by metastatic melanoma. The lead point is a 3 cm smooth polypoid mass (large black arrow). The infolding walls of the intussusceptum (small black arrows) are identified. Barium refluxes back into the intussuscipiens to outline its mucosal folds (thin white arrow). The narrowed intussusceptum is identified (thick white arrow). (Reproduced with permission from reference 6, Fig. 5.9B.)

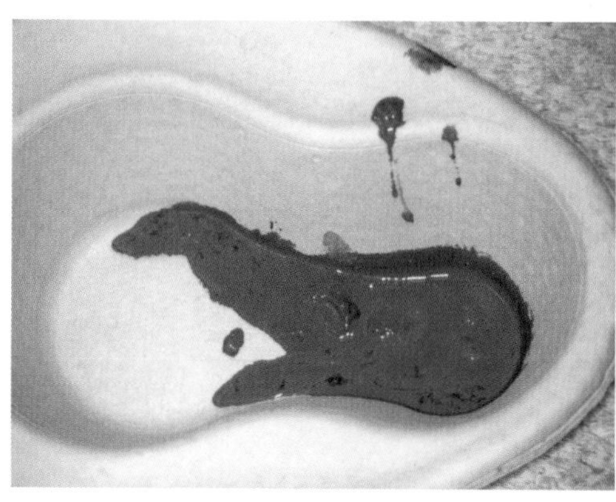

Fig. 4.29 The appearance of a steatorrheic stool. Note the visible fat globules and the evident difficulty that the patient has had in achieving a 'clean' evacuation.

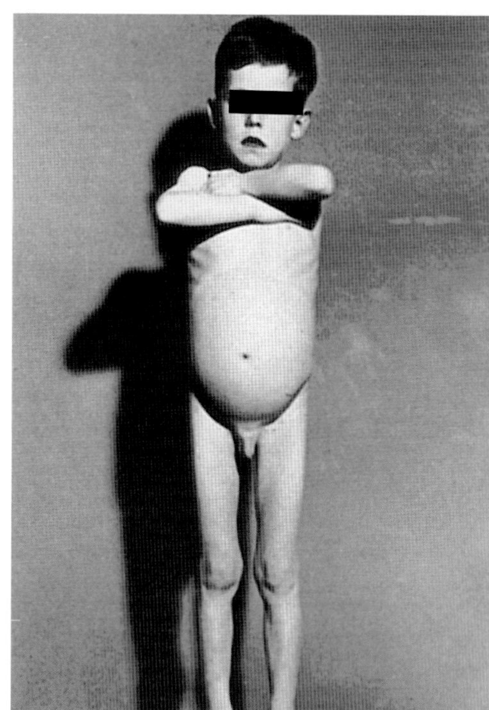

Fig. 4.30 A 7-year-old with untreated celiac disease. Courtesy of Prof R.C. Spiller.

and in the presence of duodenitis a formal jejunal biopsy needs to be taken. This can be achieved with an enteroscope or with the now almost historic Crosby or Watson biopsy capsule (Fig. 4.38). The capsule is no longer passed orally, but 'muzzle-loaded' through a standard diagnostic endoscope, which is then passed to the duodenum, the capsule then being pushed further on before being fired by suction to obtain the biopsy. At endoscopy, the typically smooth dilated bowel with prominent submucosal vessels may be observed (Fig. 4.39), while use of a dye-scattering technique further highlights the villous abnormalities (Fig. 4.40).

In untreated cases of celiac disease biopsy almost always shows a flat mucosa – the confusingly termed 'subtotal' villous atrophy (see below). The changes are most severe proximally, a villous pattern reappearing towards the terminal ileum. The mucosa is often thickened as a result of crypt hyperplasia. The enterocytes are abnormal, with

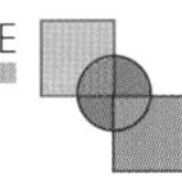

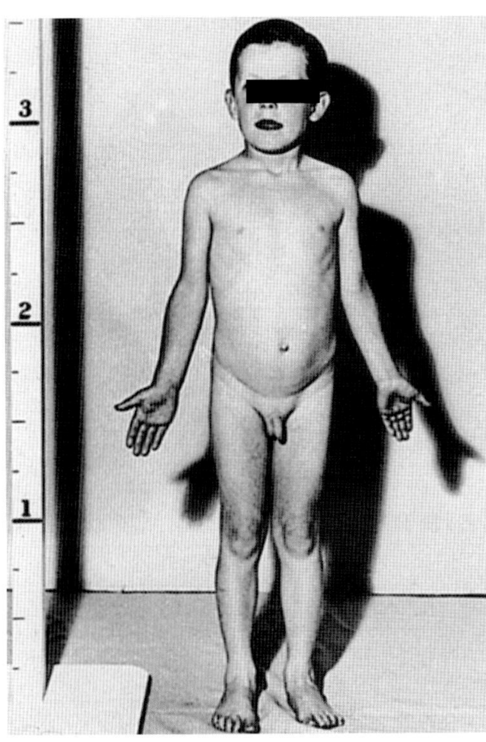

Fig. 4.31 The same child as shown in Fig. 4.30, 1 year after commencing a gluten-free diet. Courtesy of Prof R.C. Spiller.

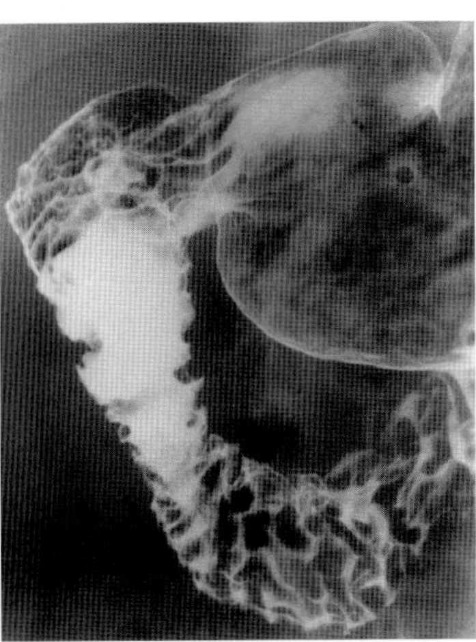

Fig. 4.34 Diffuse duodenitis in celiac disease. The folds of the second and third portions of the duodenum are enlarged and nodular. The mucosa of the duodenal bulb is nodular. The duodenum is the only portion of the small intestine where visualization of thick folds in celiac disease does not elicit a diagnosis of lymphoma or ulcerative jejunoileitis.

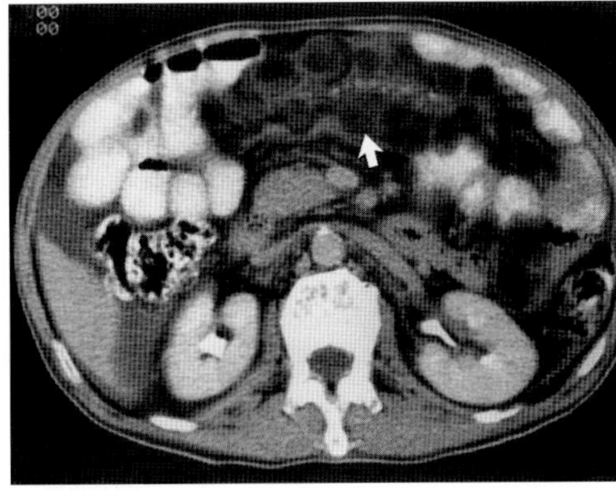

Fig. 4.35 CT demonstrating low-attenuation lymphadenopathy in celiac disease. Numerous near-fat attenuation lymph nodes (representative lymph node identified by arrow) expand the small bowel mesentery. This patient later developed cavitary mesenteric lymph node syndrome.

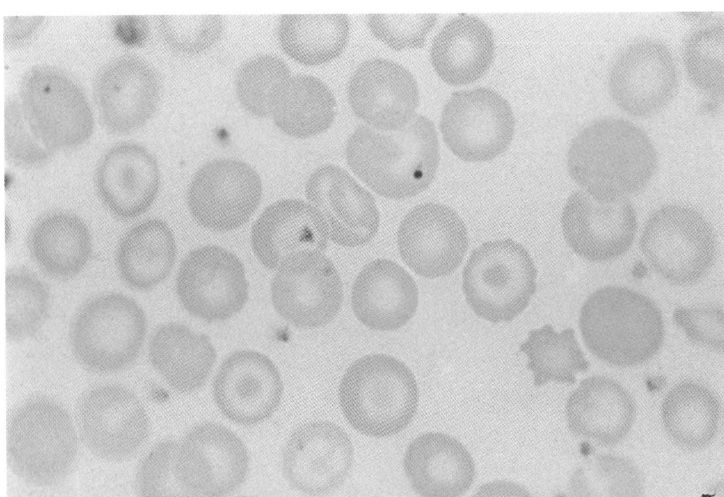

Fig. 4.32 Blood film showing Howell–Jolly bodies. Courtesy of Dr Chanarin.

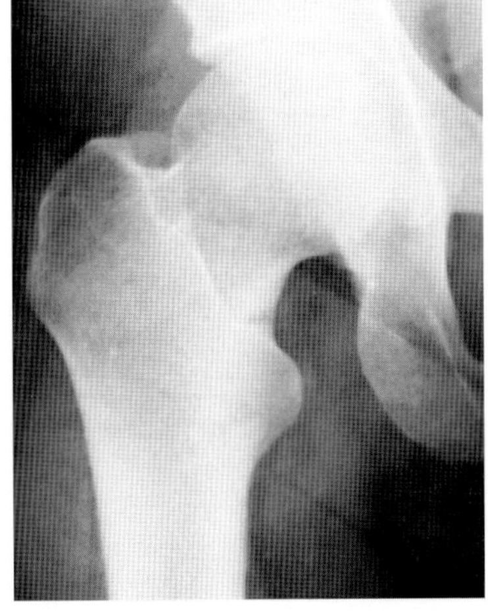

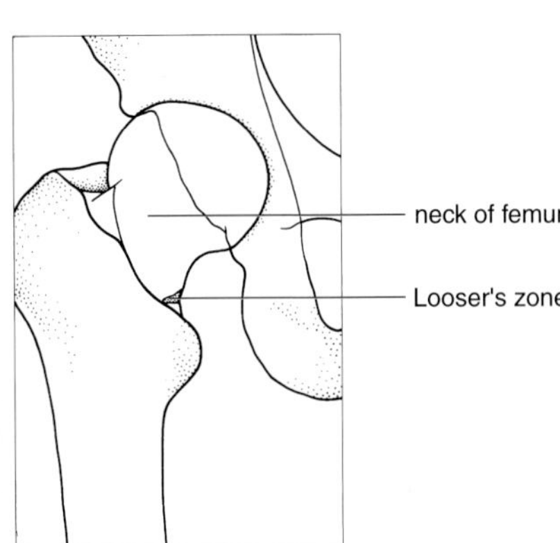

Fig. 4.36 Radiograph showing a Looser's zone in the femoral neck secondary to osteomalacia.

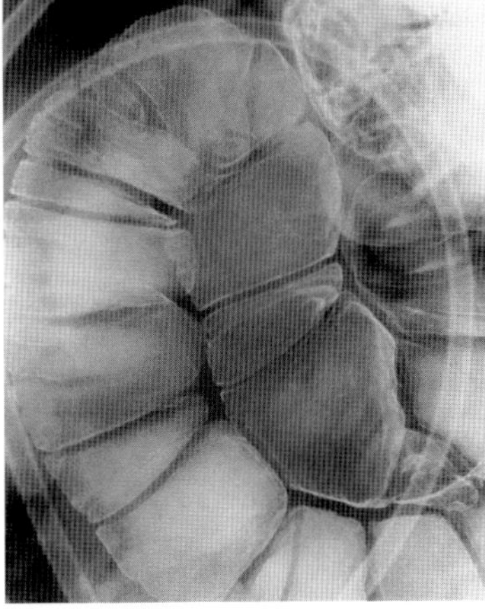

Fig. 4.33 Small bowel enema demonstrating celiac disease. Two to four valvulae conniventes are seen every 5 cm in the jejunum. Loss of folds is due to mucosal atrophy. (Reproduced with permission from reference 4, Fig. 5.)

a squashed, cuboidal shape and irregular nuclei, and there is a substantial increase in the intraepithelial lymphocyte count. There is also an increase in plasma cells, and fewer Paneth cells in the crypts. Scanning electron microscopy shows dramatic changes from normal (Figs 4.41, 4.42).

Clinical assessment of the effect of treatment is often obvious, but when there is a need to assess progress at a cellular level this is best monitored from the appearance of the villi (Figs 4.43–4.47, see also Fig. 4.10). Morphometric analysis of the villous height, and quantitative estimation of intraepithelial lymphocytes are helpful when improvements are minor.

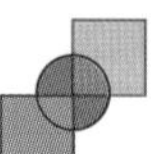

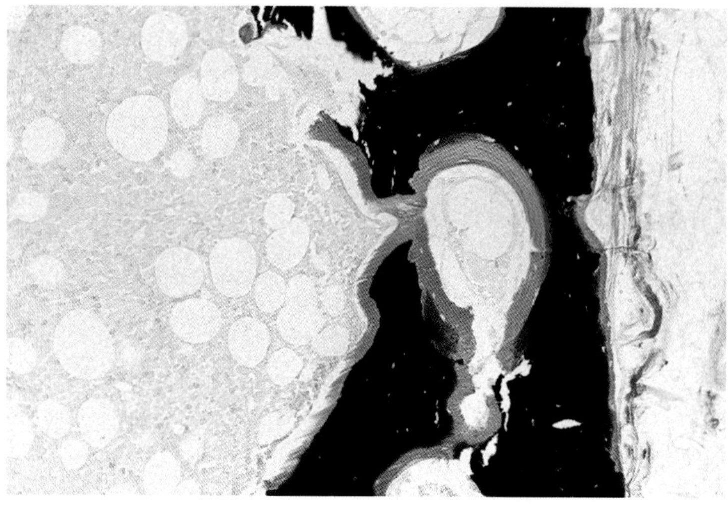

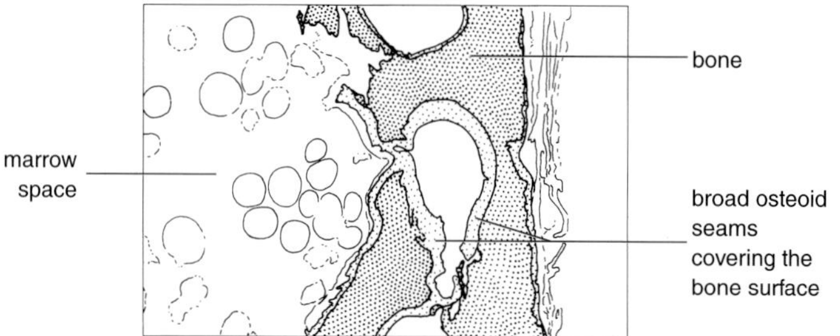

■ **Fig. 4.37** Bone biopsy in osteomalacia. Osteoid seams covering the bony trabeculae are abnormally extensive and thickened, diagnostic of the condition. Von Kossa stain (x 240). Courtesy of Dr P.J. Gallagher.

The incidence rates of intestinal lymphoma, small bowel carcinoma and esophageal carcinoma are substantially increased in celiac disease (see below). There is potential for confusion where lymphoma and celiac disease present concurrently; although this certainly occurs, an apparent celiac syndrome may also 'mask' a lymphoma, itself responsible for villous atrophy (see below). This should be considered particularly in the middle-aged patient who has no previous suggestion of disease. It is probable that lifelong compliance with a strict gluten-free diet reduces the risk of lymphoma in the celiac patient almost to control rates, and the same may also apply to esophageal and small bowel carcinoma. These judgments have major implications, given the high frequency of apparent resolution of gluten intolerance during adolescence and the natural desire of patients to return to a normal diet.

DERMATITIS HERPETIFORMIS

Dermatitis herpetiformis is a pruritic papulovesicular skin eruption usually distributed symmetrically over the scapulae, sacrum, buttocks, elbows, and knees (Figs 4.48, 4.49). IgA is deposited at the epidermodermal junction (Fig. 4.50). Most patients have enteropathy on intestinal biopsy, but in only a minority is this marked, and overt malabsorption is quite unusual. The villous abnormalities respond to a gluten-free diet and, in some patients, the skin changes also improve during gluten exclusion.

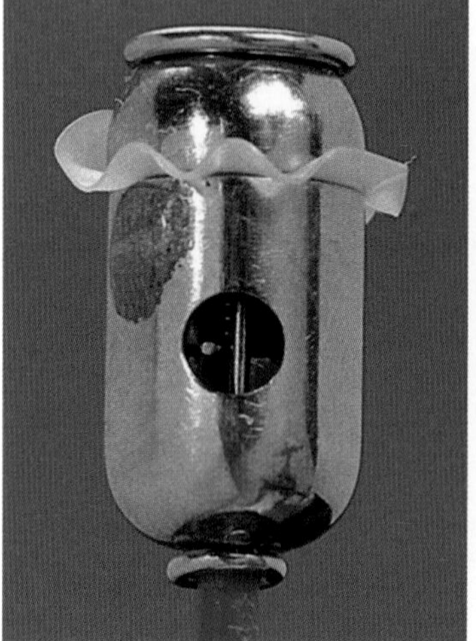

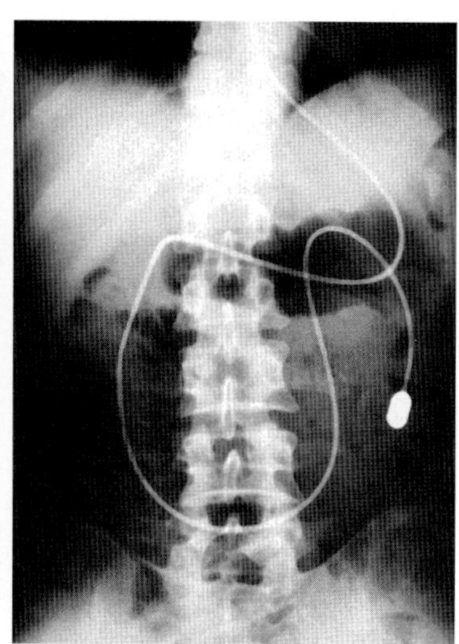

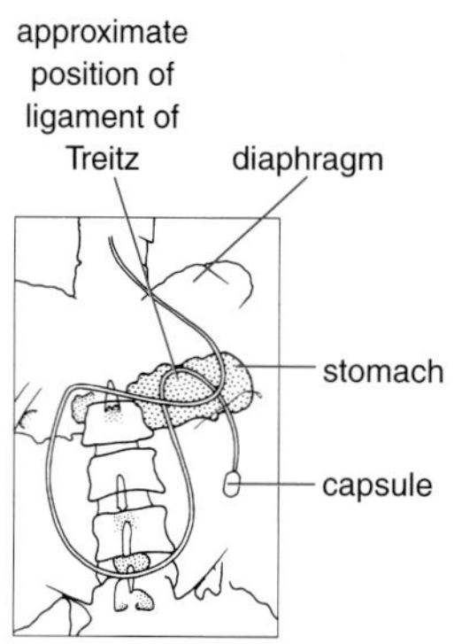

■ **Fig. 4.38** A small intestinal biopsy capsule open and ready to be fired once passed to the jejunum as subsequently seen radiographically. Courtesy of Dr J.S. Stewart.

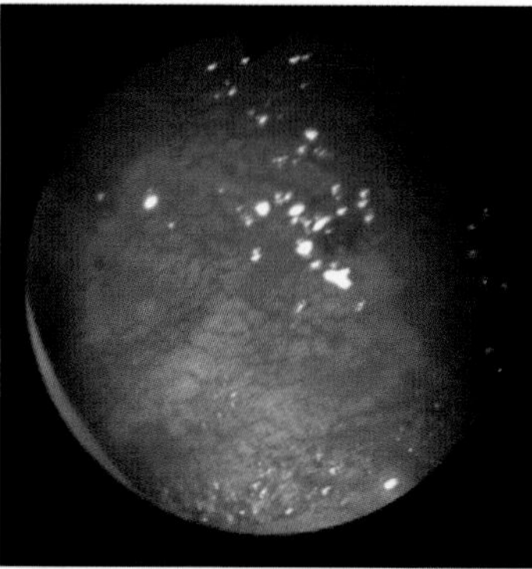

■ **Fig. 4.39** Endoscopic appearance of the distal duodenum in a patient with celiac disease. Mucosal atrophy, loss of folds, and a prominent erythema mosaic pattern are notable.

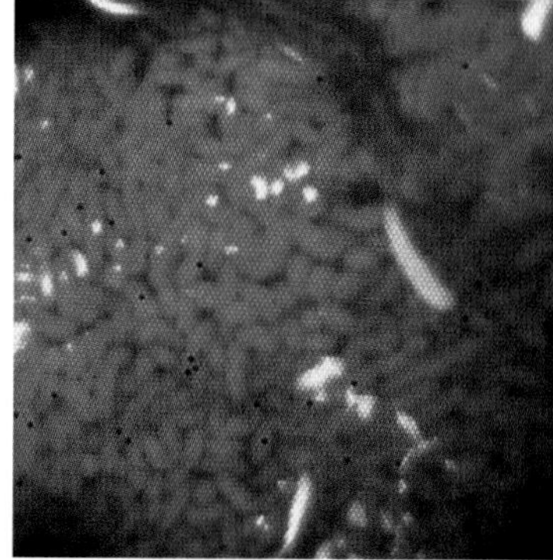

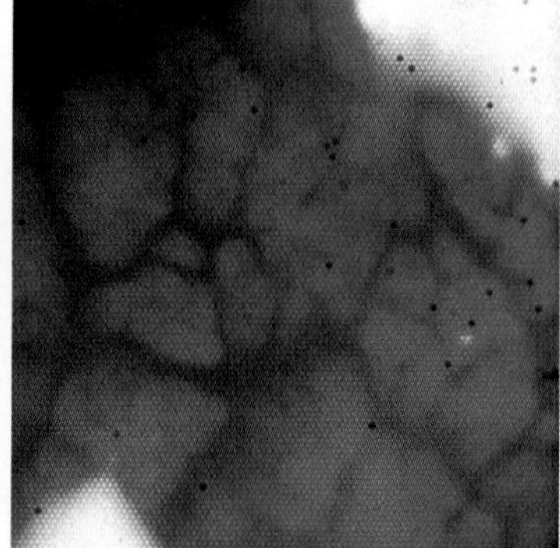

■ **Fig. 4.40** Villous abnormality in celiac disease. The distal duodenal mucosa has been outlined by spraying indigo carmine (5 ml x 0.4%) on the surface. The normal appearance (left) is replaced (right) by a mosaic, with dye outlining clefts and vestibules at the mouths of the crypts of Lieberkühn. Courtesy of Dr F.M. Stephens.

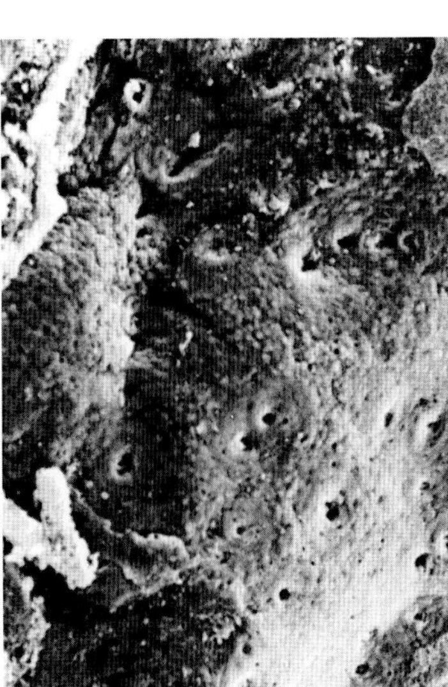

■ **Fig. 4.41** Scanning electron micrograph showing flat mucosa in untreated celiac disease (x 140).

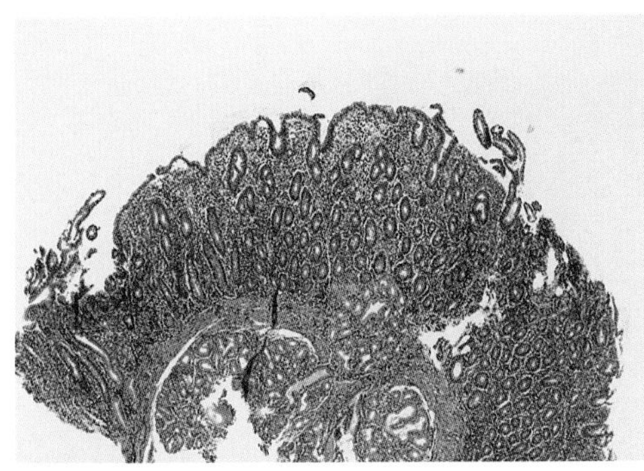

■ **Fig. 4.44** Celiac disease (gluten enteropathy): Marsh type 3c lesion. Duodenal biopsy showing the characteristic flattening of the villi, which results in a flat mucosal contour.

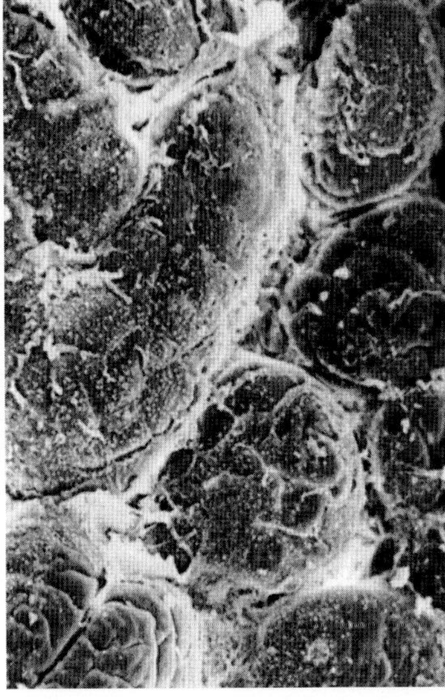

■ **Fig. 4.42** Electron micrograph showing partial villous atrophy as seen in a partially treated celiac patient (x 140).

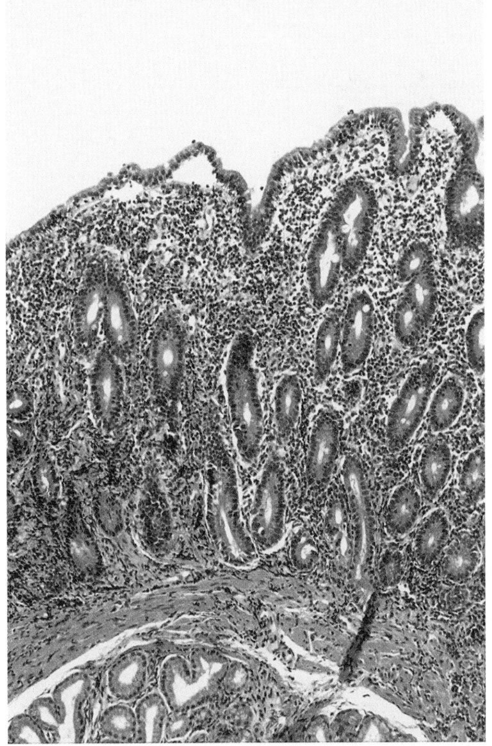

■ **Fig. 4.45** Celiac disease (gluten enteropathy): Marsh type 3c lesion. Higher magnification showing the elongation (reactive hyperplasia) of the crypts, which preserves the overall mucosal thickness despite the loss of villi and the intense plasmacytic infiltration of the stroma. The surface epithelium shows severe absorptive cell injury and complete loss of goblet cells.

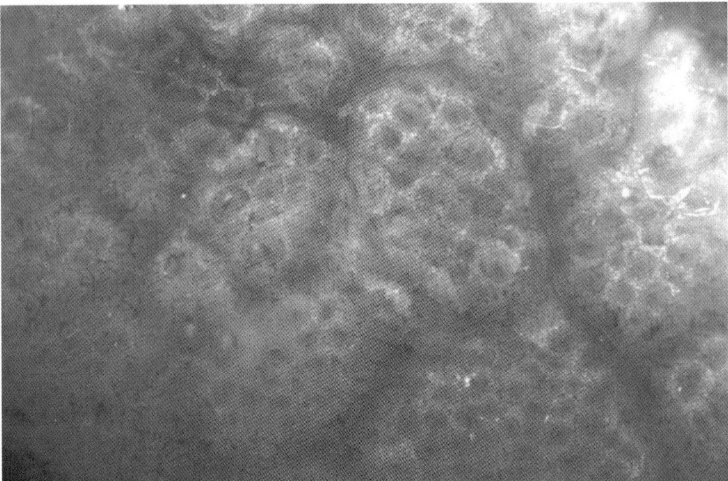

■ **Fig. 4.43** Dissecting microscope appearance of subtotal villous atrophy showing the mosaic pattern.

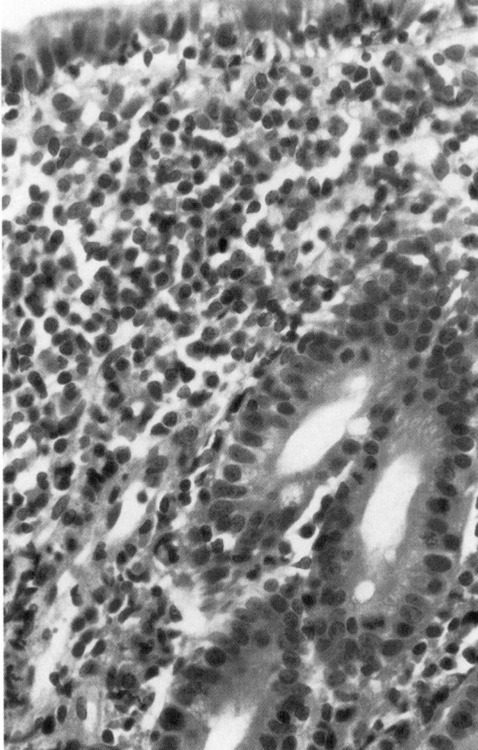

■ **Fig. 4.46** Celiac disease (gluten enteropathy): Marsh type 3c lesion. High magnification of the mucosal surface showing greatly increased numbers of intraepithelial lymphocytes in the surface (greater than 40 per 100 enterocytes) and superficial aspects of the crypts, the features that are the *sine qua non* of celiac disease.

NODULAR LYMPHOID HYPERPLASIA

Intestinal nodular lymphoid hyperplasia occurs in healthy adults and is frequent in normal children, where it should not be confused with inflammatory bowel disease (Fig. 4.51). An association with immunological disorders including celiac disease, and probably

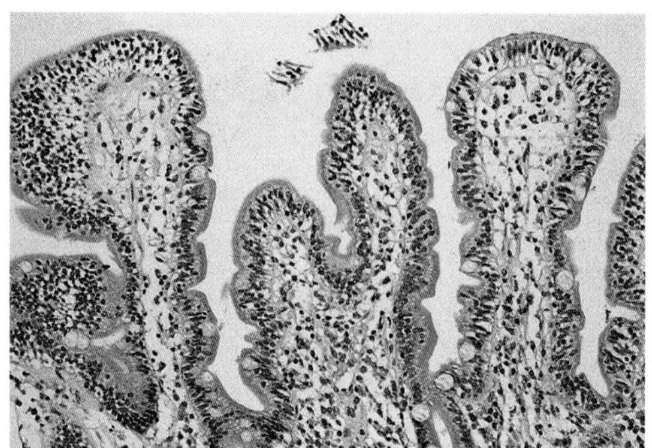

■ **Fig. 4.47** Celiac disease (gluten enteropathy): Marsh type I lesion. Microscopic appearance of an infiltrative lesion of the small bowel mucosa in gluten sensitivity showing greatly increased numbers of intraepithelial lymphocytes without significant villus injury or crypt hyperplasia as may occur in celiac patients ingesting small amounts of gluten, in patients with dermatitis herpetiformis, or family members of celiac patients.

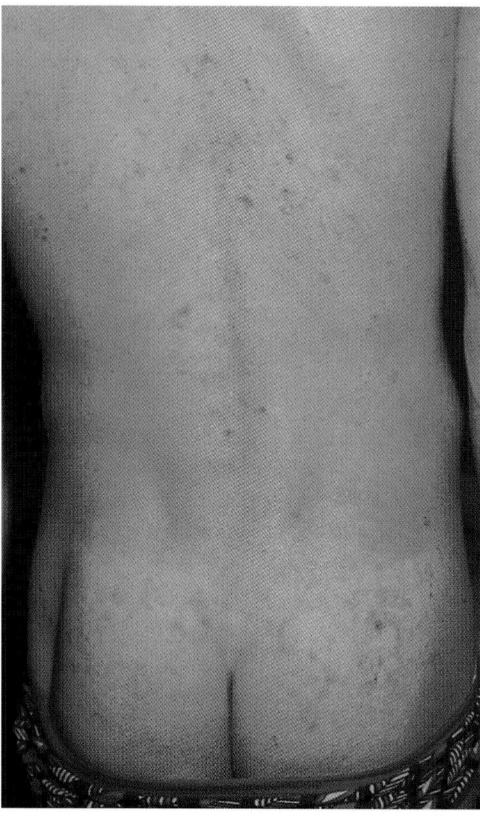

■ **Fig. 4.48** Dermatitis herpetiformis. The lesions are typically grouped and distributed over the scapulae, sacrum, buttocks, elbows, and knees. Courtesy of Dr S. Goolamali.

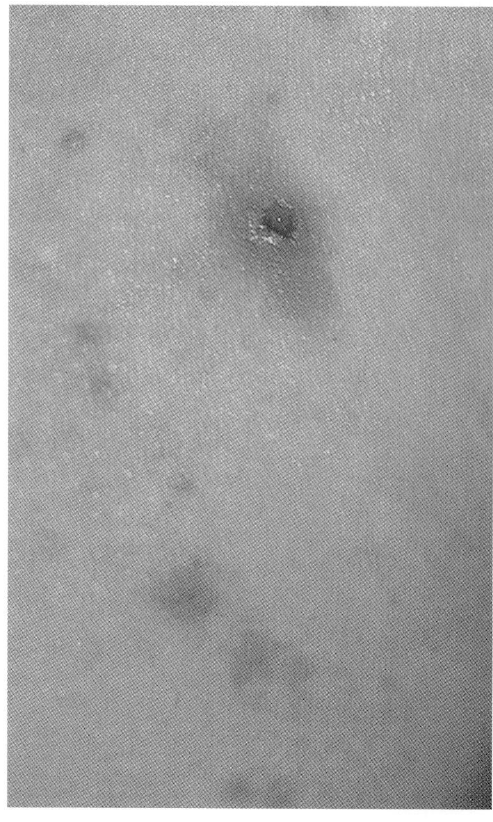

■ **Fig. 4.49** Dermatitis herpetiformis. Severe pruritus results in much excoriation and excavated lesions. Courtesy of Dr S. Goolamali.

lymphoma, also exists (Fig. 4.52). Small nodules, 1–3 mm in diameter, occur just below the epithelial cells of the intestinal mucosa; it is when the changes are sufficiently marked to cause radiological changes that difficulties in interpretation may arise (see also Chapter 3). In many cases, serum IgA and IgM (but not IgG) are reduced or undetectable. Diarrhea and malabsorption may occur and are often associated with intercurrent infection (e.g. with giardiasis). Histologically, there are abnormal mucosal aggregates of lymphoid cells, often forming follicles, which may have germinal centers (Figs 4.53, 4.54). Villous atrophy is rarely severe unless celiac disease is the underlying cause. Plasma cells are markedly reduced in number and may be absent.

INTESTINAL LYMPHANGIECTASIA

The primary form of this condition is a rare disorder of unknown etiology characterized by dilated lymphatic vessels in the small bowel. It generally affects children and young adults, and, though usually sporadic, has been reported with a familial pattern. Mild diarrhea and edema with growth retardation in children are usual, the gastrointestinal symptoms rarely being marked. Laboratory investigations demonstrate lymphopenia, hypoalbuminemia, and steatorrhea. Radiological appearances include variable degrees of thickening and enlargement of the valvulae conniventes, and diffuse dilatation of the bowel (Figs 4.55, 4.56). Dilatation of the lacteals and lymphatics are seen histologically (Fig. 4.57). The possibility that the disorder is a generalized abnormality of the lymphatic system is supported by the frequent presence of lymphatic hypoplasia on lymphangiography.

Secondary lymphatic obstruction, usually occurring in later life, but with similar clinical and radiological features, may complicate constrictive pericarditis, abdominal tuberculosis, Crohn's disease, or abdominal malignancy (Fig. 4.58). Isolated lymphangiectatic cysts are present in the jejunum in up to one-fifth of autopsy specimens, but have no known clinical significance.

ABETALIPOPROTEINEMIA

Abetalipoproteinemia (Bassen–Kornweig syndrome) is a rare disorder of lipoprotein synthesis inherited as an autosomal recessive condition of incomplete penetrance. In the first months of life, abdominal distention, steatorrhea, and failure to thrive are characteristic. In later childhood, neurological symptoms, including nystagmus, ataxia, athetosis, and weakness, demonstrate involvement of the cerebellum and basal ganglia; there is also an association with retinitis pigmentosa and cardiomyopathy.

The blood film shows the characteristic acanthocytes (Fig. 4.59), and beta-lipoprotein is absent from the blood. The villous archi-

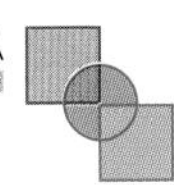

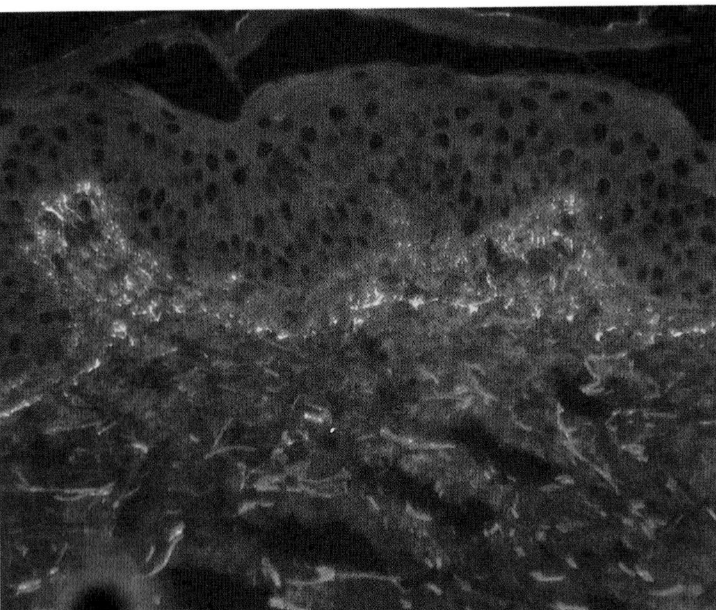

■ **Fig. 4.50** Immunofluorescence showing IgA staining in the papillary dermis of a skin biopsy from a patient with dermatitis herpetiformis. Courtesy of Professor J. Holbrow.

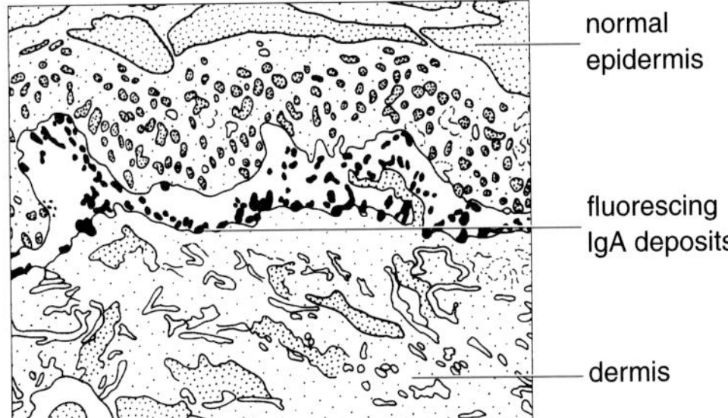

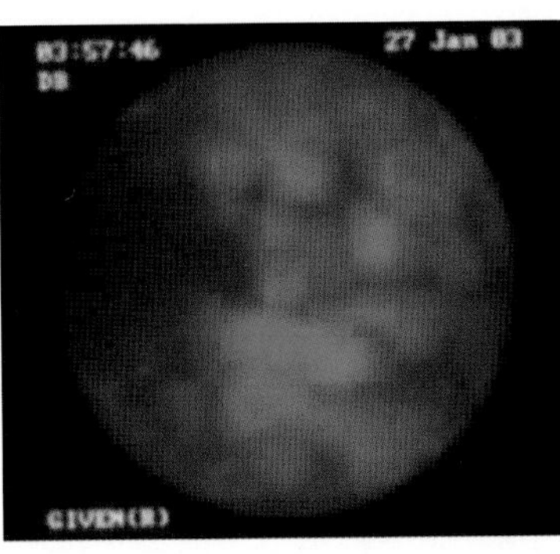

■ **Fig. 4.51** Lymphoid hyperplasia as demonstrated on capsule endoscopy in a young patient who proved to have no other pathology. Courtesy of Dr N. Kalantzis.

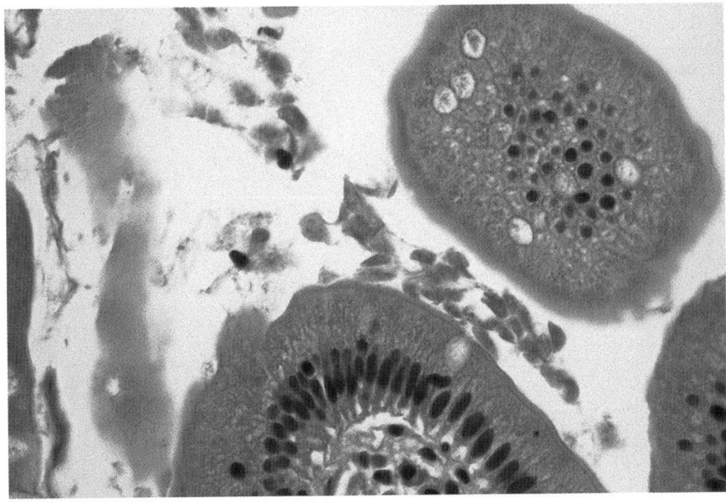

■ **Fig. 4.54** Nodular lymphoid hyperplasia with associated giardiasis. High magnification of the small bowel mucosa reveals associated parasitic infection by *Giardia lamblia* as a consequence of the underlying immunodeficiency state. Clusters of crescent-shaped organisms are seen between the tips of two villi.

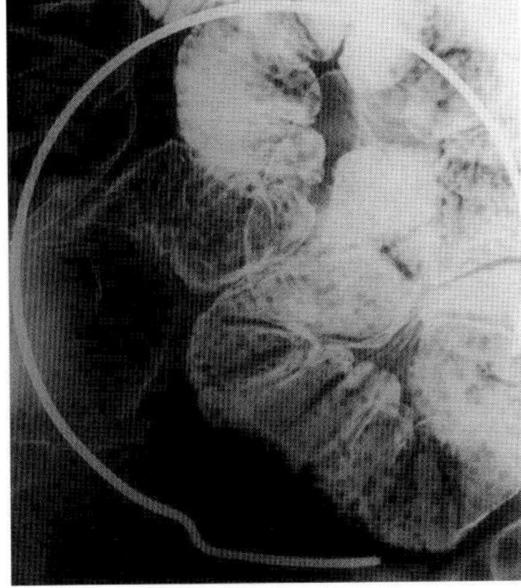

■ **Fig. 4.52** Lymphoid hyperplasia in patient with common variable immunodeficiency. Per-oral pneumocolon shows numerous 1–2 mm round radiolucent filling defects in the shallow barium pool separated by normal, smooth mucosa.

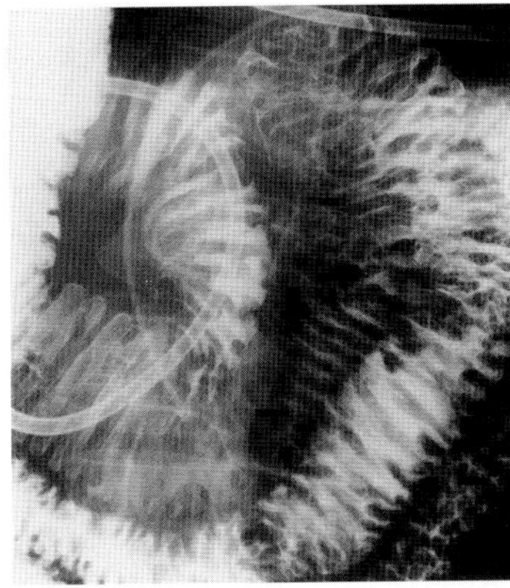

■ **Fig. 4.55** Enteroclysis in patient with lymphangiectasia. The folds of the proximal jejunum are moderately thick (3–4 mm).

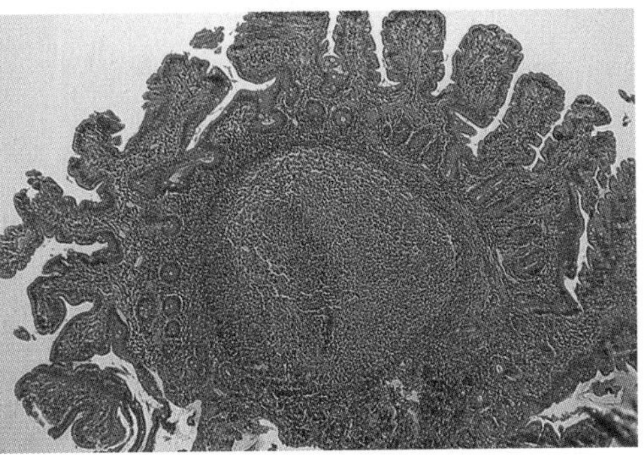

■ **Fig. 4.53** Histological appearance of the ileum with nodular lymphoid hyperplasia associated with immunodeficiency showing a greatly enlarged Peyer's patch (germinal center) in the submucosa causing polypoid projection of the mucosa.

tecture is morphologically normal but the terminal enterocytes develop large cytoplasmic vacuoles that contain neutral fat (Figs 4.60, 4.61). Although similar vacuolation may be seen in celiac disease and tropical sprue, it is then always associated with other villous abnormalities.

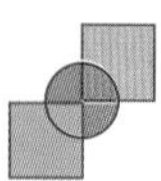

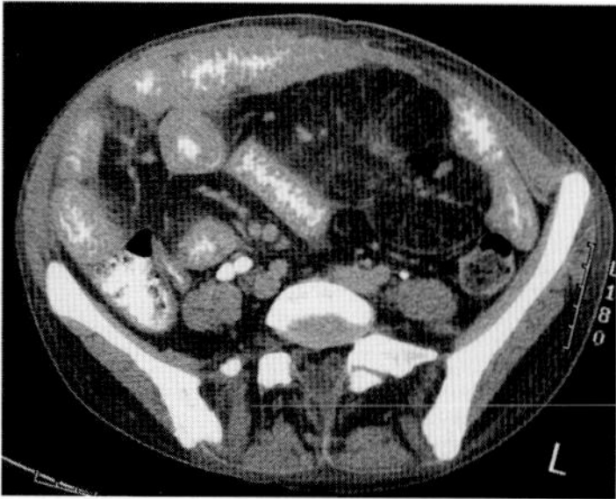

■ **Fig. 4.56** CT demonstrating a diffusely thickened small bowel wall in a patient with lymphangiectasia.

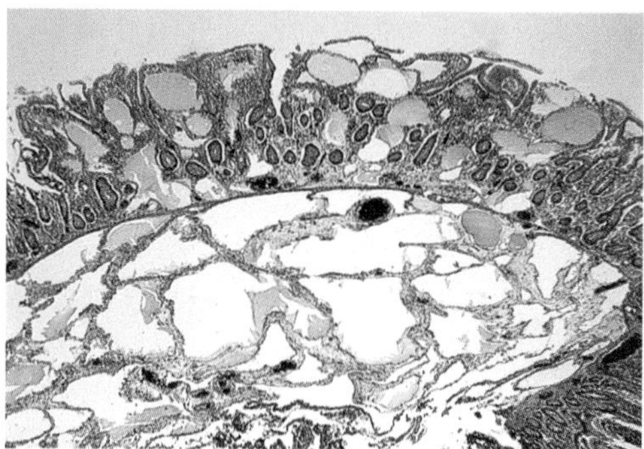

■ **Fig. 4.57** Microscopic appearance of primary intestinal lymphangiectasia showing greatly dilated mucosal lacteals and submucosal lymphatics, all distended with palely eosinophilic lymph.

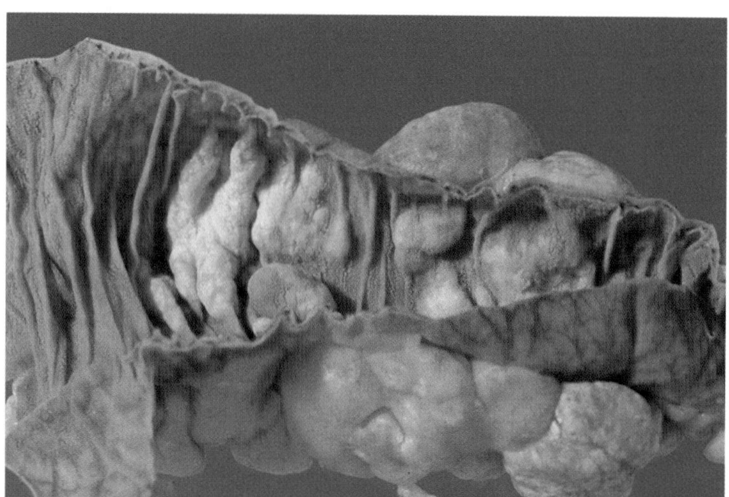

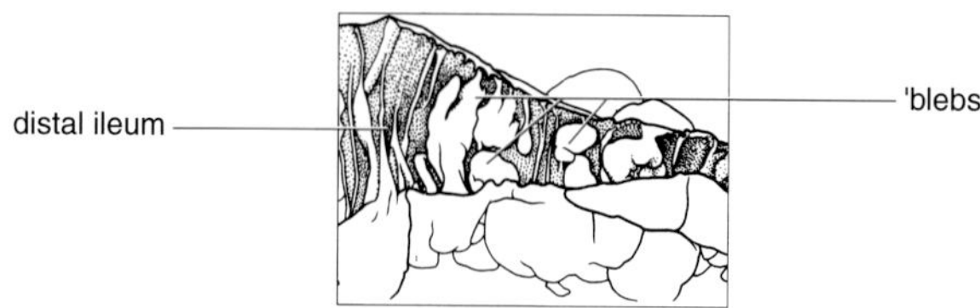

■ **Fig. 4.58** Yellow blebs produced by lymphangiectasia in the ileal mucosa, in this case secondary to a large mesenteric lymphangioma.

LYMPHOMA AND RELATED CONDITIONS

The abundant lymphoid tissue of the small intestine may become a focus of malignant transformation. Gastrointestinal lymphoma may be localized (with or without involvement of the adjacent mesenteric nodes), or part of a systemic process. Long sections of small bowel may be involved. Symptoms are often non-specific, with pain, partial obstruction, or (less often) malabsorptive syndromes, variously combined with anorexia, weight loss, and other systemic features. The characteristics of intestinal lymphoma are arguably best illustrated by a combination of CT scanning with luminal contrast studies (Figs 4.62–4.63). A number of distinctive radiological patterns are

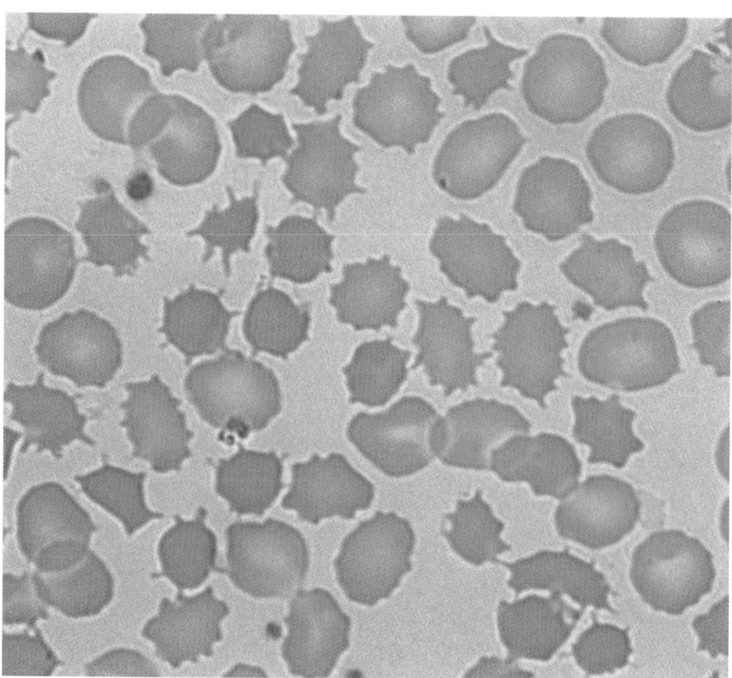

■ **Fig. 4.59** Acanthocytosis of red cells, characteristic of abetalipoproteinemia (x 400). Courtesy of Dr I. Hann.

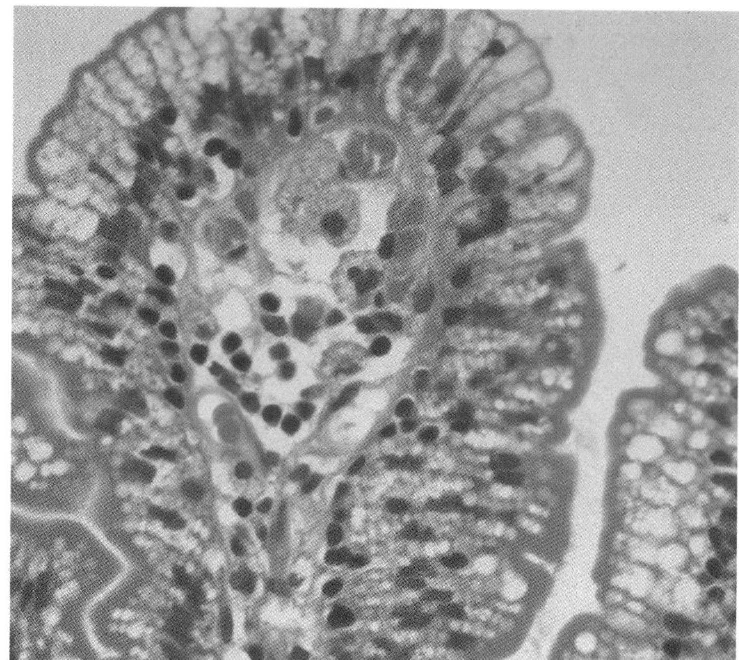

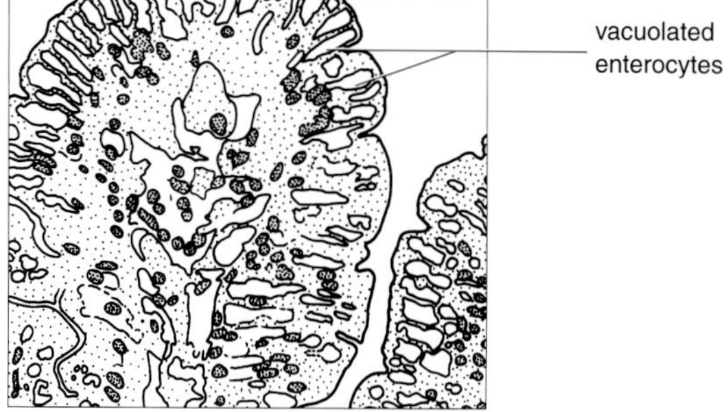

■ **Fig. 4.60** Marked vacuolation of enterocytes at tips of the villi in abetalipoproteinemia. H&E stain (x 480).

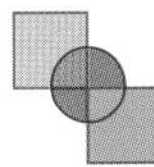

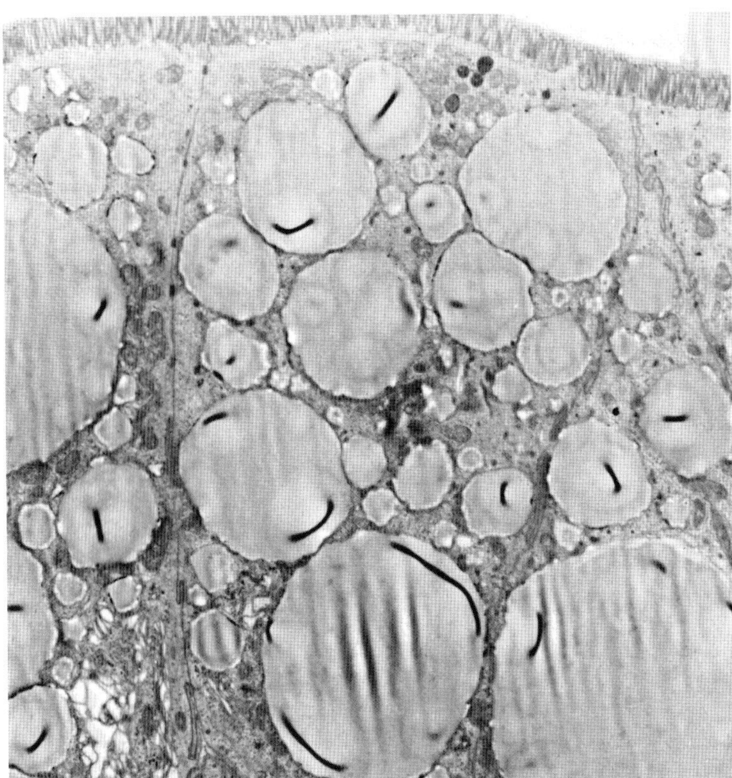

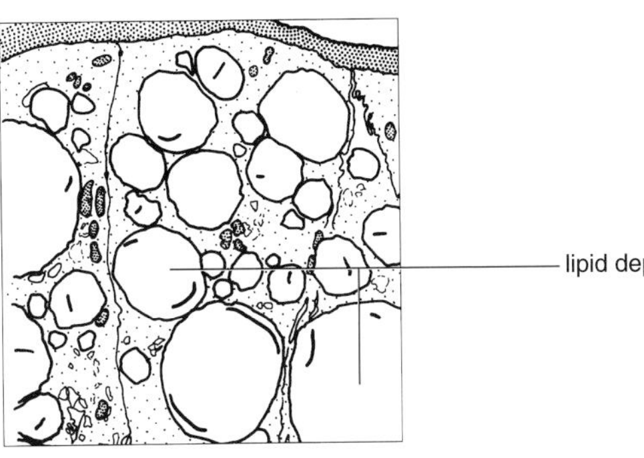

Fig. 4.61 Electron micrograph of enterocytes in abetalipoproteinemia showing large lipid droplets that are so large that they create some artefacts during sectioning (x 850). Courtesy of Dr W.O. Dobbins.

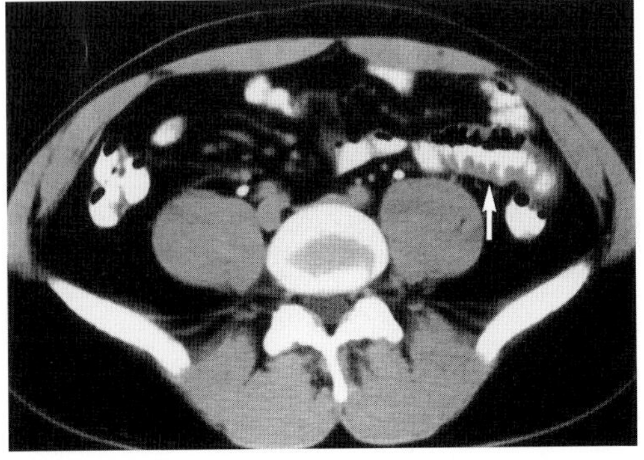

Fig. 4.62 Primary small bowel lymphoma manifested by thick folds. CT shows focal fold thickening (arrow) in mid jejunum.

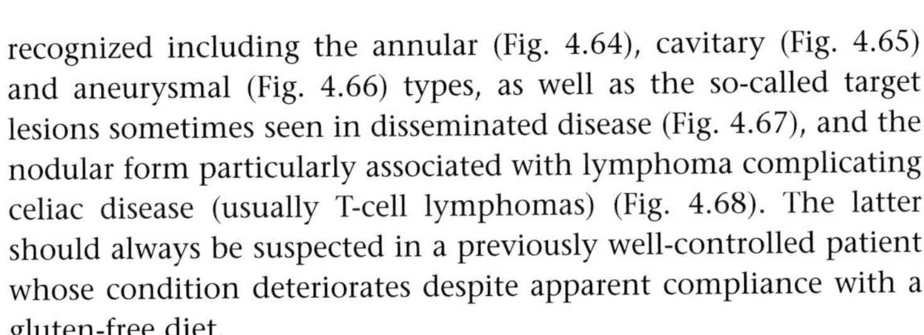

recognized including the annular (Fig. 4.64), cavitary (Fig. 4.65) and aneurysmal (Fig. 4.66) types, as well as the so-called target lesions sometimes seen in disseminated disease (Fig. 4.67), and the nodular form particularly associated with lymphoma complicating celiac disease (usually T-cell lymphomas) (Fig. 4.68). The latter should always be suspected in a previously well-controlled patient whose condition deteriorates despite apparent compliance with a gluten-free diet.

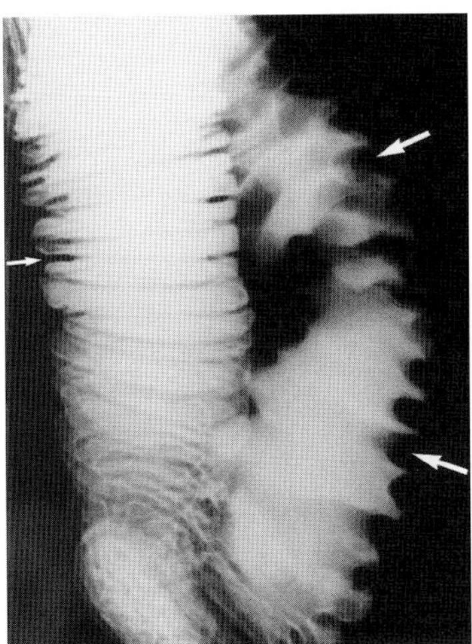

Fig. 4.63 Enteroclysis performed several days later in the patient of Fig. 4.61 shows markedly thickened folds (large arrows) in a focal small bowel loop. Compare the enlarged folds with normal width folds (small arrow).

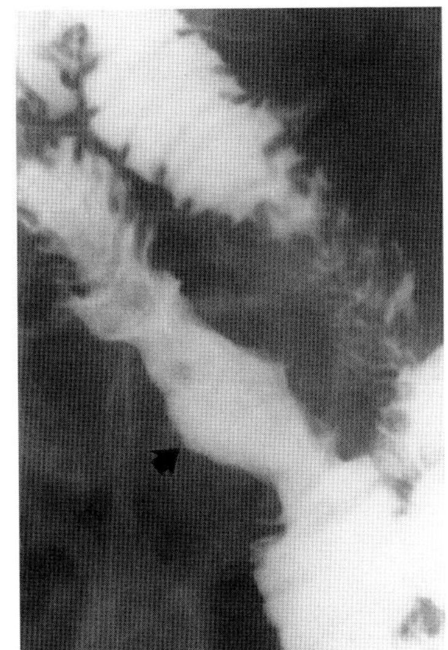

Fig. 4.64 Enteroclysis demonstrating the annular form of primary small intestinal lymphoma. Despite the circumferential extension (arrow), little luminal narrowing is seen. The valvulae conniventes have been effaced. (Reproduced with permission from reference 2, Fig. 2A.)

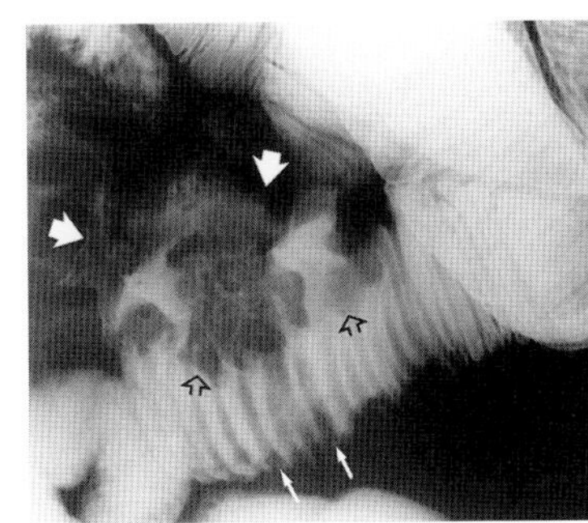

Fig. 4.65 Enteroclysis showing the cavitary form of lymphoma. A large barium-filled cavity (thick arrows) lies on the mesenteric border of a jejunal loop. Smooth, large nodules (open arrows) are present on the mesenteric border. Thick folds (thin arrows) radiate to the cavity. (Reproduced with permission from reference 6, Fig. 5.33.)

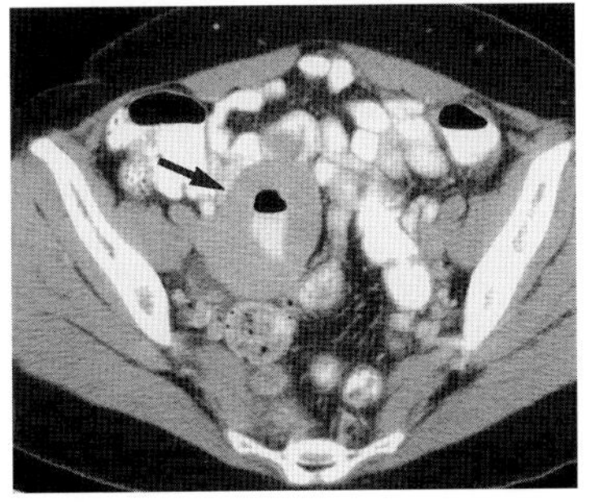

Fig. 4.66 CT demonstrating the aneurysmal form of lymphoma. The lumen of a bowel loop is surrounded by a homogeneous, thick-walled tumor (arrow).

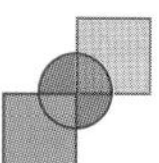

Lymphoma may itself cause a gluten-sensitive enteropathy, with response to gluten withdrawal, in the absence of celiac disease, and the index of suspicion should be high, especially in older patients. Intestinal lymphoma is also seen frequently in the late stages of AIDS, and both should be included in the differential diagnosis of the patient with diffuse abdominal pain, weight loss, and fevers, particularly when other investigations have failed to provide a diagnosis. A high index of suspicion, early CT scanning, and a readiness to perform laparoscopy or laparotomy to provide tissue are crucial in the diagnosis of intestinal lymphomas; nonetheless distal duodenal biopsies may provide histological confirmation when diffuse involvement includes the proximal small bowel.

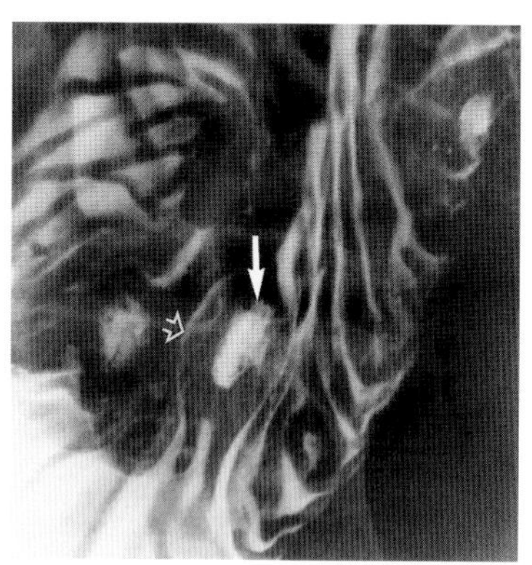

Fig. 4.67 Small bowel follow-through demonstrating target lesions in a patient with disseminated lymphoma. Five smooth surfaced, well-circumscribed masses are seen in the duodenum, four with central cavities. A representative target lesion (open arrow) with central ulceration (large arrow) is identified. (Reproduced with permission from reference 2, Fig. 12B.)

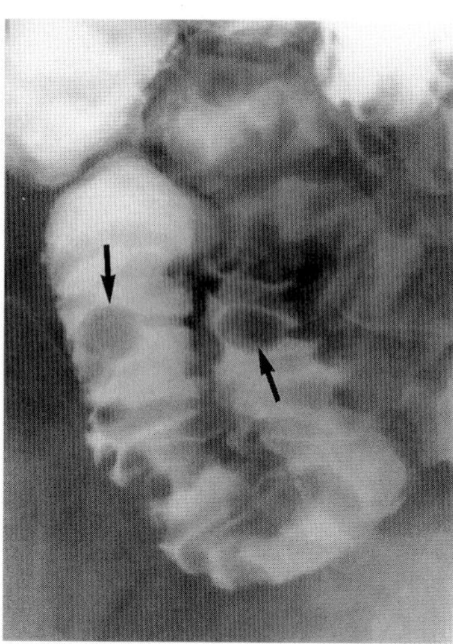

Fig. 4.68 Lymphoma arising in celiac disease. A loop of jejunum shows smooth, thick folds. Smooth ovoid nodules (arrows) splay and enlarge the folds. (Reproduced with permission from reference 2, Fig. 6.)

Focal lymphomas are commoner in the ileum (Figs 4.69, 4.70), and are more likely to be complicated by perforation or fissuring ulceration. Intestinal lymphomas are classified following standard criteria for lymphoma elsewhere in the body (Fig. 4.71). Most are of B cell lineage. In celiac patients however, complicating lymphoma is usually of the 'histiocytic' type, but this is a misnomer since the tumor is now recognized to be of T-cell origin: the preferred term is enteropathy-related T-cell lymphoma. These preferentially affect the jejunum.

Mediterranean lymphoma affecting the small bowel is seen mainly in patients from the eastern Mediterranean area and the Middle East in whom it is the commonest site of extranodal lymphoma. The term is not ideal, since immunoproliferation within the intestine may be unassociated with lymphoma, and because some of these patients have alpha heavy chain disease (see below). Immunoproliferative small intestinal disease (IPSID), which encompasses the lymphomatous and non-lymphomatous forms of this condition, is perhaps a more appropriate term.

Alpha heavy chain disease is really another variant of IPSID rather than a separate condition. Proliferation of lymphoid tissue predominantly involving the IgA secretory system leads to the production of incomplete immunoglobulin molecules. It is found most often in poor populations in the Middle East, the eastern Mediterranean, and southern Africa. The clinical features are predominantly gastrointestinal and include severe malabsorption; some patients present with finger clubbing (Fig. 4.71), and there may be respiratory

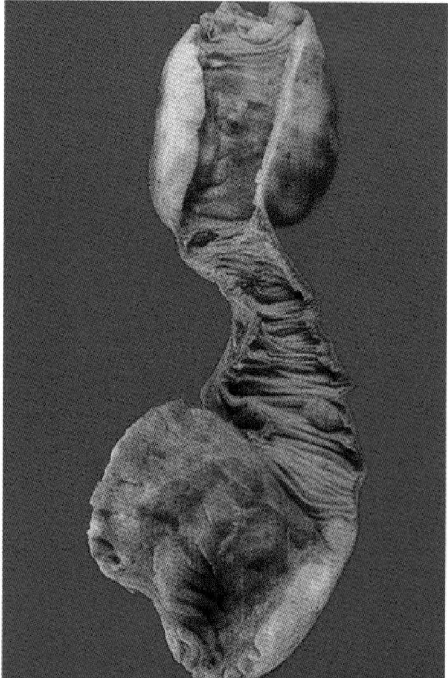

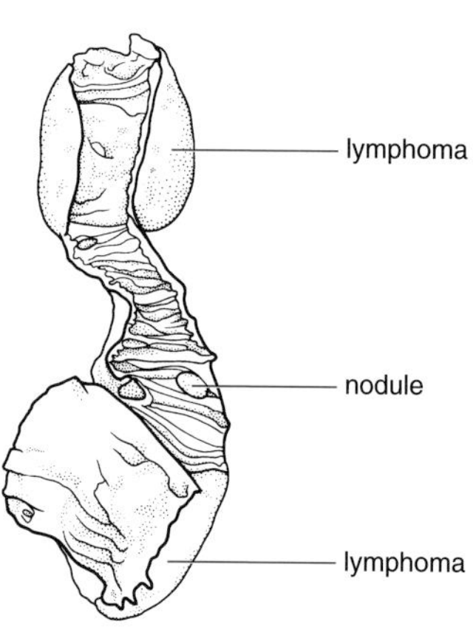

Fig. 4.69 Macroscopic view of low-grade B cell lymphoma of the jejunum showing ulceration and petechial hemorrhage of the luminal surface and thickening of the intestinal wall, the surface of which shows the characteristic pale white-tan glossy 'fish-flesh' appearance of lymphoma.

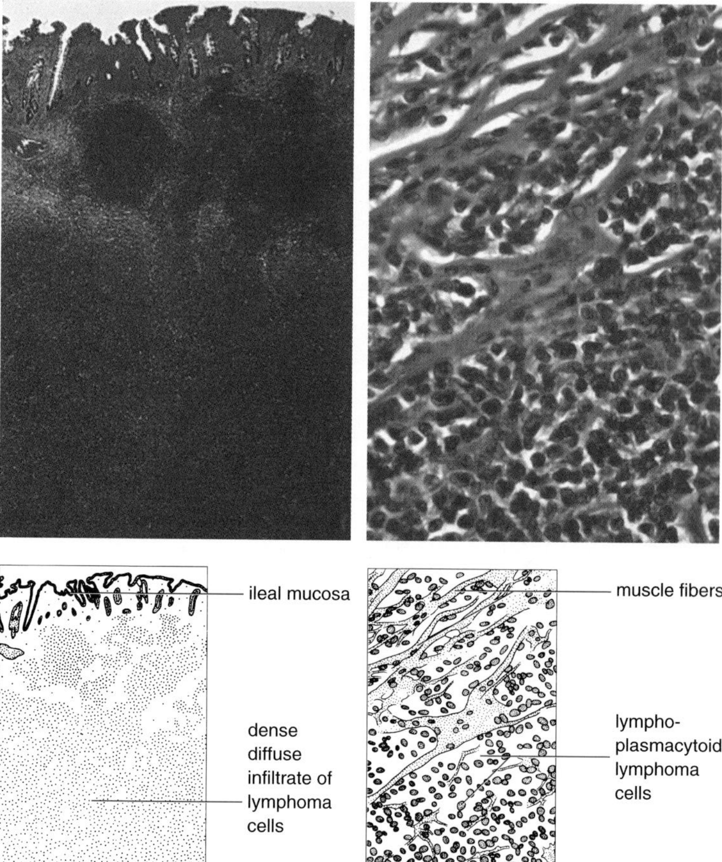

Fig. 4.70 Histological appearance of small bowel lymphoma. There are sheets of tumor cells (left) infiltrating the submucosa and muscle with relative sparing of the mucosa. H&E stain (x 15). Lymphoplasmacytoid lymphoma cells (right) infiltrating between the muscle fibers of the ileal wall. H&E (x 320).

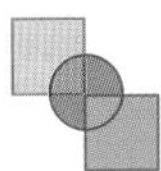

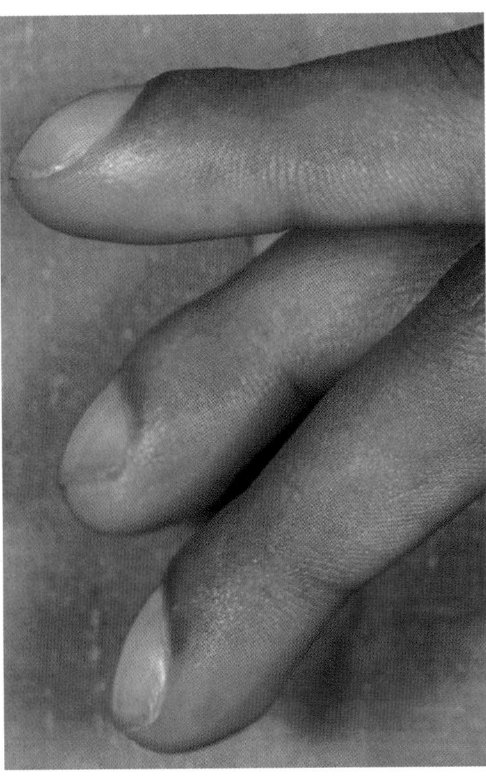

■ **Fig. 4.71** Severe finger clubbing in patient with alpha-chain disease.

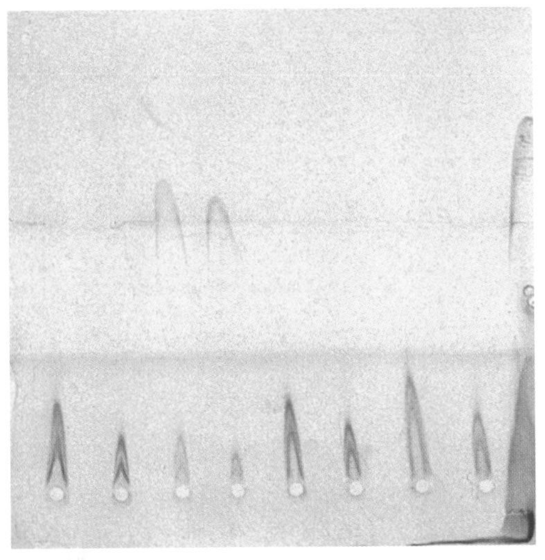

■ **Fig. 4.72** Gel electrophoresis in alpha-chain disease (patient 2) with accompanying positive control (lane 9). Patients 1 and 3 are normal. Serum containing heavy chains is precipitated in the distal third of the gel by anti-alpha chain antibodies. Normal light chains are precipitated in the proximal third of the gel by anti-kappa and anti-lambda antibodies. Courtesy of Dr A. Howard.

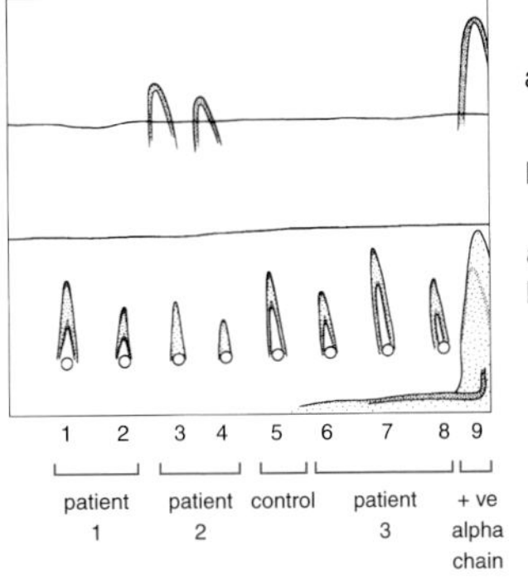

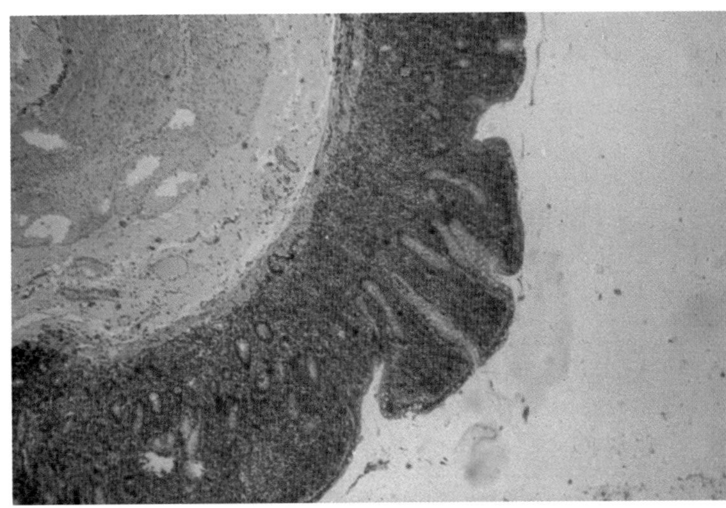

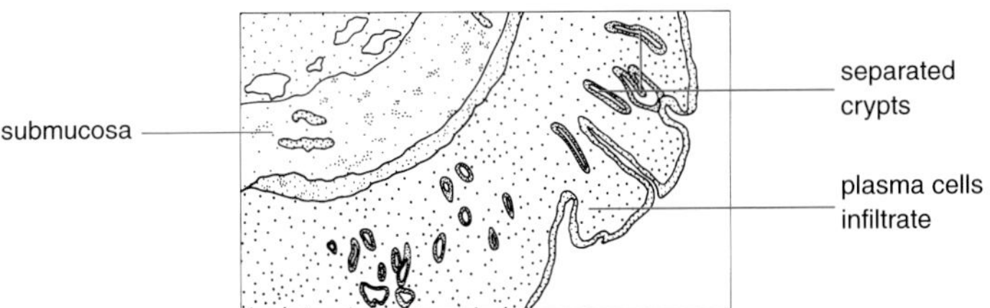

■ **Fig. 4.73** Histological appearance in alpha chain disease. Prior to the appearance of frank tumor, the mucosa shows diffuse infiltration, with mature plasma cells pushing the crypts apart. H&E stain (x 30).

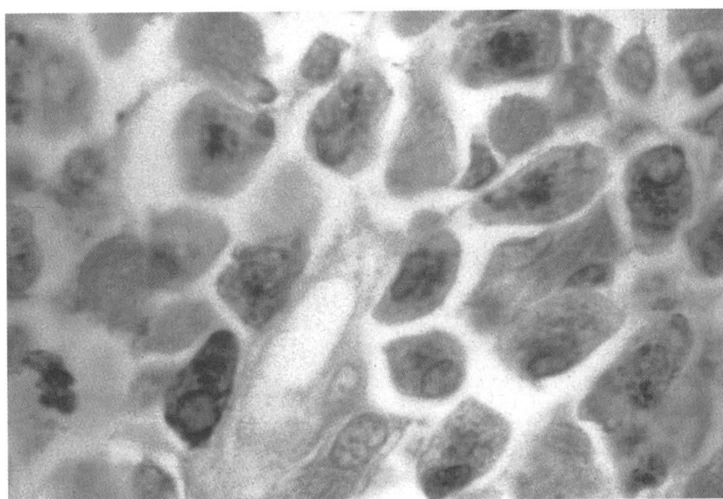

■ **Fig. 4.74** Peroxidase staining of IgA (staining brown) in plasma cells, and the absence of light chains, are demonstrable (right) (x 480).

disease. There are increased numbers of plasma cells in intestinal biopsies, but the IgA molecules produced are incomplete, comprising alpha heavy chains in considerable relative excess. These molecules are readily detectable in blood, urine, and jejunal secretions, by gel electrophoresis (Fig. 4.72).

Intestinal plasma cell proliferation also involves the mesenteric nodes and is followed by the development of overt lymphoma in most cases. In the early stages, the epithelium is intact, with crypts widely separated by the plasma cell infiltrate (Fig. 4.73). A variety of lymphomatous morphologies are recognized, the malignant infiltrate being diffusely scattered, or aggregated within nodules in the deep lamina propria. Ultimately, the muscle is infiltrated and the crypts destroyed, and at this stage, tumor masses are usually apparent. Immunohistological staining demonstrates the alpha chains (Fig. 4.74) until advanced stages of disease (Fig. 4.75) when these are lost.

ULCERATIVE JEJUNOILEITIS

Attention should also be given to the unusual condition of ulcerative jejunoileitis, which may occur in isolation or as a component of celiac disease. Essentially it is a syndrome of diffuse small bowel ulceration with accompanying malabsorption. The imaging confirms

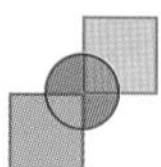

thickening of the intestinal folds and the ulcerated mucosal surface, the jejunum generally being much more affected than the ileum (Figs 4.76, 4.77). Histologically there is a partial villous atrophy. It is likely that this also is a form of IPSID. It seems to have a relatively poor prognosis, representing a low-grade malignancy of a lymphomatous nature.

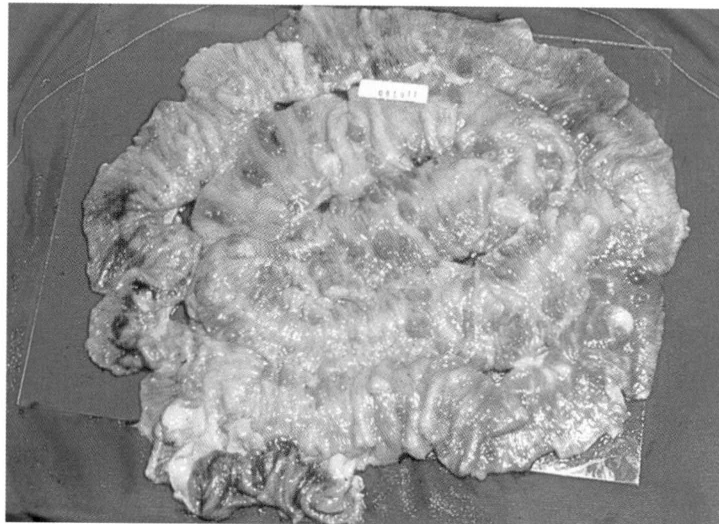

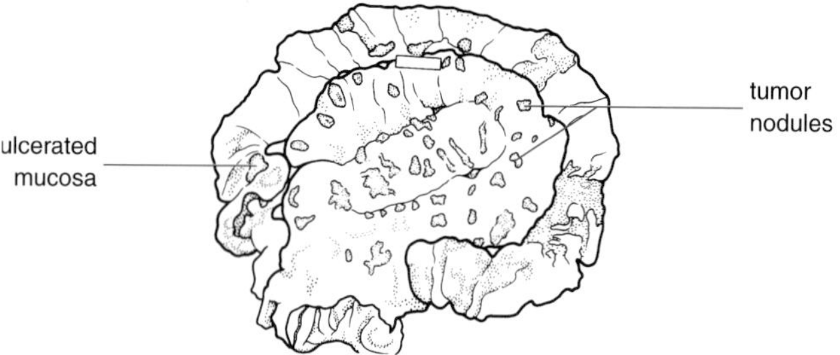

■ **Fig. 4.75** Resected ileum in alpha chain disease with frank tumor nodules visible in the mesentery and ulcerating the mucosa. Courtesy of Dr F. Asselah.

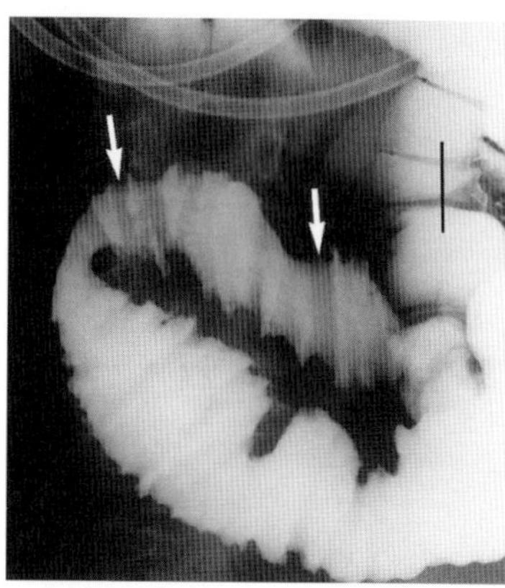

■ **Fig. 4.76** Small bowel enema demonstrating ulcerative jejunoileitis arising in celiac disease. A loop of distal jejunum has thick, undulating folds (arrows). The presence of celiac disease is diagnosed by decreased number of valvulae conniventes proximally (1 inch is identified by the black bar and demonstrates one–two folds per inch). These findings are indistinguishable from lymphoma arising in celiac disease. (Reproduced with permission from reference 4, Fig. 7.)

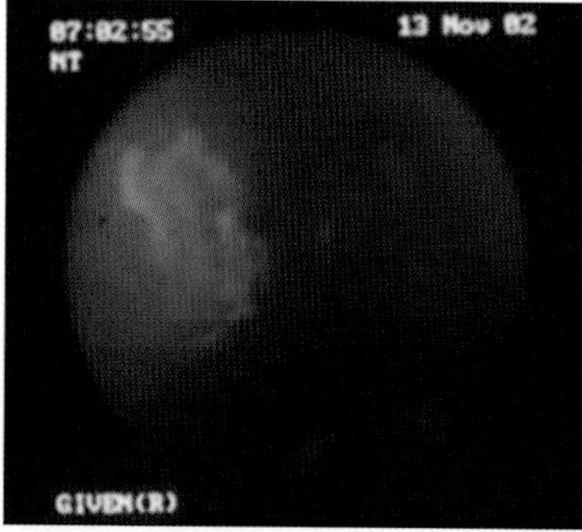

■ **Fig. 4.77** Ulcerative jejunitis with no associated condition, seen here as viewed by the endoscopy capsule. Courtesy of Dr N Kalantzis.

KAPOSI'S SARCOMA

The increased incidence of cutaneous Kaposi's sarcoma was a key feature in the recognition of AIDS. It is now clear that the human immunodeficiency virus is not solely responsible for this, and co-infection with another viral agent has been found to be present in almost 100% of cases. This is now known to be a gamma herpes virus, closely related to Epstein–Barr virus, and has been designated HHV-8. It is also found in 'classic' non-AIDS Kaposi's. HHV-8 infection is necessary, but not sufficient, to cause Kaposi's, hence the link with the immunosuppression of HIV infection. The gastroenterological manifestations of Kaposi's sarcoma are usually minor (Fig. 4.78), but lesions affecting the buccal mucosa may cause difficulties with mastication. Gastrointestinal involvement, however, is not rare, and autopsy studies have indicated that patients with ten or more cutaneous lesions should be assumed to have visceral involvement too (Figs 4.79, 4.80). Occasionally, Kaposi lesions will be responsible for upper gastrointestinal bleeding (see Chapter 2). Involvement of the small intestine may also cause blood loss (usually presenting as iron-deficiency anemia), and larger, polypoid, tumors may also cause partial obstruction. Intussusception also occurs and can then lead to complete obstruction.

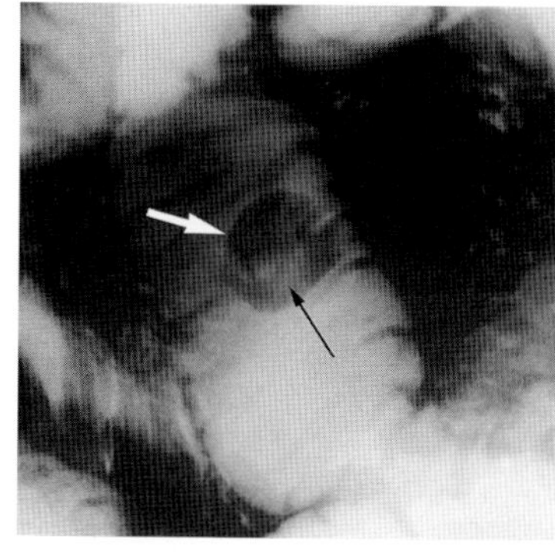

■ **Fig. 4.78** Small bowel follow-through demonstrating Kaposi's sarcoma in a patient with AIDS. A 1 cm smooth-surfaced polypoid mass (white arrow) with a central ulcer (black arrow) is seen in the mid small bowel.

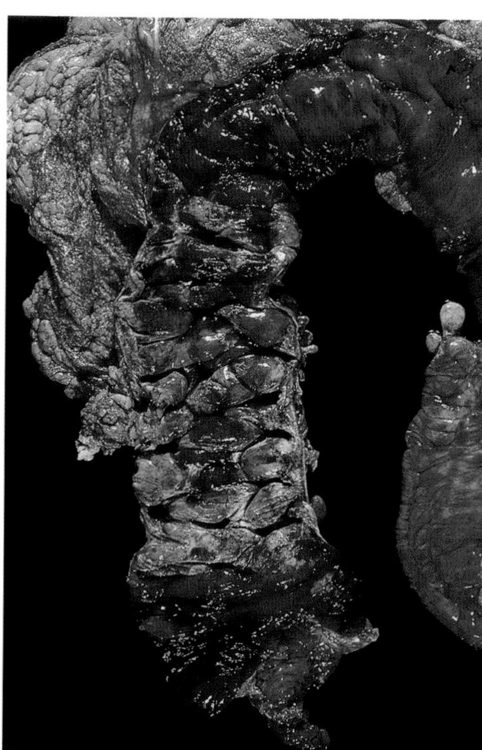

■ **Fig. 4.79** Segmental small bowel resection showing Kaposi's sarcoma involving the small intestine of an AIDS patient. The mucosal folds are distended with metastatic tumor-associated hemorrhage giving the lesions a characteristic red-maroon color.

SMALL BOWEL STROMAL TUMORS

A wide range of very rare gastrointestinal stromal tumors can affect the small bowel. There is a tendency for these to be responsible for thickening of the bowel wall, and in the example shown a leiomyosarcoma variant is the cause of fairly dramatic changes readily apparent on CT scanning (Fig. 4.81). The nature and distribution of the changes help in the differentiation from other neoplastic conditions (Figs 4.82, 4.83), and from Crohn's disease, which is the other main differential diagnosis (see Chapter 5).

SMALL BOWEL CARCINOMA

Adenocarcinomas of the small bowel constitute less than 2% of all gastrointestinal malignancies. The duodenum is most often affected, and 90% of carcinomas occur within 20 cm of the ligament of Treitz. A number of conditions predispose to intestinal carcinoma, the most important of which are celiac disease (see above) and familial adenomatous polyposis (see Chapter 7). There is an increased frequency of carcinoma in Peutz–Jeghers syndrome (see below) and possibly also in Crohn's disease (see Chapter 5).

Presentation is usually in the 6th and 7th decades, with symptoms similar to those of patients with intestinal lymphoma. Bleeding is, however, somewhat commoner, and the presence of a focal abdominal mass more likely. The diagnosis may be deduced from barium studies (Figs 4.84, 4.85), CT scan, or capsule endoscopy.

Macroscopically, a polypoid pattern is commonest, and this often leads to intussusception or bleeding, but sessile, stenosing, and ulcerating tumors are also seen (Fig. 4.86). The histological appearances are those of gastrointestinal adenocarcinoma (Fig. 4.87).

Secondary carcinoma of the small bowel

Metastases to the small intestine are relatively common, but rarely of clinical significance in their own right. They usually involve the serosal surface of the bowel, but when submucosal or mucosal involvement occurs, differentiation from primary tumors of the intestine is difficult if the true primary site is not obvious. Single or multiple polypoid masses, which may have surface ulceration, are seen radiologically (Fig. 4.88).

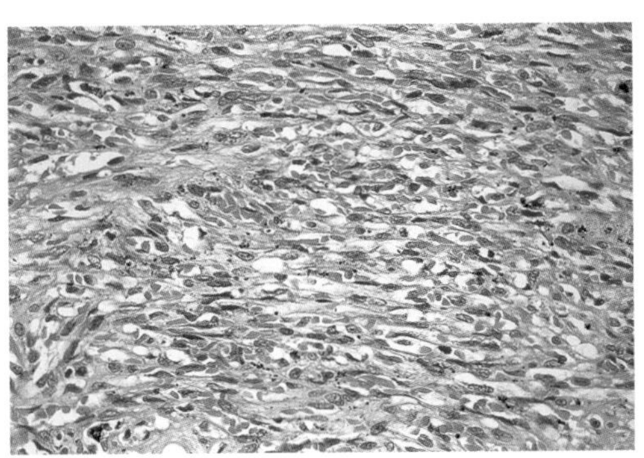

Fig. 4.80 Kaposi's sarcoma. Microscopic appearance showing typical spindle cell proliferations within which numerous narrow slits containing erythrocytes and deposits of hemosiderin are seen.

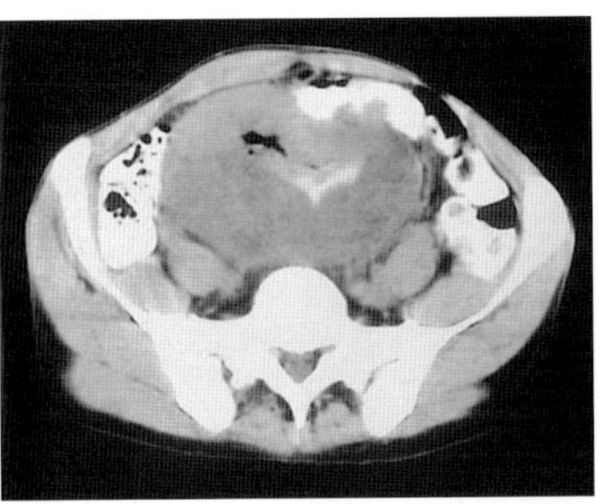

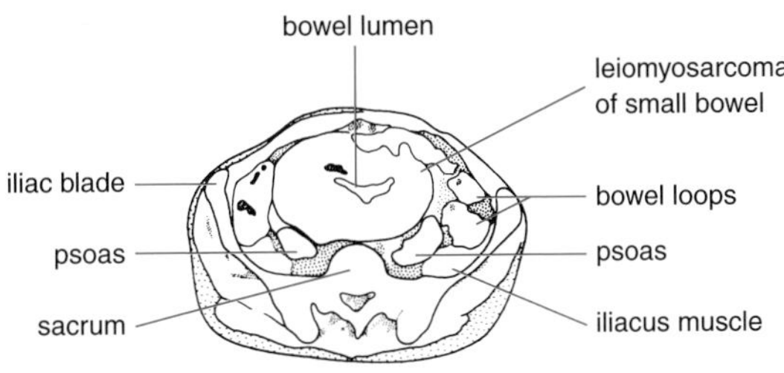

Fig. 4.81 CT scan showing gross thickening of the small bowel wall in an immunocompetent patient with a gastrointestinal stroma tumor (of the leiomyosarcoma type).

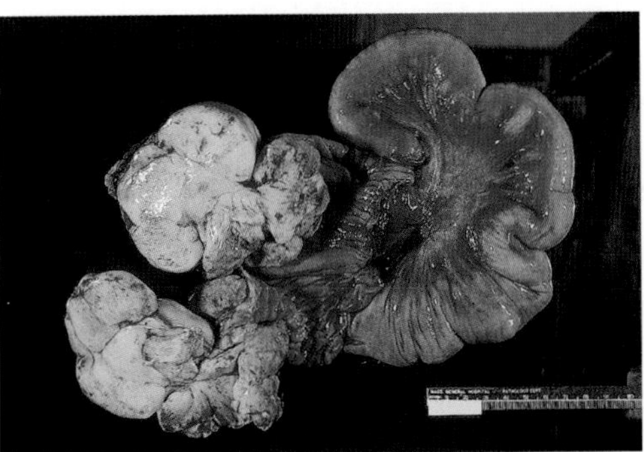

Fig. 4.82 A segmental resection of the jejunum showing the typical whorled, bulging cut surface of a gastrointestinal stromal tumor (GIST) arising from the wall and growing into the mesentery.

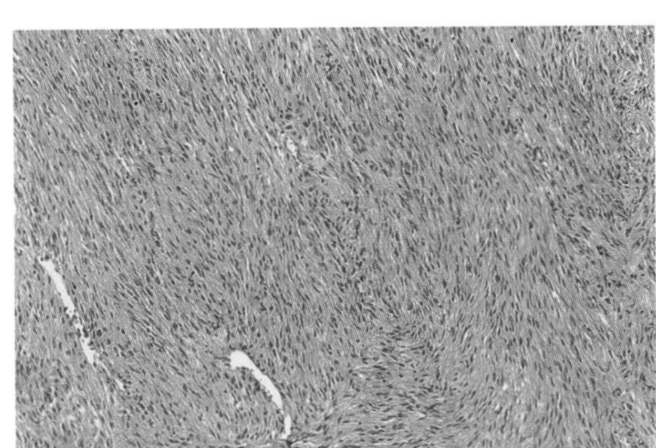

Fig. 4.83 Microscopic view of a low-grade jejunal GIST showing a densely cellular spindle cell sarcoma with a low mitotic rate.

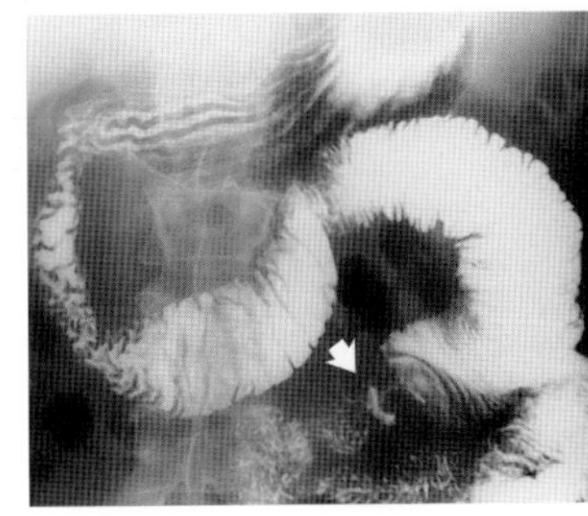

Fig. 4.84 Small bowel follow-through demonstrating small bowel adenocarcinoma. In the second loop of the jejunum, there is a 2 cm in length annular lesion with a shelf-like margin proximally and a central ulcer (arrow). Obstruction is manifested as dilatation of the distal duodenum and jejunum proximal to the tumor. (Reproduced with permission from reference 7, Fig. 46.34A.)

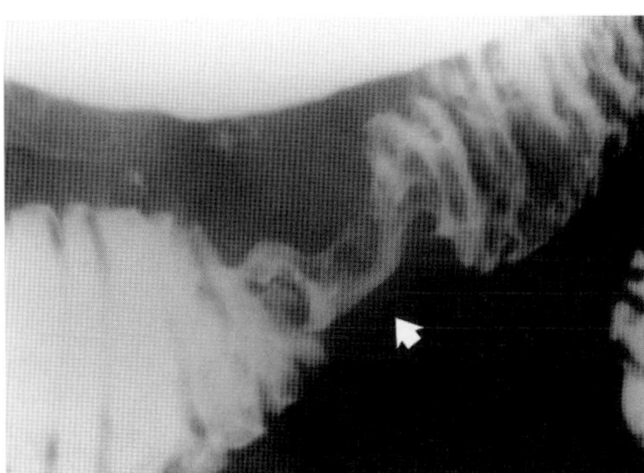

Fig. 4.85 Small bowel follow-through showing adenocarcinoma of the jejunum. A 3 cm annular lesion (arrow) has shelf-like borders and nodular mucosa.

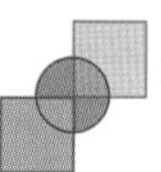

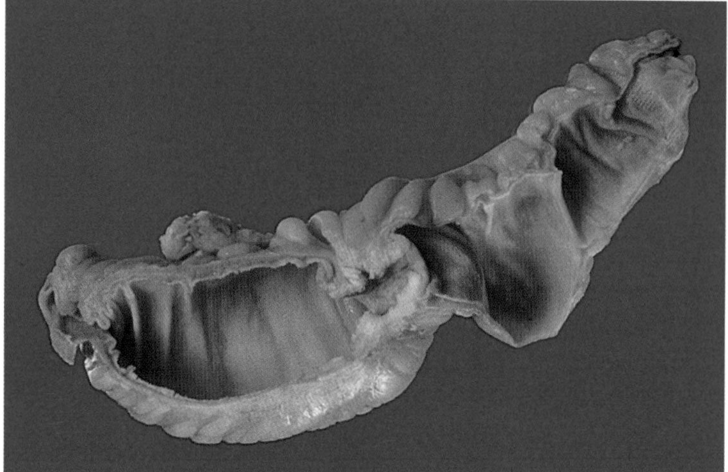

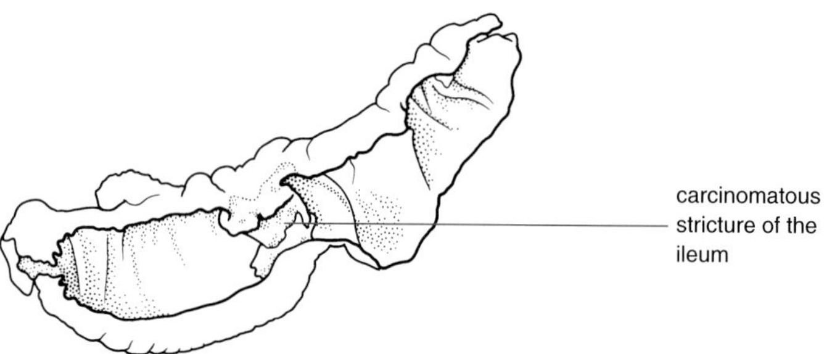

■ **Fig. 4.86** Macroscopic appearance of a resected annular carcinoma in the mid-ileum.

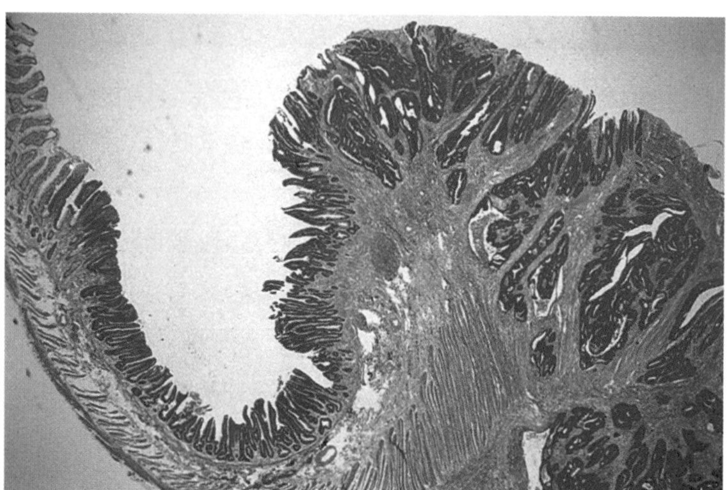

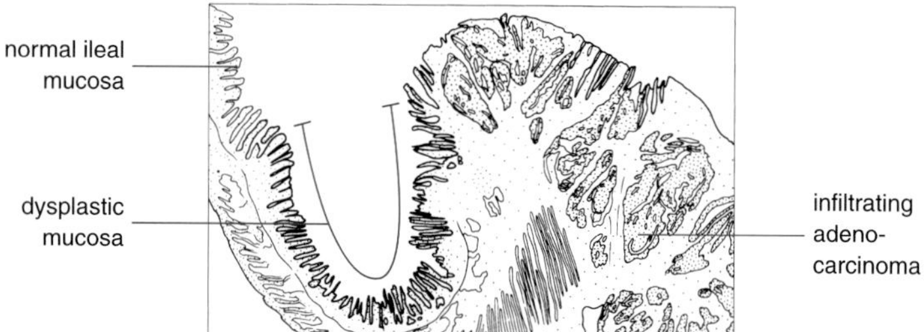

■ **Fig. 4.87** Histological appearance of primary carcinoma of the small bowel showing the gradual transition between normal mucosa, through dysplasia to invasive adenocarcinoma. H&E stain (x 10).

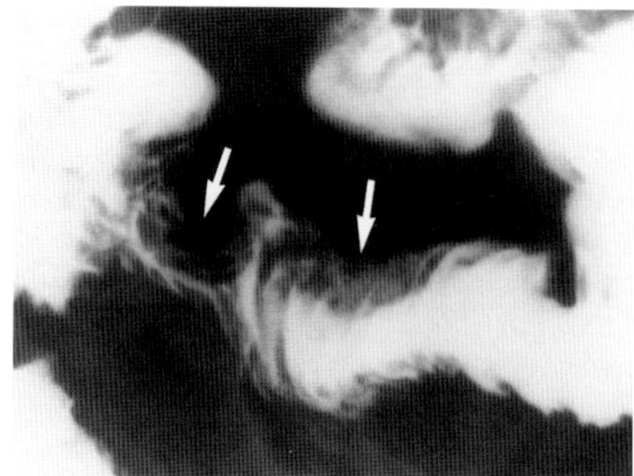

■ **Fig. 4.88** Small bowel follow-through depicting intraperitoneal metastasis from metastatic breast carcinoma. Spot image of the distal ileum shows several smooth-surfaced, broad-based masses (arrows) on the mesenteric border.

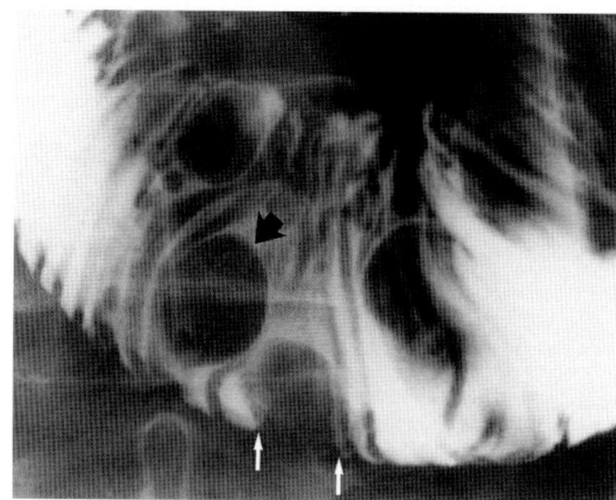

■ **Fig. 4.89** Enteroclysis demonstrating numerous hematogenous metastases in patient with occult gastrointestinal bleeding and history of metastatic melanoma. Five smooth-surfaced, well-circumscribed masses (representative mass identified by black arrow) are seen in the mid small bowel. One tumor is seen in profile and has abrupt angulation (white arrows) with luminal contour. These are typical submucosal masses. (Reproduced with permission from reference 6, Fig. 5.17.)

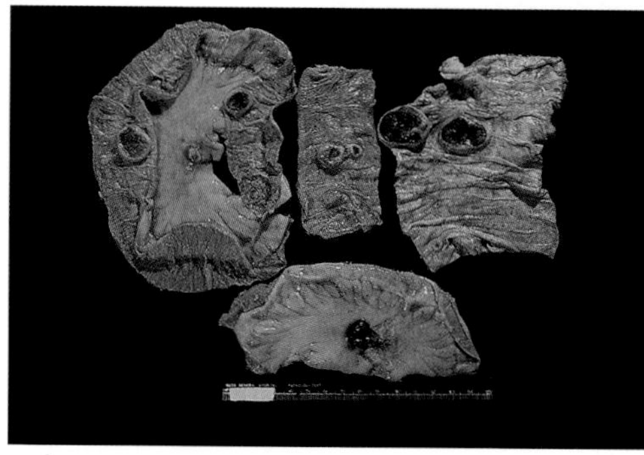

■ **Fig. 4.90** Metastatic melanoma. Segmental small bowel resection for metastatic melanoma showing numerous darkly pigmented lesions with central necrosis in the mucosa and mesenteric fat.

SECONDARY MELANOMA OF THE SMALL BOWEL

Melanomatosis is particularly prone to involve the small bowel, and while the radiological and macroscopic features are generally characteristic (Figs 4.89, 4.90), it can be difficult to make a histological diagnosis without the assistance of immunohistochemistry, given a strong overlap with the appearances of poorly differentiated carcinoma (Figs 4.91–4.94).

CARCINOID TUMORS OF THE SMALL BOWEL

Carcinoid tumors occur most often in the ileum and appendix, and are usually chance findings at appendectomy (see Chapter 7). The tumors arise from the argentaffin or Kulchitzky cells which lie deep in the crypts of Lieberkühn and are derived from neural crest tissue. Like other APUD tumors, carcinoids contain numerous neurosecretory granules. Large tumors (Fig. 4.95) may cause obstruction or intussusception, but symptoms are otherwise rare unless metastases to the liver are responsible for the carcinoid syndrome. Intestinal biopsy shows solid groups of regular polyhedral cells spreading through the submucosa and muscle; the specific neuro-

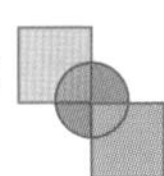

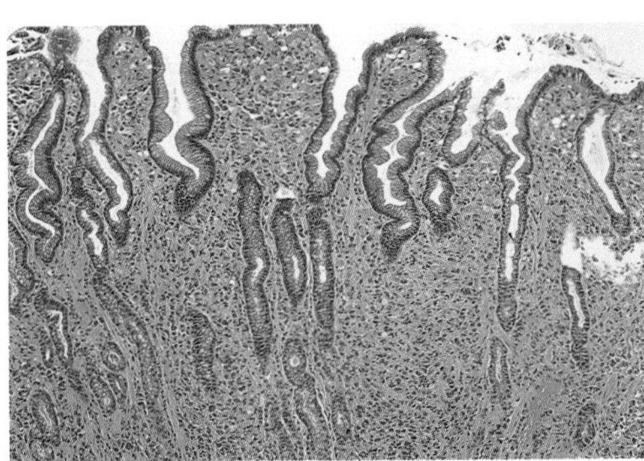

■ **Fig. 4.91** Metastatic melanoma. Microscopic appearance of the small bowel mucosa with normal epithelium infiltrated by masses of non-cohesive pleomorphic malignant cells that fill the lamina propria and focally efface crypts.

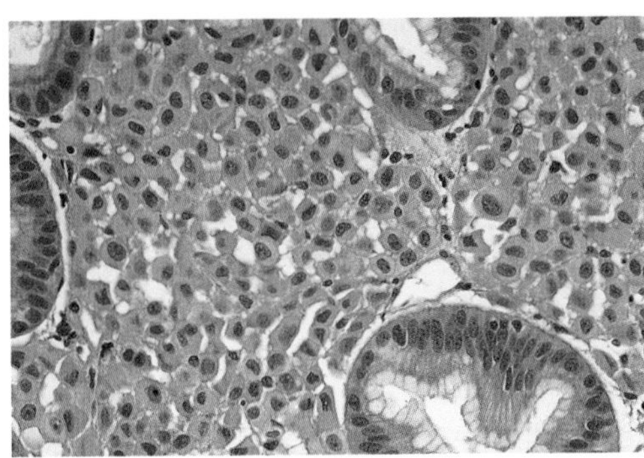

■ **Fig. 4.92** Metastatic melanoma. High-magnification appearance showing plump non-cohesive tumor cells containing varying amounts of pale brown pigment.

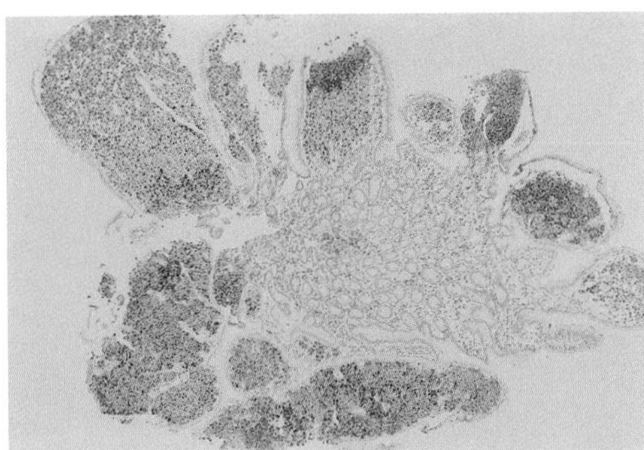

■ **Fig. 4.93** Metastatic melanoma. Immunohistochemical stain of the small bowel mucosa for HMB45, a protein characteristic of melanoma, showing staining of the infiltrating cells in the stroma.

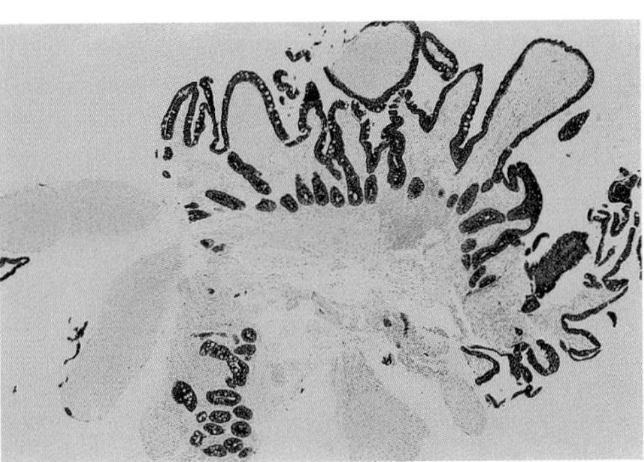

■ **Fig. 4.94** Metastatic melanoma. Immunohistochemical stain of the small bowel mucosa for cytokeratins showing strong staining of the normal epithelium and non-staining of the invading melanoma cells distinguishing them from poorly differentiated carcinoma which they resemble.

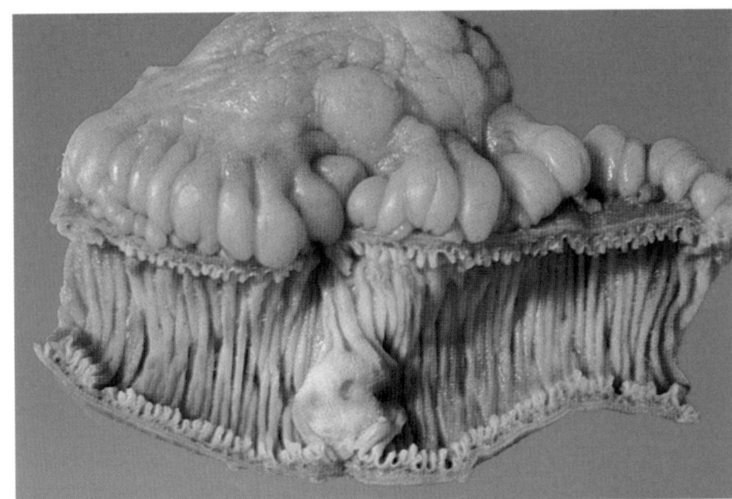

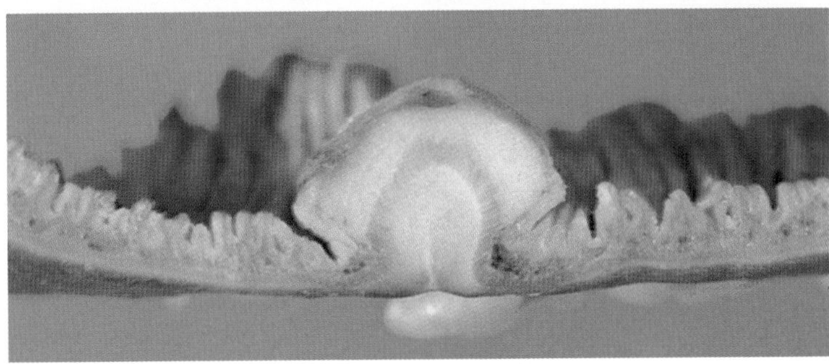

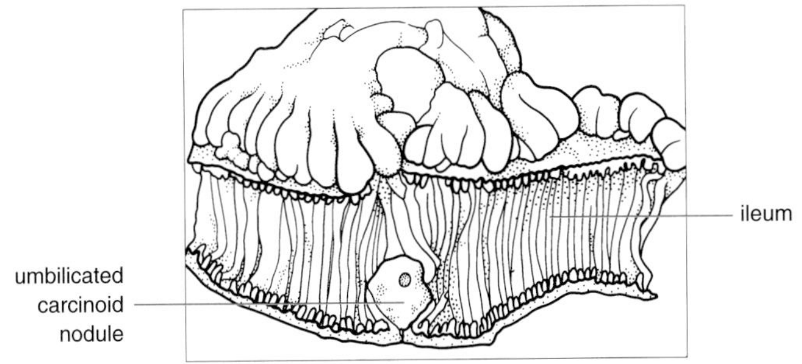

■ **Fig. 4.95** A carcinoid tumor of the ileum (above), and (below) the cut surface of the same specimen demonstrating the submucosal position. The yellow coloration is the result of formalin fixation.

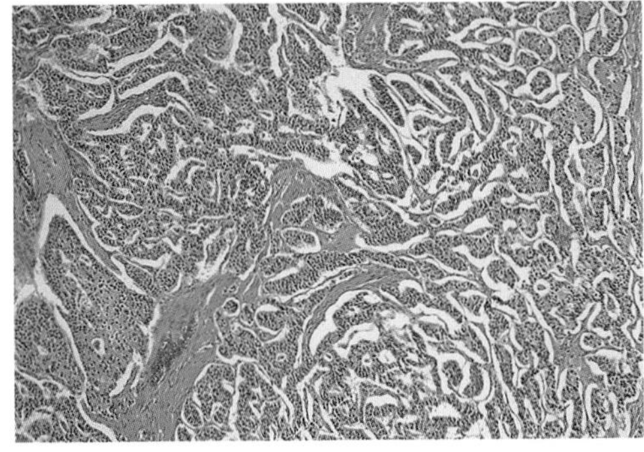

■ **Fig. 4.96** Ileal carcinoid tumor. Microscopic appearance showing an insular growth pattern with small, monomorphic tumor cells arranged in cords, solid nests with peripheral pallisading, and rosette-like acini.

endocrine characteristics may be determined from immunocytochemical stains and electron microscopy (Figs 4.96–4.98). Appendiceal tumors very rarely metastasize, but primaries from other sites derived from the mid-gut – though much less common – are more prone to disseminate once they do occur. The carcinoid syndrome is due to the excessive production of a variety of gut hormones – particularly 5-hydroxytryptamine, but also histamine, kinins, catecholamines, and prostaglandins.

Typically, patients present with episodic facial flushing, watery diarrhea, and abdominal cramps, and may have pellagra-like skin lesions as a result of niacin deficiency. Involvement of the right side of the heart is also well recognized, and there may be bronchial lesions. Examination confirms flushing (which with time becomes fixed) (Fig. 4.99), and hepatomegaly, and auscultation may indicate pulmonary and/or tricuspid valve lesions.

Barium studies may show tumor masses, dilatation or generalized thickening of the folds, and there is often a characteristic tethering of folds radiating towards the mesentery; there may also be focal calcification (Figs 4.100–4.102). The primary tumors are themselves generally small, but the liver may be almost completely replaced by metastases (see also Chapter 13).

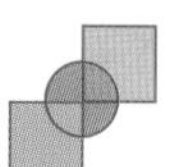

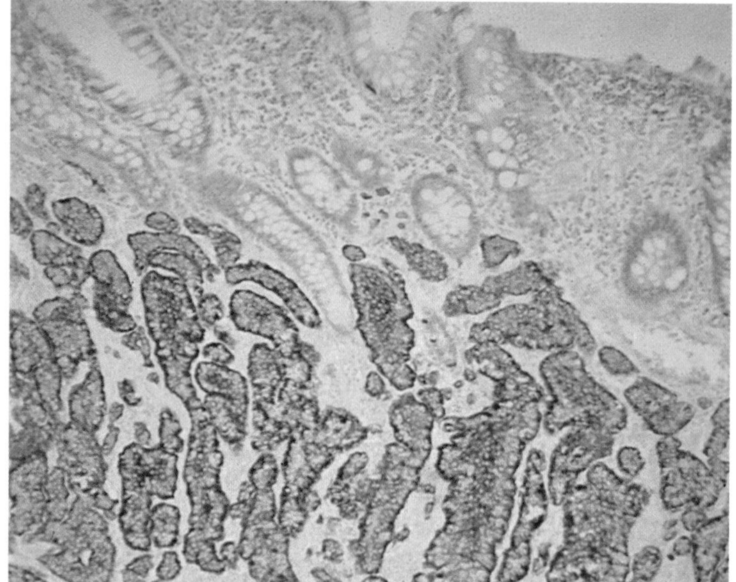

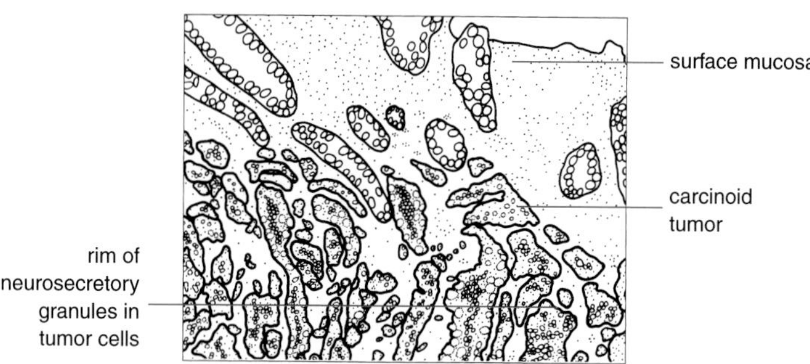

Fig. 4.97 Carcinoid tumor. Argyrophillic stain (Gremelius) stain at the periphery of a carcinoid tumor showing the brown-black granular staining of neurosecretory granules in the tumor cells.

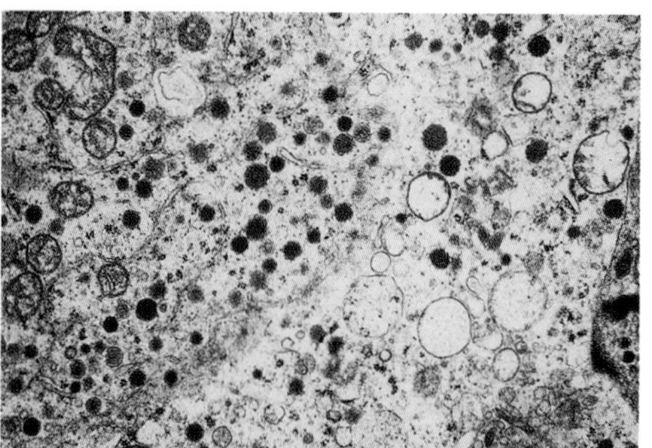

Fig. 4.98 Carcinoid tumor. Electron microscopic view of the cytoplasm of a carcinoid tumor cell showing abundant dense-core neurosecretory granules.

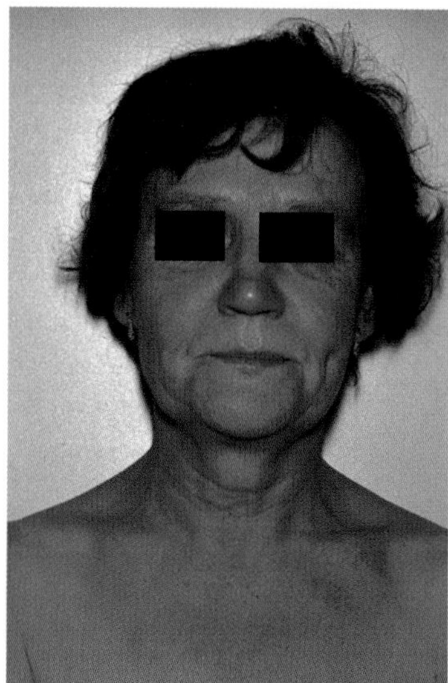

Fig. 4.99 Patient with fixed facial flushing as a result of advanced carcinoid syndrome.

INTESTINAL LIPOMATOSIS

Lipoma of the small bowel may appear as a discrete mass lesion on contrast imaging (Fig. 4.103), but involvement of the ileocecal region by lipomatosis may give rise to diagnostic confusion, with barium images sometimes suggesting inflammatory bowel disease. CT scanning, which demonstrates the high fat content clearly, usually clarifies the situation (Fig. 4.104).

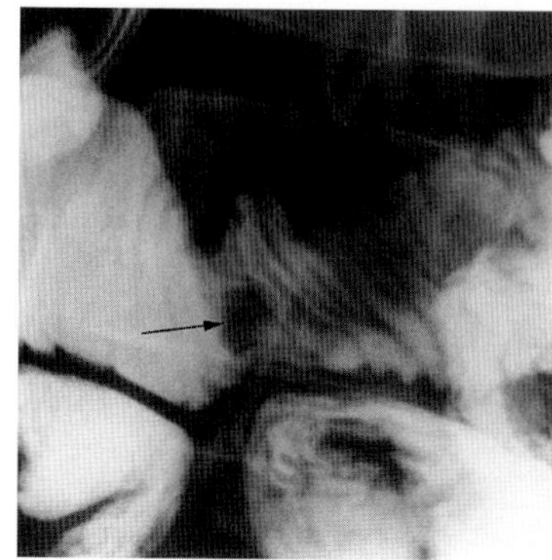

Fig. 4.100 Small bowel follow-through demonstrating a carcinoid tumor in the mid ileum. A 6 mm smooth-surfaced sessile polyp (arrow) is associated with a focally narrowed lumen. This small lesion had microscopic metastases to mesenteric lymph nodes. (Reproduced with permission from reference 1, Fig. 23.12.)

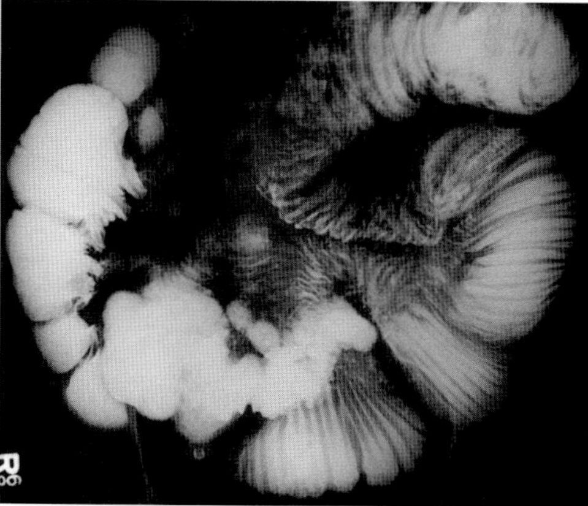

Fig. 4.101 Small bowel follow-through demonstrating carcinoid tumor. The folds of many small bowel loops are tethered toward the central small bowel mesentery. The loops are focally dilated. (Reproduced with permission from reference 8, Fig. 52.36B.)

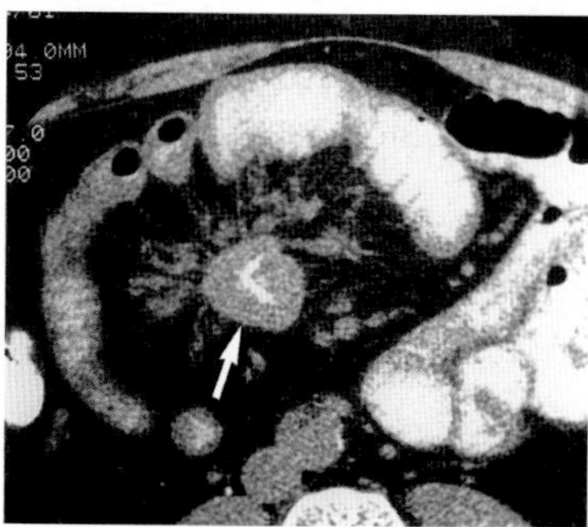

Fig. 4.102 CT scan in carcinoid syndrome. CT shows a 2 cm centrally calcified small bowel mesenteric mass (arrow). Thick strands radiate from the small bowel toward the mass, representing tumor infiltrating along vascular bundles and intrinsic vascular changes.

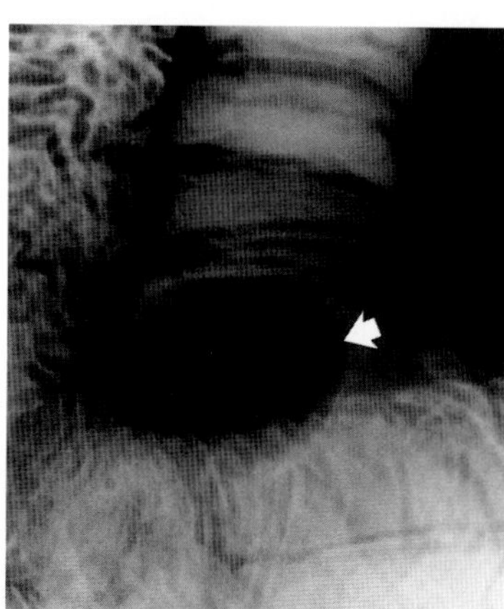

Fig. 4.103 Enteroclysis demonstrating lipoma of mid ileum. A submucosal mass is manifest as a smooth-surfaced mass (arrow) with borders having abrupt angulation with the luminal contour. (Reproduced with permission from reference 1, Fig. 23.8.)

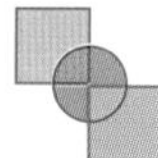

PEUTZ–JEGHERS SYNDROME

Peutz–Jeghers syndrome is inherited as an autosomal dominant condition. Multiple hamartomatous polyps occur throughout the gastrointestinal tract (see also Chapters 2 and 6) (Figs 4.105, 4.106), and are accompanied by pigmentation of the lips and buccal mucosa (Fig. 4.107). Occasionally, the face or fingers also exhibit increased pigmentation. Symptoms are relatively unusual, but are most likely from small bowel polyps, which may bleed or cause obstruction or intussusception (Figs 4.108, 4.109) (see also Chapter 7). Histologically, the lesions have a lobulated surface with a core of muscle fibers (derived from the muscularis mucosae) which arborizes around the crypts and mucosal glands, thinning out towards the surface (Fig. 4.110). Although there may be mild architectural irregularity, the glandular elements of the hamartoma remain cytologically normal. There is an associated increased risk of malignancy in the small intestine and other sites, and enteroscopic and radiological surveillance of the small bowel is widely practiced; it is possible that capsule endoscopy will soon be able to assume part of this mantle of responsibility (Fig 4.106).

JUVENILE POLYPOSIS

Isolated juvenile polyps have little consequence once removed, but there is increasing recognition that patients with multiple lesions and true juvenile polyposis have an increased risk of intestinal adenocarcinoma. As in the case of Peutz–Jeghers syndrome there is some difficulty in management of lesions in the mid small bowel where there is little access for therapeutic endoscopes. (See also Chapter 7.)

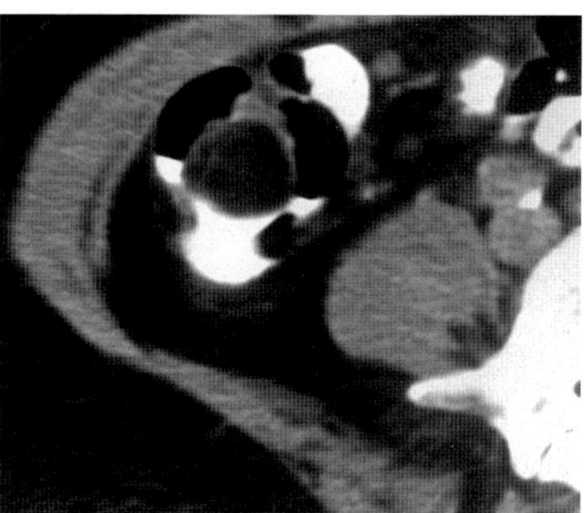

Fig. 4.104 CT scan demonstrating the low attenuation of fat within ileocecal lipomatosis.

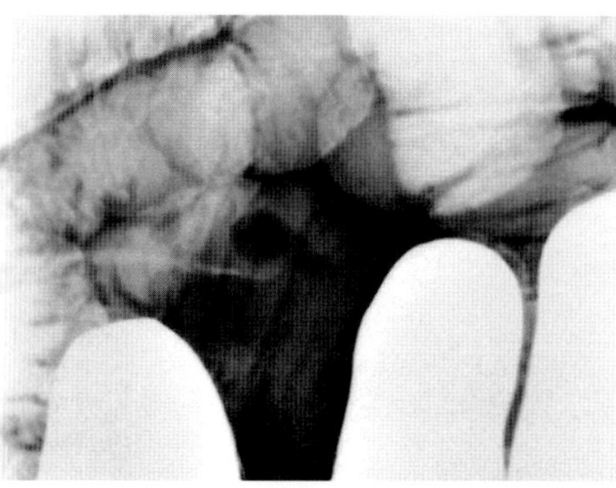

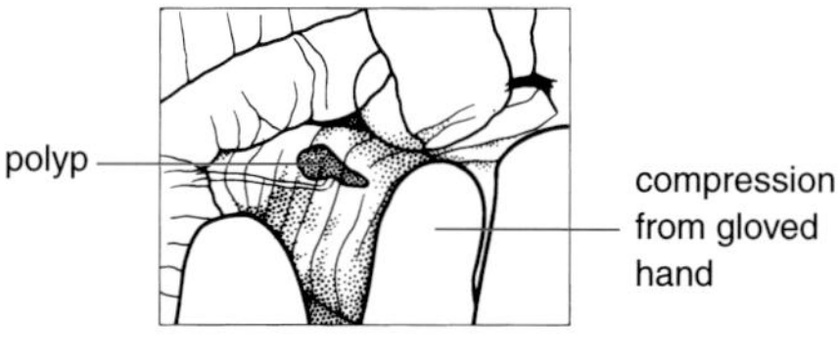

Fig. 4.105 Compression view during small bowel enema examination, revealing a 1 cm pedunculated Peutz–Jeghers polyp in the proximal ileum.

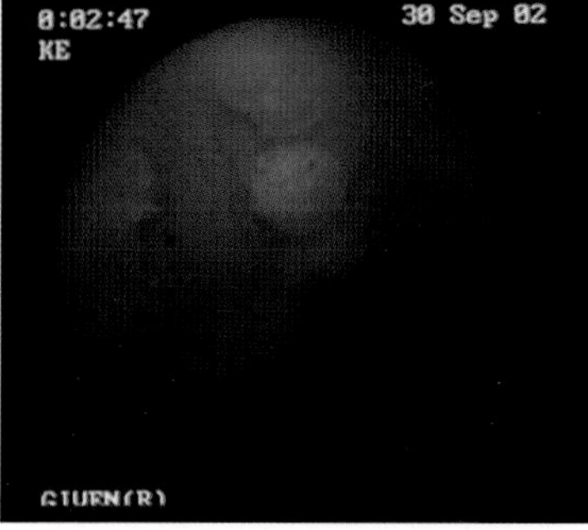

Fig. 4.106 Peutz–Jeghers hamartomatous polyp seen at capsule enteroscopy. Courtesy of Dr N. Kalantzis.

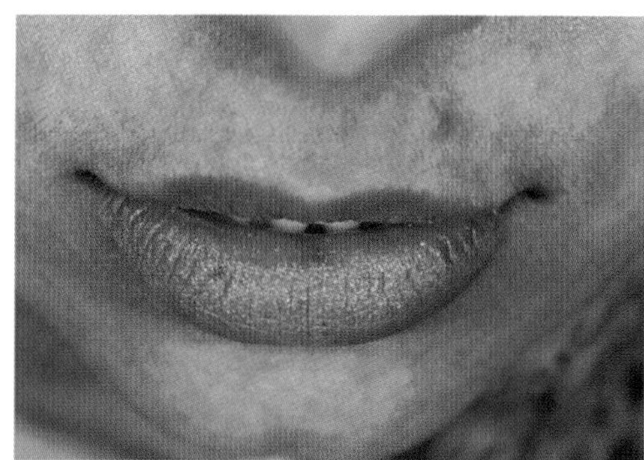

Fig. 4.107 Blue macules on the lip in Peutz–Jeghers syndrome.

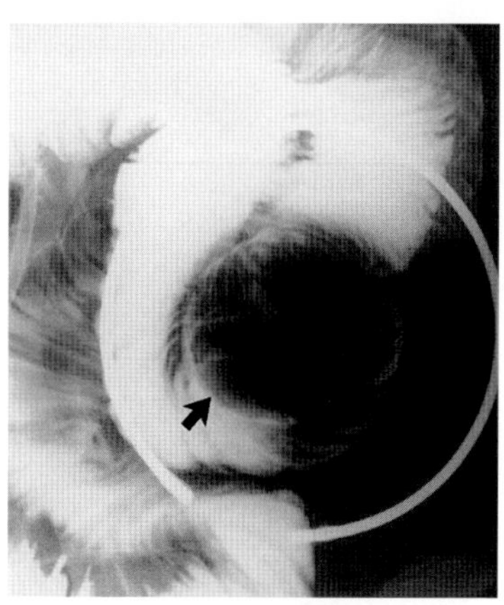

Fig. 4.108 Enteroclysis showing jejunal hamartoma in a patient with Peutz–Jeghers syndrome. A smooth surface polypoid mass (arrows) is causing a transient intussusception of the small bowel. (Reproduced with permission from reference 7, Fig. 46.41.)

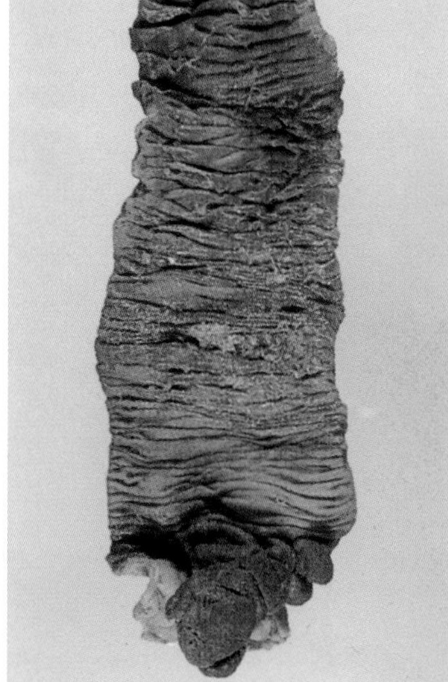

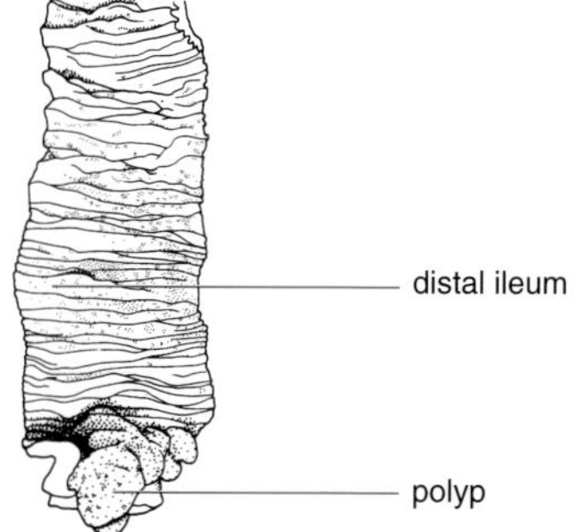

Fig. 4.109 A Peutz–Jeghers polyp in the ileum that had intussuscepted through the ileocecal valve into the colon and caused obstruction. Courtesy of Dr J. Newman.

MECKEL'S DIVERTICULUM

The Meckel's diverticulum is the most common congenital anomaly of the gastrointestinal tract, and affects approximately 2% of normal Caucasians. It represents the remains of the embryonic vitelline duct, which connects the yolk sac to the mid gut, and therefore arises from the antimesenteric border of the ileum, 50–100 cm proximal to the ileocecal valve (Fig. 4.111). It is usually about 5 cm in length and wide-mouthed (Fig. 4.112). In approximately 50% of cases, the mucosa is ileal, but duodenal, colonic, pancreatic, and/or gastric mucosa may be present (Fig. 4.113).

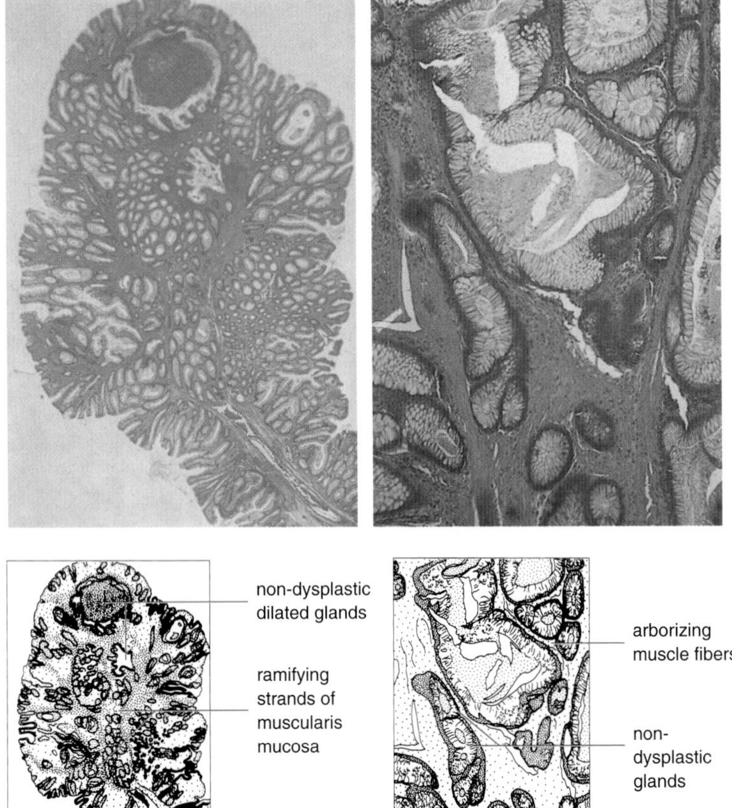

■ **Fig. 4.110** Histological appearance of a Peutz–Jeghers hamartoma. (a) The characteristic intermingling of glands and muscularis is seen. H&E stain (x 12). (b) At higher magnification, the absence of dysplasia is demonstrated. H&E stain (x 50).

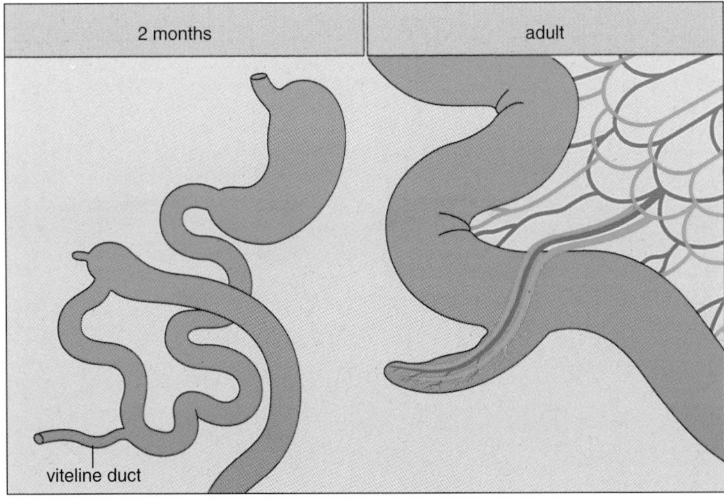

■ **Fig. 4.111** Diagram illustrating the developmental origin of a Meckel's diverticulum.

Most remain asymptomatic and undiagnosed throughout life, or are found incidentally at barium examination (Fig. 4.114), but bleeding and intestinal obstruction do occur. Bleeding is usually the result of ulceration in gastric mucosa (Fig. 4.115) and this allows the possibility of diagnosis by scintigraphy, which will usually identify tissue containing parietal cells (Fig. 4.116). Obstruction is usually a consequence of intussusception (Fig 4.117).

JEJUNAL DIVERTICULOSIS AND SMALL BOWEL BACTERIAL OVERGROWTH

Diverticula of the small intestine are not uncommon, affecting perhaps 5% of those over 60 years; they tend to be most numerous proximally (particularly around the duodeno-jejunal junction)

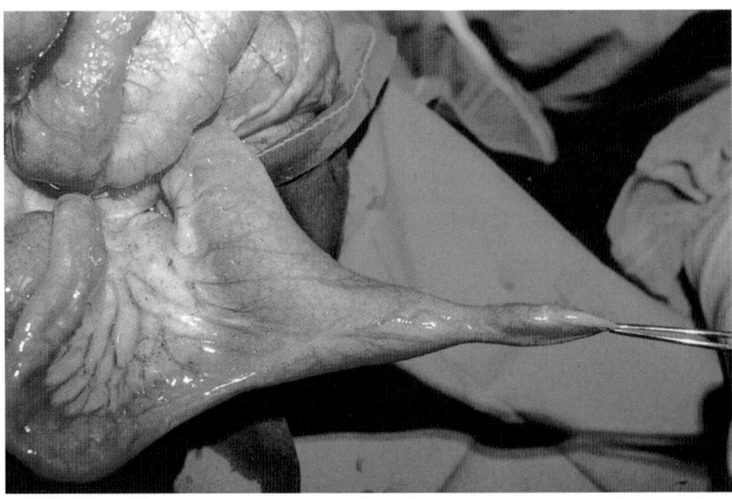

■ **Fig. 4.112** Laparotomy appearance of a Meckel's diverticulum. Courtesy of Miss V. Wright.

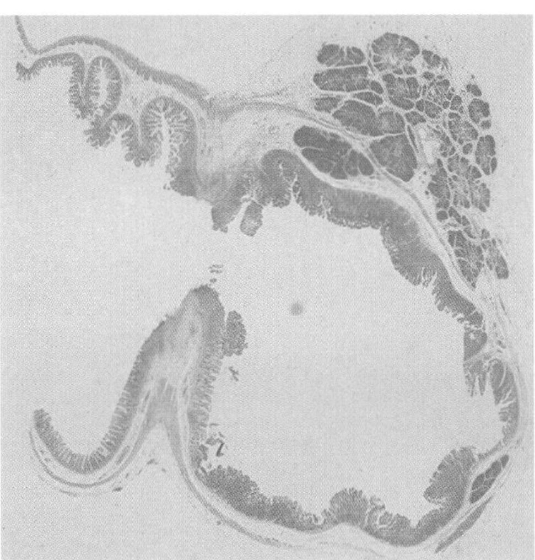

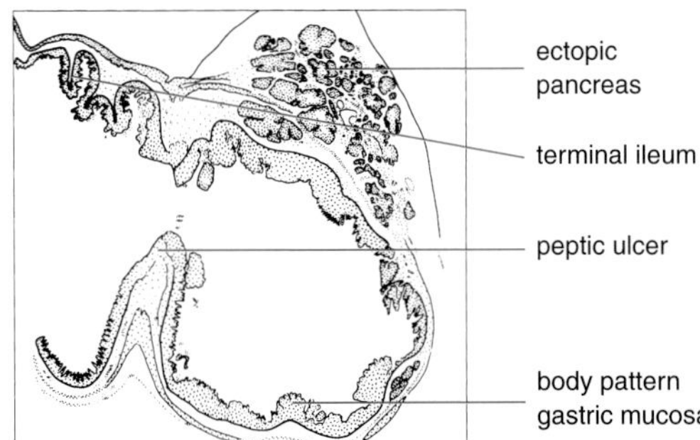

■ **Fig. 4.113** Histological appearance of a Meckel's diverticulum. H&E stain (x 3).

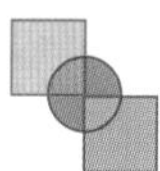

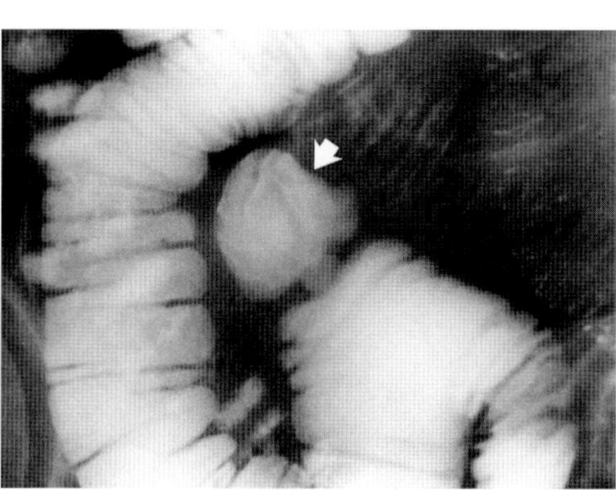

■ **Fig. 4.114** Enteroclysis demonstrating Meckel's diverticulum. A 2 cm sac (arrow) arises from the antimesenteric border of the distal ileum.

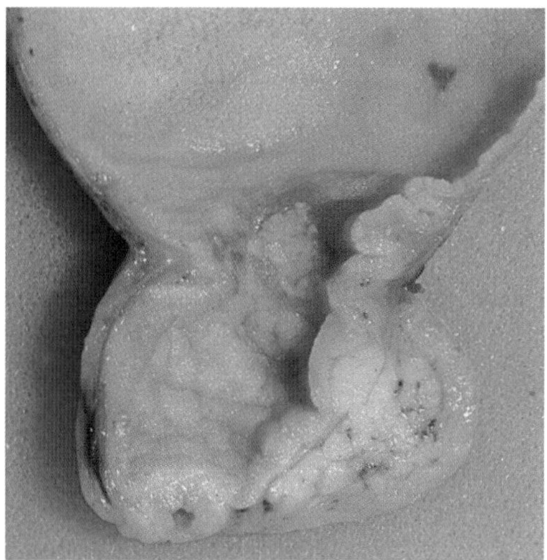

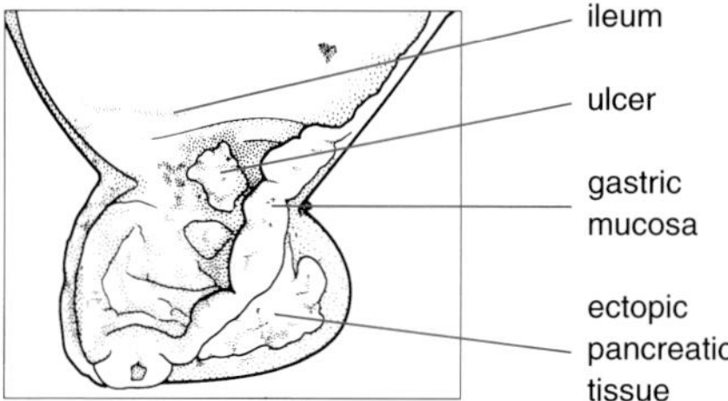

■ **Fig. 4.115** Macroscopic appearance of an opened Meckel's diverticulum showing gastric mucosa, a peptic-type ulcer, and ectopic pancreatic tissue (see also Fig. 4.113).

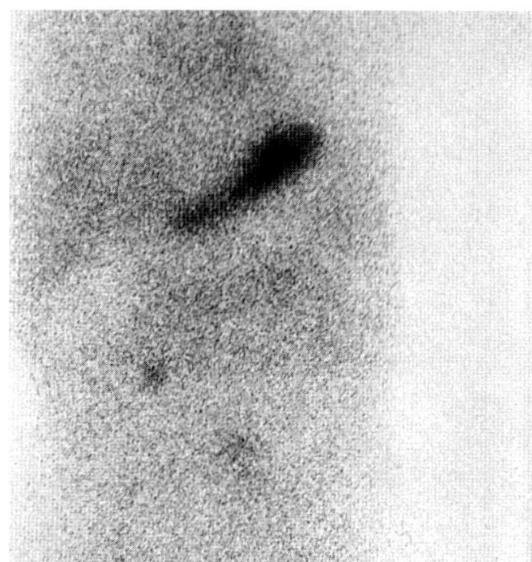

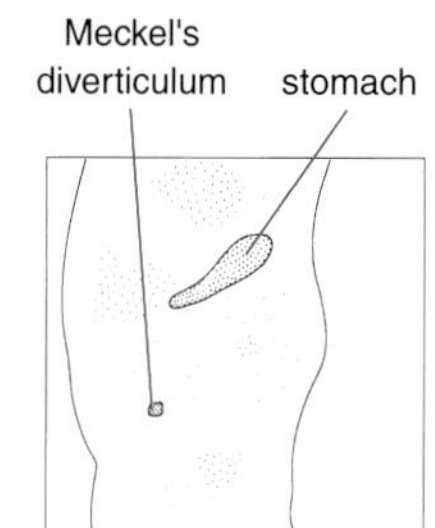

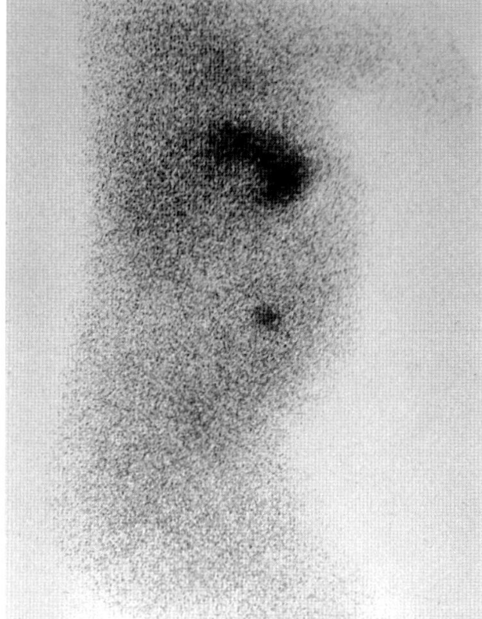

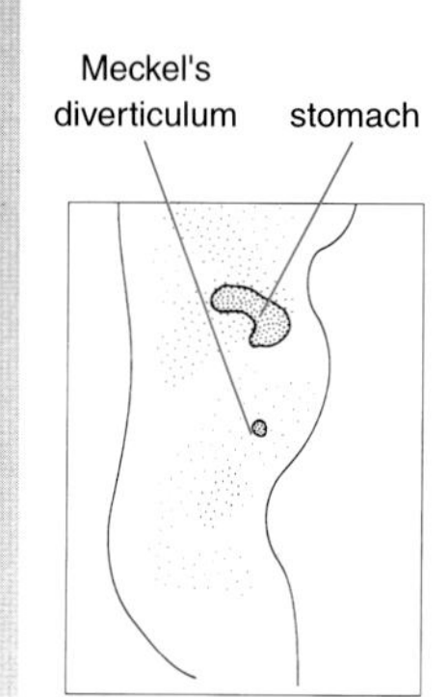

■ **Fig. 4.116** Technetium scan demonstrating a Meckel's diverticulum: isotope is apparent in the stomach and on the gastric mucosa in the diverticulum, as demonstrated on the AP and lateral views.

(Fig. 4.118) (see also Chapter 3). Most remain asymptomatic; hemorrhage, diverticulitis, and perforation are all uncommon, and enterolith and cyst formation frankly rare.

The effects of bacterial overgrowth within what are effectively multiple, small, blind loops are responsible for their commonest clinical manifestations. Jejunal diverticula are therefore – indirectly – a possible cause of diarrhea and malabsorption in the elderly. Frank malnutrition is less common than megaloblastic anemia from vitamin B_{12} deficiency (usually with normal or high folate levels). Urinary markers of overgrowth include indoles, hippuric acid, and phenols. Culture of upper small bowel contents, or a positive glucose-hydrogen breath test provide firm support for the diagnosis. Lactulose-hydrogen or bile salt breath testing is less reliable, but therapeutic trials of antibiotics can be strongly indicative of the correct interpretation.

Diverticula are not however necessary for small bowel bacterial overgrowth to occur. Bacterial overgrowth is a potentially important problem in the post-gastrectomy patient, in whom the protective effects of gastric acid are lost (see Chapter 2), and may contribute to the 'post-gastrectomy syndrome.' Prolonged use of H_2-receptor blockers and proton pump inhibitors may have similar effects. The presence of a bypassed small bowel loop or a true blind loop, removed from the flow of nutrients, poses the highest risk for bacterial overgrowth, but functional disorders such as pseudo-obstruction, scleroderma (Fig. 4.119), and visceral myopathy are also prey to this complication, which can lead to considerable therapeutic difficulties (see below; see also Chapters 1 and 7). Sacculations that fall short of complete diverticula are seen as a further feature of scleroderma (Fig 1.120).

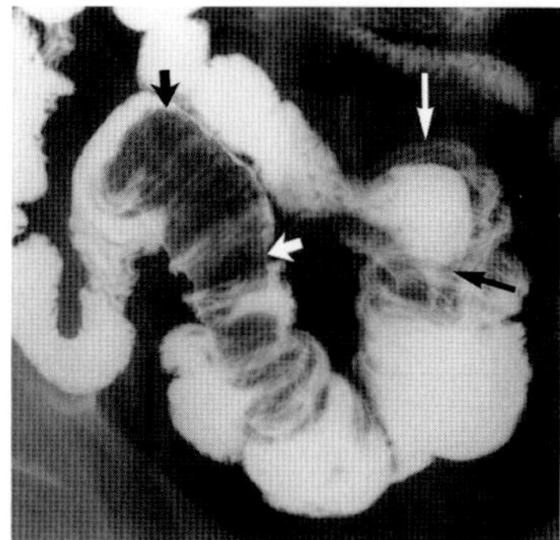

■ **Fig. 4.117** Small bowel follow-through showing inverted Meckel's diverticulum. A long polypoid mass (short arrows) is seen in the distal ileum. The mass is causing intussusception (long white arrow identifies wall of intussuscipiens; long black arrow identifies lumen of intussusceptum). (Reproduced with permission from reference 5, Fig. 1.)

HEREDITARY HEMORRHAGIC TELANGIECTASIA (OSLER–WEBER–RENDU SYNDROME)

This disorder is inherited as an autosomal dominant condition with high penetrance. Lesions usually appear in childhood and tend to increase in size and number with advancing age. Telangiectasiae are commonly found on the lips, tongue, and oral mucosa (Figs 4.121, 4.122), and less often on conjunctivae, ears, and digits. Lesions in the gastrointestinal mucosa often lead to a low-grade iron deficiency, and may be responsible for troublesome hemorrhage (Figs 4.123, 4.124), not least because their number and extensive distribution throughout the intestine often makes a surgical approach impractical (see also Chapters 2 and 7) (Figs 4.125–4.127). Associated aortic valve stenosis is important to seek, as resolution of gastrointestinal hemorrhage will often follow valve replacement in

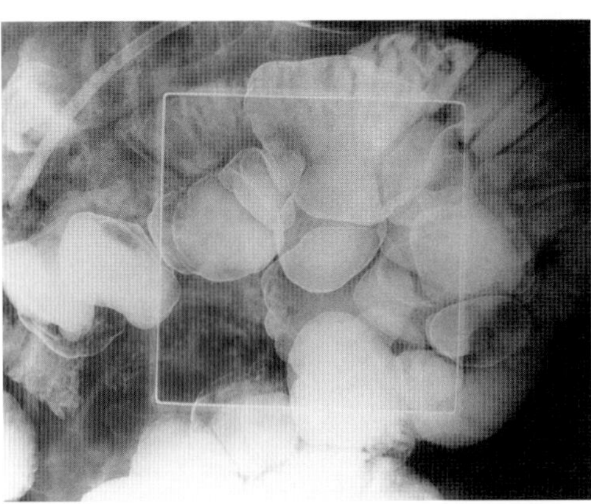

Fig. 4.118 Enteroclysis demonstrating jejunal diverticulosis. Numerous broad-based sacculations are seen in the proximal small intestine. (Reproduced with permission from reference 4, Fig. 3.)

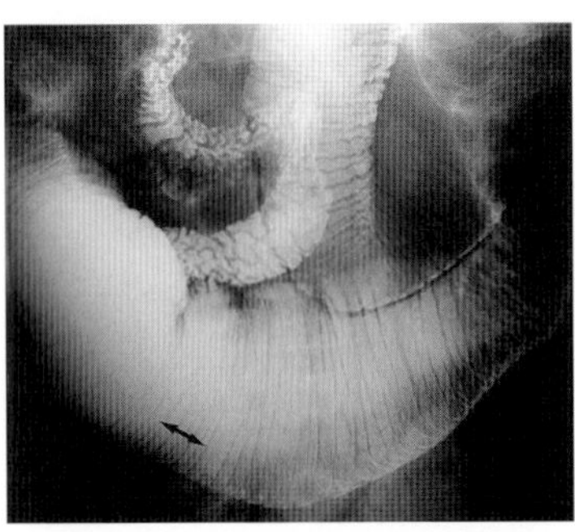

Fig. 4.119 Small bowel enema in scleroderma. The small intestine is markedly dilated. A high number of folds is seen, despite the massive luminal dilatation (the double arrow denotes 2.5 cm). (Reproduced with permission from reference 4, Fig. 4.)

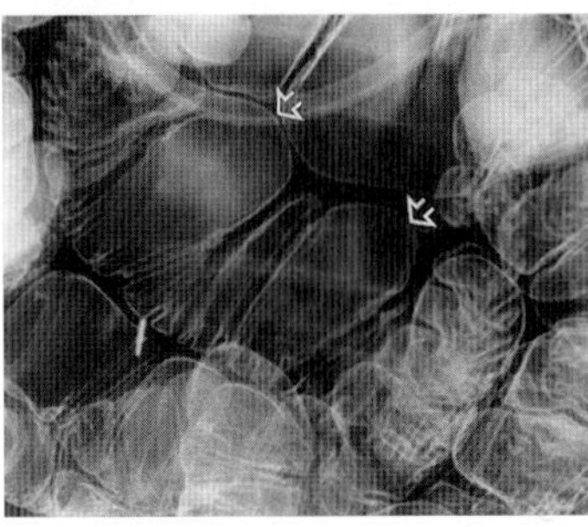

Fig. 4.120 Small bowel enema in scleroderma. Broad-based sacculations (arrows) protrude beyond the expected luminal contour, indicating focal wall weakness due to muscular atrophy and fibrosis. (Reproduced with permission from reference 6, Fig. 5.39B.)

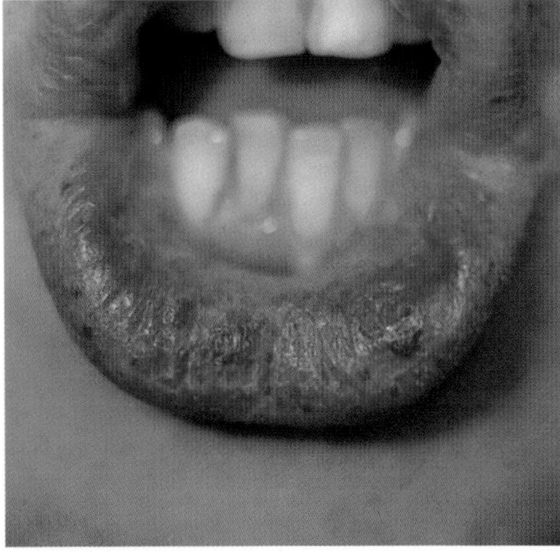

Fig. 4.121 Osler–Weber–Rendu syndrome. Labial telangiectasiae. Courtesy of Dr D.E. Sharvill.

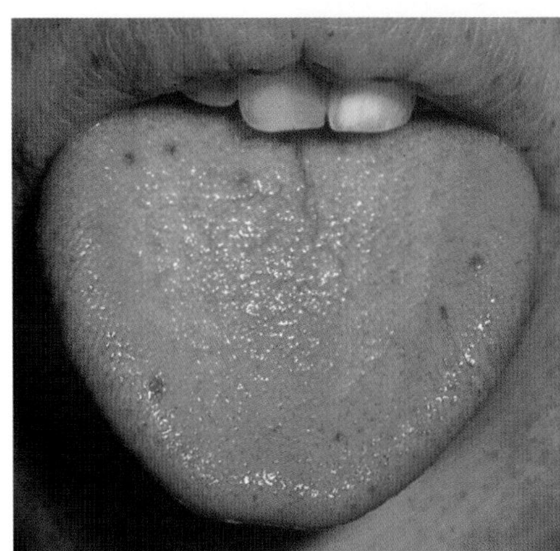

Fig. 4.122 Osler–Weber–Rendu syndrome. Lingual telangiectasiae. Courtesy of Dr D.E. Sharvill.

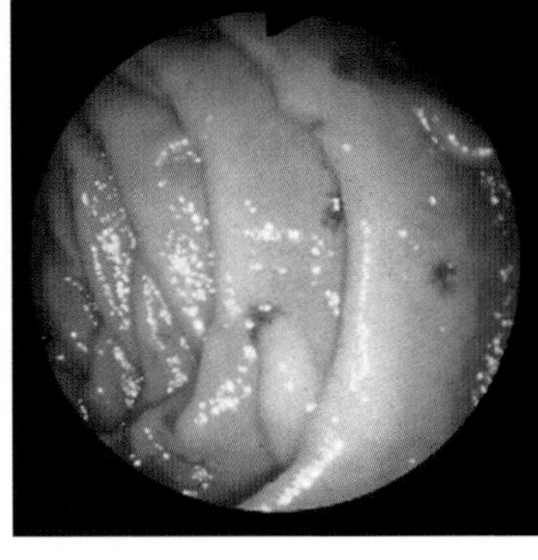

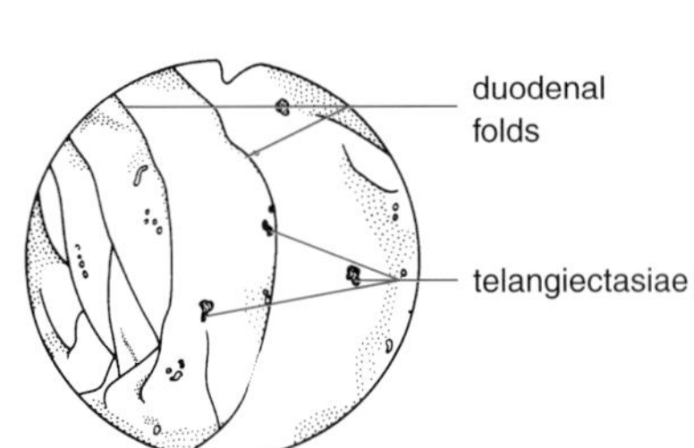

Fig. 4.123 Endoscopic appearance of distal duodenal telangiectasia in a patient with Osler–Weber–Rendu syndrome who also had multiple lesions within the more distal small bowel.

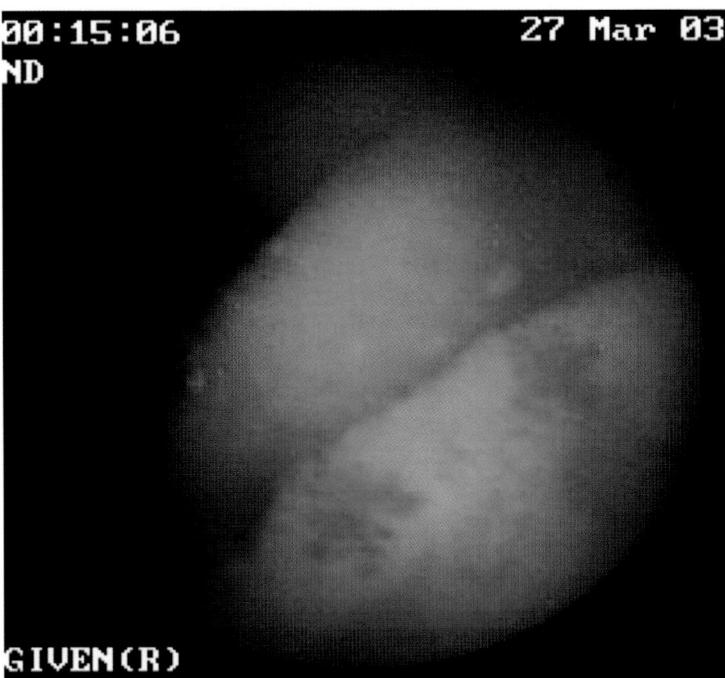

Fig. 4.124 Multiple distal jejunal lesions in a similar patient, identified here by capsule enteroscopy. Courtesy of Dr N. Kalantzis.

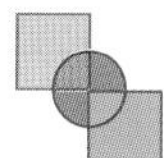

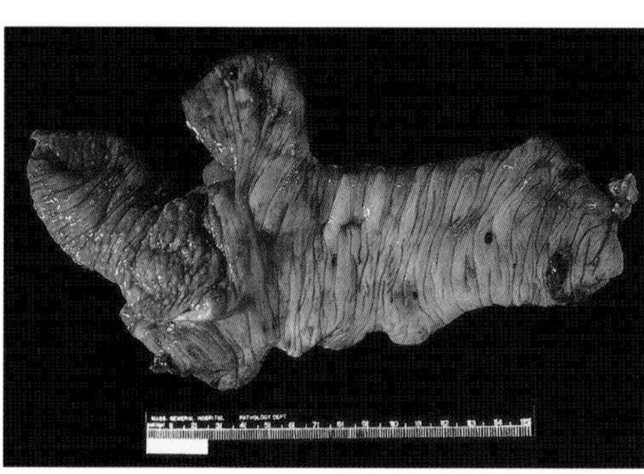

■ **Fig. 4.125** Hereditary hemorrhagic telangiectasia . Ileocolectomy specimen from a patient with occult gastrointestinal bleeding showing what resemble multiple blood-filled bullae, here affecting the cecum and right colon.

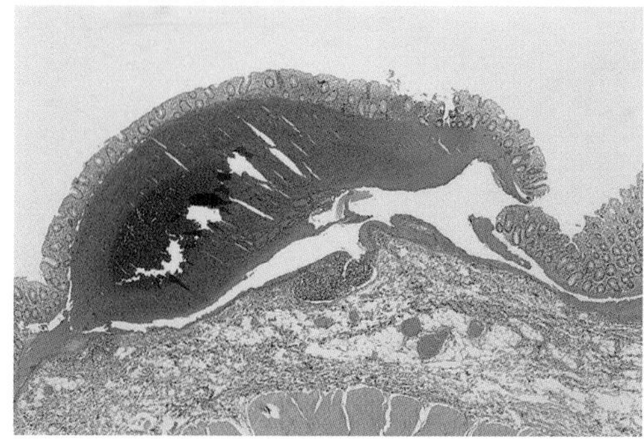

■ **Fig. 4.126** Hereditary hemorrhagic telangiectasia. Microscopic view of one of the telangiectasiae showing a blister-like lesion filled with blood that splits the muscularis mucosae and lifts the overlying mucosa.

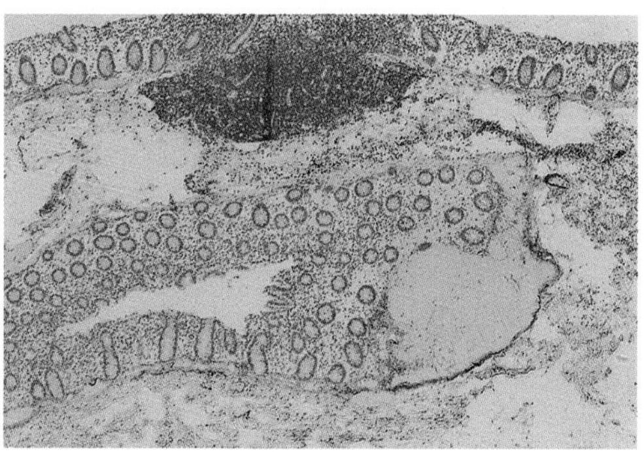

■ **Fig. 4.127** Hereditary hemorrhagic telangiectasia. An immunohistochemical stain for CD31 (an endothelial marker) revealing the endothelial lining of the abnormal ectatic vessel, which lacks a true wall.

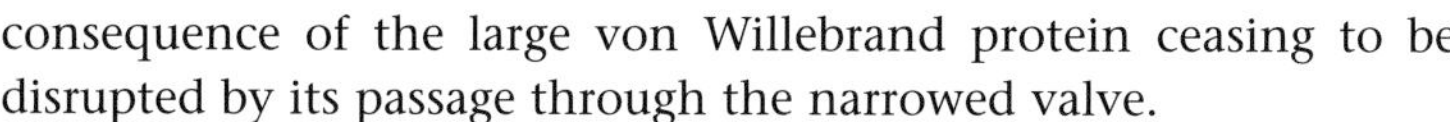

consequence of the large von Willebrand protein ceasing to be disrupted by its passage through the narrowed valve.

OCCULT GASTROINTESTINAL BLEEDING

When upper and lower gastrointestinal sites of bleeding have been excluded endoscopically and a small bowel origin is implicated, extra-intestinal manifestations, such as those of Osler–Weber–Rendu (see above) or the inherited collagen disorders such as Ehlers–Danlos syndrome (Figs 4.128, 4.129), should be sought. Investigations will at first be directed towards Meckel's diverticulum (see above), intestinal polyps such as in Peutz–Jeghers syndrome (see above), and Crohn's disease (see Chapter 5). However, contrast examination of the small bowel will usually be normal in this context.

Angiography may be diagnostic in demonstrating vascular malformations (Figs 4.130, 4.131), but has a relatively limited place, since brisk bleeding renders the examination relatively hazardous, and slow bleeding may not be detectable even in a patient anticoagulated for the procedure. Labeled red cell scanning has been proposed to fill this gap as, at least in theory, it should detect slower rates of bleeding than angiography (Fig. 4.132). Sadly, careful assessment indicates that false-negative scans result in at least 50% of cases, and falsely positive localization occurs in about 25%. The histological features are characteristic once resection is performed (Figs 4.133, 4.134).

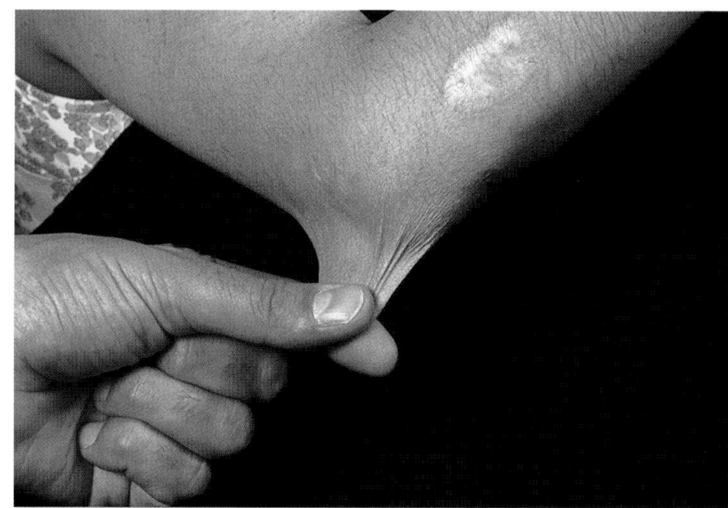

■ **Fig. 4.128** Patient with Ehlers–Danlos syndrome: the skin is hyperextensible, but recoils to its normal position when released. Courtesy of Imperial College of Science Technology and Medicine.

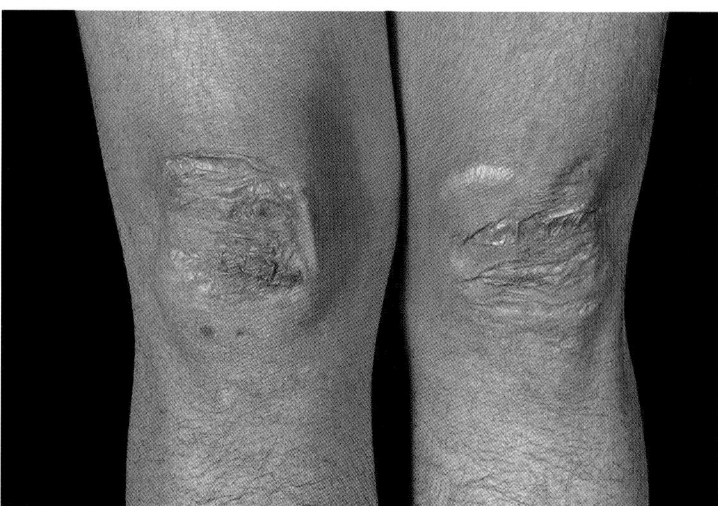

■ **Fig. 4.129** Ehlers–Danlos syndrome produces fragile skin with poor healing; similar changes in the gastrointestinal tract predispose to troublesome hemorrhage. Courtesy of Imperial College of Science Technology and Medicine.

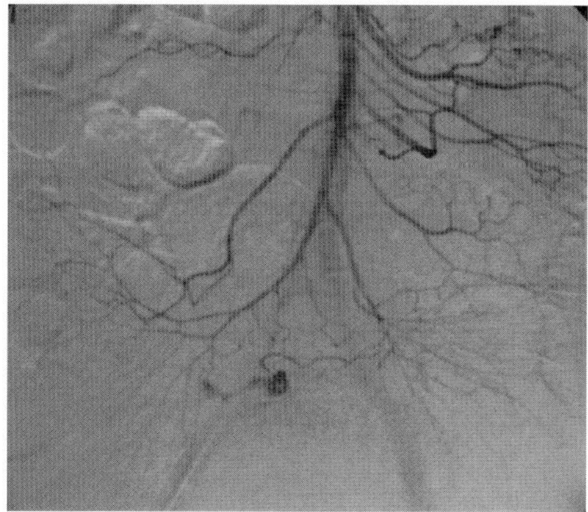

■ **Fig. 4.130** Contrast extravasation from a proximal ileal branch in a superior mesenteric arteriogram. The early arterial image shows an enlarged and somewhat tortuous vessel arising from the second ileal artery, which courses across the midline from left to right. At its distal end there is marked contrast extravasation into the small bowel. Courtesy of Dr J.E. Jackson.

Enteroscopy (once performed with pediatric colonoscopes but now with custom-built instruments) is of clear value in the patient with 'difficult' gastrointestinal bleeding, but even in the best hands it is unusual for the combination of jejunoscopy from above (Fig. 4.135), coupled with ileocolonoscopy from below, to encompass more than about 50% of the length of the small intestine. Moreover it can be quite difficult to estimate exactly which areas have been examined.

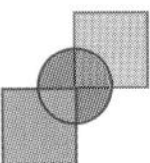

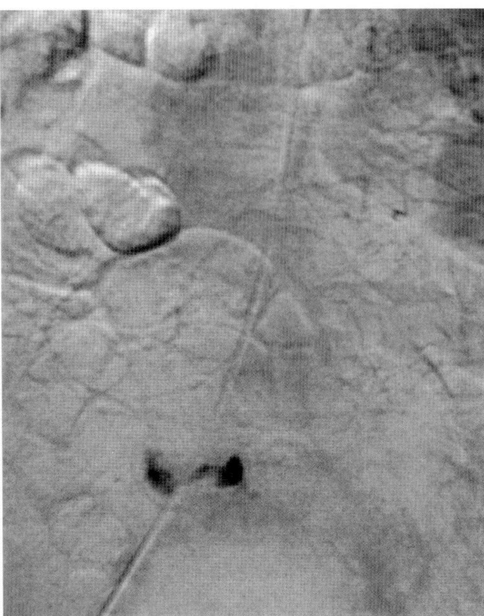

Fig. 4.131 The delayed capillary-venous phase image of the same patient as in Fig. 4.93: persistence of contrast within the bowel lumen is shown. After selective (palliative) embolization, the patient had a laparotomy at which a necrotic stromal cell tumor was found. Courtesy of Dr J.E. Jackson.

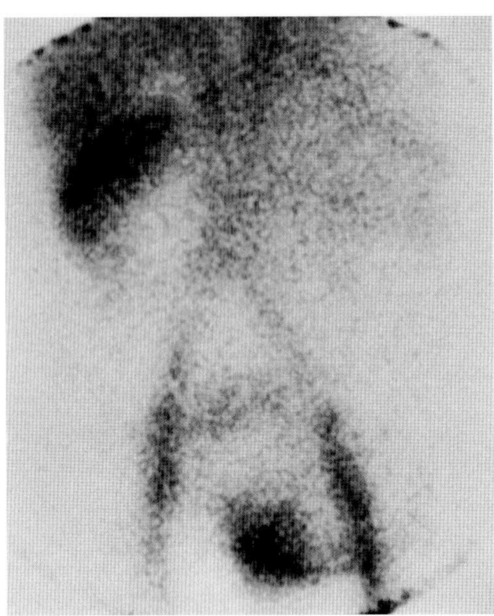

Fig. 4.132 Technetium-labeled red cell scan in a patient with rectal bleeding: this 20-minute image shows increased activity in the right upper quadrant just below the liver, which was interpreted as demonstrating extravasated red cells in the proximal transverse colon. Courtesy of Dr J.E. Jackson.

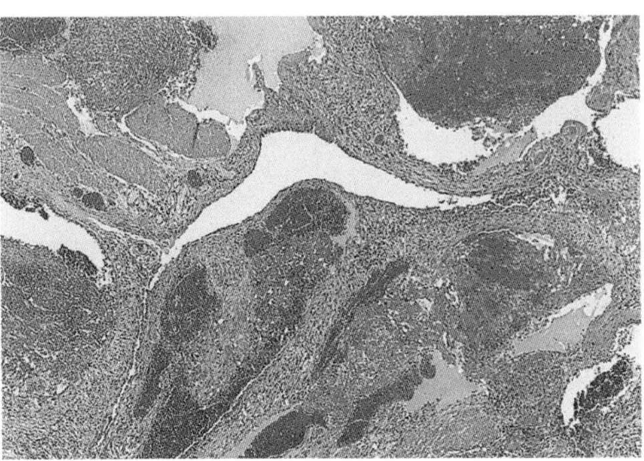

Fig. 4.133 Arteriovenous malformation of the small bowel. An elastic tissue stain demonstrating a disorganized meshwork of large thick-walled tortuous veins that, despite their hypertrophic appearance, are structurally weak. The abnormal mural structure characterized by variable wall thickness, focal absence of mural elastic tissue, and 'arteriolization' recognized by the formation of a condensed, irregularly reduplicated subluminal layer of elastic tissue resembling the internal elastic lamina of a muscular artery.

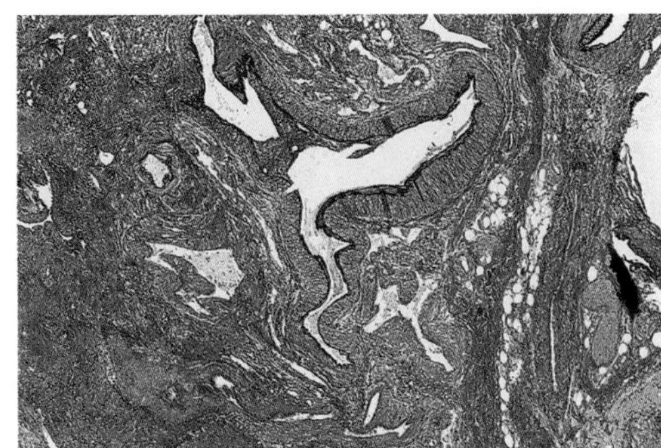

Fig. 4.134 Normal small intestinal submucosal vasculature. An elastic tissue stain demonstrating, for comparison, the configuration mural thickness and mural structure of muscular arteries and veins.

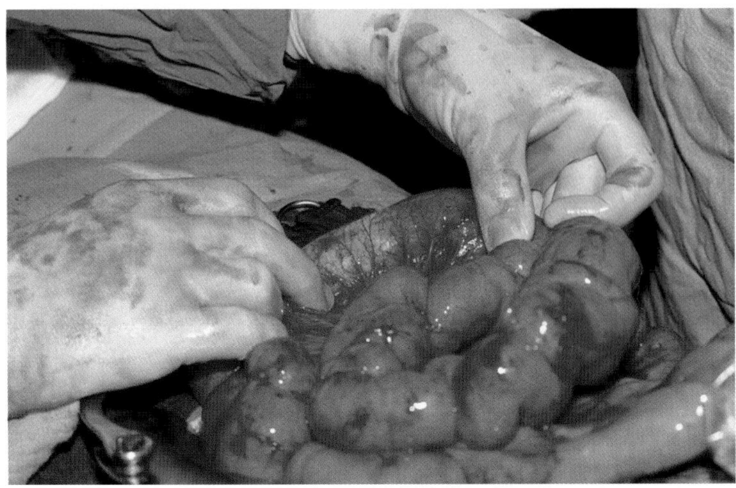

Fig. 4.135 Ileal angiodysplasia demonstrated peroperatively by transillumination from an intraluminal endoscope. Courtesy of Dr A. Van Gossum.

Greater completeness is obtained by using the 'sonde' type of instrument, which is carried (over the course of some hours) somewhat further along the small bowel by the effects of peristalsis on a balloon inflated at the tip of the instrument (Figs 4.136, 4.137). Biopsies and other interventions are not possible with the sonde endoscope. The option of per-operative enteroscopy in which the endoscope is 'milked' along the small bowel (with or without an enterotomy) has long been advocated, but the inevitable laparotomy is not desirable, particularly if numerous small lesions that preclude resection are found. Transillumination across the bowel wall may however be dramatic in angiodysplasia (Fig. 4.135).

Into this somewhat troubled arena has come the endoscopy capsule. These miniaturized endoscopes are swallowed in their entirety, and transmit their findings by radiotelemetry to a recording device similar to that used for pH monitoring (Fig. 4.138). At present the capsules have a limited battery life, which sometimes results in the signal ceasing before the cecum is reached, and even though only two images are recorded every second it takes nearly an hour to analyze each recording. The capsules are not yet steerable nor able to obtain biopsy samples, but the quality of the images already being produced and the rapid rate of technological development indicate that these are merely questions of time. It is probable that capsule endoscopy is already the investigation of choice for occult gastrointestinal bleeding. Visualization of bleeding sites and other mucosal pathology may be possible (Figs 4.139, 4.140) but there remains a small concern about stenosing lesions that have not previously been identified if careful contrast radiology has not been performed; this is most relevant to the patient who has or may have Crohn's disease. For the present, in the patient who is not currently bleeding, angiography retains the capacity to identify obvious areas

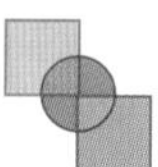

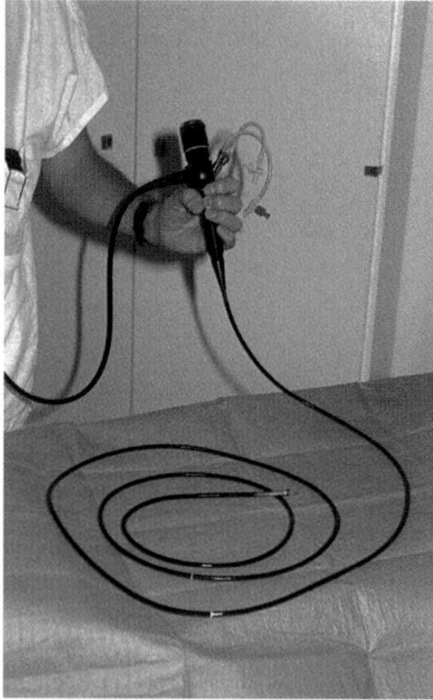

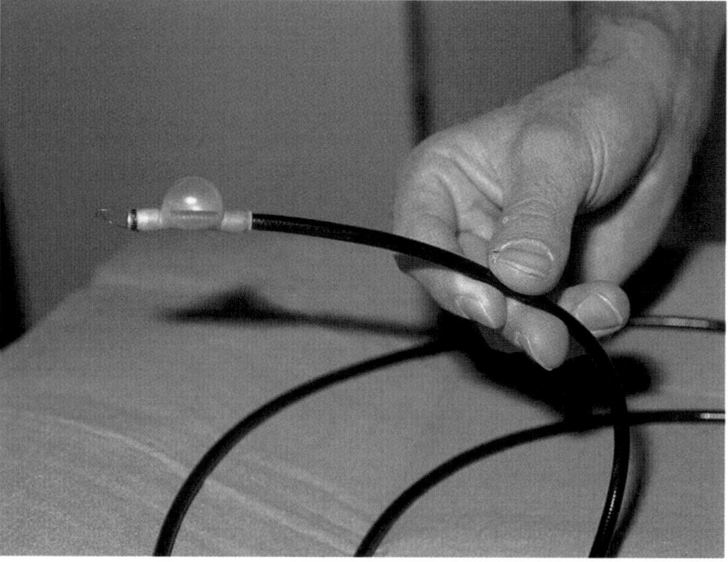

■ **Fig. 4.136** The 'sonde' type of enteroscope showing the balloon at its tip inflated. Courtesy of Dr A. Van Gossum.

of abnormal vasculature and to offer treatment by embolization: the technique should not be discarded.

INTESTINAL PSEUDO-OBSTRUCTION

Recurrent obstruction of the small intestine in the absence of a mechanical lesion is increasingly recognized (Fig. 4.141). There is considerable debate around the most suitable nomenclature and criteria for diagnosis, but it is apparent that there is a range of very specific rare conditions in which there are clear defects of the gut's muscle or neuronal networks. The visceral myopathies may be acquired or familial, and affect circular or longitudinal muscle or both, and may be degenerative or overtly inflammatory. Visceral neuropathy with clear-cut histological changes is rarer, but may also present with degenerative or inflammatory features. Patients present with pain and distention, which gradually limits their ability to eat sufficient nutrients. They may have generally dilated intestinal loops on abdominal radiography and contrast studies but this is not inevitable. These conditions are however very frequently associated with dilatation of the duodenum, which can be a very useful diagnostic pointer (Fig. 4.142). There is no specific treatment and all of these conditions tend to be progressive with increasing need for nutritional support.

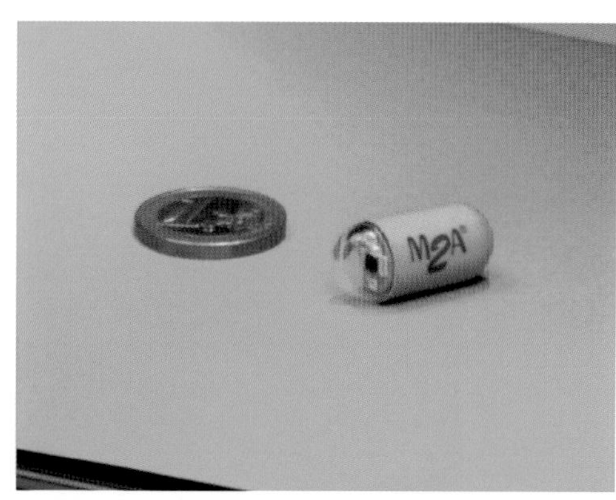

■ **Fig. 4.138** The swallowable capsule enteroscope shown alongside a 1 Euro coin (the capsule is 26 x 11 mm).

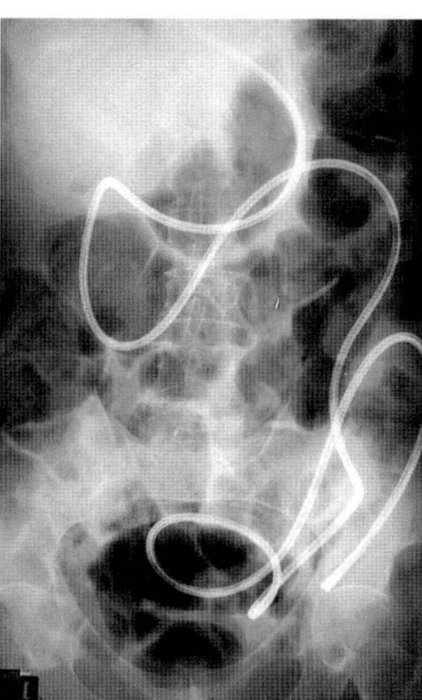

■ **Fig. 4.137** Plain abdominal radiograph showing the sonde enteroscope with its tip well advanced into the small bowel. Courtesy of Dr A. Van Gossum.

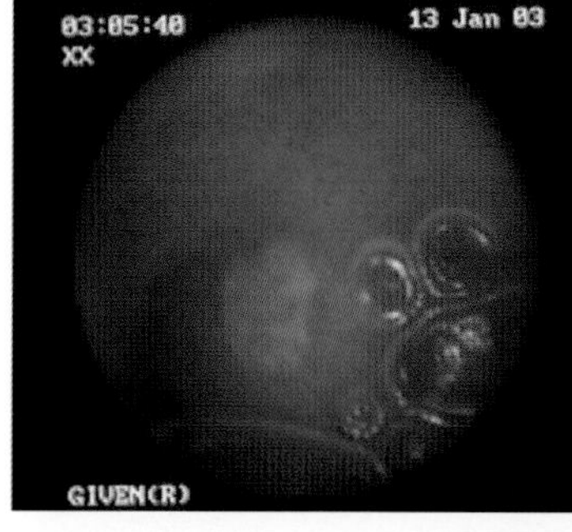

■ **Fig. 4.139** A jejunal ulcer responsible for occult gastrointestinal bleeding attributed to non-steroidal anti-inflammatory drug use (capsule enteroscopy). Courtesy of Dr N. Kalantzis.

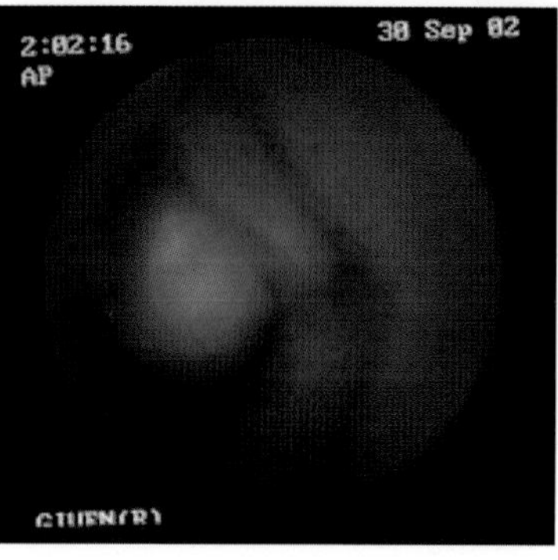

■ **Fig. 4.140** A 9 mm polyp in the small bowel which had been responsible for occult gastrointestinal bleeding, identified here by capsule enteroscopy. Courtesy of Dr N. Kalantzis.

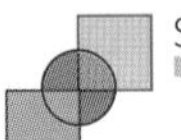

Pseudo-obstruction also occurs rarely in association with jejunal diverticula (see above) or malrotation of the gut (see below). Intestinal motility is often abnormal (see also Chapter 7). A prior diagnosis of irritable bowel syndrome is usual. Between episodes of obstruction, most patients are constipated; diarrhea, when it occurs, is usually of a malabsorptive type secondary to small bowel overgrowth (see above). Resectional and/or bypass surgery is rarely helpful, and may exacerbate the tendency to bacterial overgrowth, but histology of a resected segment may at least confirm the diagnosis.

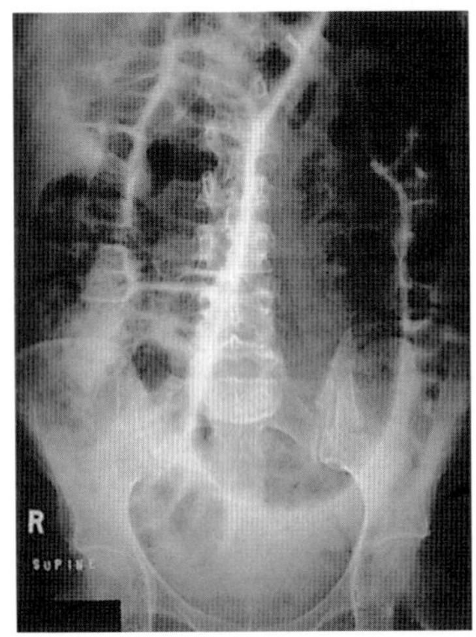

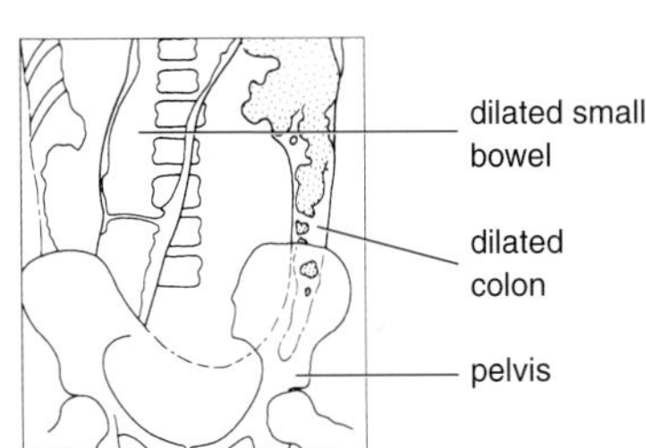

Fig. 4.141 Pseudo-obstruction. Plain radiograph showing gross distention of the small and large bowel.

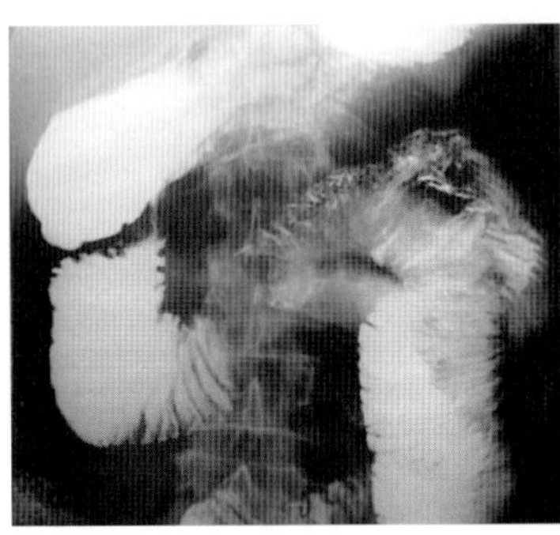

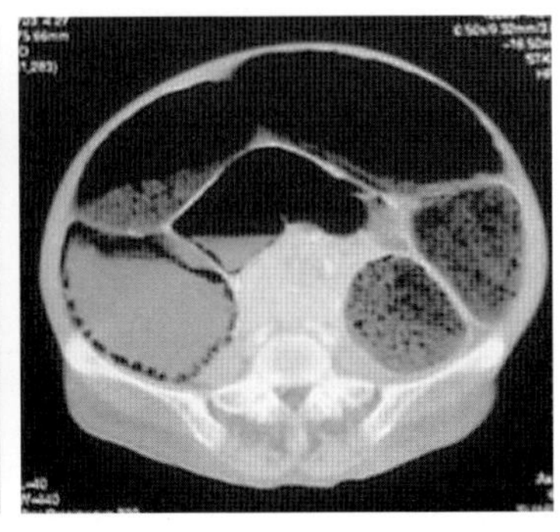

a b

Fig. 4.142a, b Characteristic massive dilatation of the duodenum, as well as the more distal small bowel, in two patients with histologically confirmed visceral myopathy, shown in the first on barium follow-through, and in the second on CT scanning (the duodenum lying near the center of the image behind the stomach).

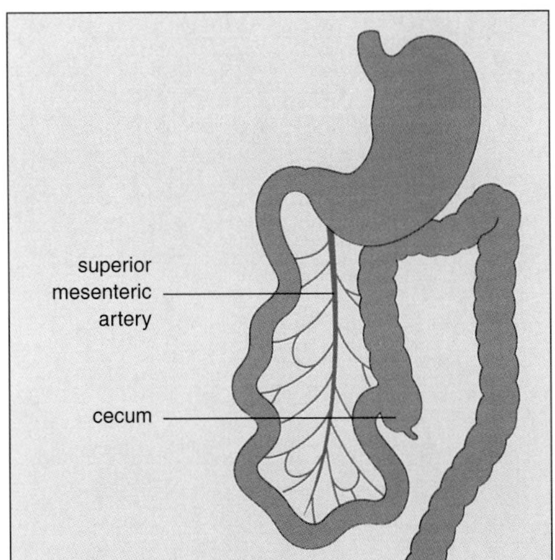

Fig. 4.143 Diagram illustrating the anatomical abnormality in complete failure of gut rotation.

MALROTATION OF THE GUT

During embryological development, the gastrointestinal tract undertakes a series of movements in the course of arriving at its normal anatomy and relationships. This occurs mainly during the 6th week of intrauterine life. Rotation of the mid gut occurs in an anticlockwise direction through 270°, about an axis formed by the superior mesenteric artery, which thus divides the gut into pre- and post-arterial segments.

If this process is incomplete or abnormal, or if it fails completely, intestinal symptoms may result. Complete failure of rotation is uncommon and causes the post-arterial segment (represented by the cecum and terminal ileum) to lie on the left side of the body (Figs 4.143–4.144). The duodenum then runs vertically on the right of the superior mesenteric artery, with the small intestine lying to the right of the abdominal cavity; the ileum enters the right of the cecum. Incomplete malrotation is commoner: the cecum is left at the splenic, or more often, at the hepatic, level (Figs 4.145, 4.146).

Problems arising from abnormal rotation may be recognized *in utero*, at birth, in infancy, or later. In exomphalos, intestine that has escaped (normally) into the umbilical cord during development then fails, either completely or in part, to return to the abdominal cavity. Coils of intestine are therefore found protruding through the umbilical ring, covered only by a jelly-like matrix of umbilical tissue. In gastroschisis, there is a defect of the abdominal wall, independent of the umbilical ring, which lies intact and to one side of the extruded abdominal organs (Fig. 4.147).

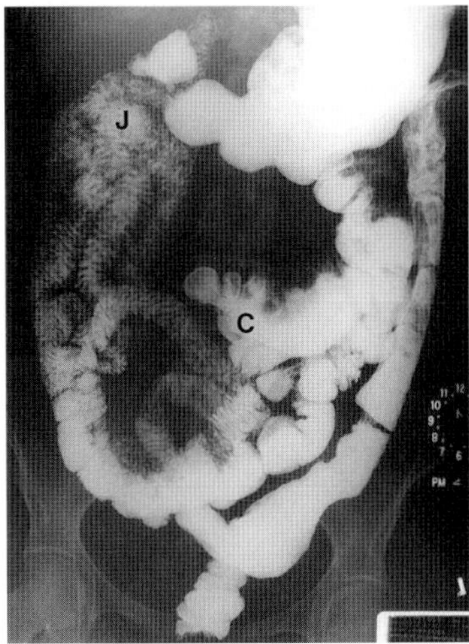

Fig. 4.144 Small bowel follow-through showing non-rotation of the bowel. The duodenum, jejunum (J) and most of the ileum lie entirely to the right of the spine. The cecum (C) is in the midline, and the remainder of the colon lies in the left abdomen.

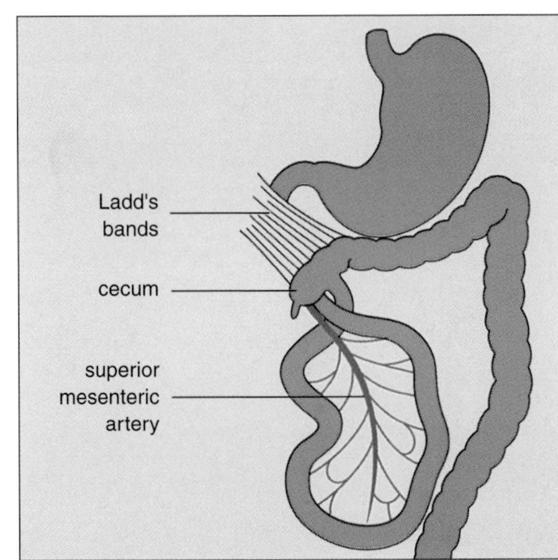

Fig. 4.145 Diagram showing the anatomical abnormality in incomplete malrotation of the gut. Ladd's bands, which may obstruct the duodenum, form across the duodenal loop if anticlockwise rotation of the colon is halted over the duodenal loop.

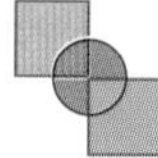

Malrotation frequently causes abnormalities of fixation, which can result in neonatal volvulus, but more often it causes recurrent abdominal pain in childhood, culminating in obstruction from intestinal volvulus (see Chapter 7) or fibrous bands. Complete transposition of the viscera – situs inversus totalis – is very uncommon and is usually asymptomatic. The diagnosis is sometimes made from a routine chest radiograph, in which the gastric gas bubble is seen on the right, with the liver and the heart both on the left; an eventration of the right hemidiaphragm is often associated.

EXTERNAL ABDOMINAL HERNIAE

External herniae are protrusions of viscus from the peritoneal cavity through openings in the abdominal wall. The most common are inguinal, femoral, umbilical, and incisional herniae. The contents are usually bowel, omentum, or both, and in general, herniae occur at sites of weakness of the abdominal wall. Congenital persistence of the peritoneal sac and defects following abdominal incisions predispose towards herniation, and any factor increasing abdominal pressure (such as chronic coughing or straining at stool) may provoke or exacerbate the problem.

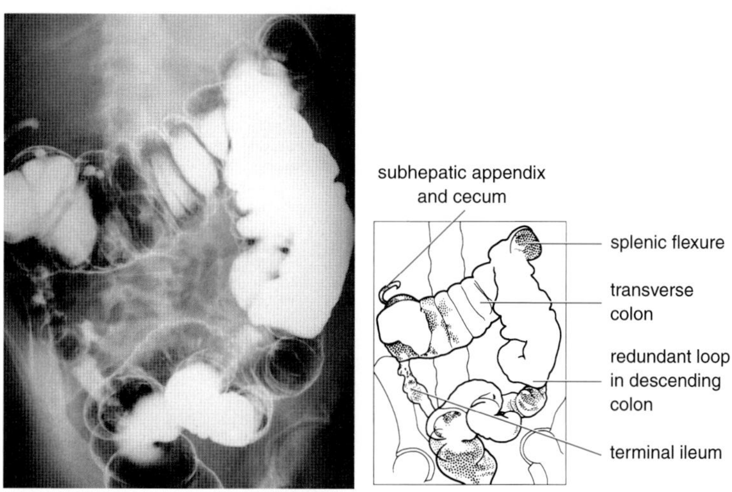

Fig. 4.146 Barium follow-through examination which shows a subhepatic cecum with the appendix lying above the colon.

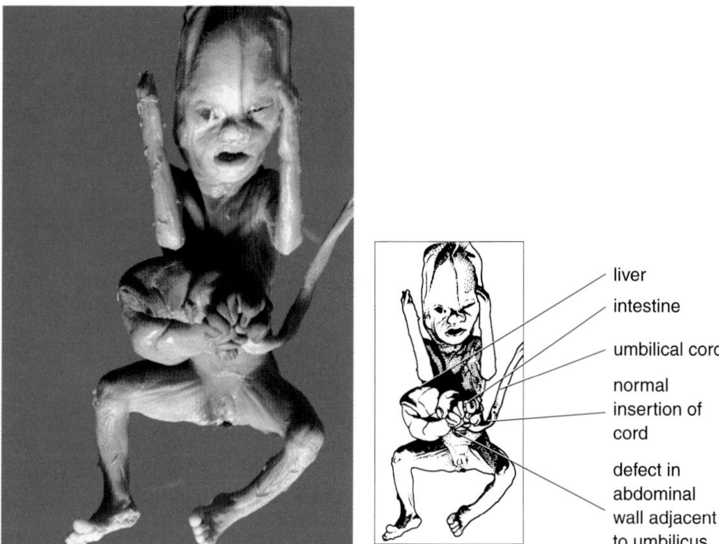

Fig. 4.147 Gastroschisis in which an extensive absence of the abdominal wall is present. The umbilical cord has a normal insertion to one side of the defect. Fetal membranes covering the organs, which would be present in an omphalocele, are absent.

INGUINAL HERNIA

The indirect inguinal hernia results from herniation of bowel or omentum through the internal inguinal ring and down the inguinal canal (Fig. 4.148); the defect is usually congenital (Fig. 4.149), although presentation may be much later in life. The direct hernia – a diffuse bulge of the medial portion of the posterior wall of the inguinal canal – arises medial to the internal inguinal ring and inferior to the epigastric vessels (Fig. 4.150); these are always acquired. If the hernia enters the scrotal sac (Figs 4.151, 4.152) it is usually indirect. If reducible, an indirect hernia is then controlled by pressure over the internal ring above the midpoint of the inguinal ligament; a direct hernia will not be. Inguinal herniae may be asymptomatic or responsible for an uncomfortable lump in the groin (Figs 4.153, 4.154). Frank pain indicates obstruction and perhaps strangulation.

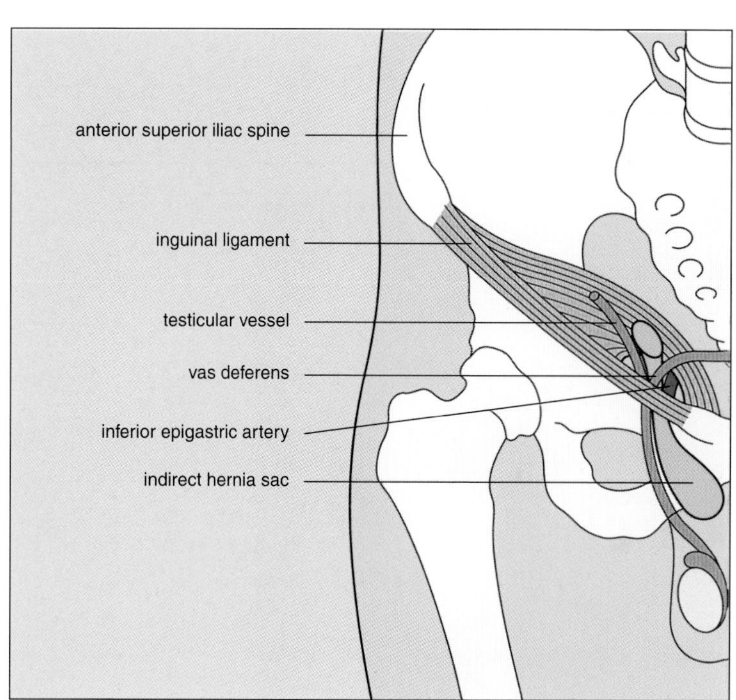

Fig. 4.148 Diagram illustrating the anatomical abnormality of an indirect inguinal hernia.

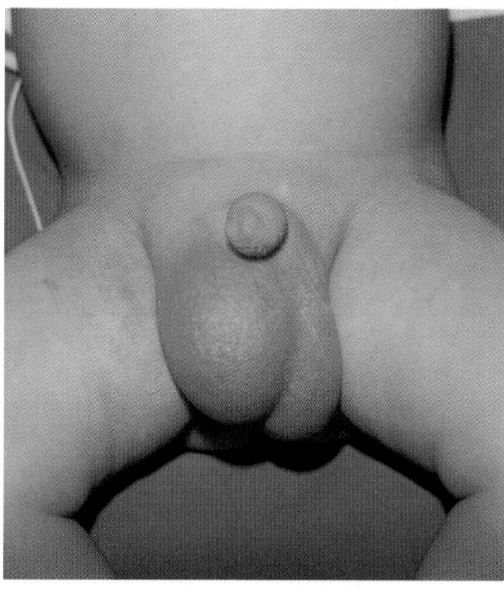

Fig. 4.149 An infant with an indirect inguinal hernia. Courtesy of Miss V. Wright.

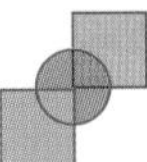

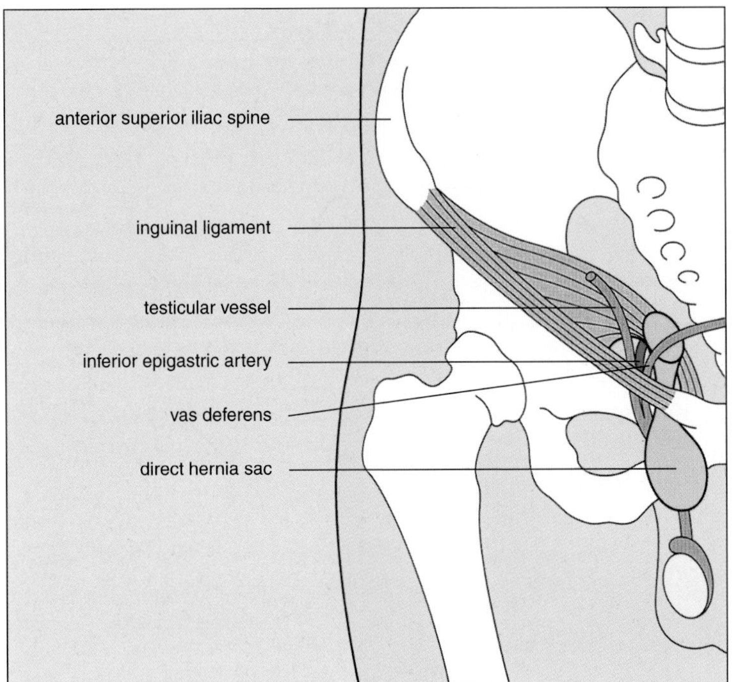

■ **Fig. 4.150** Diagram illustrating the anatomical abnormality of a direct inguinal hernia.

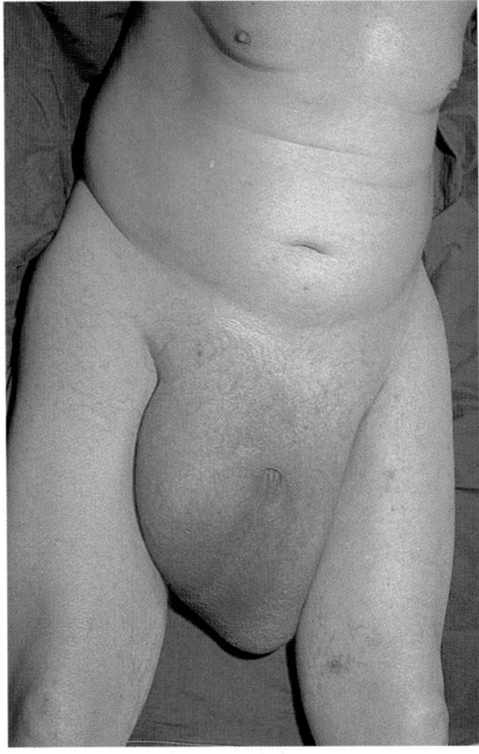

■ **Fig. 4.151** A massive non-reducible right indirect inguinal hernia.

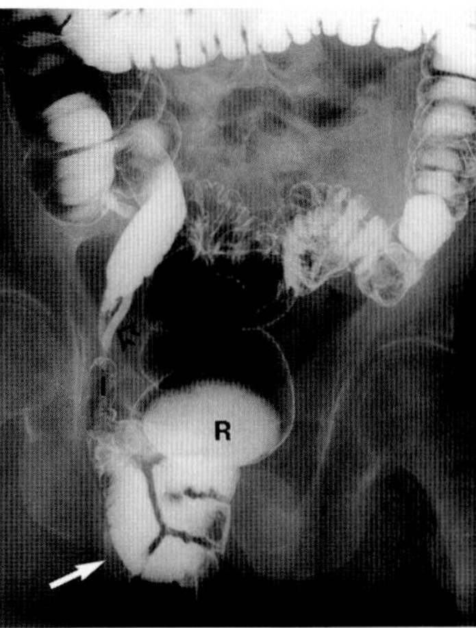

■ **Fig 4.152** Double-contrast barium enema demonstrating an inguinal hernia containing ileum and tip of the appendix. The appendix (open arrow) and terminal ileum (I) overlie the region of the inguinal canal. The distal ileum (long arrow) lies in the right side of the scrotum. The rectum is identified (R).

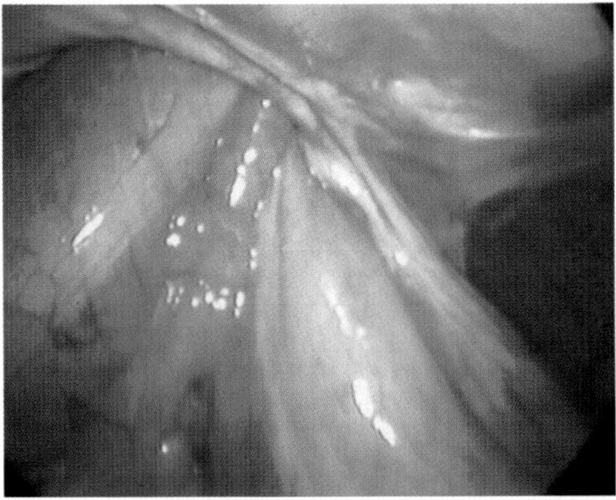

■ **Fig. 4.153** Laparoscopic view of a sliding inguinal hernia at the internal ring: a loop of bowel (with some omentum) is within the hernia. Courtesy of Mr P. Dawson.

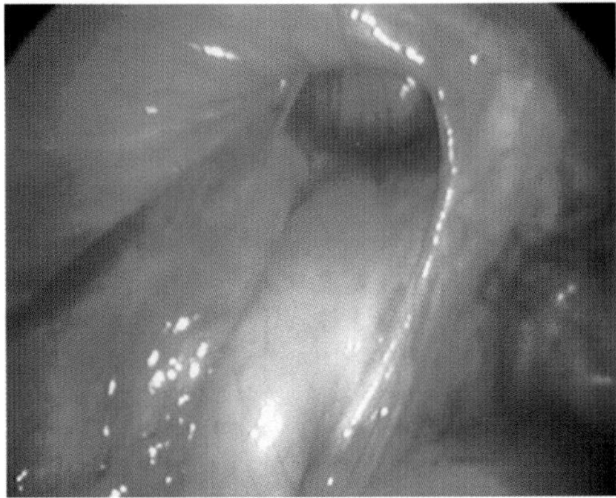

■ **Fig. 4.154** Laparoscopic view of the same hernia after its reduction. Courtesy of Mr P. Dawson.

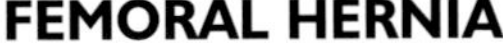

FEMORAL HERNIA

Femoral herniae are less common and are always acquired; they tend to affect middle-aged and elderly women. Herniation occurs through the femoral hernial orifice – the superficial end of the femoral canal – which lies medial to the femoral vein (Fig. 4.155). Presentation is with a lump below and lateral to the pubic tubercle (Fig. 4.156). Since the femoral ring is narrow and bounded by fairly rigid structures, there is a substantially higher risk of irreducibility, strangulation, and intestinal obstruction than in inguinal hernia.

UMBILICAL HERNIA

A true umbilical hernia is due to a defect in the umbilical ring, which has thus remained patent, and occurs during the first few days of life (Fig. 4.157). Such herniae are more apparent when the infant cries, and most resolve over 12–18 months, needing only a small pressure pad in the interim. A para-umbilical hernia is usually acquired, most commonly occurring in the elderly, the obese, the multiparous, and those with ascites. These herniae result from a small defect in the linea alba just above the umbilicus, which enlarges with the herniation and may become irreducible (Fig. 4.158). (See also sections on exomphalos and malrotation syndromes, above.)

INCISIONAL HERNIA

Incisional herniae protrude through a defect in the abdominal wall following surgery. They are more frequent in the obese, the malnour-

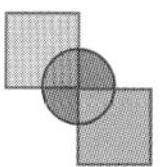

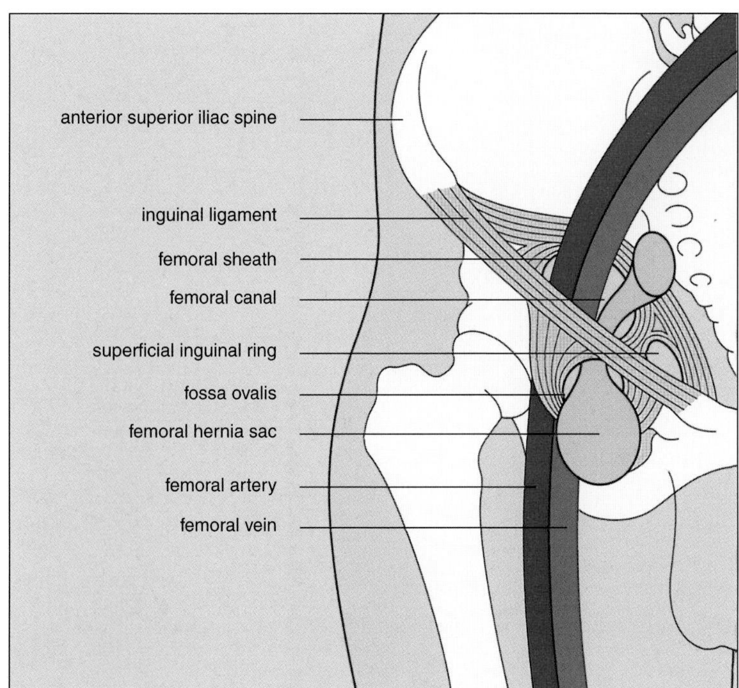

■ **Fig. 4.155** Diagram illustrating the anatomical abnormality in femoral hernia.

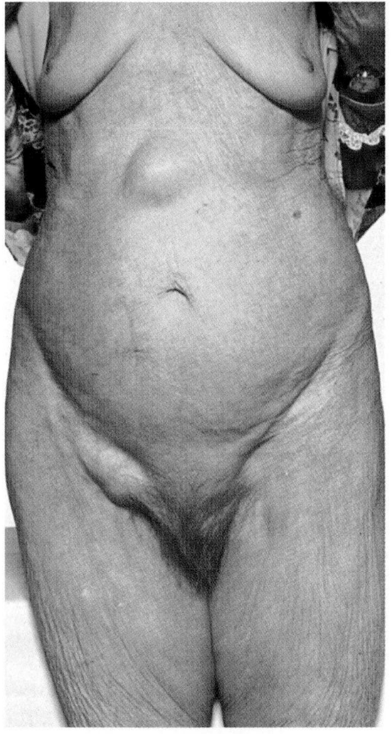

■ **Fig. 4.156** Patient with a femoral hernia. Courtesy of the Professorial Surgical Unit, King's College London.

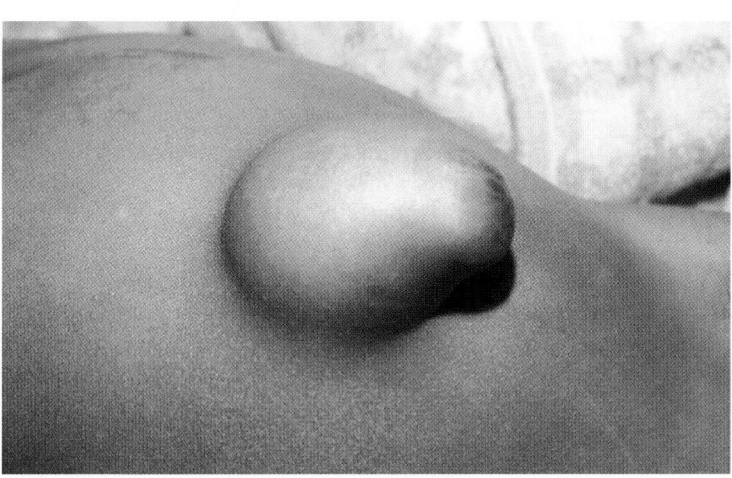

■ **Fig. 4.157** Infant with an umbilical hernia. Courtesy of Professor L. Spitz.

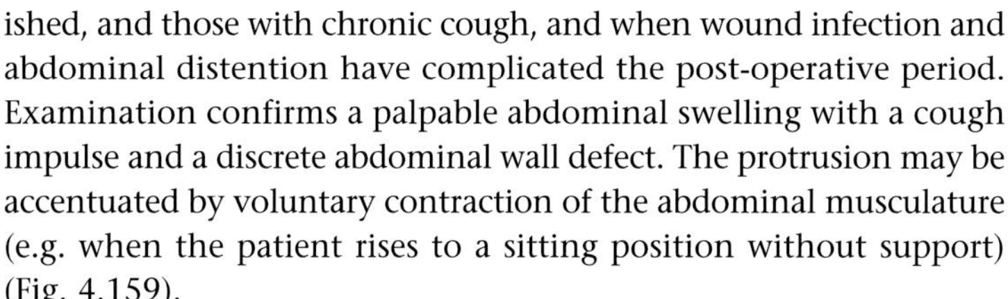

ished, and those with chronic cough, and when wound infection and abdominal distention have complicated the post-operative period. Examination confirms a palpable abdominal swelling with a cough impulse and a discrete abdominal wall defect. The protrusion may be accentuated by voluntary contraction of the abdominal musculature (e.g. when the patient rises to a sitting position without support) (Fig. 4.159).

SMALL BOWEL ISCHEMIA

Ischemic pain from the small bowel used to be considered unusual in the absence of mechanical incarceration (Fig 1.160), but it is increasingly clear that intestinal angina is also to be encountered in those with mesenteric arteriopathy. Small bowel ischemia implies pathology of the superior mesenteric artery and its branches or their draining veins, and most affected patients are smokers and have other evidence of vascular disease (such as ischemic heart disease or peripheral vascular disease) or its antecedents (such as diabetes). Since the pain is usually provoked by eating, most patients will have lost weight by the time of presentation, as they try to avoid their symptoms. When such patients present sub-acutely it is then possible to identify areas of vascular occlusion by specific imaging prior to frank infarction, and with a view to vascular reconstruction (Fig. 4.161), or semi-elective resection of limited extent (Figs 4.162, 4.163). The so-called wandering artery of Drummond may become a crucially

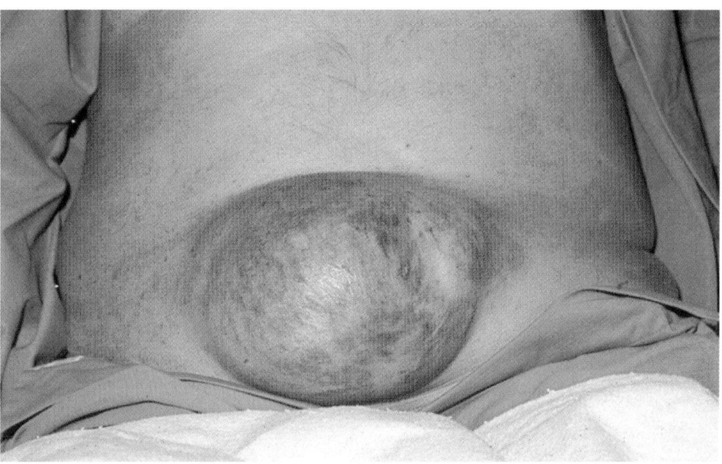

■ **Fig. 4.158** A large irreducible paraumbilical hernia. Courtesy of the Professorial Surgical Unit, King's College London.

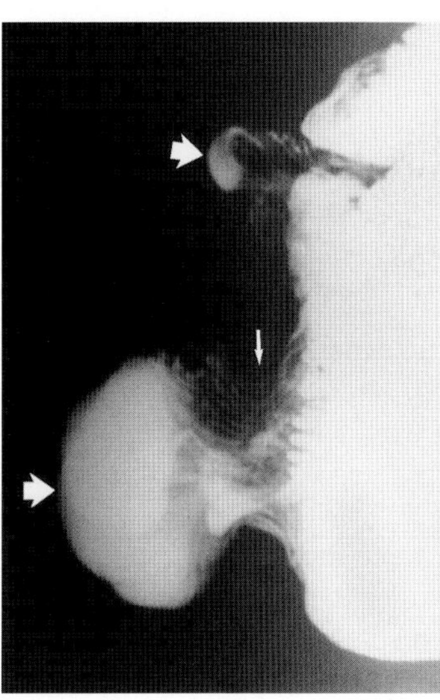

■ **Fig. 4.159** Small bowel follow-through demonstrating several loops of small bowel (thick arrows) protruding through incisional hernias of the anterior abdominal wall. In this lateral radiograph, the location of the anterior abdominal wall is identified by the thin arrow and wire sutures. (Reproduced with permission from reference 7, Fig. 46.28.)

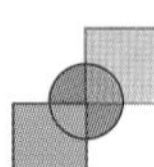

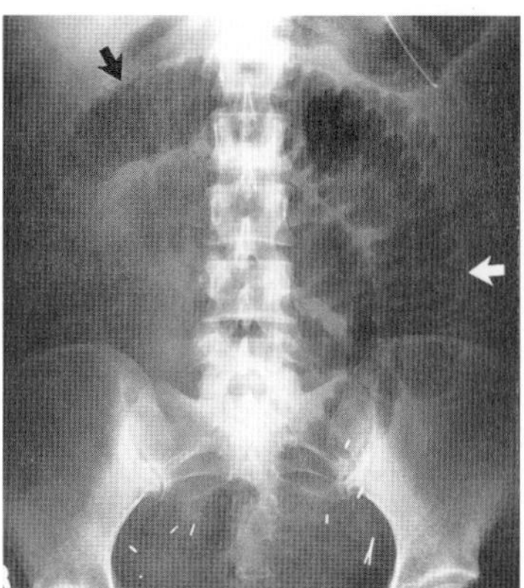

Fig. 4.160 Plain radiograph demonstrating changes suggestive of ischemia and closed loop obstruction. The mid small bowel (arrows) is dilated and has smoothly enlarged valvulae conniventes. The dilated small bowel loops are radially arranged. At surgery, adhesions were found to be the cause of this closed loop obstruction with ischemic small bowel.

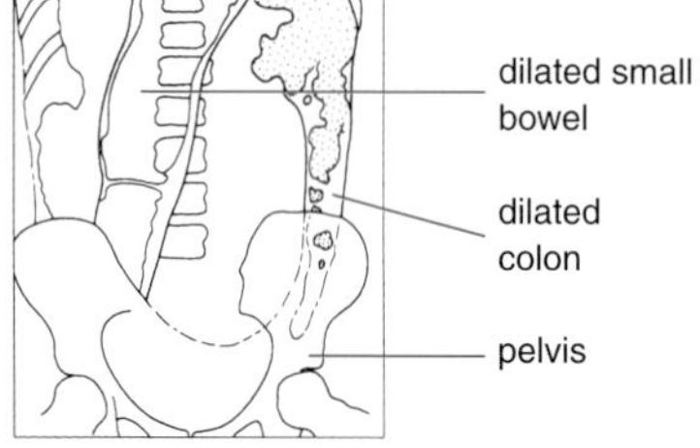

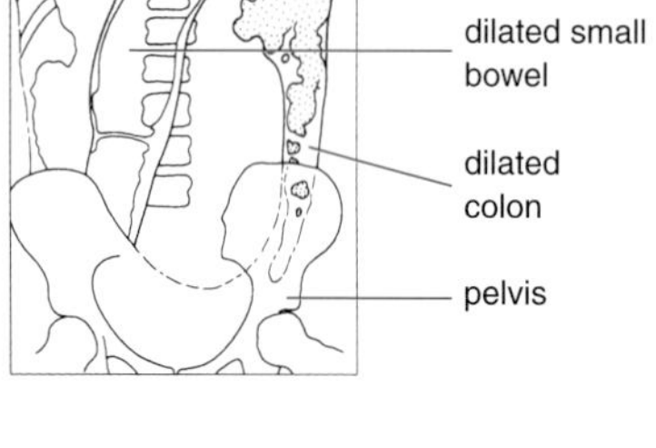

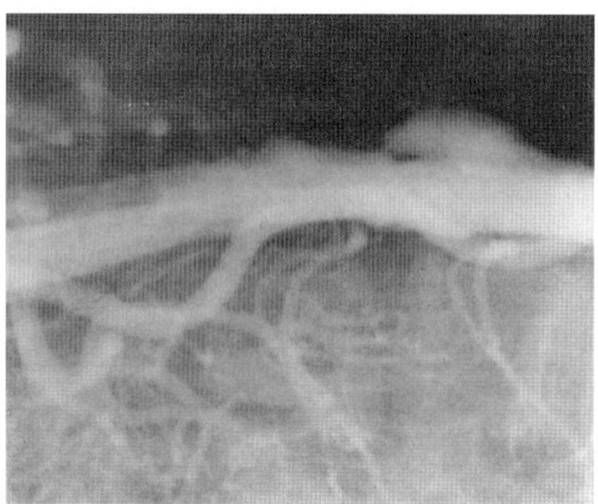

Fig. 4.161 Lateral aortogram in a patient with small bowel ischemia. The celiac axis and superior mesenteric artery are occluded (and the inferior mesenteric artery is dilated). An enlarged wandering artery of Drummond is seen below the site of the occlusion (see below).

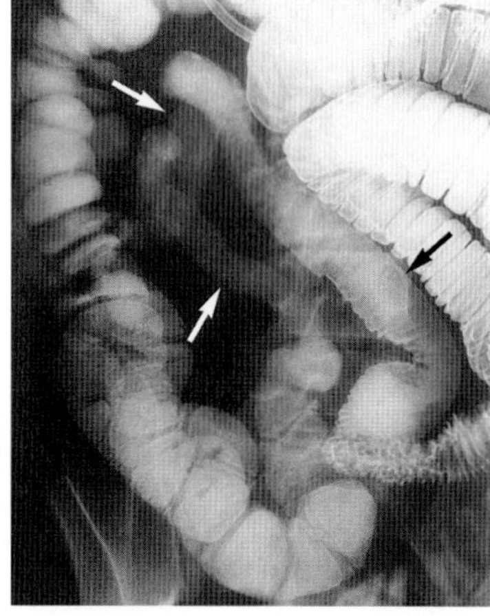

Fig. 4.162 Enteroclysis demonstrating acute and chronic ischemia. A long segment of ileum is diffusely narrowed (arrows) and its folds are mainly absent.

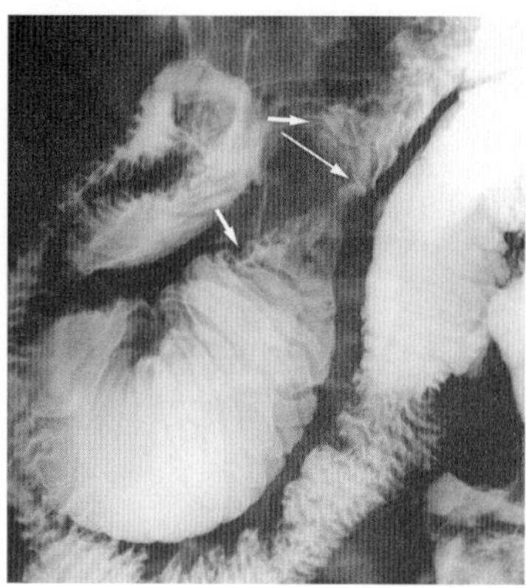

Fig. 4.163 Overhead view from small bowel enema demonstrating ischemic ulcer and stricture. A tapered narrowing (short arrows) is seen in the proximal jejunum. A small ulcer (long arrow) is seen centrally. The jejunum proximal to the stricture is dilated and partially obstructed. (Reproduced with permission from reference 1, Fig. 23.25.)

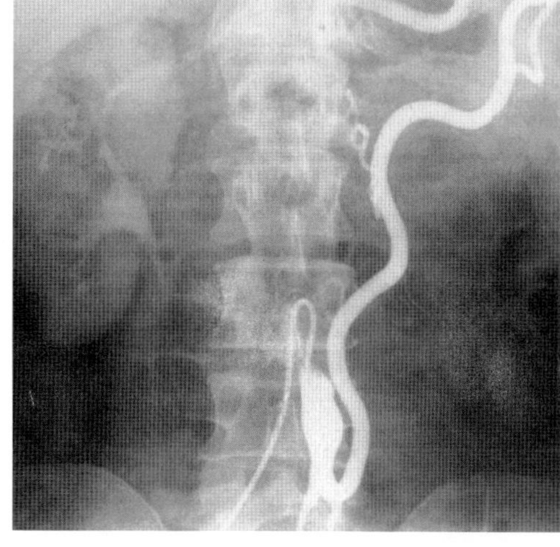

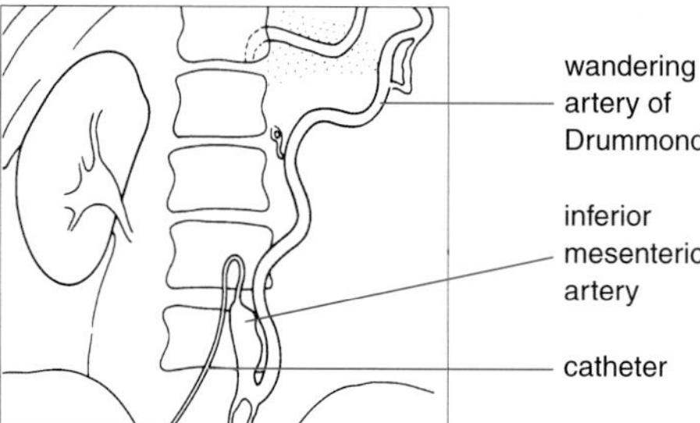

Fig. 4.164 The wandering artery of Drummond is a branch of the inferior mesenteric artery – as shown here at inferior mesenteric angiography.

important collateral supply when the superior mesenteric artery is occluded (Figs 4.161, 4.164, 4.165). Unfortunately, a very high proportion of patients presents only after catastrophe, and with no sufficient collateral system; there is then a need for major intestinal resection to preserve life.

At least half of all patients with acute mesenteric ischemia will have had arterial emboli, and it was once thought that the majority of the remainder had acute venous thrombosis. However, it is now clear that non-occlusive ischemia is the more prevalent, followed by arterial thrombosis, and that true venous thrombosis is relatively rare. Mesenteric vasculitis is identifiable radiologically by virtue of its ischemic effects (Fig. 4.166) and the damage to the small bowel from irradiation (see Chapter 5) also is mainly of ischemic nature (Fig. 4.167).

REFERENCES

1. Rubesin SE, Furth B. Differential diagnosis of small intestinal abnormalities with radiologic pathologic explanation. Herlinger H, Maglinte DDT, Birnbaum BA (eds) Clinical imaging of the small intestine, 2nd edn, pp. 527–566. New York: Springer, 1999, Figures 8, 12, 18a, 23, 25, 27, 45, 55.
2. Rubesin SE, Gilchrist AM, Bronner M, *et al.* Non-Hodgkin lymphoma of the small intestine. RadioGraphics 1990; 10: 985–998, Figs 6, 12.
3. Rubesin SE, Herlinger H, Saul S, *et al.* Adult coeliac disease and its complications. RadioGraphics 1989; 9: 1045, Fig. 15.
4. Rubesin SE, Rubin RA, Herlinger H. Small bowel malabsorption: clinical and radiologic perspectives. Radiology 1992; 184: 297–305, Figs 2.4, 5.7.

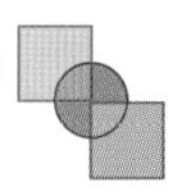

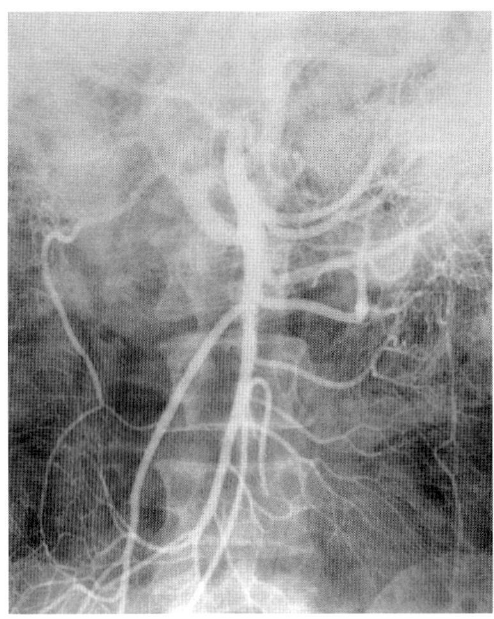

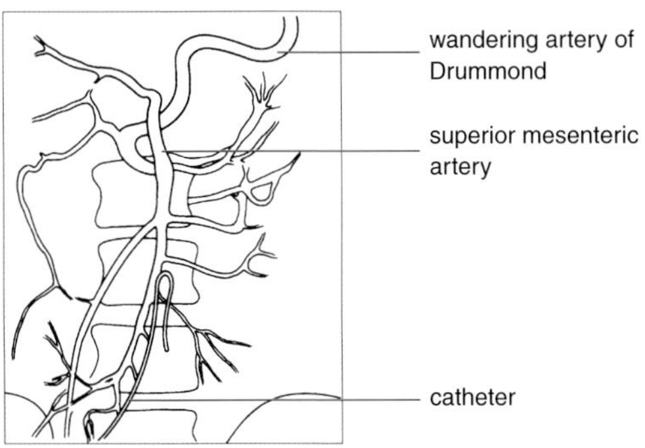

Fig. 4.165 At first glance, this examination of the superior mesenteric artery and its branches appears satisfactory – until it is realized that all the filling is through the wandering artery of Drummond.

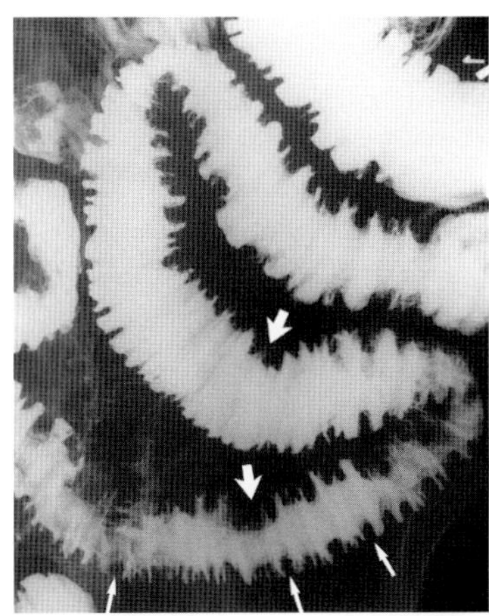

Fig. 4.166 Small bowel follow-through in patient with vasculitis and small bowel hemorrhage and ischemia. Smooth thick folds (thin arrows) lie perpendicular to the luminal contour (the so-called "stack of coins"). "Thumbprinting," radiographically indicative of either severe edema or hemorrhage, is present (thick arrows). (Reproduced with permission from reference 6, Fig. 5.38.)

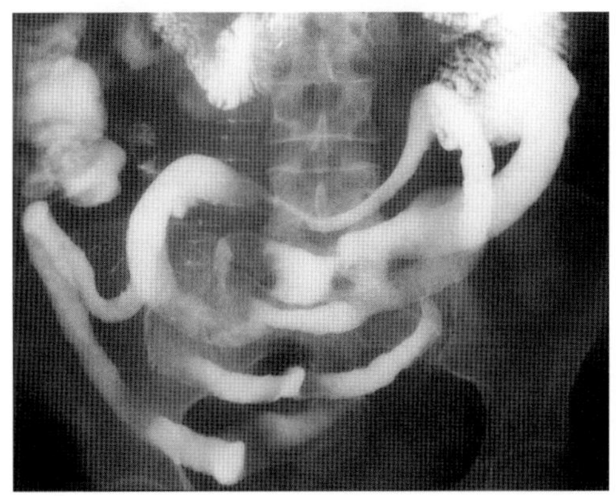

Fig. 4.167 Small bowel follow-through showing radiation-induced chronic ischemia. The small bowel in the pelvis is diffusely narrowed and has lost its valvulae conniventes. (Reproduced with permission from reference 1, Fig. 23.55.)

5. Rubesin SE, Herlinger H, DeGaeta L. Interlude: test your skills. Radiology 1990; 176: 636–644, Fig. 1.
6. Rubesin SE, Laufer I. Pictorial glossary of double contrast radiology. In: Gore RM, Levine MS (eds). Textbook of gastrointestinal radiology, 2nd edn, pp. 44–65. Philadelphia: WB Saunders Co; 2000, Fig. 5.39B
7. Herlinger H, Rubesin SE, Morris JB. Small bowel obstruction. In: Gore RM, Levine MS (eds). Textbook of gastrointestinal radiology, 2nd edn, pp. 815–837. Philadelphia: WB Saunders Co; 2000, Figs 46.28, 30, 34A, 39, 41,
8. Herlinger H, Rubesin SE. Obstruction. In: Gore RM, Levine MS, Laufer I (eds) Textbook of gastrointestinal radiology, pp. 931–966. Philadelphia: WB Saunders Co; 1994, Figs 52.30, 32, 36.
9. Marsh MN, Crowe PT. Morphology of the mucosal lesion in gluten sensitivity. Baillières Clin Gastroenterol 1995; 9: 273–293.

SMALL INTESTINE II

5

INFECTIVE DIARRHEA

In Western populations, infective diarrhea is now of bacterial cause in less than 50% of cases. Typical proportions are in the region of: *Campylobacter* 13%, clostridial species 13%, enterotoxigenic *E. coli* 8%, *Salmonellae* 7%, and *Shigellae* 4%, in northern Europe and North America. Other aggressive forms of *E. coli* are less often responsible. Viral causes probably account for most of the remainder, and rota virus infection, widely recognized in children, is now increasingly diagnosed in adult diarrhea. Traveler's diarrhea is usually the result of enteropathogenic *E. coli*. If colitis (or dysentery) exists, it is usually obvious, and infective colitis is considered further in Chapter 6. Apart from acute viral gastroenteritis and HIV infection, it is unusual for viral disease to be identified as a cause of small intestinal pathology.

TYPHOID (ENTERIC FEVER)

Typhoid is primarily a bacteremic illness caused by infection with *Salmonella typhi*. Progressive fever, malaise, anorexia, relative bradycardia, and constipation generally precede the more specific abdominal symptoms of the second week of illness. Rose spots on the abdomen and flanks (Fig. 5.1), splenomegaly, the development of a toxic state, and diarrhea follow if untreated. Intestinal perforation and bleeding from small bowel ulceration are late complications.

Involvement of the lymphoid tissue concentrates – Peyer's patches – of the small bowel produces the characteristic oval ulcers and determines their distribution along the long axis of the gut (Fig. 5.2). The changes are maximal in the distal ileum, but ulceration can extend across into the colon, and also occurs in the more proximal small intestine. The ulcers tend to be raised above and clearly demarcated from the mucosa. Histologically, typhoid ulcers demonstrate a paucity of polymorphonuclear leukocytes, the infiltrate consisting entirely of mononuclear leukocytes (Figs 5.3, 5.4). Large numbers of bacilli will usually be identifiable; earlier diagnosis (from blood culture) is naturally preferable.

YERSINIA

Infection with *Yersinia enterocolitica* or *Y. pseudotuberculosis* can cause gastrointestinal disease. The organisms are facultatively anaerobic Gram-negative rods that affect humans and animals. The mode of transmission is feco-oral from ingested liquids and solids (particularly pork).

Y. enterocolitica can be responsible for a broad range of clinical manifestations, particularly in children and young adults. It is a common cause of acute bacterial gastroenteritis in some temperate countries, but may also mimic acute appendicitis or small bowel

■ **Fig. 5.1** Rose spots on the abdomen and flanks in typhoid fever. Courtesy of Dr G.D.W. McKendrick.

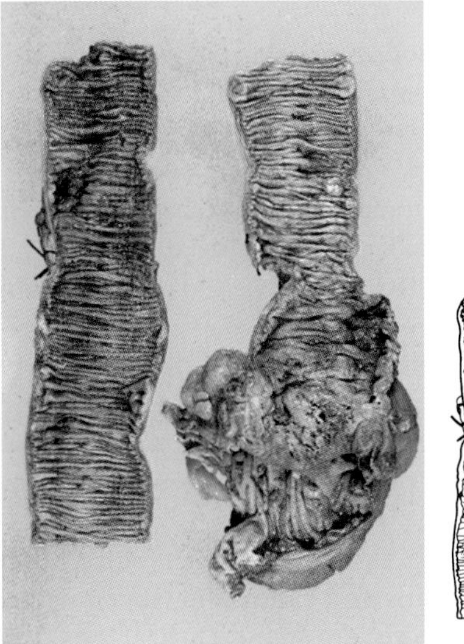

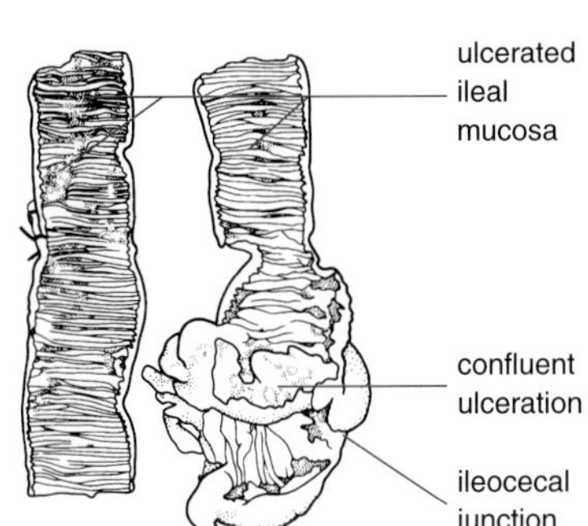

■ **Fig. 5.2** The ileocecal junction and distal ileum, with scattered ulceration in typhoid fever. The ulcers tend to be oval, and lie in the longitudinal axis of the bowel. Courtesy of Dr J. Newman.

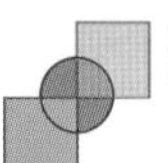

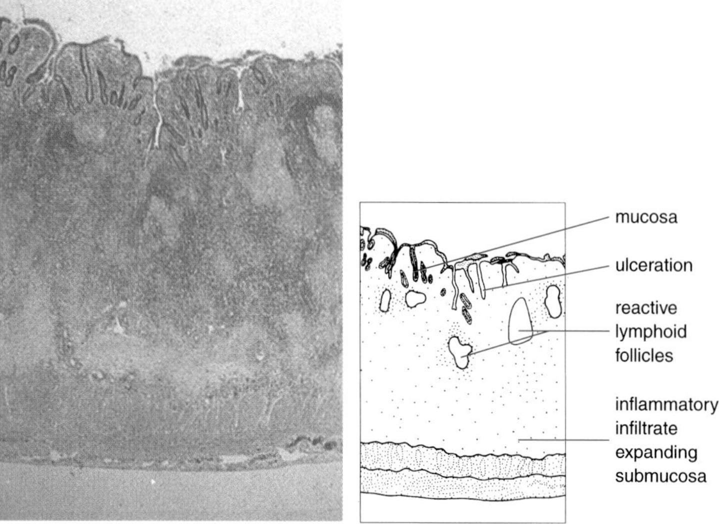

■ **Fig. 5.3** Histological appearance of the ileum in typhoid showing prominent lymphoid hyperplasia and small slit-like ulcers. At this magnification, the initial impression is one of lymphoma. H&E stain (x 10).

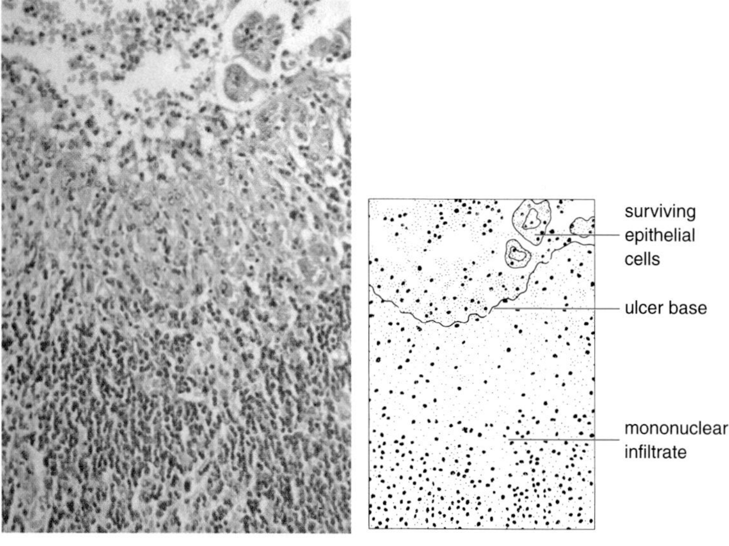

■ **Fig. 5.4** The inflammatory infiltrate in an ulcerated area in typhoid; it is characterized by many mononuclear cells and few neutrophil polymorphs. H&E stain (x 120).

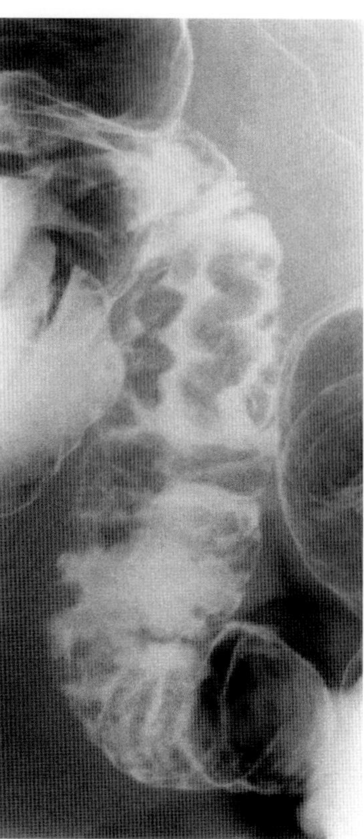

■ **Fig. 5.5** Double-contrast barium showing thick, undulating folds in the terminal ileum in a patient with *Yersinia* ileitis. (Reproduced with permission from reference 1, Fig. 5.32C.)

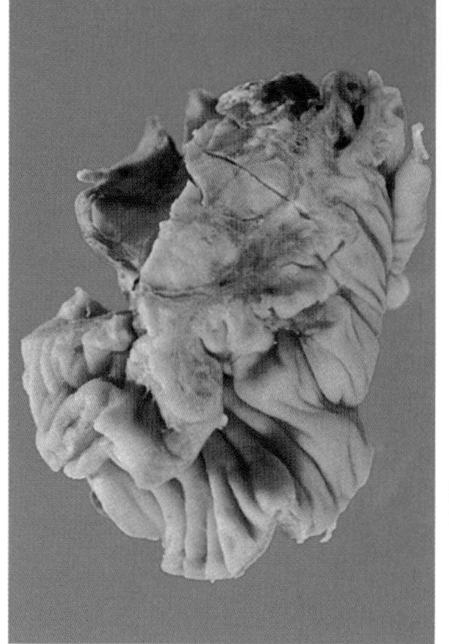

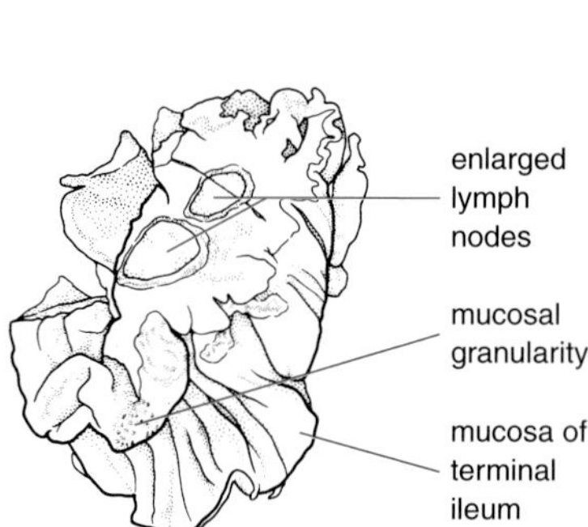

■ **Fig. 5.6** The resected ileum from a patient with yersiniosis showing two enlarged, fleshy nodes in the mesentery, and some overlying mucosal granularity.

Crohn's. Post-infective erythema nodosum or reactive arthritis predominantly affect adults. Bacteremia is unusual, however, and although the symptomatic period may last for some months, major complications such as toxic megacolon, myocarditis, and glomerulonephritis are fortunately rare. Serodiagnosis is unreliable unless very high titers are present, because of cross-reacting antibodies and because of high background population seropositivity. Early stool cultures maintained at 25°C on appropriate media should be diagnostic. In patients with chronic yersiniosis, small bowel radiology shows nodularity and shallow ulceration (Fig. 5.5). Granulomas are unusual, and histological examination of the characteristic small ulcers in the terminal ileum and proximal colon generally show non-specific changes.

Infection with *Y. pseudotuberculosis* occurs mostly in children, and is responsible for mesenteric adenitis and can mimic appendicitis. The organism can be identified from culture and serological tests. The histopathological appearances are those of epithelioid giant cell granulomas. Distinction from Crohn's disease and abdominal tuberculosis may be difficult in the absence of microbiological information, but the presence of the yersinial central micro-abscess, in which there is central necrosis with large numbers of surrounding polymorphs, is helpful (Figs 5.6–5.9).

ABDOMINAL TUBERCULOSIS

Tuberculous enteritis may develop as a primary lesion within the intestine or secondary to a focus elsewhere; in these cases, the primary focus is often occult. Although secondary tuberculous enteritis is usually the result of pulmonary disease, approximately 50% of UK patients with a final diagnosis of abdominal tuberculosis have normal chest radiographs. Intestinal involvement is also a common, though not necessarily dominant, feature of miliary disease.

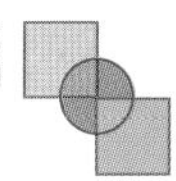

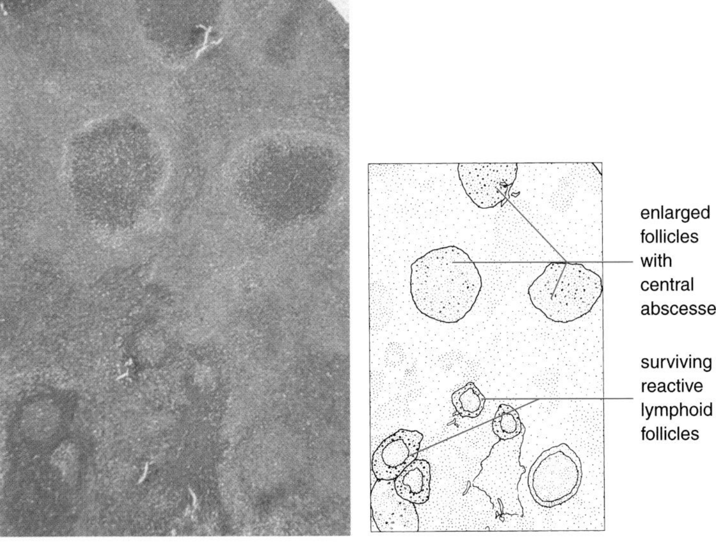

■ **Fig. 5.7** Lymph node histology in yersiniosis. The basic nodal architecture is preserved, but many of the follicular germinal centers are replaced by polymorphs, and there are tiny areas of necrosis, forming microabscesses. H&E stain (x 10).

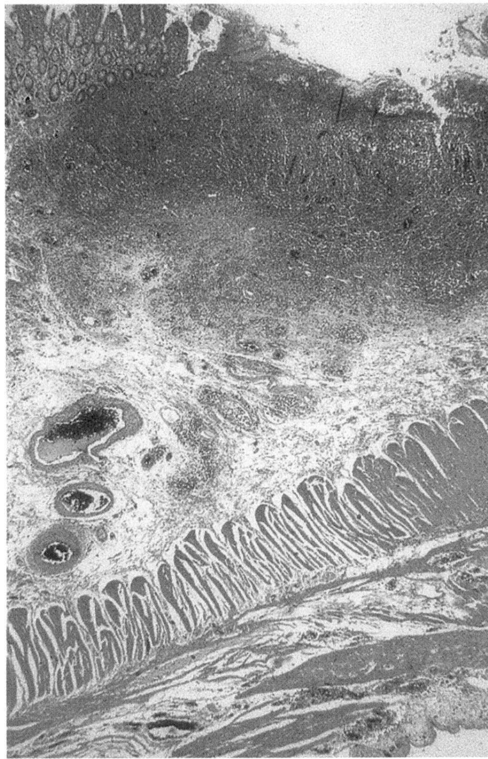

■ **Fig. 5.8** Yersiniosis. Microscopic view of early lesion in the ileum showing an aphthous ulcer cupped by collections of macrophages and a thick mantle of lymphocytes.

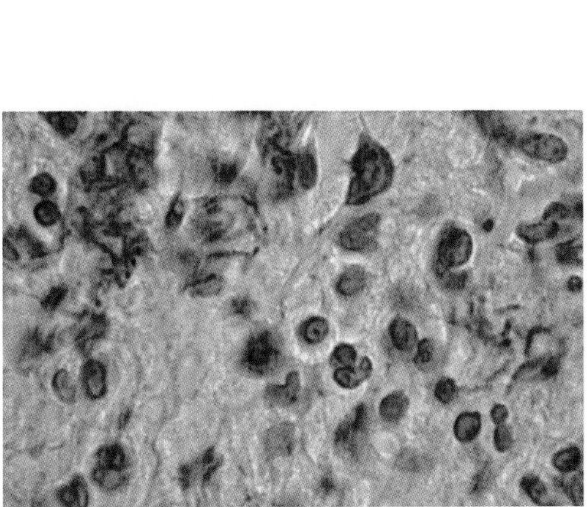

■ **Fig. 5.9** Yersiniosis. Tissue Gram stain of an aphthous ulcer showing long, thick Gram-negative bacilli within the cytoplasm of macrophages in the ulcer base.

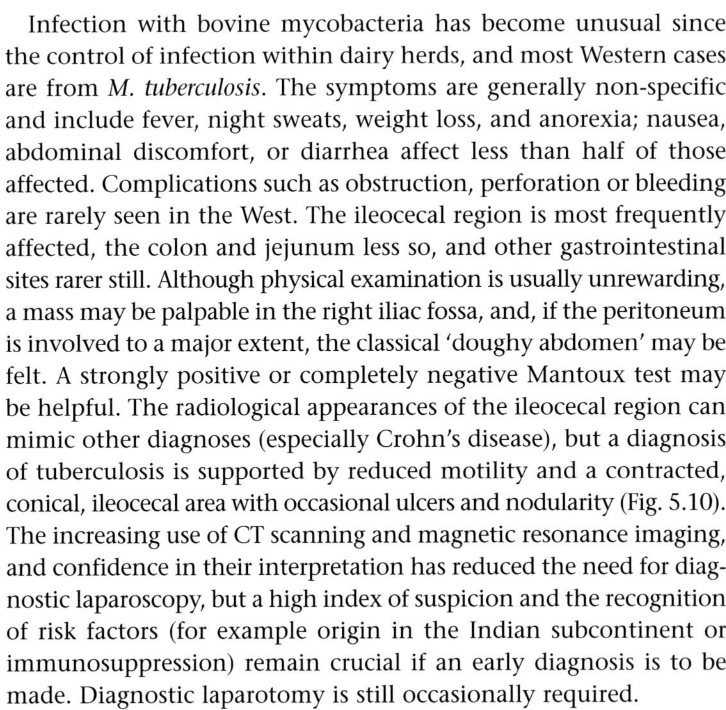

Infection with bovine mycobacteria has become unusual since the control of infection within dairy herds, and most Western cases are from *M. tuberculosis*. The symptoms are generally non-specific and include fever, night sweats, weight loss, and anorexia; nausea, abdominal discomfort, or diarrhea affect less than half of those affected. Complications such as obstruction, perforation or bleeding are rarely seen in the West. The ileocecal region is most frequently affected, the colon and jejunum less so, and other gastrointestinal sites rarer still. Although physical examination is usually unrewarding, a mass may be palpable in the right iliac fossa, and, if the peritoneum is involved to a major extent, the classical 'doughy abdomen' may be felt. A strongly positive or completely negative Mantoux test may be helpful. The radiological appearances of the ileocecal region can mimic other diagnoses (especially Crohn's disease), but a diagnosis of tuberculosis is supported by reduced motility and a contracted, conical, ileocecal area with occasional ulcers and nodularity (Fig. 5.10). The increasing use of CT scanning and magnetic resonance imaging, and confidence in their interpretation has reduced the need for diagnostic laparoscopy, but a high index of suspicion and the recognition of risk factors (for example origin in the Indian subcontinent or immunosuppression) remain crucial if an early diagnosis is to be made. Diagnostic laparotomy is still occasionally required.

The macroscopic appearances depend on the stage of the disease. In acute intestinal tuberculosis, there is usually ulceration of the terminal ileum with ulcers lying in the transverse axis (Fig. 5.11). These may be accompanied by tiny miliary tubercles on the peritoneum and mesentery. In chronic infection, fibrosis results in the so-called 'hypertrophic' or 'ulcero-constrictive' forms of disease (Fig. 5.12). Strictures are often short and multiple and this feature can help in the distinction from Crohn's disease. Tuberculosis, but also Crohn's and lymphoma, may be responsible for a short length of ulcerated, narrowed bowel with a thick wall (Fig. 5.13). Histological specimens in acute infection show confluent caseating granulomas (Fig. 5.14) with acid-fast bacilli (Figs 5.15, 5.16). With chronicity, fibrosis destroys the normal bowel architecture, and ultimately the granulomas are replaced by hyalinized fibrous tissue. Colonic tuberculosis is further considered in Chapter 6.

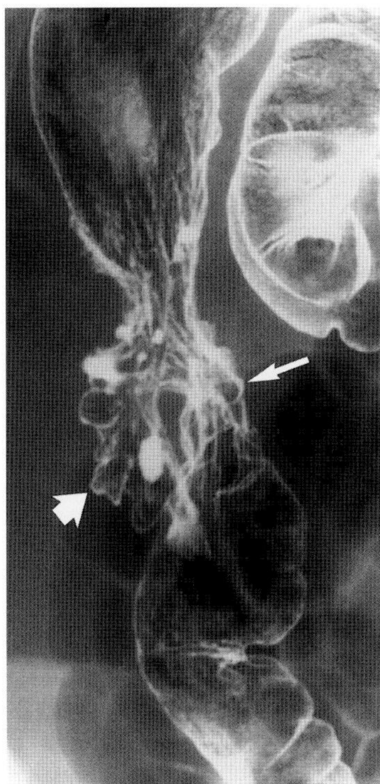

■ **Fig. 5.10** Double-contrast barium enema showing tuberculosis of the terminal ileum and ascending colon. The cecum (short arrow) is markedly contracted and sacculated. The ascending colon is narrowed and has a finely nodular mucosa. The ileocecal valve and distal-most terminal ileum (long arrow) has nodular mucosa. (Reproduced with permission from reference 2, Fig. 1.95.)

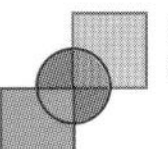

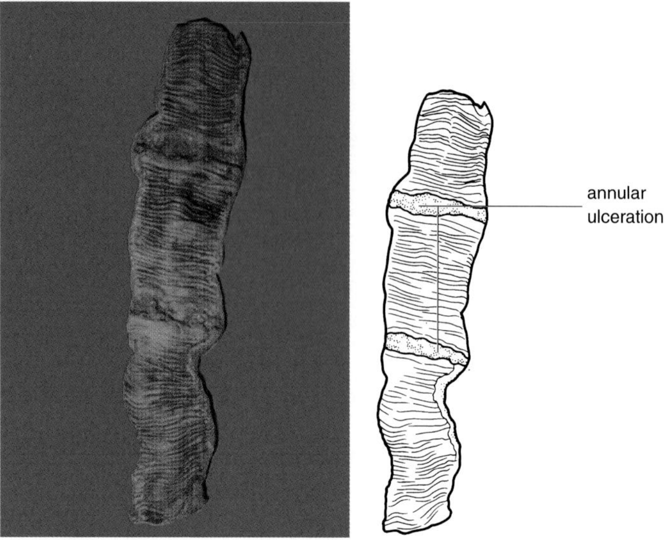

■ **Fig. 5.11** Typical, multiple, short annular areas of ulceration in ileal tuberculosis.

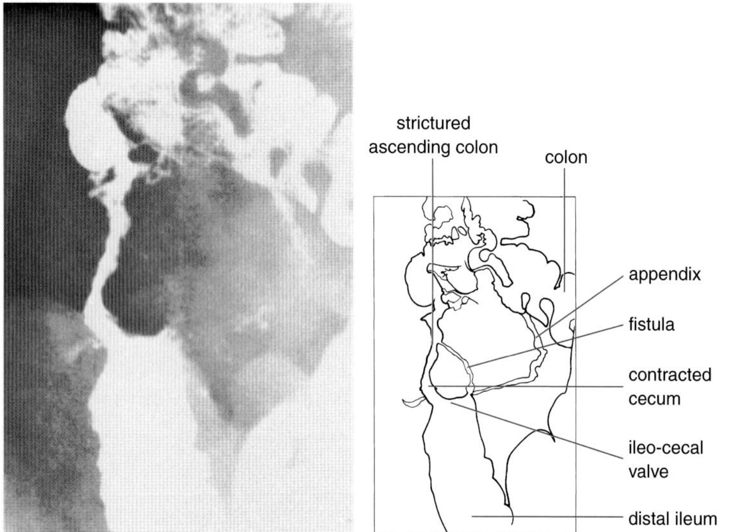

■ **Fig. 5.12** Barium study in hypertrophic tuberculosis, showing a dilated distal ileum leading into a contracted cecum and strictured ascending colon.

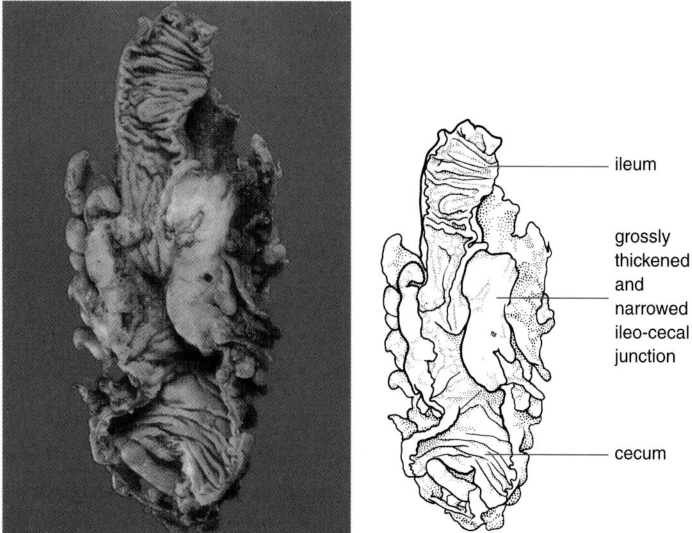

■ **Fig. 5.13** Ileocecal tuberculosis of greater chronicity, with thickened stricture giving appearances more similar to Crohn's disease.

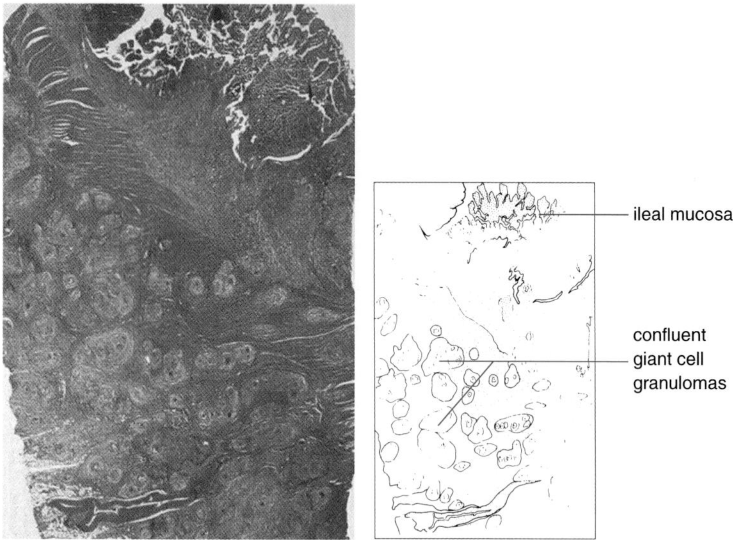

■ **Fig. 5.14** Confluent giant cell granulomas penetrating the full thickness of the intestinal wall in tuberculosis. The granulomas are larger and more multiple than usually seen in Crohn's disease. H&E stain (x 10).

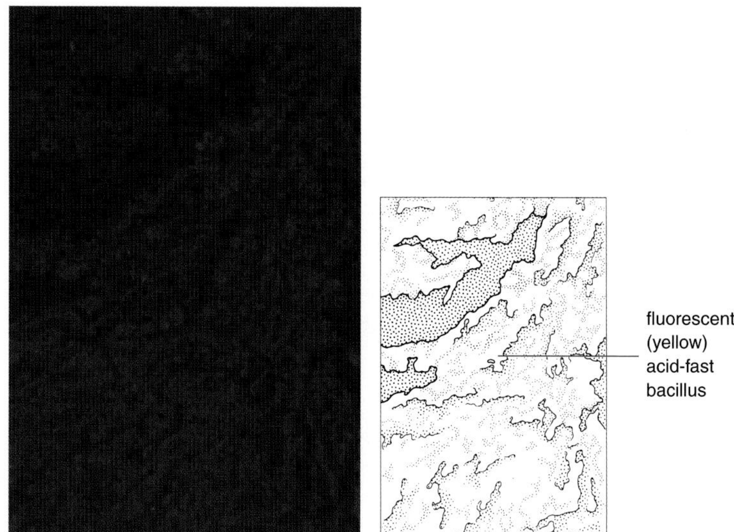

■ **Fig. 5.15** Acid-fast bacilli in tuberculosis. Initial positive screening with fluorescent microscopy using auramine-O staining (x 320).

ATYPICAL MYCOBACTERIAL INFECTION

Atypical mycobacteria of the avium intracellulare complex were once considered non-pathogenic, but it is clear that this is not the case. Nonetheless most affected patients are substantially immunosuppressed, AIDS sufferers constituting a substantial proportion of all cases. The clinical presentation is usually with pyrexia, weight loss, and diarrhea. Barium radiology may reveal apparent mass lesions (Fig. 5.17), and the organisms can be demonstrated in appropriately stained stool samples and on selective culture (Figs 5.18, 5.19). The hypothesis that these organisms are also the cause of Crohn's disease has not found general support.

WHIPPLE'S DISEASE

Whipple's disease or intestinal lipodystrophy, is a rare systemic illness that is somewhat commoner in middle-aged males. Involvement of the small intestine is almost invariable and leads to malabsorptive diarrhea, abdominal pain, and weight loss, but the clinical manifestations also include fever, lymphadenopathy, and arthritis.

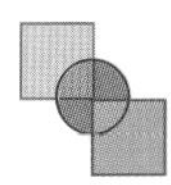

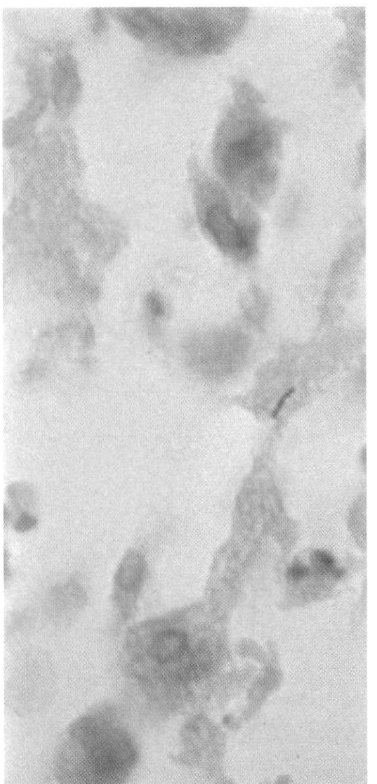

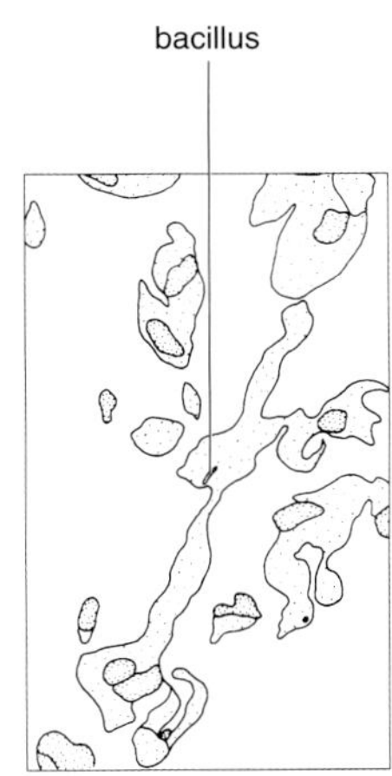

■ **Fig. 5.16** Ziehl–Neelsen stain showing an acid-fast mycobacterium (x 1200).

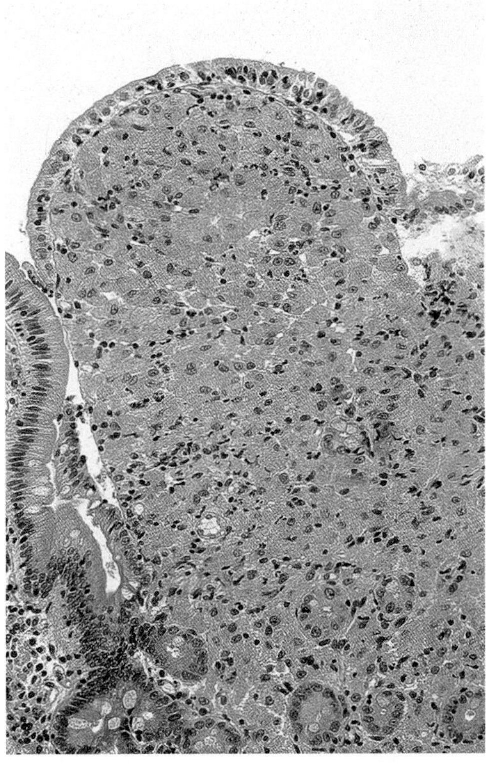

■ **Fig. 5.18** *Mycobacterium avium* complex (MAC) infection. Microscopic view of the small bowel mucosa in an AIDS patient showing large collections of macrophages with abundant pink cytoplasm in the lamina propria of the villi.

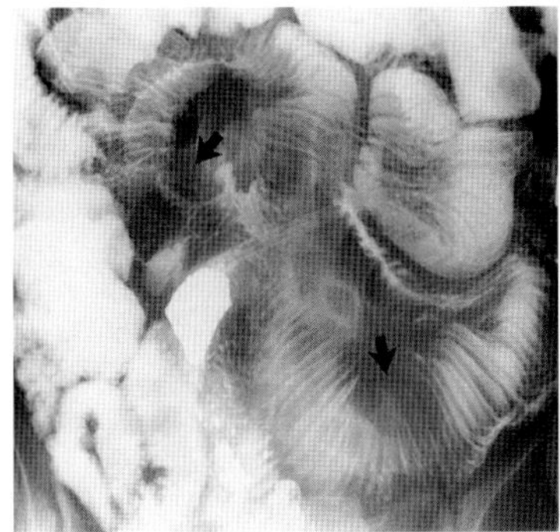

■ **Fig 5.17** Enteroclysis in patient with AIDS and peritonitis due to *Mycobacterium avium intracellulare*. Several smooth extrinsic mass impressions (arrows) are seen on the mesenteric border of the mid small bowel. The normal small bowel folds are tethered toward the mesentery. (Reproduced with permission from reference 3, Fig. 46.31.)

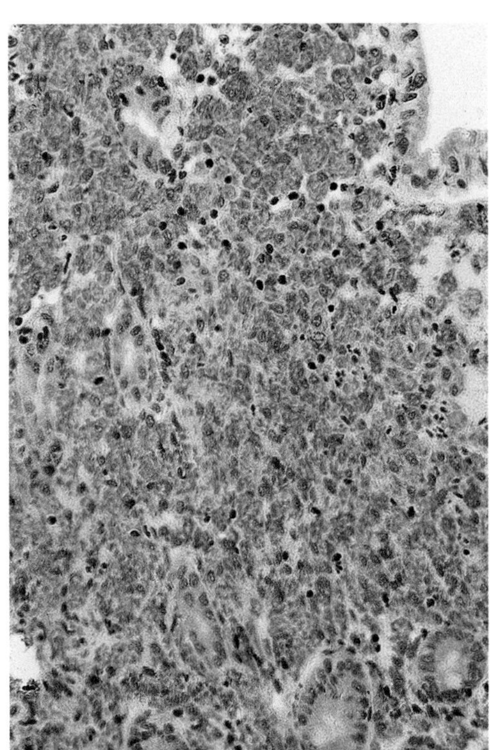

■ **Fig. 5.19** *Mycobacterium avium* complex (MAC) infection. Ziehl–Neelsen stain shows numerous long, acid-fast bacilli within the cytoplasm of the stromal macrophages.

Dermatological (Fig. 5.20), respiratory, cardiac, and neurological features can occur. Radiological examination usually reveals thickened mucosal folds, particularly in the duodenum and proximal jejunum (Fig. 5.21), and CT may indicate lymphadenopathy (Fig. 5.22). The differential diagnoses include sarcoid and a range of chronic infections including tuberculosis. Diagnosis of Whipple's usually comes initially from endoscopic small bowel biopsy which shows villous atrophy and vacuolation, but careful examination reveals characteristic PAS-staining of foamy macrophages and monocytes (Figs 5.23–5.25). Electron microscopy shows that there are rod-shaped bacilli within membrane-bound vesicles in the lamina propria, and it is the incorporation of these into lysosomal complexes that leads to the PAS positivity (Figs 5.26, 5.27). Molecular amplification techniques using polymerase chain reaction on other tissues and body fluids can also be diagnostic. The causative organism is *Tropheryma whipplei*, an actinomycete member of the Actinobacteria family, and the diagnosis should now be confirmed bacteriologically. Although the organisms disappear on vigorous antibiotic treatment, the cellular changes remain for many months (Fig. 5.28).

INTESTINAL WORMS

Ascariasis

Most cases of human ascariasis are caused by *Ascaris lumbricoides*. Infection with the pig roundworm *A. suum* occurs only occasionally. Most of the life cycle of both occurs within the small intestine (Fig. 5.29). An adult female ascarid may reach 30 cm in length and is capable of producing 200 000 eggs daily. Infection is most prevalent in areas of poor sanitation where human excrement is used as fertilizer; perhaps as much as 25% of the world's population is affected, but most are asymptomatic. Pulmonary symptoms may occur

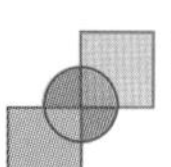

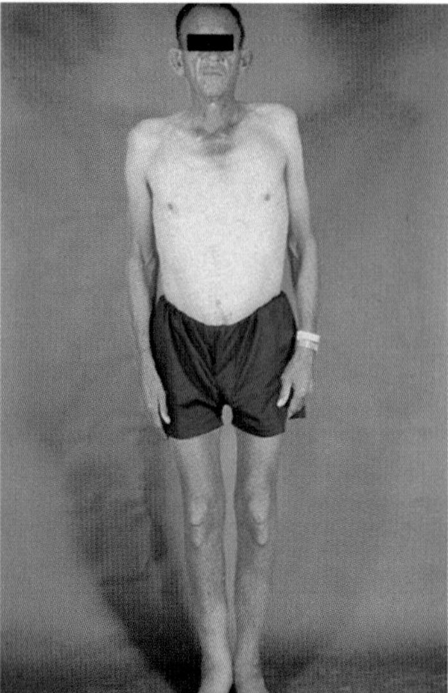

■ Fig. 5.20 A 53-year-old man with Whipple's disease, demonstrating increased pigmentation, wasting, abdominal distension, and peripheral edema from hypoalbuminemia. Both the pre-patellar nodules and the intestinal biopsy had the typical histology of the disease.

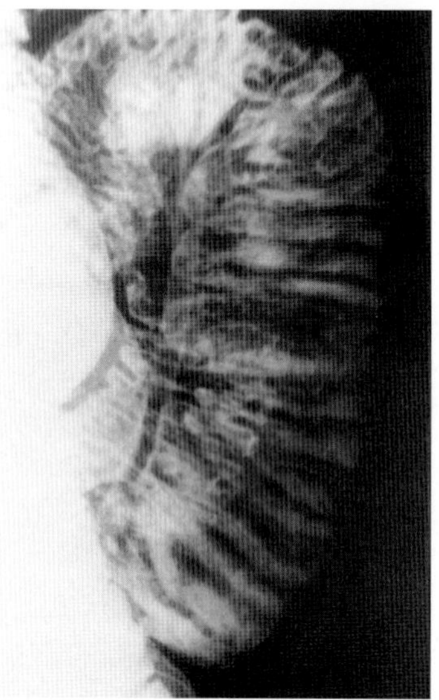

■ Fig. 5.21 Enteroclysis a in patient with Whipple's disease. Numerous tiny nodules disrupt the normally smooth surface of a loop of proximal jejunum. The nodules represent villi distended by macrophages. (Reproduced with permission from reference 1, Fig. 5.1C, courtesy of E. Salomonowitz, Vienna, Austria.)

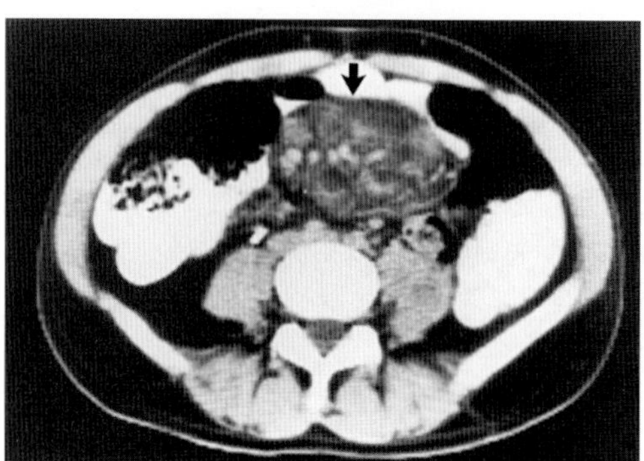

■ Fig. 5.22 CT in patient with Whipple's disease. Enlarged lymph nodes (arrow) of low attenuation expand the small bowel mesentery. The low attenuation is due to fat in the villi and stasis of lymph.

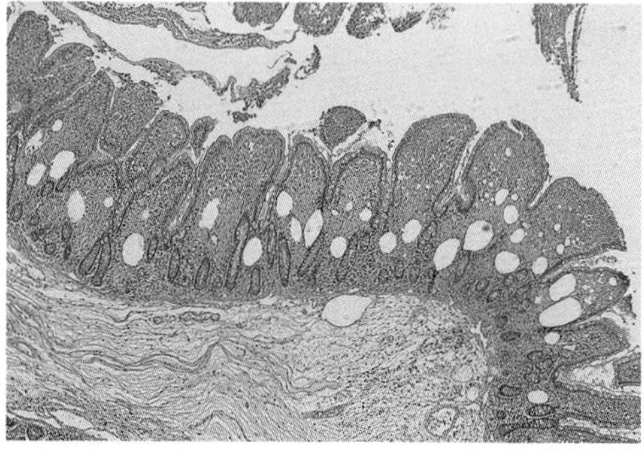

■ Fig. 5.23 Whipple's disease. Low-magnification appearance of the small intestine showing bulbous, blunted villi that are expanded with eosinophilic cells and show large lipid vacuoles (clear spaces) in the lamina propria due to lymphatic blockage.

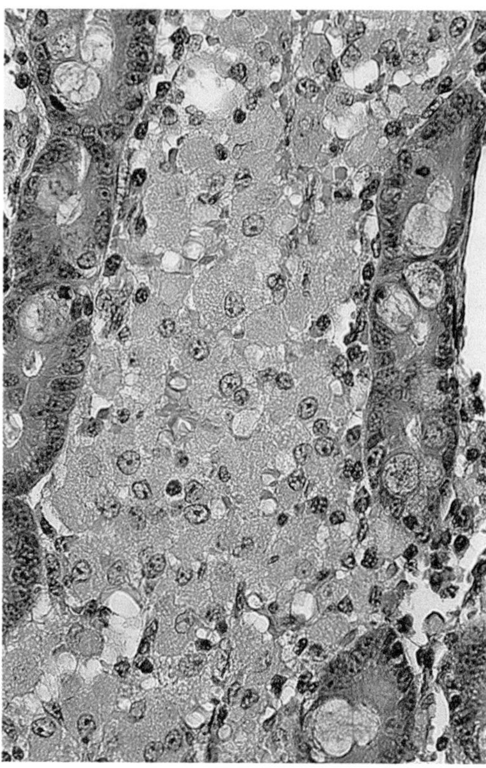

■ Fig. 5.24 Whipple's disease. High-magnification appearance of a villus showing a dense collection of stromal macrophages with eosinophilic granular cytoplasm.

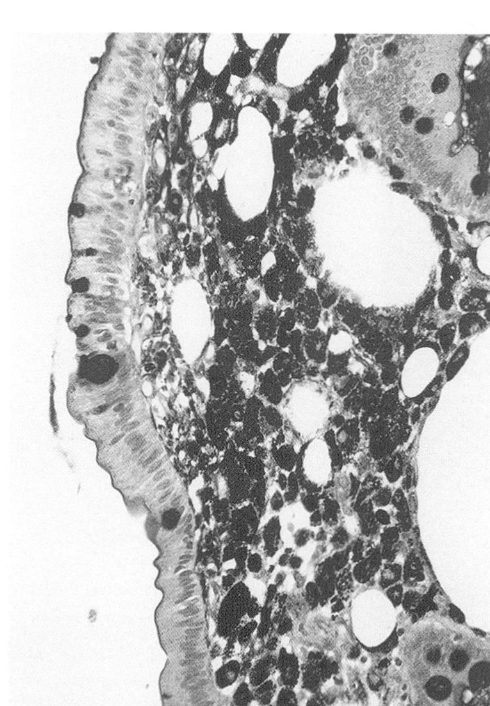

■ Fig. 5.25 Whipple's disease. A PAS stain demonstrating intense staining of the macrophage cytoplasmic granules that correspond to individual organisms *(Tropheryma whipplei)* visible on electron microscopy.

at the time of larval transpulmonary migration, other symptoms depending mainly on the parasite load and the general nutritional state of the patient. Ascariasis is generally very well tolerated with few symptoms, but contributes to malnutrition in the undernourished, and the sheer number of eggs excreted may represent a significant nitrogen loss to the host. Contrast studies of the bowel demonstrate adult worms within the lumen (Fig. 5.30), but the diagnosis is usually made from finding eggs or worms in the stools (Fig. 5.31). Intestinal obstruction from a bolus of adult worms (Fig. 5.32), and intestinal perforation are most unusual, but cholangitis or pancreatitis from migration of worms into the biliary tree (Fig. 5.33) are sometimes seen.

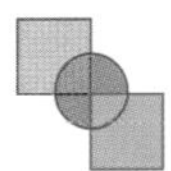

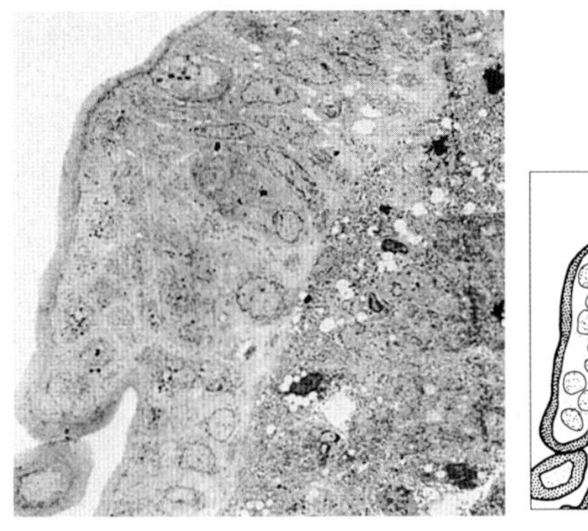

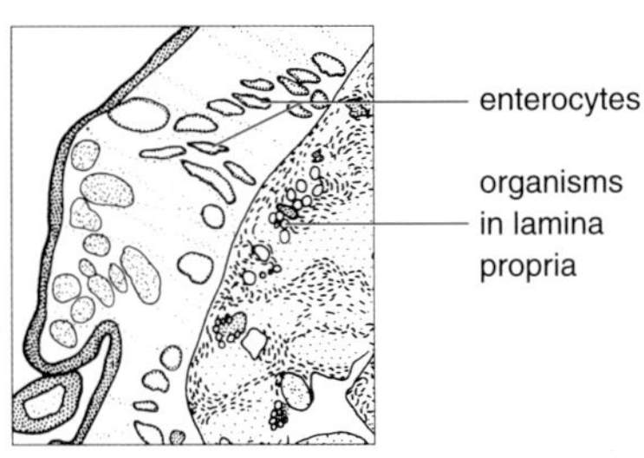

■ **Fig. 5.26** Electron micrograph of a small intestinal biopsy in Whipple's disease. Large numbers of rod-shaped organisms lie free in the lamina propria (x 700).

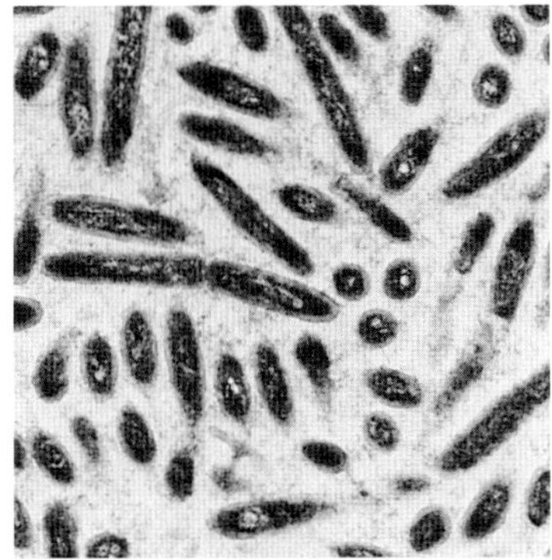

■ **Fig. 5.27** Individual organisms under high power (x 14 000).

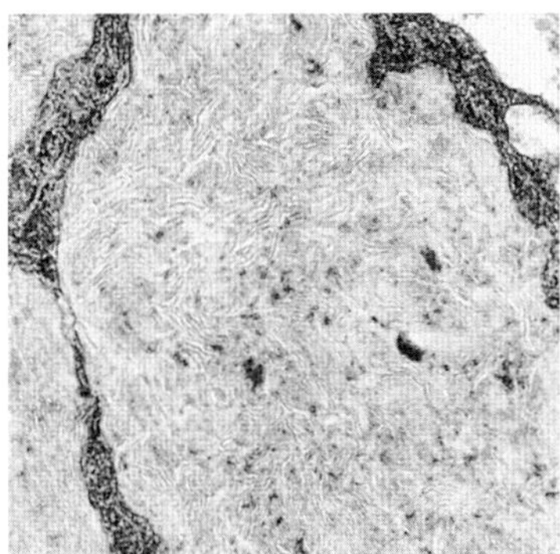

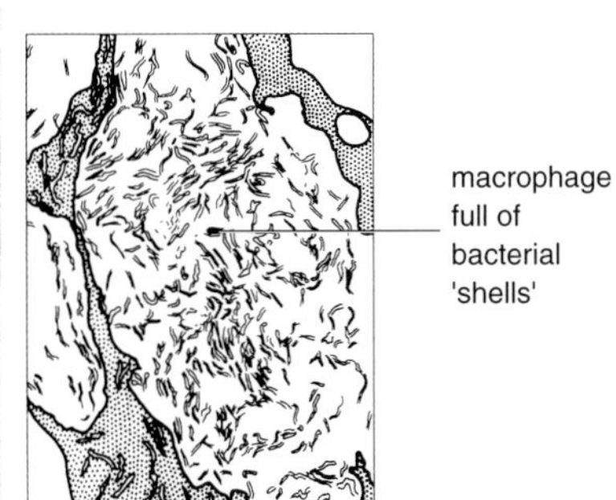

■ **Fig. 5.28** Macrophage containing the empty shells of bacteria; these cells persist long after the active disease state (x 4000).

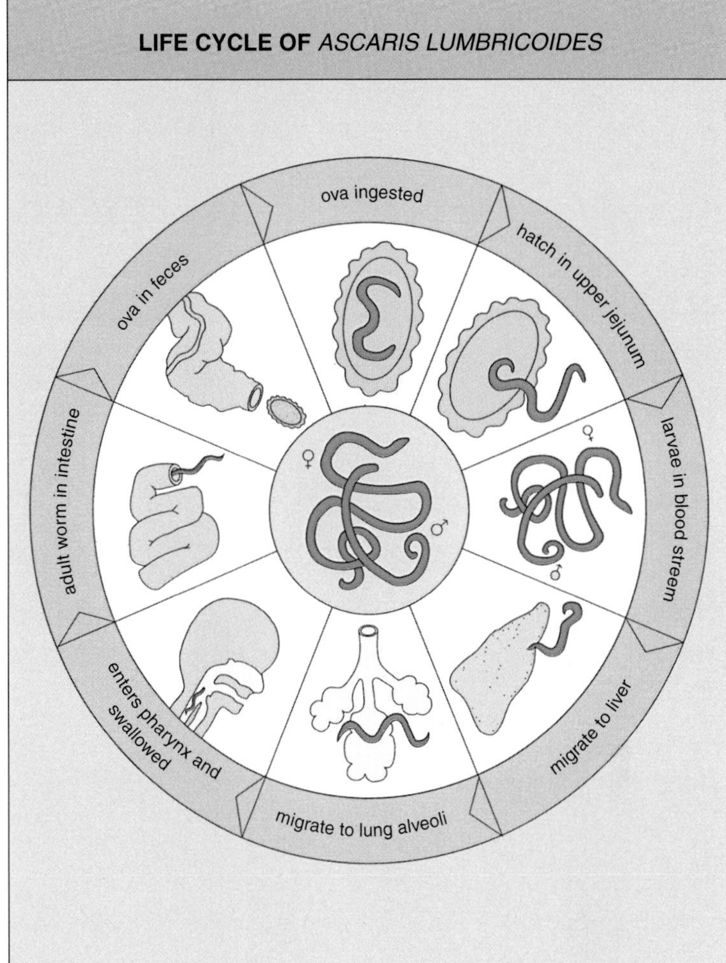

■ **Fig. 5.29** Life cycle of *Ascaris lumbricoides*. Transmission of ova from soil to man is by ingestion, with no vector. Larvae hatch in the small intestine and are carried via the blood to the liver, and thence to the lungs, trachea, throat, and esophagus, before returning to the intestine. Maturation to adult worms then occurs over 2–3 months. The adults live in the lumen for 12–18 months, and infection does not therefore persist in the absence of re-exposure. Eggs are passed in the feces when single celled, and they may then survive for many months if the temperature and humidity of soil are suitable. Courtesy of Dr J. Taverne.

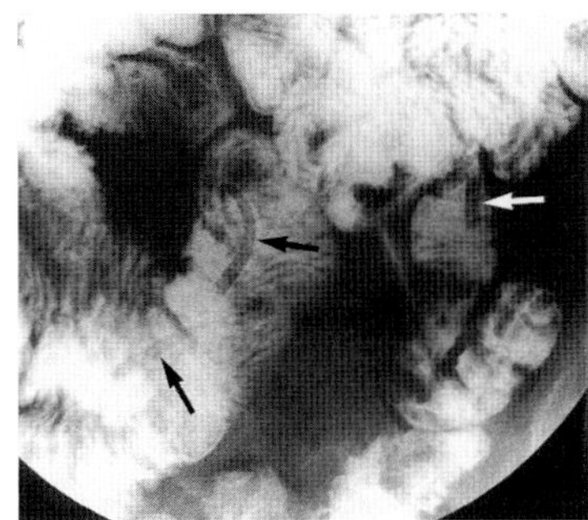

■ **Fig. 5.30** Small bowel follow-through demonstrating adult forms of *Ascaris* (arrows) in the pelvic ileum.

Hookworm

Around one quarter of the world's population is infested with one of the two soil-transmitted hookworms – usually *Ancylostoma duodenale* in Asia, and *Necator americanus* in the Americas (Fig. 5.34). *N. americanus* infects more successfully via the skin, and *A. duodenale* more so orally. Adult worms, which measure up to 15 mm in length, attach firmly to the upper intestinal mucosa (Fig. 5.35). Chronic iron deficiency is usual as each worm consumes around 0.3 ml of blood a day, but significant disease is usually seen only in those with a very high parasite load or when there is also another cause for anemia. Clinical features may include skin changes (where this is the portal of entry), pneumonitis from migration through the lungs, and non-specific upper gastrointestinal symptoms usually relieved by eating. Diagnosis depends on the demonstration of eggs in the stools (Fig. 5.36). Distinction between the two species is made from minor differences in the morphology of larvae grown from fecal smears.

Strongyloidiasis

Strongyloidiasis has a worldwide distribution but is of greatest prevalence in tropical areas. Human disease is usually caused by *Strongyloides stercoralis*. Contact with free-living filariform larvae permits their penetration of the skin or buccal mucosa, and subsequent carriage to the lungs, where the larvae rupture into the alveoli and develop into adolescent worms; these then migrate via the trachea and are swallowed. Males are not tissue parasites and are soon eliminated in the feces. Females, however, burrow into the mucosa of the small bowel (usually the jejunum) (Figs 5.37, 5.38). Symptoms

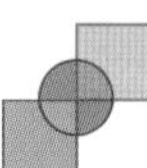

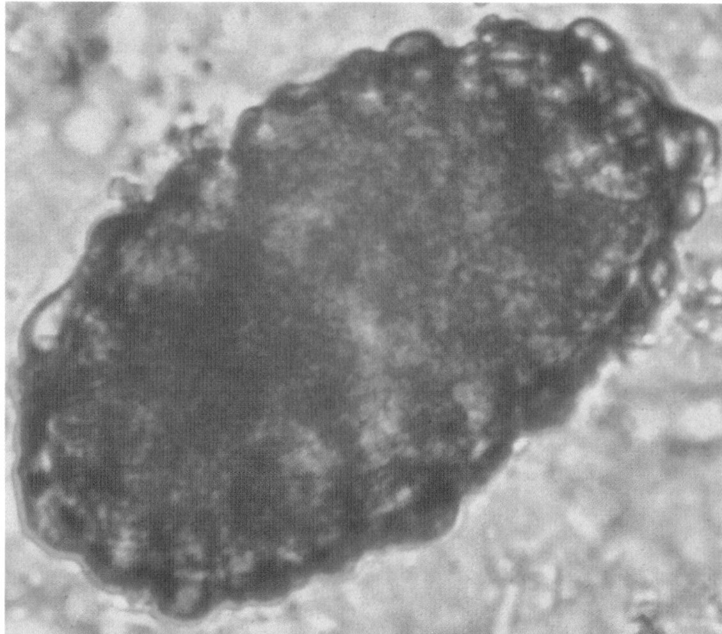

■ **Fig. 5.31** Unfertilized egg of *Ascaris lumbricoides* in a fecal smear. Courtesy of Dr T.W. Holbrook.

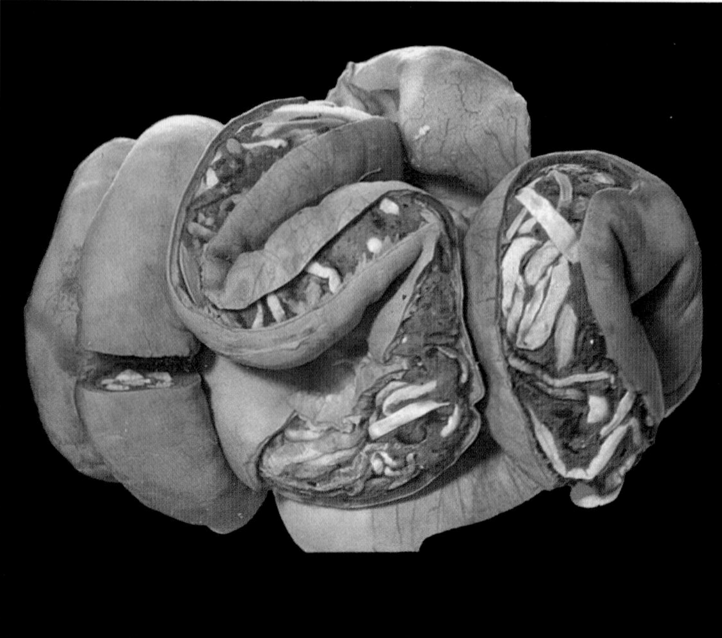

■ **Fig. 5.32** Bolus of *Ascaris* worms in the gut causing intestinal obstruction. Courtesy of Dr D.R. Davies.

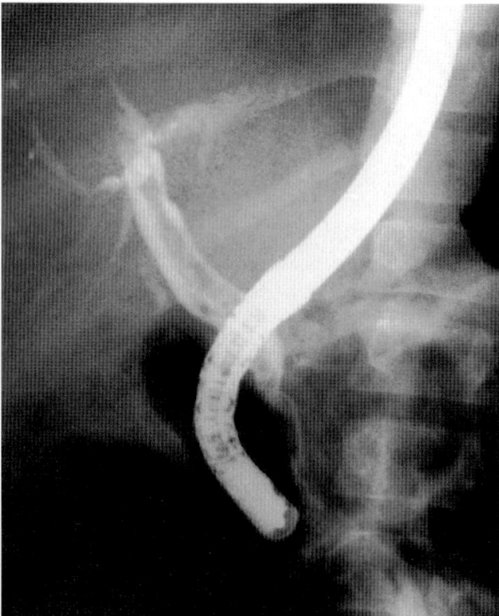

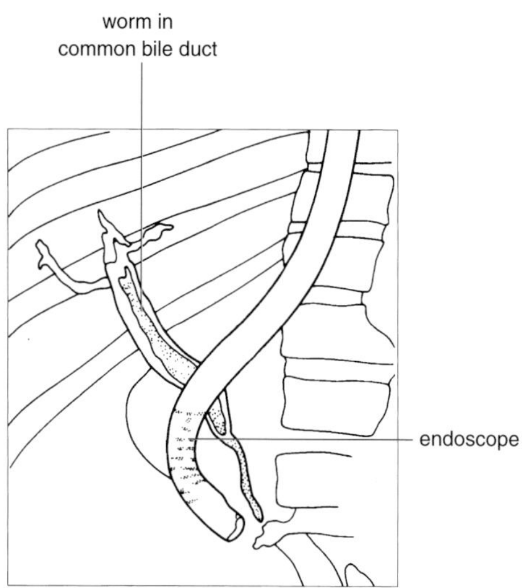

■ **Fig. 5.33** ERCP showing ascariasis affecting the common bile duct of a young African patient presenting with acute pancreatitis and cholangitis. Courtesy of Dr A. Hatfield.

include transient dermatological and pulmonary manifestations; only in severe infestations are there gastroenterological symptoms, but profuse diarrhea, which may be bloody or steatorrheic, can then occur. Auto-reinfection is frequent. Chronic asymptomatic infection may be reactivated by immunosuppression (including the therapeutic use of steroids), and this may be responsible for overwhelming anaphylactoid crisis. Diagnosis is usually established from finding larvae in duodenal secretions, this being more reliable than stool examination, as both eggs and larvae are usually absent.

Trichuriasis

Infection with the whipworm, *Trichuris trichiura*, is commonest in poor tropical countries, where it may affect 90% of the population, but probably around 1% of the US population is also affected. When stool-contaminated soil is ingested the fertilized eggs are digested by intestinal enzymes to release larvae in the small intestine. Adult worms are 3–5 cm in length and burrow into the mucosa of the cecum and proximal colon, extending to the terminal ileum (Fig. 5.39), and elsewhere in the colon in heavy infestations. Their popular name derives from their appearance, with thin, attenuated anterior, and thicker, handle-like, posterior portions. Most infestations are asymptomatic, but non-specific allergic symptoms such as urticaria are also seen. In heavy infestations, there is abdominal discomfort and diarrhea, which may be blood-stained. Diagnosis is readily made from the finding of characteristic barrel-shaped ova in the stools.

Enterobial infestation

Enterobius vermicularis (the thread- or pin-worm) infection is endemic worldwide, occurring most often in school-aged children. Unlike most other parasites it is more common in temperate than tropical climates. Poor personal hygiene and sexual transmission are implicated. Ingested ova hatch in the upper small bowel, and

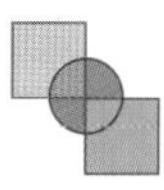

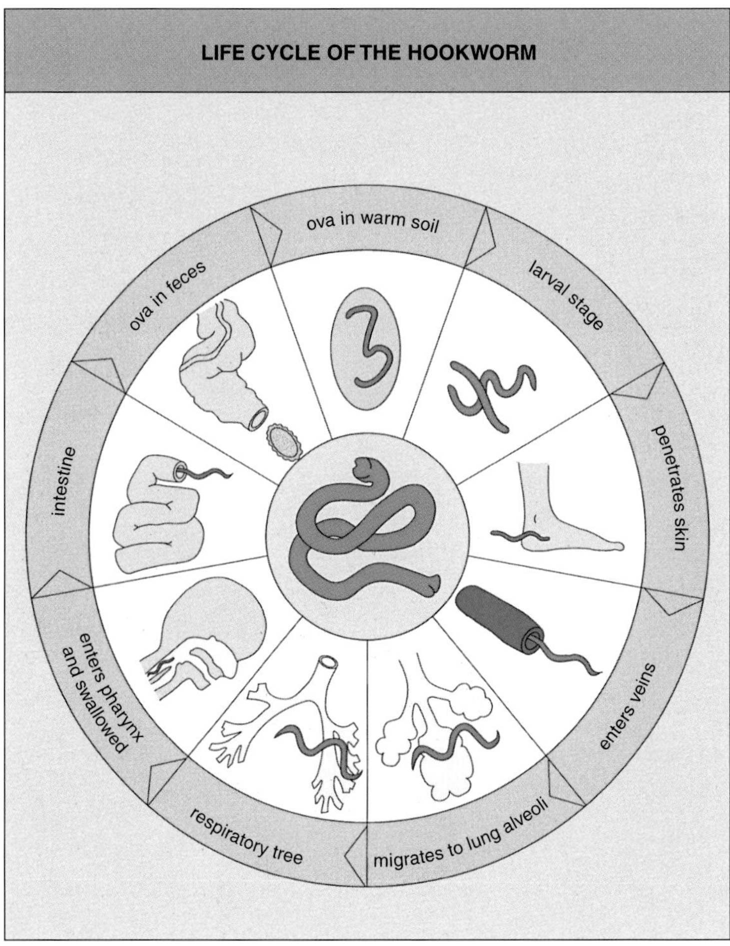

■ **Fig. 5.34** Life cycle of the hookworm. In moist soil, the ova develop into infective larvae that can penetrate the skin. They enter the bloodstream and are carried to the lungs from where they move via the trachea to be swallowed, maturing into adult worms in the small intestine. Adult females produce up to 10 000 eggs per day to be passed in the feces. Courtesy of Dr J. Taverne.

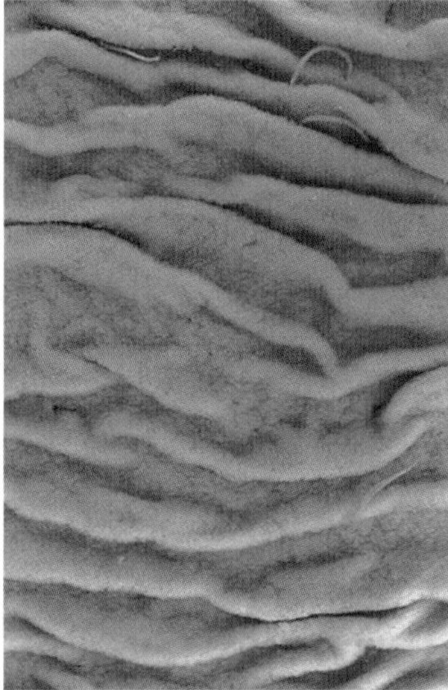

■ **Fig. 5.35** Short section of intestine infected with hookworm. Courtesy of Dr D.R. Davies.

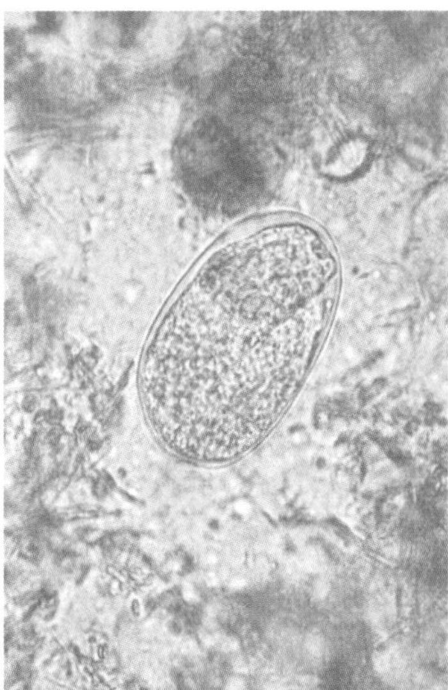

■ **Fig. 5.36** Fecal smear showing the egg of *Necator americanus*. Courtesy of Dr T.W. Holbrook.

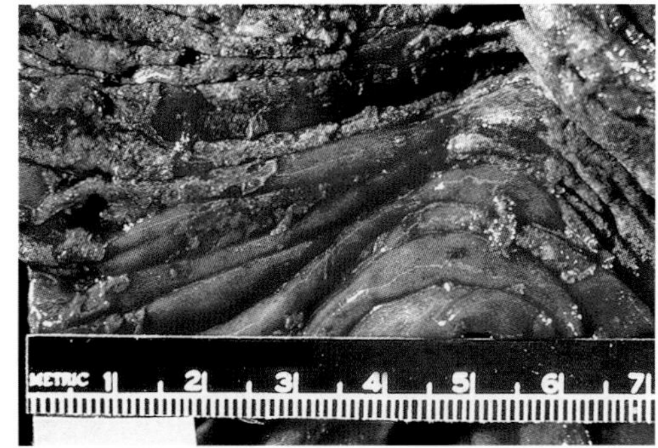

■ **Fig. 5.37** Strongyloidiasis. Segmental resection of small bowel with strongyloidiasis showing patchy mucosal ulceration with pseudomembranous exudate.

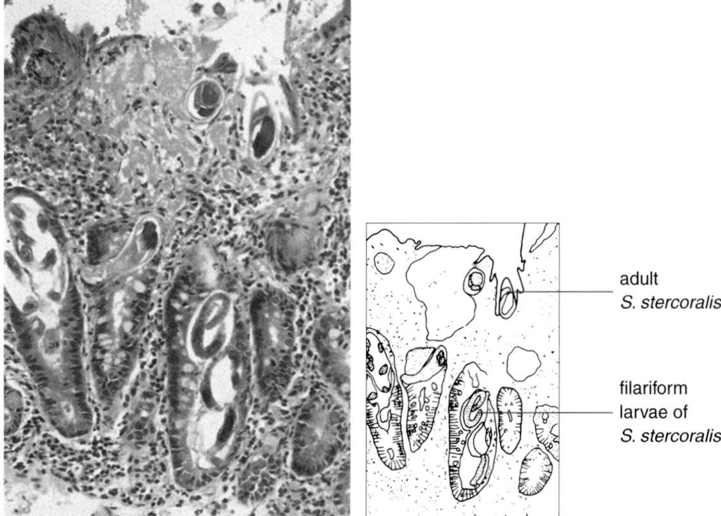

■ **Fig. 5.38** Strongyloides. Ulcerated jejunal mucosa showing adult and larval forms of *Strongyloides stercoralis*. No eggs are visible. H&E stain (x 120).

larvae mature during their passage to the colon (Fig. 5.40). An affected individual may be host to thousands of worms. There are usually no symptoms apart from intense pruritus around the anus. This occurs as the mature female (which lives for about 3 months) migrates to lay eggs (which have a sticky proteinaceous coat) in the perianal area, and has led to the use of the 'Sellotape test' in procuring eggs for microscopic diagnosis.

CESTODE INFESTATION

Taenia saginata

Humans are the only definitive hosts for this tapeworm, which inhabits the small intestine and can grow to more than 10 m in length (Fig. 5.41). Symptoms, however, are uncommon. Diagnosis usually comes from the detection of cestode segments (proglottids) or eggs in the stools. Infection follows ingestion of poorly cooked beef bearing the cystic stage of the parasite (cattle being the intermediate hosts) (Fig. 5.42), and is frequent where sanitation is poor.

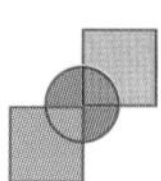

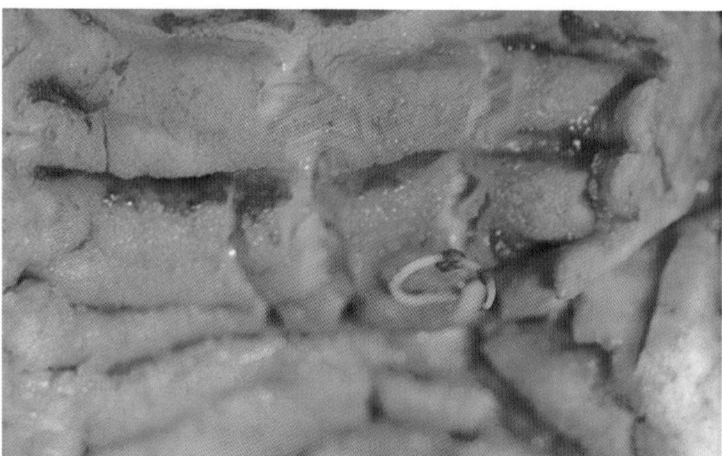

■ **Fig. 5.39** A whipworm *(Trichuris trichiura)* with its head buried in the ileal mucosa.

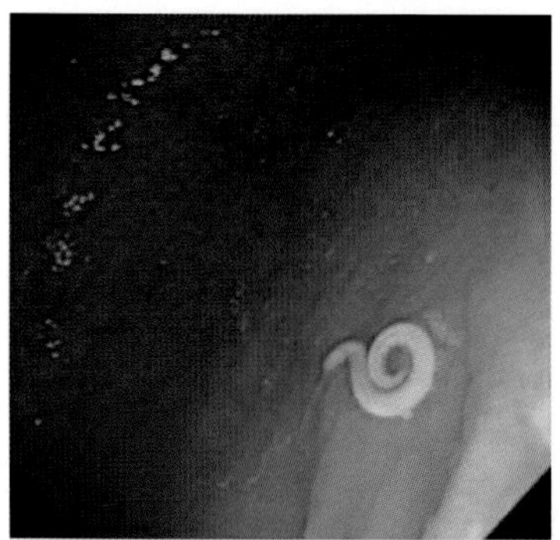

■ **Fig. 5.40** Colonoscopic view of adult *Enterobius vermicularis* in the cecum.

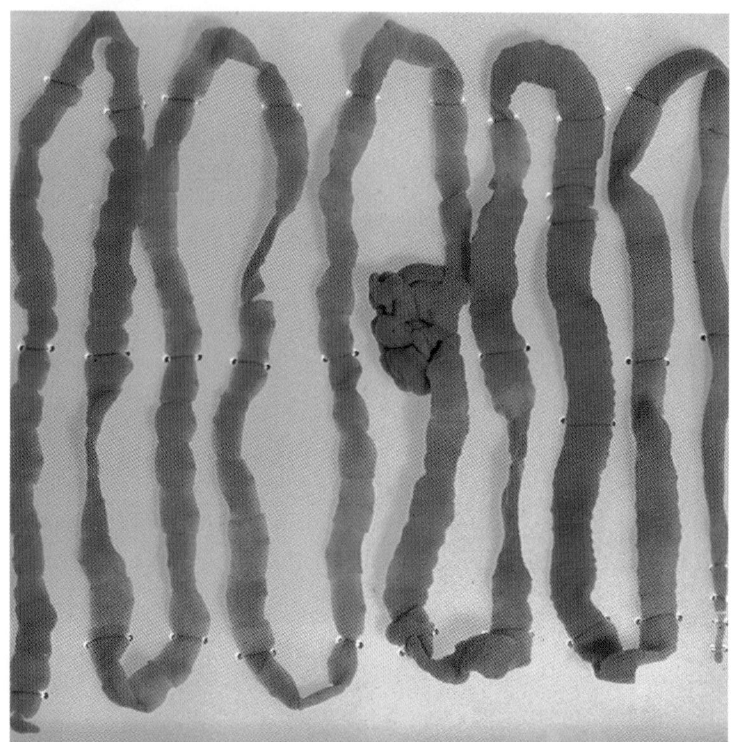

■ **Fig. 5.41** Beef tapeworm. Courtesy of Dr D.R. Davies.

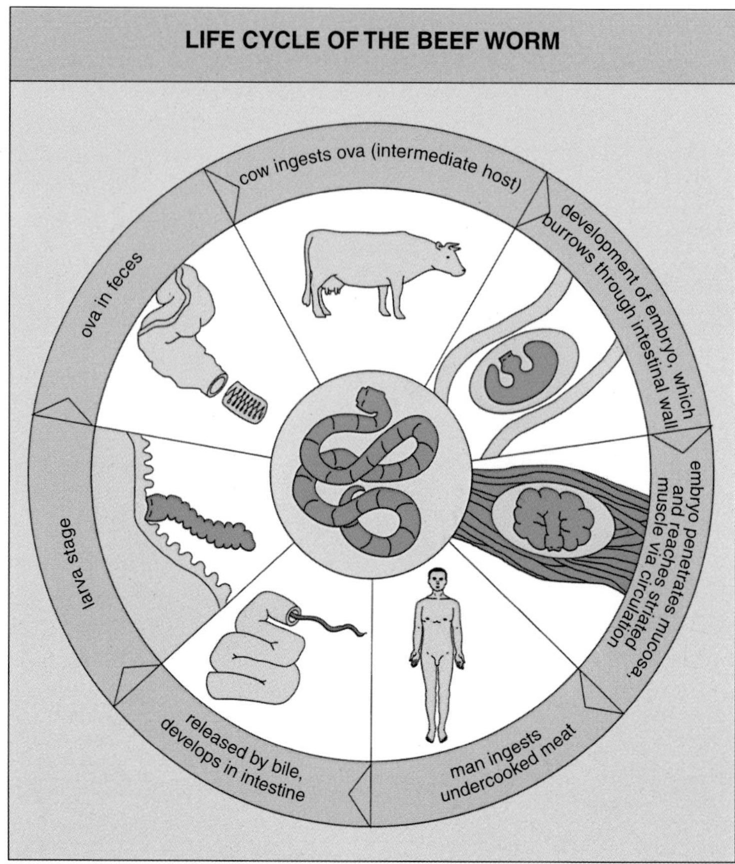

■ **Fig. 5.42** Life cycle of the beef tapeworm, *Taenia saginata*. Man becomes infected by eating undercooked, infected beef. The parasite is released by bile, enters the small intestine, and matures over 2–3 months into a long, segmented worm, attached to the intestinal wall by the suckers on its scolex. As segments of the tail mature, they are released into the lumen and are shed with the stools. Each segment contains thousands of eggs, which may then be swallowed by cattle, especially when human sewage is used as fertilizer. Swallowed eggs develop into oncospheres which then penetrate the bovine gut wall and enter the circulation, before developing in striated muscle into the cysticercus, the stage infective for man. Courtesy of Dr J. Taverne.

Although the eating of raw meat is especially risky, prior freezing of the meat is protective, as freezing generally kills cestodes. In the bowel lumen, bile salts trigger excystation, thereby releasing larvae, which develop into adult worms over approximately 8 weeks. Four muscular suction cups on the head, or scolex, attach the worm to the small intestinal mucosa, the rest of the body being divided into the proglottids. Eggs passed in the stool are largely harmless if ingested by man, but infect cattle, and only very rarely there is saginata cysticercosis analogous to the *T. solium* cysticercosis described below.

Taenia solium

Taenia solium, the pork tapeworm, shares many of its attributes with *Taenia saginata*, the intermediate host being, in this case, the pig, with infection from poorly cooked pork. If eggs are ingested by man, however, there is the additional risk that they rupture in response to gastric acid releasing oncospheres, which penetrate through the gastric wall and into the portal blood stream. These become cysticerci and can take up residence as damaging cysts in muscle, eyes, brain, and heart.

Diphyllobothrium latum

Diphyllobothrium latum infection is increasing because of the consumption of raw salmon (one of the intermediate hosts) in Japanese dishes such as sushi. Symptoms are rare unless the parasite's use of vitamin B_{12} causes megaloblastic anemia.

Hymenolepis nana

Hymenolepis nana (the dwarf tapeworm) affects rats and human children, in whom it is asymptomatic or responsible for intermittent

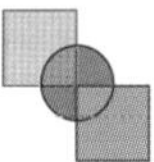

mild diarrhea. There is no intermediate host and auto-reinfection can occur.

Echinococcus

Man is the intermediate host for *Echinococcus* infection, and clinical disease is virtually confined to hydatid disease (see Chapter 11).

INTESTINAL PROTOZOAL INFECTION

Giardiasis

Giardiasis is caused by the flagellate protozoan *Giardia lamblia*. It is endemic in much of the world. Infection is spread by the feco-oral route, and epidemics are usually due to contamination of water by sewage. The trophozoites are pear-shaped disks that are pointed posteriorly and are about 15 mm long. The ventral surface is concave and carries a large adhesive organ anteriorly, with which it attaches to the enterocyte villous border (Figs 5.43, 5.44). Encystation occurs within the gut lumen, but then allows the organism to survive outside the host for some weeks. In symptomatic patients, the trophozoite form may be present in large numbers in the stools. Abdominal discomfort, borborygmi, and the passage of loose and sometimes steatorrheic stools are common. Diagnosis is confirmed serologically or by finding trophozoites or cysts in the stools; duodenal aspirates and biopsies are no longer necessary but will provide the diagnosis when less invasive investigation has been over-looked (Figs 5.45, 5.46). The villous histology is usually only slightly abnormal, but a subtotal villous atrophy may also occur. Chronic, intractable infection is a considerable problem in the immunosuppressed.

Cryptosporidiosis

Cryptosporidiosis is a self-limited diarrheal illness that occurs in the community setting, but which can often be a serious and chronic infection with uncontrollable watery diarrhea in the immunocompromised. This property led to its eventual recognition as a human pathogen in 1976. Outbreaks are usually associated with water-borne transmission, and a wide range of responsible species has now been identified, most of which are resistant to standard water chlorination methods. *C. parvum* is the commonest human pathogen. Ingestion of the cystic form of the organism is followed by luminal excystation and ileal invasion (Figs 5.47, 5.48). Methods for detecting this protozoan parasite in infected individuals and environmental samples

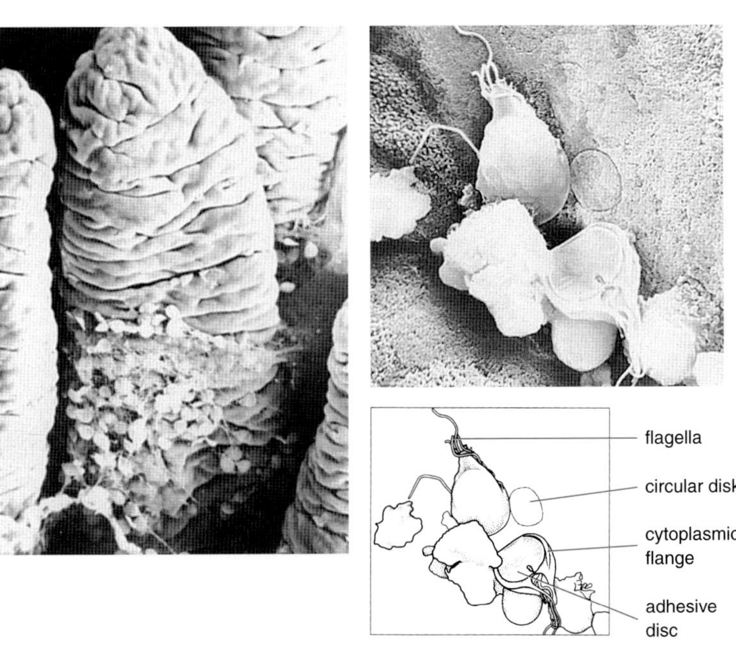

■ **Fig. 5.43** Electron micrograph showing villi of the mouse jejunum showing *Giardia* trophozoites adherent to the surface near the villous bases, wedged into furrows, and lying in mucus (x 2500). Courtesy of Dr R.L. Owen.

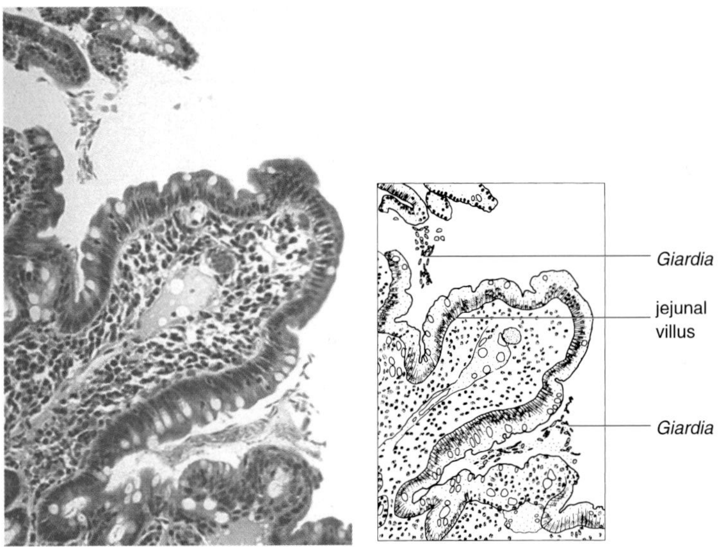

■ **Fig. 5.45** *Giardia* in a jejunal biopsy. It is important to look carefully at all material in a section since the organisms are easily obscured by debris. H&E stain (x 130).

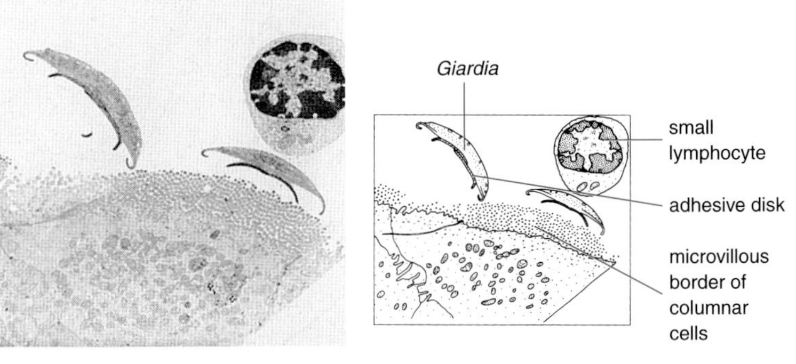

■ **Fig. 5.44** Electron micrographic study of *Giardia*. Dorsal and ventral aspects of trophozoites (a). The ventral surface exposes the adhesive disk, cytoplasmic flange and flagella. A circular adhesive disk is also seen adjacent to the adherent trophozoite (x 2200). Two *Giardia* (b) in sagittal section (and a small lymphocyte) above the microvillous border of columnar cells (x 2000). Courtesy of Dr R.L. Owen.

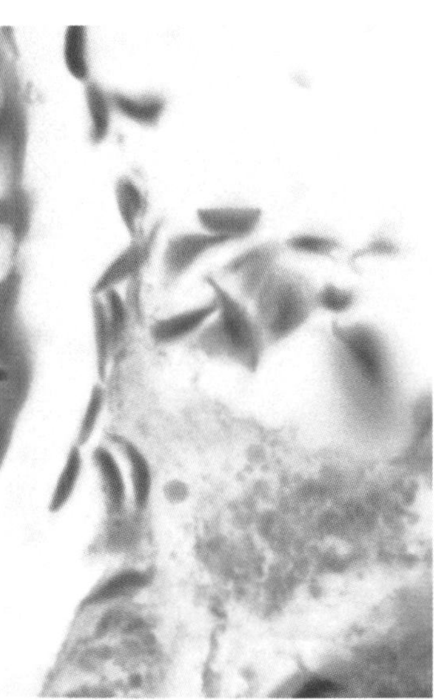

■ **Fig. 5.46** Higher power view of *Giardia* in a jejunal biopsy. H&E stain (x 860).

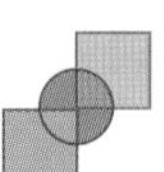

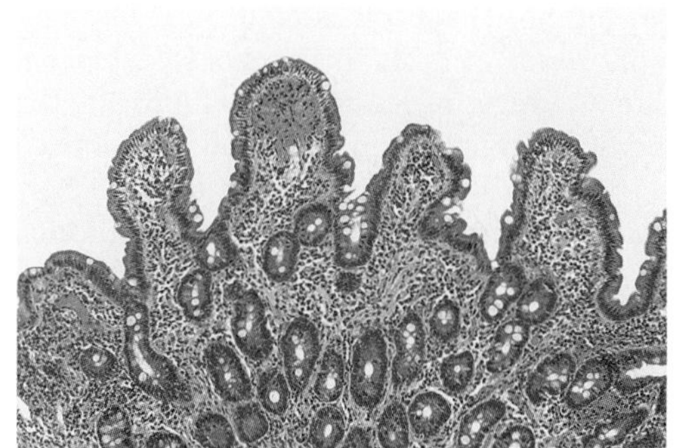

■ **Fig. 5.47** Small intestinal cryptosporidiosis. Microscopic view of the small intestinal mucosa in an AIDS patient with intestinal cryptosporidiosis showing mixed inflammatory infiltrates of the lamina propria and enterocyte injury (mild flattening and disarray) without ulceration.

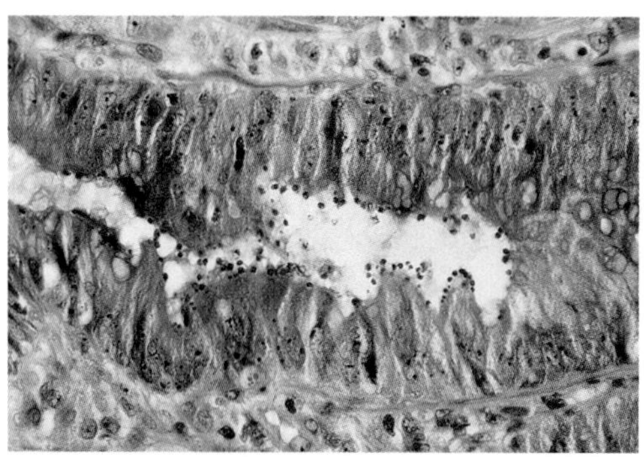

■ **Fig. 5.48** Small intestinal cryptosporidiosis. High-magnification view of a crypt studded with basophilic cryptosporidial sporozoites adherent to the enterocyte surfaces. The protozoans are shed in the stool and can be visualized on modified acid-fast stain.

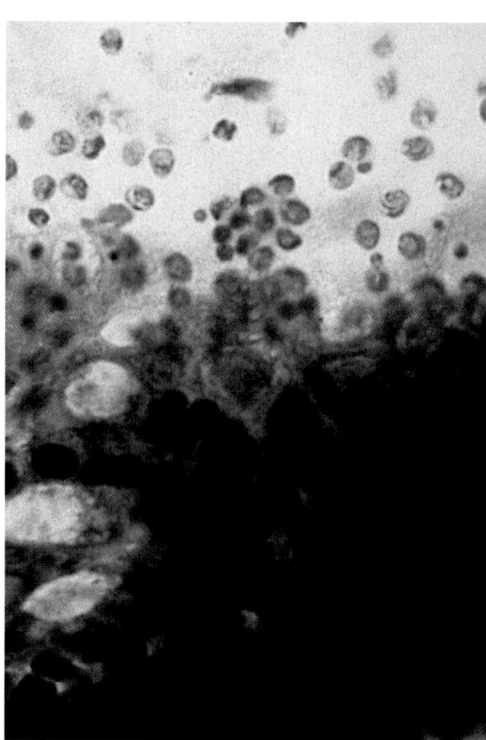

■ **Fig. 5.50** H&E stain demonstrating numerous cryptosporidia adherent to the duodenal brush border and free in the lumen, in a patient with HIV infection and profuse diarrhea (x 400). Courtesy of Dr S.A. Morse.

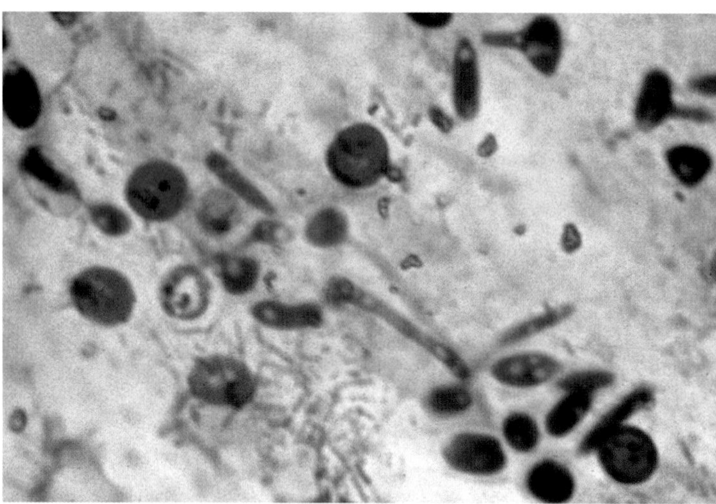

■ **Fig. 5.49** *Cryptosporidium parvum*, demonstrated by modified Ziehl–Neelsen staining of the stools; oocysts, which measure 4–6 mm, are acid fast (and therefore red), whereas yeasts and fecal material are not (x 1000). Courtesy of Dr S.A. Morse.

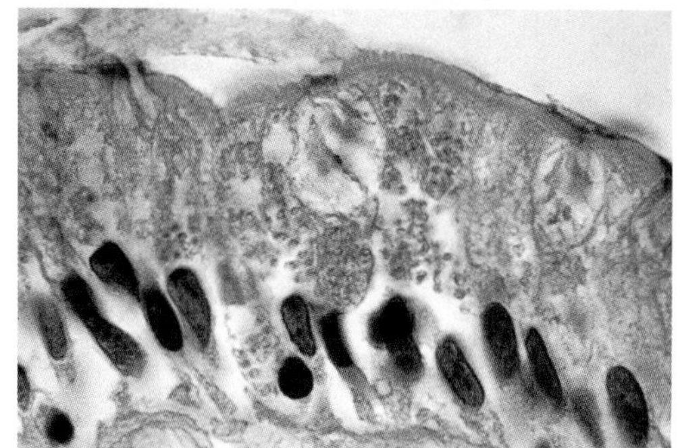

■ **Fig. 5.51** Small intestinal microsporidiosis. High-magnification view showing enterocytes at the tip of a villus containing clusters of minute, palely basophilic *Enterocytozoon bieneusi* spores in the supranuclear cytoplasm.

have progressed from technically demanding acid-fast staining of fecal smears (Fig. 5.49) or duodenal biopsies (Fig. 5.50) to identify oocysts, to antibody-based systems (enzyme immunoassays and immunofluorescent assays). Newer molecular methodologies based on PCR are being developed; each of the newer techniques is also able to identify cases in which few cysts are being excreted.

Microsporidiosis

Microsporidia are obligate intracellular protozoan parasites, and were rarely considered human pathogens until the late 1980s, when their association with chronic diarrhea in AIDS patients was recognized; they are responsible for diarrhea approximately as often as cryptosporidia. Most disease is due to *Enterocytozoon bieneusi* species. Although techniques for detection of spores in the stool exist, diagnosis is usually from histological examination of biopsies (Fig. 5.51). The experienced pathologist now rarely misses microsporidia on H&E stains, despite earlier suggestions that electron microscopy was necessary (Fig. 5.52); calcofluor fluorescent stains may also be used.

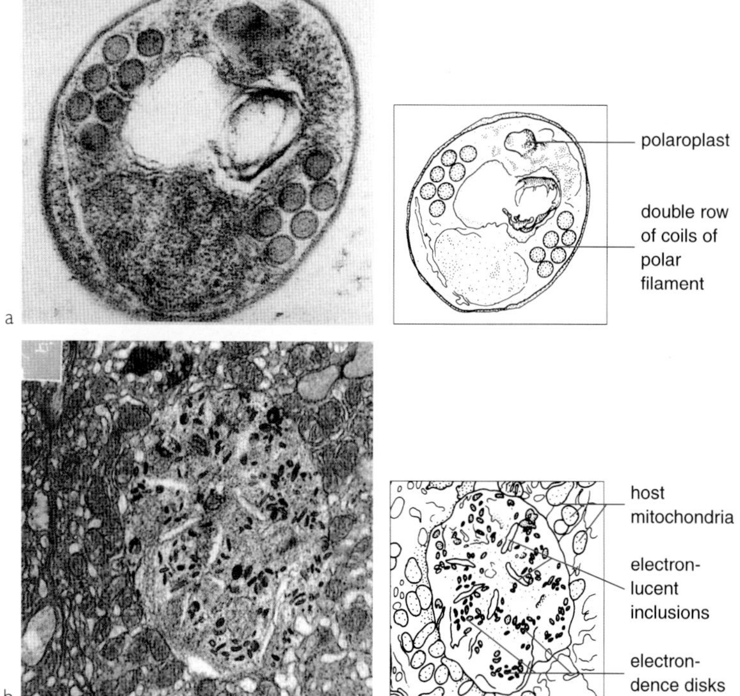

■ **Fig. 5.52** Spore of *Enterocytozoon bieneusi* demonstrated at EM (x 50 000) (a); and EM appearance of *Enterocytozoon bieneusi* – microsporidial sporont in direct contact with the host cell cytoplasm and surrounded by host mitochondria (x 50 000) (b). Courtesy of Dr C. Blanshard.

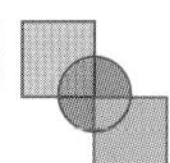

TROPICAL SPRUE

Tropical sprue is a malabsorptive condition characterized by anorexia, weight loss, and diarrhea. If untreated, it may resolve spontaneously or progress inexorably to profound emaciation with hypoalbuminemia, and deficiencies of folic acid, vitamin B_{12}, and calcium. The disorder occurs amongst natives of the tropics, but is more commonly seen in visitors from temperate climates (Fig. 5.53), particularly in those returning home after living in an endemic area for a year or more. In children it can result in severe growth retardation. All forms are less common than in previous decades. The most common cause is intestinal infection, especially by protozoa which target the small intestine, such as *Giardia intestinalis*, *Cryptosporidium parvum*, *Isospora belli*, *Cyclospora cayetanensis*, and the microsporidia. In a proportion, the pathogenesis remains unknown, but in these too there may be a response to broad-spectrum antibiotics. The radiological features are relatively non-specific (Fig. 5.54). The histological changes in the small intestine vary from mild epithelial damage with increased intraepithelial lymphocytes, to moderate but incomplete villous atrophy (Figs 5.55, 5.56). It is distinguished from gluten-sensitive enteropathy by its lesser severity, by the absence of subtotal villous atrophy, and its generally rather more patchy involvement of the proximal small bowel.

CROHN'S DISEASE

An infective etiology for Crohn's disease was postulated from the time of its initial description in the early part of the last century, but proof for this has not emerged. There is however confirmation of an unequivocal genetic association between some forms of the disease and mutations in the *CARD15* gene. The function of *CARD15* is not yet certain but it has the capacity to modulate the response of the cell to bacteria. It now seems most probable that Crohn's arises from an aberrant response to essentially normal gut flora in the genetically predisposed individual.

Crohn's disease is a chronic inflammatory condition which may affect any part of the gastrointestinal tract. It most commonly occurs in the ileocecal region, small bowel, and colon. The disease was seen mainly in Western populations, but is now increasingly prevalent in Japan and the industrialized Far East, and its annual incidence is increasing (already >4 per 100 000 in northern Europe). It tends to present in the second and third decades of life, but no age is exempt.

Despite its genetic linkage it is clear that Crohn's disease is not a single homogeneous entity, and it is accordingly classified according to its anatomical site, extent (diffuse or localized), its behavior (primarily fibrostenotic, inflammatory, or penetrating), and as to

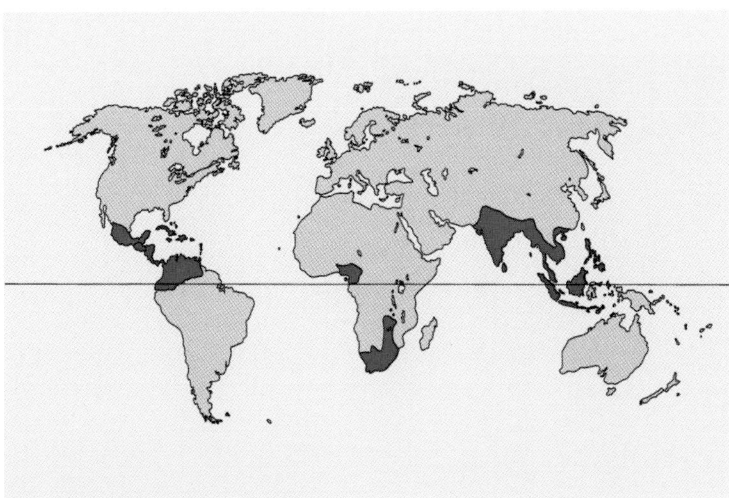

Fig. 5.53 Map showing the distribution of tropical sprue and disorders resembling sprue.

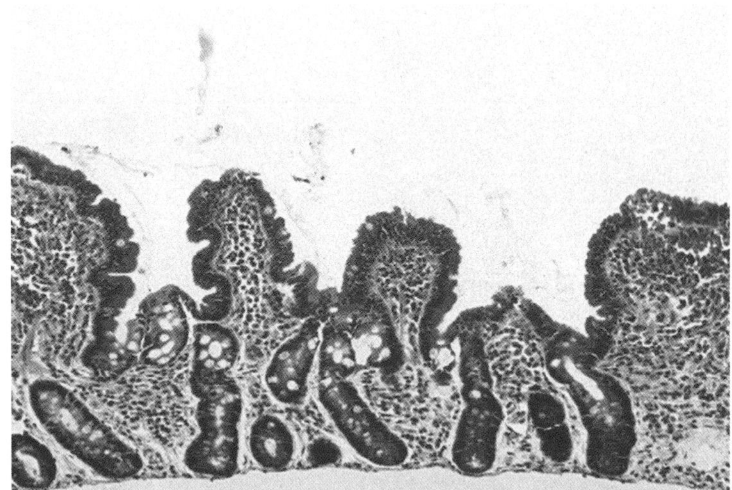

Fig. 5.55 Tropical sprue. The jejunal biopsy shows moderate, partial villous atrophy, with squat villi and a villus-height to crypt-depth ratio approaching unity. H&E stain (x 70).

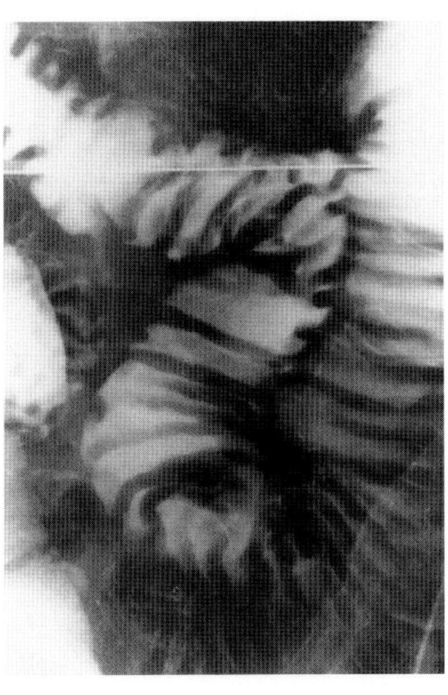

Fig. 5.54 Small bowel enema in patient with tropical sprue. There are smooth, thick folds in the proximal jejunum.

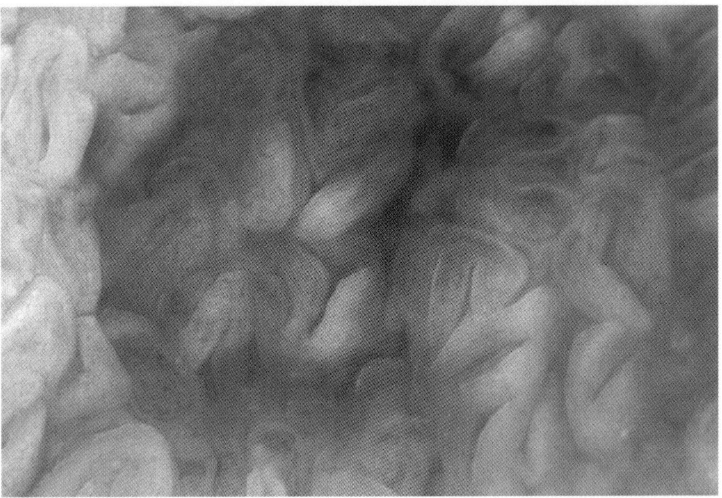

Fig. 5.56 Dissecting microscope appearance in the partial villous atrophy of tropical sprue. A pattern of convolutions and ridges is clearly abnormal.

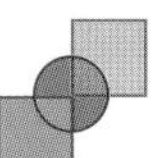

whether the patient has required surgery for Crohn's. The age of the patient is also crucial, since growth failure (which may be the only feature) is so important in children (Fig. 5.57). Small bowel disease is usually responsible for abdominal pain and diarrhea without overt blood loss, and may present with frank malabsorption with iron-, folate-, or vitamin B_{12}-deficient anemia, hypoalbuminemic edema and clubbing (Fig. 5.58). Pyrexia and weight loss are common. Inflammatory edema and the formation of fibrous strictures may cause obstruction. Roughly speaking, one third of patients have ileal disease, one third colonic, and one third both – with perianal disease in 15–20% of the total. A tender mass may be palpable in the right iliac fossa. Occasionally an acute presentation mimicking acute appendicitis or *Yersinia* ileitis occurs (see above).

To retain the anatomical organization of this Atlas, features of Crohn's disease peculiar to the colon and anorectal areas are considered in Chapters 6 and 8.

Crohn's disease runs an unpredictable course, with spontaneous remissions and relapses. Active disease may be associated with a number of extraintestinal lesions such as oral aphthous ulceration (Fig. 5.59), erythema nodosum (Fig. 5.60), pyoderma gangrenosum (see Chapter 6), iritis (Fig. 5.61), and episcleritis. Non-specific arthropathy affects as many as one third of patients, and about half

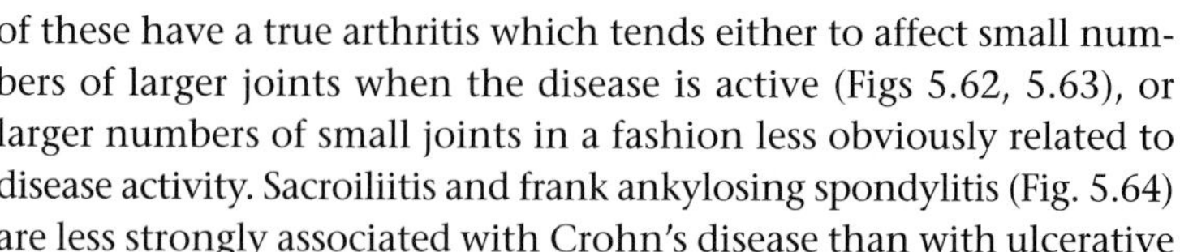

of these have a true arthritis which tends either to affect small numbers of larger joints when the disease is active (Figs 5.62, 5.63), or larger numbers of small joints in a fashion less obviously related to disease activity. Sacroiliitis and frank ankylosing spondylitis (Fig. 5.64) are less strongly associated with Crohn's disease than with ulcerative

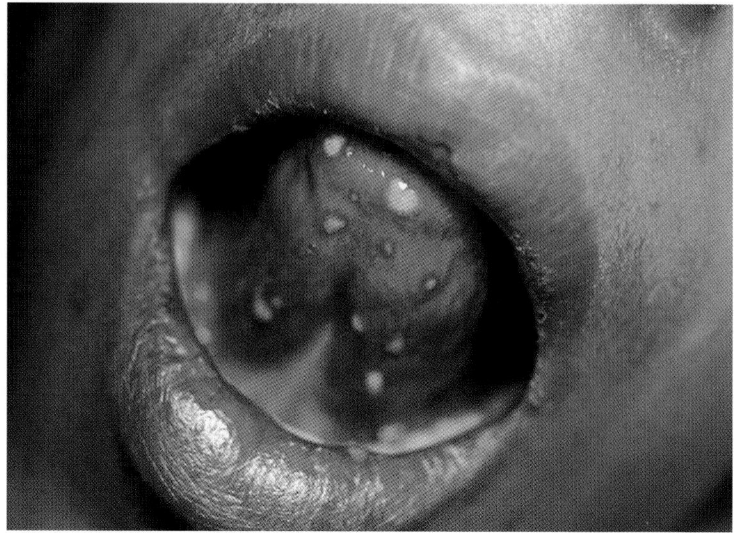

■ **Fig. 5.59** Oral aphthous ulceration in Crohn's disease.

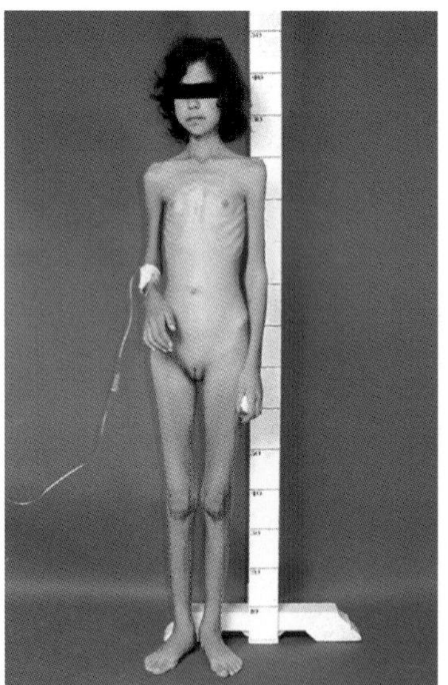

■ **Fig. 5.57** Growth failure in Crohn's disease. This 15-year-old girl had a 3-month history of diarrhea, and had height and weight both below the 3rd percentile. Secondary sexual characteristics are absent and the bone age was only 10.

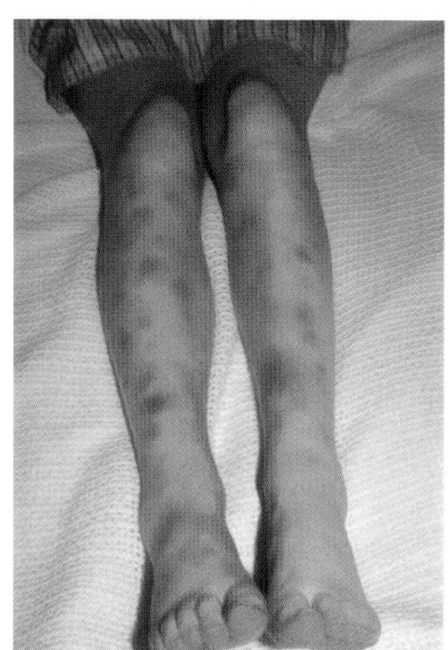

■ **Fig. 5.60** Erythema nodosum. Courtesy of Dr A. Bamji.

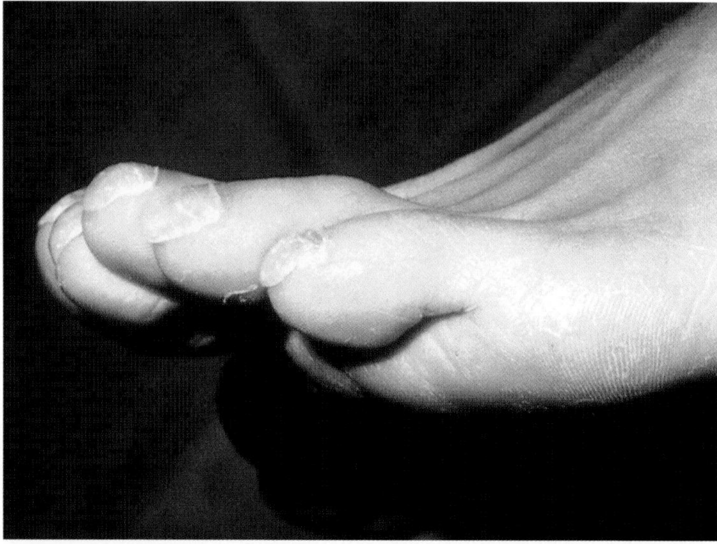

■ **Fig. 5.58** Clubbing of the toes in Crohn's disease.

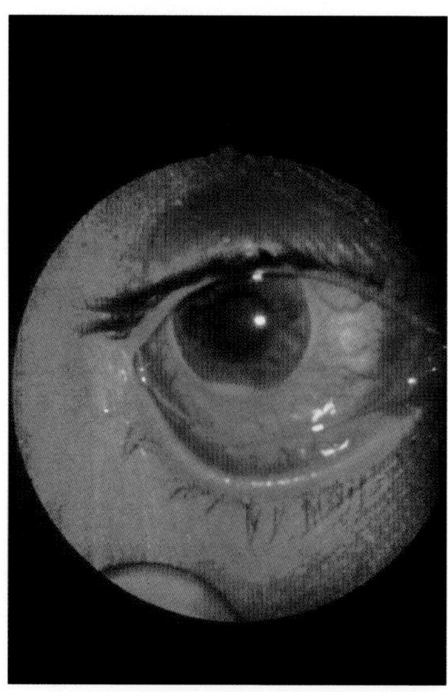

■ **Fig. 5.61** Iritis in Crohn's disease; in this case there is considerable conjunctival injection and hypopyon. Courtesy of Dr I Haslock.

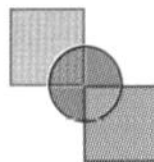

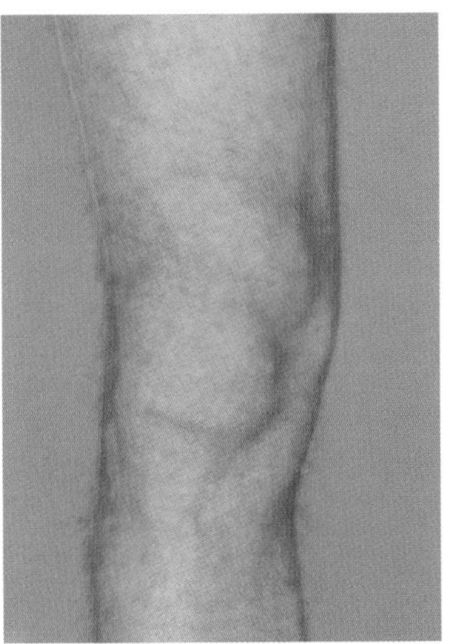

■ **Fig. 5.62** Arthropathy of the knee showing an effusion in the suprapatellar pouch. Courtesy of Dr P. Dieppe.

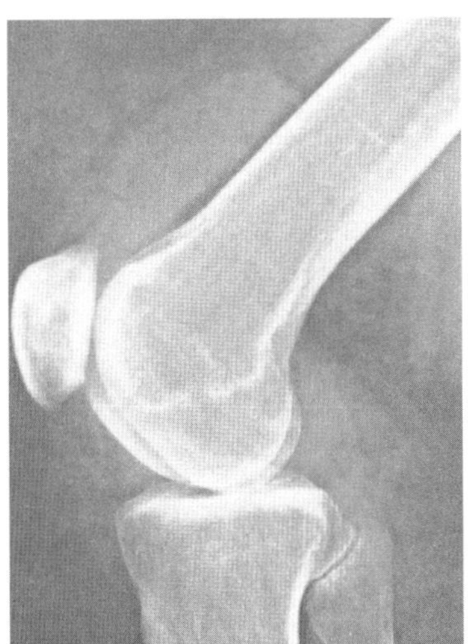

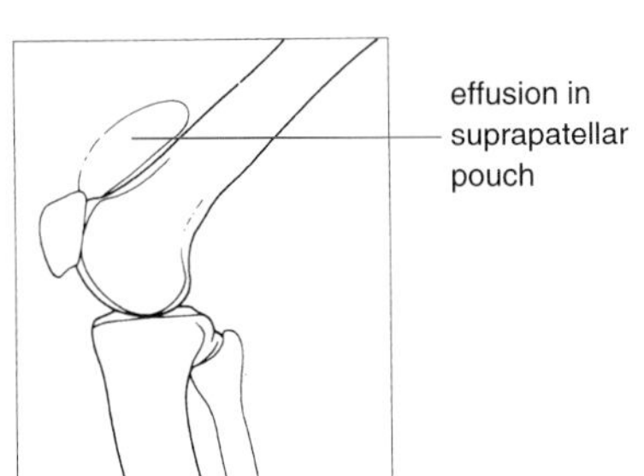

■ **Fig. 5.63** Radiological appearance of the same knee as in Fig. 5.58. Courtesy of Dr P. Dieppe.

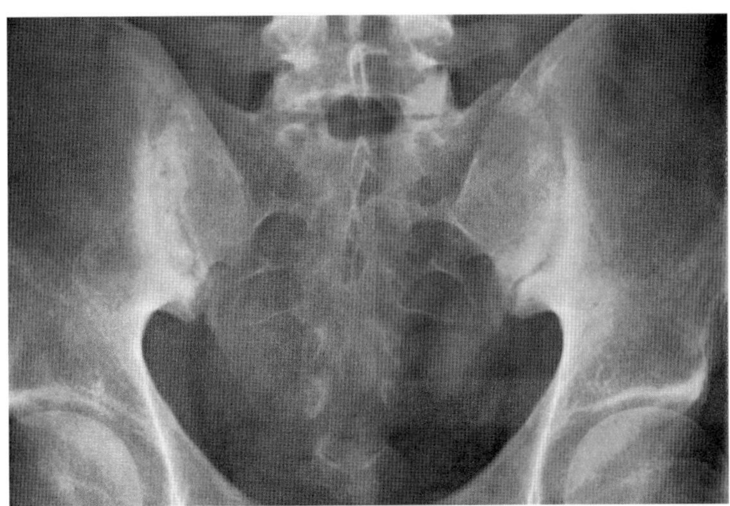

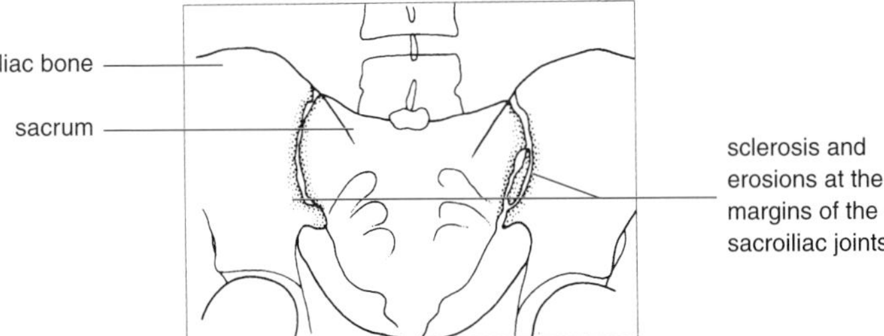

■ **Fig. 5.64** Pelvic radiograph showing bilateral sacral iliitis in Crohn's disease. The lumbar spine was normal and there was no evidence of ankylosing spondylitis.

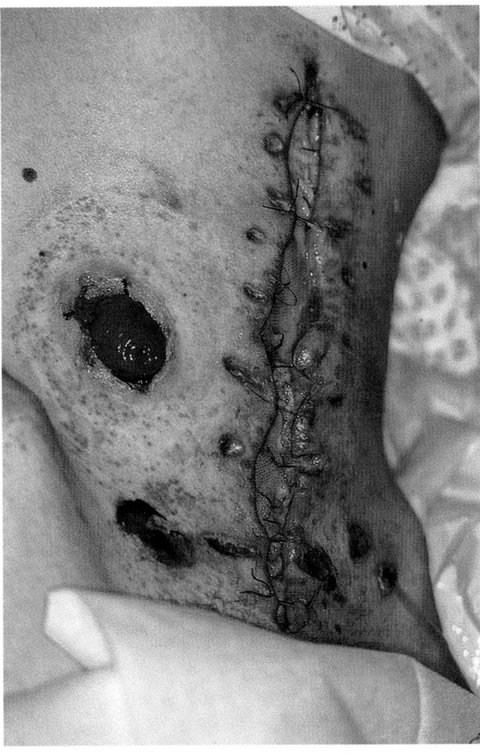

■ **Fig. 5.65** Appearances of post-operative enterocutaneous fistulae in Crohn's disease. The surgical wound has partially broken down and in addition to fistulous drainage via the main wound there are four fistulae from the lower part of the abdomen at the sites of previous surgical drains (the stoma is healthy).

colitis (see Chapter 6) but also occur in excess. Fistulae in Crohn's disease usually occur after surgery, but are sometimes seen spontaneously. Enterocutaneous fistulae, in particular, rarely occur other than through a previous operative scar (Fig 5.65). Internal fistulae may involve any combination of small or large bowel with themselves or each other, the bladder, or the vagina. Perianal fistulae are considered in Chapter 8. Although active medical therapy with azathioprine or infliximab may be sufficient, many fistulae still require resectional surgery.

In ileal disease, failure of reabsorption of bile salts results in a more lithogenic bile and a predisposition to cholesterol gallstones. Oxalate renal stones are also seen at greatly increased frequency as a result of preferential complexing of calcium with malabsorbed fatty acids in the intestinal lumen which allows excessive free oxalate absorption by the colon (see Chapter 6).

Radiological techniques remain the mainstay for investigation of the small bowel in Crohn's disease, but visualization of the mucosa of the terminal ileum at colonoscopy and, more recently, per-oral enteroscopy have challenged this to some extent (Figs 5.66, 5.67). The endoscopy capsule is also beginning to be used in the assessment of Crohn's disease (Fig 5.68), but this is not without considerable hazard should the capsule become lodged above a previously unsuspected stricture.

There is no single radiological sign pathognomonic of Crohn's, individual changes being seen in other inflammatory conditions such as intestinal tuberculosis or yersiniosis (see above). The diagnosis therefore rests on a combination of radiological features and their distribution, taken together with clinical, laboratory, and histological findings. Ultrasound scanning may reveal characteristic thickening of the bowel wall and alterations in the normal lamellar echo pattern (Fig. 5.69). It is also possible to identify areas of stenosis and upstream dilatation. It has been a relatively neglected investigation

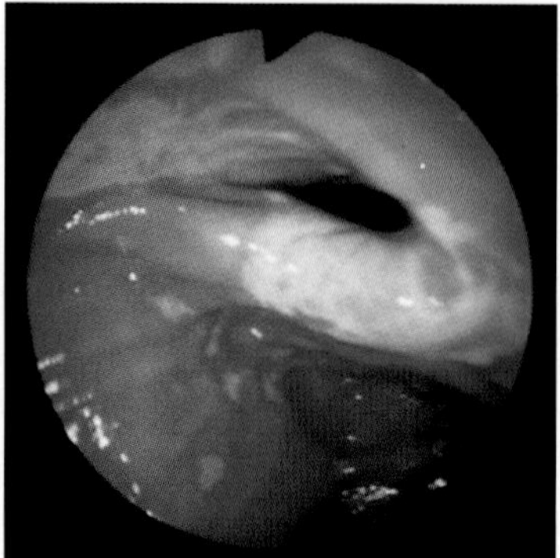

■ **Fig. 5.66** Appearance of terminal ileal Crohn's disease at colonoscopic ileoscopy.

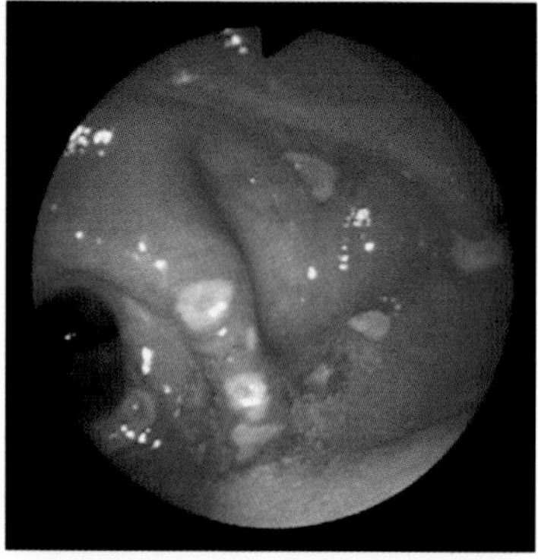

■ **Fig. 5.67** Crohn's disease recurrent after previous resection, affecting the neoterminal ileum.

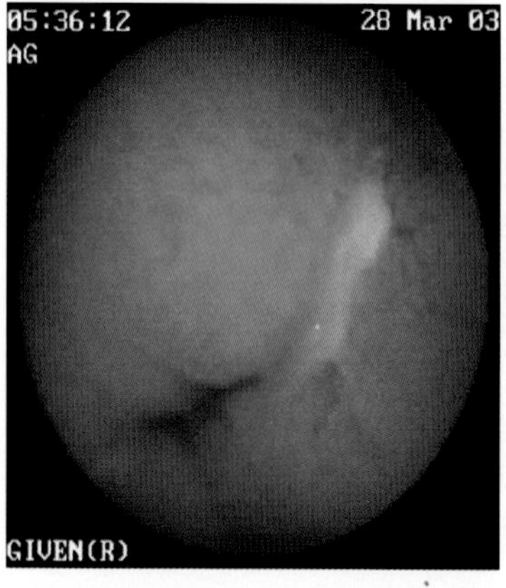

■ **Fig. 5.68** Crohn's ulcer in the jejunum demonstrated by capsule enteroscopy. Courtesy of Dr N. Kalantzis.

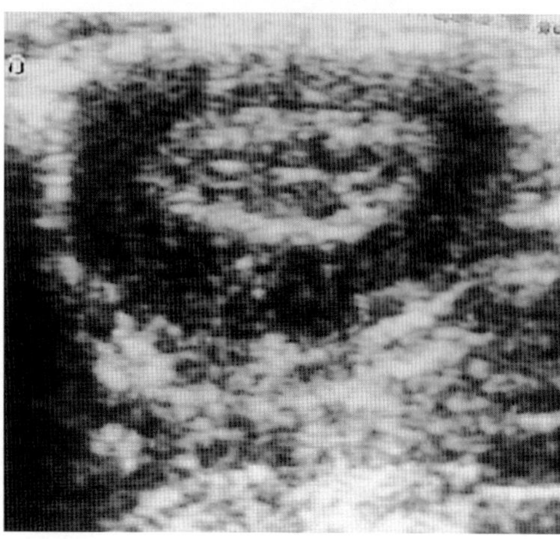

■ **Fig. 5.69** Ultrasound scan of the right iliac fossa in a patient with abdominal pain and some obstructive features. Gross thickening of the small bowel wall is seen, pointing to a diagnosis of Crohn's disease.

despite its ability to provide diagnostic information and a great deal of indication of the progress of complications such as associated abscesses. CT scanning has been more developed and is becoming a first-line radiological tool in Crohn's disease (Figs 5.70, 5.71). At present the role of magnetic resonance imaging is still evolving, but it is highly likely that its great ability to provide images in multiple planes, its ready identification of areas of inflammation and the absence of radiation, will combine to make this the radiological method of choice very soon as it has already become in pelvic imaging (see Chapter 8). Nonetheless, intraluminal contrast radiology currently remains of crucial importance in most units.

The radiological features of Crohn's disease may be quite subtle (Fig. 5.72), moving through more obvious aphthous ulceration with stenosis (Fig. 5.73) to cobblestoning (Fig. 5.74) and to the demonstration of extensive (Fig. 5.75) or complicated disease. Aphthous ulceration, pseudo-diverticula, deep fissuring ulceration, skip lesions (where segments of obviously diseased bowel are separated by apparently normal intestine) and asymmetrical wall involvement (Fig. 5.75) are all strongly suggestive of Crohn's disease. There may be confusion with the changes of radiation enteritis (Fig. 5.76), but this will normally be suggested by the history of previous abdominal radiotherapy (albeit often many years before). The combination of linear ulceration and transverse fissuring, with submucosal edema and inflammation produces the characteristic 'cobblestone' appear-

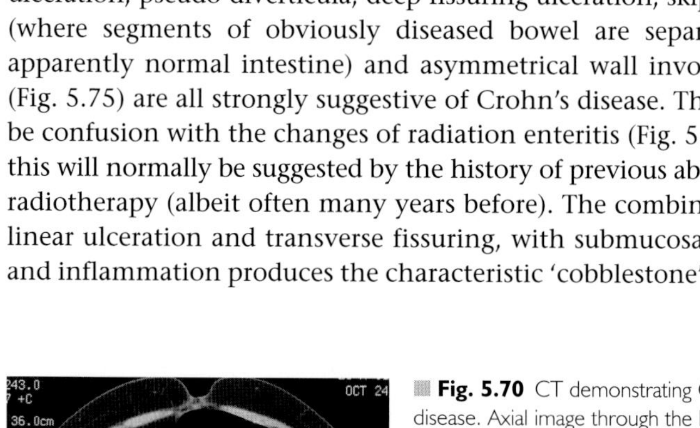

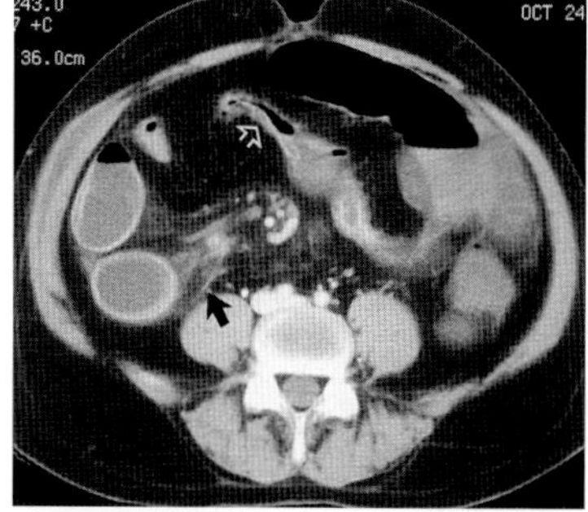

■ **Fig. 5.70** CT demonstrating Crohn's disease. Axial image through the level of the umbilicus. A segment of ileum shows luminal narrowing and mild wall thickening (open arrow). Inflammatory stranding (black arrow) of the small bowel mesentery is present.

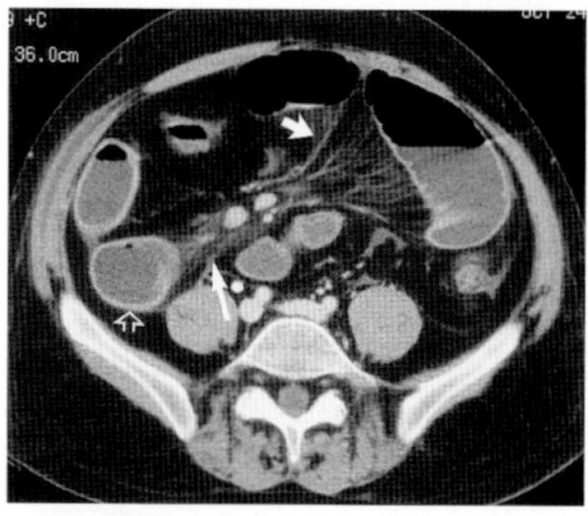

■ **Fig. 5.71** At the level of the iliac crest in the same patient as in Fig 5.70, two loops show mild bowel wall thickening (open arrow). There is inflammatory stranding in the prominent small bowel mesentery (long arrow). Stranding in the mesentery resembling a 'comb' (short arrow) reflects either vascular changes or perilymphatic inflammation.

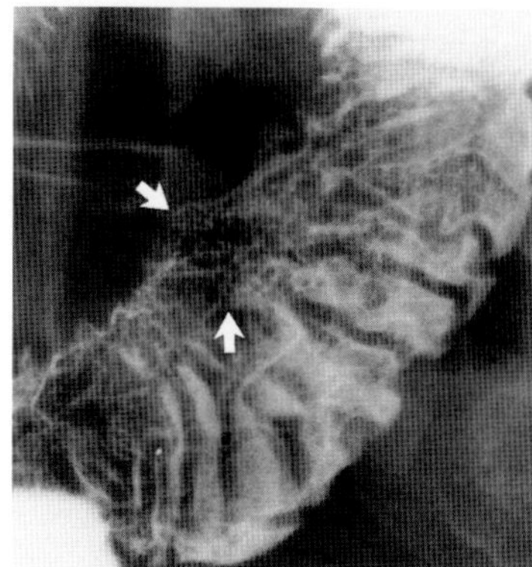

■ **Fig. 5.72** Enteroclysis demonstrating enlarged villi in Crohn's disease. Fine nodules (representative nodules identified by arrows) are seen in the distal ileum, a manifestation of villi enlarged by edema and an inflammatory infiltrate. (Reproduced with permission from reference 4, Fig. 3.)

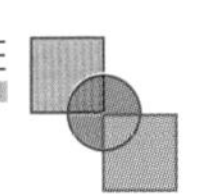

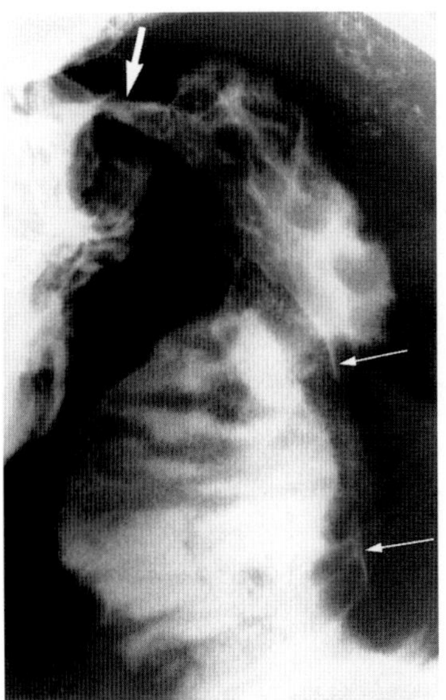

Fig. 5.73 Barium study showing Crohn's disease of the terminal ileum. A long mesenteric border ulcer is manifested as a thin, linear barium-filled groove (thin arrows) surrounded by edematous elevated radiolucent mucosa. The distal most terminal ileum has nodular mucosa. The ileocecal valve is narrowed (thick arrow). (Reproduced with permission from reference 4, Fig. 4.)

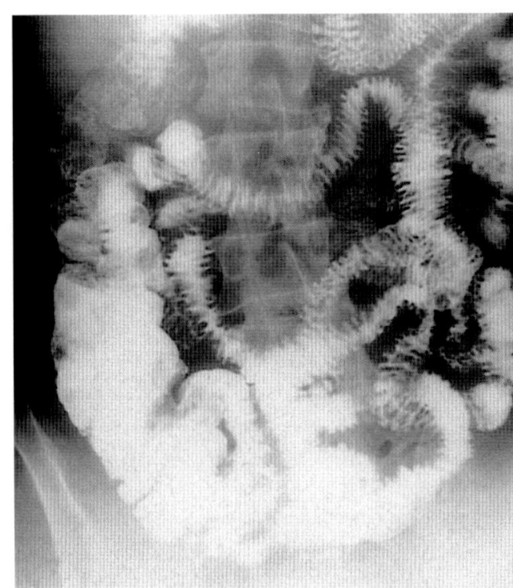

Fig. 5.76 Barium follow-through showing the changes of extensive radiation enteritis following otherwise successful treatment of lymphoma. Courtesy of Dr R.A. Parkins.

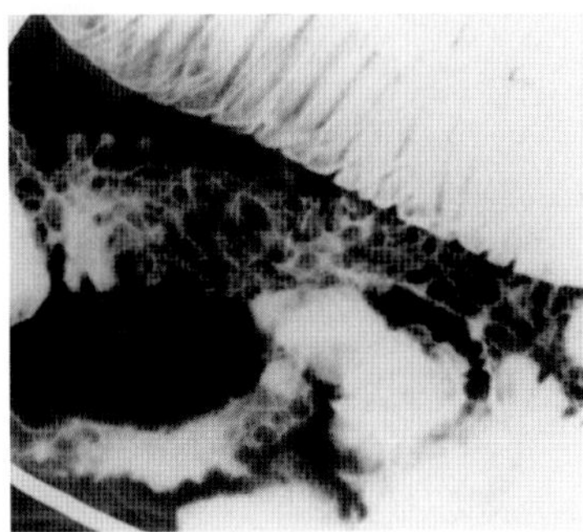

Fig. 5.74 Enteroclysis demonstrates two areas of cobblestoning (the ulceronodular pattern) in Crohn's disease. The cobblestones are the radiolucent islands of relatively spared mucosa between barium-filled transverse and longitudinally oriented knife-like clefts. The luminal narrowing reflects the transmural inflammation. (Reproduced with permission from reference 4, Fig. 16.)

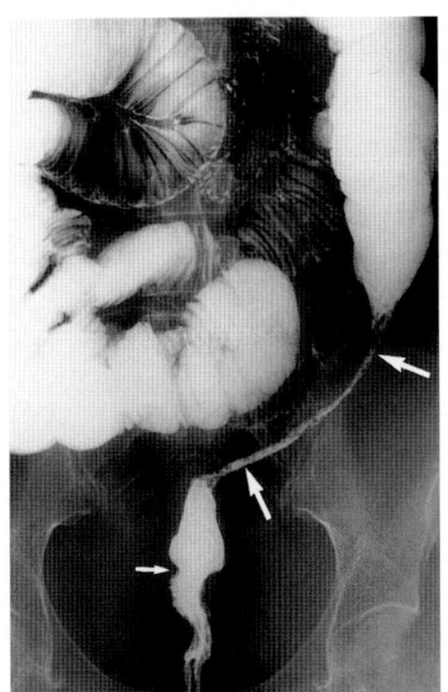

Fig 5.77 Small bowel follow-through demonstrating recurrent Crohn's disease involving the neo-terminal ileum. Marked narrowing (long arrows) of the small intestine proximal to the ileorectal anastomosis (short arrow) is seen. This is the so-called 'string sign.' (Reproduced with permission from reference 1, Fig. 5.33.)

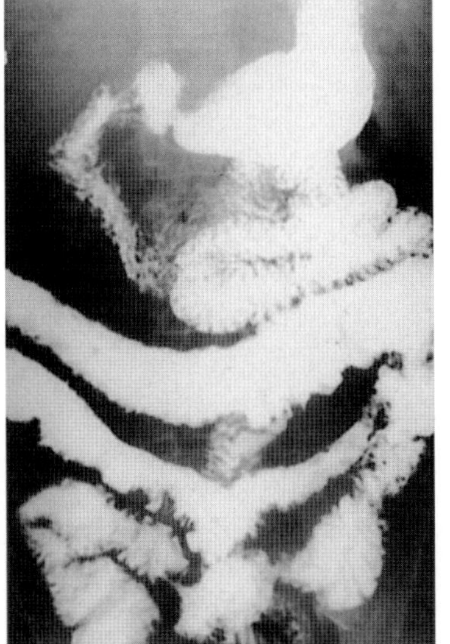

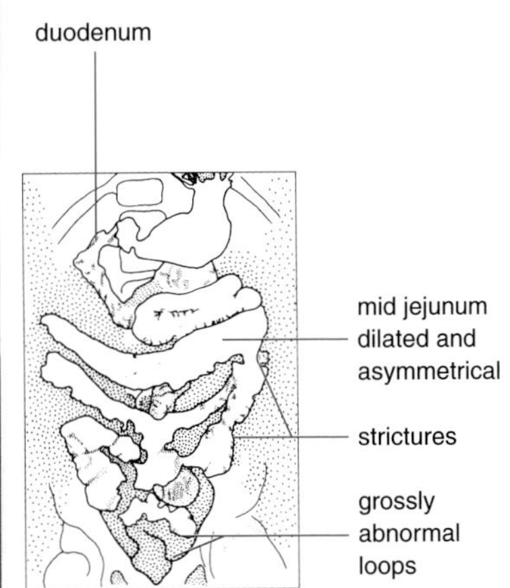

Fig. 5.75 Follow-through study showing extensive involvement of the jejunum by Crohn's disease in a young patient who had already had multiple resections. There is asymmetrical wall thickening and multiple areas of stenosis and fissuring ulceration.

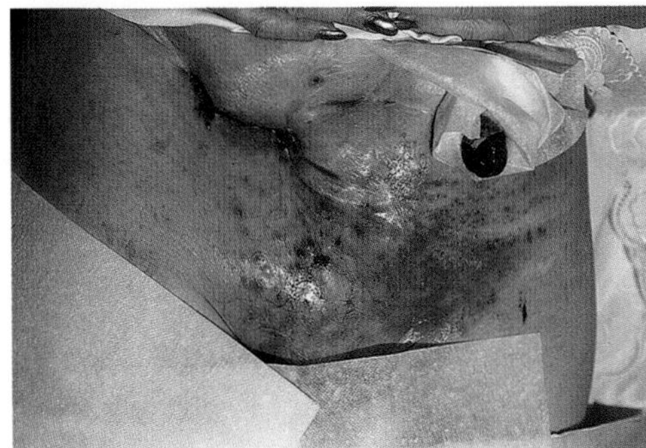

Fig. 5.78 Enterocutaneous fistula in the right iliac fossa in a patient with Crohn's disease. As is often the case, there is a great deal of excoriation of the skin below the fistulous opening. The left-sided stoma is also somewhat inflamed.

ance (Fig. 5.74), and this, with the presence of strictures and fistulae, is almost diagnostic of Crohn's disease. Ulceration may be extensive or limited to discrete superficial ulcers surrounded by normal mucosa. Any of these features may be seen in the small bowel, large bowel, or both (see Chapter 6). Ileocecal involvement often produces a thickened ileocecal valve (Fig. 5.73) with deformity of the cecum itself, and is commonly associated with terminal ileal disease. The classical 'string sign' is less often seen with better medical therapy (Fig. 5.77).

The radiological assessment of Crohn's-related abscesses and fistulae (Fig 5.78) is essential for optimal surgical management, and fistulography using a balloon occlusion catheter, ultrasound, CT, magnetic resonance imaging, and enteroscopy will all be contributory in individual cases (Figs 5.79–5.81). It is unusual for the esophagus, stomach, or duodenum to be involved without obvious disease elsewhere (see Chapters 1, 2, and 3) but ulcers similar to those seen in the proximal gastrointestinal tract may occur in the jejunum and be responsible for major complications (Fig. 5.82).

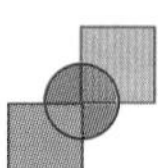

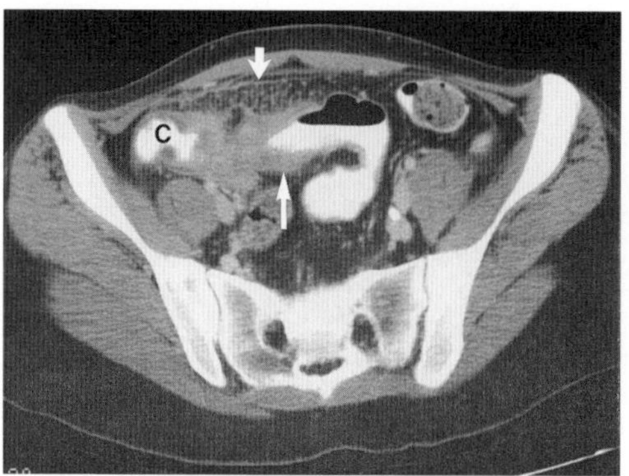

■ **Fig. 5.79** CT demonstrating complicated Crohn's disease. Axial image through the upper sacrum. Small bowel wall is normally barely perceptible on CT. There are numerous areas of mild to marked thickening of the terminal ileal wall (long arrow). The cecal wall is thick (C identifies cecal lumen), with a mural stratification pattern. There is moderate inflammatory stranding of the mesenteric fat (short arrow).

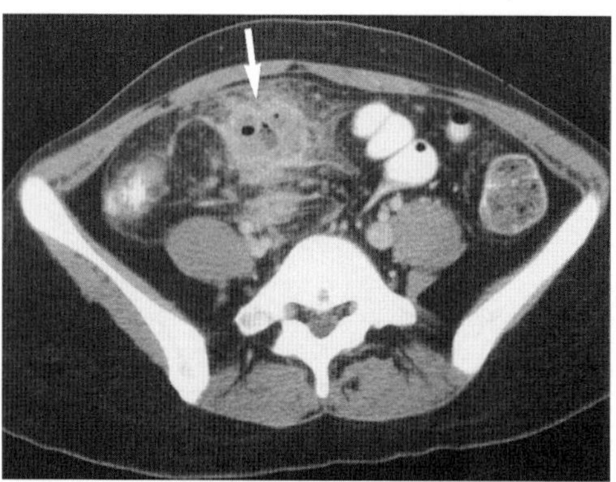

■ **Fig. 5.80** A more caudal axial image in the same patient demonstrates an abscess as a heterogeneous mass (arrow) with focal areas of fluid, air bubbles and soft tissue stranding. The wall of the ascending colon is mildly thickened. (Reproduced with permission from reference 2, Fig. 13.47A and B.)

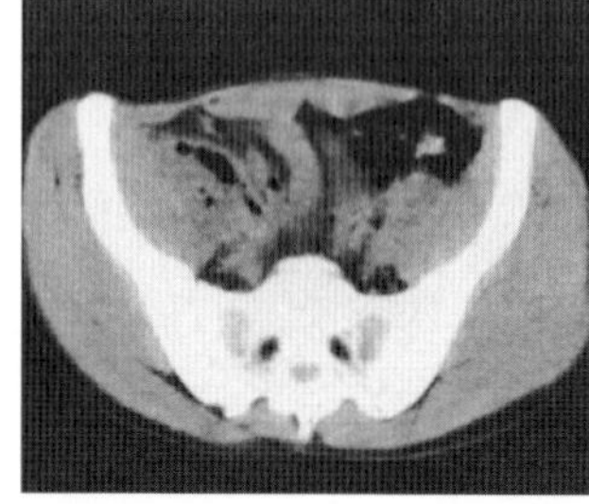

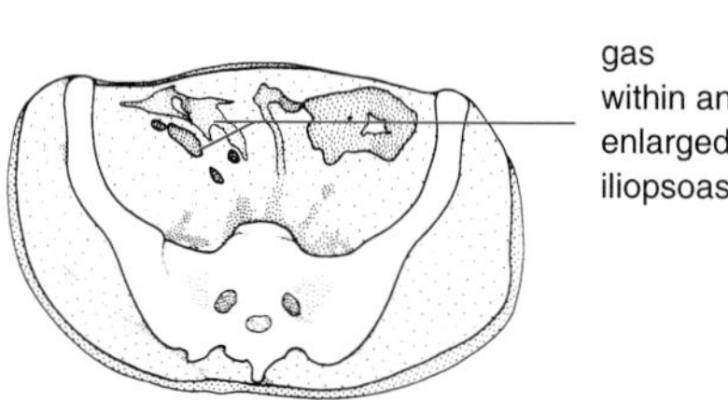

■ **Fig. 5.81** CT scan of a patient with iliopsoas abscess complicating newly diagnosed Crohn's disease affecting the terminal ileum without colonic disease. Note the considerable paucity of body fat in this malnourished patient.

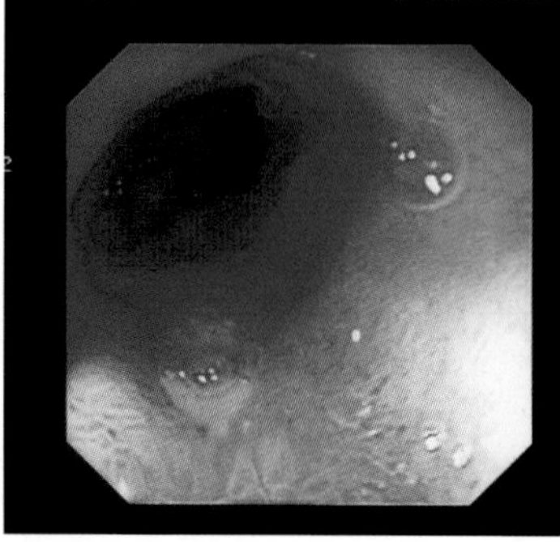

■ **Fig. 5.82** Investigation of a patient with unexplained major gastrointestinal bleeding led to the eventual discovery of an ulcer with endoscopic appearances similar to those of a peptic ulcer. It was, however, seen by push enteroscopy in the mid-jejunum, and the patient proved to have Crohn's disease.

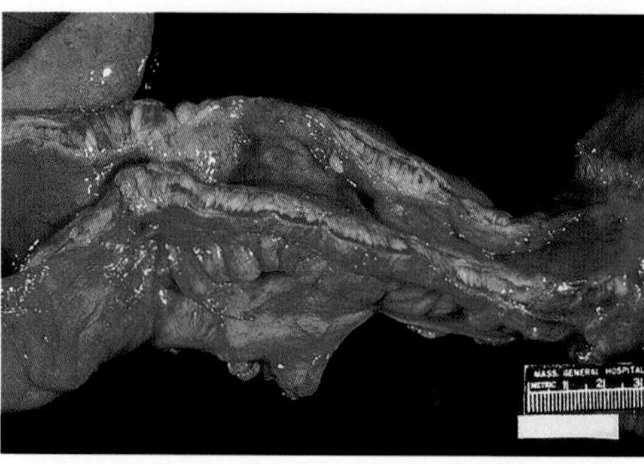

■ **Fig. 5.83** Crohn's disease. Macroscopic view of Crohn's disease showing mural thickening and stenosis of the distal ileum due to chronic transmural inflammation and fibrosis.

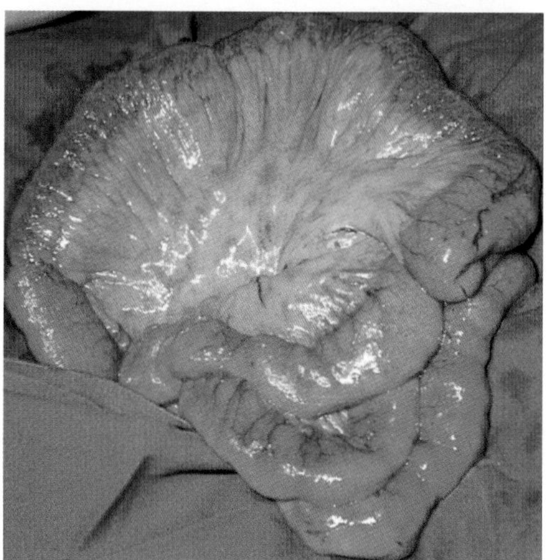

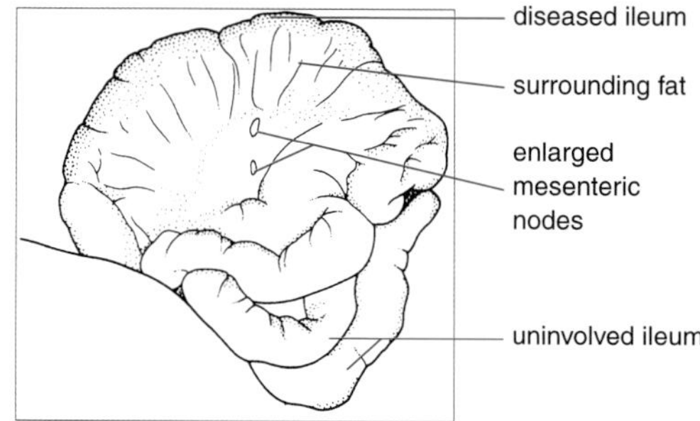

■ **Fig. 5.84** Laparotomy in florid Crohn's disease of the mid-ileum, showing a section of inflamed bowel, large mesenteric nodes and 'fat wrapping.' Courtesy of Mr J. Alexander-Williams.

Pathology

All layers of the bowel wall are involved in Crohn's disease, which can result in narrowing and thickening of involved segments; classically the segment involved is the distal 10–20 cm of the ileum (Figs 5.83, 5.84). Strictures vary greatly in length, are often multiple, and in involved areas, whether strictured or not, the mucosa tends to exhibit linear ulceration, with submucosal edema raising the surviving mucosa into the cobblestone appearance recognized radiologically. The presence of skip lesions (Fig. 5.85), or intestinal fistulae points firmly to a macroscopic diagnosis of Crohn's (Fig. 5.86).

Histological examination shows discrete granulomas (in at least 50% of cases if sufficient sections are cut), with fissuring ulceration, submucosal fibrosis, and transmural inflammation (Fig. 5.87). In addition to obvious mucosal inflammation, aggregates of lymphocytes are scattered through the bowel wall, and often appear as 'beads' of inflammation along the serosa. It is usual for the microscopic changes to be patchy, in common with the macroscopic tendency to skip lesions.

The granulomas, which do not caseate, may be seen at any site in the gut wall (Fig. 5.87). Fissuring ulceration usually extends into the submucosa, and, less often, through the full thickness of muscle. These may constitute the origins of fistulae, but loops of bowel are also bound together by fibrosis in the absence of intervening fistulae. Crohn's strictures are associated with submucosal fibrosis, reduplication, and disorganization of the muscularis mucosae. Further examples are given in Chapter 6. Crohn's disease can be diagnosed with confidence if there is characteristic rectal histology in the

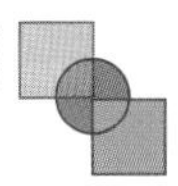

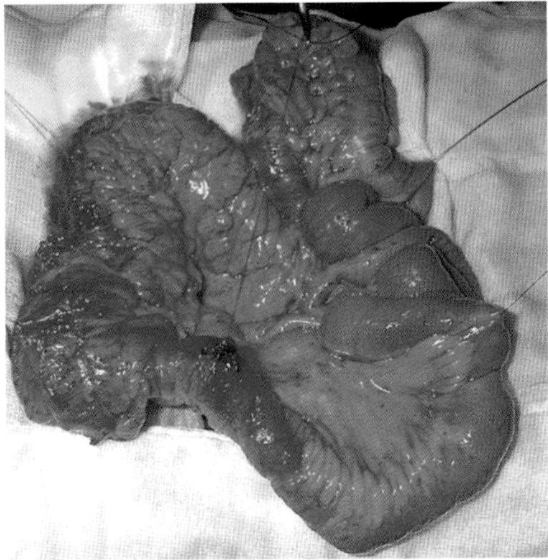

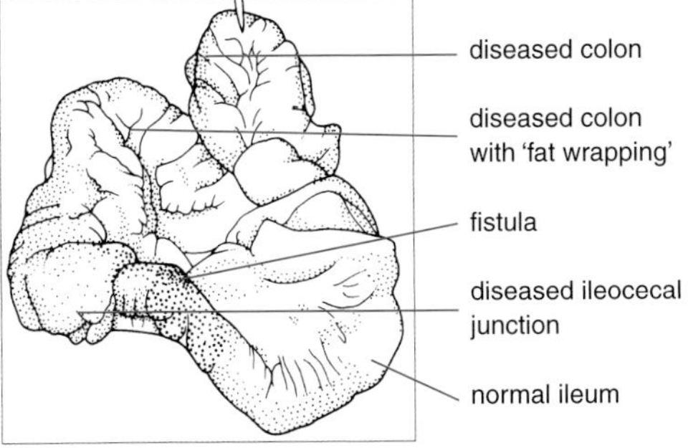

■ **Fig. 5.85** Laparotomy appearance in Crohn's ileocolitis, where a skip lesion and fistulae may be seen. Involved bowel has a prominent fat wrapping. Courtesy of Mr J. Alexander-Williams.

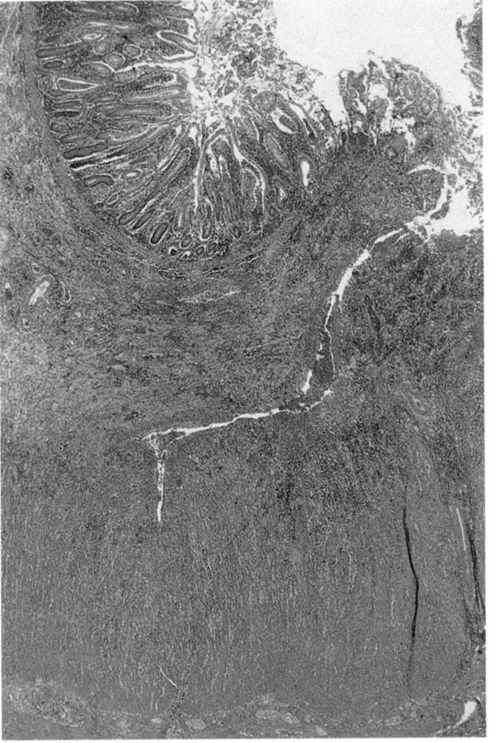

■ **Fig. 5.86** Crohn's disease. Microscopic view of a fissuring ulcer in active ileal Crohn's disease showing a characteristic deep narrow ulcer cleft flanked by intense inflammation and lined by granulation tissue.

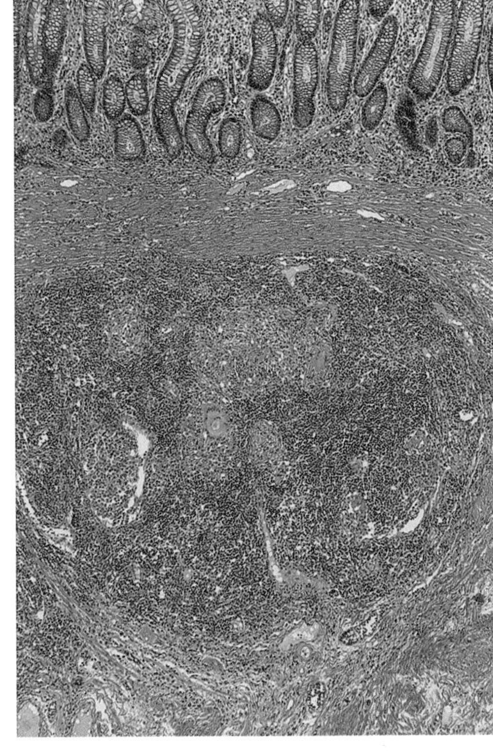

■ **Fig. 5.87** Crohn's disease. Microscopic view of the ileal submucosa showing a cluster of non-caseating granulomata surrounded by a dense lymphocytic infiltrate.

presence of suggestive small bowel radiology, even in patients with an apparently normal sigmoidoscopy. Extraintestinal manifestations are associated with a higher than average frequency of granulomas on histological assessment.

REFERENCES

1. Rubesin SE, Laufer I. Pictorial glossary. In: Gore RM, Levine MS, Laufer I (eds) Textbook of gastrointestinal radiology, pp. 50–80. Philadelphia: WB Saunders, 1994, Figs. 5.1C, 5.32C, 33.
2. Rubesin SE, Bartram C, Laufer I. Inflammatory bowel disease. In: Levine MS, Rubesin SE, Laufer I (eds) Double contrast gastrointestinal radiology, 3rd edn, pp. 417–470. Philadelphia: WB Saunders, 2000, Figs 13.47 A and B, 13.95.
3. Herlinger H, Rubesin SE, Morris JB. Small bowel obstruction. In: Gore RM, Levine MS (eds) Textbook of gastrointestinal radiology, 2nd edn, pp. 815–837. Philadelphia: WB Saunders Co, 2000, Fig. 46.30.
4. Rubesin SE, Bronner M. Radiologic-pathologic concepts in Crohn's disease. Advances in gastrointestinal radiology. Chicago: Mosby-Year Book, 1991; 1: 27–55, Figs 3, 4, 8.
5. Herlinger H, Rubesin SE, Furth EE. Mesenteric border ulcers in Crohn's disease: historical, radiologic and pathologic perspectives. Abdominal Imaging 1998; 23: 122–126, Figs 6D and 6E.

COLON I

6

NORMAL COLON AND RECTUM

The colon is commonly considered to consist of five segments: the cecum, with the vermiform appendix at its base and the orifice of the ileocecal valve a little more distally; then the ascending, transverse, descending, and sigmoid portions (Figs 6.1–6.9), leading into the rectum.

The junction of the ascending and transverse colon – the hepatic flexure – is angulated and lies close to the undersurface of the liver (Fig. 6.4). A second angulation between the transverse and descending colon – the splenic flexure – lies close to the hilum of the spleen, usually at a somewhat higher level than the hepatic flexure.

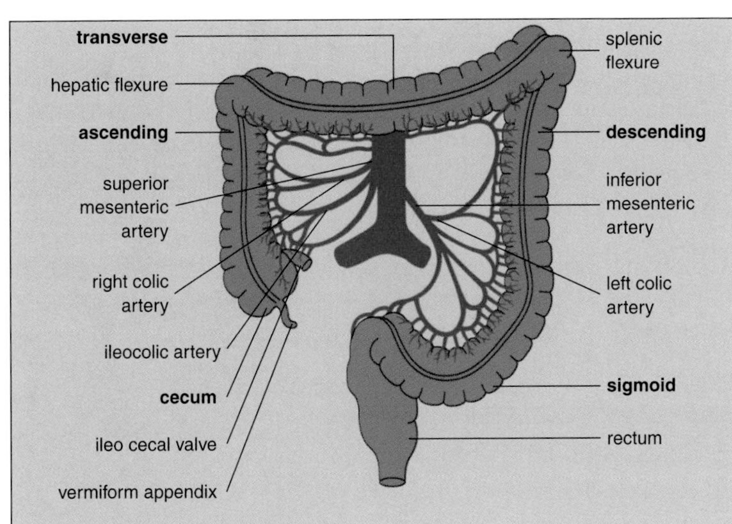

■ **Fig. 6.1** Diagram showing the anatomy of the colon and its blood supply.

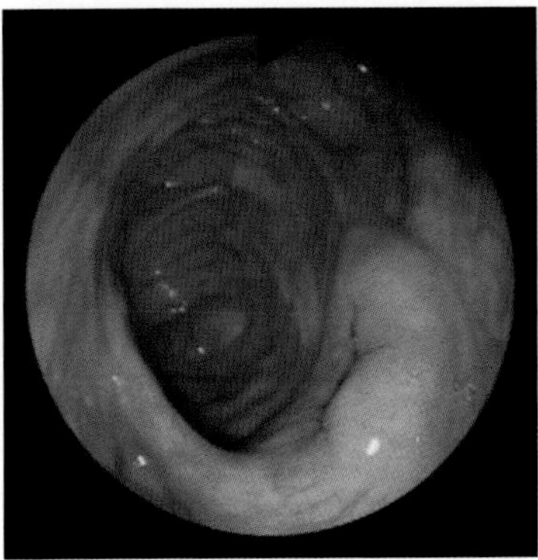

■ **Fig. 6.2** Colonoscopic view of the normal ileocecal valve and cecum.

The proximal colon, extending to the distal transverse colon, is derived from the embryonal midgut and shares its blood supply (from the superior mesenteric artery) with the small intestine (Fig. 6.1). The more distal colon arises from the embryonal hindgut and is supplied by the inferior mesenteric artery. The colon is mainly concerned with absorption of water and electrolytes, and to a lesser extent with reabsorption of bile acids; it has less absorptive capacity as one moves distally, and the lowermost parts function more as a storage site for feces prior to their evacuation. In health the colon has only a minimal nutritional role, but the bacterial fermentation of undigested carbohydrate releases butyrate, which is an important colonocyte nutrient.

The rectum, the proximal third of which is intraperitoneal, is about 18 cm in length, connecting the sigmoid colon to the anal canal. The beginning of the rectum is not defined histologically, but the rectosigmoid junction lies at the level of the sacral promontory and forms a moderately acute angle, which is usually obvious to the sigmoidoscopist. The rectum is supplied by the superior rectal artery –

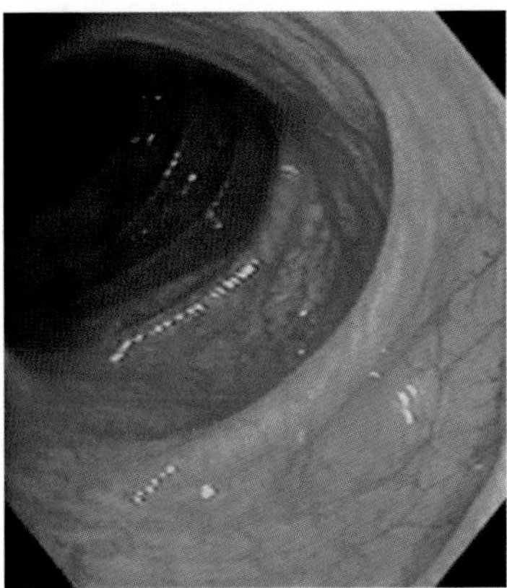

■ **Fig. 6.3** Colonoscopic view of the normal ascending colon.

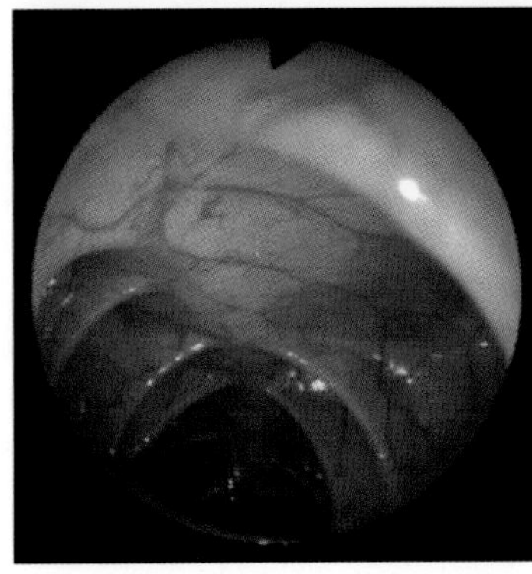

■ **Fig. 6.4** Colonoscopic appearance of the hepatic flexure showing the bluish impression formed by the adjacent liver.

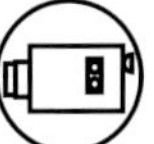

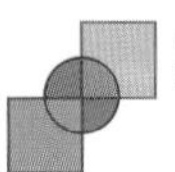

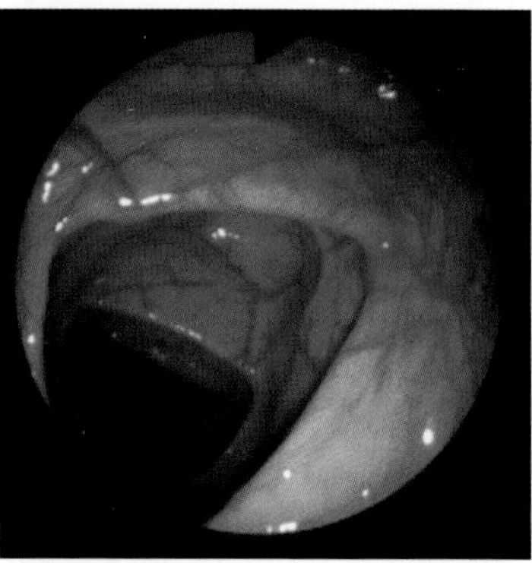

Fig. 6.5 Colonoscopic appearance of the normal transverse colon showing the triangular plicae semilunares.

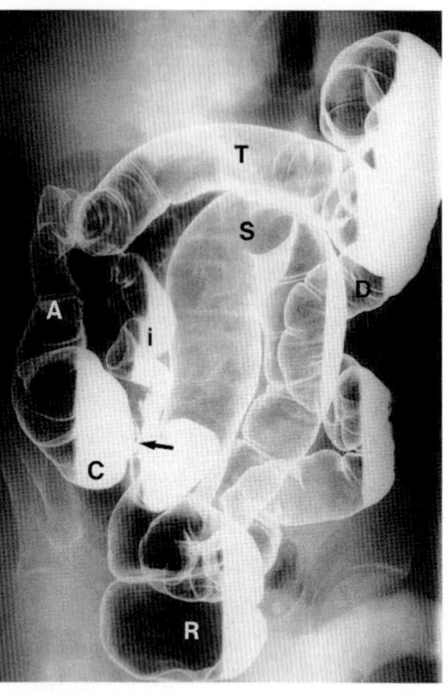

Fig. 6.6 Double-contrast barium enema demonstrating normal colon. The radiograph was obtained with the patient left-side down and the X-ray beam in a 'cross-table' position. The cecum (C), transverse colon (T), and sigmoid colon (S) are intraperitoneal. Portions of the ascending (A) and descending (D) colon are usually retroperitoneal. The rectum (R) is identified. In this patient, the sigmoid and descending colon are redundant. The appendix is identified by an arrow. Barium and air have refluxed back into the terminal ileum (i). (Reproduced with permission from reference 1, Fig. 11.31.)

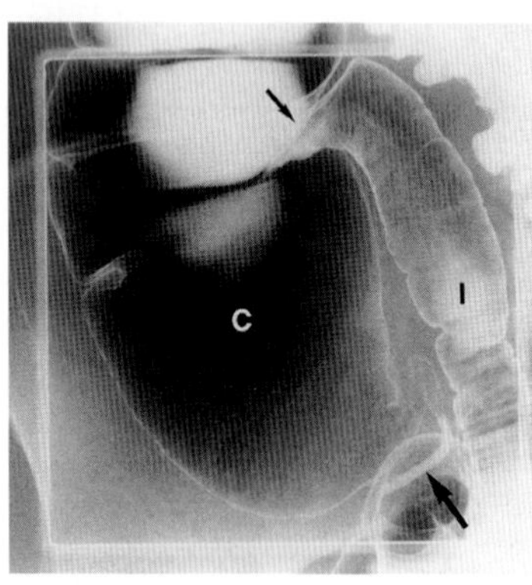

Fig. 6.7 Double-contrast barium enema demonstrating normal cecum (C), appendix and terminal ileum (I). The appendix (long black arrow) lies on the same side of the colon as the ileocecal valve (short black arrow). (Reproduced with permission from reference 1, Fig. 11.22.)

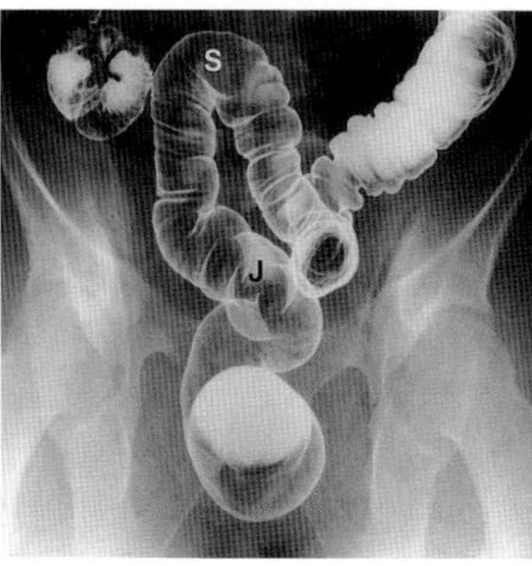

Fig. 6.8 Double-contrast barium enema demonstrating normal sigmoid colon (S) and rectosigmoid junction (J).). (Reproduced with permission from reference 1, Fig. 11.25.)

the final branch of the inferior mesenteric artery – and venous drainage is via the superior rectal vein to the inferior mesenteric vein. Lymphatic drainage is upwards unless obstructed, when lymph may drain to nodes on the pelvic side walls.

The colon and rectum are, together, a little over 1 m in length, and the diameter diminishes from cecum to sigmoid, increasing again

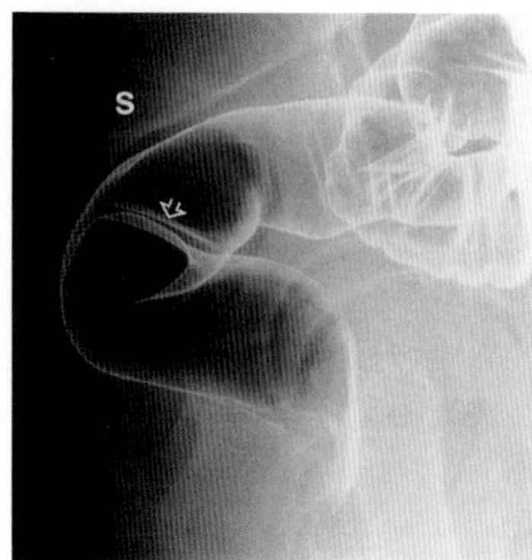

Fig. 6.9 Double-contrast barium enema demonstrating normal rectum in a lateral view. The posterior wall of the upper rectum parallels the sacrum (S) and coccyx. One valve of Houston (arrow) is seen. (Reproduced with permission from reference 3, Fig. 15.)

in the rectum. Most of the outer longitudinal muscle coat is gathered into three distinct bands – the teniae coli – 6–10 mm in width. These run from the tip of the cecum to the rectum, where they merge to form a more continuous covering. The teniae are shorter than the colon and therefore 'gather' it into sacculations, or haustra (Fig. 6.6). The mucosa of the colon is thrown into folds, the plicae semilunares, which take on a triangular appearance in the transverse colon (see Fig. 6.5).

Unlike the small intestine, the colon is relatively fixed, particularly the ascending and descending segments. The more mobile transverse colon has a short mesentery, whilst the sigmoid, with a broader, longer mesentery is generally the most mobile. Fatty structures arising within the mesentery and known as the appendices epiploicae cover the serosal surface of the colon; harmless calcification of these may occur with advancing years.

The histological architecture of the colon is similar to that of the more proximal bowel (Figs 6.10, 6.11). The mucosa comprises parallel rows of epithelial tubules or crypts, surrounded by the connective tissue framework of the lamina propria. The crypts are lined by goblet cells, and have undifferentiated cells at the base; the surface epithelium between the crypts is mostly composed of columnar absorptive cells with occasional goblet cells. The goblet cells produce glycoproteins; in health, these are predominantly sulfomucins at the crypt bases with some sialomucins more superficially. The colonic muscularis mucosae and the submucosa have fewer lymphatic channels than the small bowel – an important feature when considering the metastatic potential of neoplastic mucosal lesions.

INFECTIVE COLITIS

Most cases of infective diarrhea are unassociated with overt colitis and are therefore considered in Chapter 5, but a number of organisms, particularly *Shigella* species and *Entamoeba histolytica*, usually cause a frank colitis. Blood and mucus with large numbers of fecal leukocytes are seen, and although the rectal imaging and appearance in infective colitis is usually non-specific (Figs 6.12–6.14), standard microbiological investigation of the stools will generally provide a specific diagnosis. When this is negative, rectal biopsy becomes essential to assess for non-infective inflammatory bowel disease. The histology of infective colitis confirms the acute nature of the inflammation, with associated edema and with no major architectural changes (Fig. 6.15).

Amebic colitis

Amebiasis results from infection with *Entamoeba histolytica* (Figs 6.16, 6.17); it is most prevalent in the tropics and in areas of poor sanitation. Infection usually first becomes established in the colon, but it may subsequently affect a number of other organs. Cysts ingested

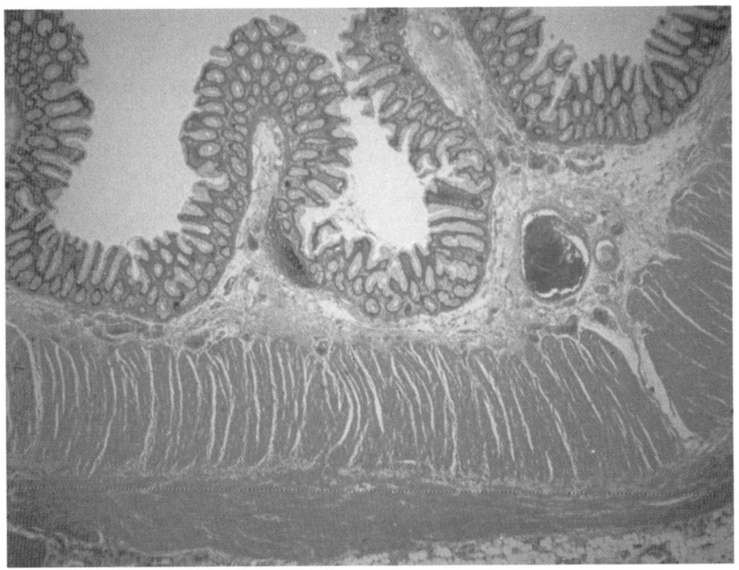

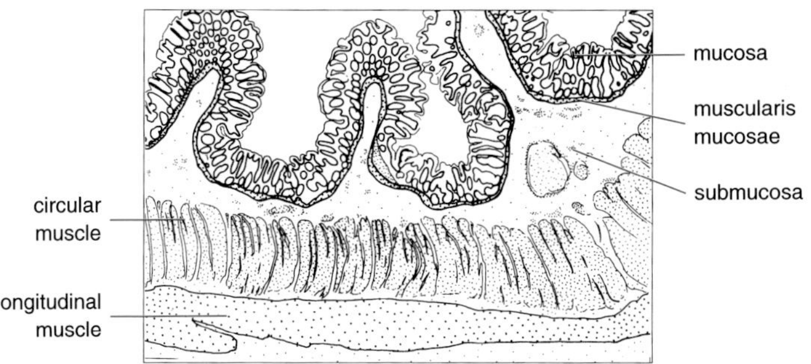

■ **Fig. 6.10** Histological appearance of the large intestine showing the relationship of the mucosa to the muscle layers. H&E stain (x 30).

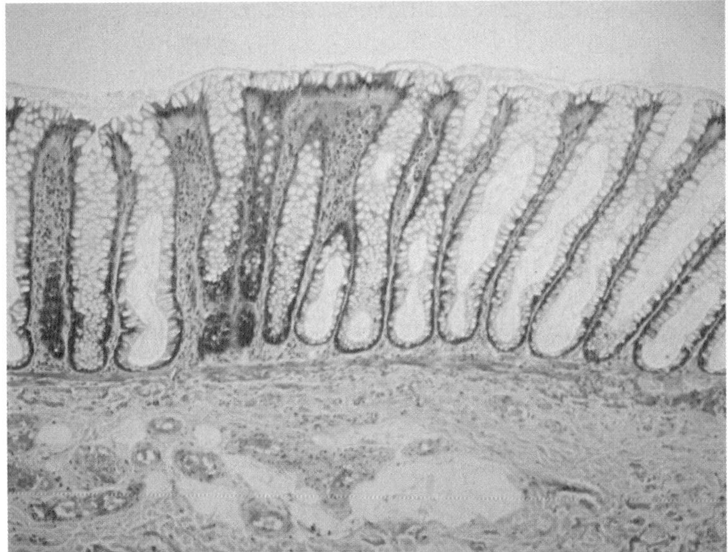

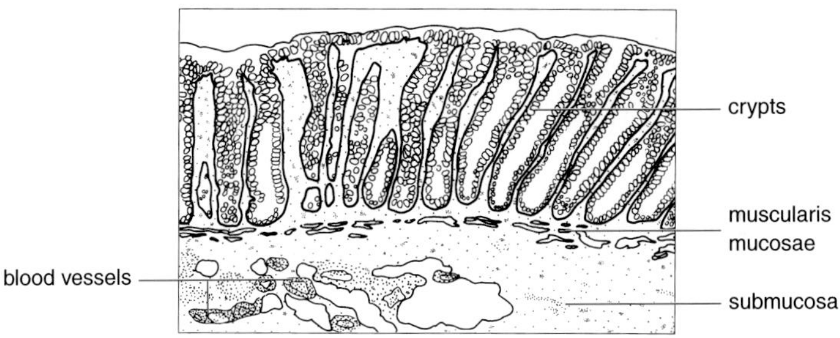

■ **Fig. 6.11** Higher-power view showing the regular arrangement of crypts occupying the full thickness of the mucosa. H&E stain (x 75).

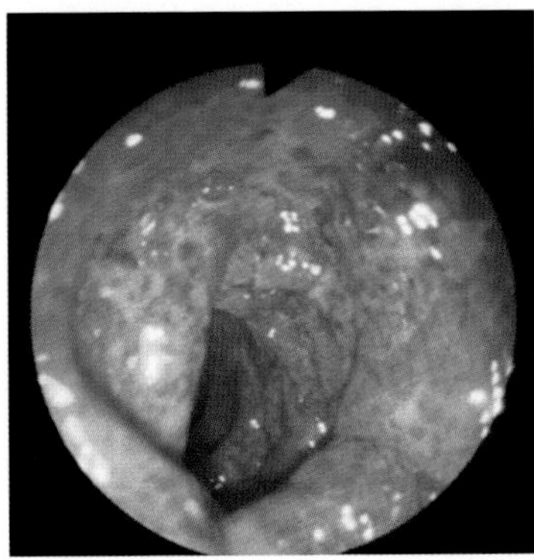

■ **Fig. 6.12** Endoscopic appearance of hemorrhagic colitis, the result of a verotoxin-producing strain of *E. coli*.

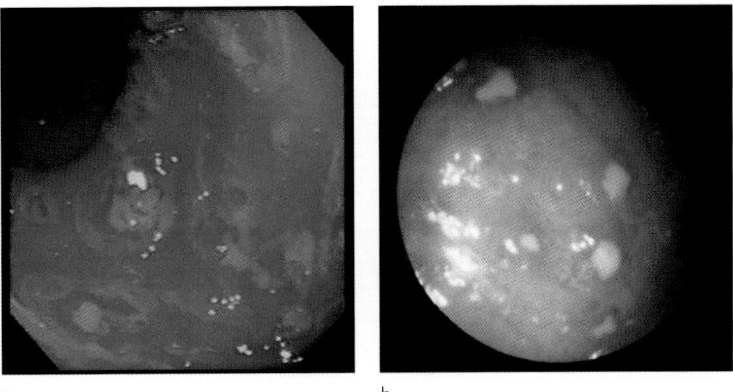

■ **Fig. 6.13** Endoscopic appearances of infective colitis – viral (a); *Campylobacter jejuni* (b).

with contaminated water or food change within the bowel into their motile trophozoite forms, which are responsible for disease. Cysts may, however, remain unconverted and then cause no symptoms. Amebiasis thus comprises a clinical spectrum from asymptomatic carrier to severe acute colitis with complicating abscesses in the liver or elsewhere (see Chapter 11). Overt colitis, with cramping lower abdominal pain and watery small volume stools streaked with blood and mucus (Fig. 6.18), may progress to an overwhelming illness and, rarely, to colonic perforation (Fig. 6.19), or it may run a more chronic course, with marked malaise and weight loss. Barium studies and endoscopy show mucosal ulceration in about 85% of cases (Fig. 6.20). The ulcers are typically in the cecum or rectum, or along the transverse axis of the bowel; they begin as shallow aphthous ulcers but become rounded or punched out, and may expose underlying muscle. They tend to be surrounded by a narrow rim of hyperemia and edema, with mucosa of relatively normal appearance in between (Fig. 6.21). Up to one fifth of patients have diffuse ulceration with abnormal background mucosa (Fig. 6.22). Scrapings from the ulcer base, blood-stained exudate, and liquid feces all show the confirmatory presence of trophozoites. Amebae can also be shown on the surface of a rectal biopsy, but this test is less reliable. The cysts of *E. histolytica* can usually be distinguished easily from those of the non-pathogenic *Entamoeba coli* (see Figs 6.16, 6.17). Serological tests are increasingly relied upon.

With chronicity, strictures and a characteristically conical cecum with an irregular mucosal surface occur (Fig. 6.23), and in a few patients, an ameboma may develop (Fig. 6.24). Typically found in the cecum, at the flexures, or in the rectosigmoid area, amebomas comprise large ulcerative granulomatous masses (Fig. 6.25). A rapid response to metronidazole helps in distinguishing them from carcinoma. Typhlitis is also described in this context (Fig. 6.26).

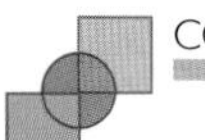

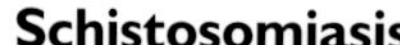

On histological examination, amebae are demonstrated (best by PAS stain) close to the surface beneath a typically overhanging mucosal edge. However, they may be present only in the overlying debris and it is therefore important to process any tissue fragments received with a biopsy (Figs 6.27–6.29). The observation of ingested erythrocytes within amebae helps in the distinction from *Entamoeba coli*, which is not erythrophagocytic (Fig. 6.30; see also Figs. 6.16, 6.17). When no organisms are demonstrated, the histology is non-specific. A post-dysenteric colitis with persistent histological changes (and functional symptoms) may persist for some months and can then be difficult to distinguish from idiopathic ulcerative colitis.

Schistosomiasis

Schistosomiasis probably affects more than 200 million people in the developing world, and both *Schistosoma mansoni* and *S. japonicum* can cause proctocolitis. Since the egg-laying female of *S. japonicum* resides in the superior mesenteric venous system, and that of *S. mansoni* in the inferior mesenteric venous system, colitic features are

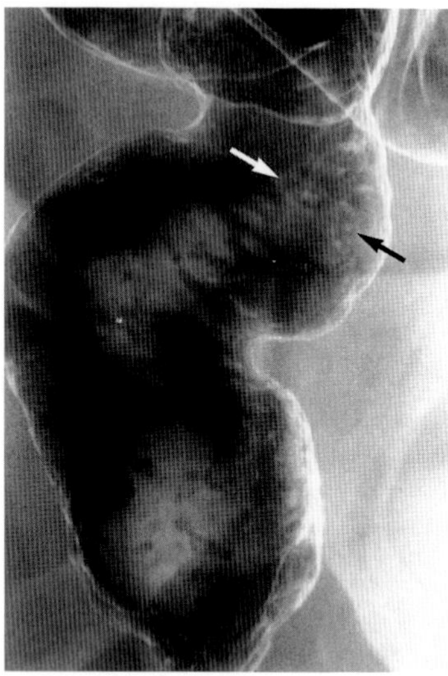

Fig. 6.14 Double-contrast barium enema demonstrating viral colitis. Numerous small ulcers (representative ulcers identified by arrows) are seen on the left lateral wall of the rectum. A biopsy revealed viral inclusion bodies. (Reproduced with permission from reference 4, Fig. 68.49C.)

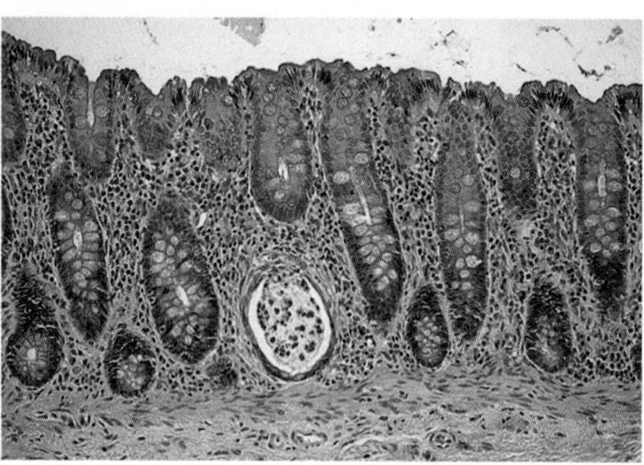

Fig. 6.15 Microscopic appearance of infectious colitis caused by *Campylobacter jejuni* showing increased cellularity of the lamina propria, neutrophilic cryptitis, and crypt abscess formation but no glandular architectural distortion, gland shortening, or fibrosis.

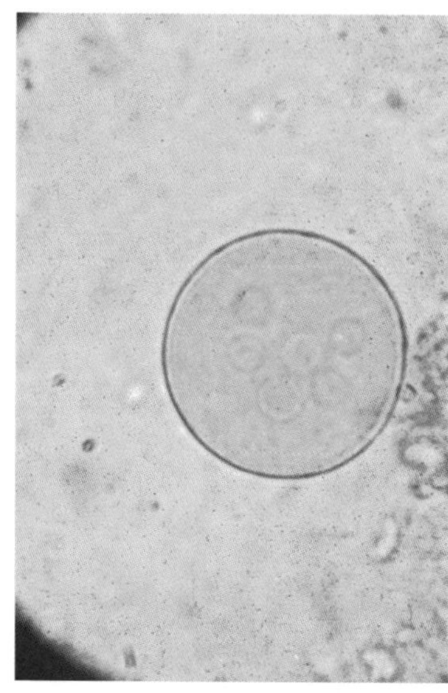

Fig. 6.16 Iodine stain of *Entamoeba coli* cyst in a fecal preparation. Courtesy of Dr D. Seal.

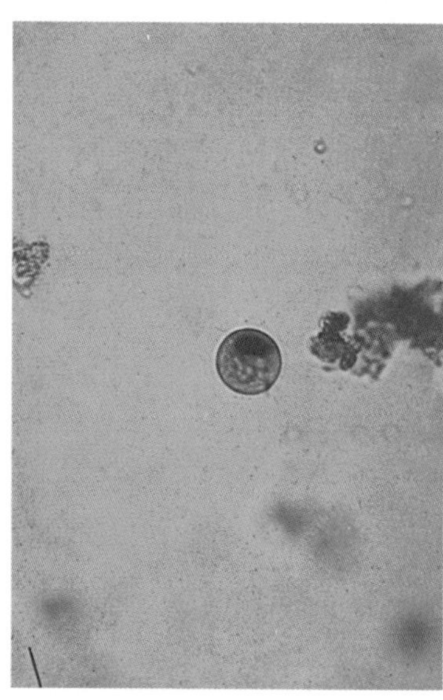

Fig. 6.17 *E. histolytica* cyst at the same magnification as Fig. 6.16. Courtesy of Dr D. Seal.

a

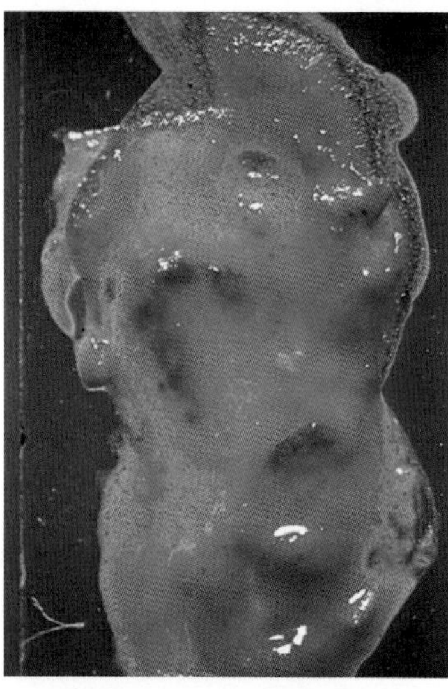

b

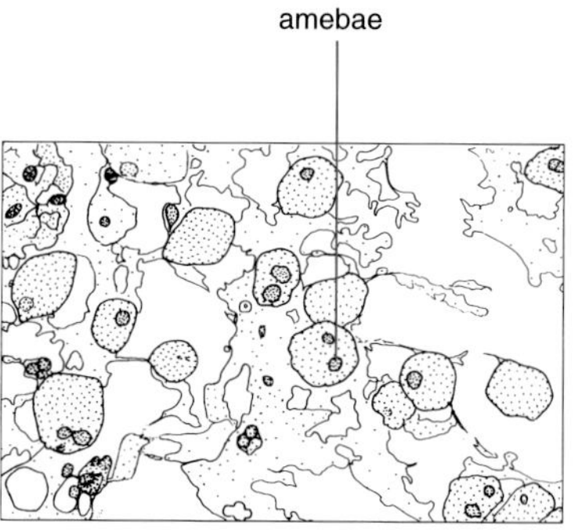

Fig. 6.18 Appearance of blood- and mucus-containing stool in amebiasis (a), and amebae in the stool smear (b); H&E stain (x 480). Courtesy of Dr S. Lucas.

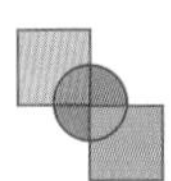

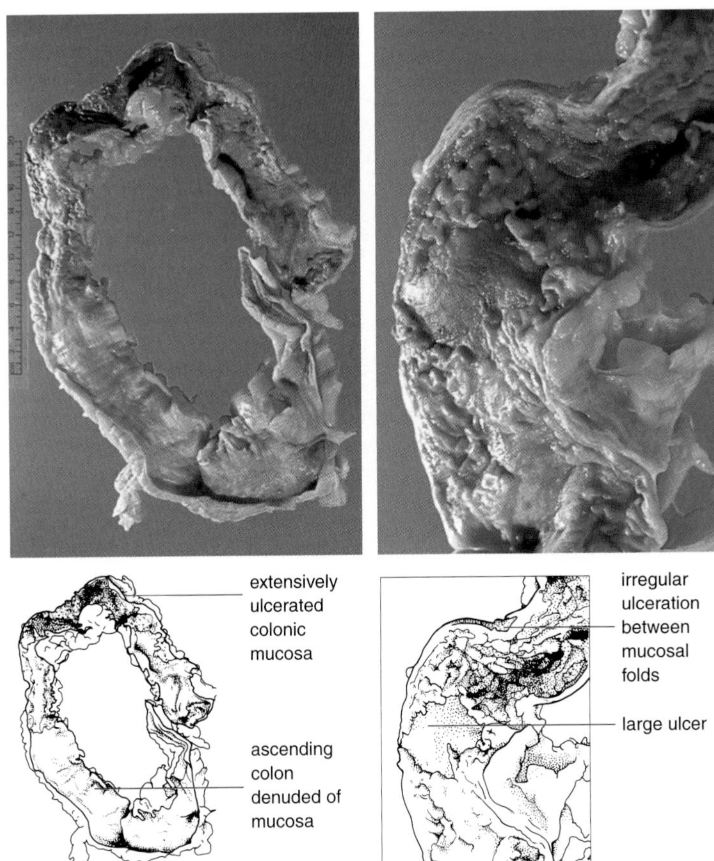

■ **Fig. 6.19** Macroscopic appearance of the colon in fatal amebiasis. Some mucosa survives, but there is extensive ulceration.

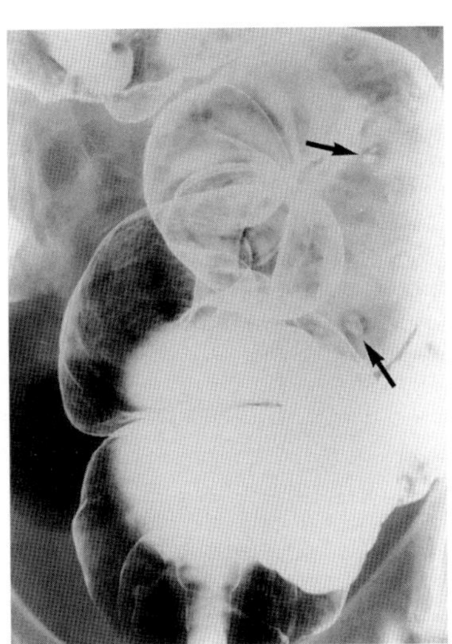

■ **Fig. 6.20** Double-contrast barium enema in patient with amebiasis. Many small aphthous ulcers are seen as round or linear barium collections surrounded by radiolucent halos (of edema) (arrows). (Reproduced with permission from reference 4, Fig. 68.48, courtesy of Harvey Goldstein, M.D., San Antonio, TX)

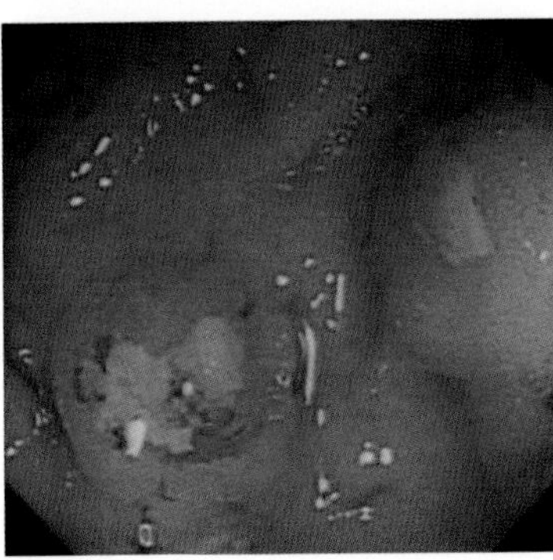

■ **Fig. 6.21** Endoscopic appearance of acute amebiasis with multiple superficial hemorrhagic ulcers.

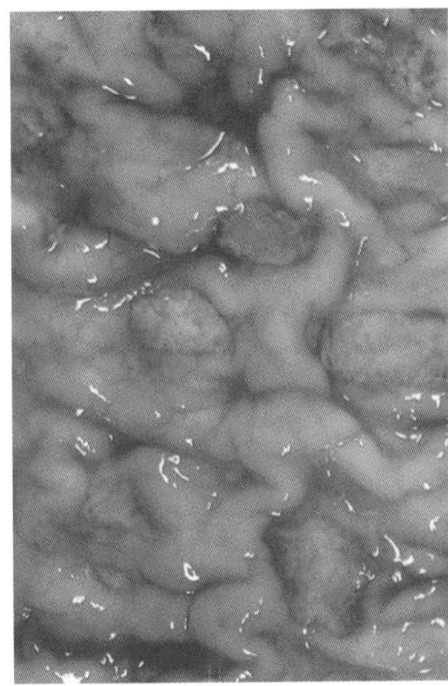

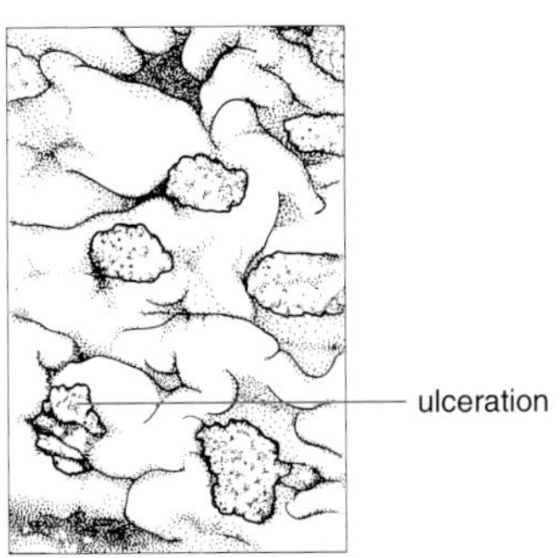

■ **Fig. 6.22** Macroscopic appearance of the colonic surface showing amebic ulcers. Courtesy of Dr S. Lucas.

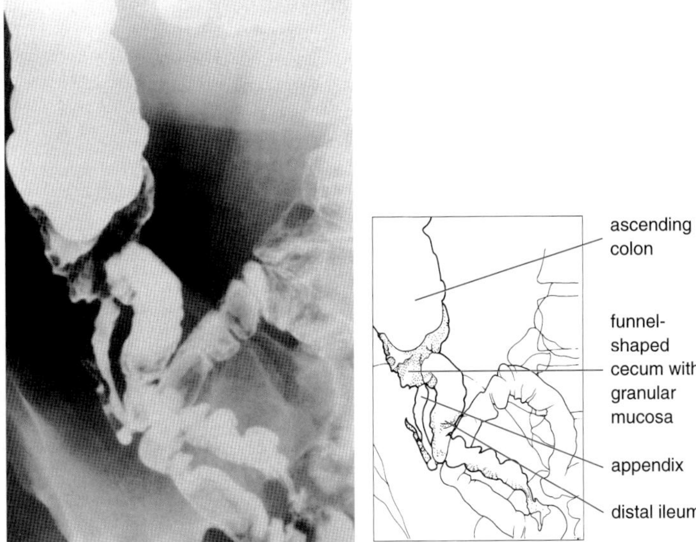

■ **Fig. 6.23** Barium enema in chronic amebic colitis showing a funnel-shaped cecum with granular deformity.

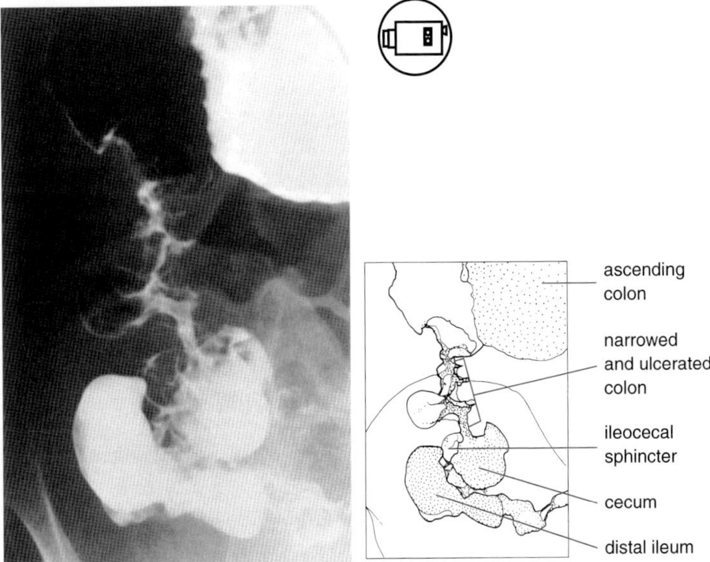

■ **Fig. 6.24** Barium enema showing an ameboma in the ascending colon.

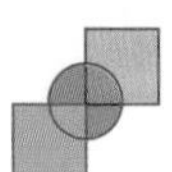

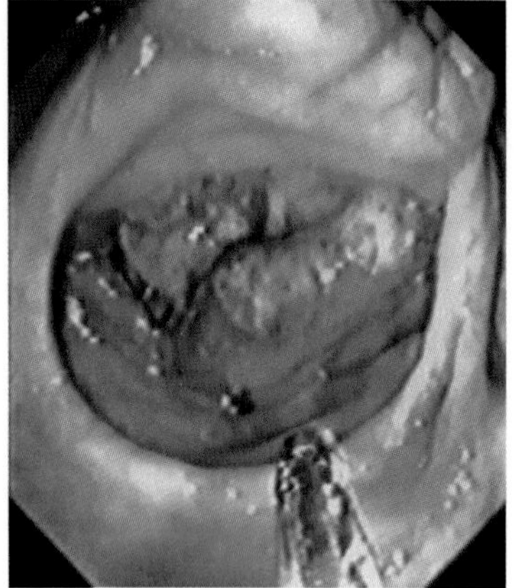

Fig 6.25 Endoscopic appearance of ameboma in the cecum.

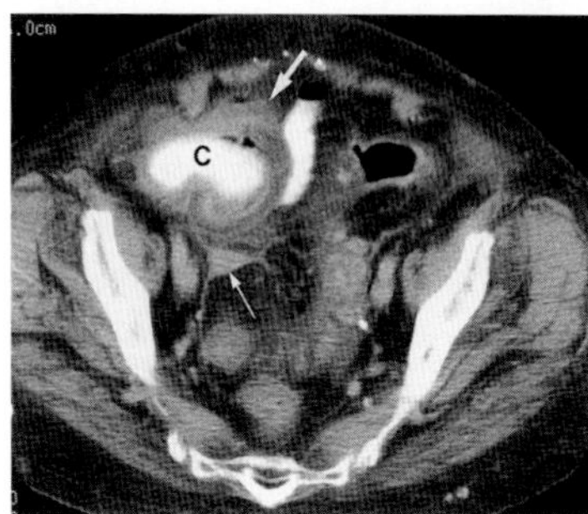

Fig. 6.26 CT in patient with typhlitis. The wall of the cecum (C) is thickened (large white arrow). Pericecal fluid is seen (thin white arrow).

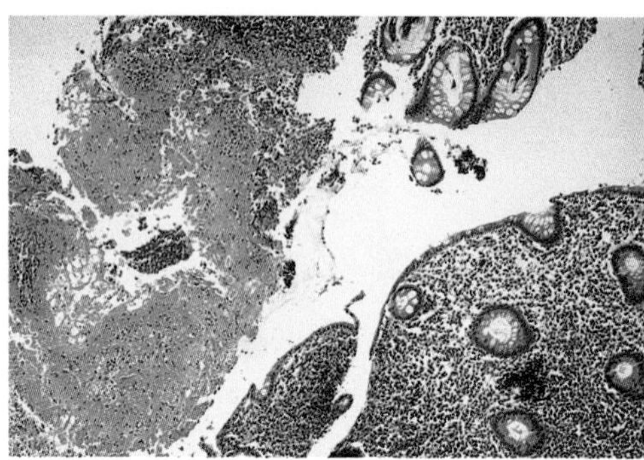

Fig. 6.27 Biopsy appearance of amebic colitis showing chronically inflamed mucosa and thick fibrinopurulent exudate originating from an ulcer, within which the trophozoites of *E. histolytica* are typically found.

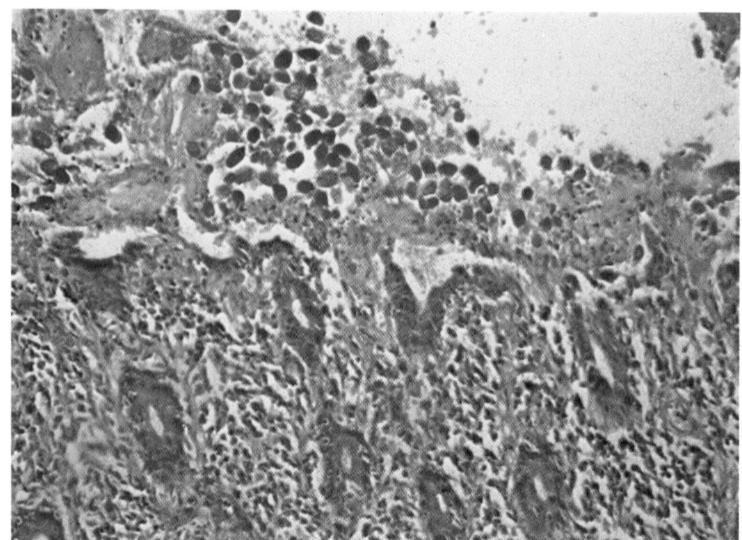

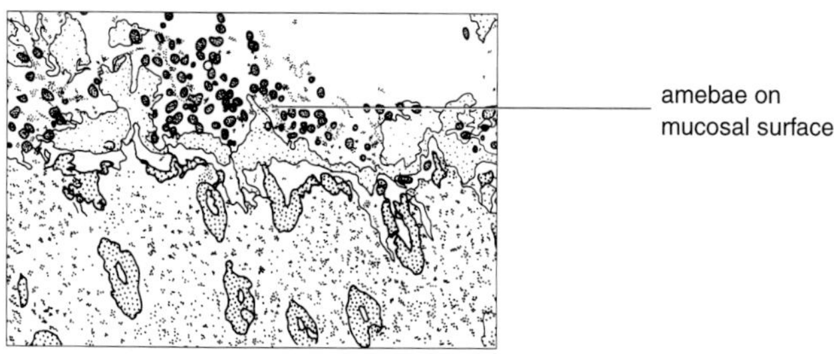

Fig. 6.28 PAS stain in amebic colitis. PAS stain (x 180) showing the characteristic bright magenta staining of amebic trophozoites within the fibrinopurulent exudate overlying the eroded mucosa.

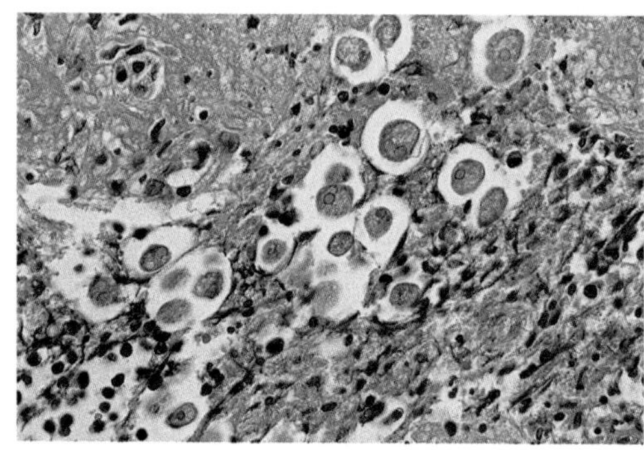

Fig. 6.29 Amebic colitis. High magnification showing amebic trophozoites with small round eccentric nuclei and abundant eosinophilic cytoplasm.

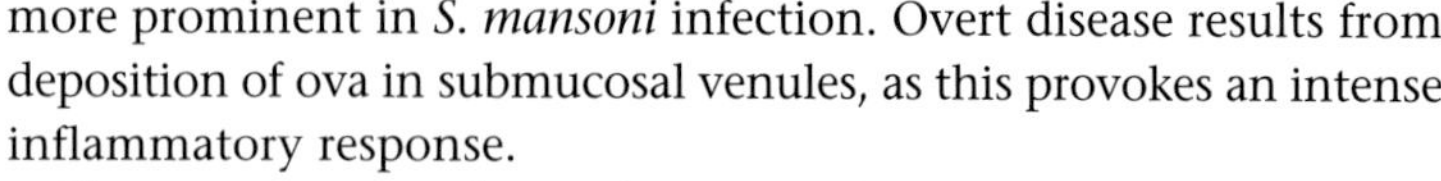

more prominent in *S. mansoni* infection. Overt disease results from deposition of ova in submucosal venules, as this provokes an intense inflammatory response.

The symptoms are those of a low-grade colitis coupled with pain, and often with pyrexia. Hypersensitivity (including urticaria and facial edema) also occurs. Hepatosplenomegaly and generalized lymphadenopathy are occasional features of the acute phase (see also Chapter 11). Peripheral eosinophilia is invariable but often mild, and sigmoidoscopy reveals a friable proctitis. In severe cases, there may also be punctuate hemorrhages and shallow ulceration.

In chronic schistosomiasis, imaging may show pedunculated papillomas, ulceration, and occasionally multiple granulomatous nodules resembling tuberculomas (Figs 6.31, 6.32). Histological examination shows the schistosomal eggs, which form the focus of granulomatous reactions in the mucosa and bowel wall (Figs 6.33–6.37), and around which other inflammatory cells accumulate to varying degrees. With time, the inflammatory response diminishes, but a possible link with carcinoma in long-standing infection exists.

Tuberculosis

Intestinal tuberculosis is usually a disease of the small bowel (see Chapter 5), but the colon may also be involved. As in the small bowel,

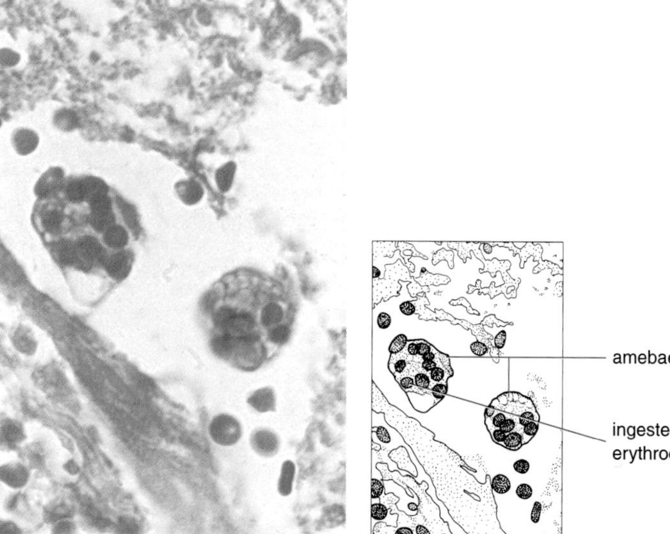

Fig. 6.30 Amebae with ingested erythrocytes. H&E stain (x 660). Courtesy of Dr S. Lucas.

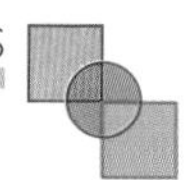

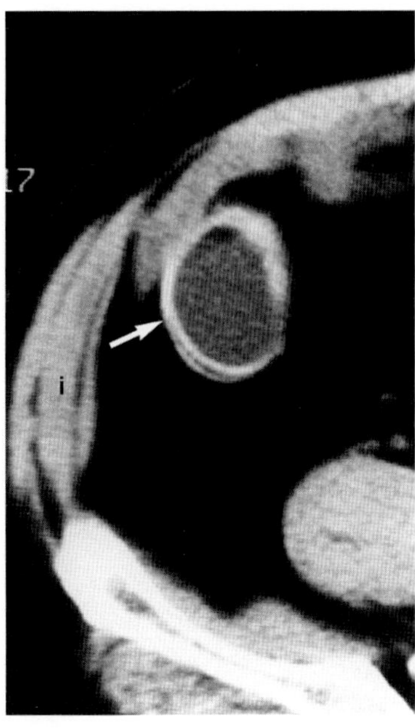

Fig. 6.31 CT demonstrating calcification of the wall in patient with chronic *Schistosoma japonicum* infection. Coned down view from an unenhanced CT shows a dense ring of calcium (arrow) in the ascending colon due to calcification of eggs embedded in the wall. Compare the density of the calcification with the soft tissue attenuation of the internal oblique muscle (i). (Reproduced with permission from reference 5, Fig. 3.)

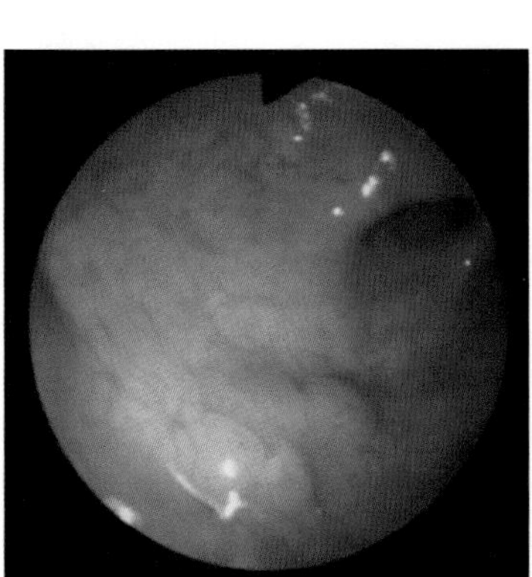

Fig. 6.32 Endoscopic appearance in chronic schistosomiasis showing irregularly thickened polypoidal mucosa.

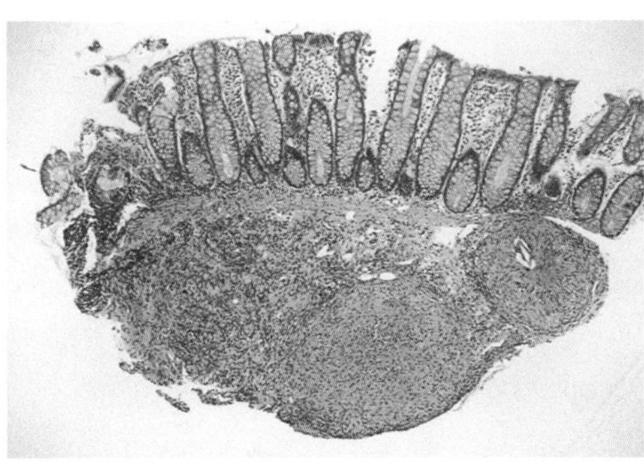

Fig. 6.33 Schistosomal colitis. Colonic biopsy in chronic colitis caused by *S. mansoni* showing large granulomas in the submucosa, the most superficial of which contains a remnant of a degenerating ovum.

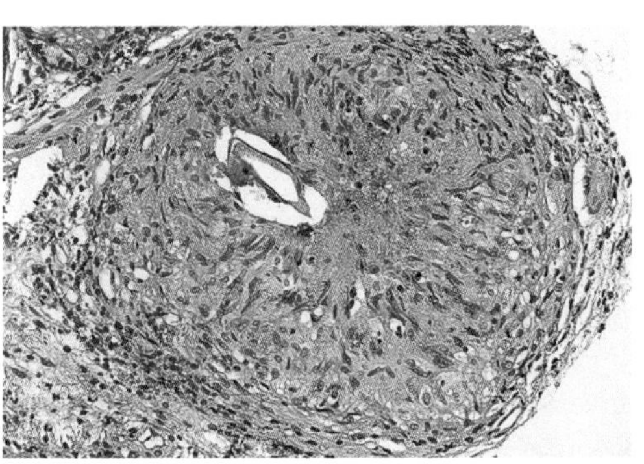

Fig. 6.34 Schistosomal colitis. High magnification of the submucosal granuloma containing the degenerating schistosome egg showing the residual shell of the ovum but no internal structure.

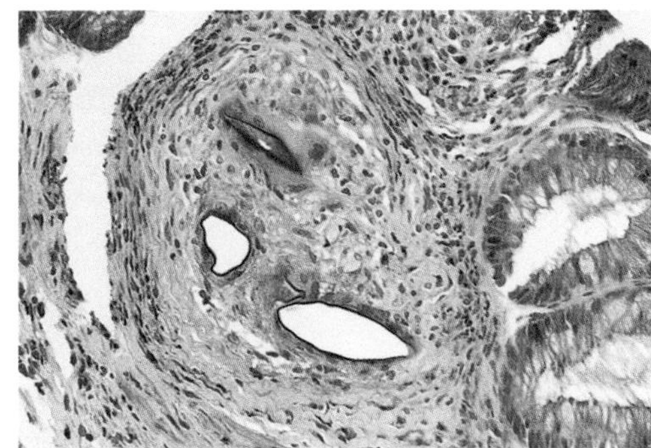

Fig. 6.35 A Ziehl–Neelsen stain of a granuloma showing the acid-fast staining and ovoid shape (although the lateral spine is not visible in this section) that are characteristic of the egg shells of *S. mansoni*.

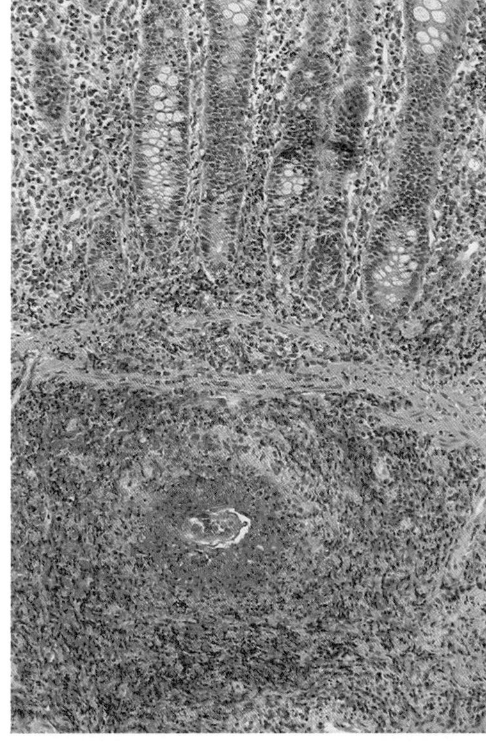

Fig. 6.36 High-magnification appearance of early schistosomal colitis characterized by massive eosinophilia associated with an ovum that contains an intact, viable miracidium.

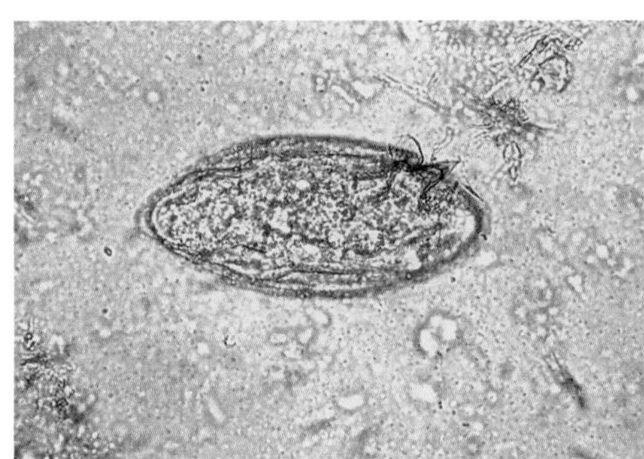

Fig. 6.37 *Schistosoma mansoni* ovum. Stool specimen showing an ovum of *Schistosoma mansoni* with the lateral spine that distinguishes it from the ova of other schistosomal species.

the disease may be hypertrophic, ulcerative, or a combination of both. Non-specific lower abdominal symptoms result, sometimes with diarrhea, but only occasionally with the passage of blood. A mass may be felt in the right iliac fossa, the commonest site involved being the cecum, often in continuity with ileal involvement. The radiological appearance may be non-specific and easily confused with those of Crohn's disease. Characteristics pointing towards tuberculosis include the circumferential plane of ulceration (Figs 6.38, 6.39), annular strictures sharply demarcated from normal bowel (Figs 6.38, 6.40, 6.41), a conically contracted cecum (Fig. 6.40) and hypertrophic masses (Fig. 6.42). (See also Chapter 5.) Unless there is a confident diagnosis from laboratory testing (e.g. PCR), endoscopy to obtain

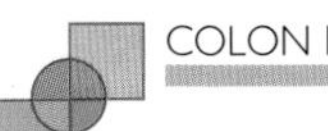

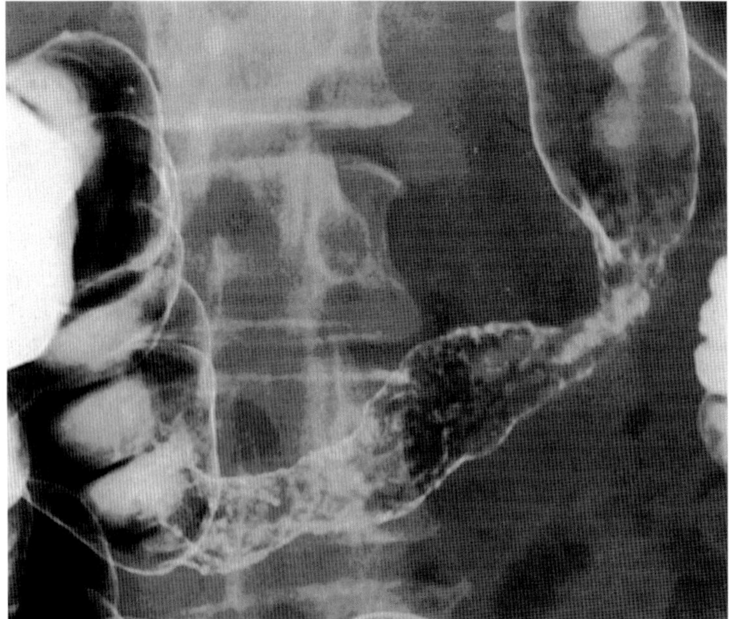

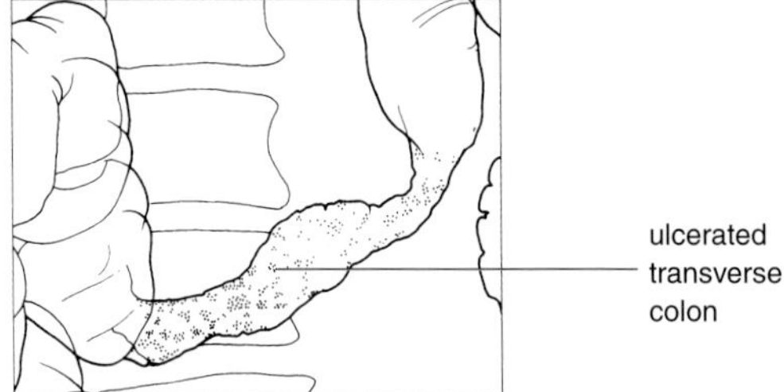

Fig. 6.38 Barium enema in tuberculous colitis showing a well-demarcated stricture in the mid-transverse colon with confluent superficial ulceration.

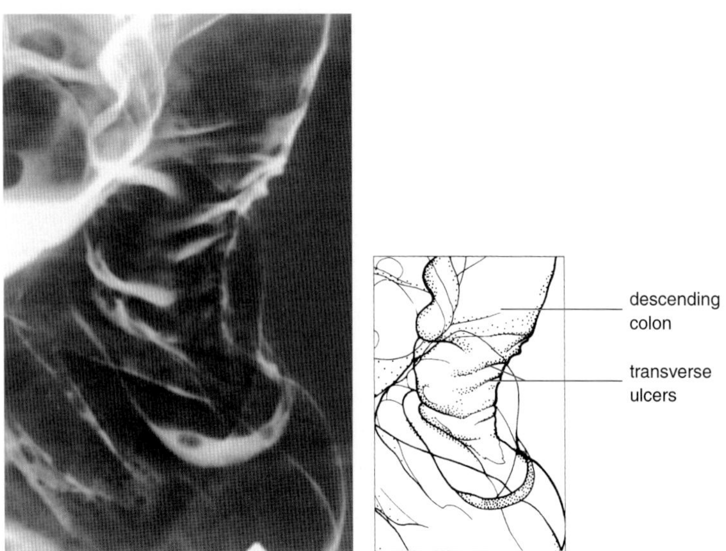

Fig. 6.39 Tuberculous transverse ulceration in the proximal descending colon.

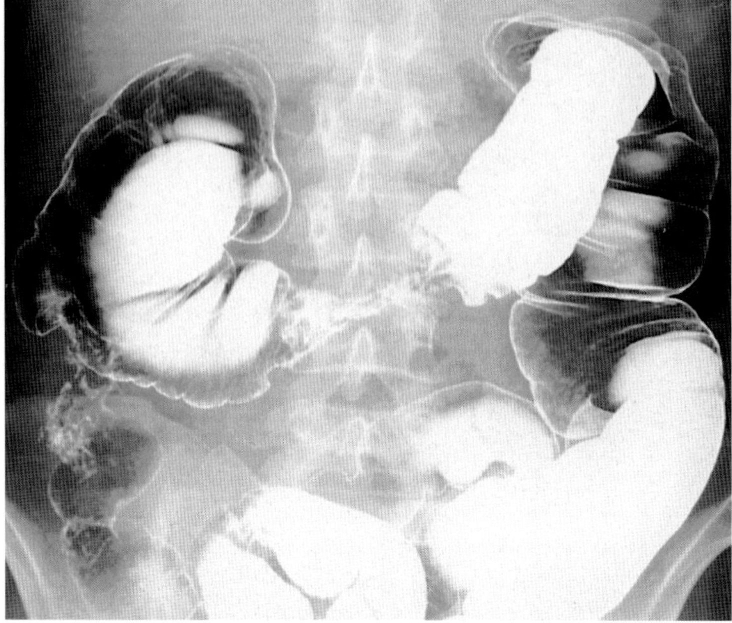

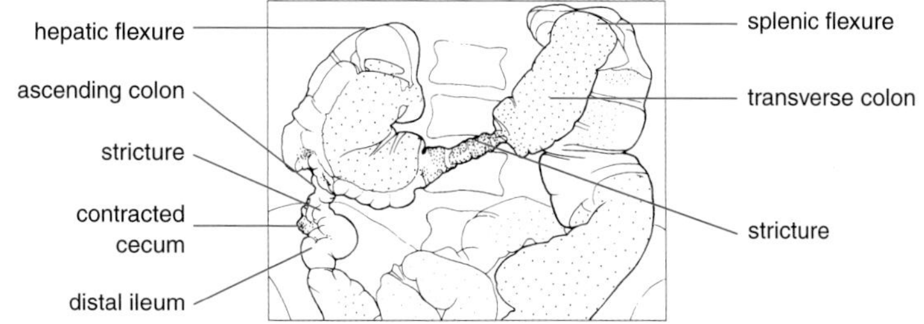

Fig. 6.40 Barium enema showing tuberculous stricturing in the transverse and ascending colon.

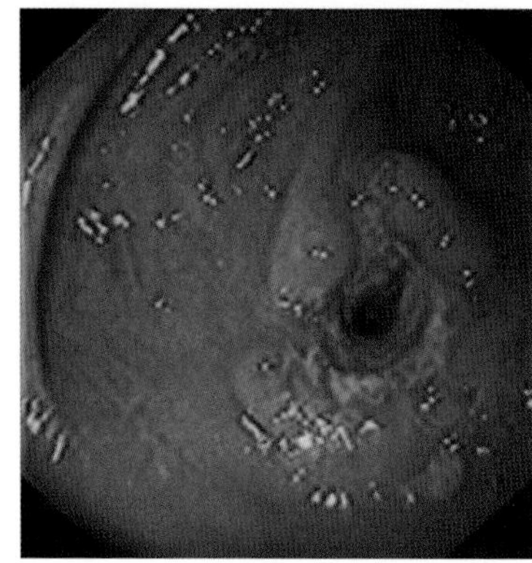

Fig. 6.41 Endoscopic view of tuberculous stricture with essentially normal adjacent tissue.

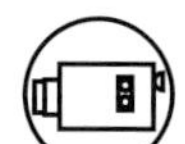

samples for histology and microbiology will be necessary (Figs 6.41, 6.43, 6.44). Full thickness biopsy requiring a surgical approach should not normally be necessary when the colon is known to be abnormal, but diagnosis may still depend on the acquisition of a peritoneal tubercle. The pathology is comparable to that in the small bowel (Figs 6.45, 6.46; see also Chapter 5). Diagnostic trials of anti-tuberculous therapy still have a place in the most difficult cases.

Actinomycosis

Actinomycosis is a rare condition caused by the fungus *Actinomyces israelii*, which is a normal oral commensal. Escape of actinomycetes from a ruptured appendix is the commonest route to infection, which therefore tends to be of the ileocecal region. Characteristically, there is a chronic inflammatory mass with induration, stricturing, and sinus formation; although marked necrosis and fibrosis occur frank peritonitis is rare. After the ileocecal region, the rectum is the most likely site to be involved. The imaging is rarely diagnostic, but at microscopy, a tangled mass of hyphae with peripherally arranged club-shaped bodies will be seen (Fig. 6.47). However, the organism may be present without causing inflammation and thus be an incidental finding; it is conventional to require an associated inflammatory reaction before considering it to be pathogenic

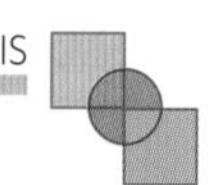

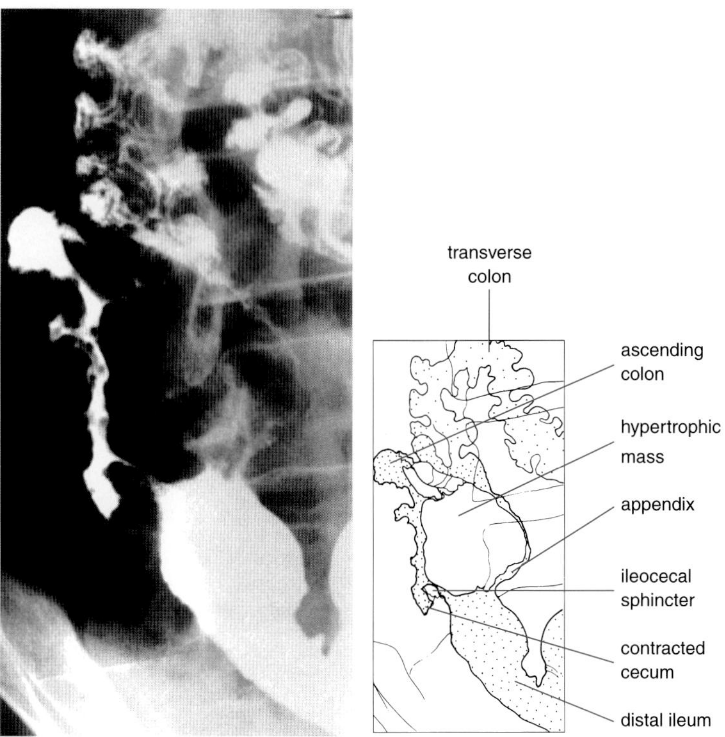

Fig. 6.42 Barium enema in hypertrophic tuberculosis affecting mainly the ascending colon in a 32-year-old Indian presenting with a large right iliac fossa mass.

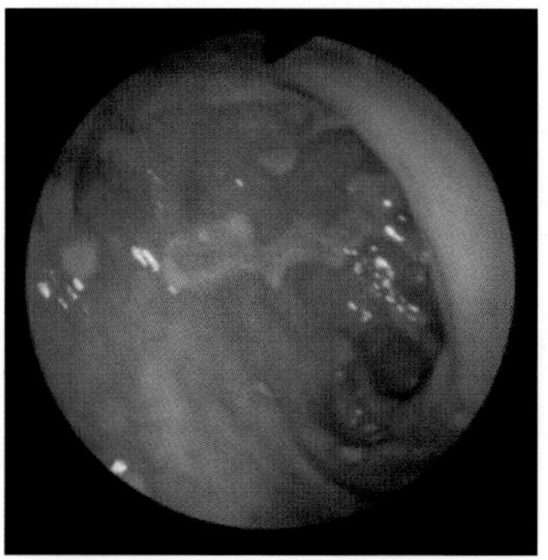

Fig. 6.43 Colonoscopic appearance of tuberculous ulceration.

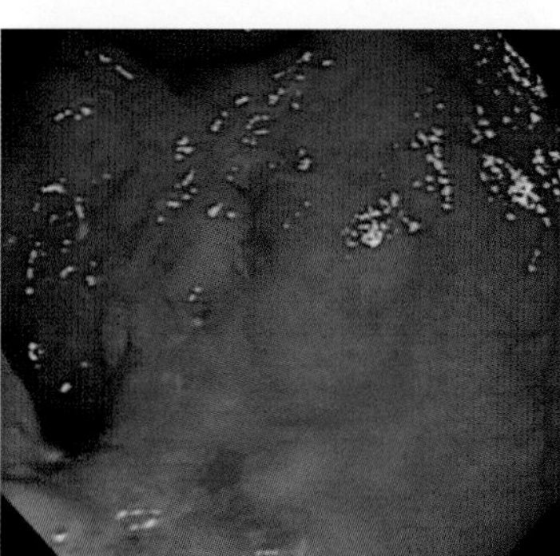

Fig. 6.44 Characteristic cecal tuberculosis.

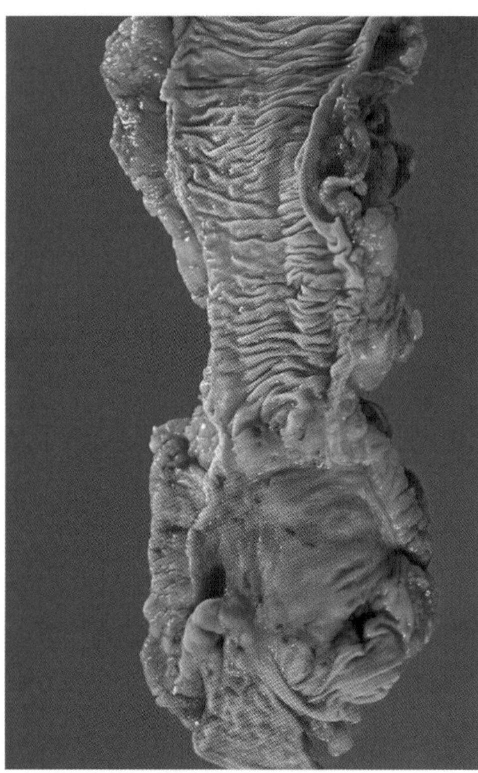

Fig. 6.45 Macroscopic appearance of ileocecal tuberculosis showing thickened, flattened mucosa and small hemorrhagic ulcers in the cecum.

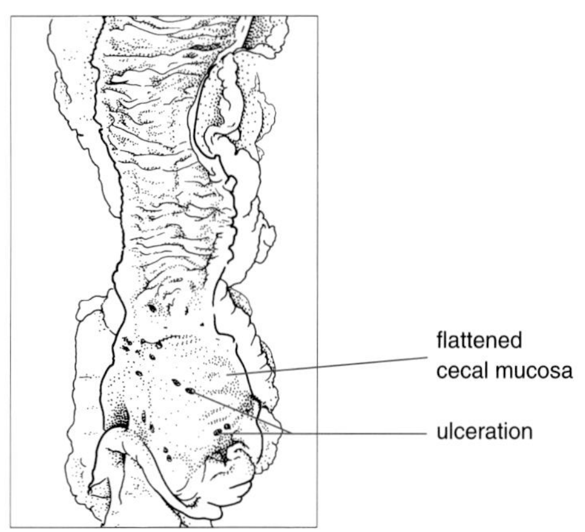

Chagas' disease

Chagas' disease is caused by *Trypanosoma cruzi* infection; the principal gastrointestinal sites affected are the esophagus (see Chapter 1) and the colon. The parasite is carried by the reduviid bug, *Triatoma magistus* (Fig. 6.48), which infects by biting its victim, thereby allowing parasites from its feces to penetrate the skin. The disease is endemic in parts of Central and South America and the southern United States. Disordered gut motor activity is a feature of patients with Chagas' disease, and colonic involvement leads to the development of megacolon proximal to a distal aganglionic segment of variable length (Fig. 6.49), and to symptoms of constipation. The resultant megacolon and associated chronic constipation is occasionally responsible for small bowel dilatation and aperistalsis, but the small bowel is not itself involved directly. It is thought that the parasite releases a neurotoxin specific to ganglion cells of the myenteric plexus. The interstitial cells of Cajal are thought to modulate gut motility, and their density in Chagasic megacolon is reduced in comparison to normal colonic tissue in the longitudinal muscle layer, the intermuscular plane, and the circular muscle layer, probably causally. The diagnosis is usually prompted by the geographical context.

Cytomegalovirus colitis

CMV very rarely causes symptomatic colitis in immunocompetent people, but in the severely immunosuppressed it can be a major and life-threatening problem, treatment of which is difficult. The virus probably causes an ischemic insult to the bowel, and deep, penetrating ulcers and perforation may result. The plain radiograph often shows dilatation, and there may be intramural gas (Fig. 6.50); at CT, thickening of the bowel wall may be dramatic (Fig. 6.51).

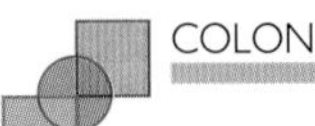

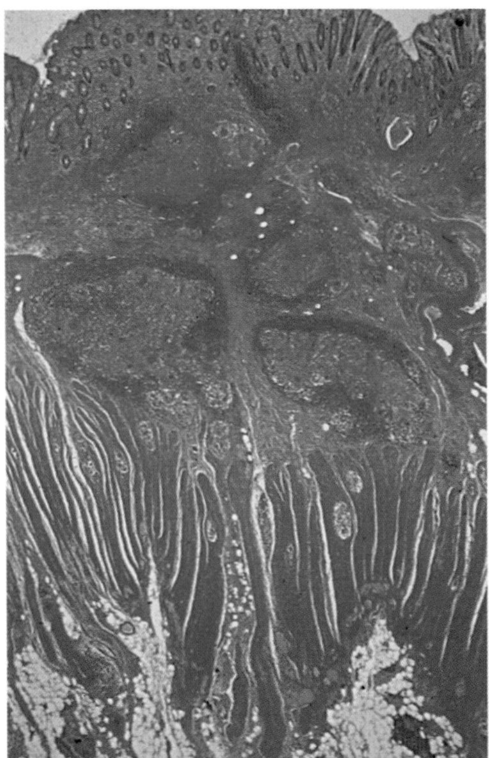

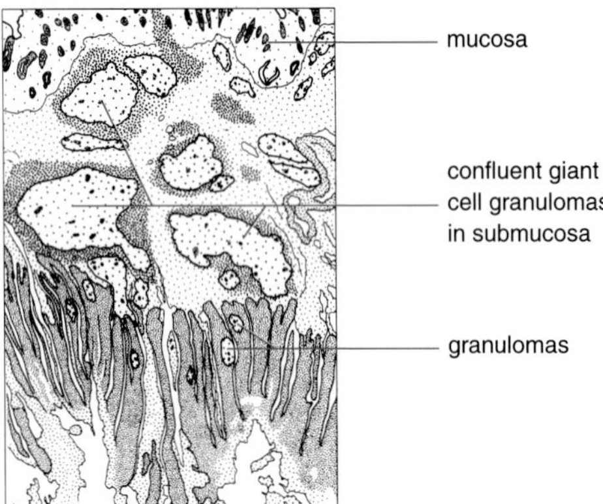

■ **Fig. 6.46** Histological appearance in colonic tuberculosis with large confluent granulomas extending into the muscle wall. The granulomas are larger than those seen in Crohn's colitis.

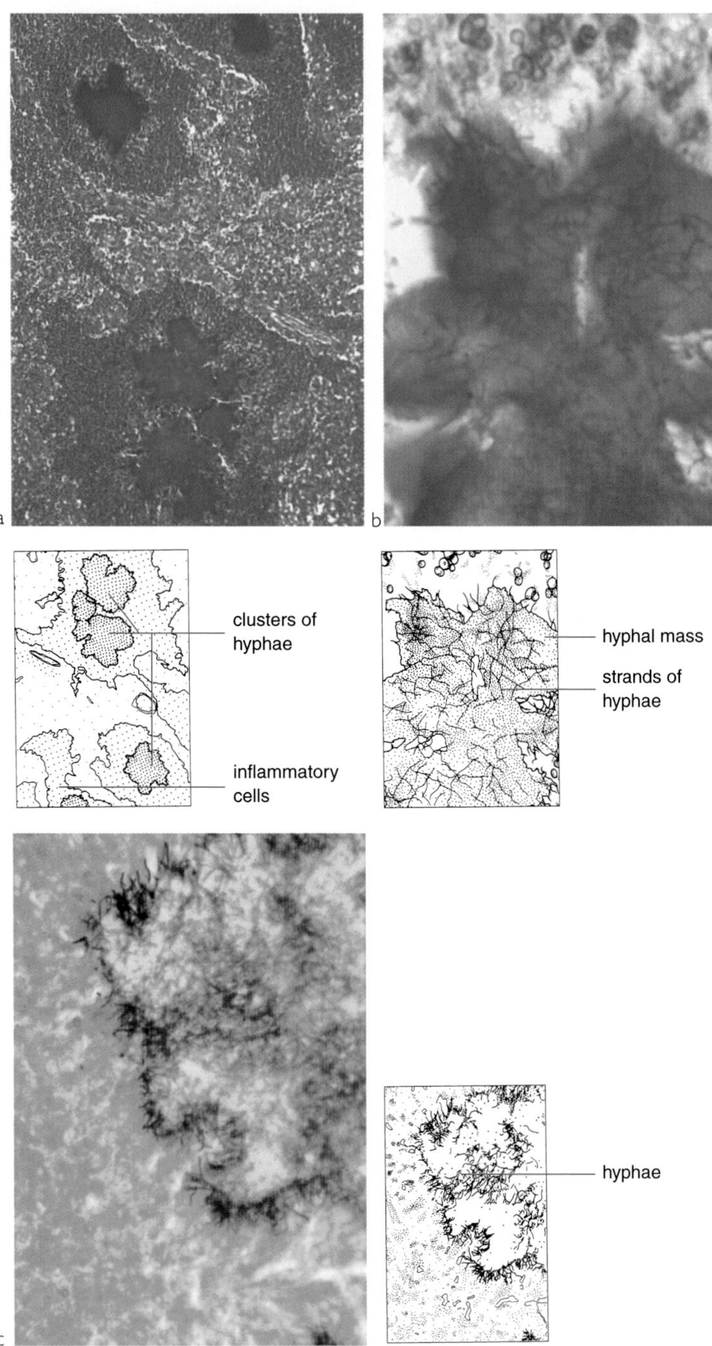

■ **Fig. 6.47** The histology of actinomycosis. (a) Basophilic clusters of hyphae (H&E stain (x 20)); (b) Periodic acid-Schiff reagent stains the actinomycetes magenta, with hyphae just visible at the margins of the colony (x 180); (c) with the Gomori–Grocott stain, the hyphae appear black (x 320).

Sigmoidoscopy and colonoscopy may reveal only non-specific inflammation, but, as in the esophagus (see Chapter 1), there may be highly suggestive almost malignant-looking ulcers (Fig. 6.52). Biopsies show inflammation and CMV inclusion bodies (Figs 6.53, 6.54). Because (like other herpes viruses) CMV may be an innocent bystander, it is conventional to diagnose CMV colitis only when viral inclusions are associated with an inflammatory response. This is a particular issue in the patient with ulcerative colitis and CMV in whom there is debate as to the magnitude of the role of the virus.

PSEUDOMEMBRANOUS COLITIS

The formation of a pseudomembrane on the colonic mucosa is a non-specific event which can occur in such diverse circumstances as mercury poisoning, intestinal ischemia, or bronchopneumonia, but is commonest in antibiotic-associated colitis (Figs 6.55–6.58). In about one third of patients, antibiotics will have been discontinued before the onset of symptoms. No particular group of antibodies seems uniquely implicated, but cephalosporins are probably the most important numerically; even metronidazole, which is often used in its treatment, can be to blame. Those unwell with other conditions

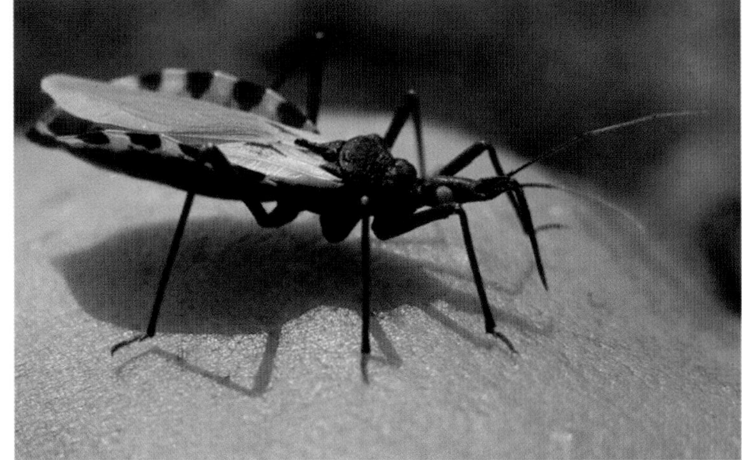

■ **Fig. 6.48** Reduviid bug. Courtesy of Dr W. Petana.

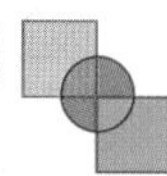

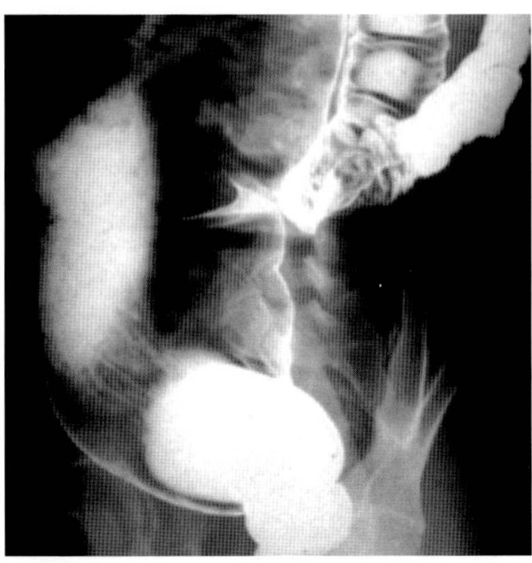

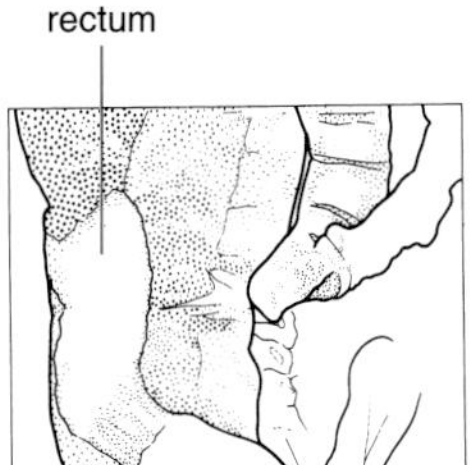

Fig. 6.49 Barium enema in Chagas' disease showing megacolon. Courtesy of Professor A. Habr-Gama.

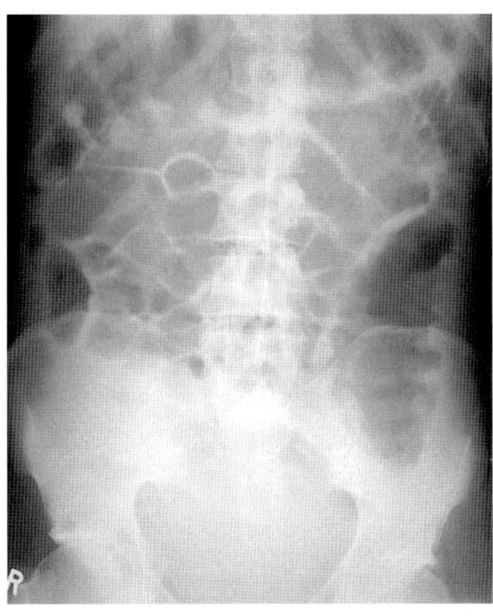

Fig. 6.50 Plain abdominal radiograph in acute CMV colitis. There is thickening of the colonic wall particularly in the transverse colon, and some degree of dilatation of both small and large bowel.

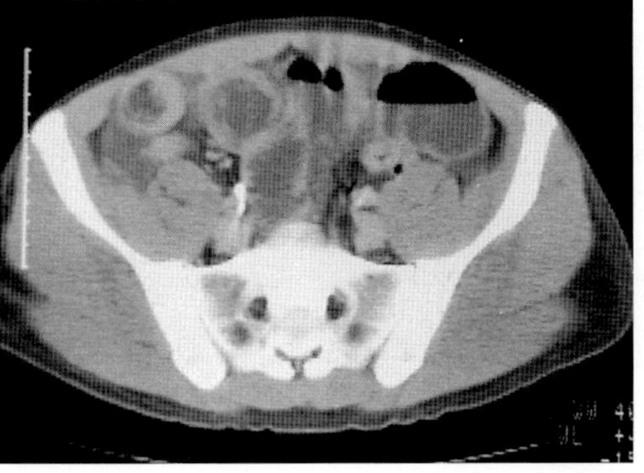

Fig. 6.51 CT scan in CMV colitis showing gross thickening of the colonic wall. Courtesy of Dr M. McCarty.

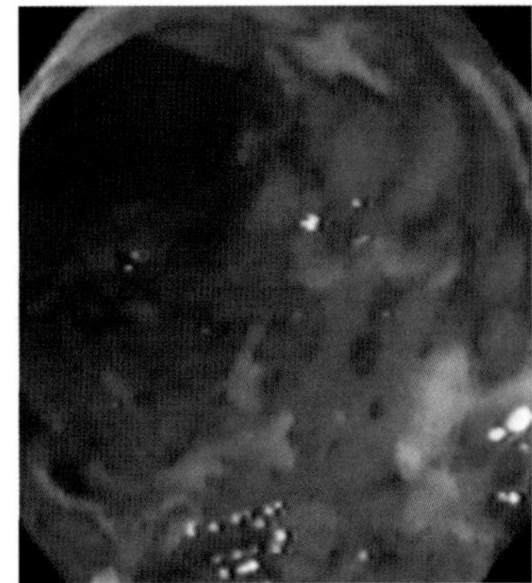

Fig. 6.52 Colonoscopic appearance of severe ulceration caused by CMV.

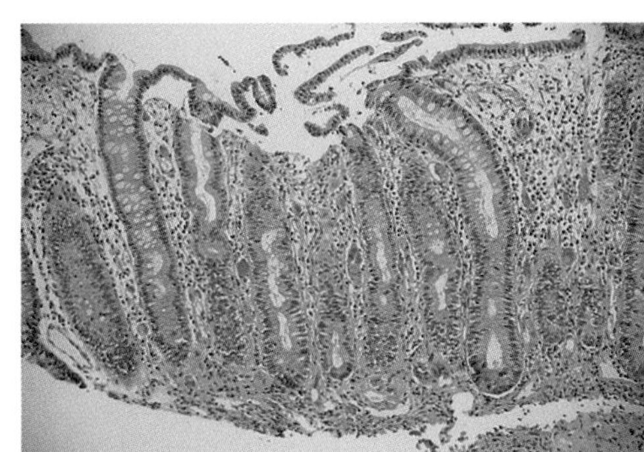

Fig. 6.53 CMV colitis. Mucosal biopsy showing epithelial injury with flattening of the cells, detachment from the basement membrane and reactive hyperplasia (elongation) of the glands accompanied by a moderate stromal inflammatory infiltrate.

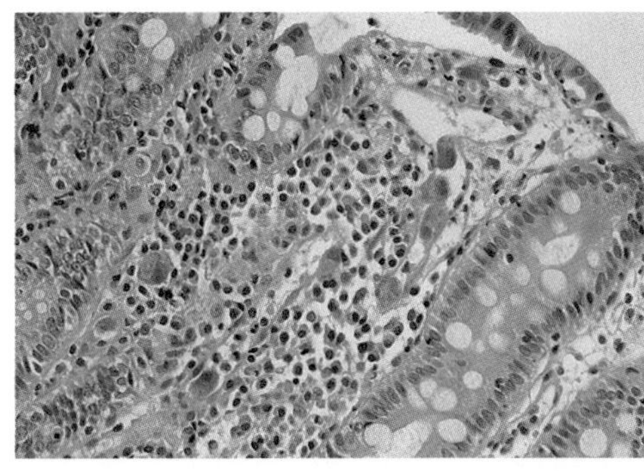

Fig. 6.54 High magnification of the colonic mucosa showing the typical massive enlargement of CMV-infected endothelial cells in the lamina propria; infected cells show both amphophilic intranuclear inclusions and granular cytoplasm inclusions.

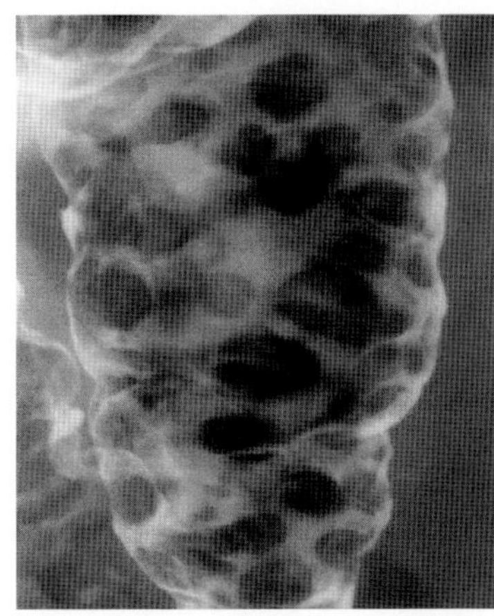

Fig. 6.55 Double-contrast barium enema in *C. difficile* colitis. Numerous radiolucent plaque-like elevations are seen in the descending colon.

and the elderly are most at risk, perhaps through a necessary disorder of the background gut microflora. Then, *Clostridium difficile* (which can be a commensal) becomes the predominant causative agent. *C. difficile* secretes at least three heat-labile toxins, and although toxins A, B, and C all cause fluid accumulation in the small intestine, and A and C cause epithelial cell shedding, only toxin A causes severe necrosis and bleeding (Fig. 6.59). Patients with pseudomembranous

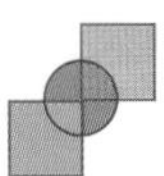

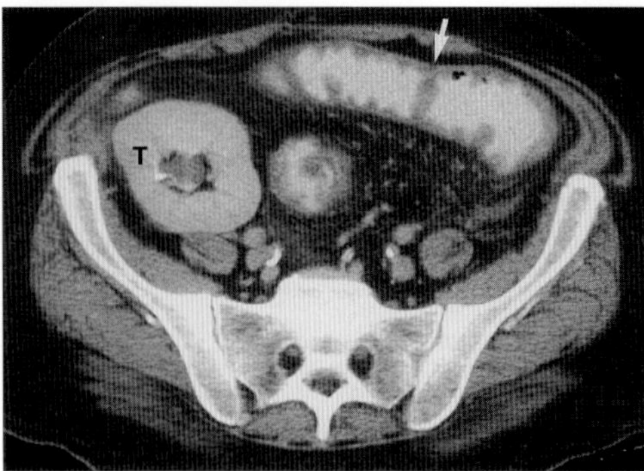

■ **Fig. 6.56** CT demonstrating thickened wall and interhaustral folds (arrow) in patient with *C. difficile* colitis. A renal transplant (T) is seen in the upper right pelvis.

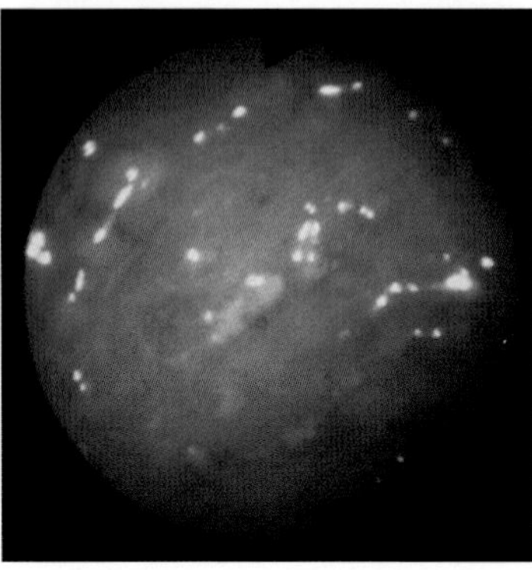

■ **Fig. 6.57** Colonoscopic appearance of mild pseudomembranous colitis. Note the yellowish pseudomembranes contrasting with the reddened colonic mucosa.

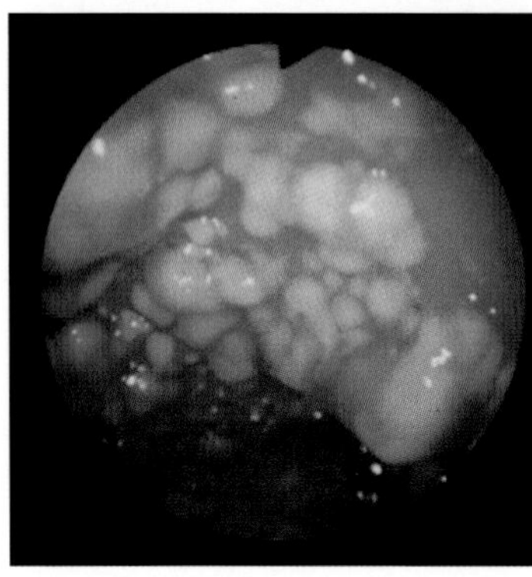

■ **Fig. 6.58** Severe pseudomembranous colitis with marked pseudomembrane formation.

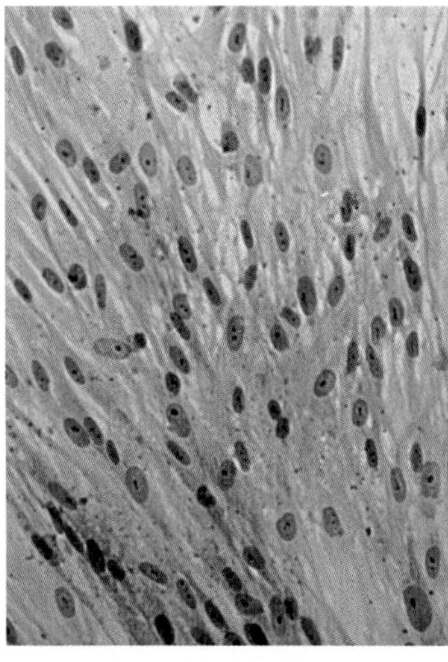

a b

■ **Fig. 6.59** Demonstration of the cytopathic action of *Clostridium difficile* toxin. Normal lung tissue growing on culture medium (a) has its fibroblasts regularly aligned, whereas the culture to which toxin has been added (b) shows gross disruption and marked nuclear changes.

colitis are often pyrexial, with profuse diarrhea, abdominal cramping and lower abdominal tenderness. The diarrhea is usually free of blood or mucus, except in extreme cases, when even perforation may occur.

Plain radiographs of the abdomen may show an irregular mucosal outline (Fig. 6.60) and blunting of edematous haustra, but this, like the barium enema appearance, is non-specific. The diagnosis is usually considered confirmed by the presence of *C. difficile* toxin. A firm macroscopic or histological diagnosis depends on the presence of pseudomembranes, but these may be present only too proximally for rigid sigmoidoscopic access. The pseudomembrane is formed by the coalescence of a characteristic series of small yellow plaques (Figs 6.61–6.63; see also Figs 6.57, 6.58), the appearances of which become progressively less diagnostic with increasing severity. On biopsy, there are multiple discrete foci or disrupted crypts, and the spray of cellular debris and inflammatory cells originating from the

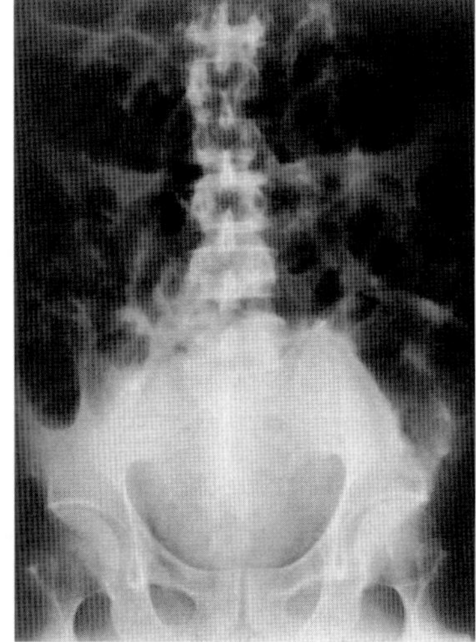

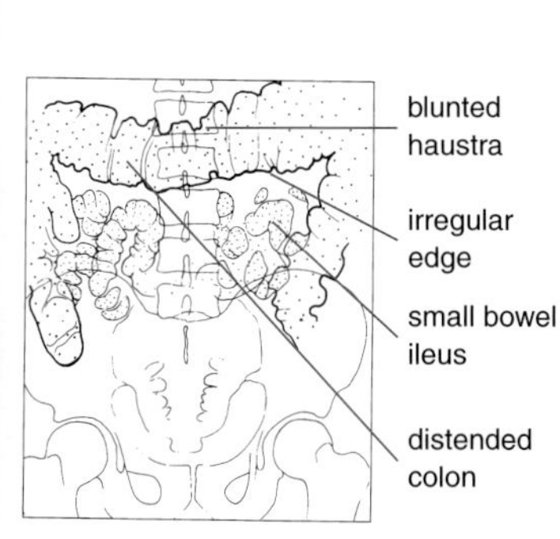

■ **Fig. 6.60** Plain abdominal radiograph in pseudomembranous colitis.

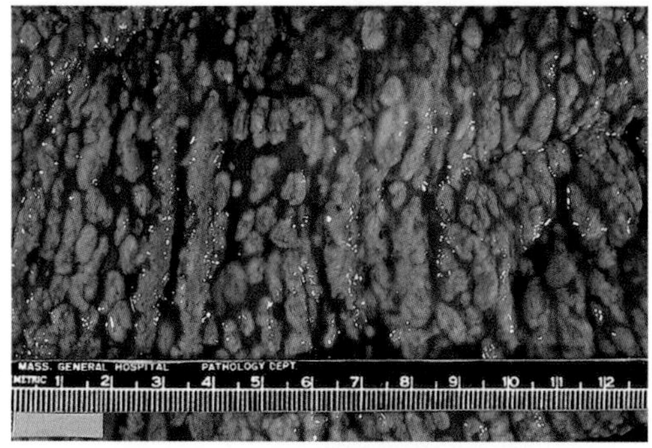

■ **Fig. 6.61** Macroscopic appearance of the colonic mucosa in the late plaque-forming stage of antibiotic-associated *Clostridium difficile* pseudomembranous colitis.

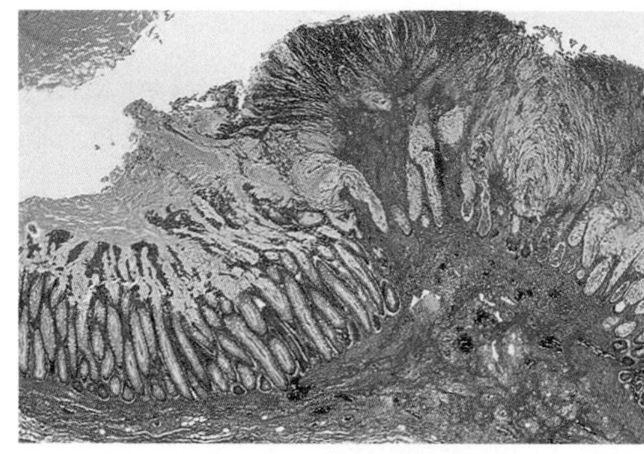

■ **Fig. 6.62** Antibiotic-associated *Clostridium difficile* pseudomembranous colitis. Microscopic view of the colonic mucosa showing the focality of the destructive lesions caused by the organisms' toxin-production. Typically, during the evolving stages of the disease, normal unaffected mucosa is seen between foci of injury (typically six to ten glands abreast).

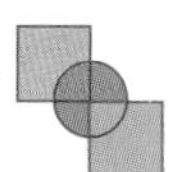

crypt surface which forms the pseudomembrane may give the appearance of an erupting volcano (Figs 6.62, 6.63). Between such foci, the intervening mucosa is virtually normal.

NECROTIZING ENTEROCOLITIS

Necrotizing enterocolitis (NEC) is an important problem in neonatal intensive care units, usually affecting premature infants (>95% in those delivered at <37 weeks), and the average US annual incidence is around 0.7 cases per 1000 live births, but is higher in the urban poor. It usually occurs shortly after oral feeding commences, and although it is probable that it has an infective cause, fewer than half of affected infants have positive blood cultures. Protection from breast milk indicates that it is at least partly the result of immuno-deficiency. When microbiology is positive there is a predominance of Gram-negative enteric micro-organisms, and infections with *E. coli*, *Klebsiella*, *Enterobacter*, and *Clostridium* species are each strongly associated with elevated concentrations of endotoxin in stool filtrates. Clostridia are the most strongly associated with NEC disease. Staphylococcal infection is less strongly implicated than reported in the older literature. The clinical features include bloody diarrhea with systemic sepsis, and pneumatosis intestinalis on abdominal radiography (Fig. 6.64). Portal venous gas may be seen but this does not necessarily indicate a hopeless prognosis as it does in other situations. Nonetheless this is an important cause of widespread ischemia, which can lead to the need for massive intestinal resection; it is the commonest cause of intestinal failure in the neonatal period.

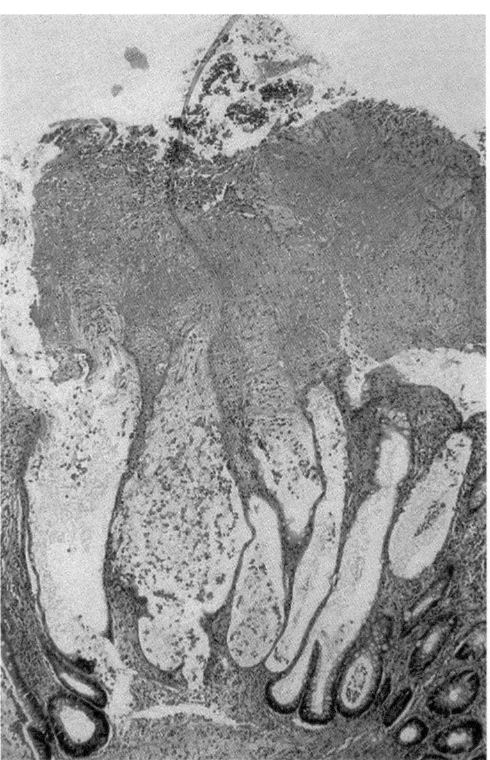

Fig. 6.63 Antibiotic-associated *Clostridium difficile* pseudomembranous colitis. Microscopic view of a single eruptive, necrobiotic ('volcanic') lesion showing the destruction of the superficial aspect of the glands with streaming of necrotic epithelium, neutrophils, and fibrin into the lumen creating a 'pseudomembranous' cap over the injured focus.

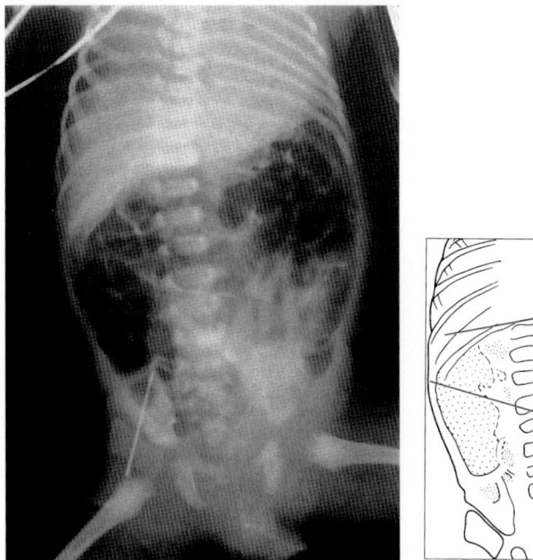

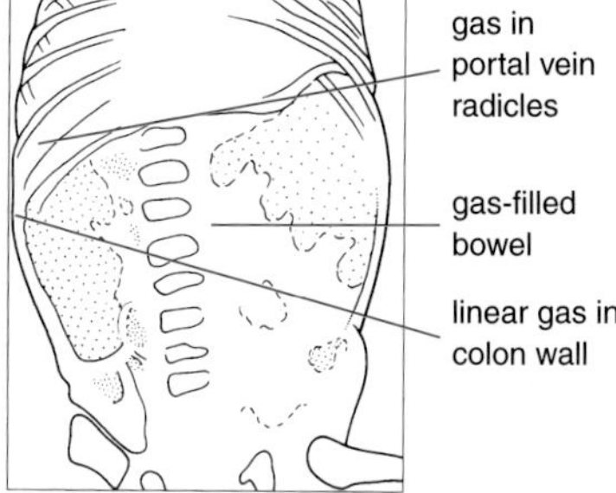

Fig. 6.64 Plain abdominal radiograph in an infant with necrotizing enterocolitis. The bowel is dilated with gas and there is pneumatosis intestinalis apparent at the right costal margin where there is a linear gas shadow in the colonic wall. There is also gas in the portal vein radicals.

CROHN'S COLITIS

The general manifestations of Crohn's disease are considered in Chapter 5, but in at least 40% of cases, the colon is overtly involved, and in these patients bloody diarrhea is proportionately more likely. Perianal disease is considered in Chapter 8.

The sigmoidoscopic appearance in Crohn's is often normal despite more proximal colonic involvement, but there may be small aphthous ulcers with normal intervening mucosa (Fig. 6.65), or more diffuse inflammatory changes, similar to those seen in ulcerative colitis (with granularity, contact bleeding, and ulceration). Colonoscopy will usually allow a more confident diagnosis, particularly when multiple and discrete shallow linear ulcers, cobblestoning, or clear-cut skip lesions are demonstrated (Figs 6.66–6.70).

As in the small bowel, radiological evidence of aphthoid ulceration (Figs 6.71–6.74), fissuring ulcers (Fig. 6.74), skip lesions, asymmetrical wall involvement, and the formation of strictures (Fig. 6.75), and post inflammatory polyps (Figs 6.76, 6.77) point to a diagnosis of Crohn's disease. Rectal sparing is frequent and only infrequently is there a total colitis 'in continuity.'

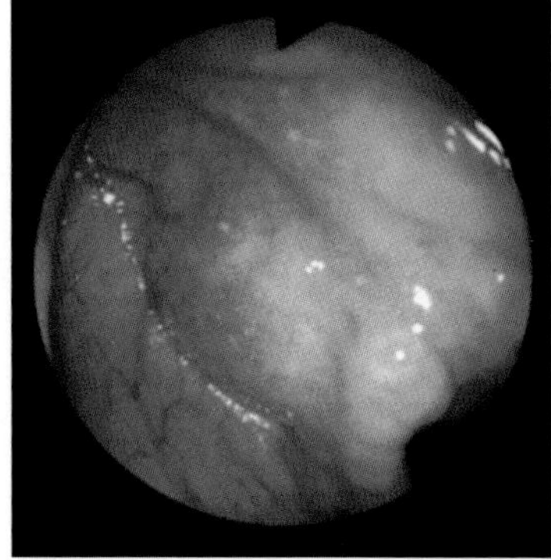

Fig. 6.65 Discrete aphthoid lesions in the rectum in Crohn's disease.

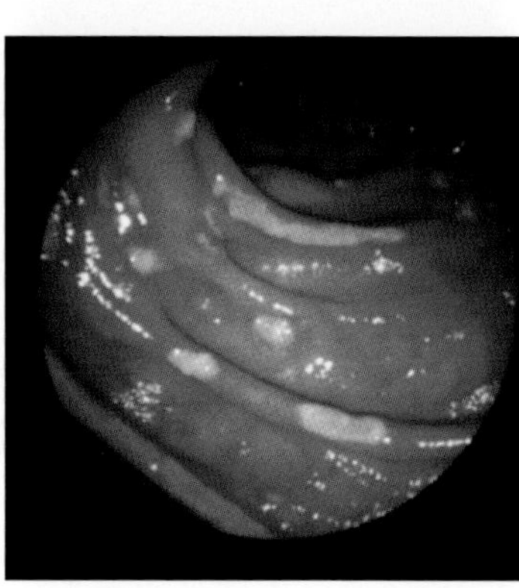

Fig. 6.66 Multiple aphthoid ulcers at colonoscopy.

Complicating fistulae are very characteristic of advanced Crohn's (Figs 6.78–6.81), but toxic dilatation is much less common than in uncontrolled ulcerative colitis. Colitis-associated colorectal carcinoma probably occurs to a similar frequency to that in long-standing extensive ulcerative colitis (see below) when a major proportion of the colon has been involved by Crohn's for more than 10–15 years. Following resolution of acute episodes, post-inflammatory polyps (Figs 6.76, 6.77) and marked scarring deformity may be seen (Fig. 6.82), and when fibrous strictures are left without apparent inflammation, balloon dilatation may be indicated to relieve obstructive symptoms (Fig. 6.83).

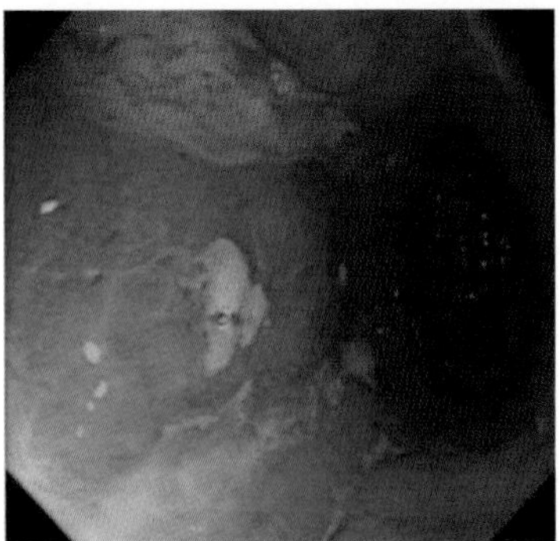

Fig. 6.67 Characteristic linear ulcers in Crohn's colitis.

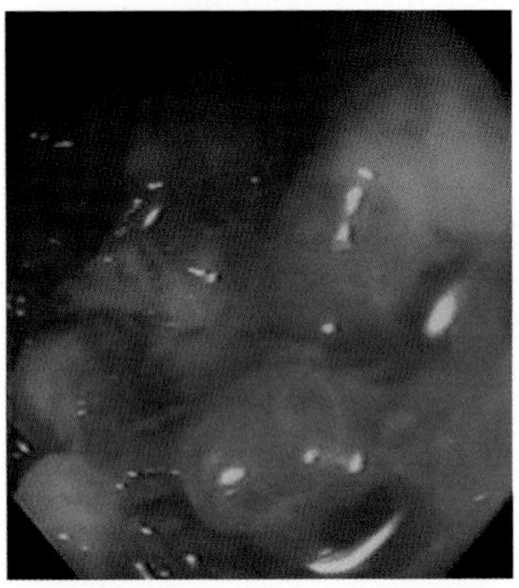

Fig. 6.68 Characteristic cobblestoning with relatively little surface ulceration.

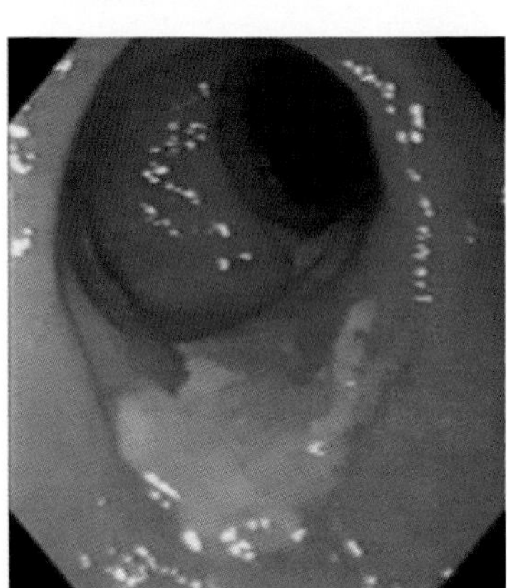

Fig. 6.69 Large Crohn's disease ulcer.

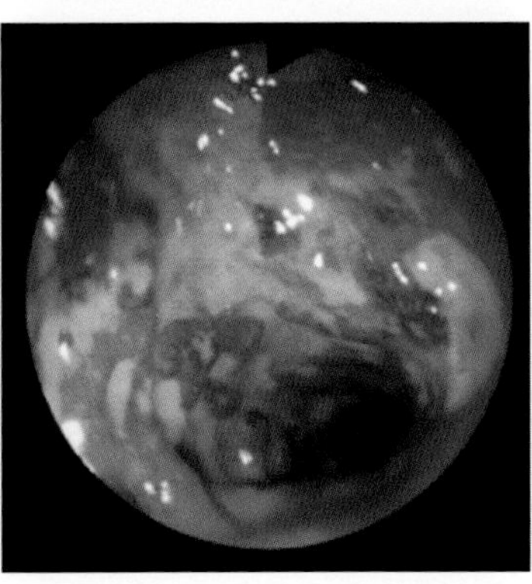

Fig. 6.70 Confluent, severe ulceration in Crohn's disease.

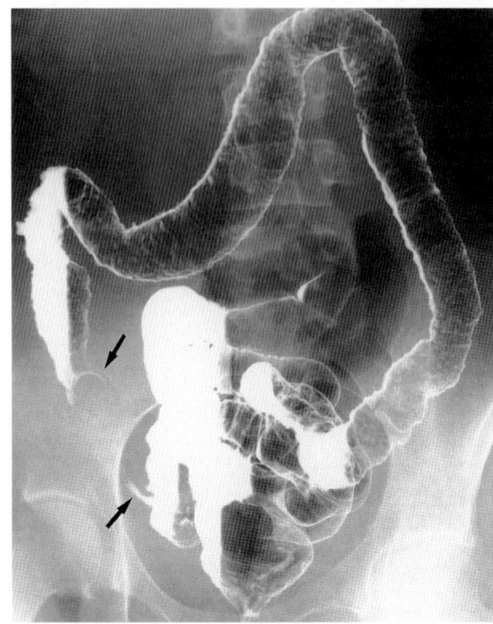

Fig. 6.71. Double-contrast barium enema demonstrating Crohn's disease. The terminal ileum is narrowed (arrows). Innumerable aphthoid ulcers are seen in the ascending, transverse and descending colon. The rectum has a normal-smooth mucosa. (Reproduced with permission from reference 2, Fig. 70.)

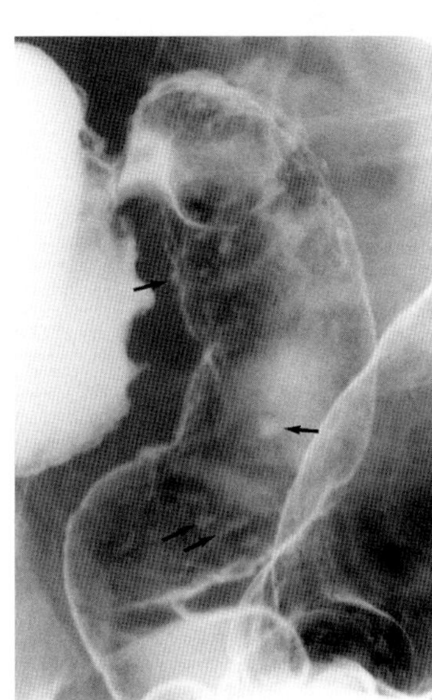

Fig. 6.72 Double-contrast barium enema in Crohn's disease. Numerous aphthoid ulcers are manifested as punctate and linear barium collections surrounded by radiolucent halos (black arrows). (Reproduced with permission from reference 4, Fig. 8.)

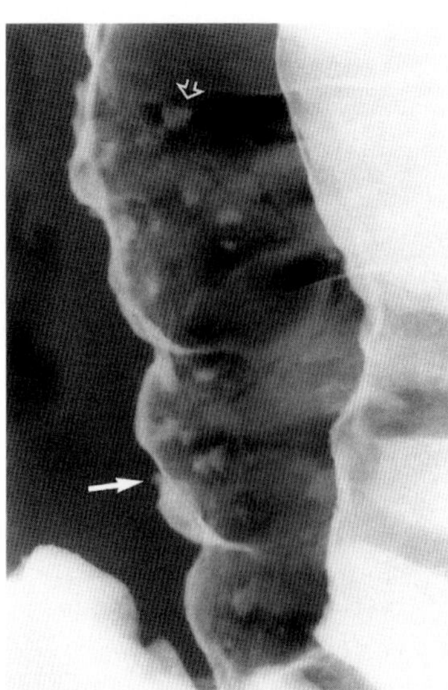

Fig. 6.73 Double-contrast barium enema demonstrating aphthoid ulcers in a patient with Crohn's disease. Small, barium-filled collections are surrounded by radiolucent halos (representative ulcer seen *en face* identified by open arrow). In profile, aphthoid ulcers are punctate collections of barium (arrow) surrounded by a mound of edema. The mucosa between ulcers is smooth and normal. (Reproduced with permission from reference 2, Fig. 30.)

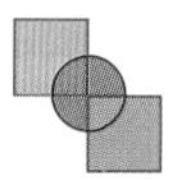

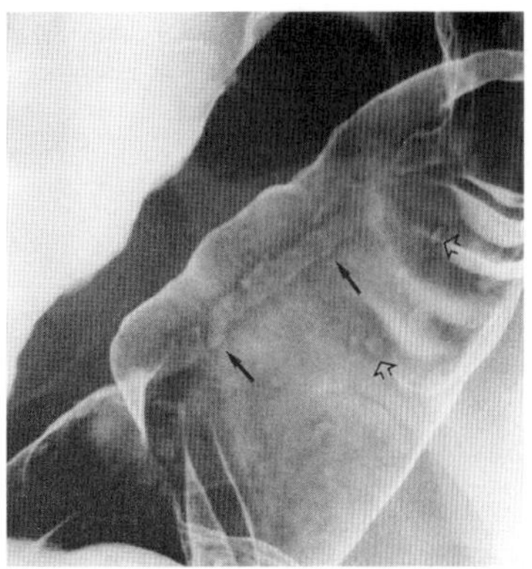

Fig 6.74 Double-contrast barium enema in Crohn's disease. A long ulcer is manifest as a shallow, longitudinal barium collection surrounded by a radiolucent edge (arrows). Many small aphthoid ulcers are also seen (open arrows). (Reproduced with permission from reference 2, Fig. 36).

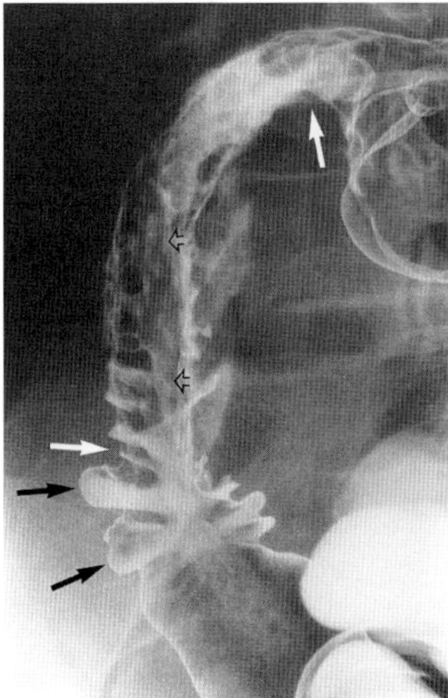

Fig. 6.75 Double-contrast barium enema in a patient with Crohn's disease. Focal narrowing of the sigmoid colon (white arrows) reflects the transmural inflammatory process. A long shallow ulcer (open arrows) is seen *en face*. The mucosa is focally nodular. Sacculations are seen distally (black arrows). (Reproduced with permission from reference 2, Fig. 49.)

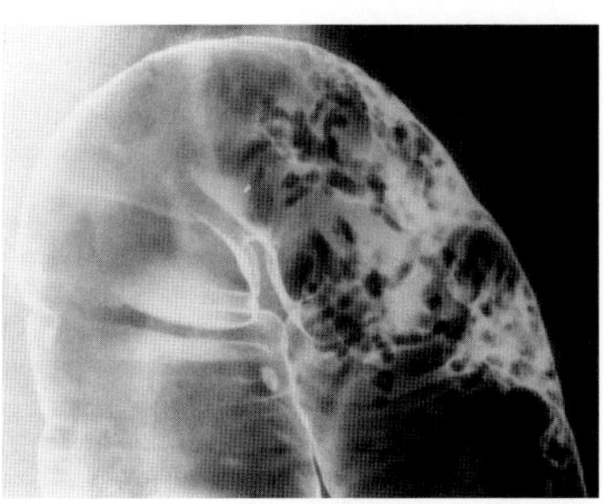

Fig. 6.76 Filiform polyps in patient with Crohn's colitis. Numerous tubular radiolucent filling defects are seen in the splenic flexure.

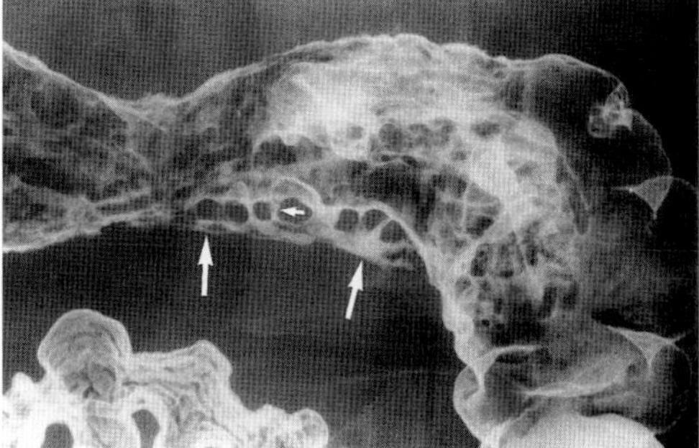

Fig. 6.77 Double-contrast barium enema in a patient with Crohn's disease. Barium fills a long pericolonic track (arrows) adjacent to the splenic flexure. Tiny fissures (one fissure identified by small arrow) extend to the pericolonic track. The colonic mucosa is nodular and inflammatory polyps are seen. (Reproduced with permission from reference 2, Fig. 52.)

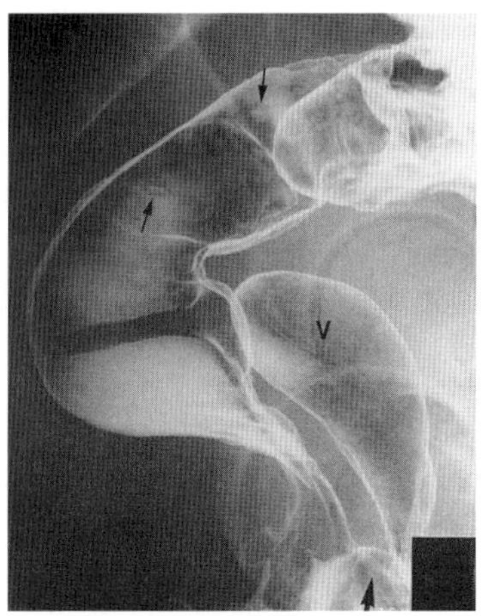

Fig. 6.78 Double-contrast barium enema demonstrating anovaginal fistula in a patient with Crohn's disease. Numerous aphthoid ulcers (thin arrows) are seen in the rectum. Barium outlines a fistula (thick arrow) from the proximal anal canal to the vagina. The vagina (V) is distended by air insufflated into the rectum. (Reproduced with permission from reference 2, Fig. 55.)

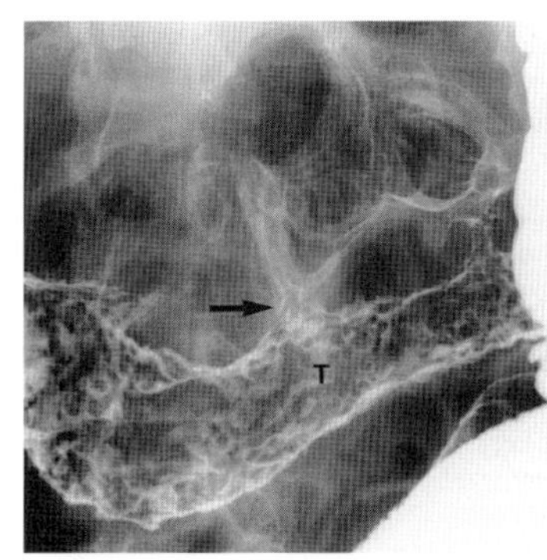

Fig. 6.79 Double-contrast barium enema demonstrating colo-enteric fistula in Crohn's disease. The transverse colon (T) has a tubular configuration and is covered by a diffusely abnormal mucosa. A fistula (arrow) results in barium and air entering a small bowel loop. (Reproduced with permission from reference 2, Fig. 59.)

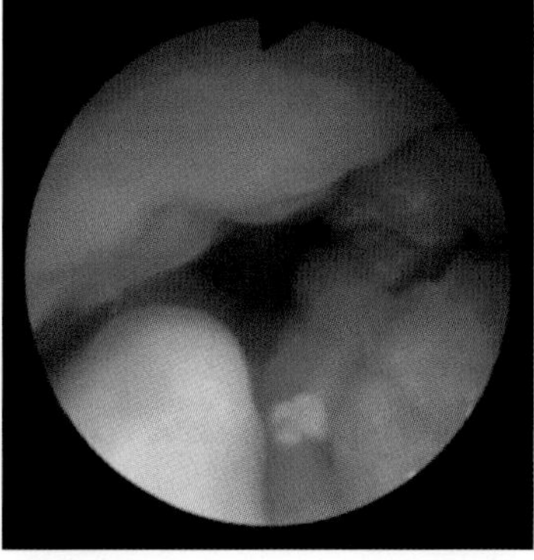

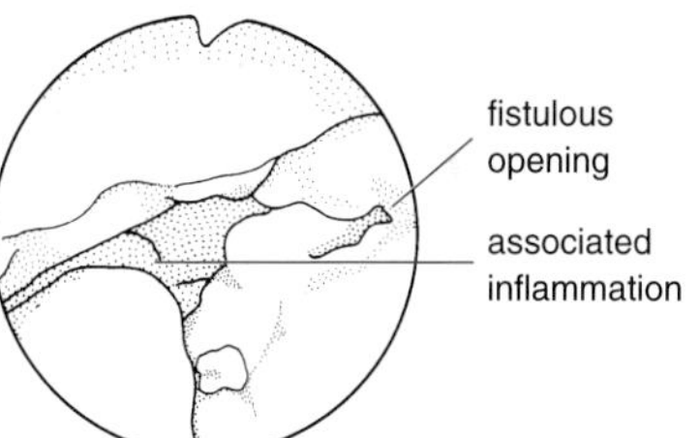

Fig. 6.80 Colonoscopic appearance of an internal fistula at the site of active inflammation, as is typical.

The macroscopic appearance of the large bowel may be dramatic in Crohn's disease (Figs 6.84–6.87). Histologically, the aphthoid ulcers are found to represent tiny ulcerated lesions overlying lymphoid follicles (Fig. 6.88). The histology is generally similar to that seen in the small bowel (see Chapter 5) (Figs 6.89–6.92).

ULCERATIVE COLITIS

Ulcerative colitis is a chronic disorder of still unknown etiology, characterized by inflammation limited to the colonic mucosa, and by an intermittent, relapsing clinical course. It has a prevalence of around 0.1% in the West. It affects the rectum, and extends in continuity to involve a variable extent of the proximal colon, so that the patient may have proctitis alone, proctosigmoiditis, left-sided disease (usually defined as from the splenic flexure), or subtotal or total colitis. Endoscopic detection is more sensitive than radiological, and histological sampling still more so. It is therefore logical to

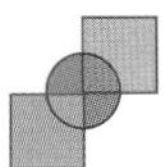

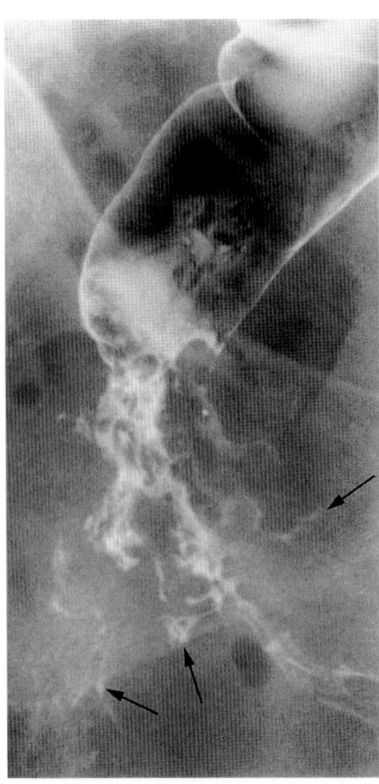

■ **Fig. 6.81** Double-contrast barium enema demonstrating distal rectal and anal Crohn's colitis. The distal rectum is narrowed and has a nodular mucosa. Several barium-filled tracks (arrows) extend deeply into perirectal and perianal tissue. (Reproduced with permission from reference 6, Fig. 28.)

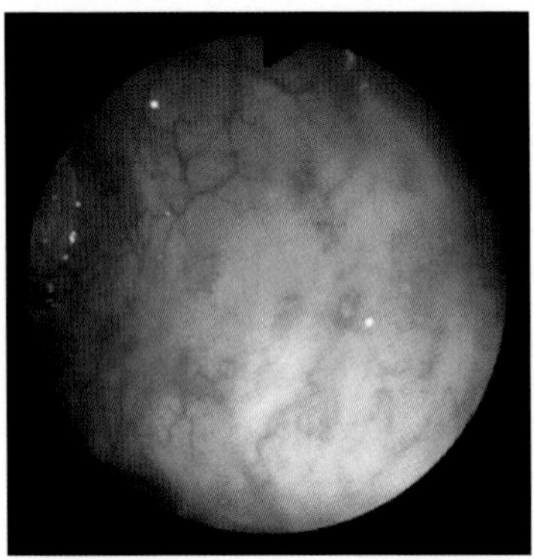

■ **Fig. 6.82** Widespread scarring (and several small aphthoid lesions) in a patient recovering from an acute exacerbation of Crohn's colitis.

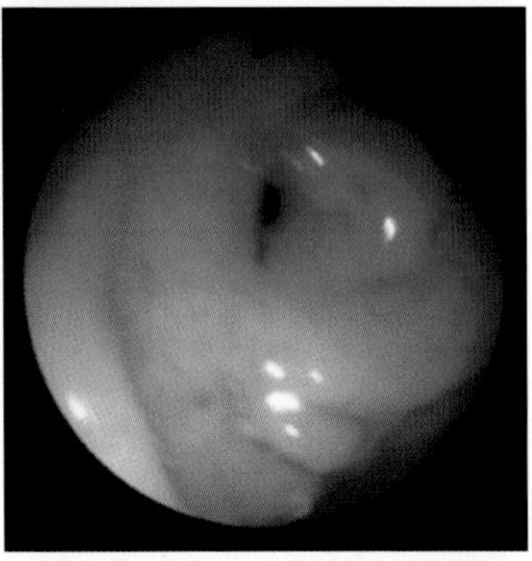

■ **Fig. 6.83** Tight fibrous stricture at the site of anastomosis in a patient with inactive Crohn's disease.

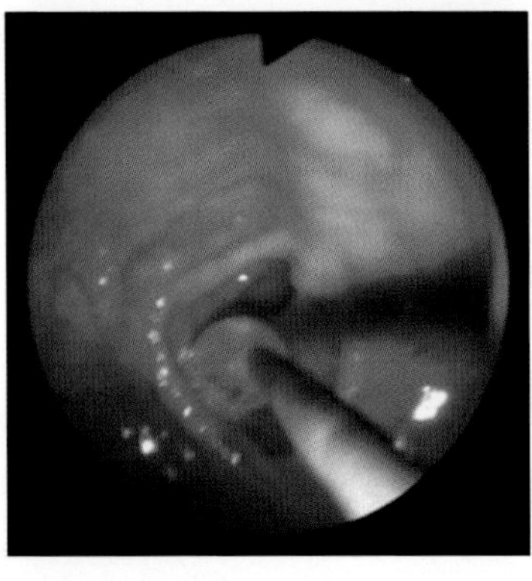

■ **Fig. 6.84** Colectomy specimen in Crohn's disease. The entire colon was involved by granulomatous colitis. Courtesy of Mr J. Alexander-Williams.

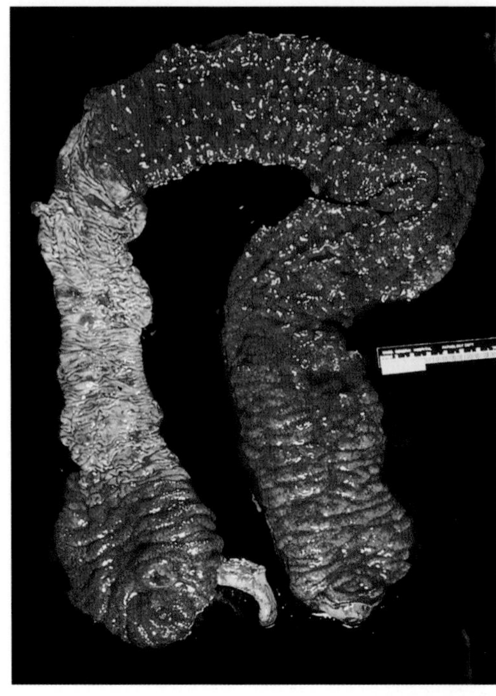

■ **Fig. 6.85** Total abdominal colectomy for Crohn's colitis showing a typically segmental pattern of involvement with active inflammation of the cecum, transverse and left colon but sparing the right colon, between.

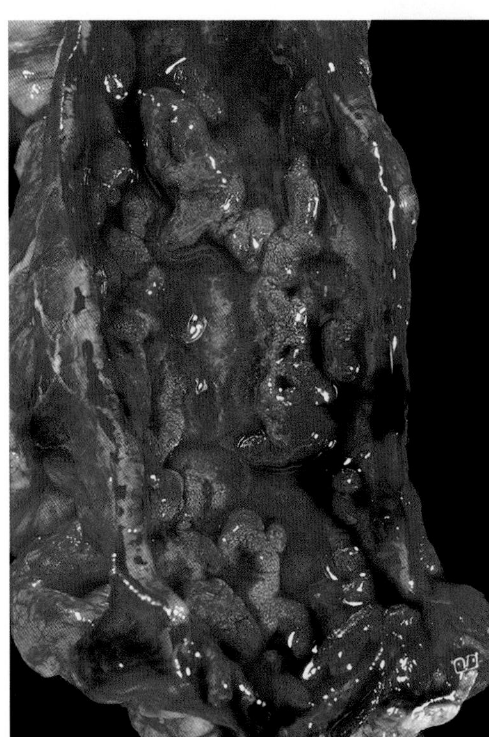

■ **Fig. 6.86** Macroscopic view of Crohn's colitis showing the typical 'cobblestone' appearance created by serpiginous ulcers (healed or active) traversing edematous, hyperemic, and hemorrhagic (severely inflamed) mucosa.

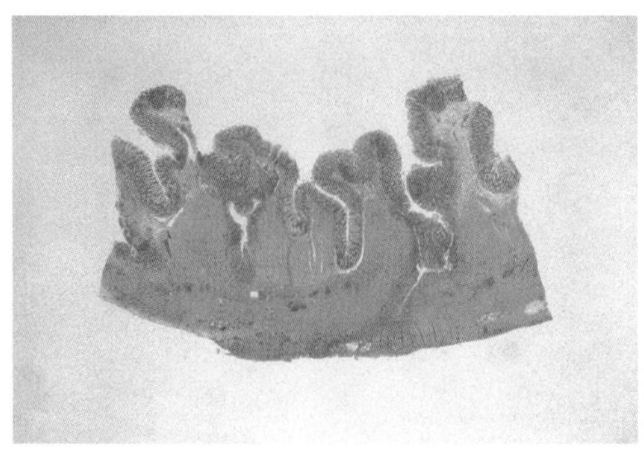

■ **Fig. 6.87** Whole-mount microscopic section through a cobblestoned colonic segment in Crohn's colitis.

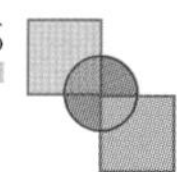

define a patient's disease on the basis of its extent macroscopically and microscopically since they may not be the same. Although the colonic manifestations of ulcerative colitis and Crohn's disease do not differ greatly, there are features of ulcerative colitis that help in the clinical distinction of the two conditions: the absence of small bowel involvement, the limitation of the disease to the mucosa, and the subsequent freedom from deep ulceration and fistula formation. There is a familial tendency to ulcerative colitis, and there are several possible gene loci including those responsible for HLA associations (the latter particularly in patients with concurrent sacroiliitis).

The clinical presentation of ulcerative colitis depends on the length of colon involved and the severity of the episode. It is semi-

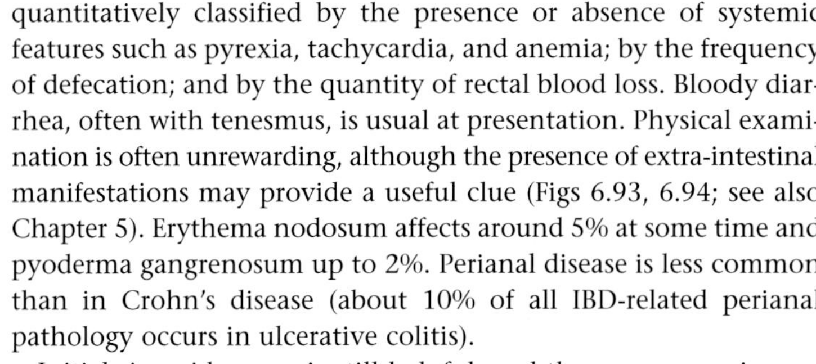

quantitatively classified by the presence or absence of systemic features such as pyrexia, tachycardia, and anemia; by the frequency of defecation; and by the quantity of rectal blood loss. Bloody diarrhea, often with tenesmus, is usual at presentation. Physical examination is often unrewarding, although the presence of extra-intestinal manifestations may provide a useful clue (Figs 6.93, 6.94; see also Chapter 5). Erythema nodosum affects around 5% at some time and pyoderma gangrenosum up to 2%. Perianal disease is less common than in Crohn's disease (about 10% of all IBD-related perianal pathology occurs in ulcerative colitis).

Initial sigmoidoscopy is still helpful, and the appearance is conveniently graded on a 4-point scale from normal, through mild hyperemia and mucosal granularity, and more marked inflammation with contact bleeding, to grade III proctitis in which there is extensive ulceration and spontaneous bleeding (Figs 6.95–6.97). Investigation will include rectal biopsy and stool culture to exclude infective causes, and a plain abdominal radiograph, which may give an indication of the extent of the colonic involvement (Fig. 6.98). A complete absence of colonic gas and fecal residue suggests active disease of the whole colon (Fig. 6.99). Larger amounts of intraluminal gas correlate with severity of the colitis; dilatation to more than 6 cm diameter – toxic megacolon – indicates deep penetration of ulcers into colonic muscle and carries a high risk of colonic perforation if not promptly treated. Barium radiology is relatively

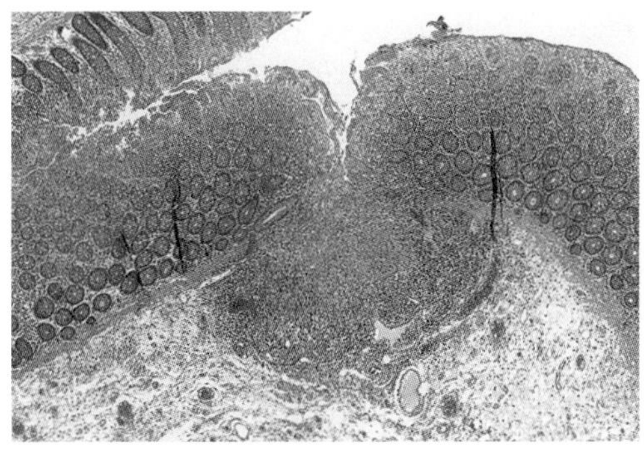

■ **Fig. 6.88** Microscopic view of an aphthous ulcer in Crohn's colitis showing the typically narrow and shallow mucosal defect flanked by active inflammation and cupped basally by a lymphoid aggregate.

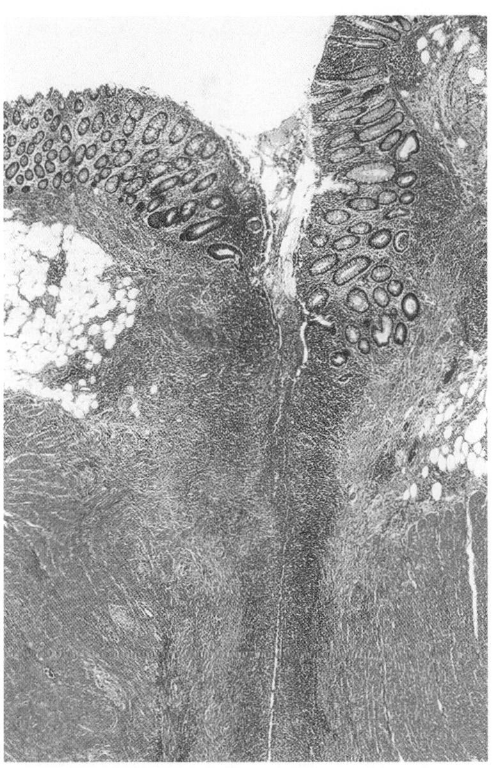

■ **Fig. 6.89** Microscopic view of a fissure in Crohn's colitis showing the typical deep, narrow ulcer cutting through the mucosa, submucosa, and muscularis propria.

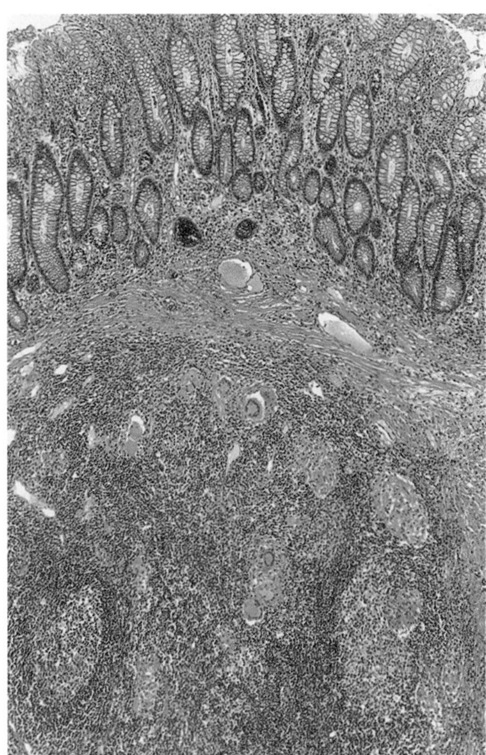

■ **Fig. 6.91** Microscopic view of Crohn's colitis with numerous well-formed non-caseating granulomata and dense lymphoid aggregates with germinal centers in the submucosa.

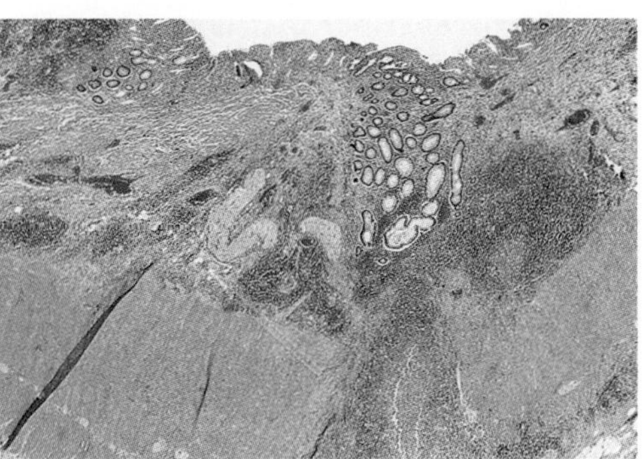

■ **Fig. 6.90** Typical microscopic features of Crohn's disease including mucosal glandular disarray, submucosal fibrosis, submucosal neural hypertrophy, transmural fissuring ulceration cuffed by chronic inflammatory infiltrates, and transmural lymphoid hyperplasia (germinal center formation throughout all bowel wall layers).

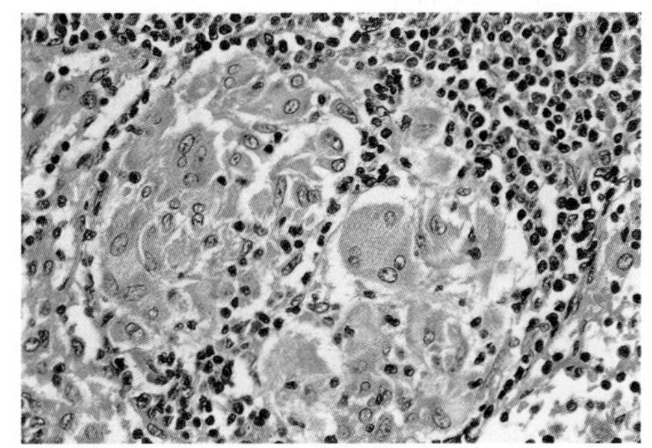

■ **Fig. 6.92** High-magnification appearance of a submucosal granuloma in Crohn's disease showing tight, nodular aggregates of unicellular and syncytial (giant cell) macrophages with abundant eosinophilic cytoplasm surrounded by small lymphocytes; no central necrosis (caseation) is seen.

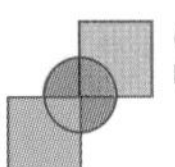

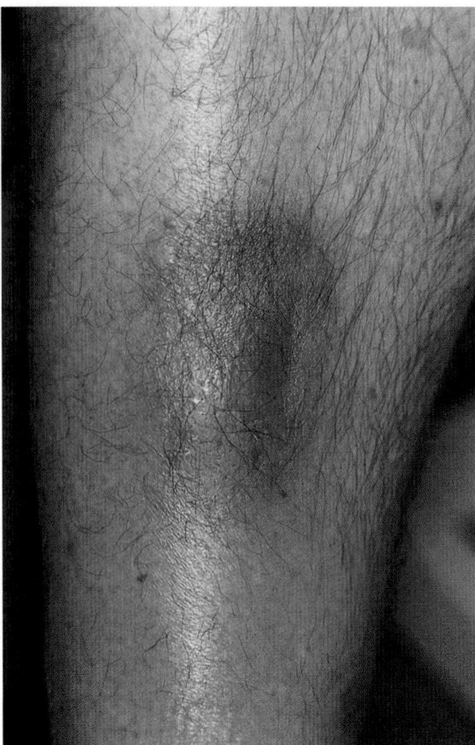

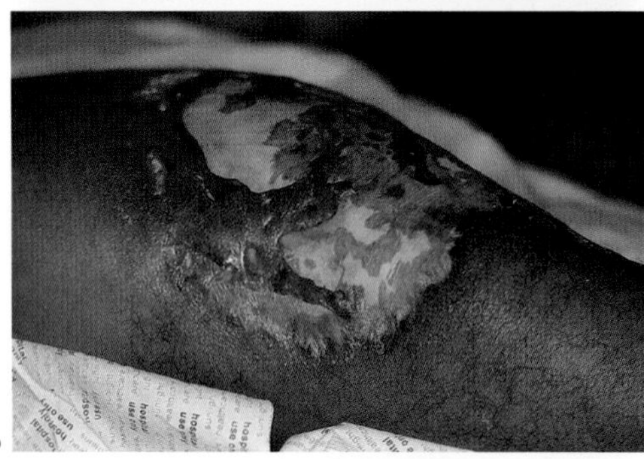

■ **Fig. 6.93** Pyoderma gangrenosum at characteristic sites on the leg. In the first case this is very early and preceded frank ulceration (a), whereas in the second there is profound ulceration with typical undermining of the skin edges (b).

■ **Fig. 6.94** Pyoderma gangrenosum adjacent to a stoma in a patient with Crohn's disease.

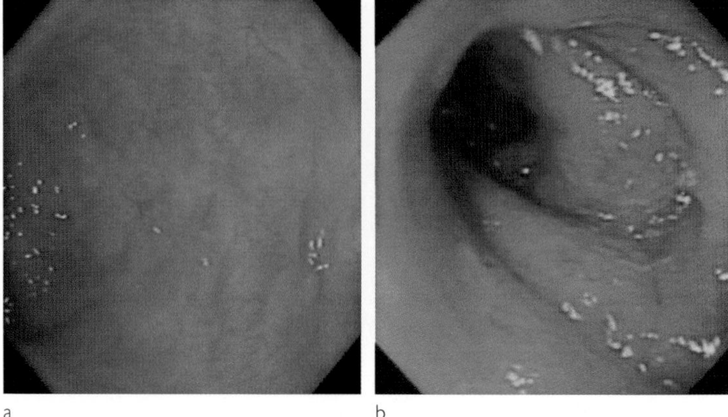

■ **Fig. 6.95** Colonoscopic appearances in early ulcerative colitis; the first image shows only hyperemia and loss of the normal vascular pattern (a) while in the second there is also some mucosal granularity and edema (b).

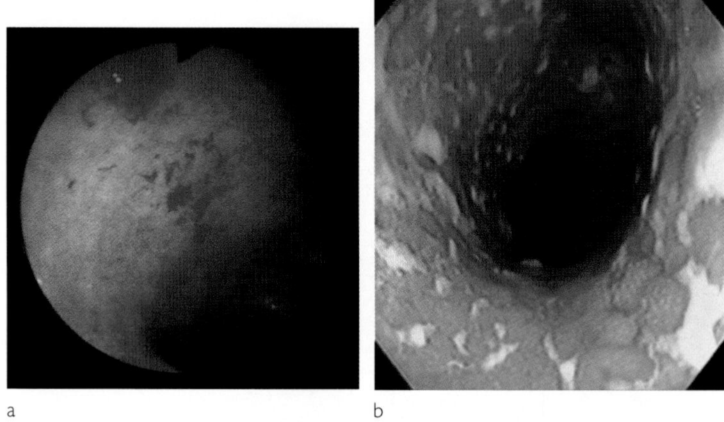

■ **Fig. 6.96** Colonoscopy in more severe ulcerative colitis. Contact bleeding (Baron grade II) (a), and more diffuse ulceration (b) .

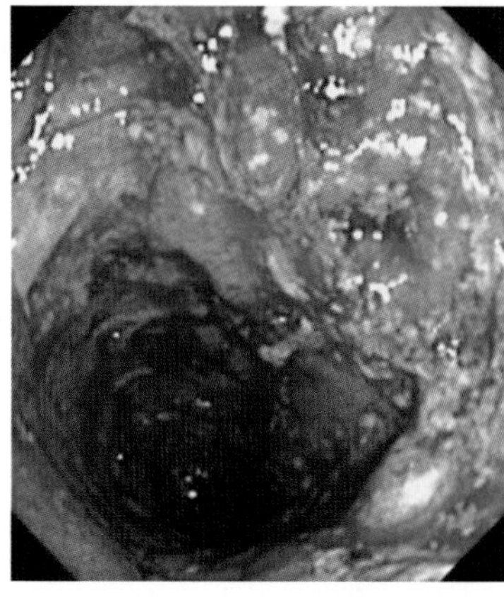

■ **Fig. 6.97** Colonoscopy showing extensive ulcerative changes with edema and congested folds with spontaneous and contact bleeding (Baron grade III).

contraindicated in acute disease, but the so-called 'instant' enema in which a contrast study is performed without prior preparation may be contributory (Fig. 6.100). Rectal balloon catheters should not, however, be used, and in fulminant colitis, radiology should be restricted to plain films. In more chronic disease, conventional double-contrast barium enema demonstrates mucosal granularity (Figs 6.101–6.104). CT scanning does not have a huge role in ulcerative colitis but is able to demonstrate the key features (Figs 6.105, 6.106) and may be useful in the more severe episode.

The definitive investigation is, without question, the colonoscopy, which permits a detailed examination of the whole colon and the ability to obtain histological samples. The disease activity can be recorded for each colonic segment to the same criteria as described above for sigmoidoscopy. The peculiar phenomenon of the cecal patch may also be discerned; some patients with otherwise distal colitis have an isolated area of inflammation near or around the appendiceal opening. The cecal patch does not seem to have special significance as the patient remains at the same risk of complications as one with equivalent distal colitis without the cecal inflammation.

When ulceration is extensive in colitis (Fig. 6.107), the remaining intact, but edematous, mucosa may go on to assume a pseudopolypoid appearance (Figs 6.108, 6.109) or to form mucosal bridges (Fig. 6.110). Healing after ulceration may leave a residuum of post-inflammatory polyps and/or benign stricturing (Fig. 6.111). Total colitis may be

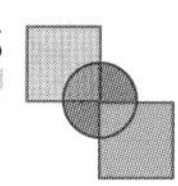

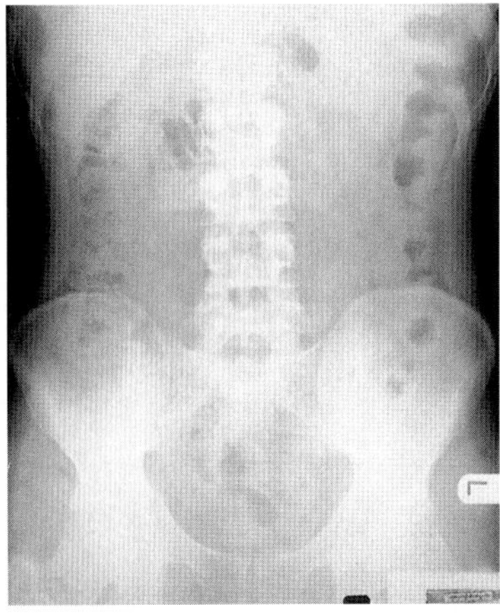

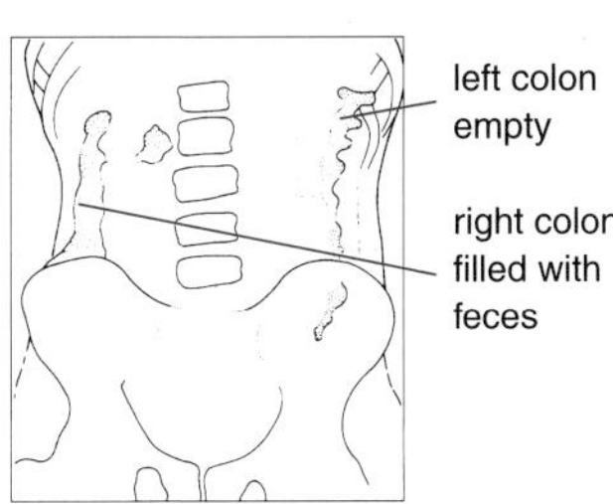

Fig. 6.98 Plain abdominal radiograph in acute colitis. The left colon is empty with a blunted haustral pattern indicative of inflammation, but the right side of the colon is filled with feces. The impression of disease limited to the left side was later confirmed colonoscopically.

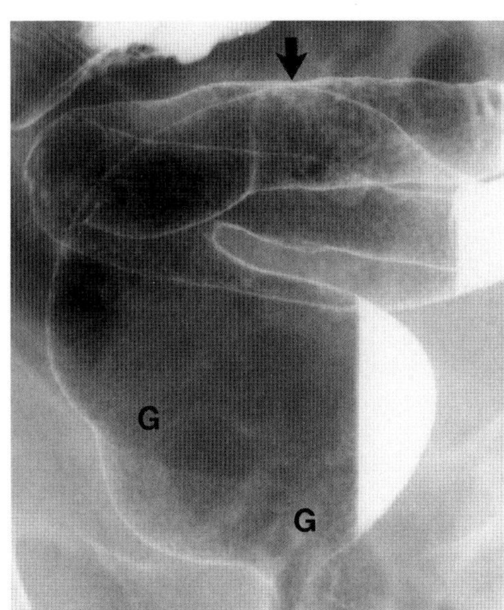

Fig. 6.101 Double-contrast barium enema in patient with ulcerative colitis. The distal rectal mucosa has a finely granular appearance (G); the distal sigmoid mucosa has a coarsely granular appearance (arrow). The rectosigmoid colon has a tubular configuration. (Reproduced with permission from reference 2, Fig. 13.11.)

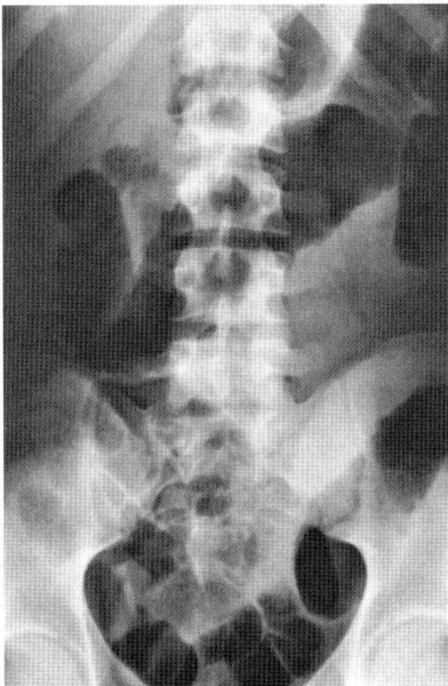

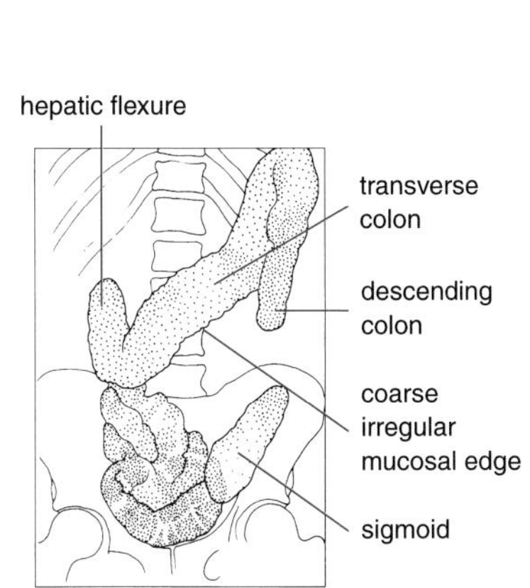

Fig. 6.99 Plain abdominal radiograph in severe active colitis showing extensive gas in the colon and small bowel with no formed fecal residue. The transverse colon is dilated with a coarse mucosal edge without haustra. At histological examination after colectomy, early changes of toxic megacolon were found.

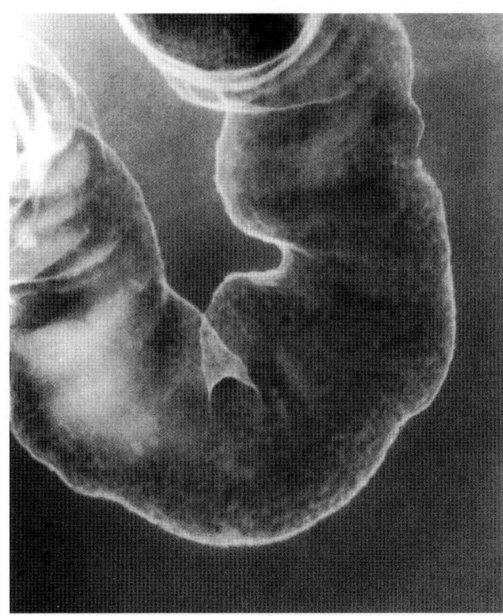

Fig. 6.102 Double-contrast barium enema demonstrating coarsely granular mucosa in ulcerative colitis. (Reproduced with permission from reference 7, Fig. 5.3A.)

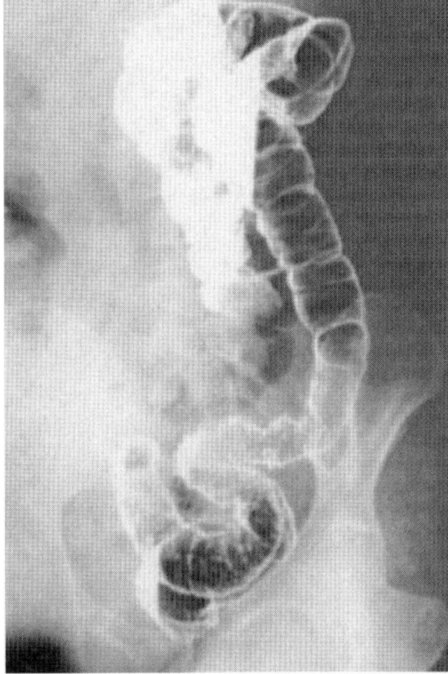

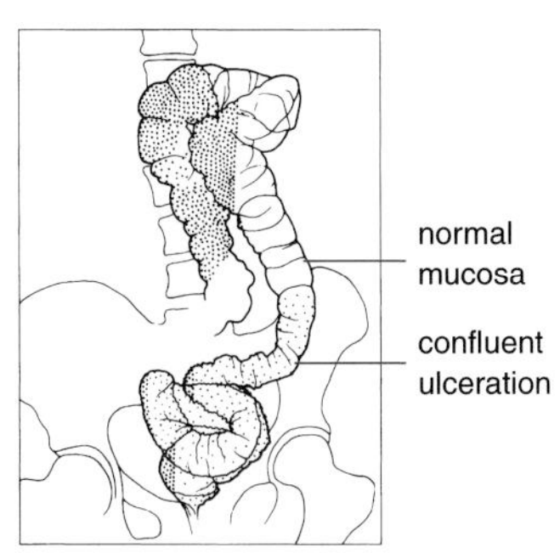

Fig. 6.100 Instant enema in acute ulcerative colitis with distal ulceration. The ulcers are shallow and confluent, and there is an abrupt transition to normal mucosa in the lower descending colon.

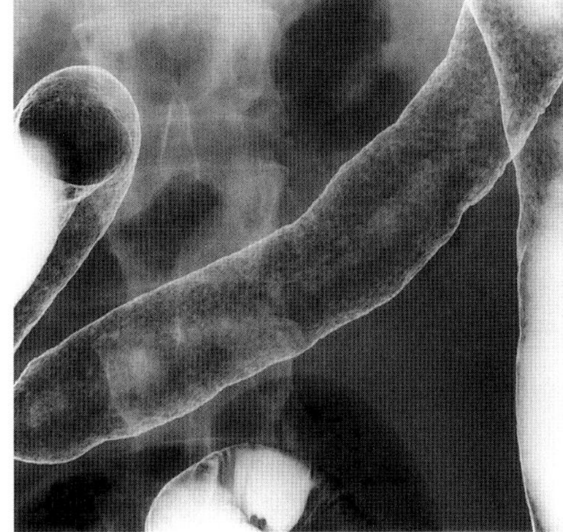

Fig. 6.103 Double-contrast barium enema demonstrating finely nodular mucosa in ulcerative colitis. The transverse colon has lost its haustral sacculations and interhaustral folds. The mucosa is coarsely granular/finely nodular. (Reproduced with permission from reference 8, Fig. 25.35.)

associated with inflammation of the terminal ileum – known as backwash ileitis – if the ileocecal valve is incompetent (Fig. 6.112).

Complications

Severe acute colitis may be complicated by intractable hemorrhage or to toxic megacolon which may lead on to perforation: all are sur-

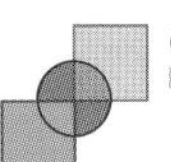

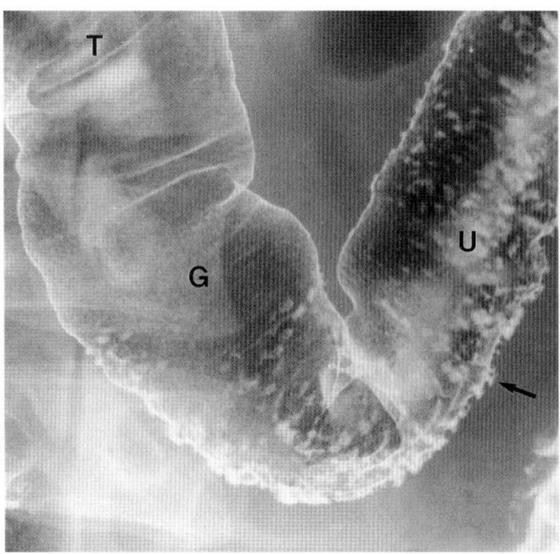

Fig. 6.104 Double-contrast barium enema demonstrating the transition between normal mucosa, mild colitis, and moderate ulcerative colitis. Just distal to the smooth, proximal transverse colon (T), the mucosa becomes finely granular (G). Numerous small ulcers (U) are then seen in the mid and distal transverse colon. An ulcer resembling a 'collar button' is seen in profile and identified by an arrow. (Reproduced with permission from reference 8, Fig. 25.36.)

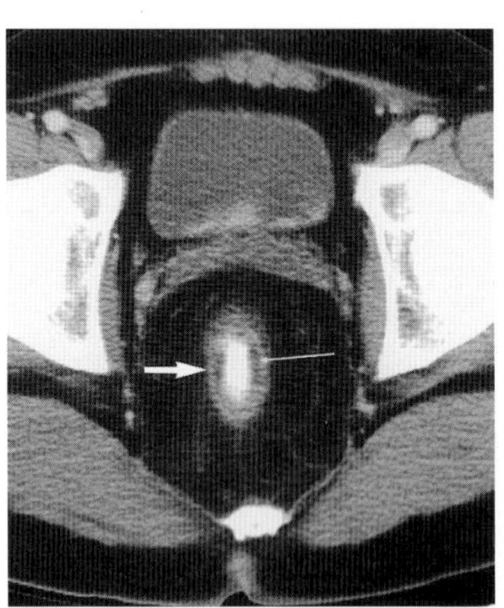

Fig. 6.105 CT demonstrating ulcerative colitis in the rectum. CT through the level of the urinary bladder and seminal vesicles shows that the rectum has a narrowed, tubular configuration (thick arrow). The submucosa is of fluid attenuation (thin arrow), creating a 'mural stratification' pattern.

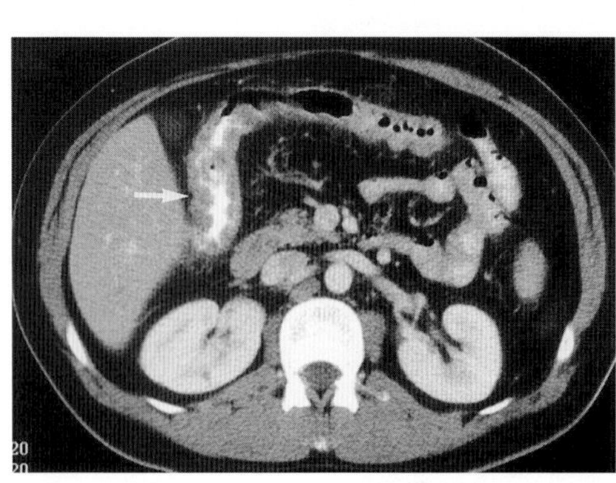
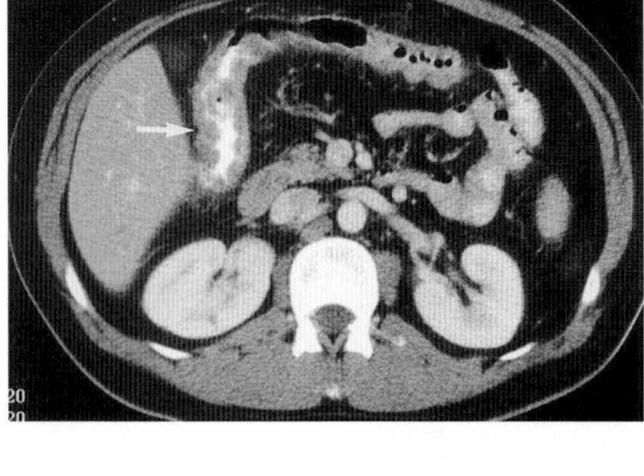

Fig. 6.106 CT demonstrating ulcerative colitis in the transverse colon. The transverse colon has a tubular configuration. The wall is thickened in the hepatic flexure (arrows).

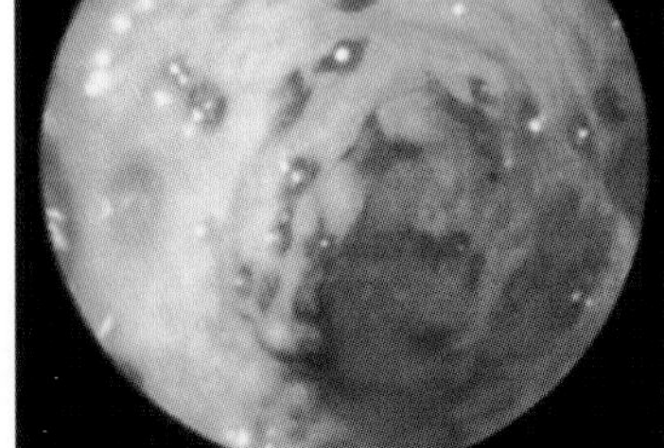

Fig. 6.107 Colonoscopic appearance of severe ulcerative colitis with almost complete slough of the mucosa.

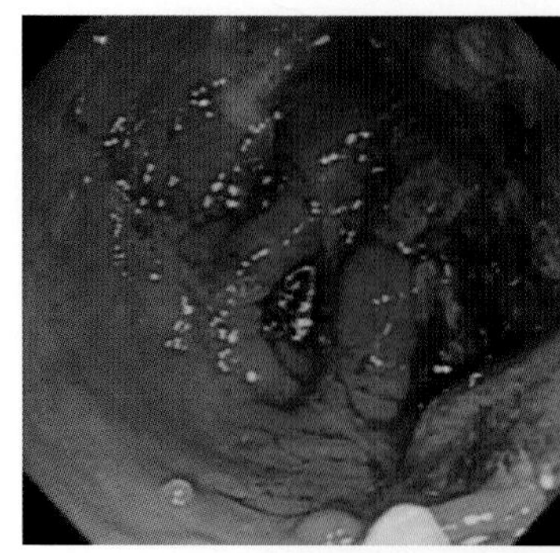

Fig. 6.108 Previously severe ulcerative colitis with numerous prominent inflammatory pseudopolyps.

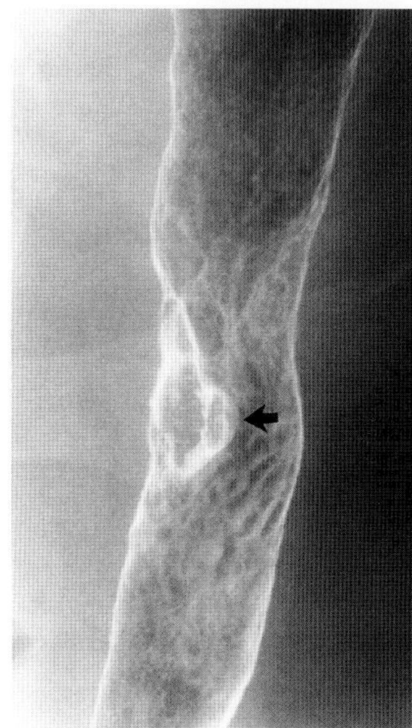

Fig. 6.109 Double-contrast barium enema demonstrating an inflammatory polyp in a patient with ulcerative colitis. A 2-cm polypoid lesion (arrow) is seen on the medial wall of the descending colon. The background mucosa has a granular and finely nodular appearance indicative of chronic ulcerative colitis. (Reproduced with permission from reference 8, Fig. 25.37.)

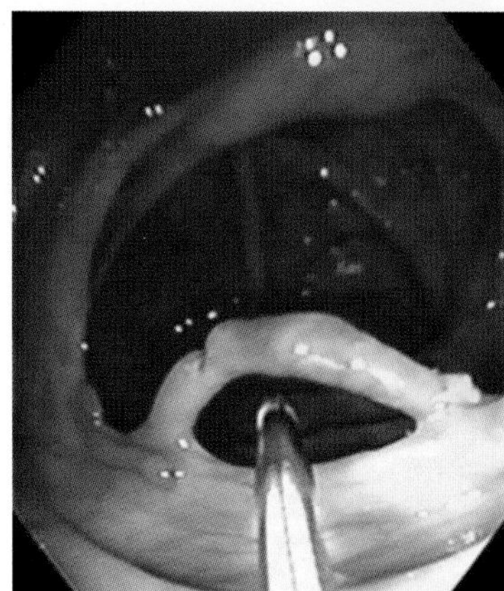

Fig. 6.110 Colonoscopic appearance of previously severe ulcerative colitis with post-inflammatory bridging (a biopsy forceps passes 'under' the bridge).

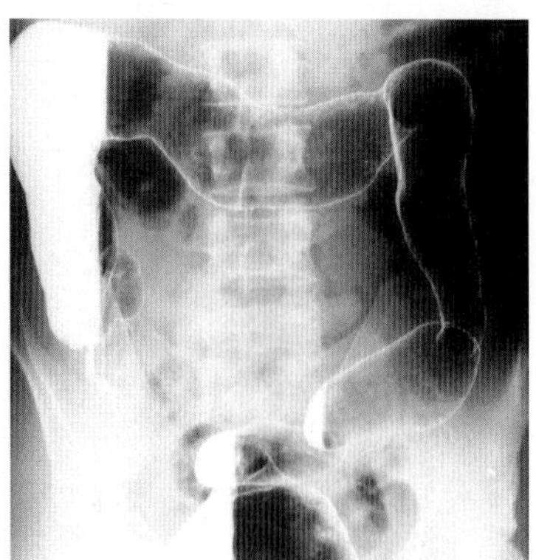
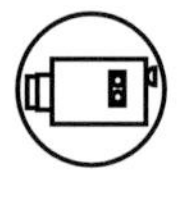
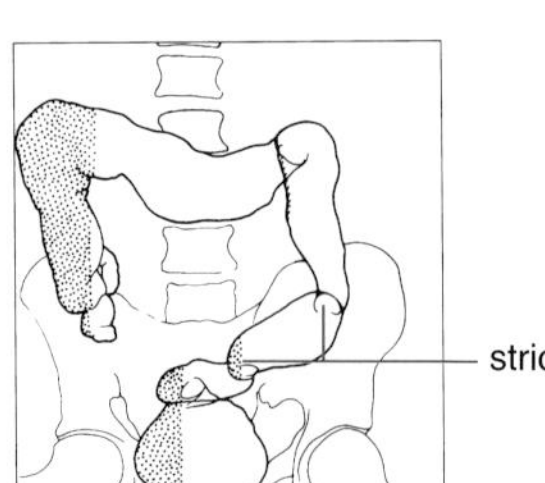

Fig. 6.111 Barium enema showing the granular mucosa and complete absence of haustra, which confirm total colitis. Two short strictures are present in the descending colon, but there were no malignant features radiologically: colonoscopy with biopsy confirmed their benign nature.

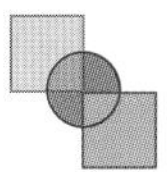

gical emergencies. The development of toxic megacolon (Fig. 6.113) may be preceded by deterioration in physical signs, but also by an increasing diameter of the transverse colon on serial plain abdominal radiographs. The radiological identification of 'mucosal islands,' which are apparently raised areas but are in fact the only surviving mucosa in a bowel otherwise stripped to the muscle layers (Fig. 6.114), or of small bowel dilatation (Fig. 6.115) are especially important adverse prognostic indicators (Fig. 6.116).

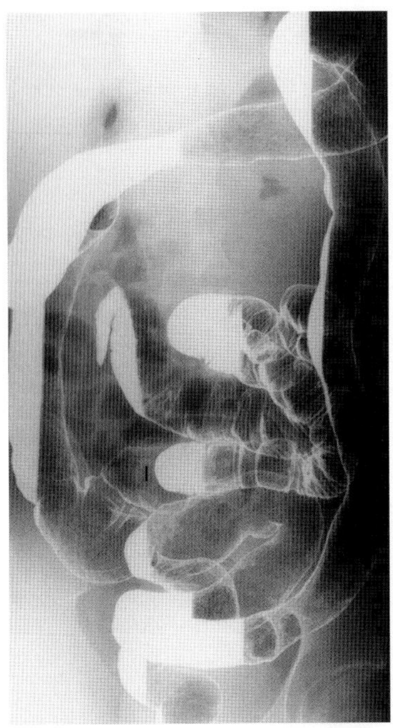

Fig. 6.112 Double-contrast barium enema in a patient with diffuse ulcerative colitis. The colon has a tubular configuration. The haustral sacculations and interhaustral folds have disappeared. Backwash ileitis (I) is manifest by terminal ileal dilatation and loss of valvulae conniventes. (Reproduced with permission from reference 8, Fig. 25.40.)

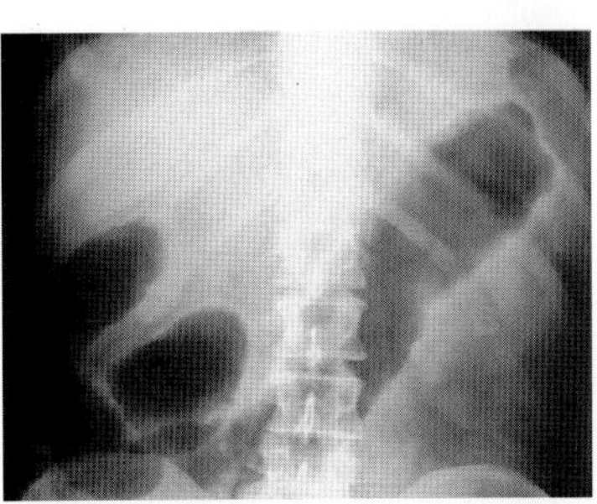

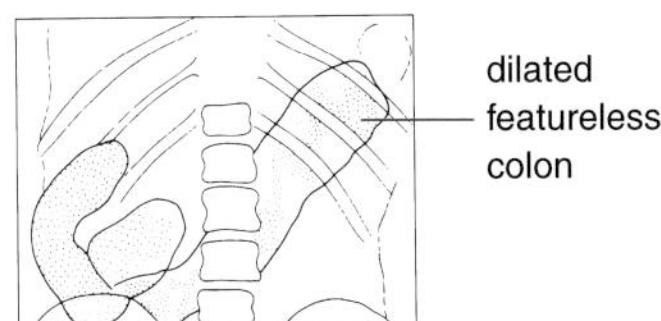

Fig. 6.113 Plain abdominal film showing dilatation of a featureless colon in toxic megacolon complicating ulcerative colitis.

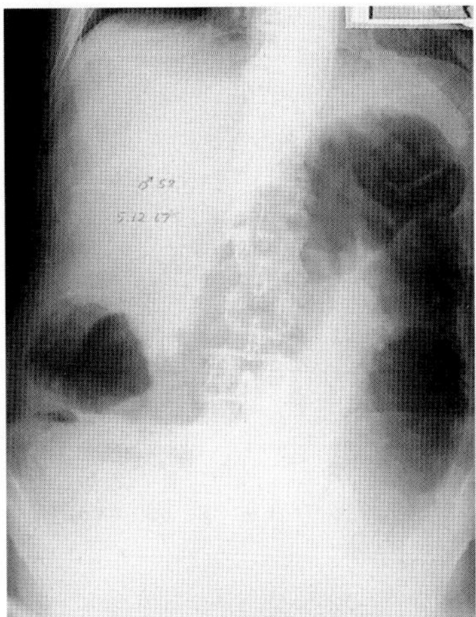

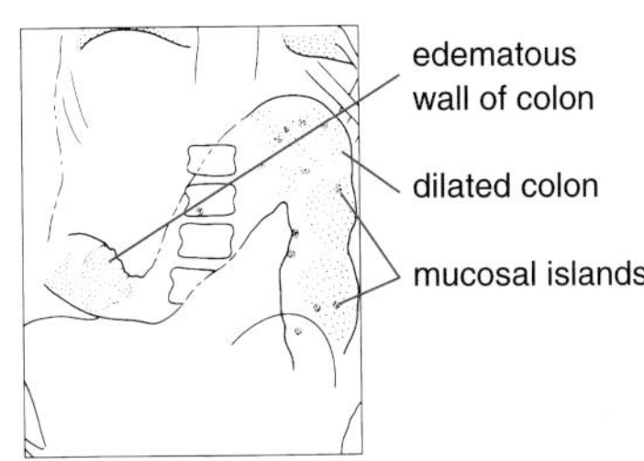

Fig. 6.114 Toxic megacolon demonstrating the mucosal islands indicative of small areas of preserved and relatively normal mucosa amidst an otherwise virtually denuded colon.

The most sinister long-term complication of ulcerative colitis is colonic carcinoma. The risk is directly related to the duration of colitis and to the extent of colon involved. In patients with total colitis, the cancer risk approaches 15% at 20 years from the first symptoms and constitutes about a six-fold lifetime increase relative to controls. Surveillance colonoscopy is therefore widely considered appropriate for the majority of patients with extensive colitis of 10 or more years standing. Confirmed mucosal dysplasia (see below), even of low grade, is almost certainly premalignant, and any confirmed dysplasia will lead to a call for colectomy. On the occasion that barium studies are necessary because of poor tolerance of colonoscopy or strictures preventing access to the proximal colon dysplastic areas may be demonstrable (Fig 6.117).

Colitis-associated carcinomas tend to develop as shallow plaque-like tumors, and the more obvious annular or polypoid tumors probably occur only quite late (Figs 6.118–6.120). There are more right-sided lesions than for colorectal carcinoma in general but the majority of tumors are still left-sided.

In addition to the extra-intestinal manifestations of inflammatory bowel disease mentioned above, ulcerative colitis may be complicated by primary sclerosing cholangitis (PSC). PSC generally runs a course independent of that of the colitis and is illustrated in Chapter 14. The co-existence of PSC greatly increases the risk of colorectal carcinoma in ulcerative colitis.

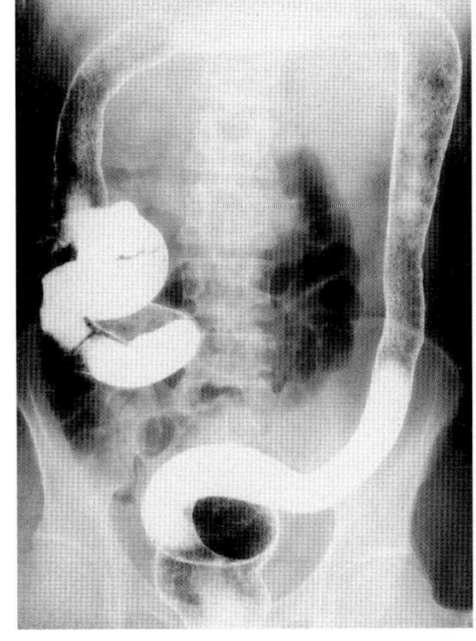

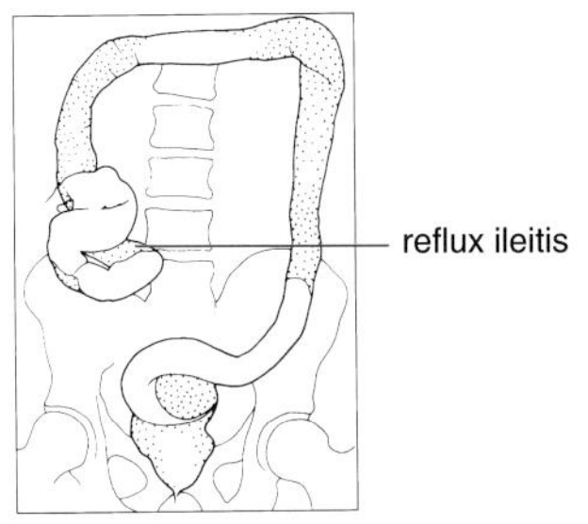

Fig. 6.115 Instant barium enema in total ulcerative colitis. The distal ileum is dilated with a granular surface typical of reflux or backwash ileitis.

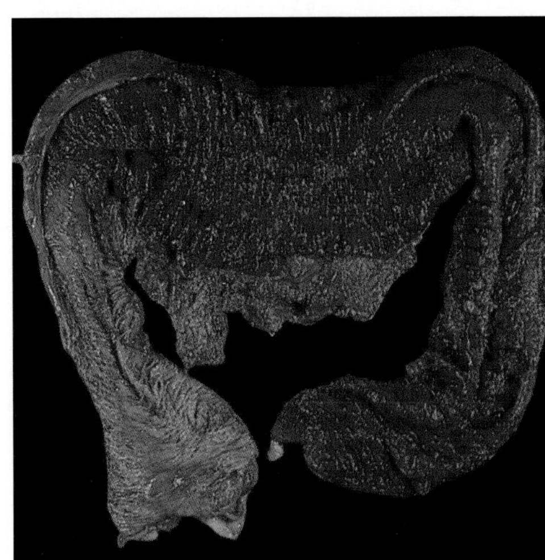

Fig. 6.116 Colectomy specimen in toxic megacolon. Courtesy of Mr J. Alexander-Williams.

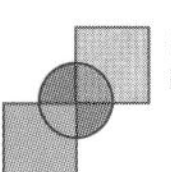

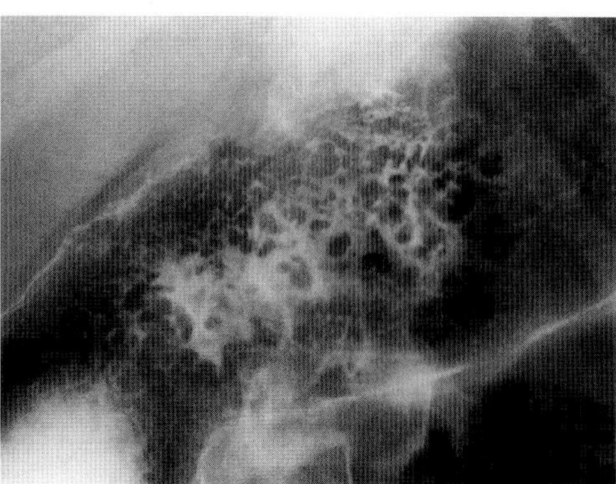

Fig. 6.117 Barium enema demonstrating a dysplasia-associated mass in ulcerative colitis. A focus of 2–5 mm polygonal nodules is seen in the mid-transverse colon.

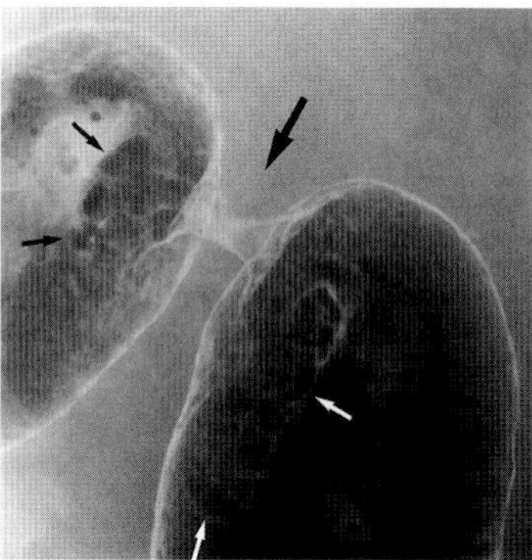

Fig. 6.118 Double-contrast barium enema demonstrating adenocarcinoma arising in dysplasia in a patient with ulcerative colitis. A smooth-surfaced tapered narrowing (large arrow) is seen in the splenic flexure. Polygonal islands of dysplastic mucosa (small arrows) are seen both proximally and distally to the carcinoma. (Reproduced with permission from reference 8, Fig. 25.41B, courtesy of Giles Stevenson, M.D., Duncan, ON, Canada)

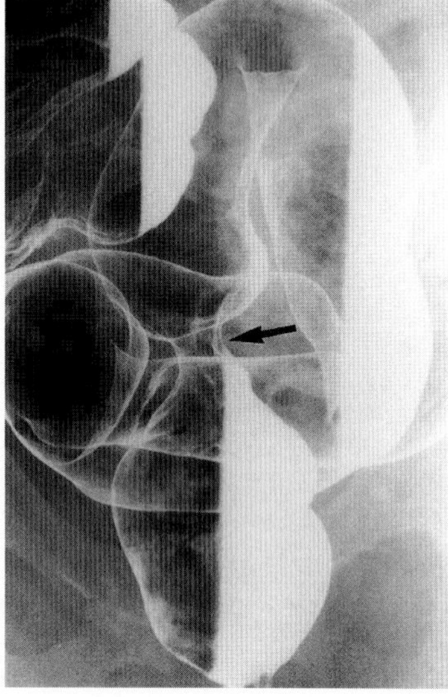

Fig. 6.119 Scirrhous carcinoma arising in ulcerative colitis. A smooth tapered narrowing (arrow) is seen at the rectosigmoid junction. Compare this smooth malignant stricture to the typical appearance of an annular colonic carcinoma. (Reproduced with permission from reference 2, Fig. 13.24.)

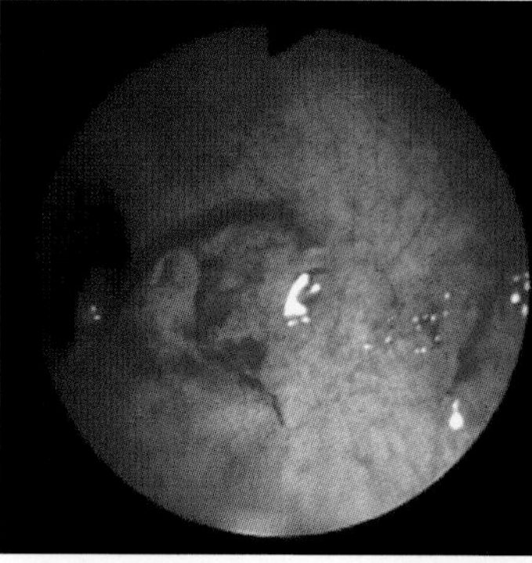

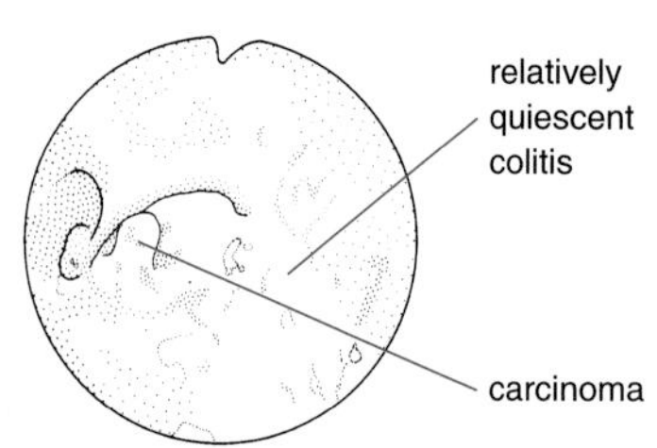

Fig. 6.120 Colonoscopic appearance of relatively early carcinoma complicating ulcerative colitis. This proved to be a Dukes' A lesion.

Pathology

In ulcerative colitis, the colon usually appears normal from the serosal aspect, apart from a generalized shortening. The mucosa has an even pattern of abnormality, which invariably involves the rectum (Figs 6.121–6.128). The precise appearance depends on the disease activity with a spectrum from minimal inflammation, through patchy granularity, to extensive ulceration with only small remnants of mucosa. Between ulcers, the mucosa is always abnormal. In more

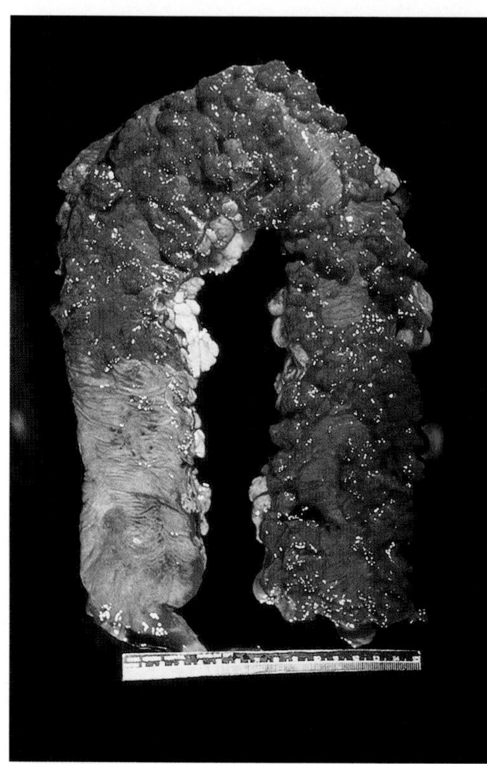

Fig. 6.121 Total abdominal colectomy specimen in ulcerative colitis showing confluent involvement of the left and transverse colon with sparing of the right colon.

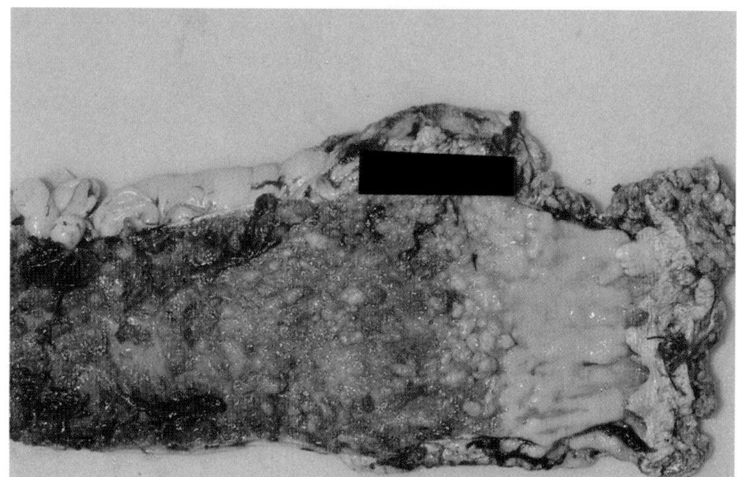

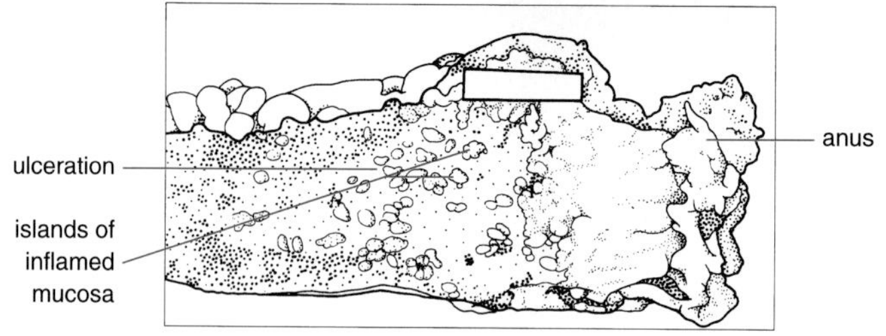

Fig. 6.122 Macroscopic appearance of the rectum in severe ulcerative colitis showing inflamed mucosa surviving as islands between intercommunicating areas of ulceration. The mucosa immediately proximal to the anal margin, although intact, is also histologically inflamed.

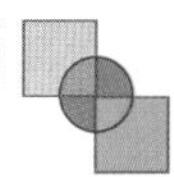

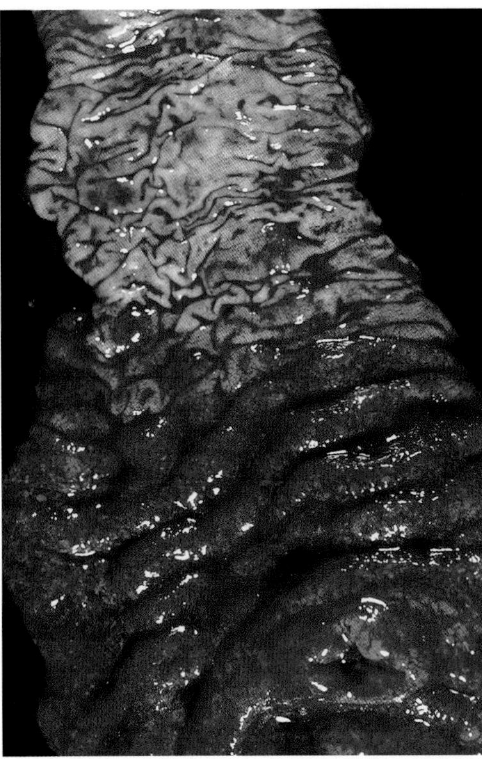

■ **Fig. 6.123** Interface between involved distal and uninvolved proximal colonic mucosa in ulcerative colitis showing the abrupt transition between the two.

quiescent phases and after treatment, the mucosa appears flat, pale, and featureless, but because not all regions of the bowel may be equally active, a misleading apparently segmental pattern of the disease may be suggested (Figs 6.125, 6.128). The presence of numerous pseudopolyps (Fig. 6.127, 6.128) (which are little more than mucosal tags) indicates healing of previous severe ulceration.

In contrast to Crohn's disease, the inflammatory changes are limited to the mucosa. Ulceration rarely extends into the submucosa, and fissuring is never present. In active disease, the intact mucosa is inflamed with prominent crypt abscesses, mucin depletion, and derangement of the normal crypt architecture (Figs 6.129–6.131). This rarely returns to normal, and, in remission, mucosal atrophy

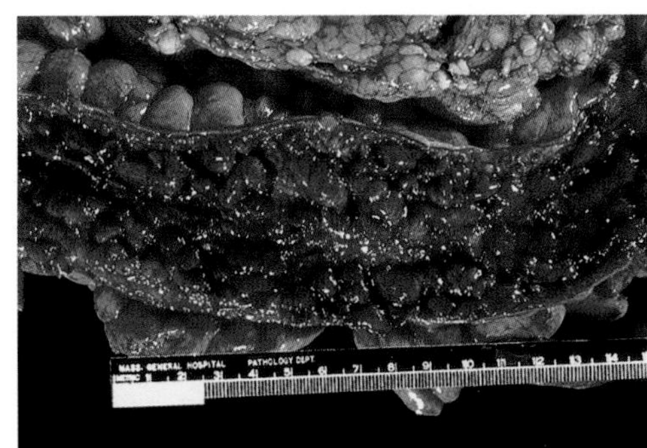

■ **Fig. 6.126** Typical gross appearance of ulcerated mucosa showing puffy projections of inflamed mucosa in relief against a network of shallow ulcers.

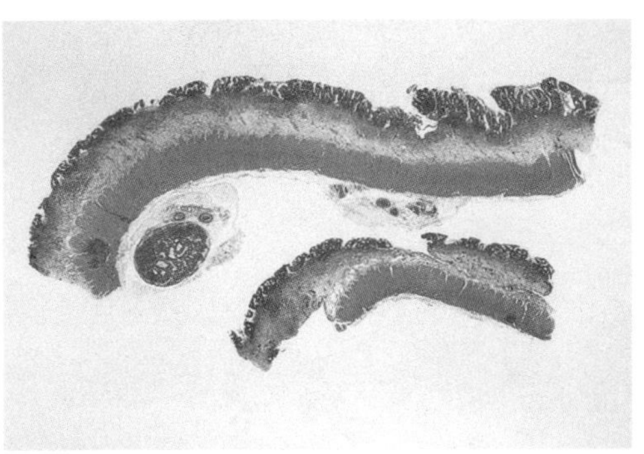

■ **Fig. 6.124** Whole-mount microscopic section of active ulcerative colitis showing confluent severe inflammation of the mucosa and superficial submucosa as well as multifocal shallow ulceration. No fissuring, transmural inflammation or normal 'skip' areas are seen.

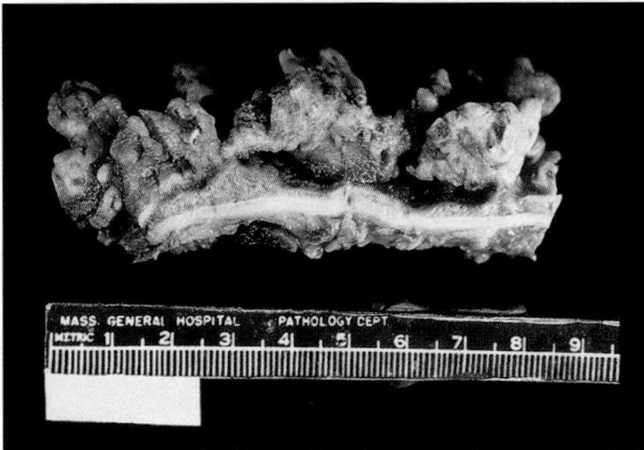

■ **Fig. 6.127** Macroscopic transmural section of colon involved by long-standing ulcerative colitis showing extensive pseudopolyp formation and the broad tangential ulcers that skim the submucosa; the muscularis propria is normal in appearance.

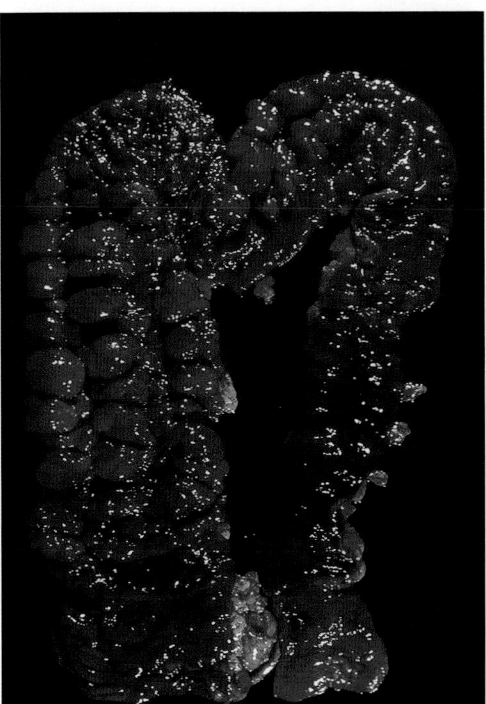

■ **Fig. 6.125** Total colectomy specimen for severe pancolitis refractory to medical management in a patient with chronic ulcerative colitis showing prominent pseudopolyp formation distally and diffusely hemorrhagic mucosa proximally.

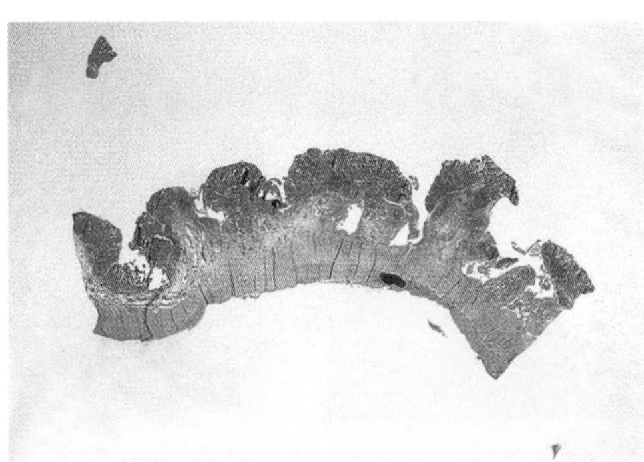

■ **Fig. 6.128** Whole-mount microscopic section of pseudopolyps in ulcerative colitis showing alternating foci of shallow ulceration and markedly inflamed mucosa.

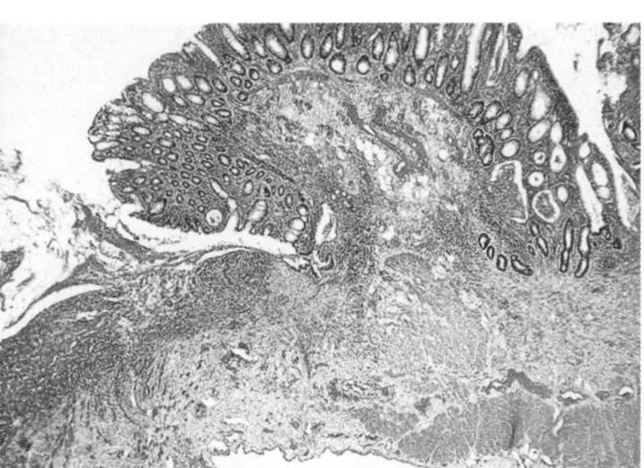

■ **Fig. 6.129** Microscopic appearance of a pseudopolyp showing the interface between an ulcer (left) and inflamed mucosa (right).

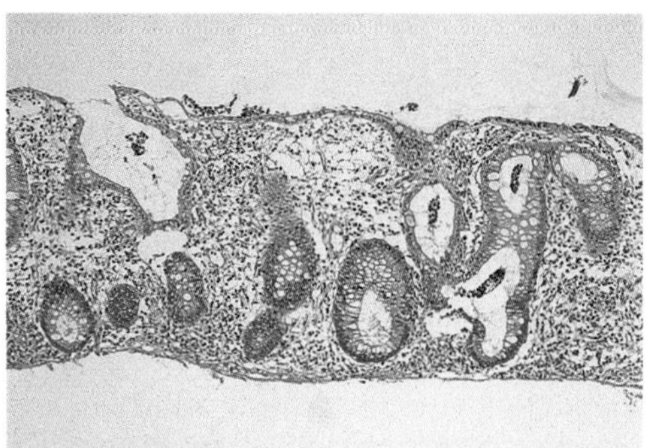

■ Fig. 6.130 Mucosal biopsy in active ulcerative colitis showing the marked glandular architectural distortion of a chronic inflammatory colitis and the numerous crypt abscesses indicative of ongoing activity. Both features are common in ulcerative colitis but neither is pathognomonic.

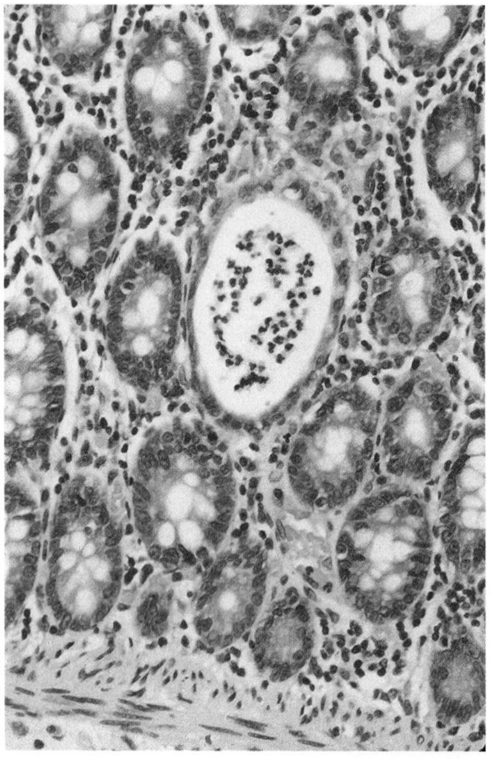

■ Fig. 6.131 High magnification of a crypt abscess showing a dilated mucosal gland filled with neutrophils.

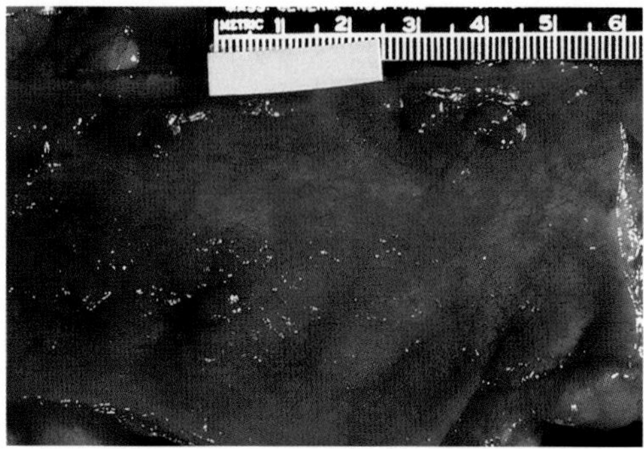

■ Fig. 6.132 Macroscopic appearance of flat, featureless mucosa of the distal colon in long-standing, ulcerative colitis which harbored flat dysplasia discovered on surveillance biopsy.

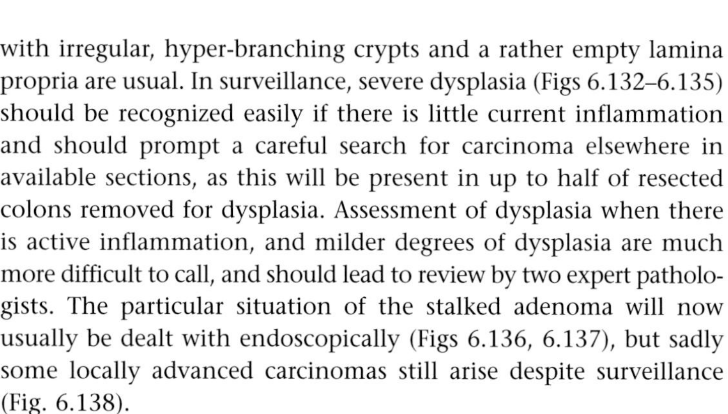

with irregular, hyper-branching crypts and a rather empty lamina propria are usual. In surveillance, severe dysplasia (Figs 6.132–6.135) should be recognized easily if there is little current inflammation and should prompt a careful search for carcinoma elsewhere in available sections, as this will be present in up to half of resected colons removed for dysplasia. Assessment of dysplasia when there is active inflammation, and milder degrees of dysplasia are much more difficult to call, and should lead to review by two expert pathologists. The particular situation of the stalked adenoma will now usually be dealt with endoscopically (Figs 6.136, 6.137), but sadly some locally advanced carcinomas still arise despite surveillance (Fig. 6.138).

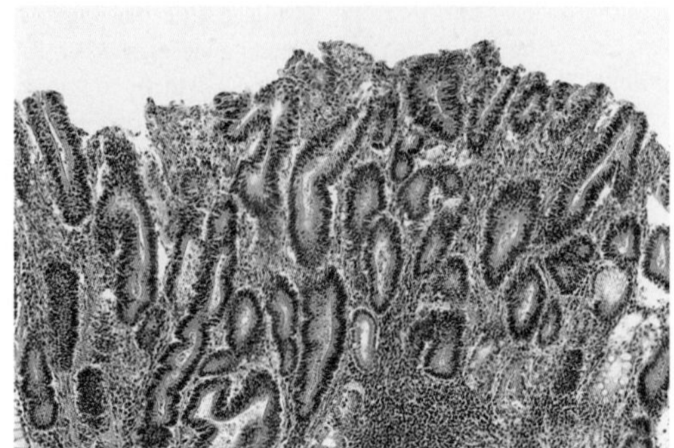

■ Fig. 6.133 Microscopic view of low-grade dysplasia in flat mucosa in ulcerative colitis showing the enlarged, hyperchromatic nuclei of the glandular epithelium that, although crowded and pseudostratified, remained confined to the basal half of the cells.

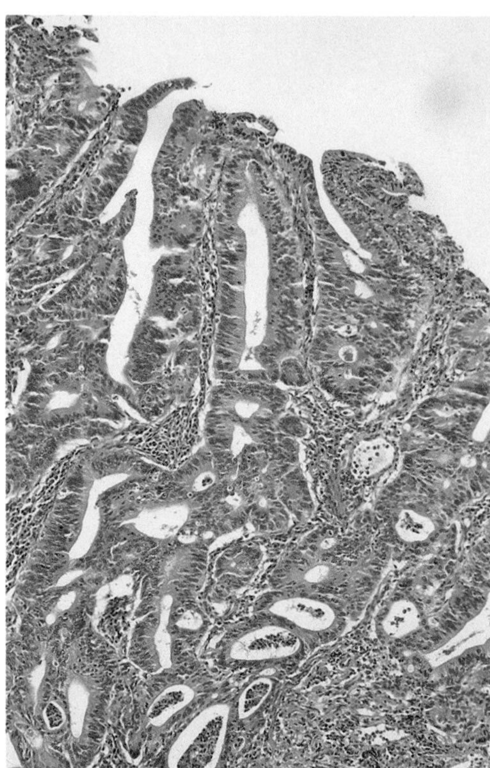

■ Fig. 6.134 Microscopic view of high-grade dysplasia/carcinoma *in situ* with focal early invasion of the lamina propria in flat mucosa in ulcerative colitis showing the complexity of the dysplastic glands with cribriform gland-within-gland formation, loss of polarity of the epithelial cells, and stratification of the dysplastic nuclei into the luminal half of the cells. Small irregular foci of epithelial extension of glands or small cell nests into the lamina propria consistent with stromal invasion are seen.

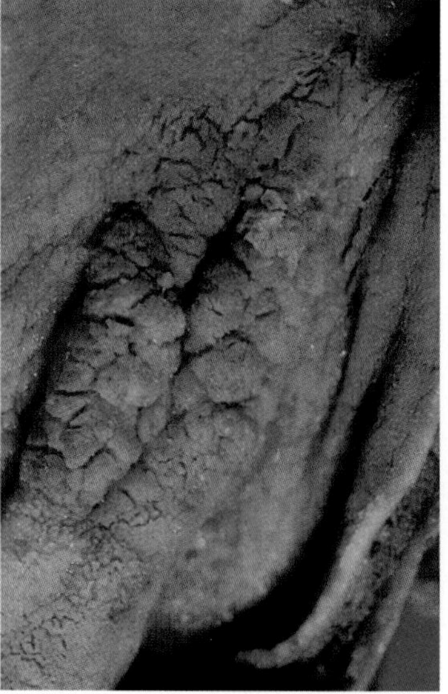

■ Fig. 6.135 Macroscopic view of high-grade dysplasia/carcinoma *in situ* in chronic ulcerative colitis showing the flat to slightly raised, roughened to finely granular appearance of the mucosa, changes that are subtle and easily overlooked.

The resected toxic megacolon shows involvement of the entire colonic wall with disintegration of the muscle coat (see Fig. 6.116). This no longer has features specific to ulcerative colitis, and is essentially an end-stage in which subtle diagnostic features are totally masked by the severity of the inflammatory and degenerative processes (Fig. 6.139).

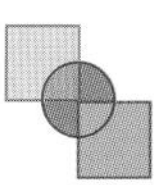

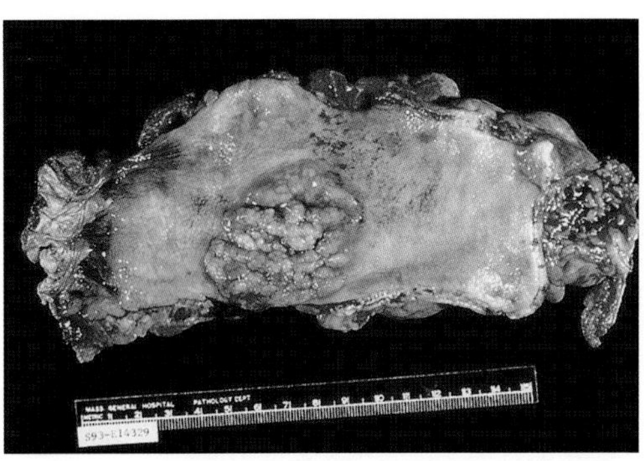

■ **Fig. 6.136** Rectal resection specimen showing a discrete, well-demarcated polypoid lesion consistent with a sessile adenoma arising from the featureless rectal mucosa of long-standing ulcerative colitis.

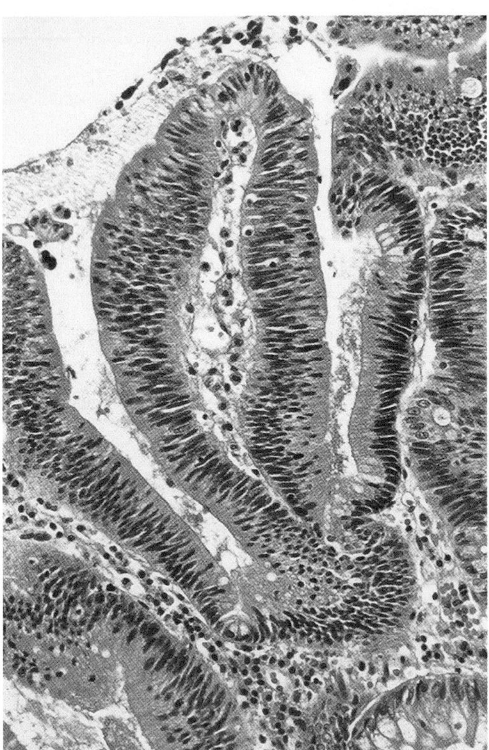

■ **Fig. 6.137** Microscopic appearance of the polyp is consistent with a tubulo-villous adenoma without malignancy. Sporadic adenomas occurring in proximal, uninvolved colonic mucosa in patients with less than pancolonic ulcerative colitis are generally treated by polypectomy alone.

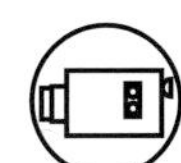

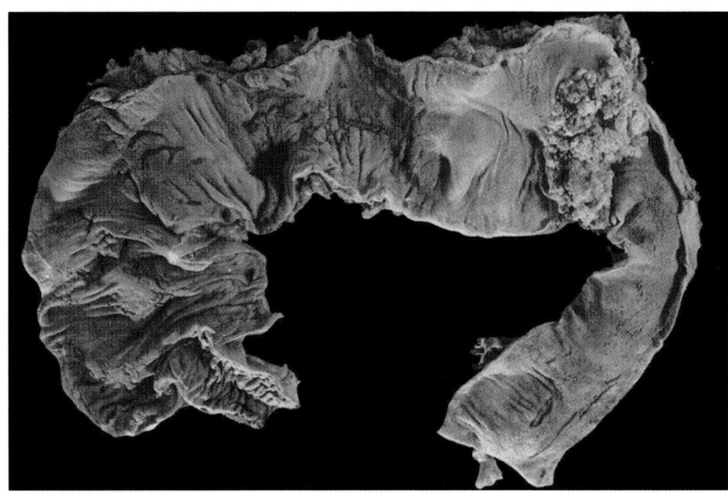

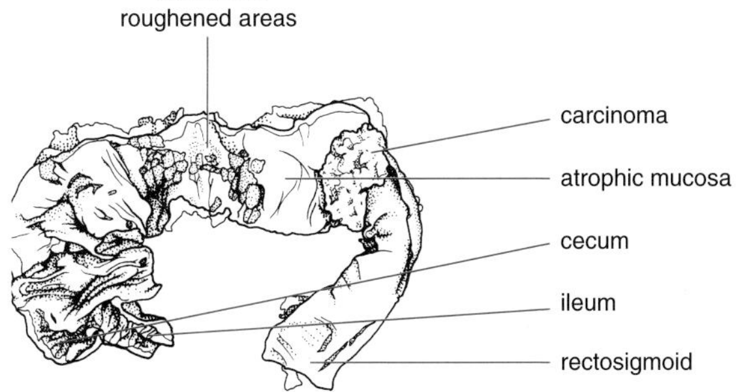

■ **Fig. 6.138** Colectomy specimen in long-standing ulcerative colitis complicated by carcinoma and also showing the raised roughened areas which are common sites of dysplasia.

Surgery for ulcerative colitis

Removal of the rectum and colon in their entirety provides a cure for ulcerative colitis. Initial preservation of a recto-sigmoid stump (particularly when colectomy has been necessary as an urgent procedure) is usual, but the risk of malignant transformation within the rectal mucosa remains. Ileorectal anastomosis is therefore no longer favored and a total panproctocolectomy, with a Brooke ileostomy (Fig. 6.140) or, increasingly often, the fashioning of a 'pouch' neorectum, is preferred. A pouch is formed from a loop of ileum, which is then anastomosed directly to the anal mucosa within a residual cuff of rectal muscle completely stripped of its mucosal lining: intestinal continuity is thereby restored (Fig. 6.141). Although good results are achieved in most patients in whom a pouch has been created, difficulties with evacuation, or the emergence of troublesome pouchitis (Figs 6.142–6.144) may occasionally prompt reversion to end-ileostomy.

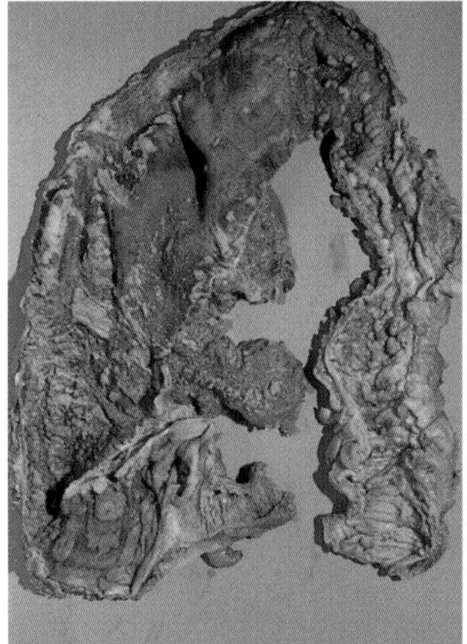

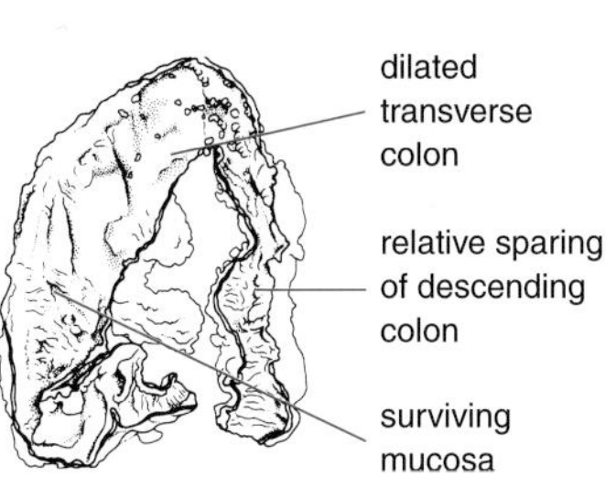

■ **Fig. 6.139** Macroscopic appearance in toxic megacolon affecting predominantly the ascending and transverse colon. The transverse colon and hepatic flexure are dilated with complete loss of the mucosa.

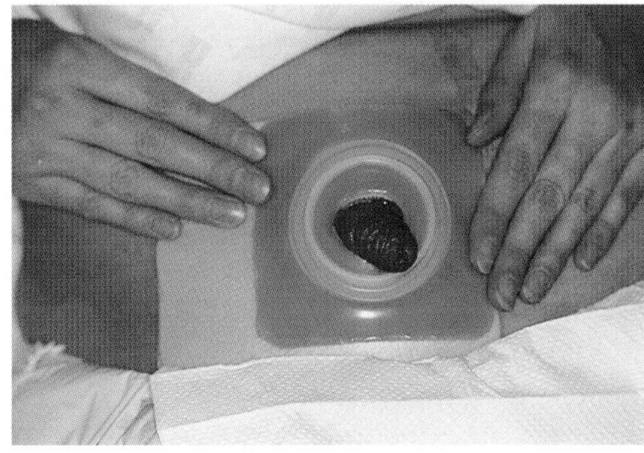

■ **Fig. 6.140** Brooke ileostomy.

INDETERMINATE, MICROSCOPIC, LYMPHOCYTIC AND COLLAGENOUS COLITIS

Although the combination of clinical, radiological, endoscopic, and histological criteria usually allows ulcerative colitis to be clearly distinguished from Crohn's, this is not always possible. These patients are sensibly held to have indeterminate colitis until (if ever) a

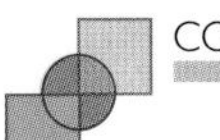

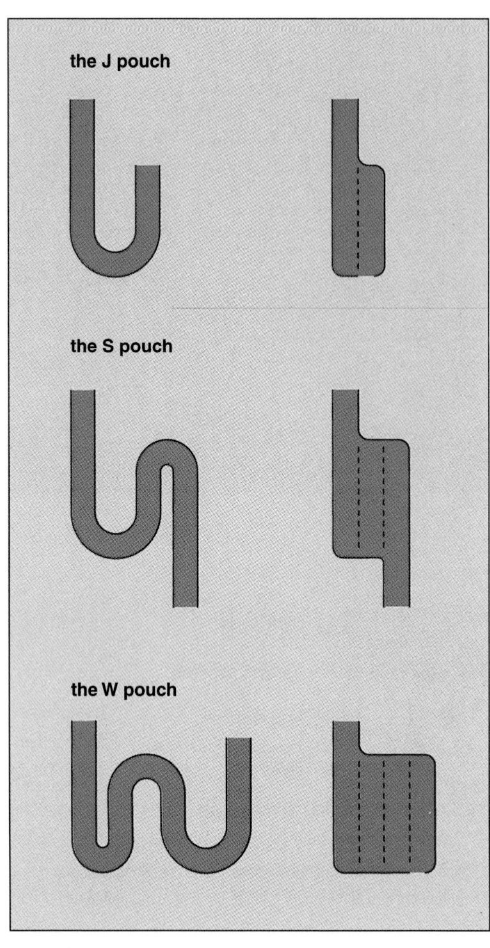

■ **Fig. 6.141** Diagrammatic representation of some of the types of ileoanal pouches devised for restorative panproctocolectomy.

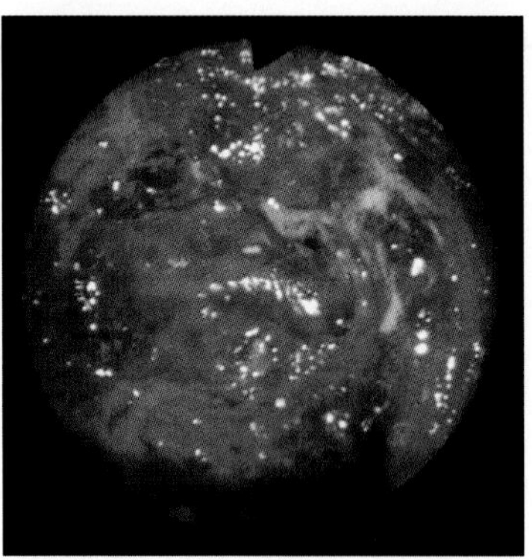

■ **Fig. 6.142** Severe inflammation in an ileal pouch (pouchitis).

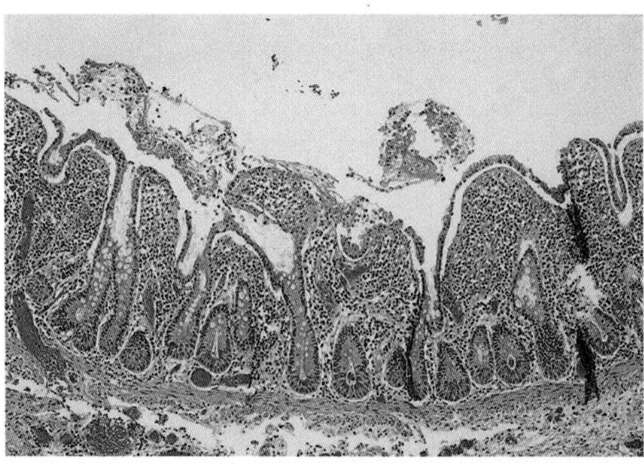

■ **Fig. 6.143** Microscopic appearance of moderate pouchitis showing subtotal atrophy of small intestinal villi, inflammatory infiltrates of the stroma, enterocyte injury with cuboidalization, vacuolization, and loss of the microvillous brush borders, and focal erosion with fibrinopurulent exudation.

defining feature emerges. Distinct from these are patients in whom there are symptoms (usually watery diarrhea) and a microscopic colitis, but no radiological or colonoscopic abnormality. Confusion may be avoided by restricting the terms appropriately, and making it clear when one is referring to ulcerative colitis, which has proximal histological changes that are not visible, above overt

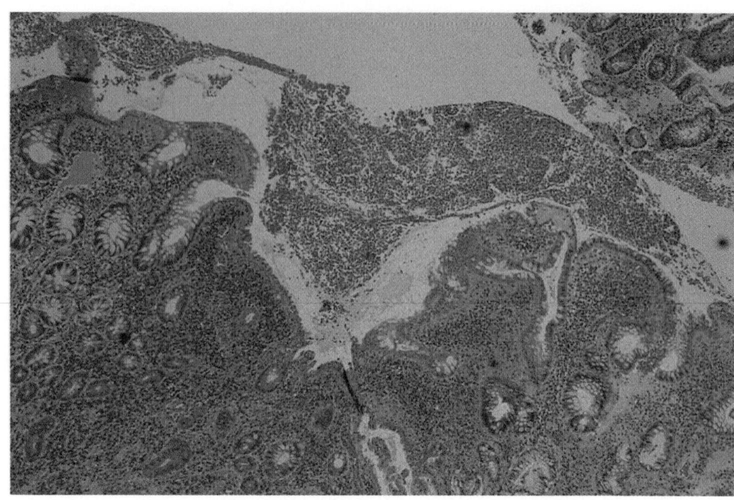

■ **Fig. 6.144** Histological appearance of pouchitis; severe inflammation and loss of the typical ileal characteristics are notable. H&E stain. Courtesy of Dr J. Sheffield.

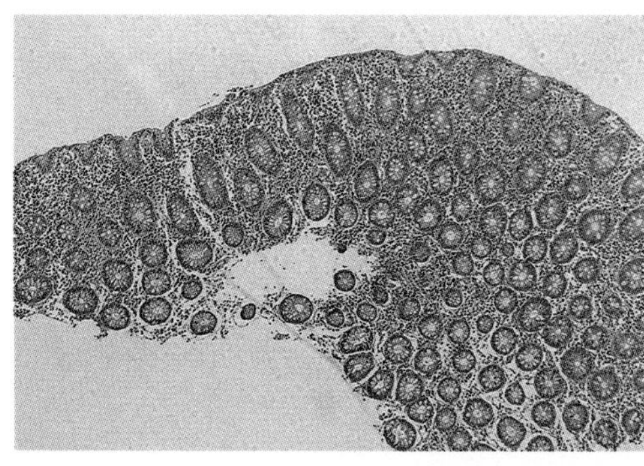

■ **Fig. 6.145** Biopsy appearance of lymphocytic colitis showing moderately increased cellularity of the lamina propria that is typical of the low-magnification appearance of the disease.

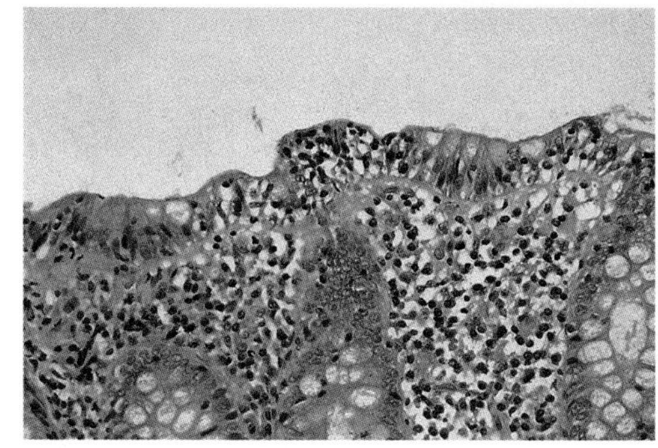

■ **Fig. 6.146** Lymphocytic colitis. High magnification of the mucosal surface in lymphocytic colitis showing the markedly increased number of intraepithelial lymphocytes (greater than 15–20 per 100 surface epithelial cells) that is the diagnostic feature of this disease. Fewer than five intraepithelial lymphocytes per 100 surface epithelial cells are present in normal colonic mucosa and fewer than ten are present in all other disease states.

distal disease. The histologist can usually distinguish two main forms of microscopic colitis both of which are commoner in women and which have an association with celiac disease. Lymphocytic (Figs 6.145, 6.146) and collagenous microscopic colitis are best recognized (Figs 6.147–6.149), but there may be some overlap between the two. Subtle endoscopic abnormalities are permitted within the definition by some authorities (Fig. 6.150).

ISCHEMIC COLITIS

Ischemic colitis arises from a failure of the blood supply to the colon and occurs most commonly in conjunction with advanced atherosclerotic disease. It is becoming steadily more common in

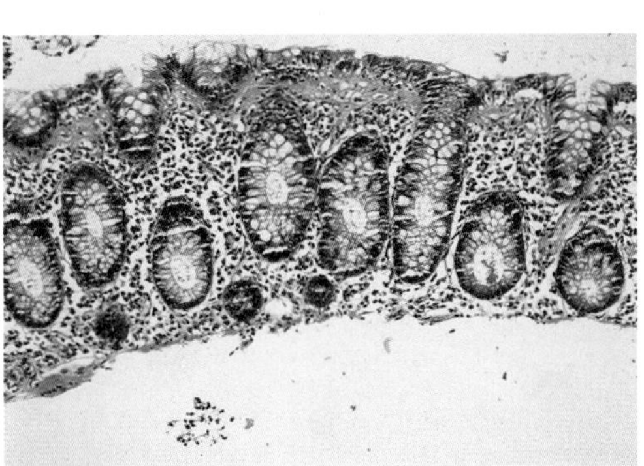

■ **Fig. 6.147** Collagenous colitis. Mucosal biopsy showing the increased stromal cellularity and prominent subepithelial collagen band that are the hallmarks of this condition.

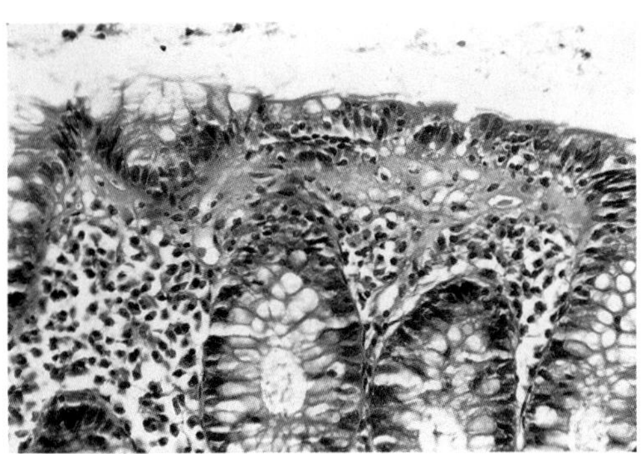

■ **Fig. 6.148** Collagenous colitis. High-magnification appearance of the mucosal surface showing the eponymous collagen band that is confined to the subepithelial zone (does not involve the pericryptal stroma), broad (greater than 10 μm in thickness), somewhat irregular, and sparsely infiltrated by lymphocytes. The surface epithelium contains increased numbers of intraepithelial lymphocytes.

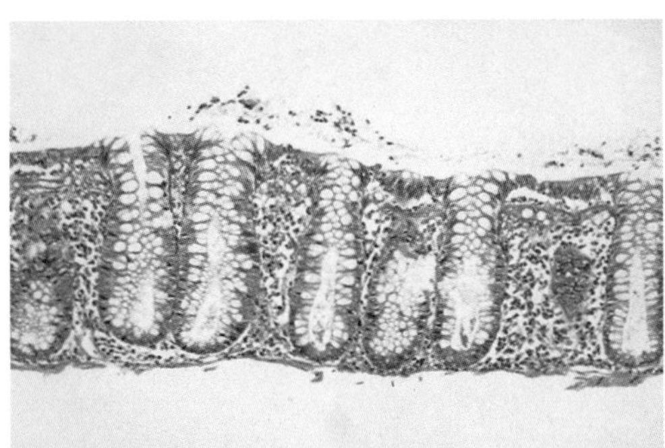

■ **Fig. 6.149** Collagenous colitis. Trichrome stain which stains type I collagen blue, highlights the distribution and thickness of the subepithelial collagen band.

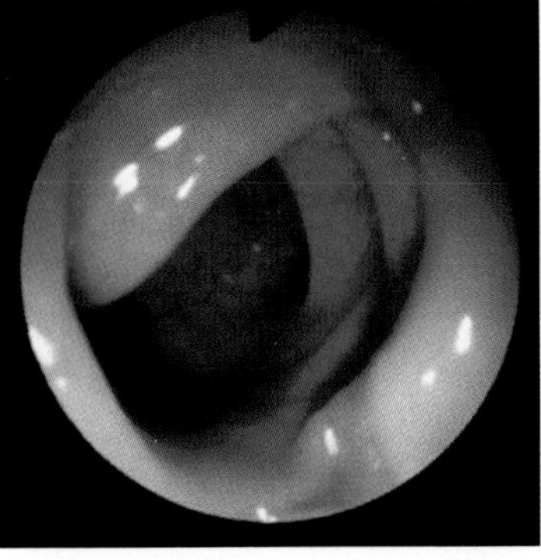

■ **Fig. 6.150** Subtle endoscopic abnormality in collagenous colitis. The loss of clarity of mucosal features contrasts with those of the normal colon (see above).

Western populations. Acute occlusion of a major artery leads to a surgical emergency with colonic gangrene (Fig. 6.151) or to a less acute syndrome typified by abdominal pain and bloody diarrhea. Arterial emboli, dissecting aortic aneurysm, and a number of rarer vasculitic cases may also be responsible. Gradual impairment – even to the extent of complete occlusion of one of the main arteries – can, however, occur without infarction, as the colon is well vascularized

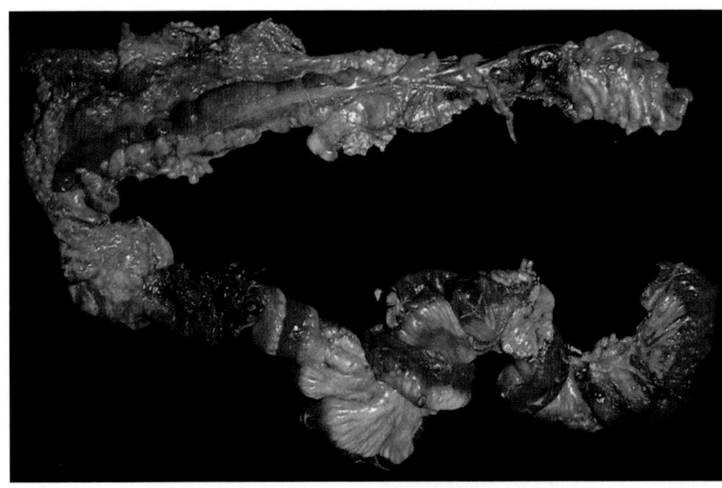

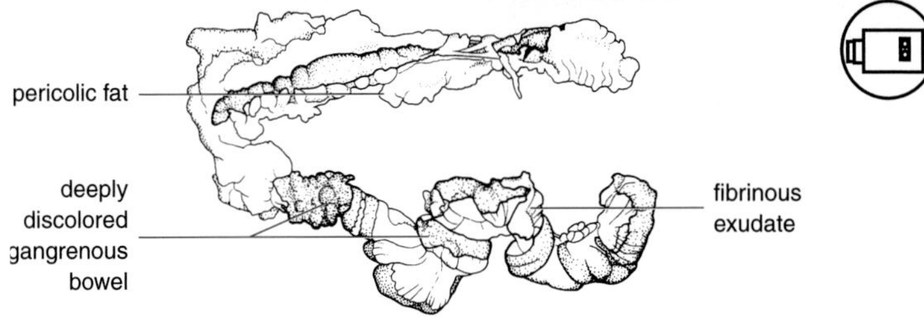

■ **Fig. 6.151** Macroscopic appearance of the large bowel in acute ischemic colitis showing gangrenous areas with overlying peritonitis.

and able to develop an adequate collateral circulation. The most vulnerable areas of the colon are around the splenic flexure, and, to a lesser extent, the rectosigmoid region, both of which lie in relatively poorly vascularized 'watershed' areas (between the superior and inferior mesenteric, and inferior mesenteric and internal iliac artery territories, respectively) (see Fig. 6.1).

It is relatively unusual for ischemic colitis to occur in the absence of generalized, previously recognized arteriopathy, but an additional trigger, such as a hypotensive episode, may initiate it. Typically abdominal pain, which is initially colicky, becomes localized to the left side, and then more severe as peritonitis develops. Bloody diarrhea, nausea, and vomiting are common. The plain abdominal radiograph may show an abnormal air pattern (Fig. 6.152) and 'thumbprinting,' representing edema of the mucosal folds, which shows better on contrast imaging (Fig. 6.153). Barium studies also show characteristic sawtooth irregularities and narrowing, but the preferred modality now is CT scanning which again confirms the abnormal air distribution and shows focal thickening of the colon (Figs 6.154–6.158). The colonoscopic features may be non-specific, but the localization to the splenic flexure and the exclusion of other causes are informative, and the presence of intramural bleeding almost diagnostic (Fig. 6.159–6.161). After spontaneous resolution, barium studies either appear normal or show persistent fibrous stricturing (Fig. 6.162). Rectosigmoid ischemia tends to cause a less dramatic illness, and peritonitis is most unusual. A non-specific proctitis or multiple discrete ulcers may be seen sigmoidoscopically.

The pathology depends on the rate of onset of ischemia, and similar changes may also be seen proximal to an obstructing carcinoma (which presumably reduces intramural blood flow as a result of raised intraluminal pressure). In acute ischemia, the involved section of bowel undergoes infarction; it is dilated and darkly congested with a friable wall, and is usually filled with blood. Mucosal ulceration and intense submucosal edema with hemorrhage and necrosis are seen, and in late cases, necrosis and hemorrhage of the muscle layers also occur (Figs 6.163–6.170). In less severe cases the histology may

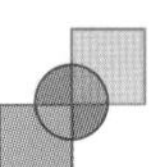

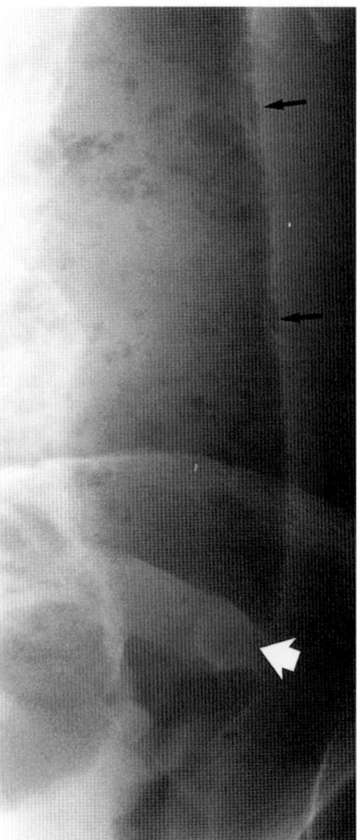

Fig. 6.152 Ischemic colitis with pneumatosis coli. Plain radiograph of the descending colon shows tiny bubbles overlying the air shadow of the colon. Bubbles of air are seen within the wall of the colon when viewed in profile (arrows). A thick fold (white arrow) crosses the lumen.

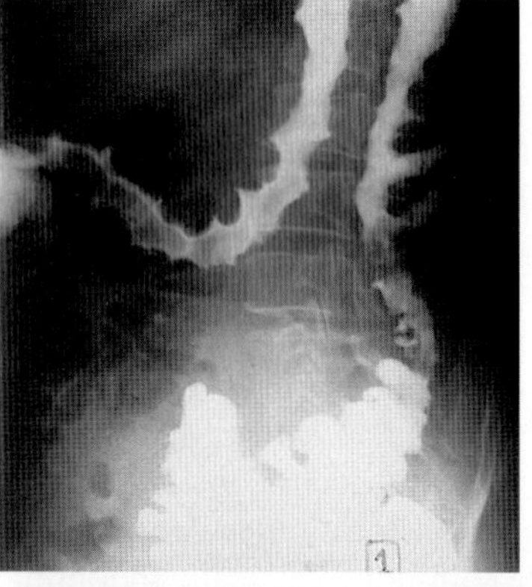

Fig. 6.153 'Thumb-printing' seen on a single-contrast barium enema in a patient with acute ischemic colitis.

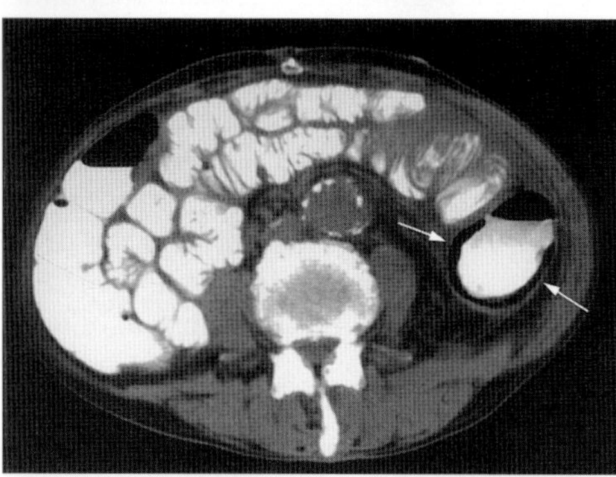

Fig. 6.154 Ischemic colitis with pneumatosis coli. CT through the descending colon shows curvilinear air (arrows) surrounding the contrast-filled lumen.

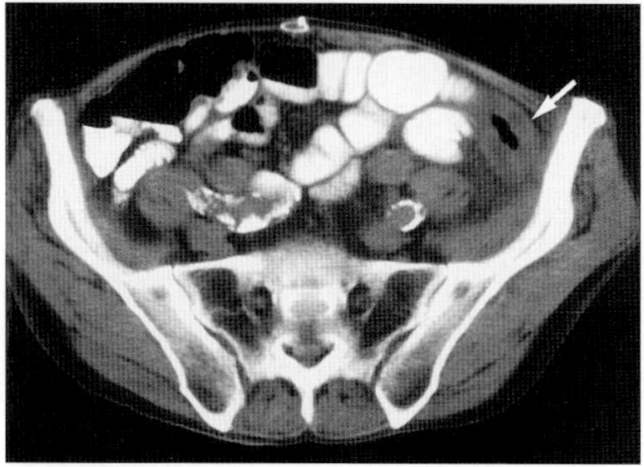

Fig. 6.155 CT through the upper pelvis shows symmetric thickening (arrow) of the lower descending colon with a subtle mural stratification pattern, corresponding to the area identified by the white arrow on the plain radiograph in Fig 6.152. (Reproduced with permission from reference 2, Fig. 13.73A–C.)

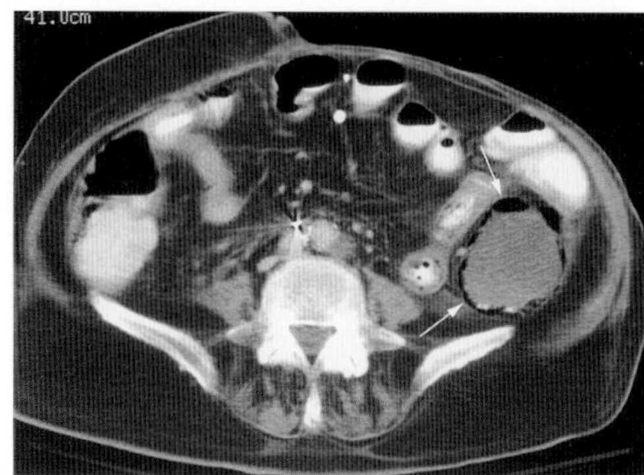

a

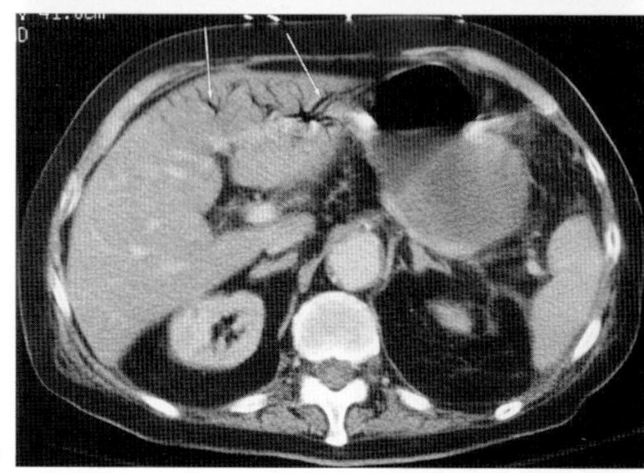

b

Fig. 6.156 CT demonstrates pneumatosis coli and portal venous gas in a patient with ischemic colitis. See also Chapter 7. (a) Pneumatosis coli is manifested as curvilinear gas (arrows) following the contour of the fluid-filled lumen of the descending colon. (b) Many 'seagull'-shaped tubular gas densities (arrows) are seen in the periphery of the left lobe of the liver. (Reproduced with permission from reference 2, Fig. 13.74.)

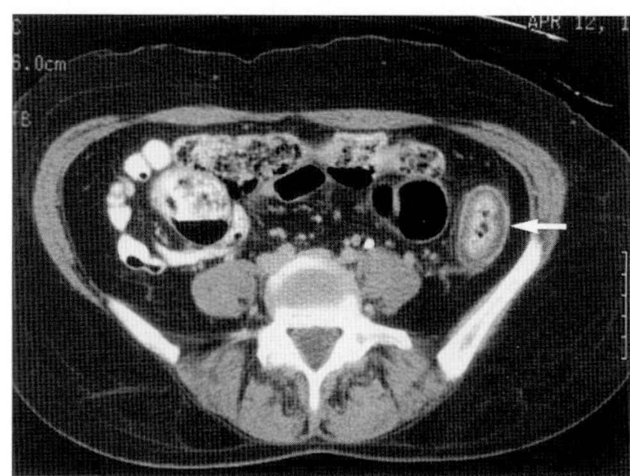

Fig. 6.157 Ischemic colitis in patient with left lower quadrant pain. CT demonstrates a thick-walled descending colon (arrow) with a mural stratification pattern. (Reproduced with permission from reference 2, Fig. 13.72.)

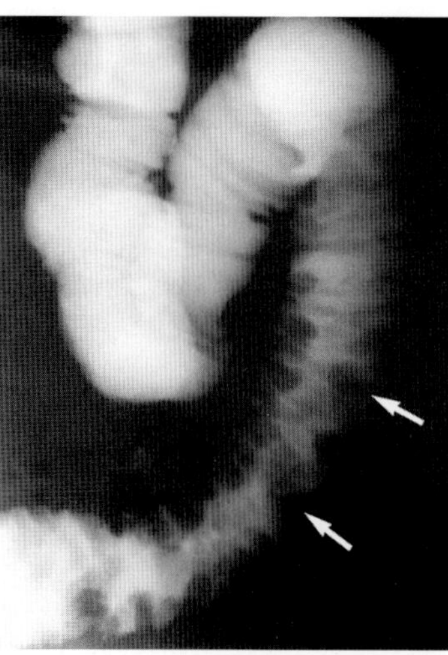

Fig. 6.158 Ischemic colitis in a patient with acute rectal bleeding. Single-contrast barium enema demonstrates numerous smooth-surfaced protrusions into the lumen (representative thumbprints identified by arrows). (Reproduced with permission from reference 2, Fig. 13.76.)

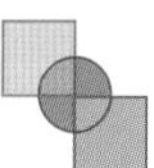

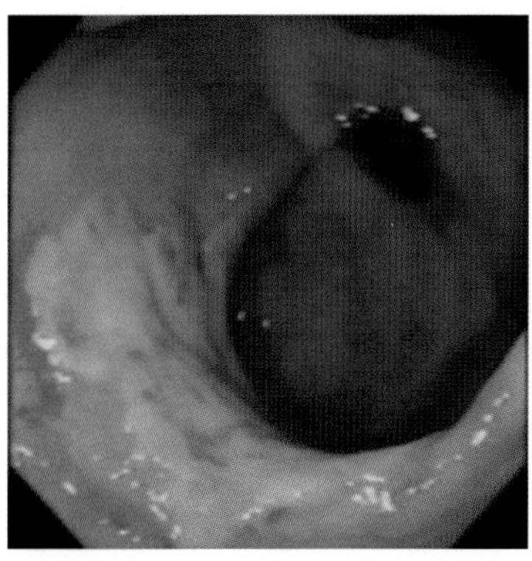

■ **Fig. 6.159** Colonoscopic appearance of an area of acute focal ischemia.

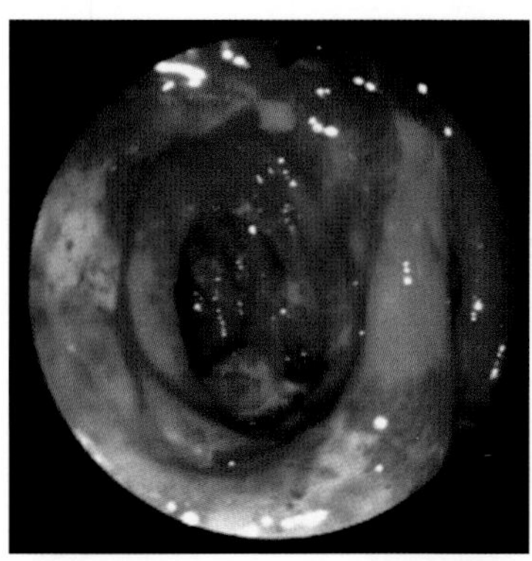

■ **Fig. 6.160** Colonoscopic appearance of ischemic colitis at the splenic flexure. The intramural bleeding is almost pathognomonic.

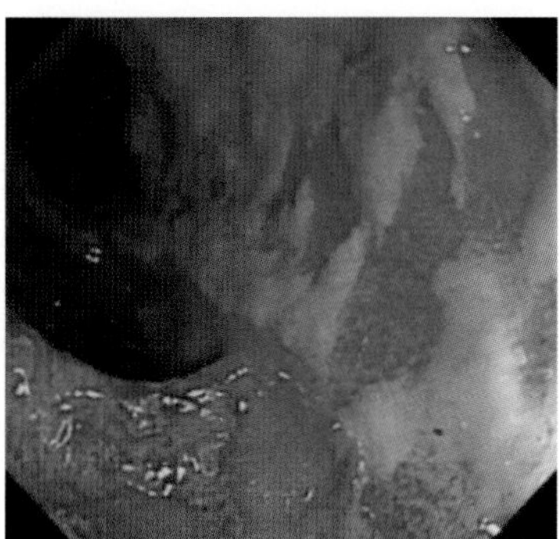

■ **Fig. 6.161** Another appearance typical of ischemic colitis, and not to be confused with pseudomembranous colitis (see Fig. 6.58).

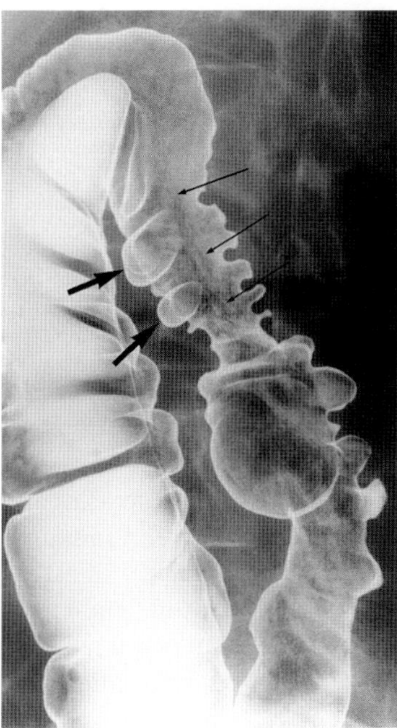

■ **Fig. 6.162** Double-contrast barium enema demonstrating healing ischemic colitis. A shallow barium-filled ulcer (thin arrows) is seen in the splenic flexure. Sacculations (thick arrows) of the colon reflect scarring. The patient had bled 1 week prior to the study. (Reproduced with permission from reference 9, Fig. 11.)

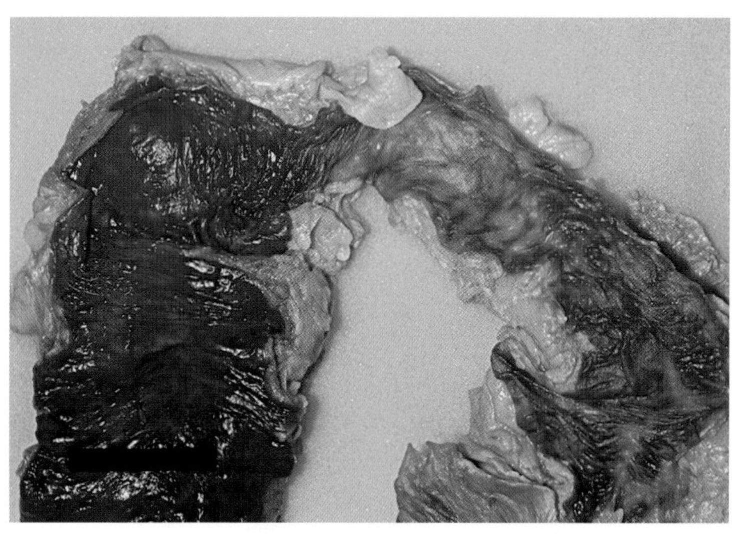

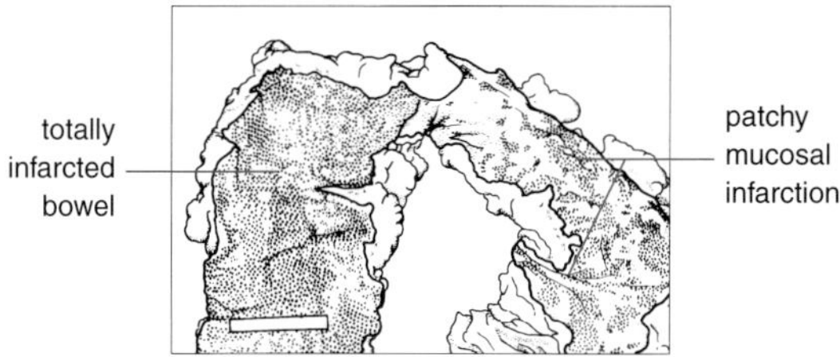

■ **Fig. 6.163** Macroscopic appearance of the colon in severe acute ischemic colitis with full thickness infarction.

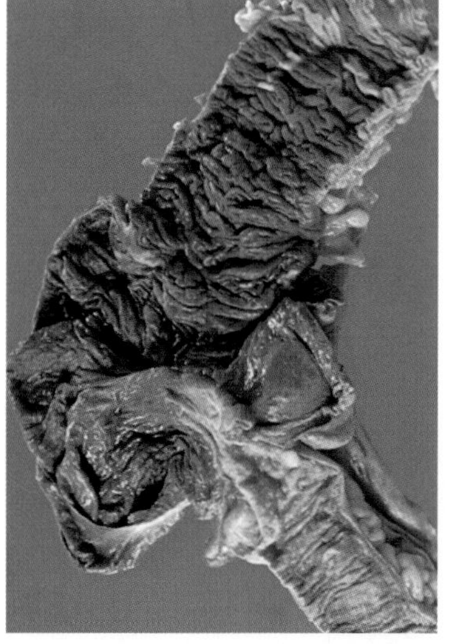

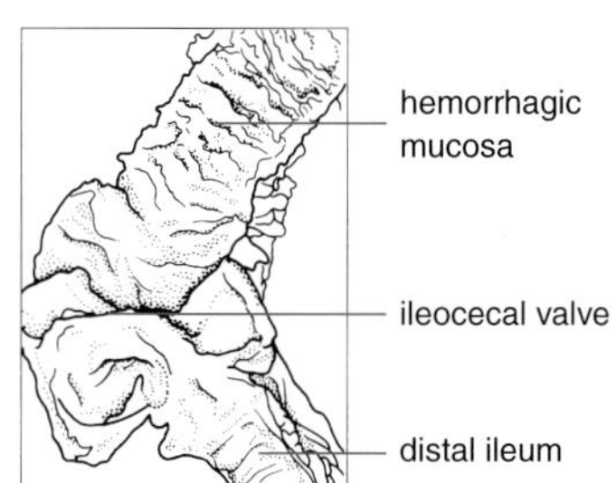

■ **Fig. 6.164** Acute ischemia of the right colon due to occlusion of a branch of the right colic artery. In this case, only the mucosa is infarcted and the muscle is still viable.

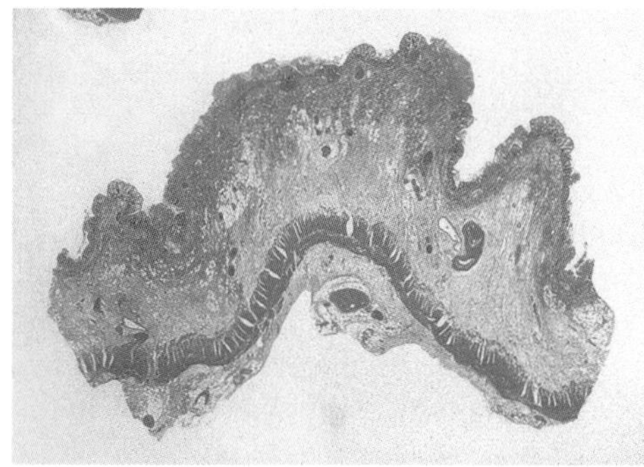

■ **Fig. 6.165** Whole-mount microscopic section in early ischemic colitis showing marked expansion of the submucosa due to edema (seen as 'thumb-printing' on barium imaging) and hemorrhagic necrosis of the mucosa. The muscularis mucosa is still viable.

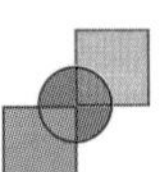

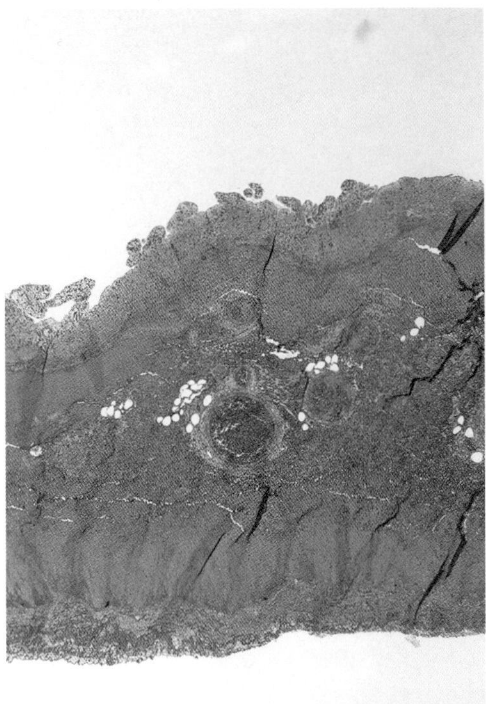

■ **Fig. 6.166** Ischemia secondary to mesenteric vein thrombosis. Microscopic appearance showing the characteristically massive accumulation of blood in the intestinal wall with necrosis of the mucosa and muscularis propria and thrombosis of submucosal veins.

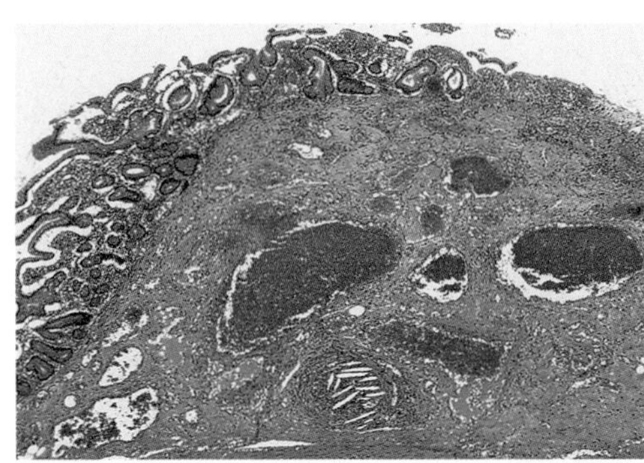

■ **Fig. 6.167** Ischemic colitis due to atheroembolus. Microscopic appearance showing massive edema of the submucosa, hemorrhage and patchy necrosis of the mucosa, and a large cholesterol embolus occluding a muscular artery in the deep submucosa (bottom center).

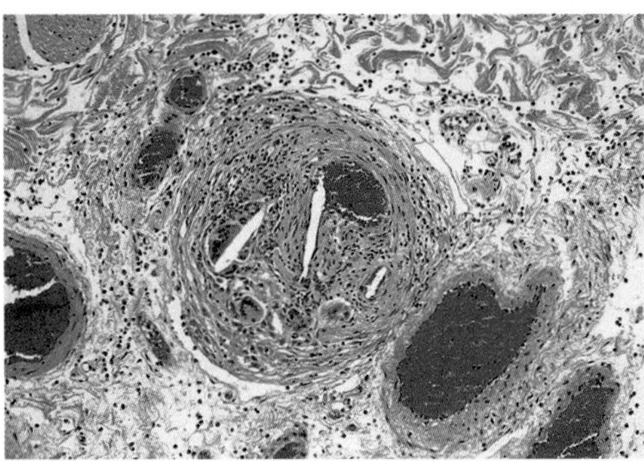

■ **Fig. 6.168** High-magnification view of an embolized atherosclerotic plaque within a submucosal artery. The shard-like cholesterol crystals and associated foreign body giant cell reaction by which the atherosclerosis can be recognized are seen plugging a submucosal artery.

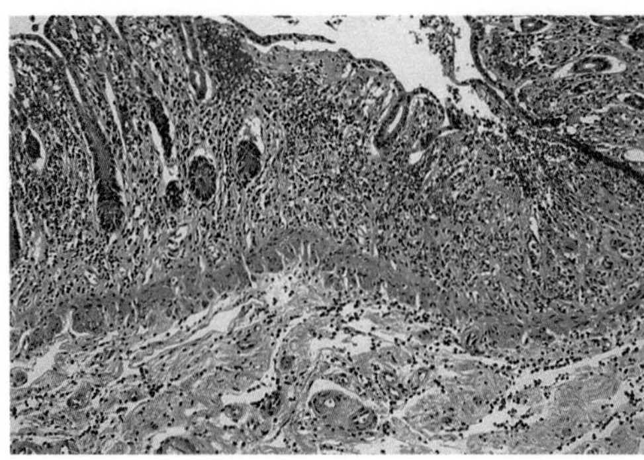

■ **Fig. 6.169** Acute ischemic colitis. Mucosal biopsy showing characteristic microscopic features including hemorrhage and fibrin exudation into the lamina propria, marked epithelial injury, and a relative paucity of acute inflammation. Ischemia injury causes epithelial cell flattening and sloughing ('gland withering'), leaving behind the slit-like outlines of denuded glandular basement membranes.

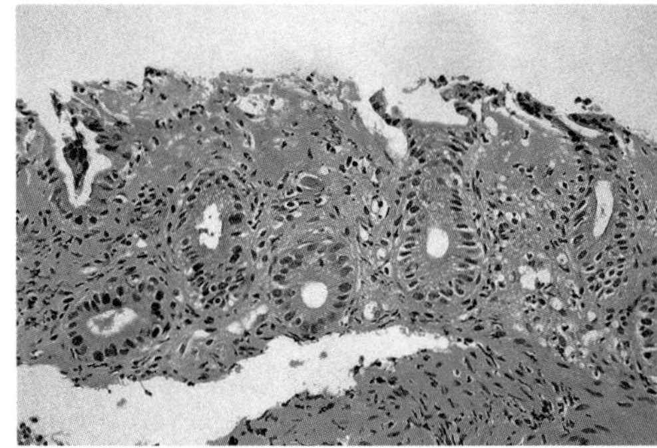

■ **Fig. 6.170** Acute ischemic colitis. High-magnification appearance of sloughing of the surface epithelium, dense, palely eosinophilic fibrin deposits in the lamina propria, and a fibrin thrombus in a mucosal capillary. The differential diagnosis of this pattern of injury includes mesenteric vascular disease, embolic disease, enteric vasculitis, drug (vasoactive, volume-depleting, and/or thrombogenic) effect, and infection by toxin-producing pathogens such as entero-hemorrhagic strains of *E. coli*.

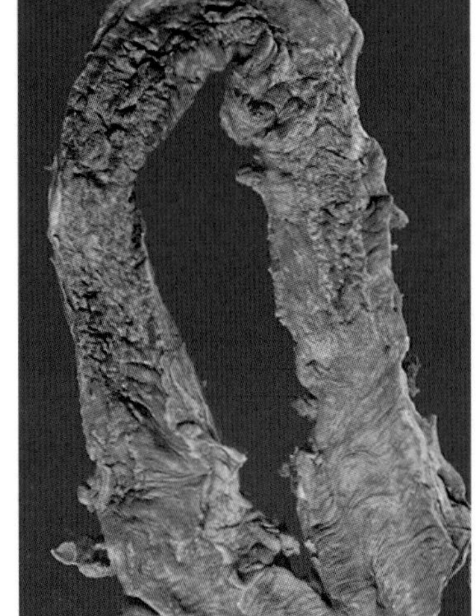

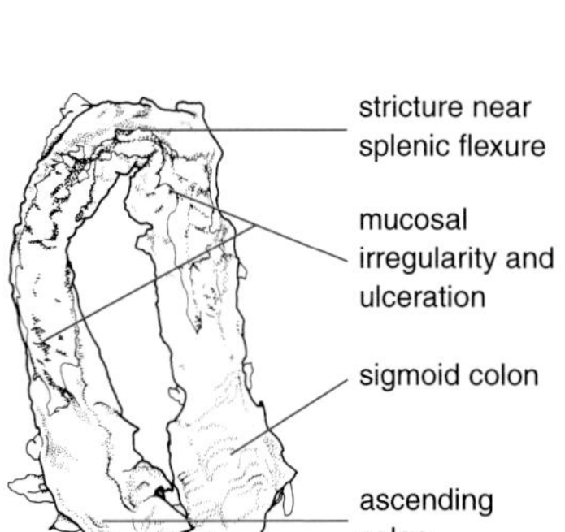

■ **Fig. 6.171** Macroscopic appearance in chronic ischemia showing narrowing and ulceration predominantly at the splenic flexure.

be almost normal despite striking endoscopic findings. In convalescence, reparative granulation tissue is formed and re-epithelialization of the mucosa begins. Granulation tissue is later replaced by fibrosis, and it is this that leads to post-ischemic stricturing. Chronic ischemia often exhibits both stricturing and ulceration with granulation tissue (Figs 6.171, 6.172). Fibrosis of the submucosa and circular muscle coat is also characteristic. Where mucosa survives, iron-laden macrophages are often prominent in the lamina propria (Figs 6.173–6.175).

A mild and transient form of ischemic colitis is seen occasionally in young women on the combined oral contraceptive. Abdominal pain and diarrhea, accompanied by the usual radiological signs, are rapidly followed by complete spontaneous resolution. The endoscopic and histological appearances are those of an acute mucosal hemorrhagic necrosis. A number of other drugs have also been implicated.

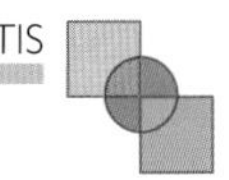

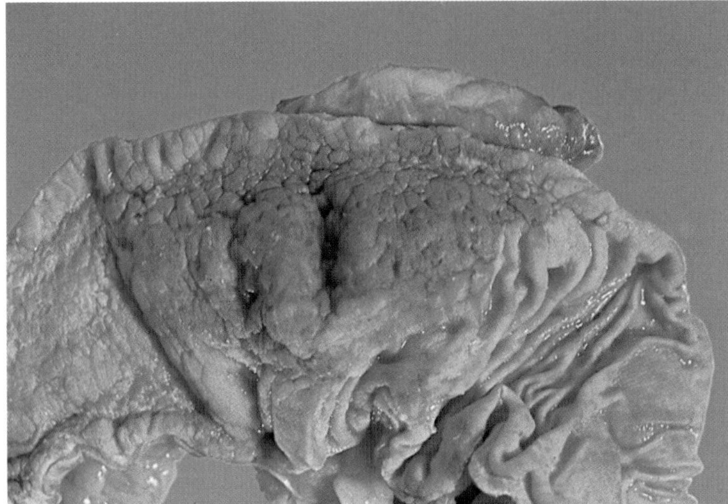

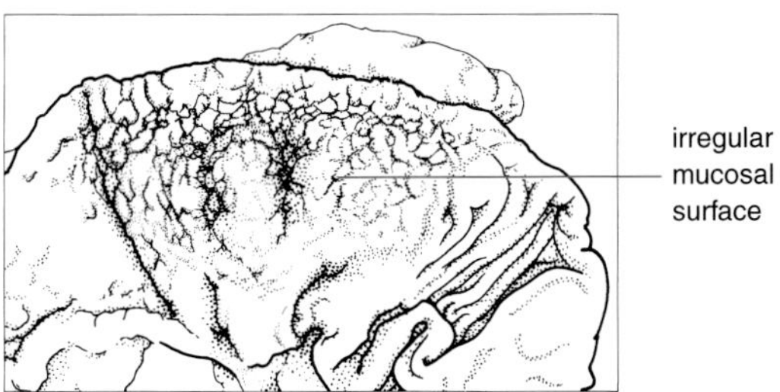

■ **Fig. 6.172** Macroscopic appearance of strictured colon (in the region of the splenic flexure) in chronic ischemia showing the irregular and thickened mucosal surface produced by re-epithelialization and granulation tissue.

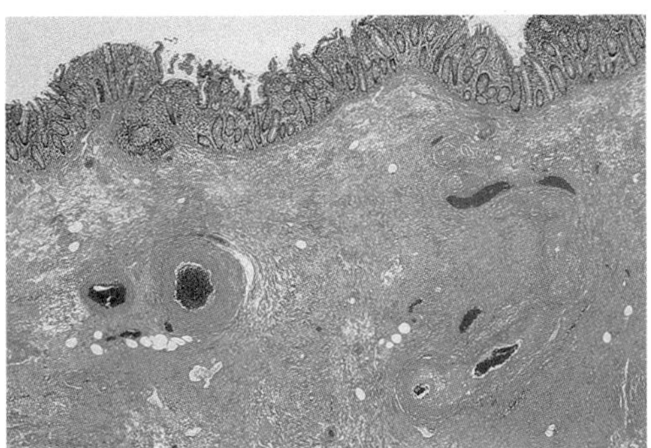

■ **Fig. 6.173** Microscopic appearance of chronic, non-occlusive ischemic colitis showing characteristic scarring of the submucosa.

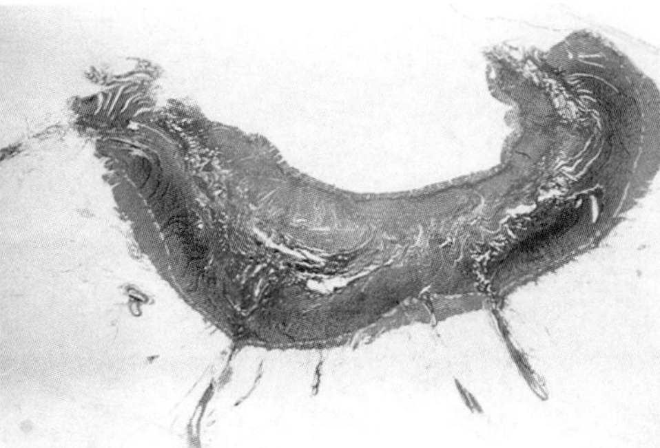

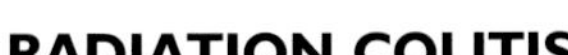

■ **Fig. 6.174** Trichrome stain of colonic stricture due to chronic ischemic colitis showing transmural fibrosis.

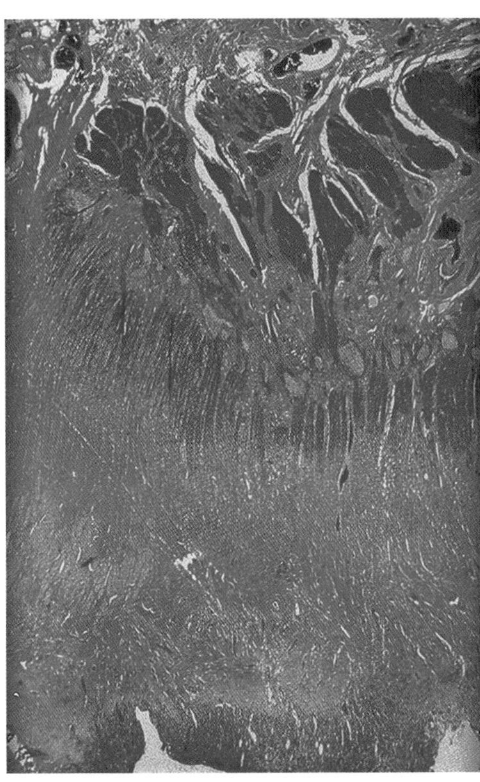

■ **Fig. 6.175** Trichrome-stained section of the colonic wall in chronic ischemia showing the dense scarring of the submucosa and the patchy fibrosis of the mucosa and the muscularis propria.

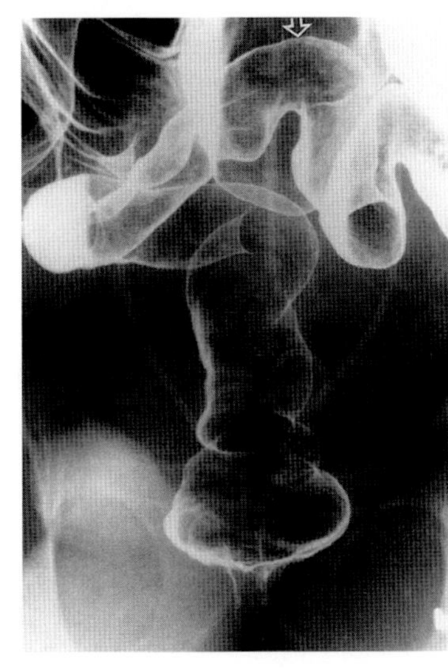

■ **Fig. 6.176** Double-contrast barium enema demonstrating radiation proctosigmoiditis. The rectosigmoid colon has a narrowed, tubular shape, with loss of the valves of Houston. Finely granular mucosa is seen in the distal sigmoid colon (arrow) and rectosigmoid junction. Ureteral stents are in place. (Reproduced with permission from reference 4, Fig. 68.61.)

RADIATION COLITIS

Radiation colitis may be acute or chronic. Historically it has mostly followed radiotherapy for gynecological malignancies, but some exposure of the relatively fixed rectum is inevitable in treatment of prostate and the rectum itself, and as radiation therapy is increasingly used for these indications more cases of radiation enteritis are to be expected. The acute form is rarely severe and is generally self-limiting. The chronic variety – which is largely of an ischemic nature – begins at least 6 months and as much as 10 years after the radiotherapy. Tenesmus and rectal bleeding are frequent presenting symptoms; radiology is sometimes helpful (Fig 6.176) but diagnosis is strongly suggested by the presence of associated telangiectasia at endoscopy (Fig. 6.177); the histology is supportive (Fig 6.178).

REFERENCES

1. Rubesin SE, Laufer I. Double contrast barium enema: technical aspects. In: Levine MS, Rubesin SE, Laufer I (eds) Double contrast gastrointestinal radiology, pp. 331–356. Philadelphia: WB Saunders, 2000, Figs 11.22, 25, 31.
2. Rubesin SE, Bartram CI, Laufer I. Inflammatory bowel disease. In: Levine MS, Rubesin SE, Laufer I (eds) Double contrast gas-

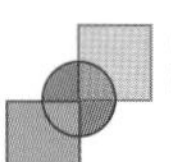

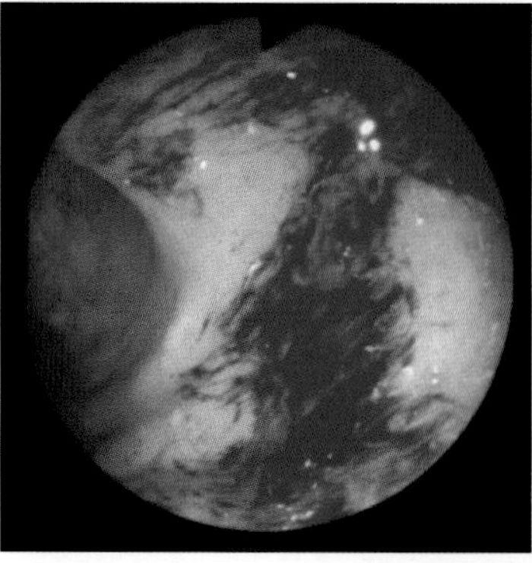

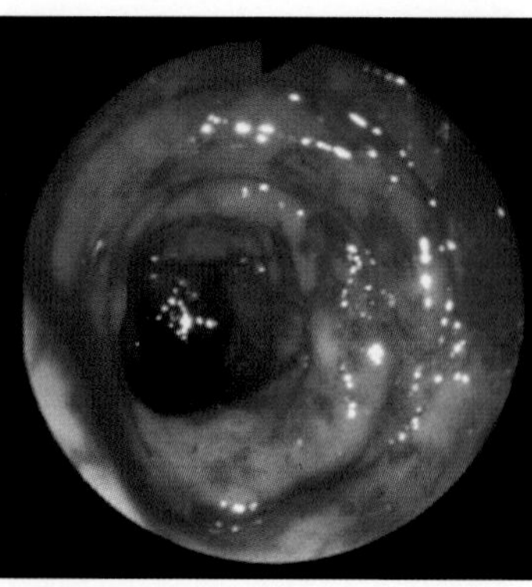

■ Fig. 6.177 Endoscopic appearance of radiation colitis. The presence of numerous telangiectatic lesions is suggestive of the diagnosis.

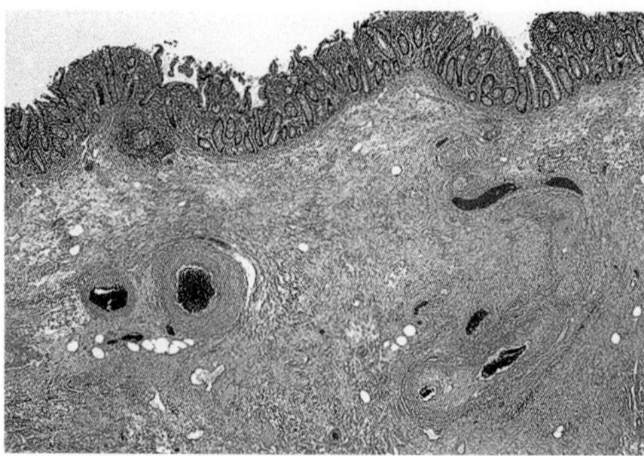

■ Fig 6.178 Histology of radiation enteritis. Submucosal fibrosis and vascular thickening are present in the absence of inflammation.

trointestinal radiology, pp. 331–356. Philadelphia: WB Saunders, 2000, Figs 13.11, 24, 30, 36, 49, 52, 55, 59, 70, 72, 73A–C, 74, 76.

3. Rubesin SE, Levine MS, Laufer I, Herlinger H. Double contrast barium enema technique. Radiology 2000; 215: 642–650, Fig. 15.
4. Rubesin SE, Schnall M. Rectum. In: Gore RM, Levine MS, Laufer I (eds) Textbook of gastrointestinal radiology, pp. 1291–1309. Philadelphia: WB Saunders, 1994, Figs. 68.48, 49C, 61.
5. Lee R-C, Chiang J-H, Chou Y-H, *et al.* Intestinal *Schistosomiasis japonica:* CT-pathologic correlation. Radiology 1994; 193: 539–542, Fig. 3.
6. Rubesin SE, Bronner M. Radiologic-pathologic concepts in Crohn's disease. Adv Gastrointest Radiol 1991; 1: 27–55, Fig. 28.
7. Rubesin SE, Laufer I. Pictorial glossary of double contrast radiology. In: Gore RM, Levine MS (eds) Textbook of gastrointestinal radiology, 2nd edn, pp. 44–65. Philadelphia: WB Saunders, 2000, Fig. 5.3A.
8. Rubesin SE *et al.* Radiologic investigation of inflammatory bowel disease. In: MacDermott RP, Stenson WF (eds) Inflammatory bowel disease, pp. 453–491. New York: Elsevier Science Publishing Co, 1992, Figs. 25.35, 36, 37, 40, 41B.
9. Rubesin SE, Levine MS, Laufer I, Herlinger H. Double contrast barium enema technique. Radiology 2000; 215: 642–650, Fig. 11.

COLON II

7

COLORECTAL CANCER

Colorectal cancer is the second commonest neoplasm in most developed countries and accounts for approximately 10% of deaths from malignancy and at least 3% of all deaths in the United Kingdom. It occurs at all ages, but is commonest in the sixth and seventh decades. Colonic cancer affects the sexes approximately equally, but rectal cancer is commoner in men. No single cause has been established but research in recognized high-risk groups has led to some important discoveries. The genetics of familial adenomatous polyposis (FAP) (see below), of hereditary non-polyposis colonic carcinoma (HNPCC), and the increasing knowledge of oncogenes, tumor suppressor genes and mismatch repair genes have shed useful light on the mechanisms operating in sporadic carcinomas. Acquired chromosomal defects are usual in patients with sporadic tumors, at sites often including the FAP locus (apc), and the p53 site on chromosome 17. Mutated in about 70% of cases, p53 is the commonest chromosomal alteration not only in colorectal carcinoma but also in many other solid tissue malignancies. In most tumors, at least two chromosomal defects are present. The loss of tumor suppression activity (e.g. p53, apc) appears of more general importance than unrestrained effects of oncogenes (e.g. c-myc, K-ras) (Fig. 7.1). HNPCC families have mutations in the mismatch repair genes, which code for the repair mechanism when DNA is damaged (see below). These mutations too are over-represented in sporadic tumors in which they appear also to engender a better than average prognosis for a given histological staging. Genetic counseling is obviously relevant for the autosomal dominant cancer families, but is also possible for families with multiple cases but in whom the risk falls short of a pure Mendelian inheritance. There is an increased incidence of carcinoma in patients with adenomatous polyps even when these have been removed, and the extra risk in ulcerative colitis is discussed in Chapter 6. Environmental factors nonetheless play an important part, and dietary fiber (from fruit and vegetables and perhaps cereals) is protective. It is highly probable that low doses of folate and of aspirin and non-steroidal anti-inflammatory agents are also protective.

In populations at average risk, about two thirds of colorectal malignancies occur in the sigmoid colon or rectum (Fig. 7.2), about 15% in the cecum, and the remainder distributed more or less evenly throughout the rest of the colon. This has the practical implication that the majority of tumors are potentially within the range of flexible sigmoidoscopy. The tumors spread by local invasion, by distant dissemination through blood vessels and lymphatics, and to a lesser extent directly into the peritoneal cavity. A system of pathological staging, described by Dukes in 1932 (Fig. 7.3), has been amended and updated, but remains widely

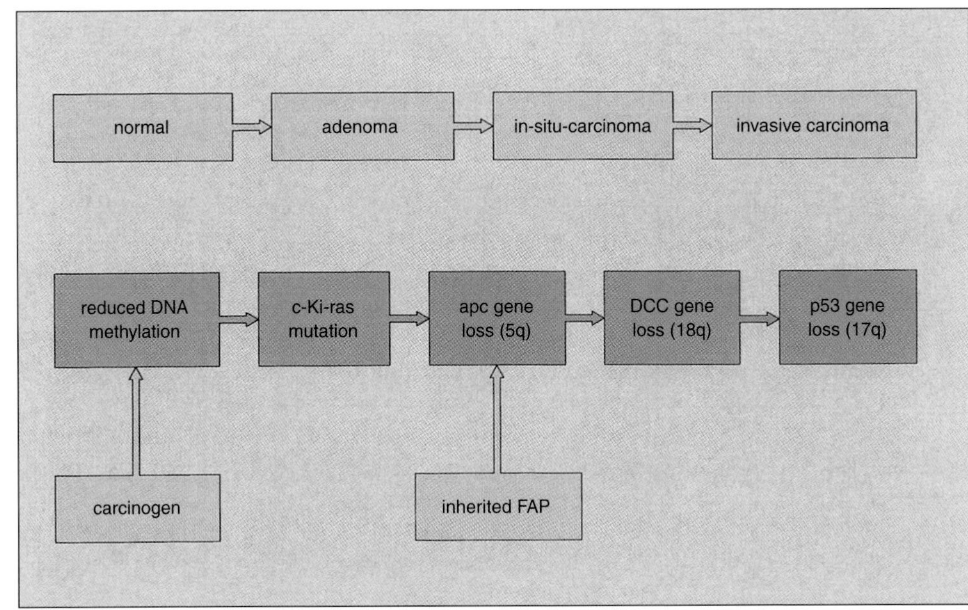

Fig. 7.1 Progression of the genetic defect leading to colonic carcinoma. Although the sequence of events is thought often to occur as shown, it does not necessarily need to involve all of the changes nor to follow this particular order.

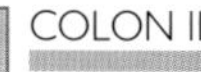

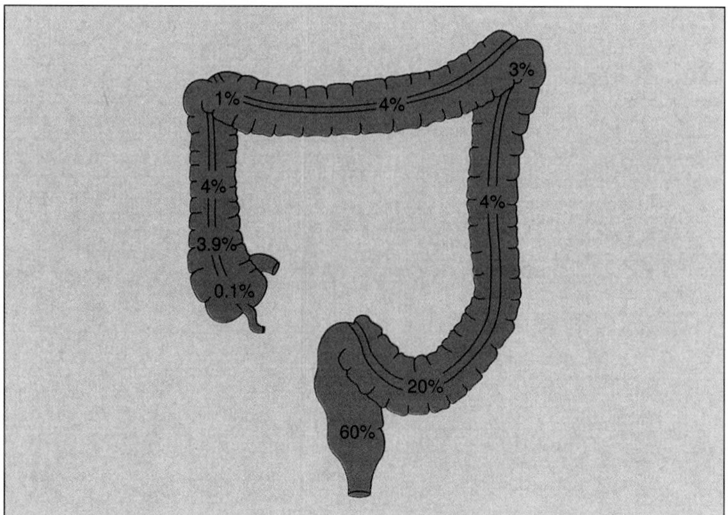

■ **Fig. 7.2** Diagram showing the incidence of carcinoma in different parts of the colon.

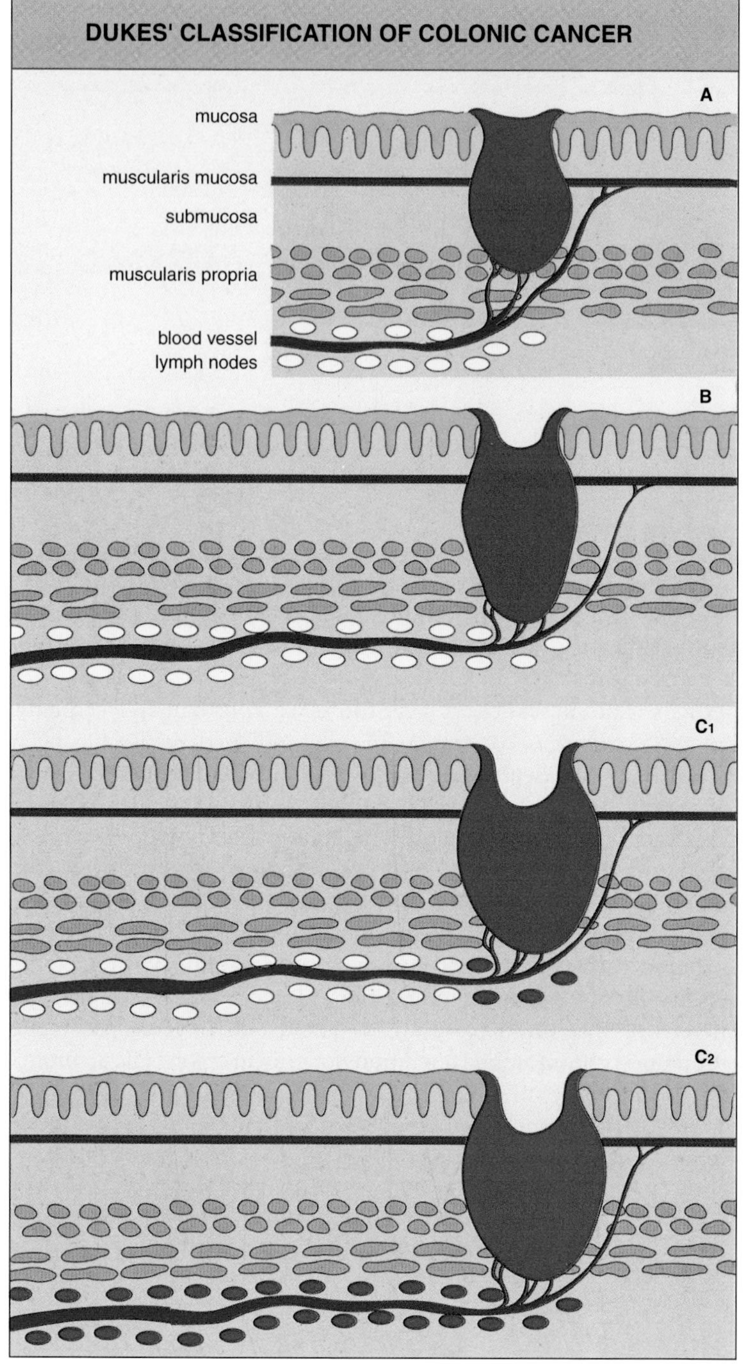

■ **Fig. 7.3** Diagram showing Dukes' grading of colonic carcinoma. In A, the tumor is confined to the bowel wall. In B, it extends through the muscle coat but does not involve lymph nodes. In C, all layers are affected, with the proximal lymph nodes affected in C1, and both the proximal and the highest resected nodes positive in C2.

used. Outside screen-ing programs, approximately 15% of tumors are stage A, 40% stage B and 45% stage C or worse. Approximately 5% of patients have multiple malignancies at presentation (synchronous carcinomas), but metachronous tumors are also well recognized.

Symptoms of colorectal carcinoma depend largely on the site of the lesion. Typically, change in bowel habit and rectal bleeding occur with the more distal tumors, while more proximal tumors tend to present later in their evolution, with obstruction, or with symptomatic anemia. Prolapse of a rectal carcinoma at the anus is occasionally seen (Fig. 7.4), and some patients first present with symptomatic metastases (Fig. 7.5). Rectal bleeding remains the most useful single symptom from a diagnostic viewpoint, and detection of occult bleeding is of proven value in population screening.

Physical examination is usually normal, but there may be anemia, a palpable abdominal mass, or hepatomegaly from metastases. Digital examination of the rectum and sigmoidoscopy may provide the diagnosis (Fig. 7.6) (confirmed by biopsy). Barium enema examines also the more proximal colon, and can identify the site of the tumor more accurately than conventional colonoscopy, but the ability of colonoscopy to provide tissue and to remove synchronous polyps makes it the clear preferred option (Figs 7.7, 7.8). Now that electromagnetic imaging techniques are becoming available the previous concerns about the accuracy of identification of tumor site can be eliminated (Fig 7.9), and the surgeon given confident anatomical guidance.

The classical 'apple-core' stricture (Fig. 7.10), irregular polypoid lesions (Fig. 7.11), the saddle-like (Fig. 7.12) and plaque forms of tumor (Fig. 7.13) are virtually diagnostic to the extent of leading to laparotomy without intervening colonoscopy in some centers, but the colonoscopist is less likely to be misled by atypical, benign strictures, malignant 'carpeting' of the colonic wall (Fig. 7.14) or co-existent sigmoid diverticular disease; the identification of recurrent anastomotic cancer may also be easier to identify colonoscopically (Fig. 7.15). In the case of an obstructing or intussuscepting lesion, which does not permit passage of the colonoscope, it is important to visualize the colon proximal to the tumor prior to surgery. This can be done by conventional barium studies (Fig. 7.16), or by standard CT scan (Fig. 7.17), but the preferred technique now should be CT colography or 'virtual colonoscopy' in which an apparent three-dimensional reconstruction of the colon is made possible with the same degree of preparation but minimal invasiveness (Fig. 7.18). So-called 'fly through' views are possible from proximal to distal or in reverse. This technique is taking on an important general diagnostic role also in many centers now. It is probable that in time this technique will be overtaken by analogous MR imaging so as to avoid the substantial radiation exposure, but for the present MRI has its major role in the staging of rectal tumors (Fig. 7.19).

At diagnosis, most colorectal tumors are apparently circumscribed and ulcerated with raised, rolled edges (Fig. 7.20), but increasingly colonoscopists are identifying adenomatous polyps with foci of malignancy (Figs 7.21, 7.22), important as these can safely be removed endoscopically with definitive resolution of the problem. Large, fungating tumors are less common and predominate in the cecum

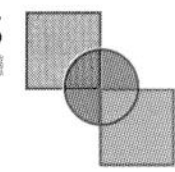

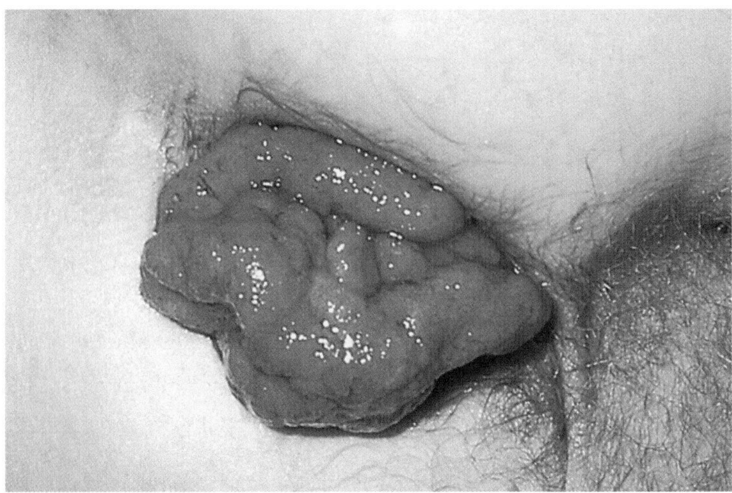

■ **Fig. 7.4** A prolapsing rectal carcinoma. Courtesy of Mr J.P.S. Thomson.

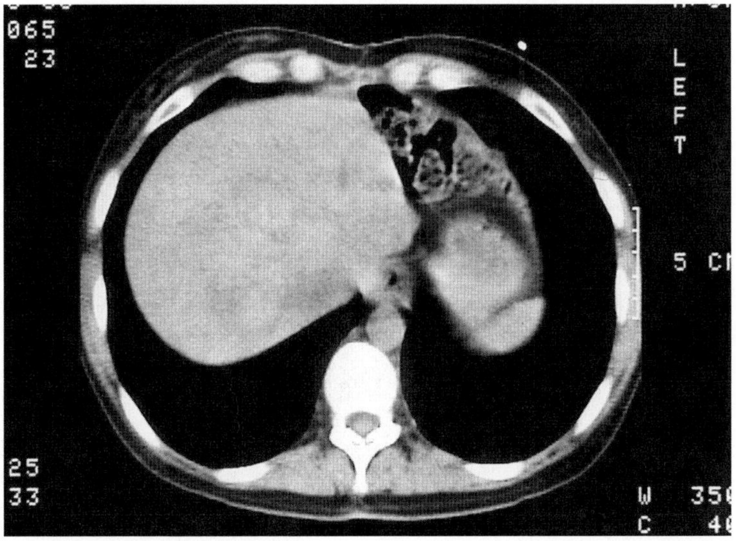

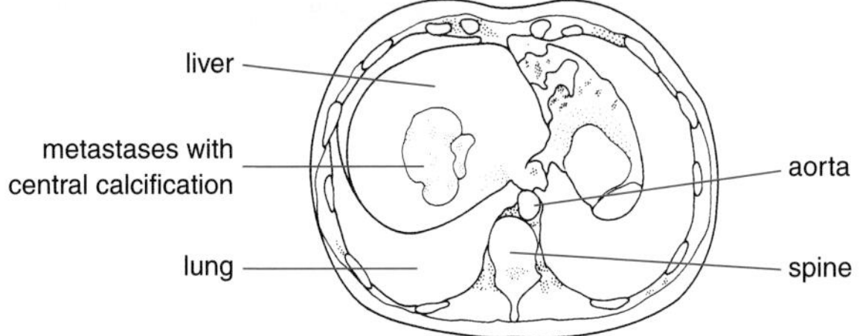

■ **Fig. 7.5** CT scan demonstrating metastases with central calcification in a patient with jaundice from disseminated colorectal carcinoma who had no bowel symptoms.

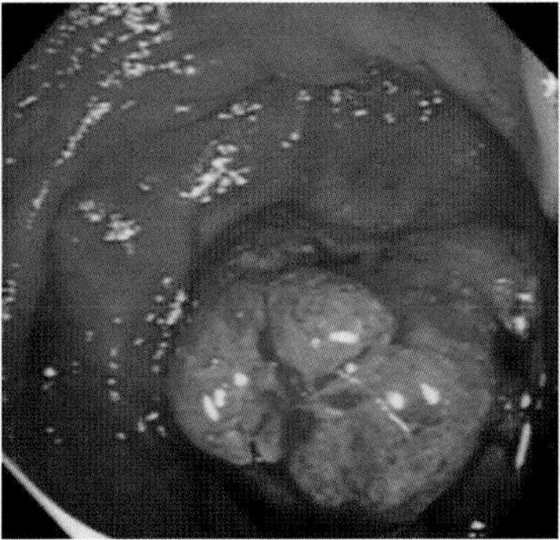

■ **Fig. 7.6** Malignant polyp seen in the lower bowel at flexible sigmoidoscopy.

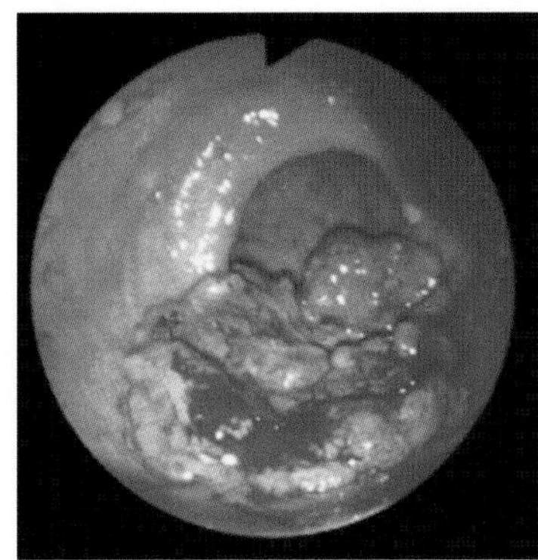

■ **Fig. 7.7** Colonoscopic appearance of hemorrhagic carcinoma in ascending colon.

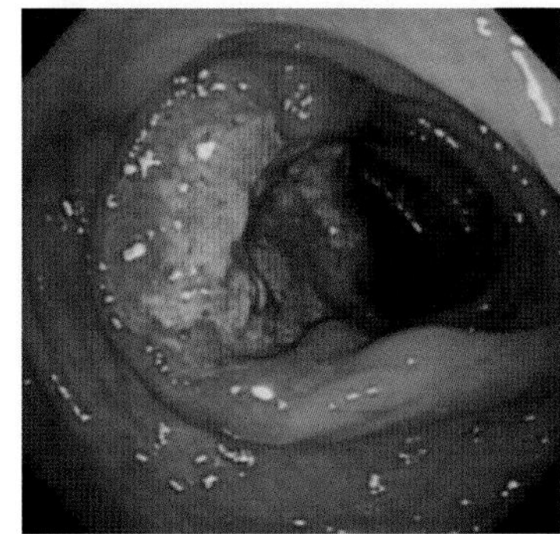

■ **Fig. 7.8** Carcinoma of the right side of the colon.

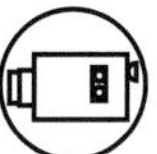

(Fig. 7.23). Annular stenosis occurs (Figs 7.24, 7.25) but a diffusely infiltrating tumor akin to a gastric linitis plastica is rare – except perhaps in ulcerative colitis (Fig. 7.26). The small proportion of tumors which are mucoid have a worse prognosis. Histologically, almost all colorectal malignancies are adenocarcinomas, with varying degrees of differentiation (Figs 7.27–7.30). Residual non-malignant adenoma will be found in at least 15% of cases. Colosonography discriminates the layers of the colonic wall (Fig. 7.31), and can contribute to the pre-operative staging of colonic tumors, but the preferred options in most leading centers now are CT scanning for colonic tumors (Fig. 7.17), and magnetic resonance imaging for those in the rectum (Fig. 7.19).

POLYPS

Colonic polyps may be neoplastic, hamartomatous, inflammatory, or hyperplastic. The majority of neoplastic lesions are adenomas, but other more unusual tumors are also seen. Hamartomatous polyps are seen in juvenile polyposis and Peutz–Jeghers syndrome (see also Chapter 4). The inflammatory polyp and hyperplastic polyp are seen in inflammatory bowel disease (see Chapter 6), and the former also in benign lymphoid polyposis.

Adenomatous polyps

Adenomatous polyps may cause rectal bleeding, or occasionally intussusception (see below), with the potential for external prolapse (see Chapter 8), but their malignant potential is of greater importance. Approximately 75% are tubular, 10% villous, and the remainder tubulo-villous in form (Figs 7.32–7.38). The risk of malignant transformation is highest in villous adenomas and increases with polyp size, rising dramatically in those over 2 cm in diameter. Although the natural history of small (<5 mm) polyps is admittedly less well established, it is wise to remove all identified adenomatous polyps. Surveillance regimes with regular colonoscopy are then advo-

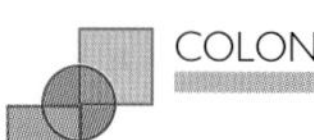

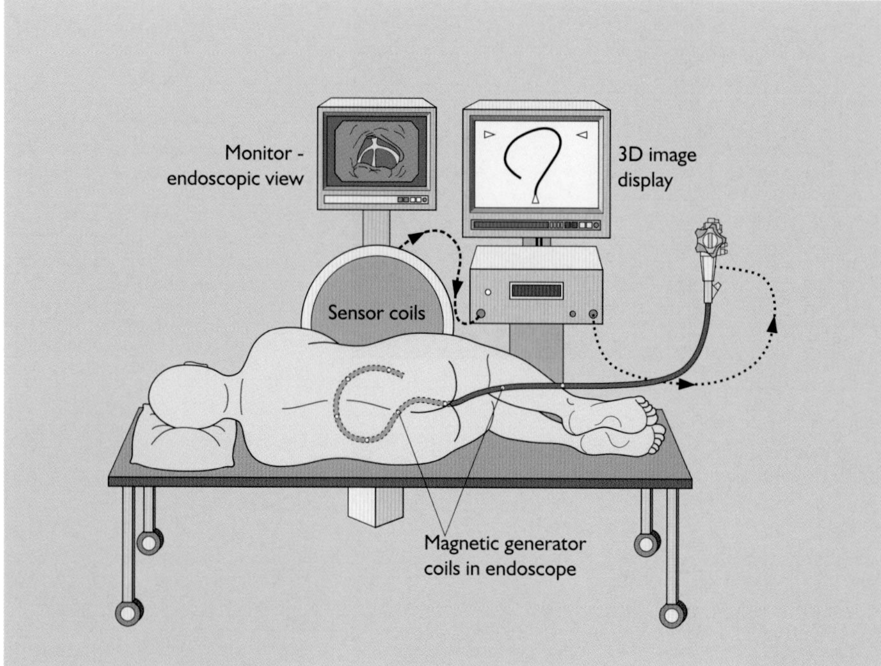

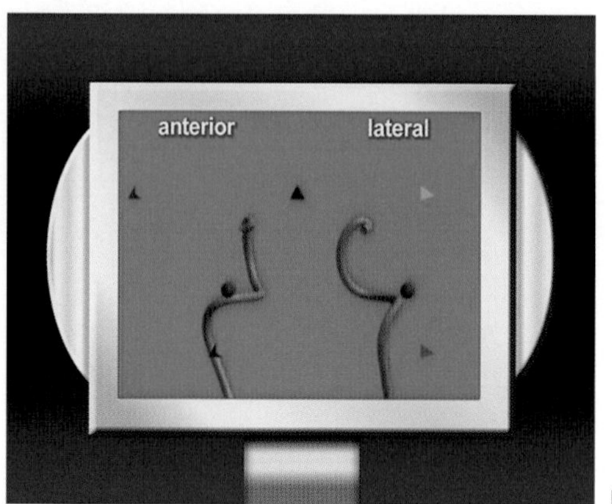

■ **Fig. 7.9** (a) The principles of the electromagnetic imager, and (b) the characteristic views to be expected in its use in colonoscopic positioning – here shown in both an antero-posterior plane and laterally. Courtesy of Dr S. Shah and Mr D. Swain.

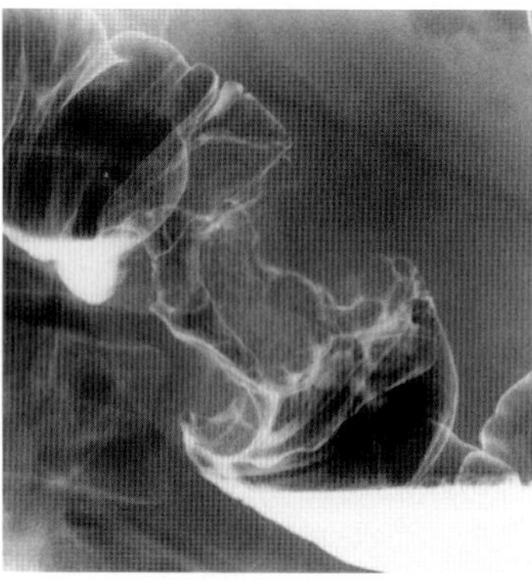

■ **Fig. 7.10** Double-contrast barium enema demonstrating an annular carcinoma of the mid transverse colon. A 4 cm in length circumferential narrowing with shelf-like margins and nodular mucosa is seen. (Reproduced with permission from reference 5, Fig. 13.)

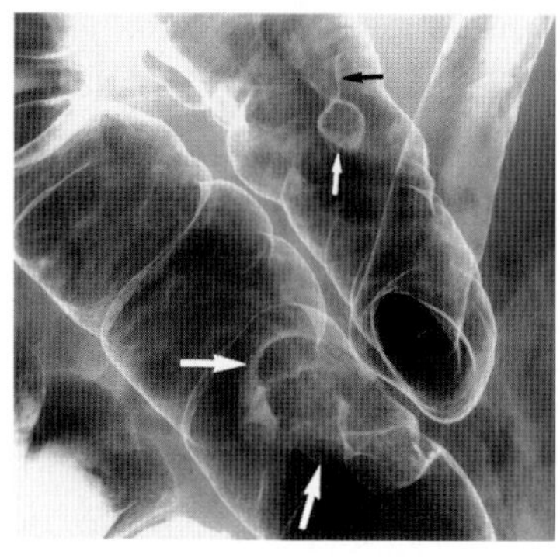

■ **Fig. 7.11** Double-contrast barium enema demonstrates synchronous adenocarcinoma and tubular adenoma. At the rectosigmoid junction, a polypoid carcinoma (large white arrows) is etched in white. The pedicle (black arrow) and head (small white arrow) of a tubular adenoma is seen in the proximal sigmoid colon. (Reproduced with permission from reference 5, Fig. 11.)

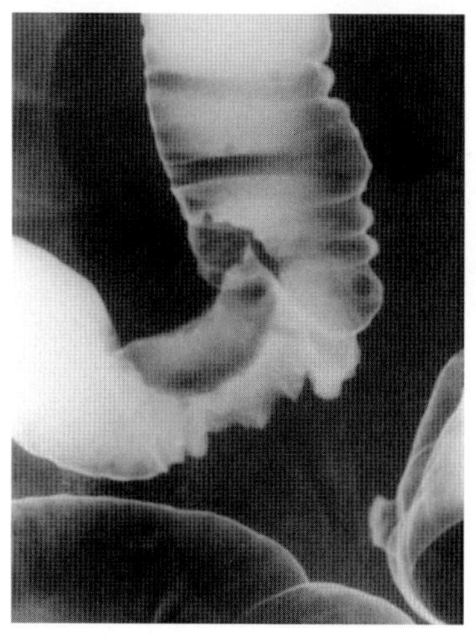

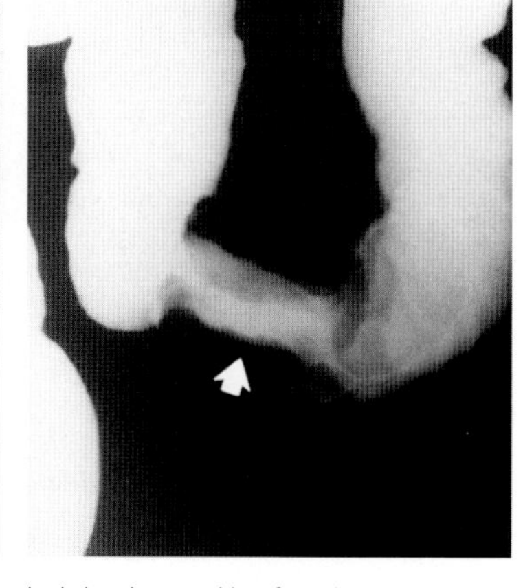

■ **Fig. 7.12** Double-contrast barium enema depicting the transition form between polypoid and annular carcinoma – a 'semi-annular' or 'saddle' lesion. In one view, a polypoid mass is seen projecting into the proximal sigmoid colon. The wall opposite (white arrows) the polypoid lesion is pulled in by partial circumferential infiltration of tumor. In an orthogonal view, the mass (arrow) is encircling the colon. (Reproduced with permission from reference 1, Fig. 12.23A and B.)

cated, the optimal arrangements for follow-up then depending on the histological characteristics and number of polyps removed.

The typical tubular adenoma is less than 15 mm in diameter and is pedunculated with a lobulated surface (Figs 7.39, 7.40). By contrast, the typical villous adenoma is larger, sessile, and with a shaggy surface (Figs 7.41–7.43). The tubulo-villous adenoma consists of closely packed, dysplastic epithelial tubules separated by lamina propria. The stalk consists of submucosa and normal mucosa (Figs 7.39–7.41). The pure villous adenoma includes numerous finger-like villi with dysplastic epithelium, over a core of lamina propria; these rest directly on the muscularis mucosa (Fig. 7.42). The degree of cytological and architectural abnormality determines the grading of dysplasia, which is, in turn, another factor determining the likelihood of malignant transformation (Figs 7.43–7.45).

It is increasingly clear that adenomas may not necessarily have a polypoid phenotype and experienced colonoscopists now actively seek the flat adenoma (Fig. 7.46). Although the great majority are visible with meticulous conventional videoendoscopy they are often more obvious when using one of the techniques of chromoendoscopy (Fig. 7.47). Magnifying endoscopy is also helpful but a full examination of the colon with the instrument set in magnification mode is rarely practicable.

Adenomas have no metastatic potential until dysplastic epithelium penetrates the muscularis mucosa and into the submucosa

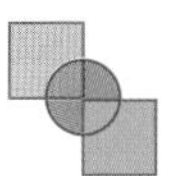

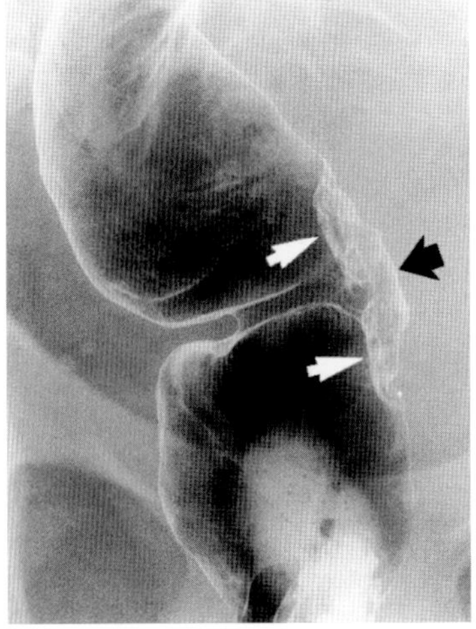

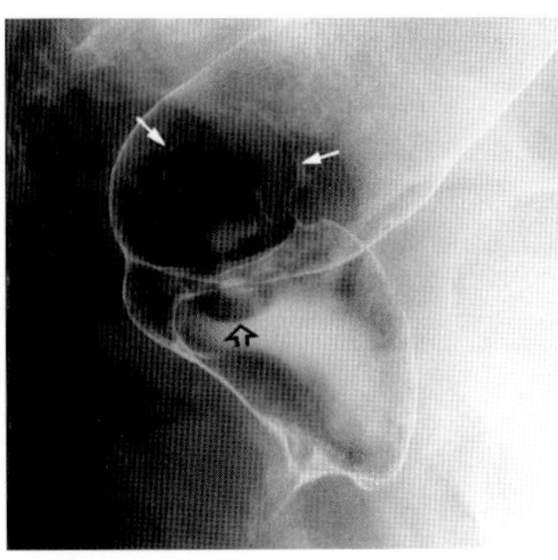

Fig. 7.13 Double-contrast barium enema showing plaque-like cancer of the rectum. A 5 cm lesion etched in white is slightly raised (white arrows) and has a central ulcer (black arrow) extending below the expected luminal contour. *En face*, the plaque-like cancer is considerably less obvious but can be seen both etched in white (white arrows) and as a radiolucent filling defect (black arrow) in the shallow barium pool. (Reproduced with permission from reference 5, Figs 12A and 12B.)

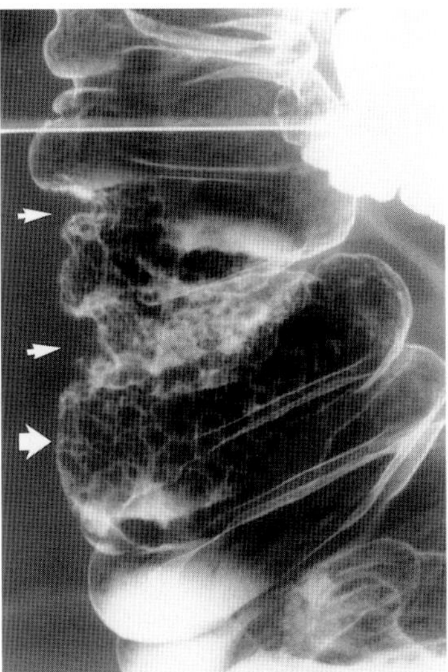

Fig. 7.14 Double-contrast barium enema demonstrating a 'carpet' lesion of the ascending colon. Barium fills the interstices between polygonal islands of tumor. In the region of tubulo-villous adenoma, the tumor does not alter the contour of the colon (large arrow). In the region of adenocarcinoma, the tumor now protrudes into the lumen (small arrows). (Reproduced with permission from reference 2, Fig. 5.20.)

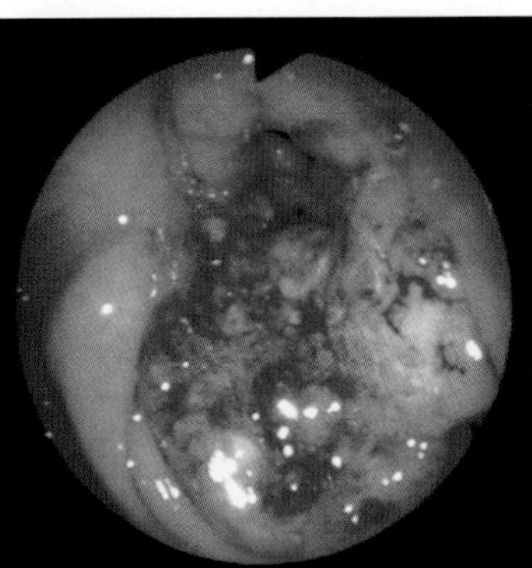

Fig. 7.15 Colonoscopic appearance of anastomotic recurrence after prior resection for rectal carcinoma.

(Figs 7.48, 7.49). In this situation, the term malignant polyp or early carcinoma is used. Provided that the base of the stalk of the adenoma is free from invasion, there is no lymphatic penetration; local excision by endoscopic polypectomy is then almost certainly adequate treatment (Figs 7.6, 7.45). The position of the uncertain lesion that is biopsied prior to attempted endoscopic excision should be marked by Indian ink tattooing in order that its site can be recognized unequivocally at surgery or repeat colonoscopy (Figs 7.50–7.52).

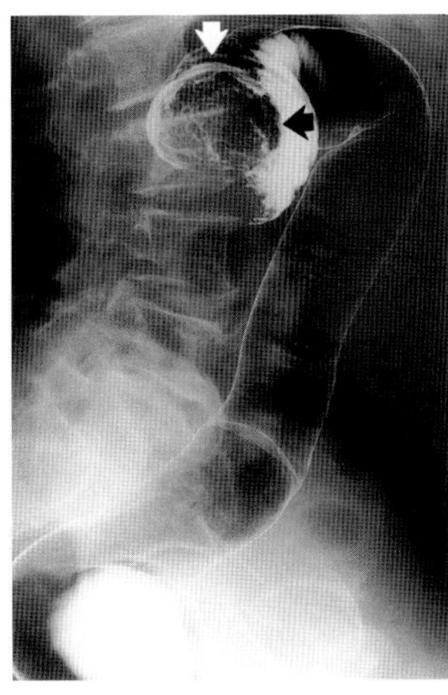

Fig. 7.16 Double-contrast barium enema showing polypoid carcinoma causing intussusception. A finely lobulated mass (arrows) is seen in the proximal transverse colon. Complete retrograde obstruction is present. (Reproduced with permission from reference 2, Fig. 5.9A.)

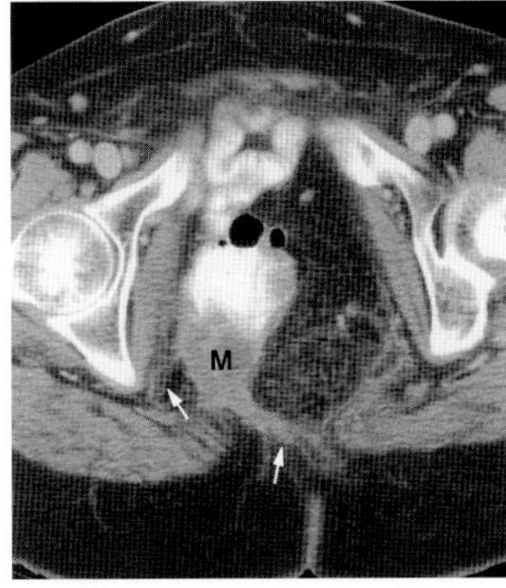

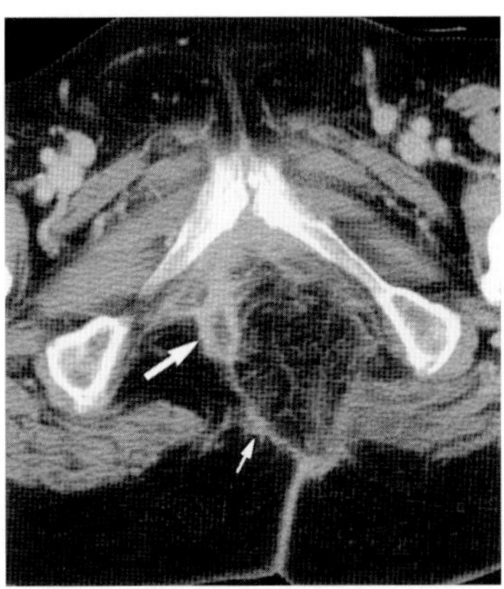

Fig. 7.17 CT demonstrating recurrent rectal carcinoma after abdominoperineal resection. Image through the acetabulae shows a 3 cm inhomogeneous mass (M) invading a dilated small bowel loop. Tumor infiltrates the right pelvic side-wall and the pelvic fat (arrows). Image through the ischiopubic ramus shows a small soft tissue mass (large arrow) and strands of tumor (small arrow) infiltrating the pelvic fat.

Studies of the adenoma–carcinoma sequence indicate that this progression normally takes at least 3 years: obviously of importance in planning surveillance programs.

Familial adenomatous polyposis

Familial adenomatous polyposis (FAP) is responsible for, at most, 1% of patients with colonic polyps, but is of critical importance to these patients and their families. At least 100 adenomas, and often vast numbers, will be found by the third decade in most affected individuals. Macroscopic lesions are however rarely apparent before the late teens. Their importance lies in the virtual certainty of progression to colorectal carcinoma at a young age if left untreated. FAP is inherited in autosomal dominant fashion (although sporadic cases also occur as new mutations) and it is associated with virtually 100% penetrance. The apc gene is on chromosome 5q and has been sequenced; although there are very many different mutations, in most families it is now possible to screen young family members and to reassure those definitely not carrying mutations.

A variety of other manifestations of the condition (previously distinguished as Gardner's syndrome) occur. Of greatest diagnostic use, because it is present in about 80% of patients from birth, is congenital hypertrophy of the retinal pigment epithelium (multiple punctate pigmented areas in the optic fundi), but careful indirect ophthalmoscopy is needed as the lesions are mainly peripheral

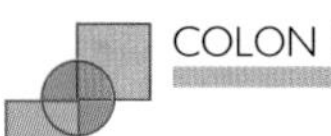

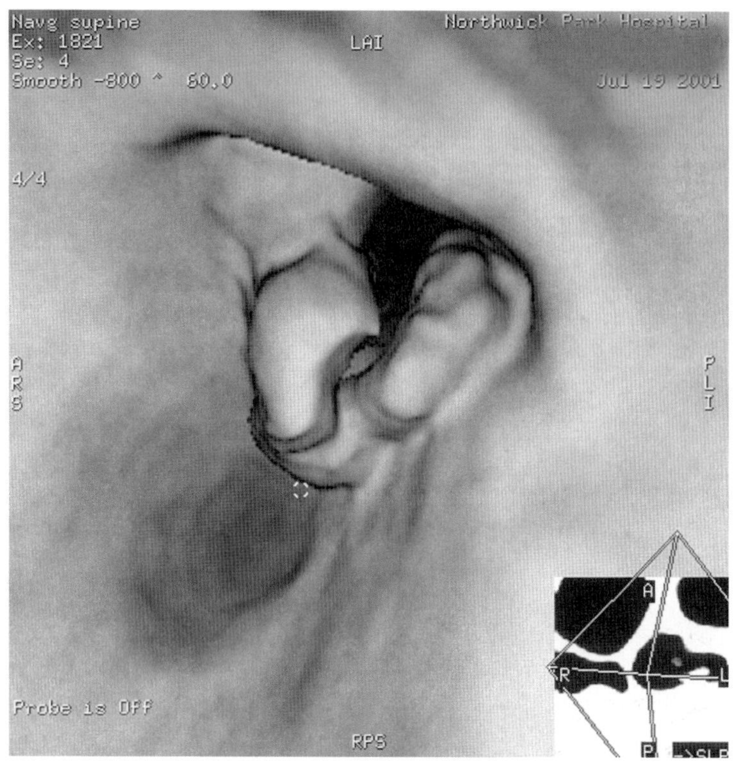

a

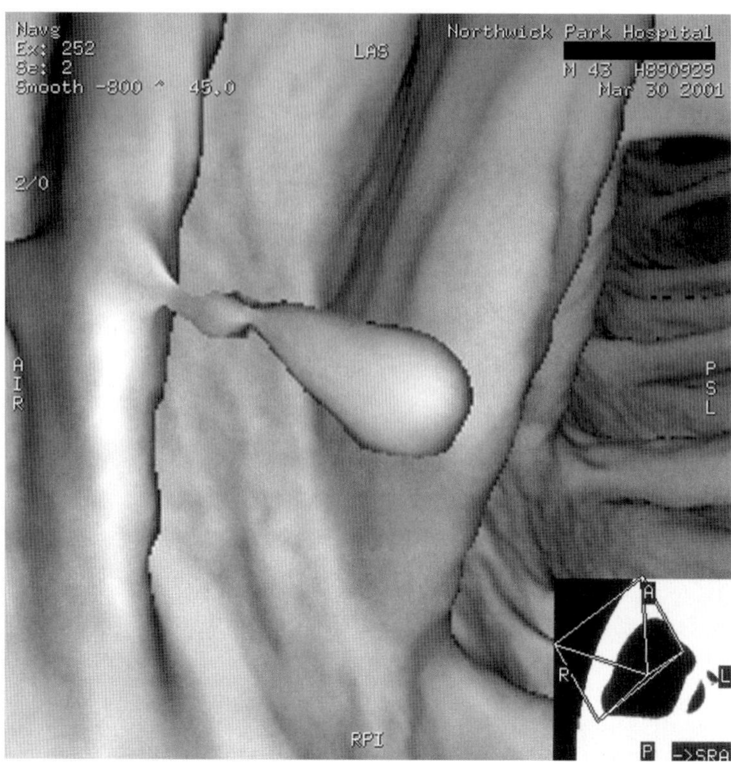

b

Fig. 7.18 Virtual colonoscopy showing (a) fairly readily identified colonic carcinoma, and (b) an obvious pedunculated polyp. Courtesy of Dr S. Halligan and Dr M. Rutter.

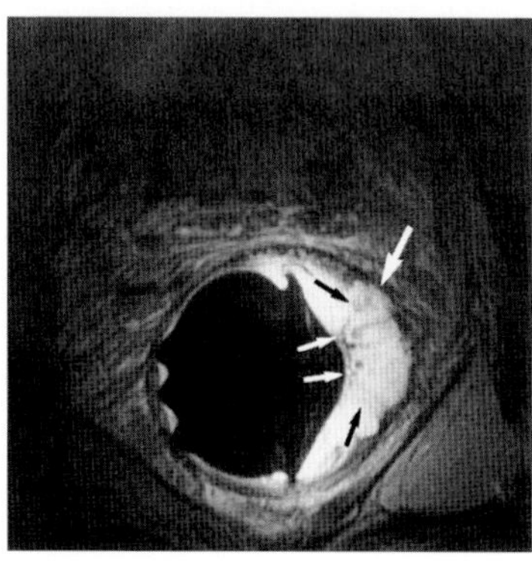

Fig. 7.19 MRI in local staging of rectal cancer. Axial T_2-weighted image shows a polypoid tumor (short arrows) of high signal due to mucinous histology. The tumor is focally invading the left lateral rectal wall (long arrow).

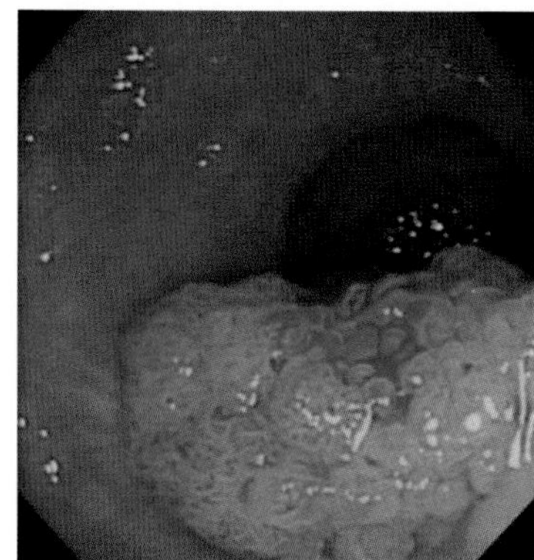

Fig. 7.21 Malignant polyp with a broad base.

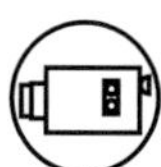

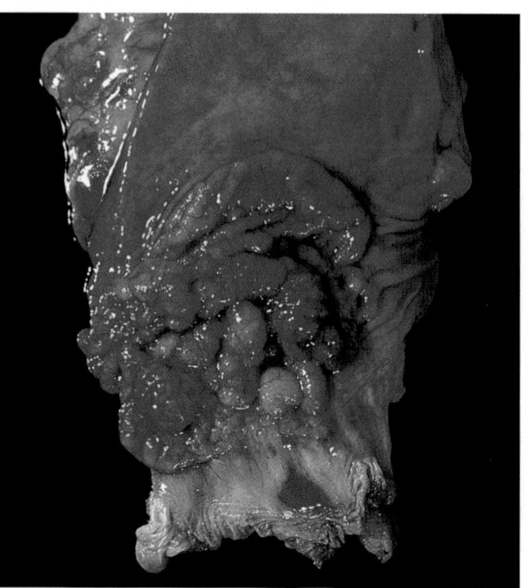

Fig. 7.20 Rectal carcinoma. Abdominoperineal resection specimen showing a fungating carcinoma of the distal rectum extending to the dentate line, well within the reach of palpation by digital rectal examination.

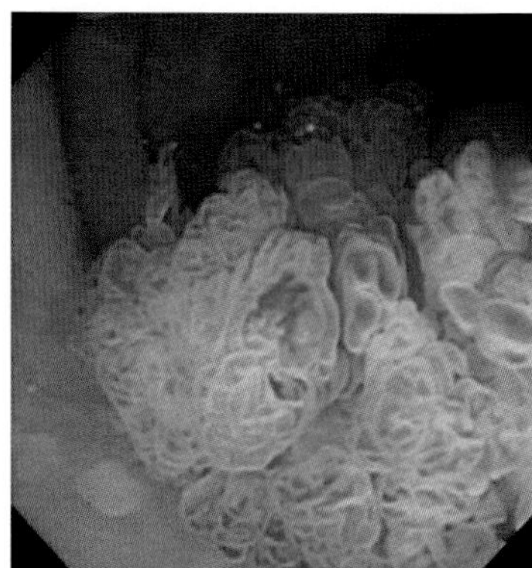

Fig. 7.22 The same polyp as in Fig. 7.21 after the lumen was filled with water.

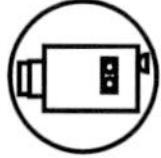

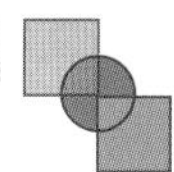

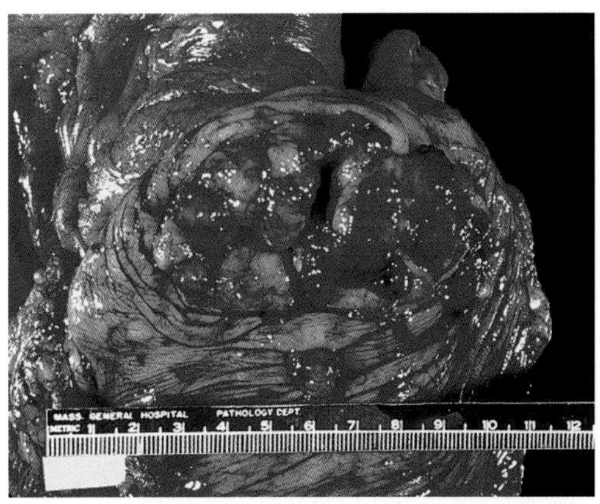

■ **Fig. 7.23** Cecal carcinoma. Right hemicolectomy specimen showing a large exophytic tumor with a nodular irregular surface filling the cecum.

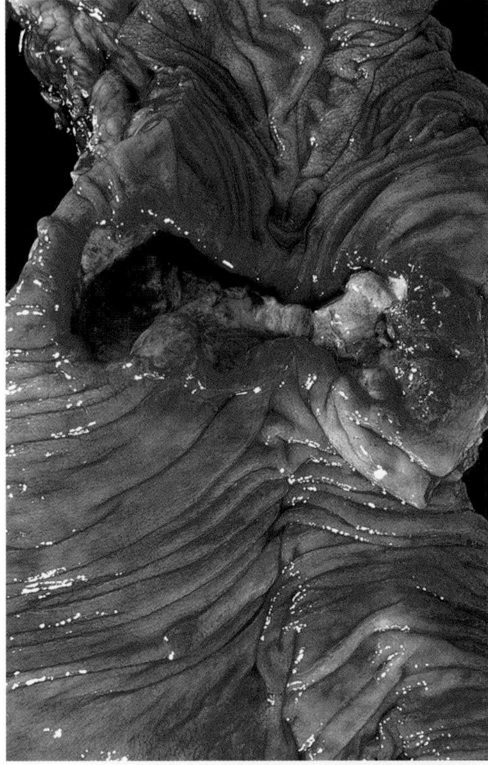

■ **Fig. 7.24** Ulcerating carcinoma of the right colon. Right hemicolectomy specimen showing an ulcerating carcinoma of the right colon with raised, irregular edges that involves 90% of the circumference of the colon.

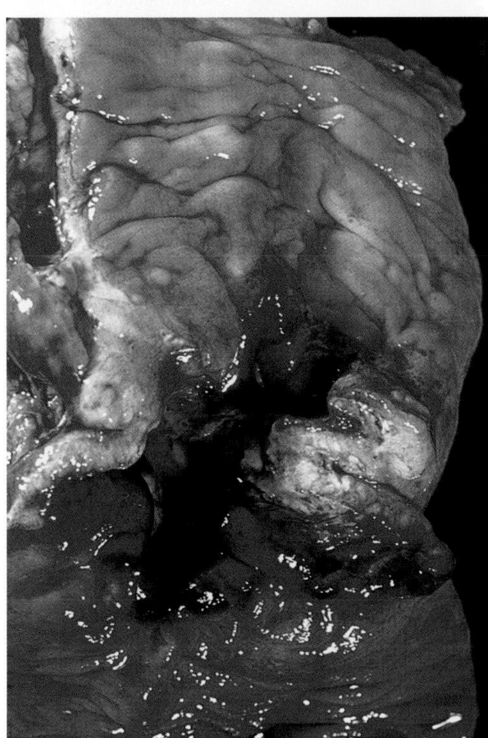

■ **Fig. 7.25** Circumferential (annular) carcinoma of the sigmoid colon. Sigmoidectomy specimen showing a centrally necrotic circumferential tumor mass that invades through the wall, seen at the cut edge of the muscularis propria, and constricts the lumen. The proximal colonic segment is dilated and dusky (congested) due to partial obstruction by the tumor.

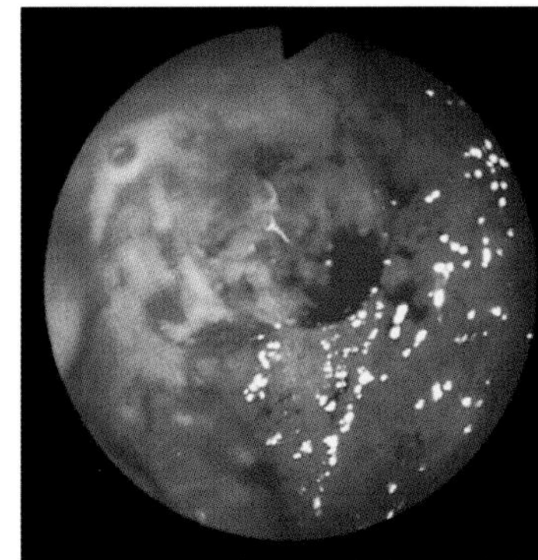

■ **Fig. 7.26** Endoscopic appearance of colonic carcinoma complicating ulcerative colitis.

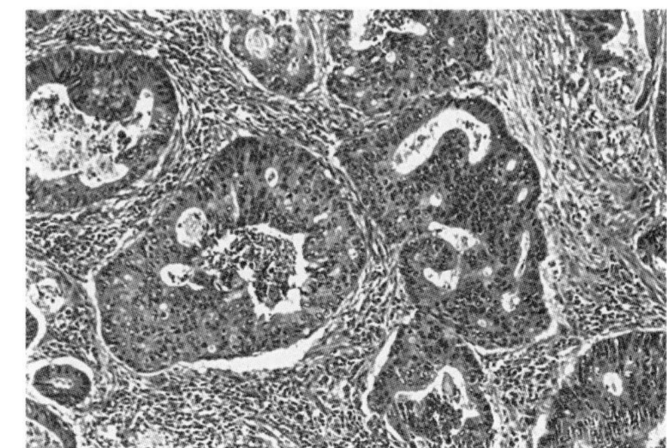

■ **Fig. 7.27** Microscopic appearance of adenocarcinoma of the colon, the most common histology type of carcinoma of the colorectum, showing well-formed malignant glands, many with central necrosis and/or mucinous content.

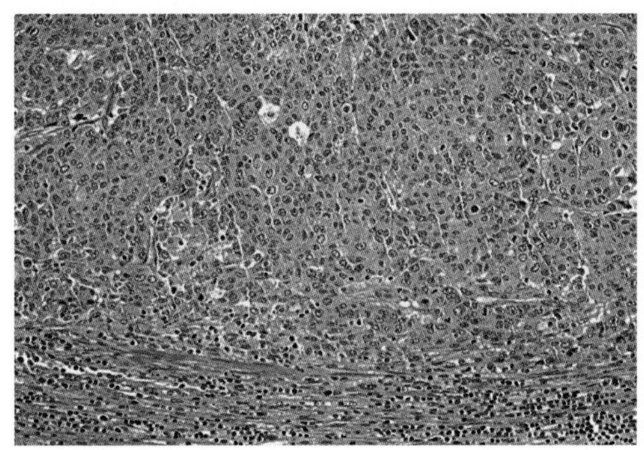

■ **Fig. 7.28** Microscopic appearance of medullary carcinoma, a rare type of undifferentiated carcinoma composed of large eosinophilic cells growing in solid masses with pushing borders and containing numerous infiltrating lymphocytes. This histological type is particularly associated with HNPCC.

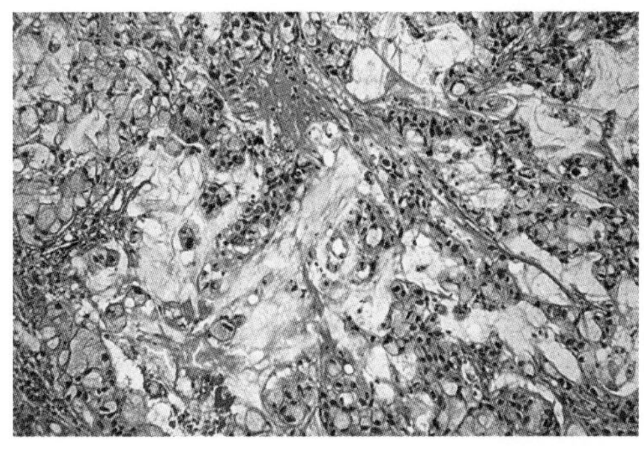

■ **Fig. 7.29** Microscopic appearance of a mucinous carcinoma of the colon showing the large pools of extracellular mucin made by the malignant cells seen floating within the mucin pools. Classification as a mucinous carcinoma requires that 50% or more of the mass of the tumor be composed of extracellular mucin.

■ **Fig. 7.30** Whole-mount microscopic view of mucinous carcinoma of the right colon, arising from a villous adenoma (visible at the mucosal surface), showing the pools of pale mucin that are disrupting and dissecting through the inner circular layer of the colonic wall and focally extending through the longitudinal layer into the pericolonic soft tissue.

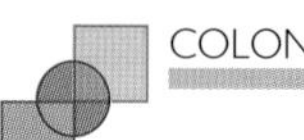

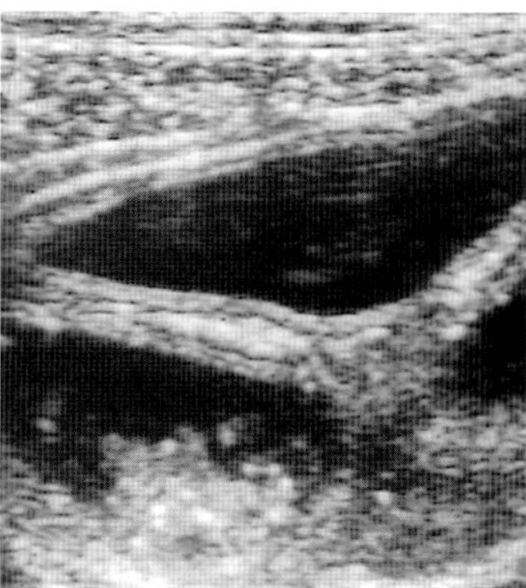

■ **Fig. 7.31** Colosonography showing the layered appearance of the colonic wall and some fecal material in the colon in a patient investigated for a palpable mass and in whom no sinister cause was demonstrable.

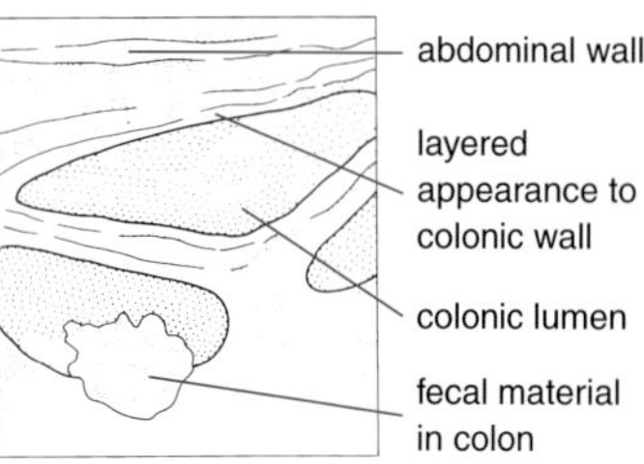

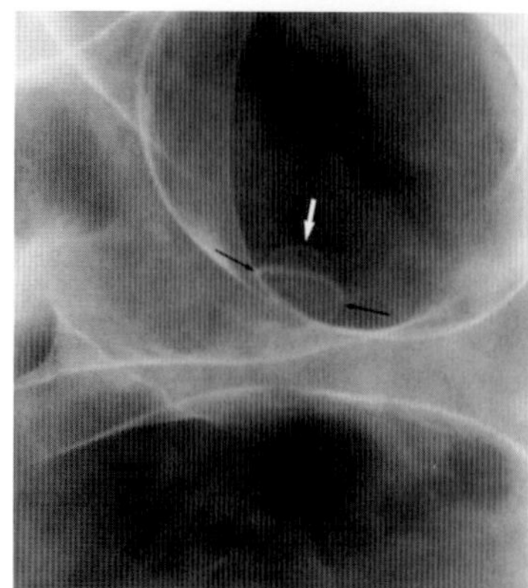

■ **Fig. 7.33** Double-contrast barium enema demonstrating 6 mm tubular adenoma, resembling a 'bowler hat.' The top of the polyp is a curved line (white arrow) – the top of the hat. A second curved line (black arrows) is etched where the pedunculated polyp is retracted against the mucosa – the brim of the hat. (Reproduced with permission from reference 7, Fig. 2.)

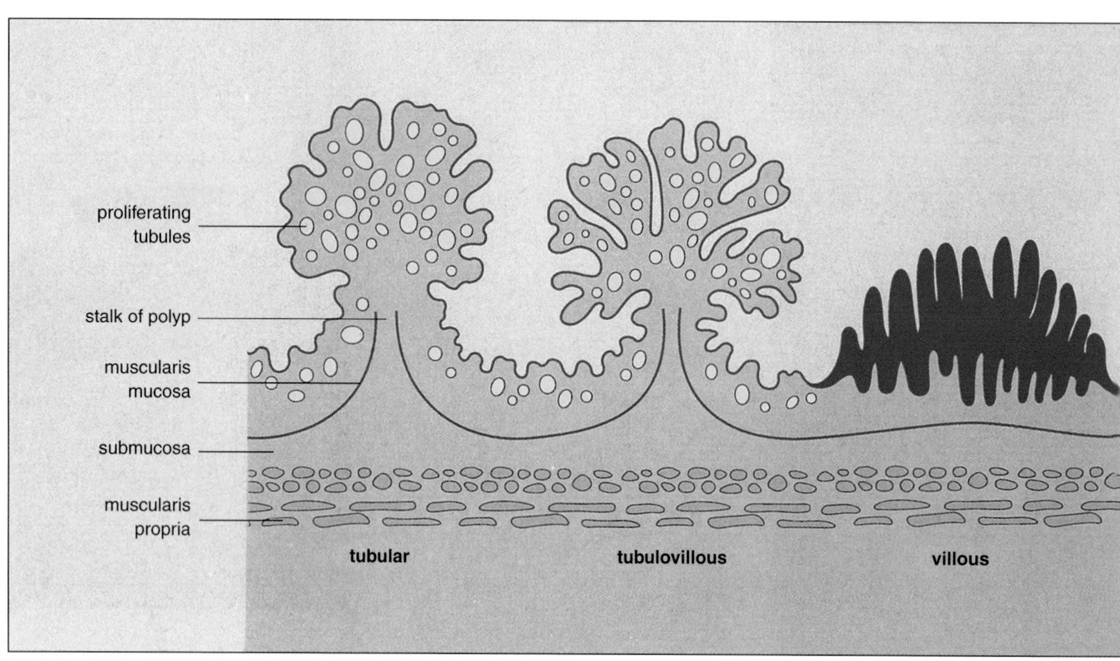

■ **Fig. 7.32** Diagram showing the different patterns of colonic adenomatous polyp.

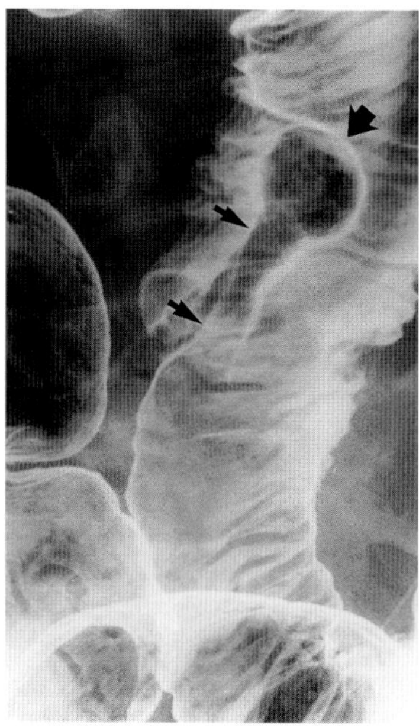

■ **Fig. 7.34** Double-contrast barium enema demonstrating pedunculated tubulovillous adenoma. The head of the polyp (thick arrow) is finely nodular. The stalk (thin arrows) is etched in white.

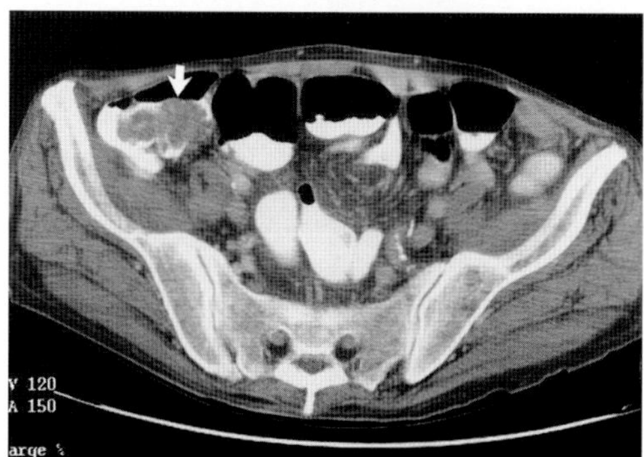

■ **Fig. 7.35** CT demonstrating villous adenoma of the cecum. A lobulated soft tissue mass (arrow) is seen in the barium pool. (Reproduced with permission from reference 10, Fig. 2A.)

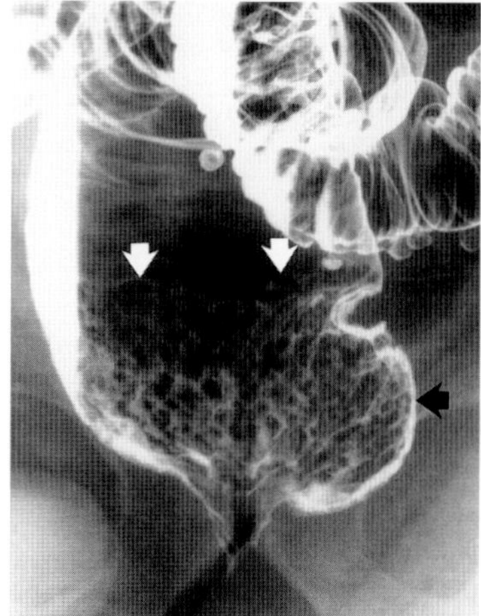

■ **Fig. 7.36** Double-contrast barium enema demonstrating villous adenoma of the rectum. Polygonal nodules of tumor (white arrows) disrupt the smooth rectal mucosa. The flat nature of the lesion is manifested as lack of change of the contour of the rectum seen in profile (black arrow). (See also Fig 7.14) (Reproduced with permission from reference 8, Fig. 1A.)

(Figs 7.53–7.56). Other features include osteomas (particularly of the skull and jaws) (Figs 7.57, 7.58), epidermoid cysts, and desmoid tumors (Fig. 7.59).

Upper gastrointestinal polyps are substantially over-represented in the FAP population (see Chapters 2 and 3), and malignant trans-

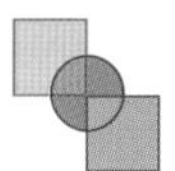

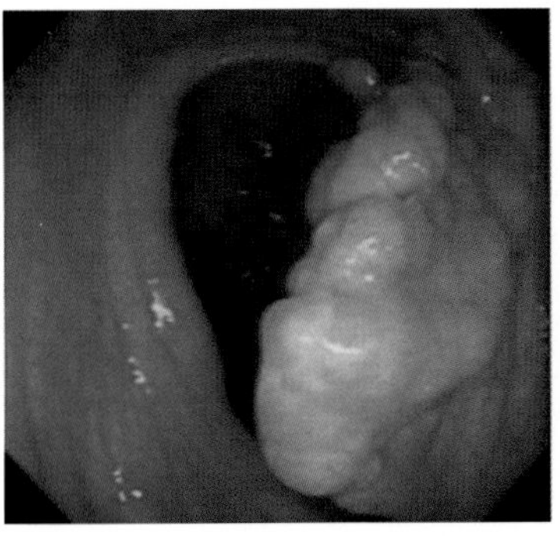

■ **Fig. 7.37** Tubulovillous adenoma.

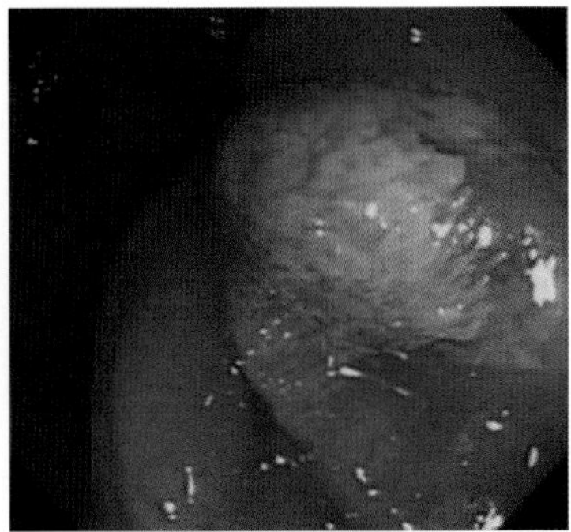

■ **Fig. 7.38** Villous adenoma.

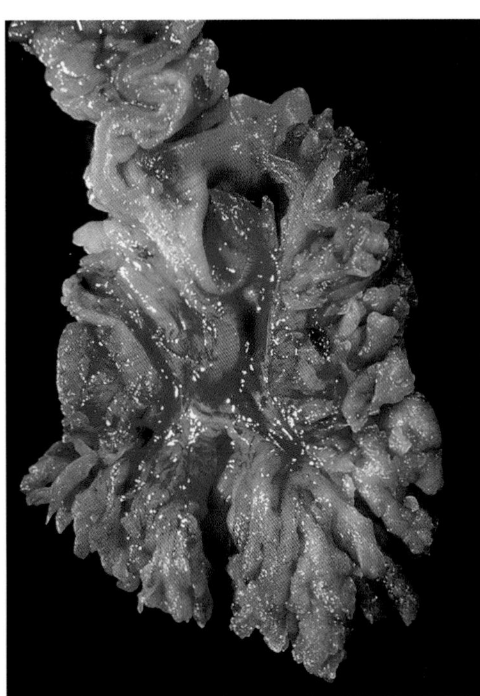

■ **Fig. 7.41** Macroscopic view of a transverse section through a pedunculated villous adenoma showing delicate tumor fronds covering the polyp head, the central core consisting of areolar submucosa tissue that is continuous with the submucosa of the stalk.

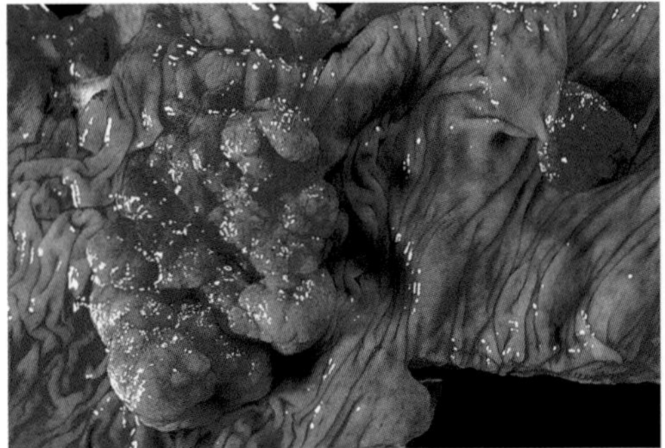

■ **Fig. 7.39** Colonic adenomas. Macroscopic view of two colonic adenomas showing a large sessile adenoma and a smaller pedunculated adenoma, the stalk of which is covered by normal mucosa.

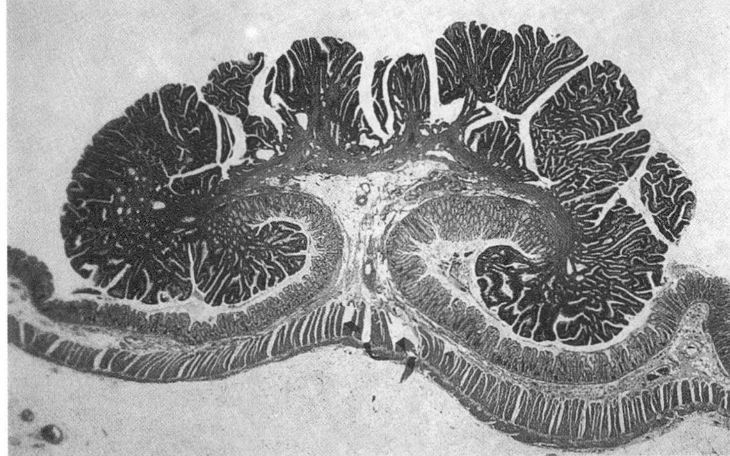

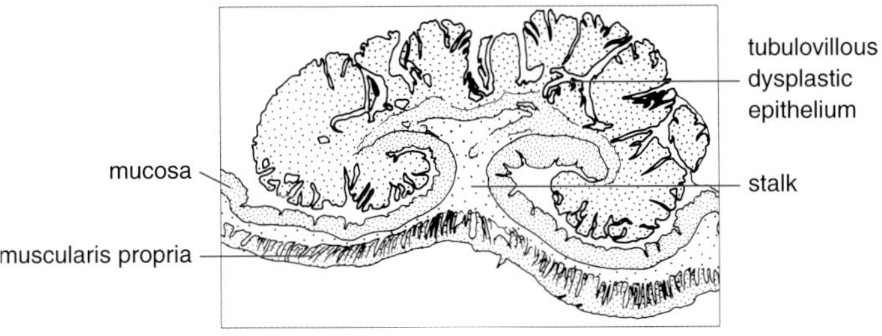

■ **Fig. 7.40** Tubulovillous adenoma. Microscopic section through a tubulovillous adenoma with a short stalk showing the thickening and splaying of the muscularis mucosae in the polyp head and the continuity of the submucosa of the polyp head, stalk, and surrounding colon.

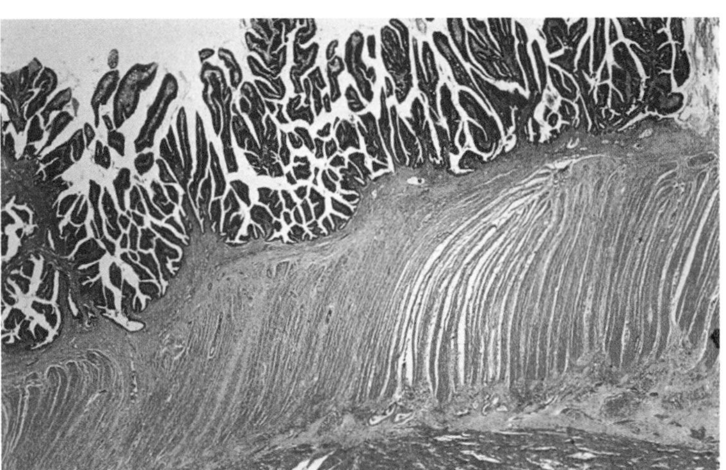

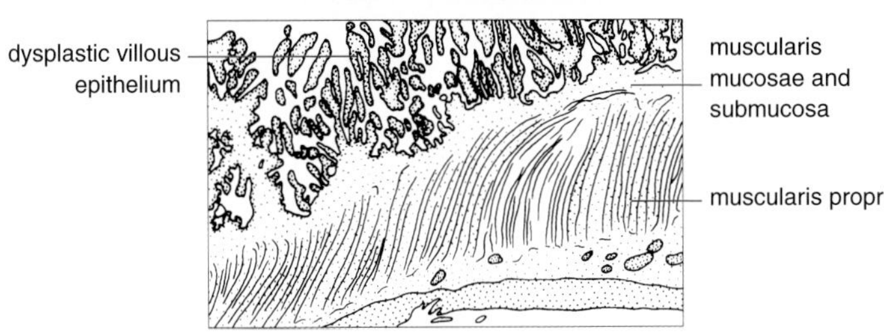

■ **Fig. 7.42** Villous adenoma. Microscopic view of a sessile villous adenoma showing replacement of the mucosa by a carpet-like growth of adenomatous villi.

formation, especially to ampullary and duodenal carcinoma, also occurs.

The colonic polyps in FAP are readily demonstrable (Figs 7.60, 7.61), and the histology is that of the sporadic adenoma (Fig. 7.62). Elective colectomy, preferably total proctocolectomy, is advised (Figs 7.63, 7.64) because, despite regular sigmoidoscopy, rectal carcinomas remain a substantial threat in patients with an ileorectal

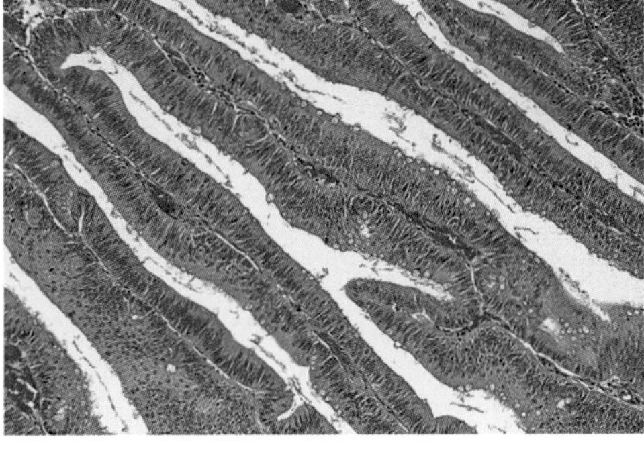

■ **Fig. 7.43** Villous adenoma. High-magnification view showing the crowded, hyperchromatic dysplastic cells with elongated nuclei oriented perpendicular to the epithelial basement membrane and the spindly stromal cores.

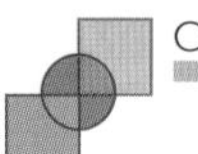

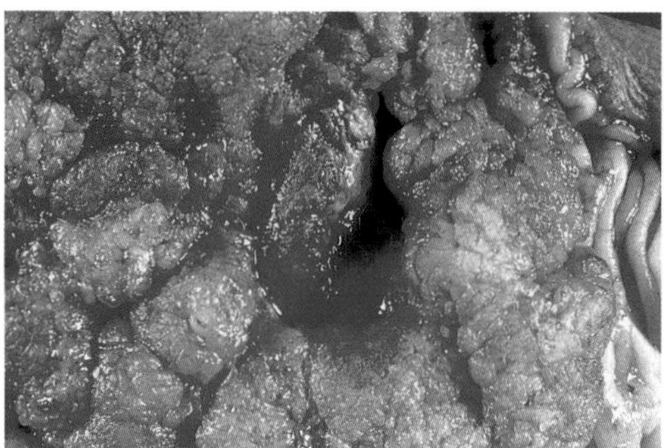

■ **Fig. 7.44** Macroscopic view of a large sessile villous adenoma showing a central focus of ulceration corresponding to an invasive adenocarcinoma arising within it.

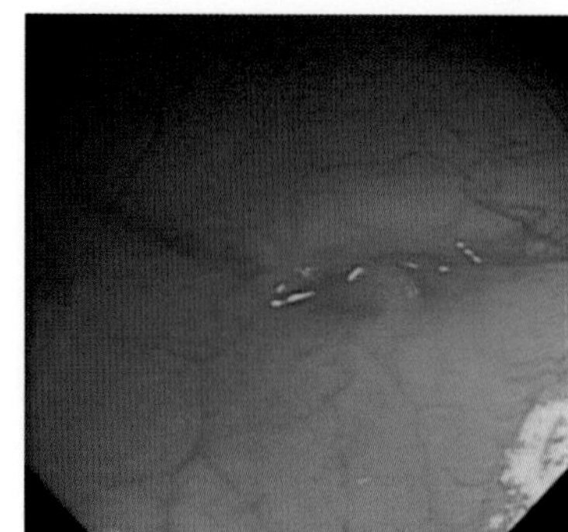

■ **Fig. 7.46** Flat adenoma.

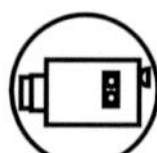

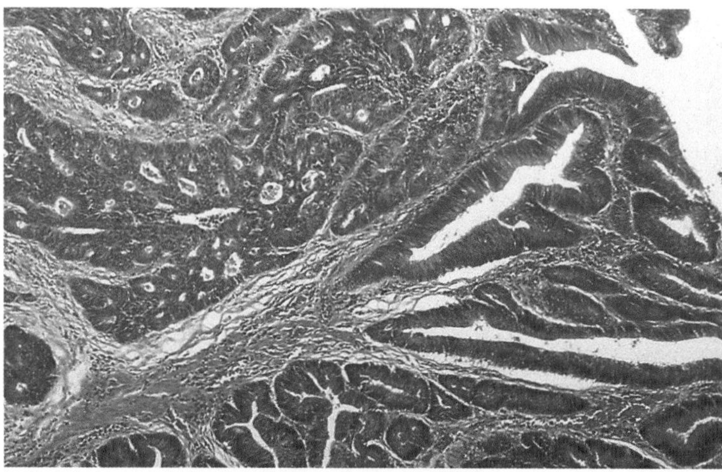

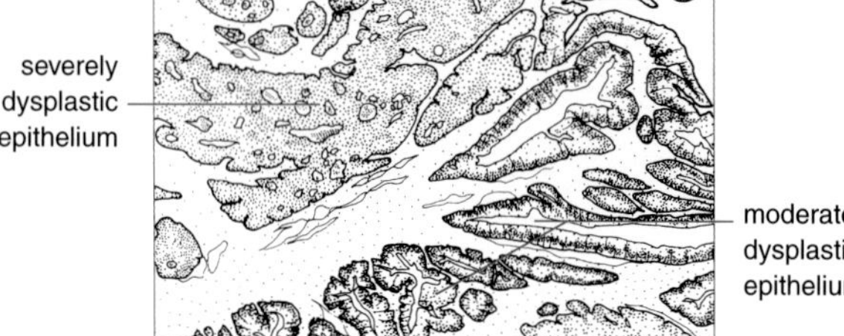

■ **Fig. 7.45** Intramucosal carcinoma arising in an adenoma. The surface of a tubulovillous adenoma (right) with a focus of well-differentiated adenocarcinoma, recognized by its cribriform glandular architecture invading the lamina propria of the polyp mucosa (intramucosal carcinoma); polypectomy was curative.

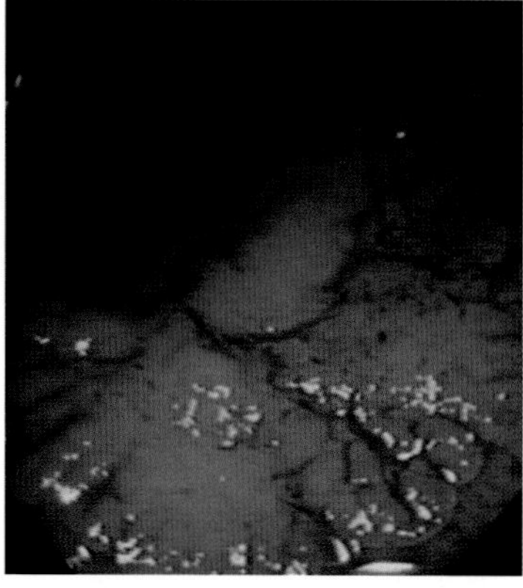

■ **Fig. 7.47** The same flat adenoma shown much more clearly after the use of indigo carmine dye-spraying.

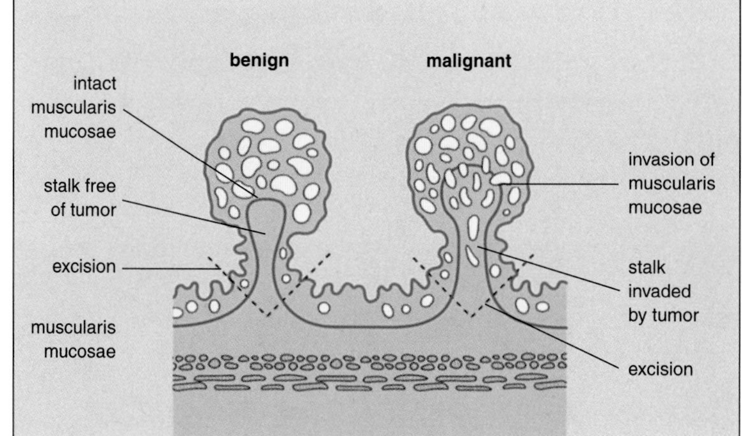

■ **Fig. 7.48** Diagram comparing the structure of benign and malignant polyps.

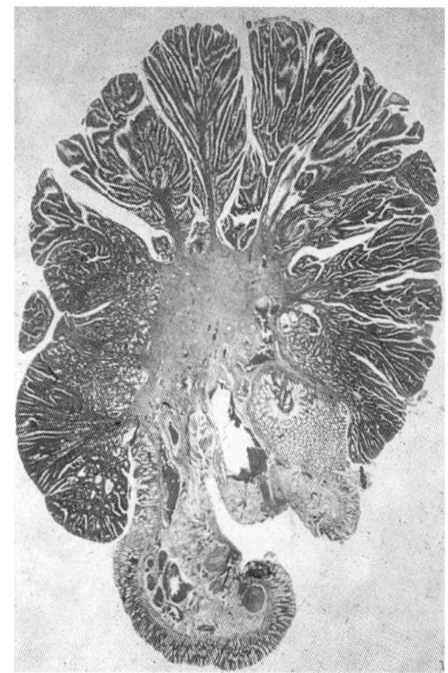

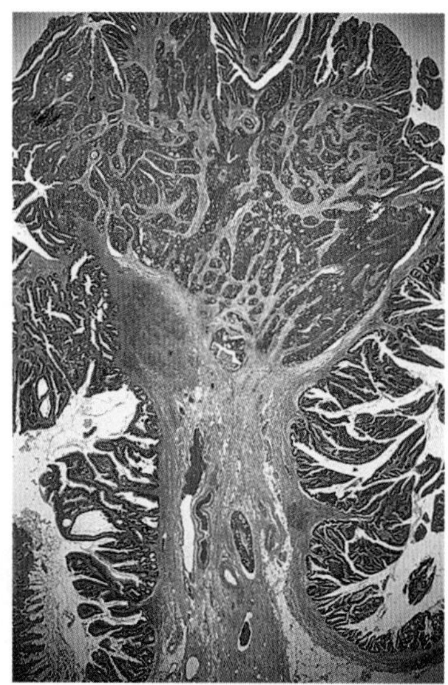

■ **Fig. 7.49** Histological appearances demonstrating the differences between benign and malignant adenomas. In the benign case (a), the muscularis is intact, whereas in the malignant lesion (b), the muscularis mucosa is obviously invaded by malignant epithelium. Malignant glands in the lymphatics are seen close to the base of the stalk. H&E stain (x 8).

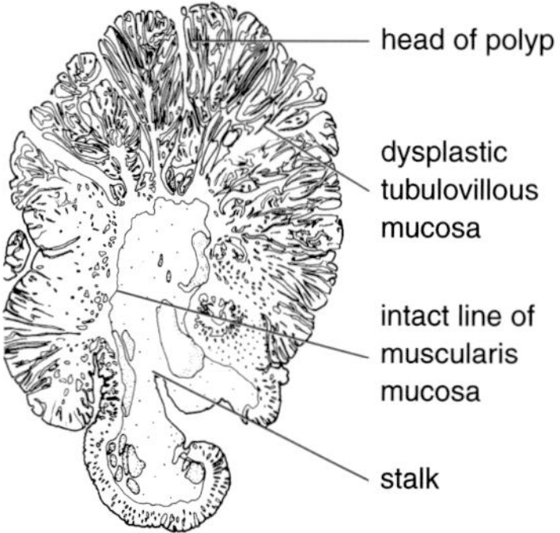

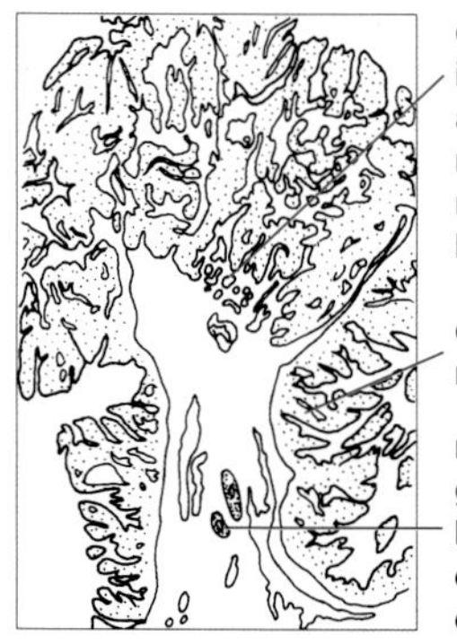

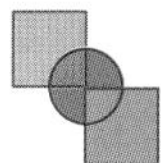

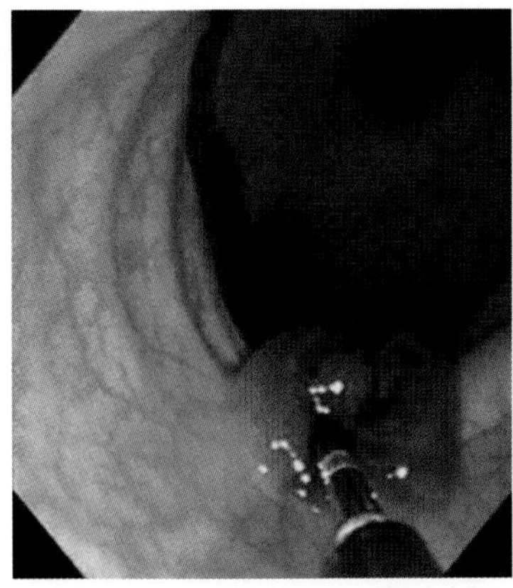

■ **Fig. 7.50** Injection of Indian ink adjacent to a suspicious lesion that was to be biopsied rather than removed.

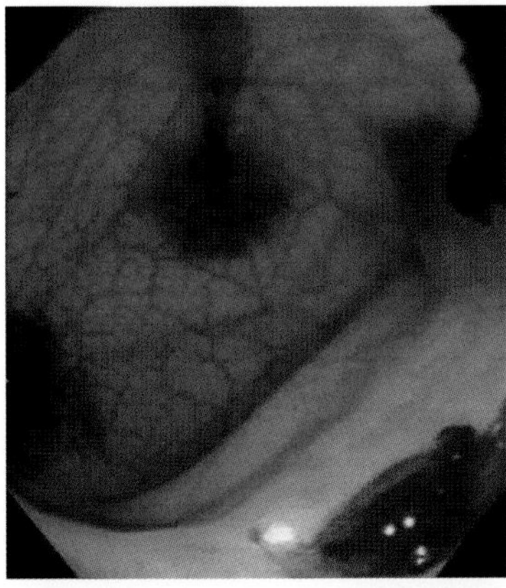

■ **Fig. 7.51** Four-quadrant tattooing. It will be a simple matter to recognize this site at laparotomy whichever orientation of the bowel presents to the surgeon.

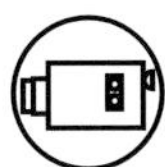

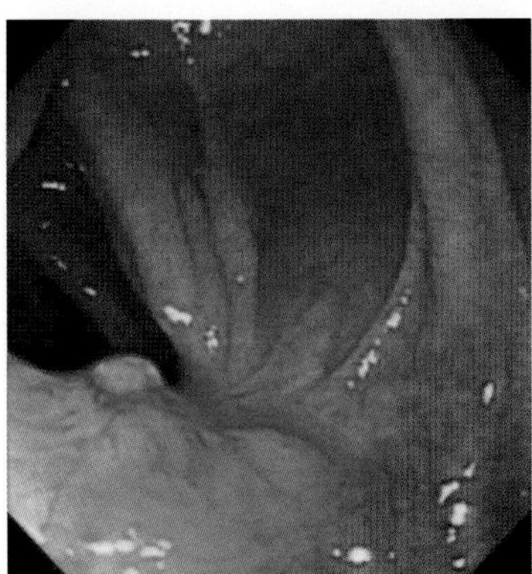

■ **Fig. 7.52** Characteristic late result showing minor deformity from a preceding polypectomy the site of which is marked by the tattoo.

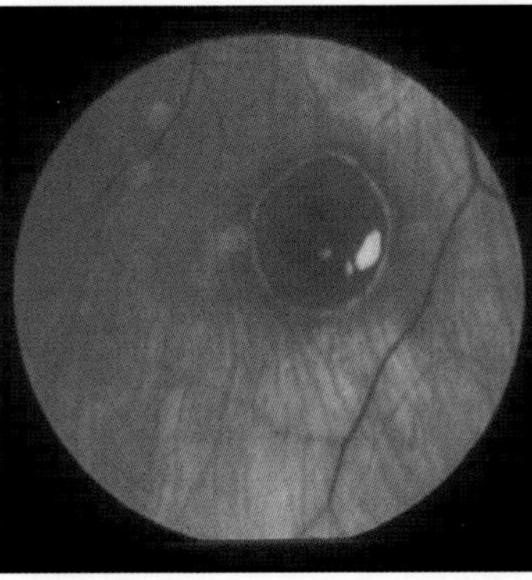

■ **Fig. 7.53** The optical fundus in congenital hypertrophy of the retinal pigment epithelium. This example was the only lesion in a normal individual unaffected by polyposis. Courtesy of Mr A.T. Moore.

anastomosis; a restorative pouch operation will often now be offered (see Chapter 6), but possibly preceded by an ileorectal anastomosis for a few years while the patient is at a lesser risk of rectal cancer. Unfortunately proctocolectomy does not protect against the extra-colonic manifestations of FAP indicated above: desmoid tumors may be particularly unpleasant (Fig 7.65).

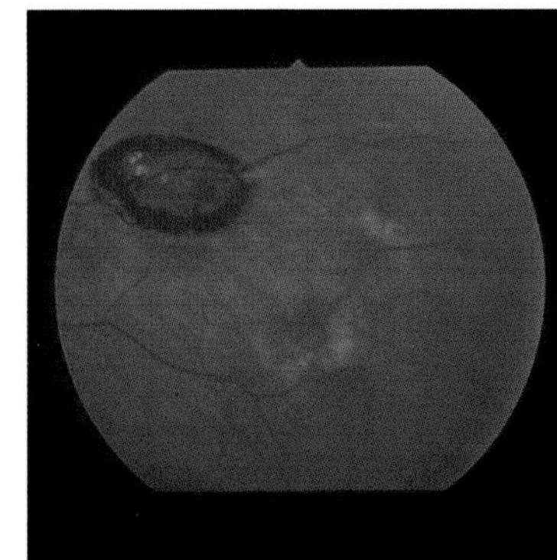

■ **Fig. 7.54** Fundal appearance in congenital hypertrophy of the retinal pigment epithelium (CHRPE) in a patient with polyposis. The pale halo around the increased pigmentation is less clear cut, and this was one of multiple lesions. Courtesy of Mr A.T. Moore.

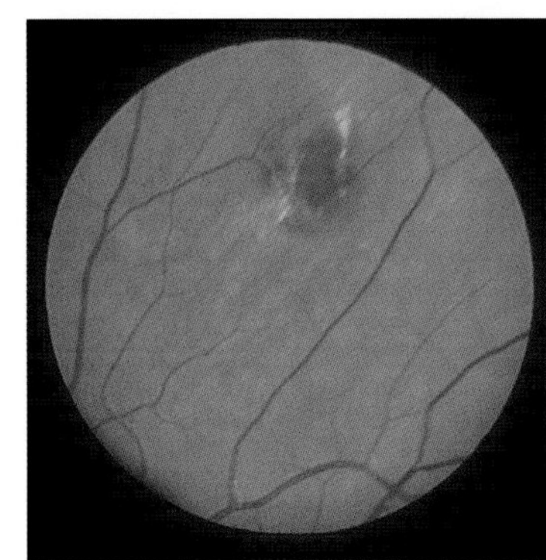

■ **Fig. 7.55** Fundal appearance of CHRPE in a patient with polyposis. The irregular borders and the varying degree of pigmentation are characteristic of the lesions seen in polyposis patients. Courtesy of Mr A.T. Moore.

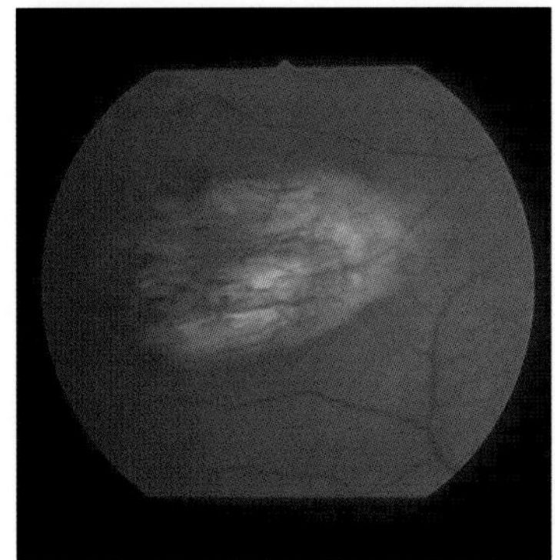

■ **Fig. 7.56** Fundal appearance of CHRPE in another patient with polyposis. Courtesy of Mr A.T. Moore.

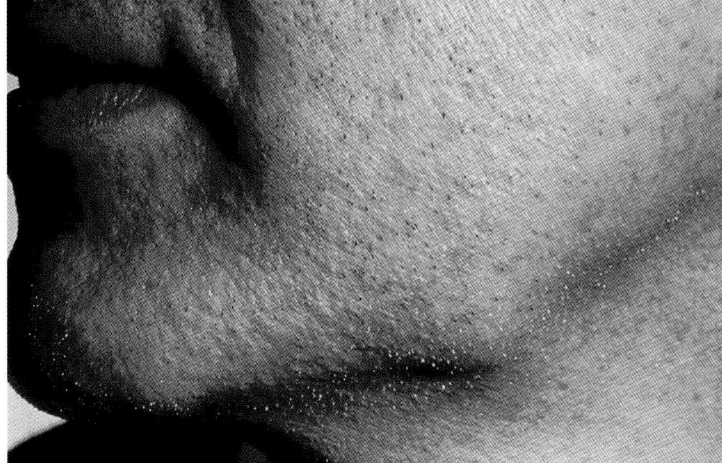

■ **Fig. 7.57** Appearance in a polyposis patient with an osteoma of the mandible. Courtesy of Ms K. Neale and the St Mark's Polyposis Registry.

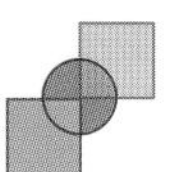

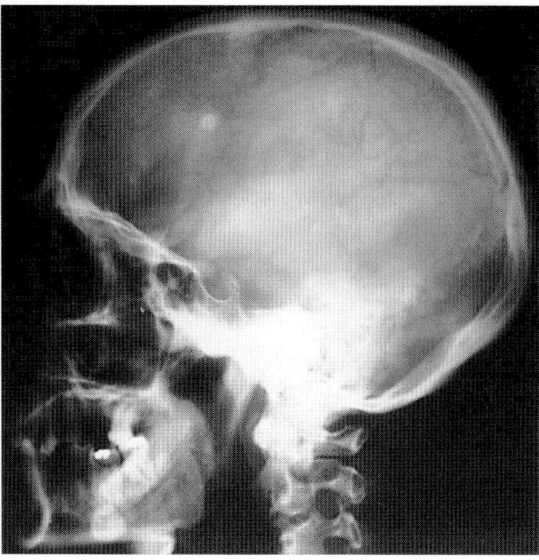

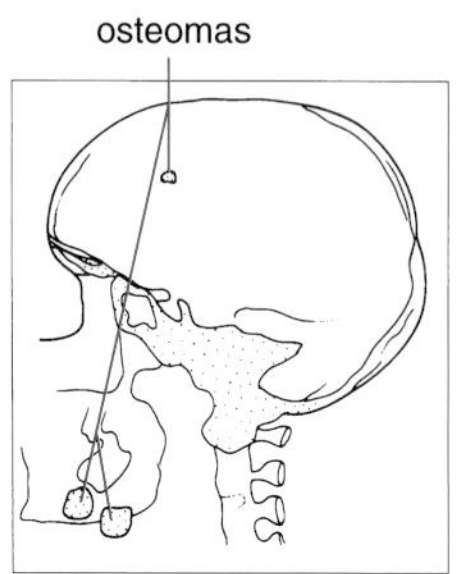

Fig. 7.58 Skull radiograph in polyposis showing osteoma in the skull vault and two further lesions in the mandible.

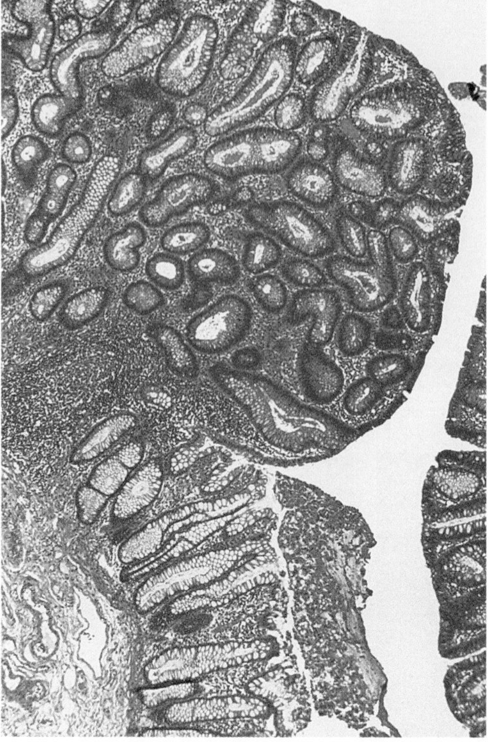

Fig. 7.62 Microscopic view of the junction between the head and stalk of a tubular adenoma in familial adenomatous polyposis showing the abrupt transition between the dysplastic mucosa of the polyp head and the normal mucosa of the stalk, features identical to those of sporadic tubular adenomas.

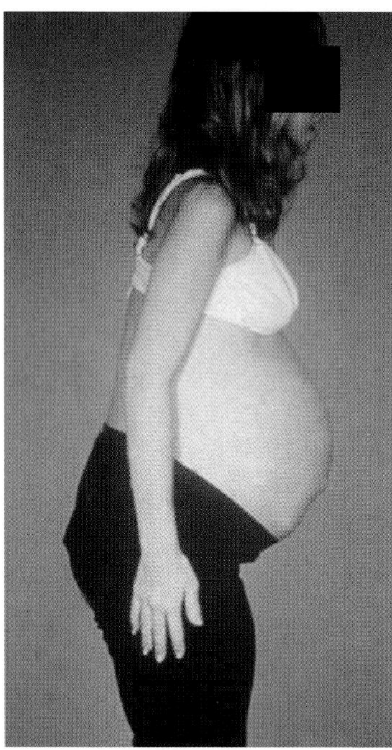

Fig. 7.59 Desmoid tumor affecting (as is usual) the abdominal wall. Courtesy of Ms K. Neale, Mr D Swain, and the St Mark's Polyposis Registry.

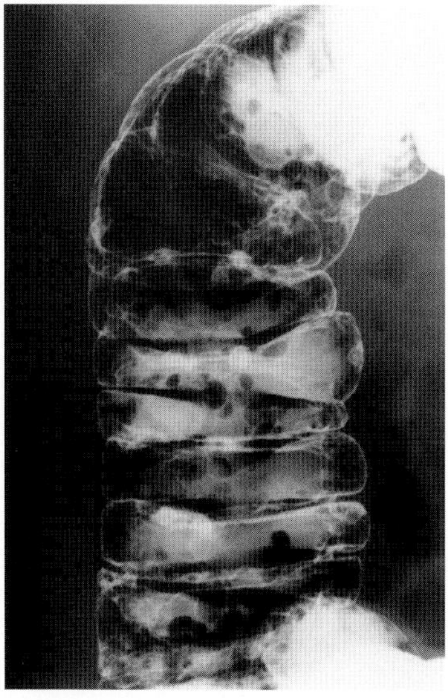

Fig. 7.60 Double-contrast barium enema demonstrating numerous tubular adenomas in a patient with familial adenomatous polyposis syndrome. (Reproduced with permission from reference 1, Fig. 12.91.)

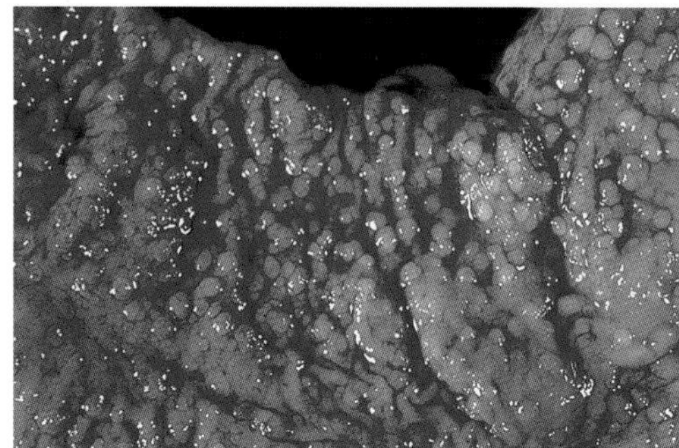

Fig. 7.63 Colectomy specimen in familial adenomatous polyposis showing innumerable small tubular adenomas of approximately equal size diffusely studding the colonic mucosa.

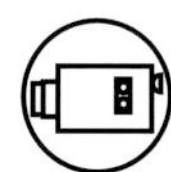

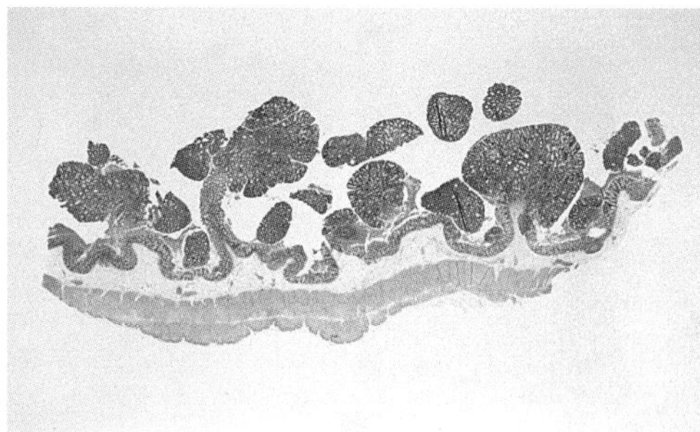

Fig. 7.64 Whole-mount microscopic section of the colon in familial adenomatous polyposis showing a forest of small tubular adenomas.

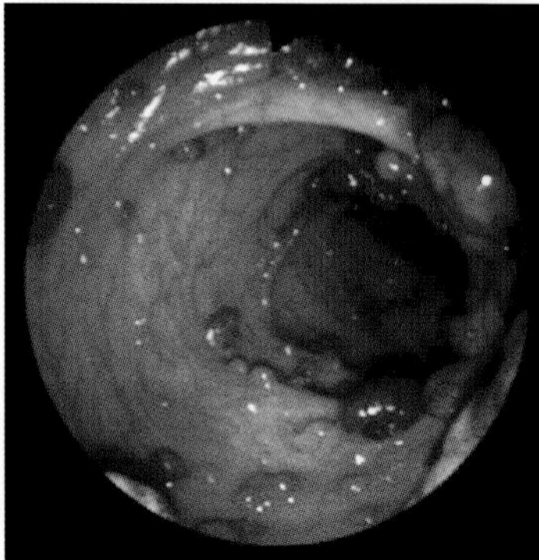

Fig. 7.61 Colonoscopic appearance of multiple small polyps in a polyposis patient.

Other polyposis syndromes

Turcot–Despres–Pierre syndrome, or glioma polyposis, in which multiple colorectal adenomas are associated with tumors of the central nervous system and endocrine neoplasia, probably includes another phenotype of the FAP gene defect in which the germline mutation is accompanied by a medulloblastoma. However, there is another group of Turcot patients in whom the genetic defect has more in common with that of HNPCC and in which the brain tumors are glioblastomas.

In the Cronkhite–Canada syndrome there are multiple colonic adenomas and alopecia, hyperpigmentation, and onychodystrophy (Fig. 7.66). Histologically, the polyps possess large cystic glands, which

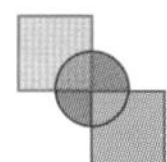

differentiate them from other forms; they do not become dysplastic and are probably without malignant potential (Fig. 7.67). Characteristic gastric polyps are also seen in this condition (Figs 7.68, 7.69).

Juvenile polyps occur most often in the rectums of children, but are occasionally seen in adults (Fig. 7.70). They are usually smooth and round with a cystic cut surface. At microscopy, they appear as dilated epithelial tubules sited in abundant stroma (Fig. 7.71). They have a similar structure to some inflammatory polyps, but no stalk, and their tendency to auto-amputate presumably explains their lack of persistence into adulthood. They have no premalignant qualities.

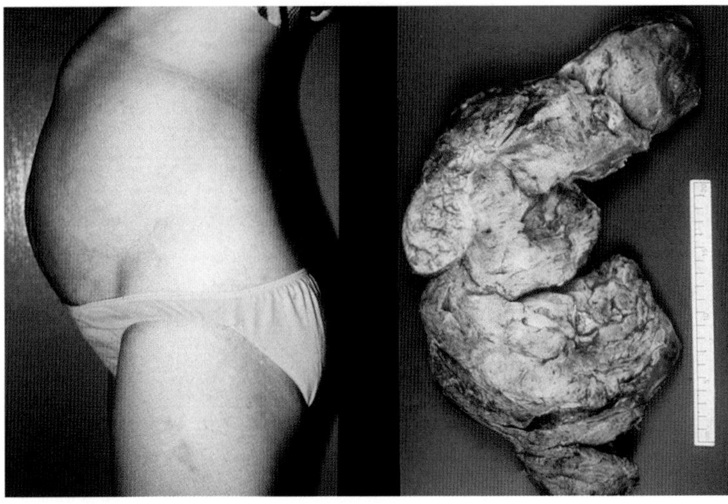

■ **Fig. 7.65** Massive abdominal wall desmoid and the consequent huge resection specimen. The patient lost small bowel within the tumor mass and is now dependent on artificial nutritional support. Courtesy of Mr D. Swain and the St Mark's Polyposis Registry.

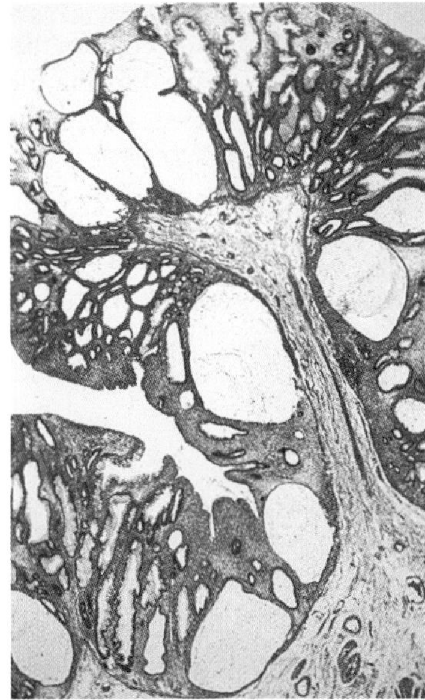

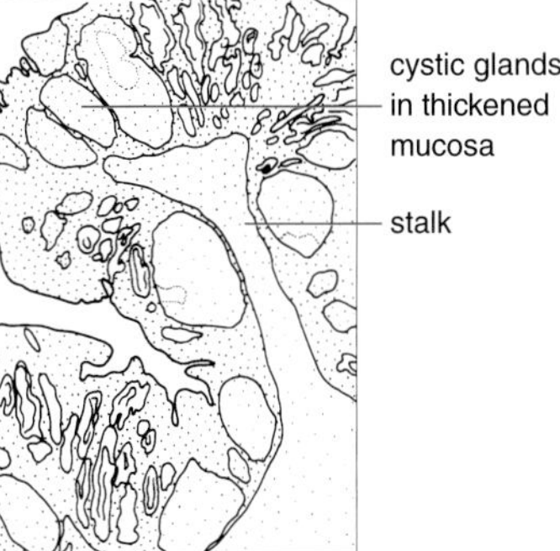

■ **Fig. 7.67** Histological appearance of the Cronkhite– Canada syndrome. The cystic glands are neither dysplastic nor accompanied by a stromal element, which differentiates them from other forms. H&E stain (x 8).

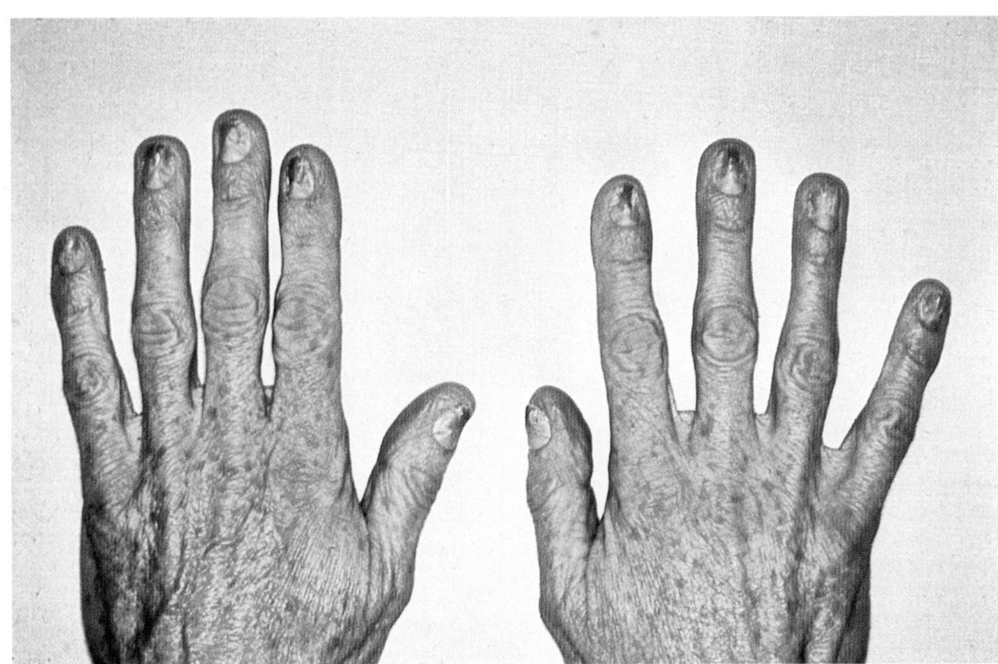

■ **Fig. 7.66** Onychodystrophy in the Cronkhite–Canada syndrome. Courtesy of Dr W.J. Cunliffe.

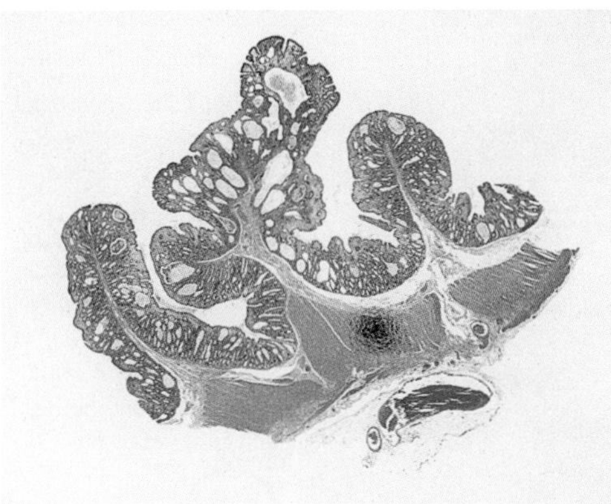

■ **Fig. 7.68** Microscopic view of the gastric mucosa in the Cronkhite–Canada syndrome showing the replacement of the normal mucosa by hamartomatous mucosa from which focal polypoid projections are seen. The confluent nature of the mucosal hamartomas in this syndrome distinguish it from all other gastro-intestinal hamartomatous syndromes.

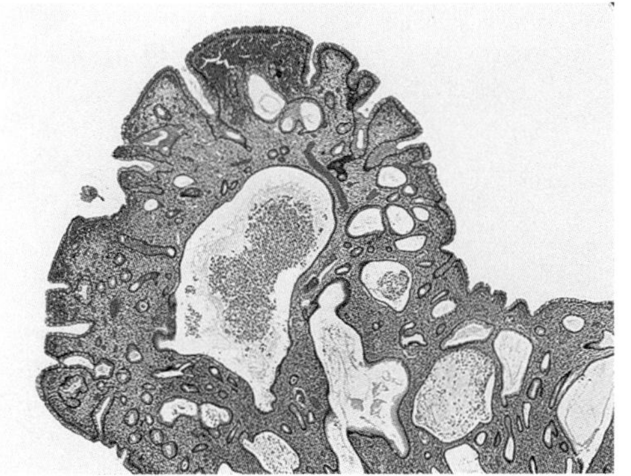

■ **Fig. 7.69** Higher-magnification view of a polypoid gastric hamartoma in the Cronkhite–Canada syndrome showing the cystically dilated pits lined by cytologically normal foveolar epithelium and the abundant edematous stroma that is devoid of smooth muscle.

Much less common is juvenile polyposis, in which there are multiple (>5) juvenile polyps (Fig. 7.72), and which does seem to be associated with an increased colon cancer risk, as supported by the discovery of associated dysplasia in some resected lesions (Fig. 7.73).

Peutz–Jeghers syndrome (hamartomatous polyposis) is discussed in more detail in Chapter 4, but it may be responsible for multiple hamartomas in the colon (Figs 7.74, 7.75). It is responsible for a substantial increase in cancer deaths (not only of colorectal origin).

Cowden's syndrome is also hamartomatous, but the colonic lesions have a characteristic pattern with disorganized muscularis mucosae and normal overlying epithelium (Figs 7.76–7.78). The other features of the syndrome include oral, upper gastrointestinal and cutaneous hamartomas, together with a higher frequency of breast and thyroid tumors.

Other forms of benign polyps and the serrated adenoma

Hyperplastic polyps are found most often in the rectum, but can occur at any colonic site (Fig. 7.79). They are nearly always multiple and usually an incidental finding, their numbers increasing with age. Macroscopically, they appear as sessile mucosal elevations rarely larger than 5 mm in diameter (Fig. 7.80). Microscopically, they comprise elongated dilated tubules, but the saw-tooth epithe-

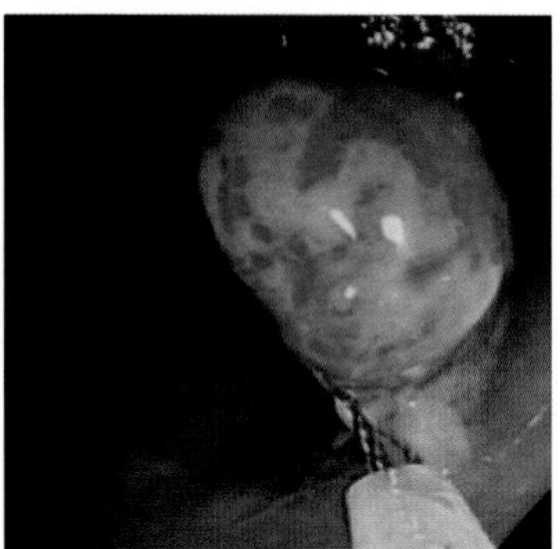

Fig. 7.70 Juvenile polyp in an adult.

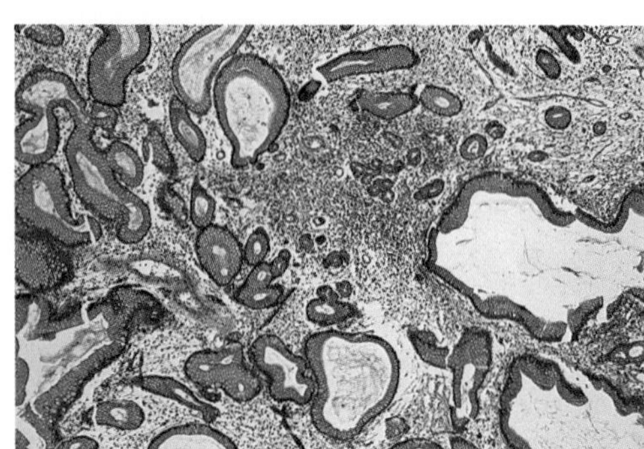

Fig. 7.71 Juvenile polyp. Microscopic view showing the characteristically abundant stroma that is delicate, edematous, mildly inflamed, and devoid of smooth muscle and the cystic dilatation of the glands lined by cytologically normal colonic epithelial cells.

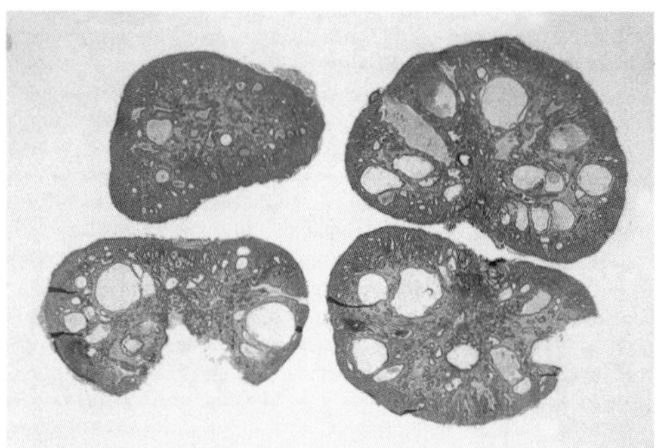

Fig. 7.72 Whole-mount microscopic view of colonic polyps in a patient with juvenile polyposis showing the smooth surface, abundant edematous stroma, and cystically dilated glands typical of these hamartomas.

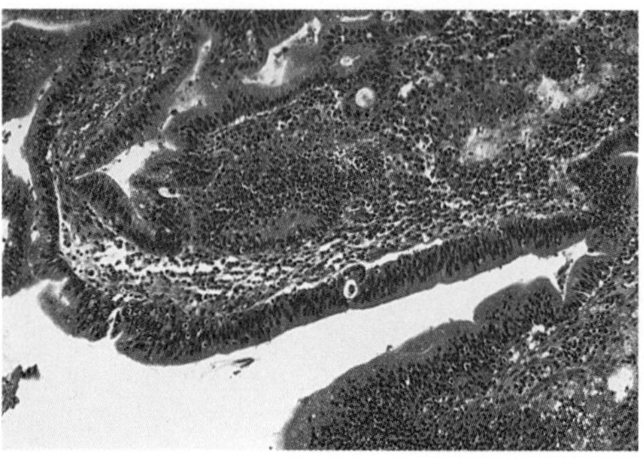

Fig. 7.73 Juvenile polyp with dysplasia. Microscopic view of a dysplastic focus in a juvenile polyp from a syndromic patient showing the enlargement, hyperchromasia, and pseudostratification of the glandular and surface epithelium.

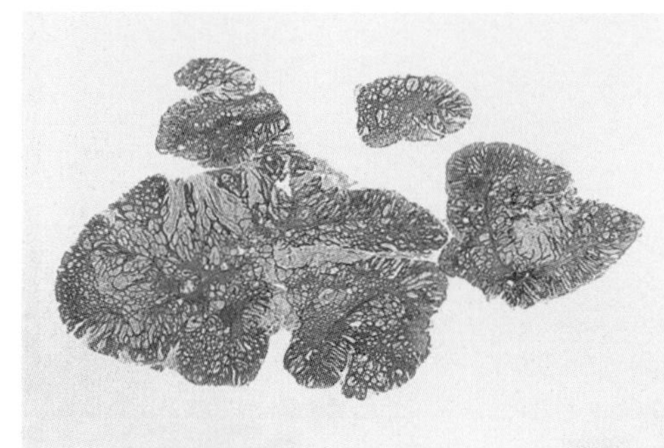

Fig. 7.74 Peutz–Jeghers polyp. Whole-mount microscopic view of a colonic Peutz–Jeghers hamartoma showing the typical lobulated, 'hydra-headed' configuration, the dense proliferation of tightly packed, highly branched glands of the mucosa, and the thick arborized bands of smooth muscle at the core of each of the lobules of the polyp head.

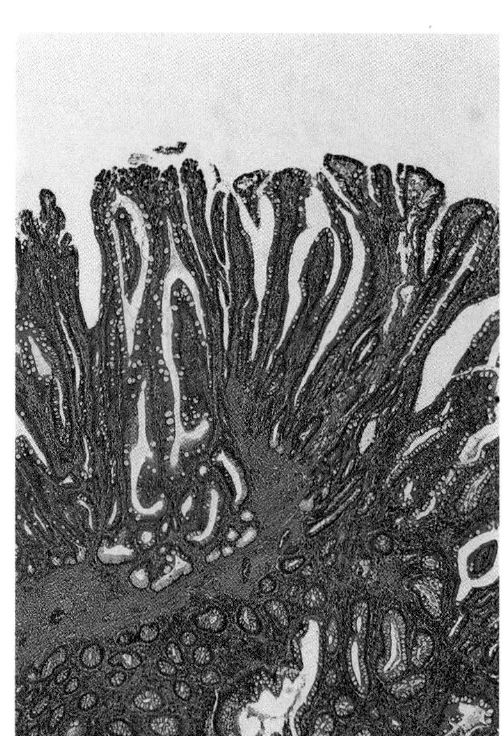

Fig. 7.75 Microscopic view of a Peutz–Jeghers polyp showing the crowding and complex architecture of the glands, the relatively sparse intervening stroma, and the thick bands of smooth muscle that course through the polyp head.

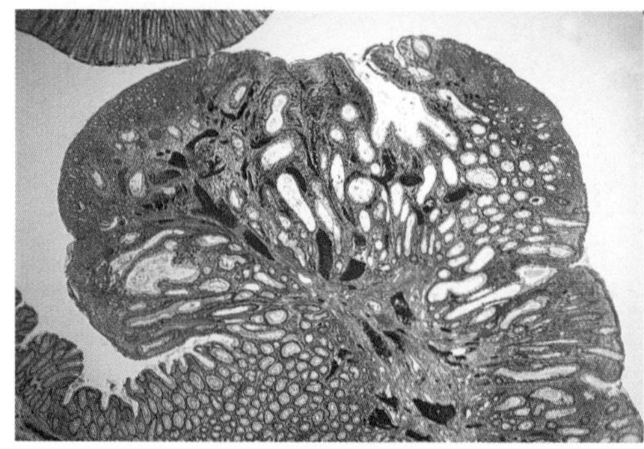

Fig. 7.76 Cowden's syndrome. Microscopic appearance of a typical mucosal hamartoma showing a proliferation of branched and focally dilated glands, with moderate amounts of inflamed stroma that may contain wisps of smooth muscle, and focal surface erosion.

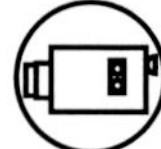

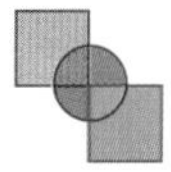

lial pattern previously thought characteristic (Fig. 7.81) is also a feature of the serrated adenoma (Figs 7.82, 7.83). Molecular evidence suggests that there is a developmental con-tinuum linking the two types of polyp, and it is now clear that dysplasia does indeed occur in conjunction with the hyperplastic polyp (Fig. 7.84), and that there is therefore malignant potential from these polyps also.

Benign lymphoid polyps are seen most often in the rectum and are usually asymptomatic despite measuring up to 3 cm in diameter. They comprise normal lymphoid tissue with a prominent follicular pattern (Figs 7.85–7.87).

Inflammatory pseudopolyps are the result of defective mucosal healing following severe ulceration, and are usually seen in chronic inflammatory bowel disease (see Chapter 6).

OTHER COLONIC TUMORS

A variety of neoplastic lesions of mesodermal and ectodermal origin may involve the colon. Lipomas are the most frequent of the gastrointestinal stromal tumors, and may produce the characteristic smooth submucosal lesions recognized elsewhere in the gastro-intestinal tract (Fig. 7.88); the characteristic 'cushion sign' is then almost diagnostic (Fig. 7.89). Lipomata typically change shape with the patient's posture (Fig. 7.90) and are readily diagnosed from the low signal returned from fat on CT scanning (Fig. 7.91). CT is also helpful in assessing the invasive potential of gastrointestinal stromal tumors (Fig 7.92).

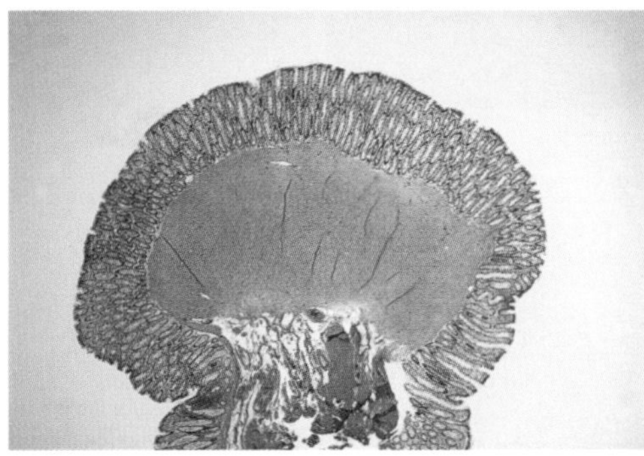

Fig. 7.77 A second type of hamartoma in Cowden's disease that is the equivalent of a leiomyoma of muscularis mucosae (see also below).

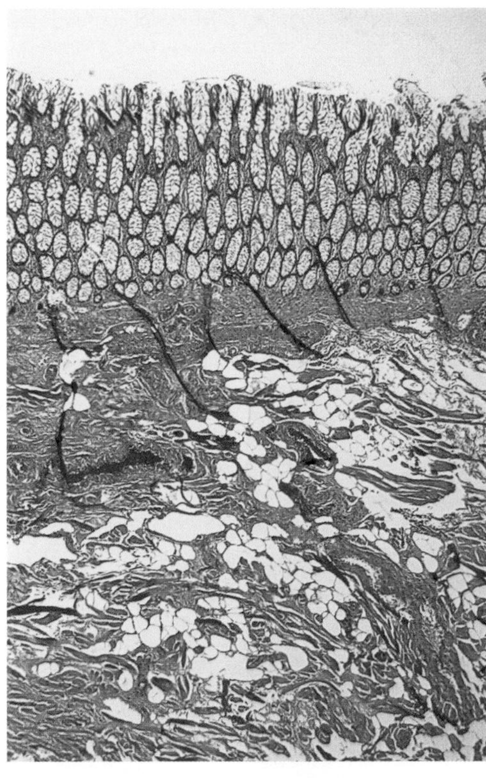

Fig. 7.78 A third variety of hamartoma in Cowden's syndrome that is the equivalent of a submucosal lipoma (see also below).

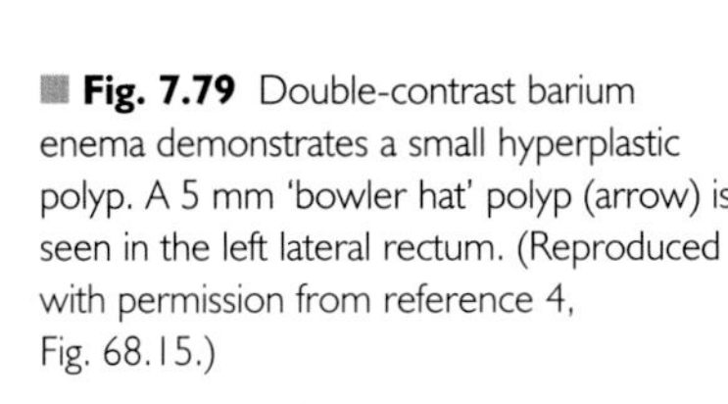

Fig. 7.79 Double-contrast barium enema demonstrates a small hyperplastic polyp. A 5 mm 'bowler hat' polyp (arrow) is seen in the left lateral rectum. (Reproduced with permission from reference 4, Fig. 68.15.)

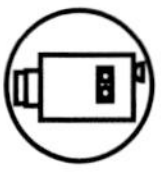

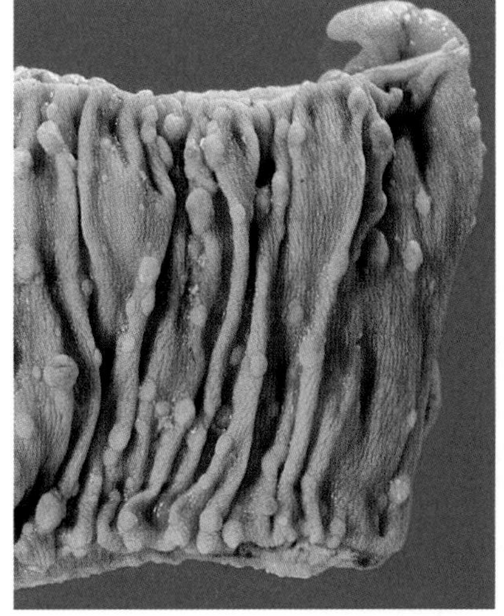

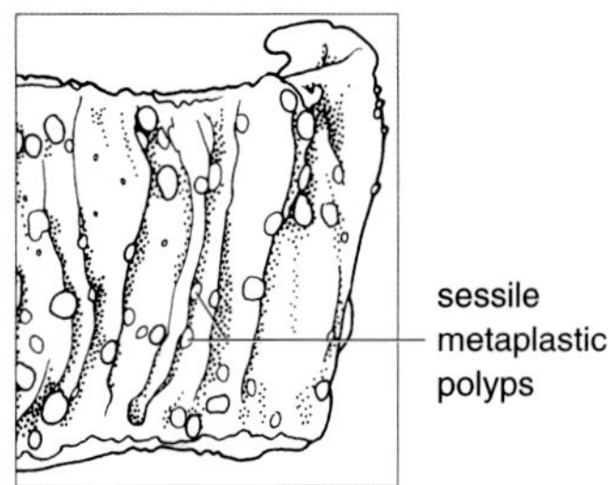

Fig. 7.80 A short length of colon covered with tiny sessile hyperplastic polyps.

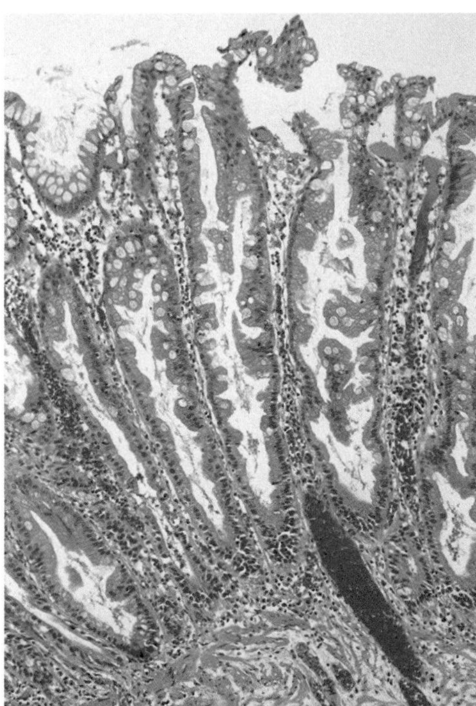

Fig. 7.81 Hyperplastic polyp. Microscopic appearance of a hyperplastic polyp showing gland elongation with expansion of the basal proliferative zone and crowding of the maturing cells with epithelial tufting (the 'saw-toothed' or serrated appearance) in the luminal half of the glands.

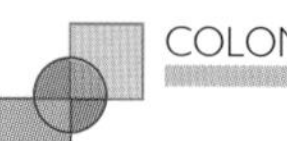

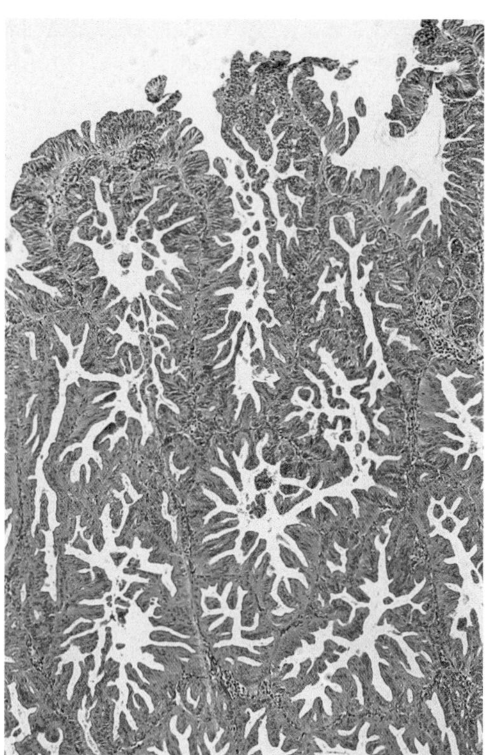

Fig. 7.82 Serrated adenoma. Microscopic appearance of a serrated adenoma showing the characteristic tufting ('saw-toothed' appearance) of the highly dysplastic epithelium that comprises the entire polyp.

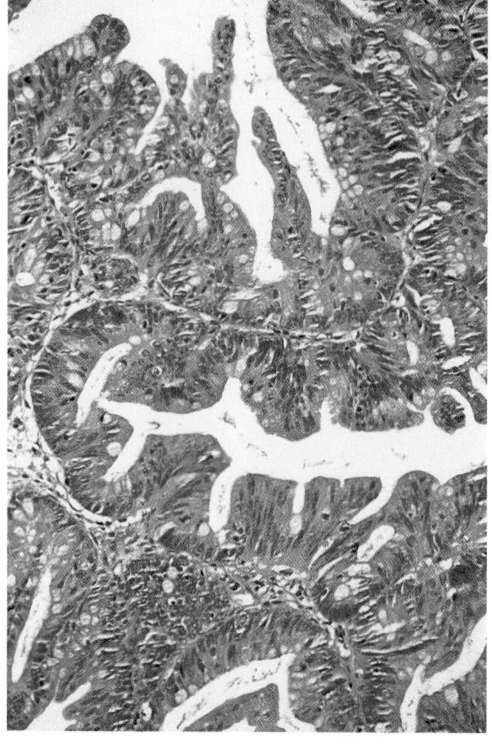

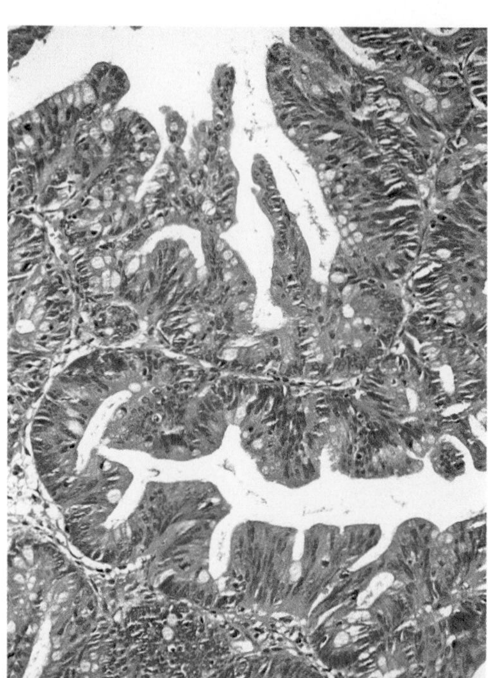

Fig. 7.83 High-magnification view of a serrated adenoma showing the adenomatous cytological features of the epithelium and the tufted growth pattern.

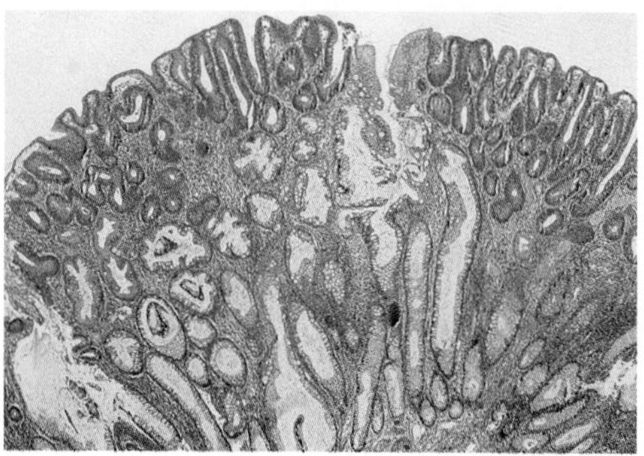

Fig. 7.84 Hyperplastic polyp with dysplasia. An otherwise typical hyperplastic polyp showing epithelial dysplasia in the superficial aspects of the glands consistent with neoplastic progression.

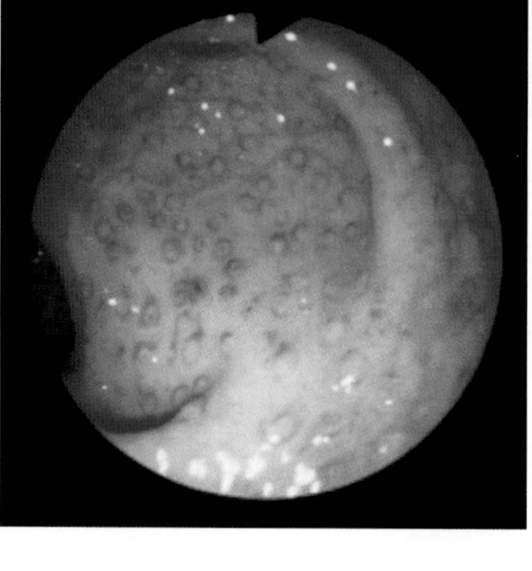

Fig. 7.85 Colonoscopic appearance of lymphoid folliculitis.

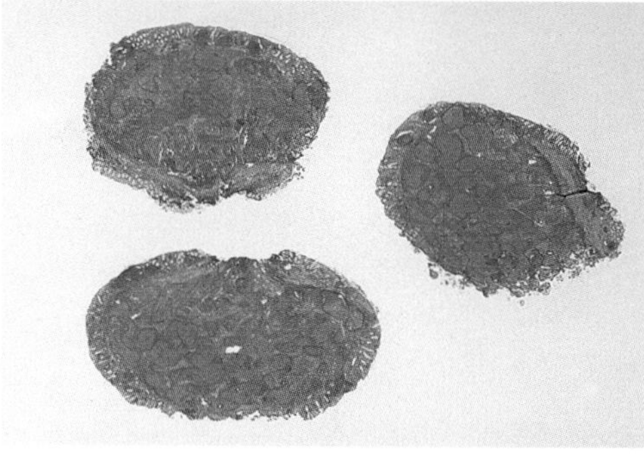

Fig. 7.86 Lymphoid polyps. Whole-mount microscopic view of four rectal polyps showing the hyperplastic lymphoid follicles that fill the submucosa of the polyp head and extend focally into the overlying mucosa. Although usually solitary, rectal lymphoid polyps may occur in small groups (two to six polyps) in about 20% of cases.

Fig. 7.87 Rectal lymphoid polyp. Microscopic appearance showing the numerous large germinal centers cuffed by small lymphocytes that fill the submucosa of the polyp head.

Von Recklinghausen's disease may have colonic manifestations (Fig. 7.93), as may the carcinoid syndrome (Fig. 7.94), and Kaposi's sarcoma (Fig. 7.95).

Colonic lymphoma is uncommon but occasionally poses an important differential diagnosis from colorectal carcinoma – imaging is usually a good guide prior to biopsy (Fig. 7.96). It is characteristic,

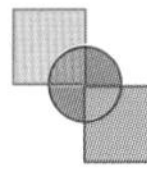

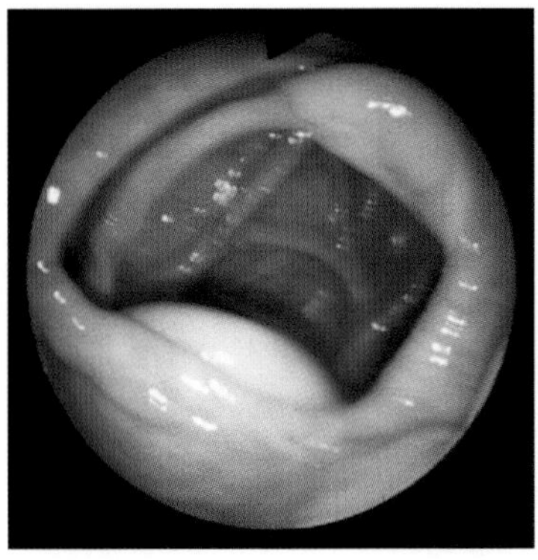

■ **Fig. 7.88** Endoscopic appearance of a colonic lipoma lying in front of the ileocecal valve.

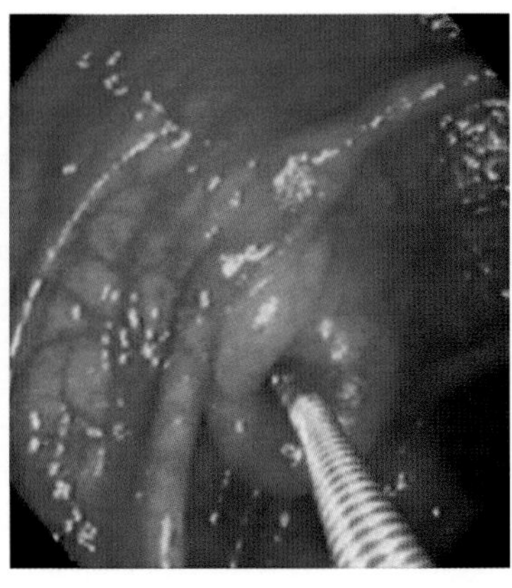

■ **Fig. 7.89** The characteristic 'cushion sign' seen when a biopsy forceps is pushed gently into a lipomatous lesion.

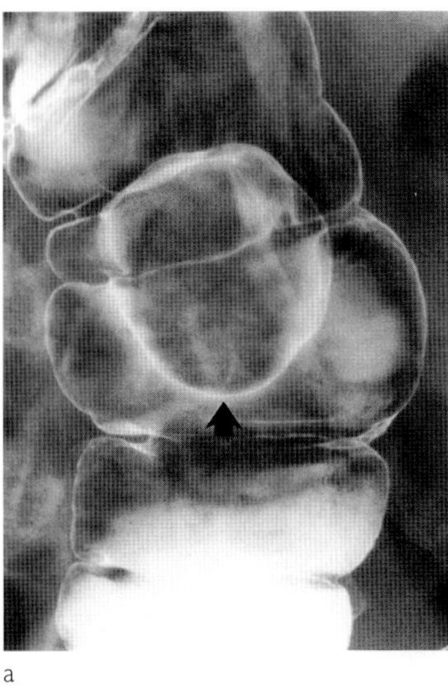

a

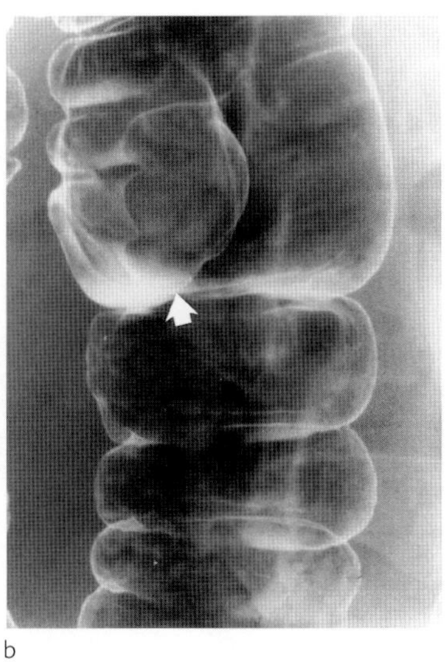

b

■ **Fig. 7.90** Double-contrast barium enema shows lipoma of descending colon. A smooth-surfaced 4 cm mass (black arrow) is shown (a). The mass (white arrow) changes position shape when the patient stands in the erect position (b). (Reproduced with permission from reference 3, Fig. 57.13.)

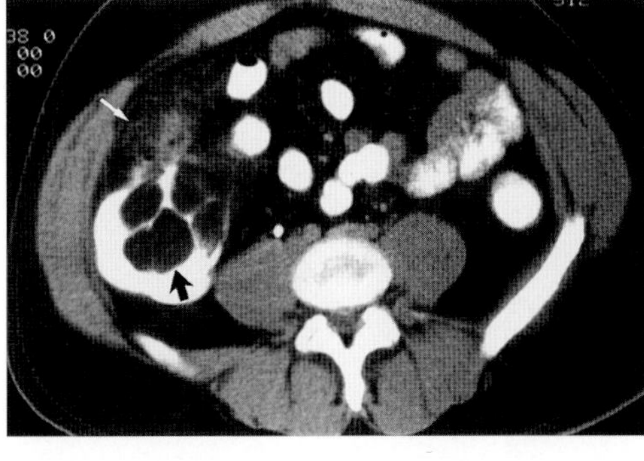

■ **Fig. 7.91** CT demonstrating lipoma in ascending colon. A lobulated mass of fat attenuation (black arrow) is seen in the barium pool. Stranding of the pericolic fat (white arrow) is due to diverticulitis of the ascending colon (not shown). (Reproduced with permission from reference 1, Fig. 12.62.)

unlike lymphoma at some sites, that this is not a diffuse infiltration, but that there is a focal lesion with a well-defined margin (Figs 7.97, 7.98).

The colon is, rarely, a site for secondary deposits from primaries sited elsewhere (Figs 7.99–7.102).

DIVERTICULAR DISEASE

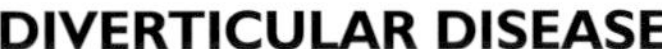

Colonic diverticula are acquired pouches of mucosa and submucosa herniating through the muscle layers of the bowel. Patients with diverticulosis have increased left-sided intraluminal colonic seg-

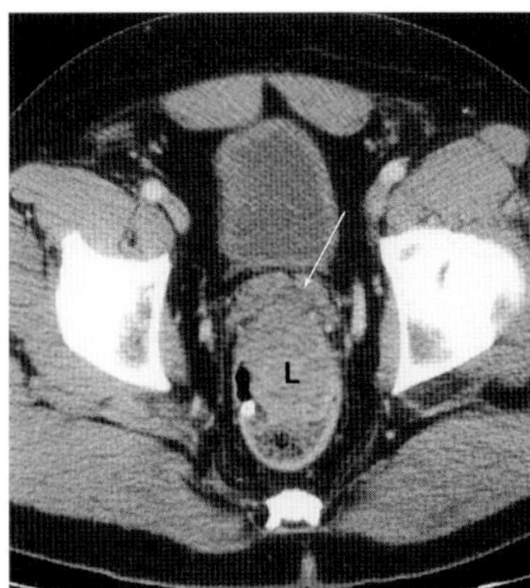

■ **Fig. 7.92** CT depicting malignant gastrointestinal stromal tumor of rectum. A 5 cm soft tissue mass (L) fills the lumen of the mid rectum. Loss of the fat plane with the seminal vesicles (arrow) is due to local tumor infiltration.

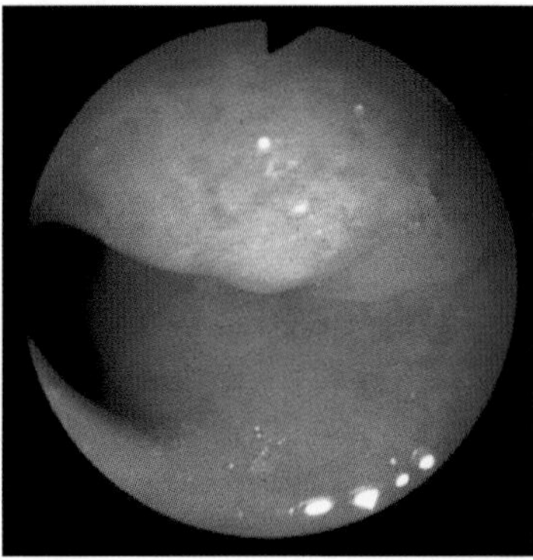

■ **Fig. 7.93** Neurofibromatosis affecting the colon in a patient with Von Recklinghausen's disease.

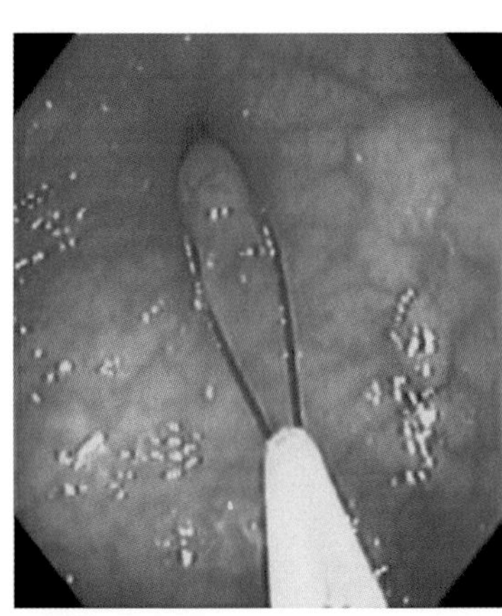

■ **Fig. 7.94** Endoscopic appearance of a rectal carcinoid tumor.

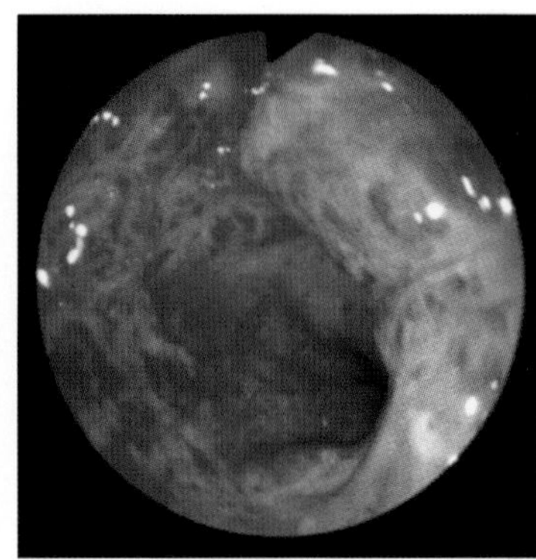

■ **Fig. 7.95** Kaposi's sarcoma affecting the colon and responsible for rectal bleeding.

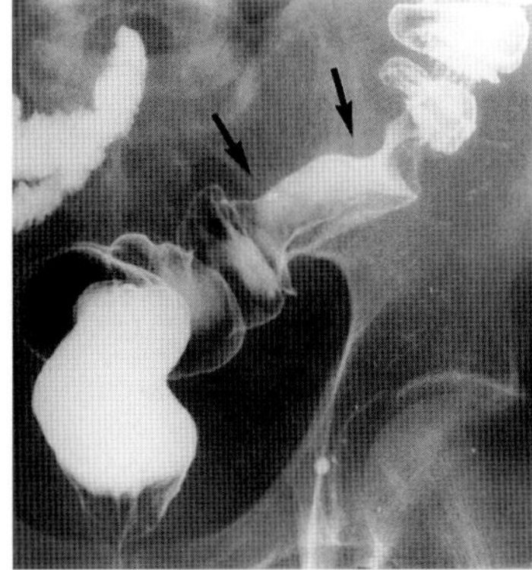

■ **Fig. 7.96** Double-contrast barium enema demonstrating lymphoma of sigmoid colon. A relatively long circumferential lesion (arrows) with a tapered border proximally and shelf-like border distally is seen. The surface of the tumor is smooth. Despite the length of the lesion, there is not much luminal narrowing or evidence of obstruction. (Reproduced with permission from reference 3, Fig. 57.3, courtesy of S.N. Glick, M.D., Philadelphia, PA)

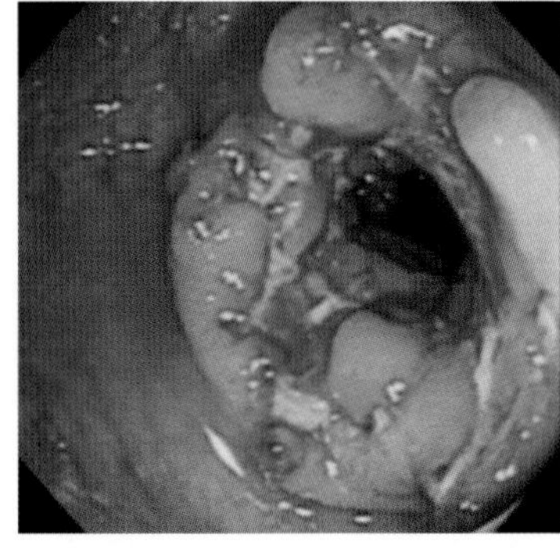

■ **Fig. 7.97** Comparable endoscopic view of colonic lymphoma.

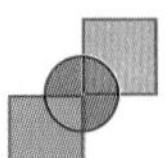

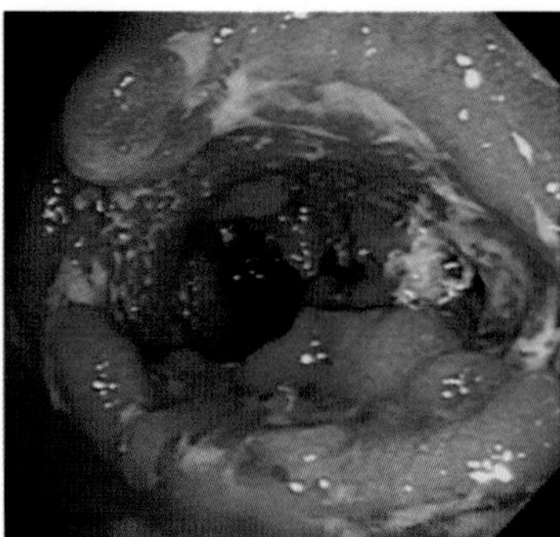

Fig. 7.98 Close-up view of the lymphoma shown in Fig. 7.97.

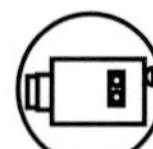

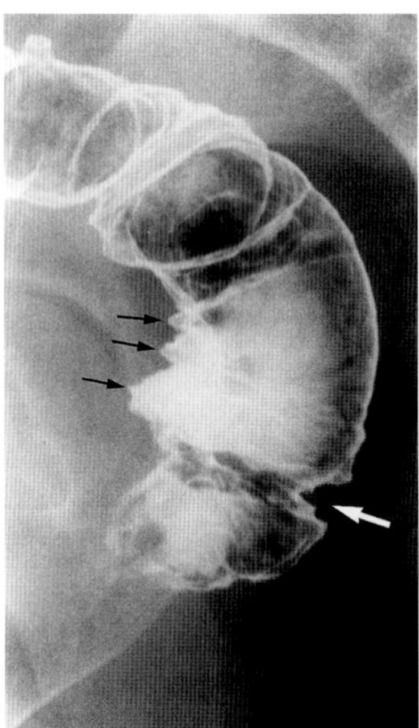

Fig. 7.99 Prostatic cancer invading the rectum. The anterior wall of the mid rectum has a spiculated contour (black arrows). Focal circumferential extension of tumor is seen (white arrow). Biopsy showed invasion of the submucosa with focal extension into the mucosa. (Reproduced with permission from reference 9, Fig. 1B.)

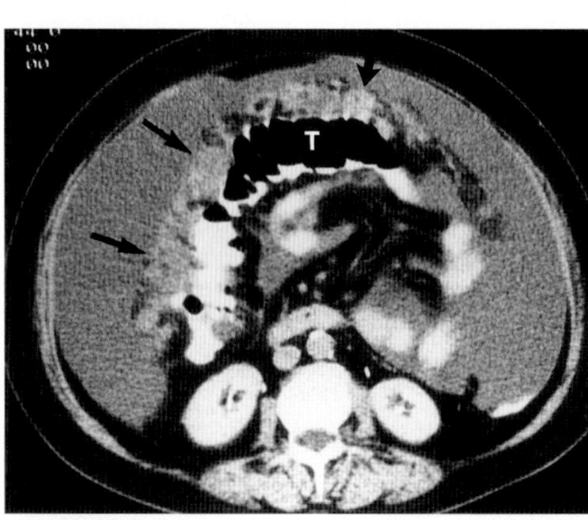

Fig. 7.100 Intraperitoneal metastases to greater omentum from ovarian carcinoma with secondary colonic involvement. CT demonstrates ascites and soft tissue masses (arrows) abutting the anterior wall of the transverse colon (T), replacing the fat of the greater omentum. (Reproduced with permission from reference 3, Fig. 57.36B.)

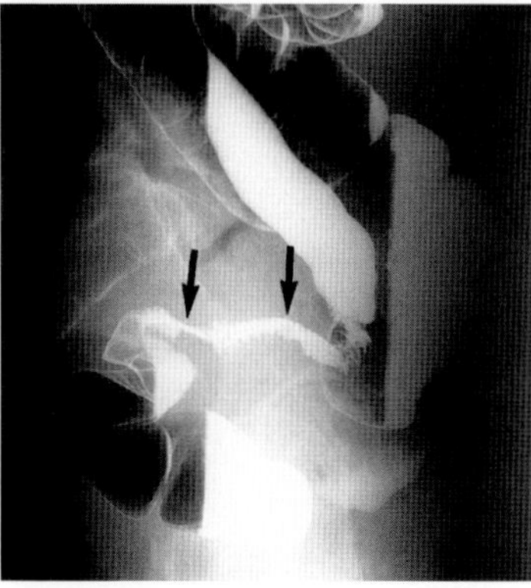

Fig. 7.101 Double-contrast barium enema demonstrates intraperitoneal metastases from ovarian carcinoma. The sigmoid colon is diffusely narrowed (arrows).

menting pressures, particularly in response to food, thus initiating herniation. The sigmoid is affected in 95% but diverticula may occur throughout the colon. They usually arise in rows between the lateral and mesenteric taenii at the site of (potential) weakness in the bowel wall, where large blood vessels penetrate the interfascicular connective tissue of the circular muscle layer. They are commoner with aging and in populations where typical diets are low in fiber content (their prevalence is at least 30% in those over 60 in the United Kingdom) (Figs 7.103–7.106). The presence of diverticula is of no consequence in most of those affected, but a related phenomenon is associated with scleroderma (Fig. 7.107). The typical pathology of diverticular disease includes a narrowed length of sigmoid colon with thickened bands of circular muscle, giving the bowel a concertina-like appearance (Fig. 7.108). The mouths of the diverticula open into the bowel lumen between the bands, and the diverticular sacs extend into the pericolic fat where they are covered

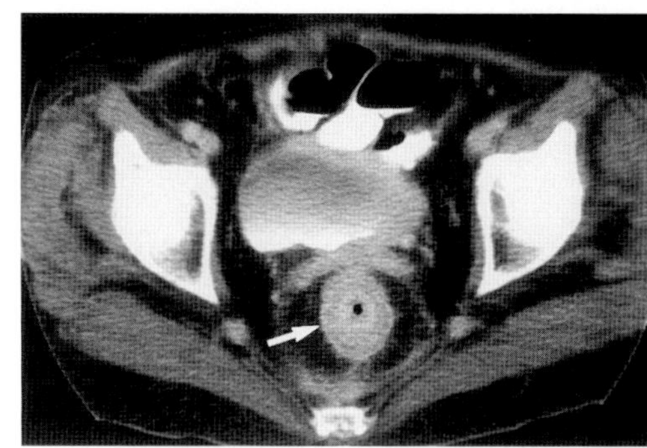

Fig. 7.102 CT showing diffuse thickening of rectum (arrow) due to hematogenous metastasis from breast carcinoma. The uniform thickening and mural stratification here mimic ulcerative colitis.

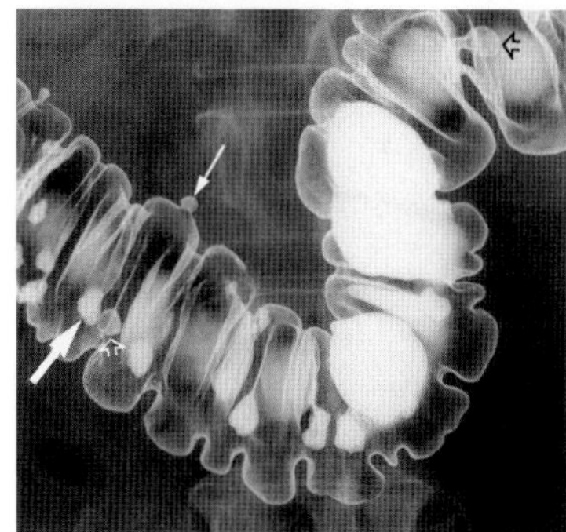

Fig. 7.103 Double-contrast barium enema demonstrating diverticulosis of transverse colon. Seen *en face*, the diverticula appear as barium-filled sacs (large white arrow) or ring shadows (open arrows). Seen in profile, the diverticula (small white arrow) protrude from the luminal contour. (Reproduced with permission from reference 6, Fig. 14.19.)

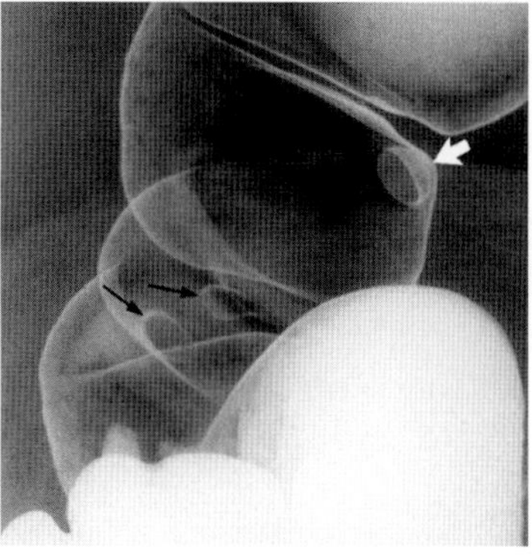

a

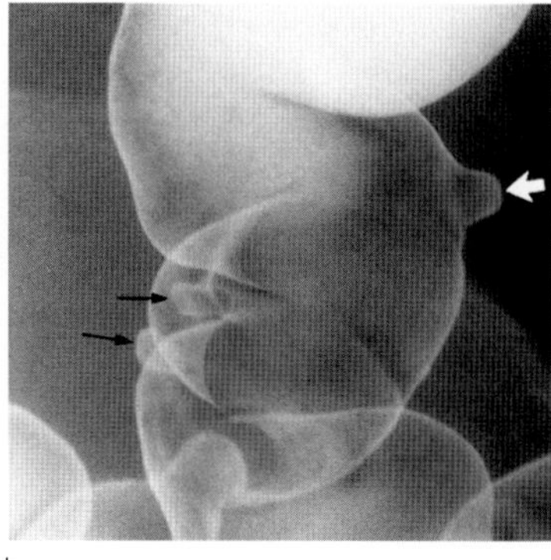

b

Fig. 7.104 Double-contrast barium enema demonstrating diverticulum resembling a 'bowler hat' (white arrow). (a) In contrast to a polyp, the apex of the bowler hat diverticulum (white arrow) protrudes away from the longitudinal axis of the lumen. Two other diverticula are manifested as ring shadows (black arrows). (b) In profile, the diverticulum (white arrow) protrudes outside of the luminal contour. The two other diverticula, these with narrow necks, are now seen in profile (black arrows). (Reproduced with permission from reference 7, Figs. 3A and 3B.)

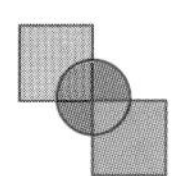

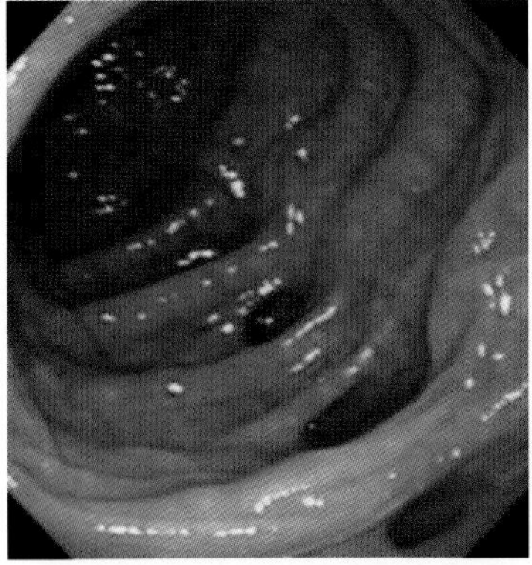

■ **Fig. 7.105** Colonoscopic appearance of diverticular disease affecting the sigmoid colon.

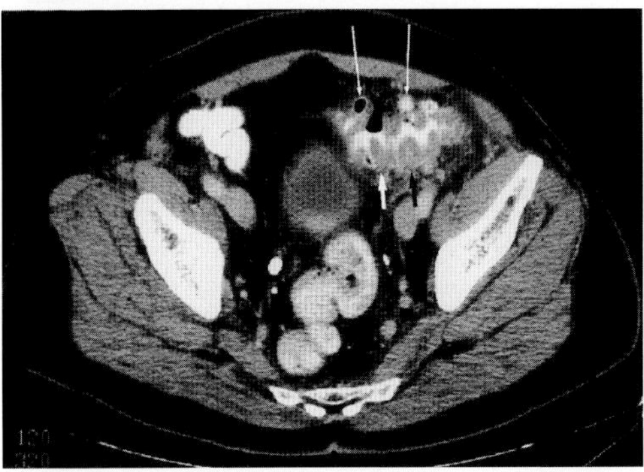

■ **Fig. 7.106** CT demonstrating circular muscle thickening and diverticulosis. The wall of the proximal sigmoid colon is thick and undulating (short arrows). Several diverticula are seen anteriorly (long arrows). (Reproduced with permission from reference 6, Fig. 14.17.)

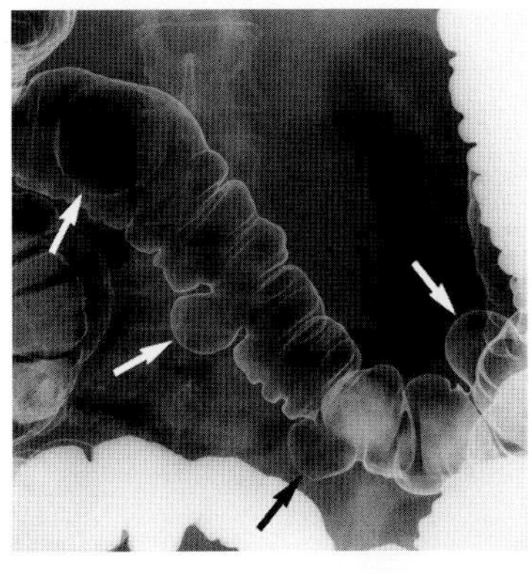

■ **Fig. 7.107** Double-contrast barium enema demonstrating sacculations caused by scleroderma. Muscular atrophy and scarring in the transverse colon result in sacculations (arrows) with wide mouths. Compare these sacculations to the diverticula in the other images, which are smaller and have narrow necks. (Reproduced with permission from reference 6, Fig. 14.18.)

only by a thin layer of longitudinal muscle (Fig. 7.109). Once formed, diverticulae generally remain for life, but may most occasionally invert (Fig. 7.110).

Hemorrhage from a diverticulum in the absence of inflammation is no longer thought to be common, but may be responsible for brisk and usually self-limiting rectal bleeding (Fig. 7.111). Associated mucosal prolapse (Figs 7.112–7.114) may also be responsible for bleeding.

A small minority of patients with diverticulosis develop diverticulitis. This may be preceded by fecal impaction within the mouths of diverticula but it is by no means certain that this is a sufficient or necessary precursor (Figs 7.115–7.117). Lower abdominal pain and tenderness with fever and leukocytosis are usual. Imaging may leave no doubt as to the diagnosis (Fig. 7.118) and may provide evidence for localized perforation (Figs 7.119, 7.120). Resection yields parallel pathology (Fig. 7.121). As well as by bleeding, diverticulitis may be complicated by frank peritonitis, or intra-abdominal

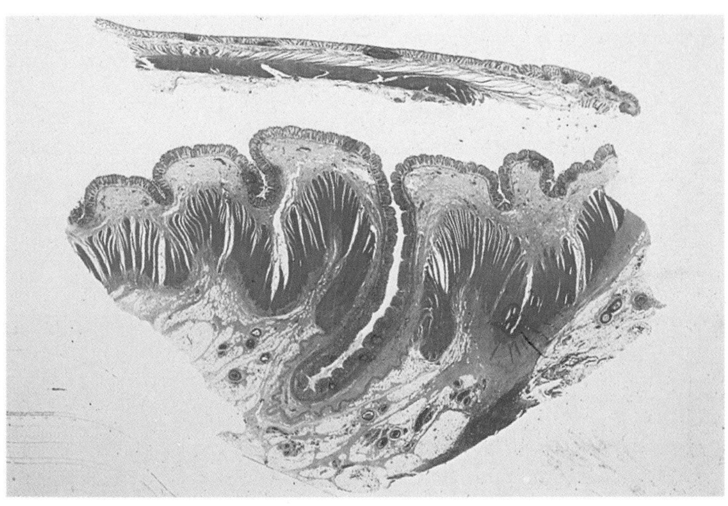

■ **Fig. 7.109** Sections of colon contrasting normal bowel wall (above) with the thickened wall in diverticular disease (below). The absence of a muscular covering to the diverticulum is apparent. H&E stain (x 12).

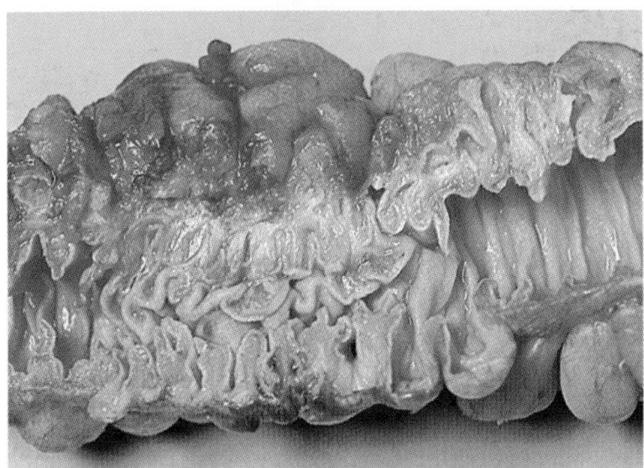

a

folds of mucosa
bowel lumen
diverticulum
bands of thickened muscle

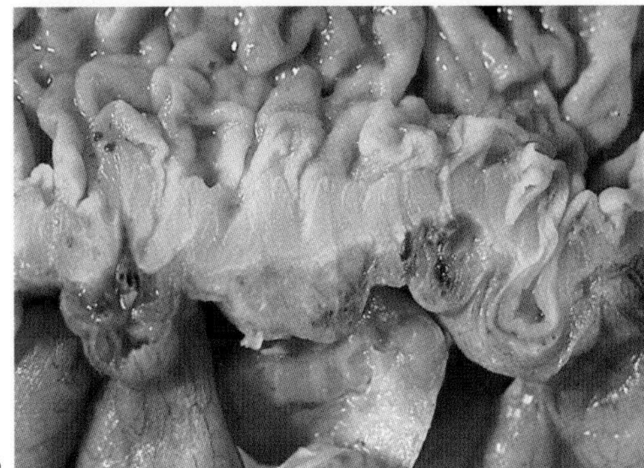

b

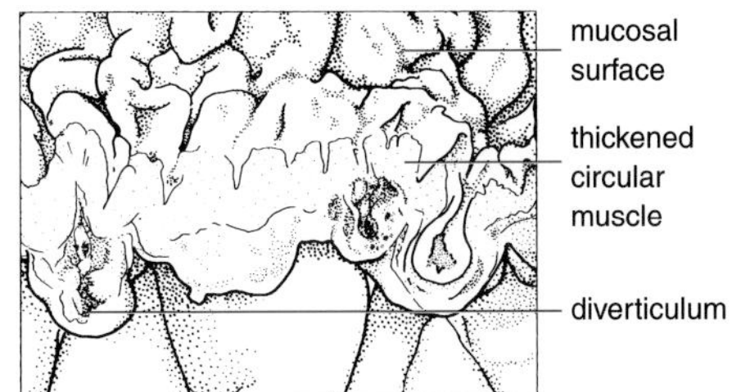

■ **Fig. 7.108** Macroscopic appearance of the colon in diverticular disease. An increase in muscle thickness and redundant mucosal folds combine (a) to occlude the lumen. A close-up view (b) shows the thick bands of circular muscle.

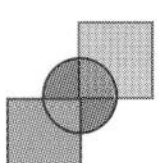

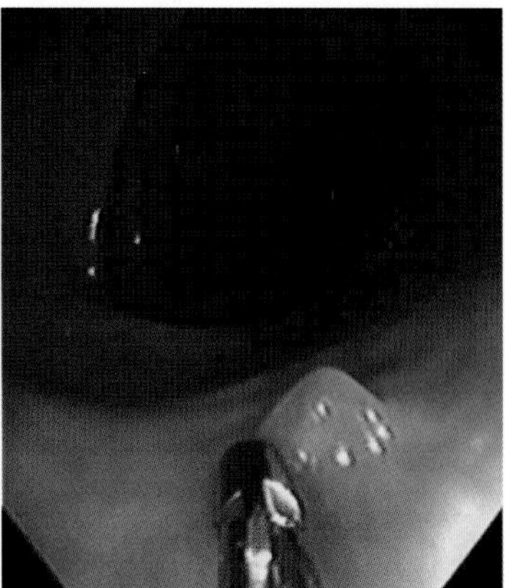

■ **Fig. 7.110** The unusual appearance caused by an inverted diverticulum. Biopsy or 'polypectomy' would obviously be dangerous.

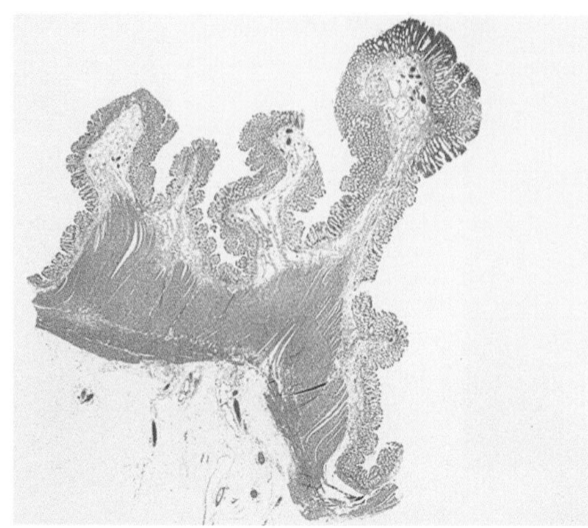

■ **Fig. 7.114** Diverticular disease-associated mucosal prolapse. Whole-mount microscopic view of a polypoid projection of prolapsed mucosa at the edge of a diverticular orifice showing congestion and erosion of the polyp head, another possible source of bleeding in diverticular disease.

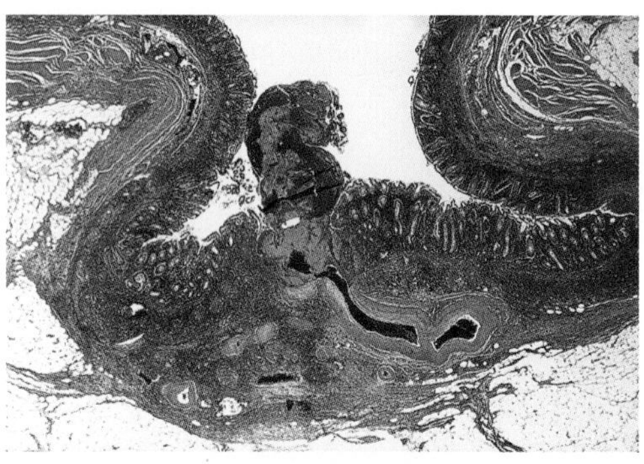

■ **Fig. 7.111** Diverticular disease complicated by hemorrhage. Eroded arterial vessel at the base of an inflamed diverticulum is identified as the source of hemorrhage.

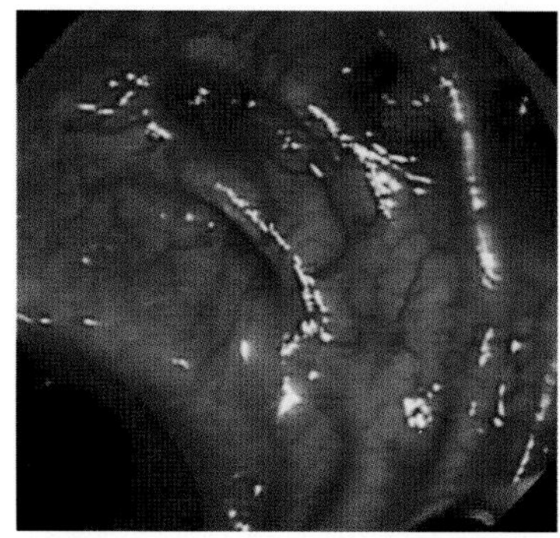

■ **Fig. 7.115** Fecoliths in diverticular disease.

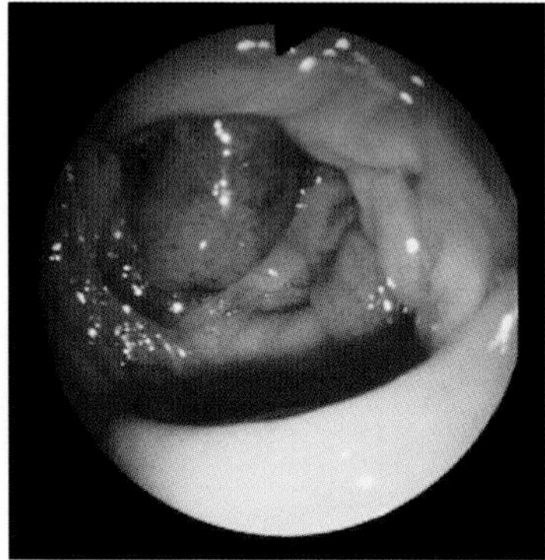

■ **Fig. 7.112** Colonoscopic appearances of mucosal prolapse in association with diverticular disease.

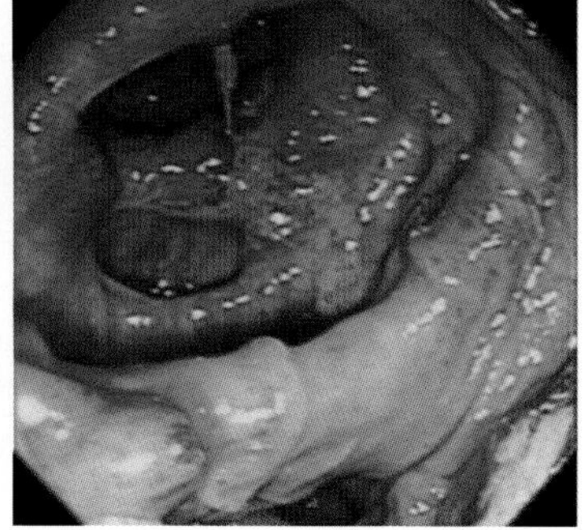

■ **Fig. 7.113** More marked mucosal prolapse which had been responsible for overt bleeding.

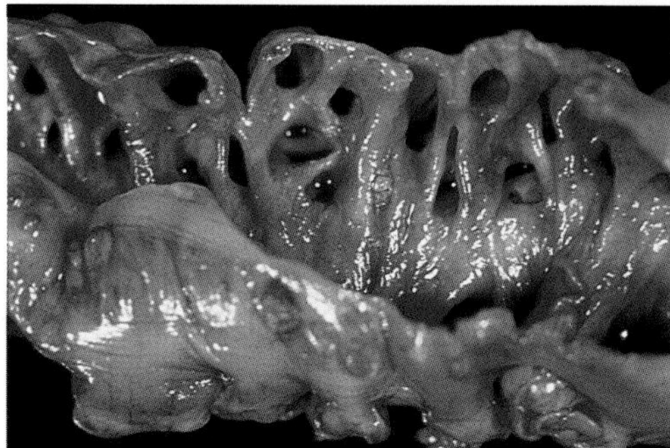

■ **Fig. 7.116** Sigmoid resection specimen showing the luminal view of massively dilated diverticular openings that had been impacted with feces (still visible in the diverticulum in the center of the photograph).

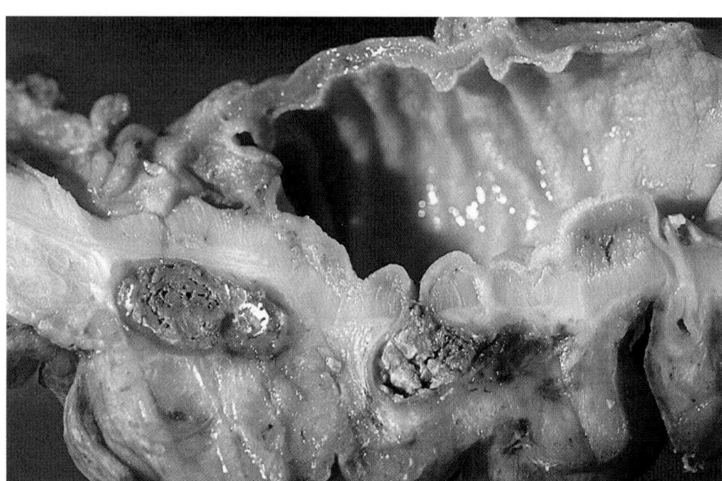

■ **Fig. 7.117** Macroscopic appearance of fecal debris trapped in a diverticulum on the peritoneal aspect of the sigmoid colon.

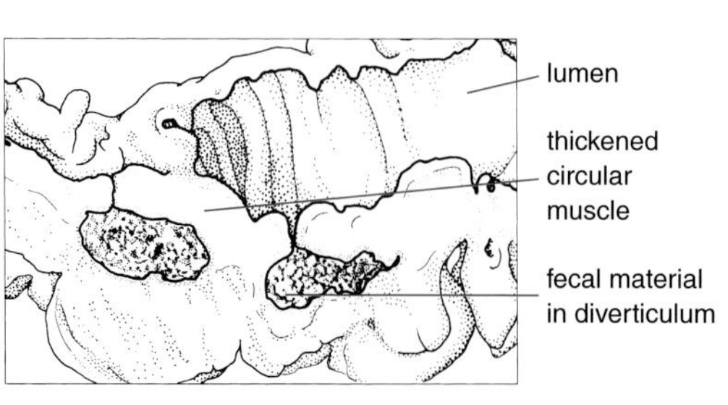

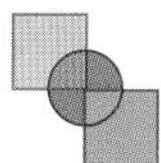

abscess (Fig. 7.122). Isotopic scanning can be most helpful when the site of an abscess is unclear (Fig. 7.123). Diagnosis and surgical planning in this group of patients are now beginning to be helped by MRI scanning which will often show the fistula and its openings (see Chapter 8). Diverticulitis may also be responsible for features of intestinal obstruction from the presence of an edematous inflammatory mass together with the associated muscle thickening. Partial obstruction may subside with antibiotic therapy, but chronic thickening and fibrosis may require surgical relief. Spontaneous and postoperative fistulae are also strongly associated with complicated diverticulitis. Symptoms vary according to the nature of the fistula, but pneumaturia, recurrent urinary tract infection, or passage of feces from the vagina will often be more indicative than routine investigations (Fig. 7.124). Although not strictly a complication of diverticulosis, the presence or development of a concurrent carcinoma is important as its features may be rendered considerably less obvious, and endoscopy is almost always indicated (Fig. 7.125).

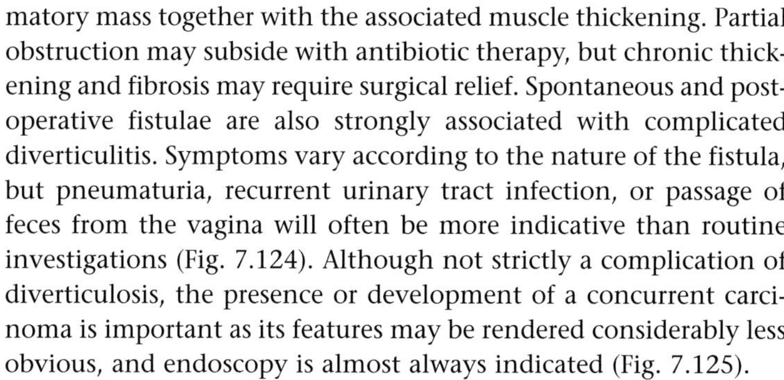

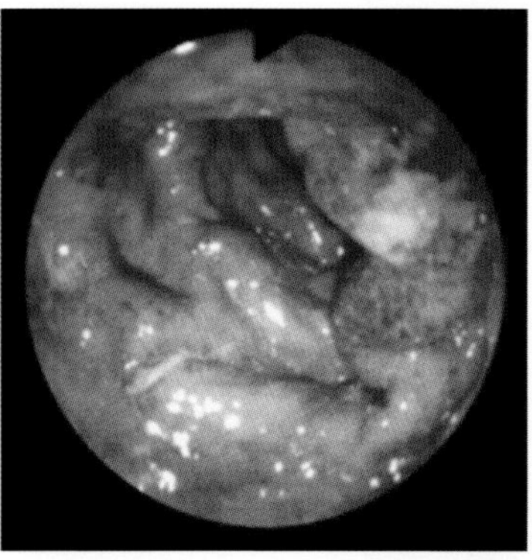

Fig. 7.118 Endoscopic appearance in diverticulitis. There is obvious inflammatory change associated with the diverticula and also visible pus.

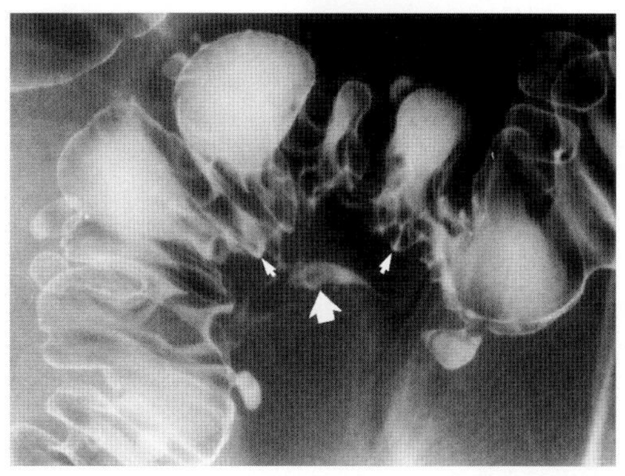

Fig. 7.119 Double-contrast barium enema demonstrating diverticulitis of the sigmoid colon. Barium fills extraluminal tracks and a flame-shaped collection (large arrow). The inflammatory process causes extrinsic mass effect and spiculation (small arrows) of the adjacent colonic wall. (Reproduced with permission from reference 6, Fig. 14.24.)

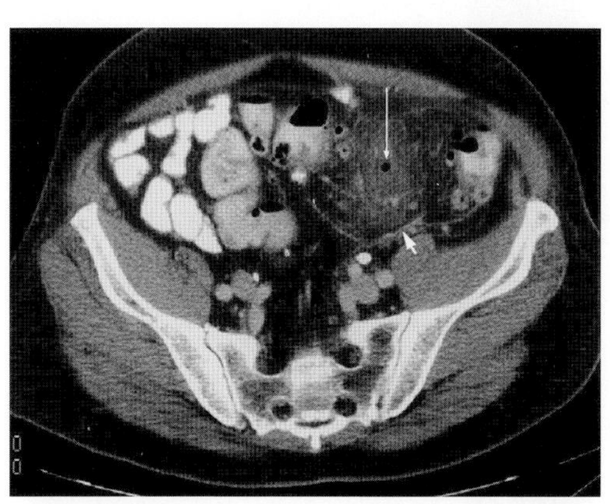

Fig. 7.120 CT demonstrating small pericolic abscess due to diverticulitis. A focal collection of extraluminal air (long arrow) is in the center of an area of soft tissue stranding of the fat adjacent to the sigmoid colon. Fluid in the sigmoid mesentery (short arrow) is identified. (Reproduced with permission from reference 6, Fig. 14.19B.)

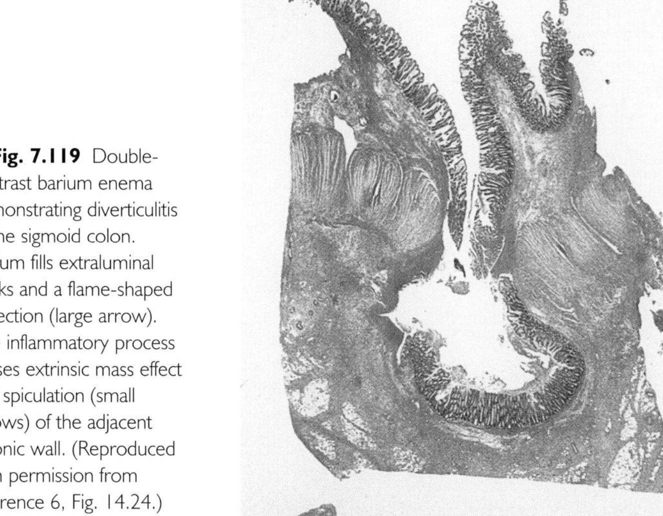

Fig. 7.121 Ulcerated diverticulum with diverticulitis. Microscopic view of a sigmoid diverticulum showing focal ulceration of the lining mucosa (seen at left) and dense inflammation of the surrounding subserosal fat.

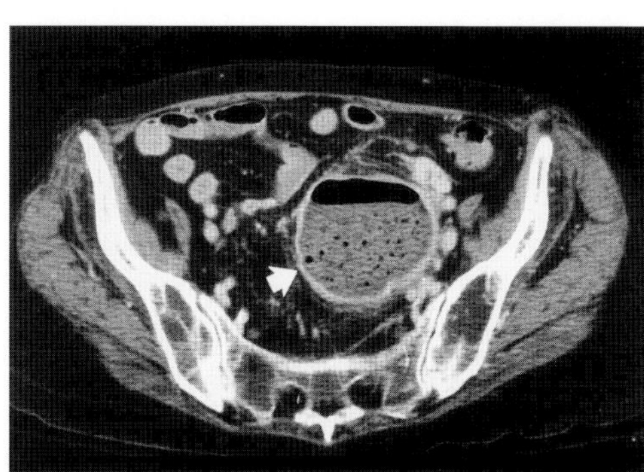

Fig. 7.122 CT demonstrating large pericolic abscess due to diverticulitis. A debris- and air-filled abscess (arrow) has a thick, contrast-enhancing wall. (Reproduced with permission from reference 6, Fig. 14.20.)

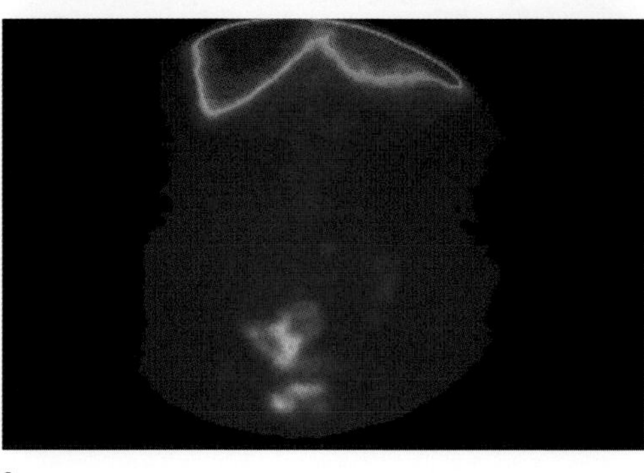

a

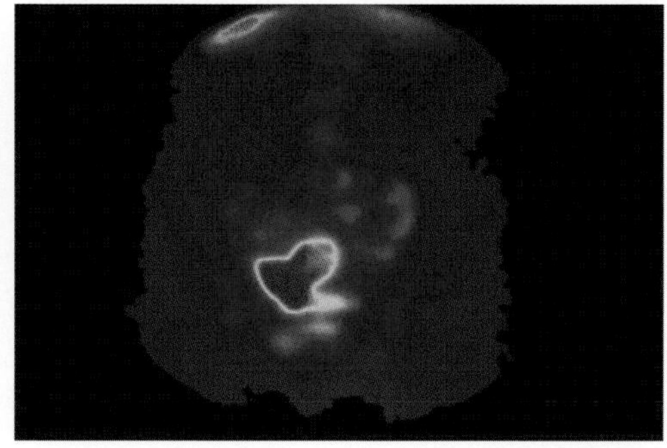

b

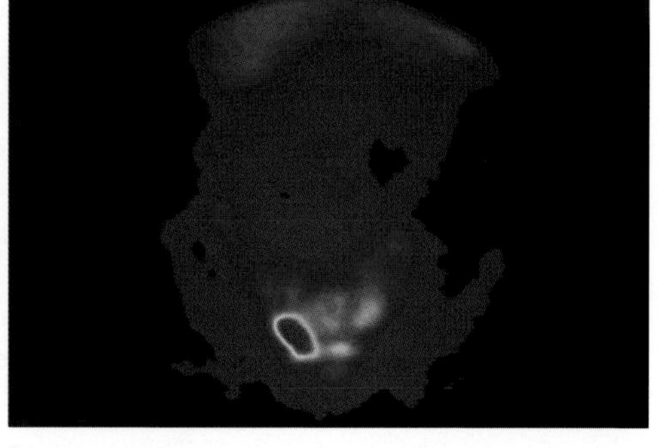

c

Fig. 7.123 ^{99m}Tc HMPAO-white cell scan in a patient with clinical evidence of sepsis but in whom the site was not obvious. At 1 hour, the isotope is normally distributed in the liver and spleen (a). At 3 hours, there is isotope within the bowel but there is also an obvious collection in the pelvis (b). By 22 hours (c), there is residual isotope almost exclusively in the pelvic abscess. Courtesy of Mr G.P. Morris and Cancer Research UK.

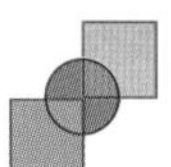

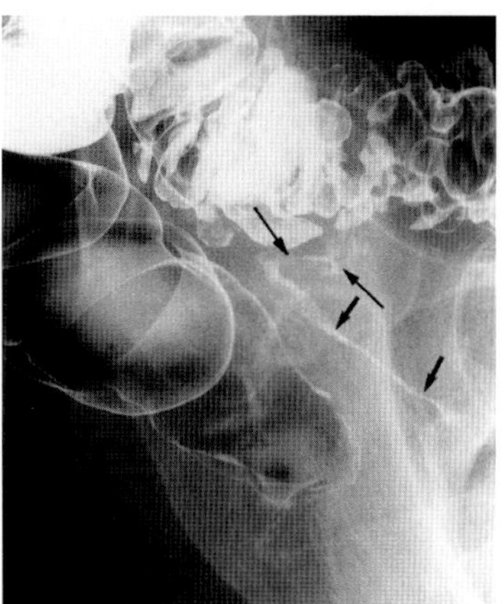

■ **Fig. 7.124** Double-contrast barium enema demonstrating rectovaginal fistula due to sigmoid diverticulitis. A fistula (thin arrows) fills the vagina (thick arrows) with barium. Deformed diverticula are seen on the inferior border of the sigmoid colon. (Reproduced with permission from reference 4, Fig. 2.)

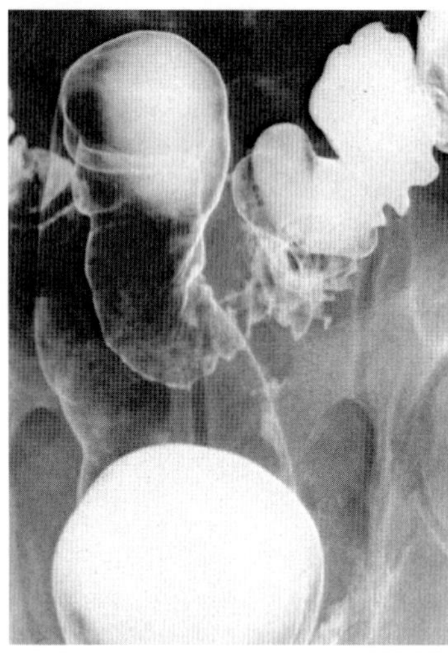

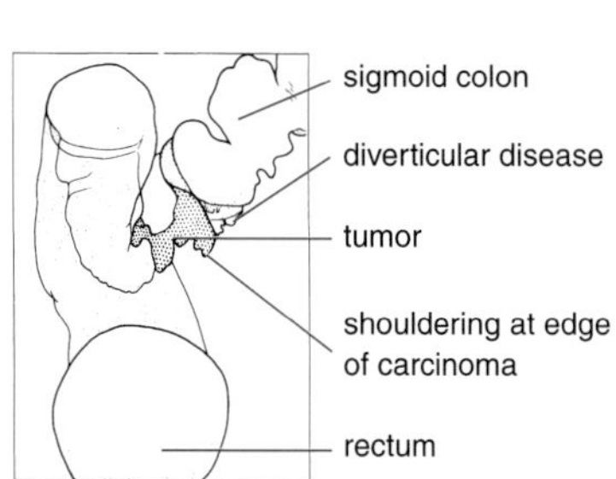

■ **Fig. 7.125** Barium enema showing diverticular disease and sigmoid carcinoma. In this example, the shouldering at the edge of the carcinoma is reasonably obvious, but this is not always the case.

APPENDICITIS

Acute inflammation of the appendix is the commonest reason for emergency abdominal surgery in the West. It is only with the greater use of emergency CT scanning (Fig. 7.126) that there is confidence not to assume that severe acute right iliac fossa pain is a strong indication for surgery. The condition is commonest in the second and third decades of life and affects around 6% of Caucasians. The precise cause remains unknown, but obstruction of the appendiceal lumen by a fecolith (Figs 7.127, 7.128), with subsequent bacterial proliferation and invasion of the hypoxic mucosa, is thought to be implicated. The higher frequency of fecoliths in populations with low dietary fiber intake fits the observed epidemiology. Typically, abdominal pain, pyrexia, guarding, and rebound tenderness in the right iliac fossa point to the diagnosis. Leukocytosis is often present, but laboratory findings are otherwise unhelpful. The pre-operative diagnosis should be obvious from CT or ultrasound scanning (Figs 7.127, 7.129). Acute appendicitis may progress from simple (Fig. 7.130), through gangrenous, to perforated if surgery is delayed (Fig. 7.131). Perforation may result in generalized fecal peritonitis or in an appendix mass with or without a frank abscess; the latter may resolve spontaneously but usually requires surgical drainage.

There is congestion of the serosal vessels followed by dilatation of the appendix, which usually involves the tip. It is the distal half that subsequently becomes swollen and covered by purulent exudate (Figs 7.132, 7.133). Later still, softening, hemorrhagic change, and

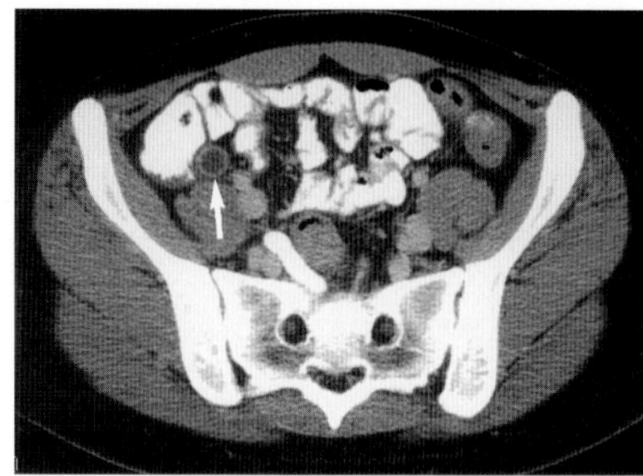

■ **Fig. 7.126** CT demonstrating appendicitis. The appendix (arrow) is mildly dilated and fluid-filled. The wall of the appendix is slightly thickened.

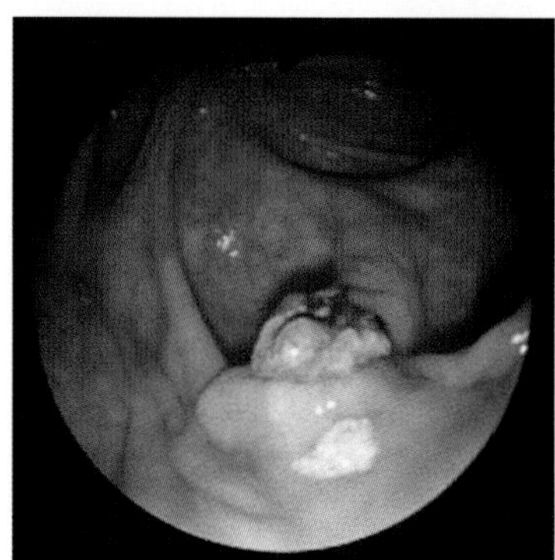

■ **Fig. 7.127** CT demonstrating an appendicolith (arrow) in the appendix.

■ **Fig. 7.128** Fecolith impacted in the appendix.

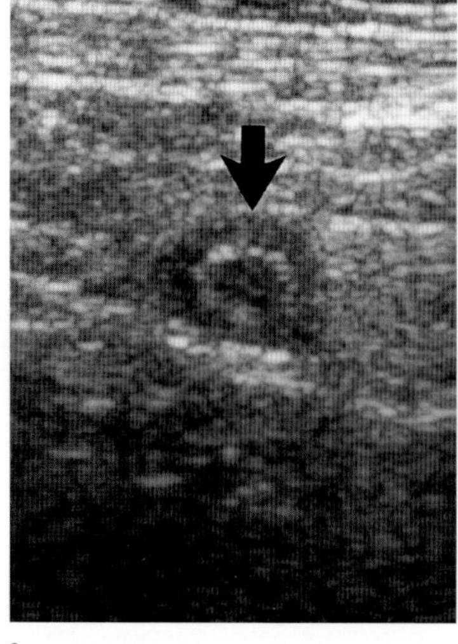

a

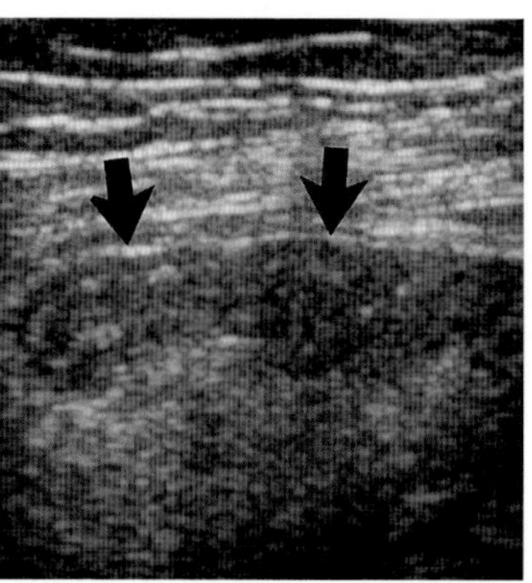

b

■ **Fig. 7.129** Ultrasound demonstrating appendicitis. Transverse (a) and longitudinal (b) scans of the right lower quadrant demonstrate that the lumen of the appendix is dilated and the appendiceal wall thickened (arrows). Courtesy of Dr J.E. Langer, Philadelphia.

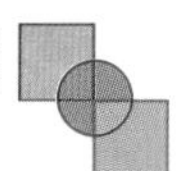

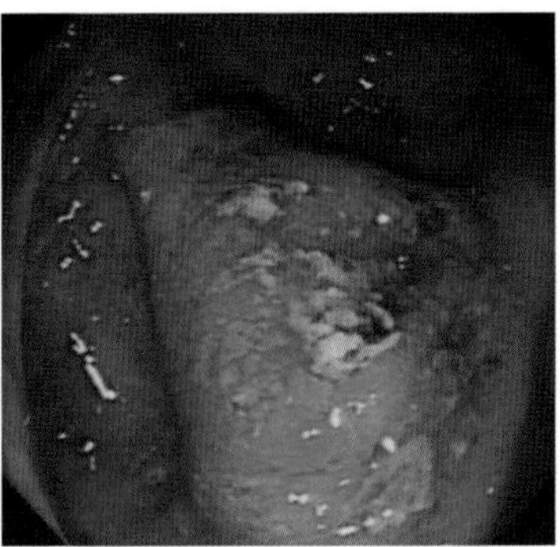

■ **Fig. 7.130** Frank appendicitis seen colonoscopically (not the recommended route to diagnosis!).

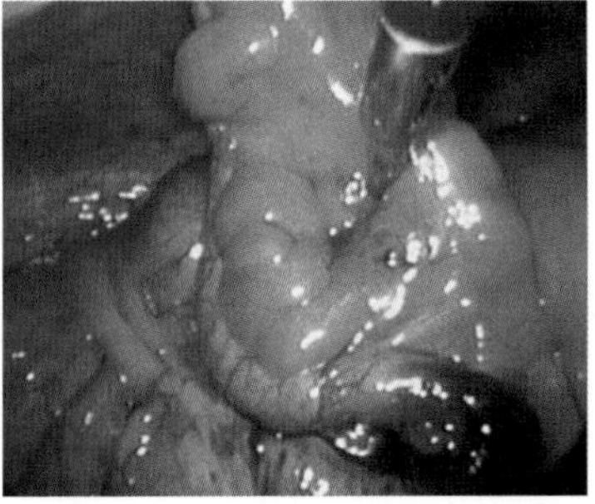

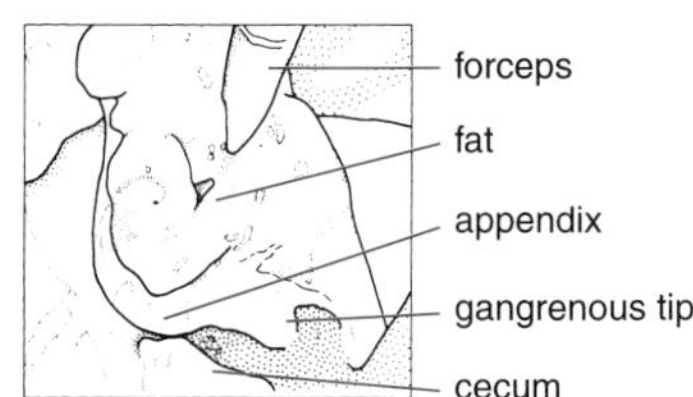

■ **Fig. 7.131** Laparoscopic appearance of gangrenous appendicitis. The pericolic fat is lifted clear of the appendix lying below the normal cecum. Courtesy of Mr P. Dawson.

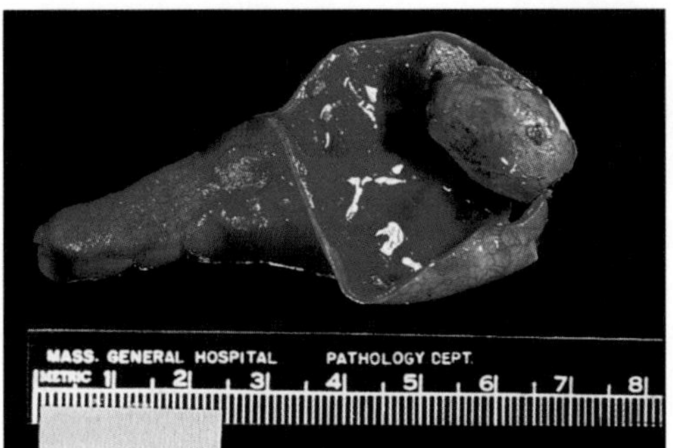

■ **Fig. 7.132** Acute appendicitis. Appendectomy specimen showing a fecolith lodged in the base and the hemorrhagic appearance of the inflamed mucosa.

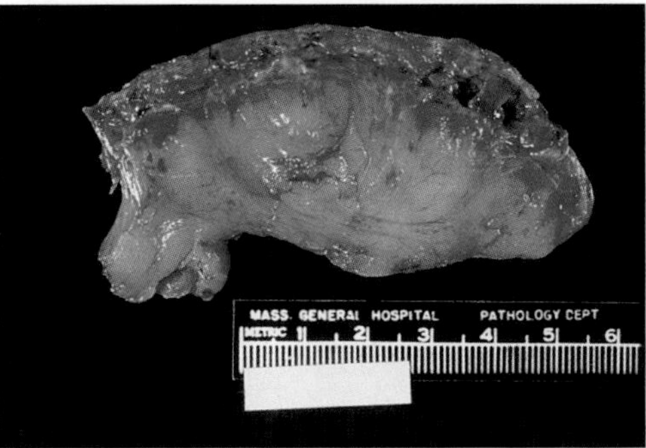

■ **Fig. 7.133** Gangrenous appendicitis. Appendectomy specimen in which the appendix has been transected longi-tudinally to reveal the hemorrhagic and purulent appearance of the gangrenous wall. The mesoappendix shows multiple foci of hemorrhage and extramural abscess formation.

necrosis supervene. Histological examination shows a progressively severe acute inflammatory infiltrate commencing in the mucosa and spreading through the full thickness of the wall (Fig. 7.134). The invagination of the base of the appendix practiced by many surgeons at open appendectomy should not lead to the erroneous diagnosis of a polyp at the cecal pole at subsequent colonoscopy (Fig. 7.135). Only rarely is a carcinoid tumor at the tip of the appendix responsible (Figs 7.136, 7.137); appendectomy is then almost always curative. The bizarre barium radiograph of appendiceal diverticulosis is probably of no clinical consequence (Fig. 7.138).

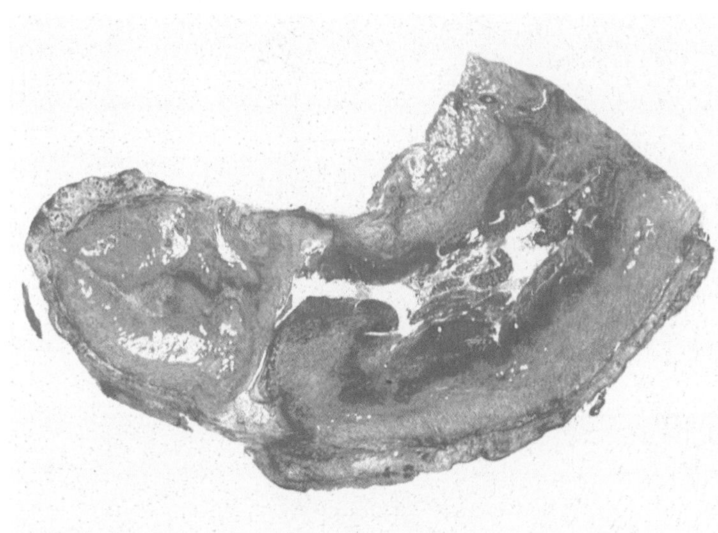

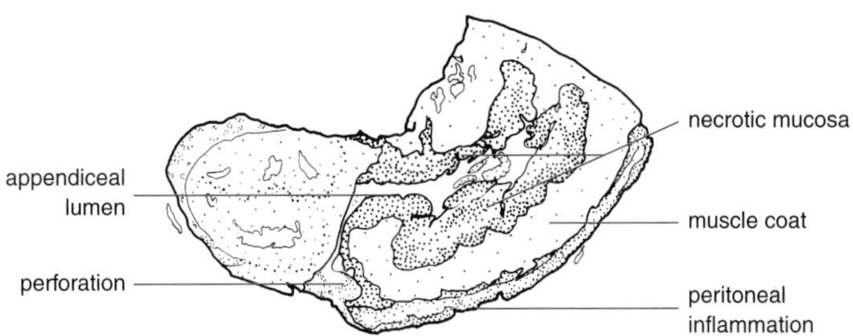

■ **Fig. 7.134** Histological appearance in acute appendicitis showing a perforation close to the tip. The mucosa is ulcerated and a florid inflammatory infiltrate is present throughout the wall and on the peritoneal surface. H&E stain (x 12).

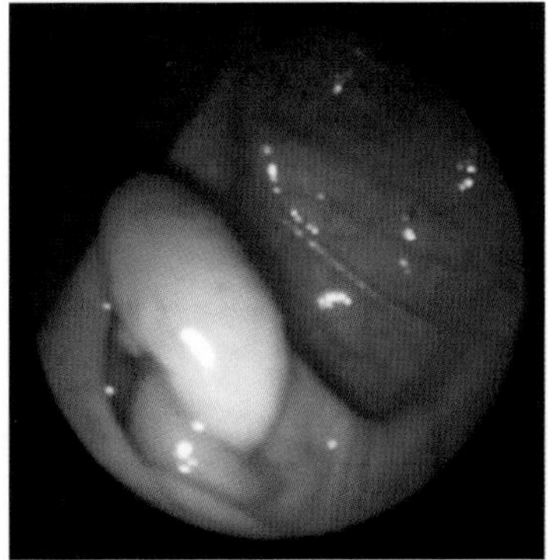

■ **Fig. 7.135** Colonoscopic appearance of a healthy invaginated appendix stump following appendectomy.

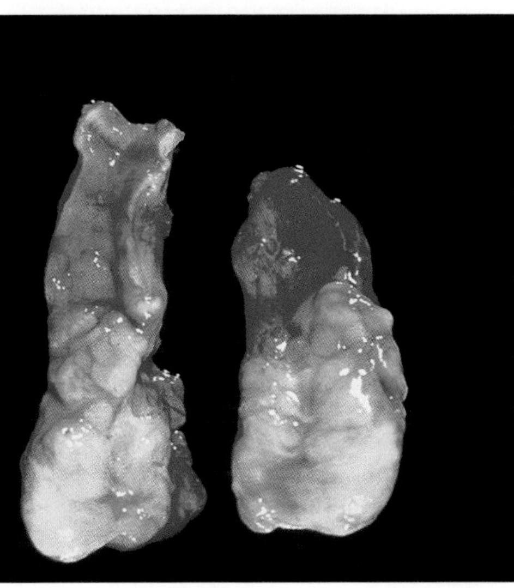

■ **Fig. 7.136** Macroscopic view of a carcinoid tumor in the tip of the appendix showing the typical pale yellow-tan, lobular cut surface and well-defined but slightly irregular borders.

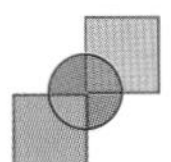

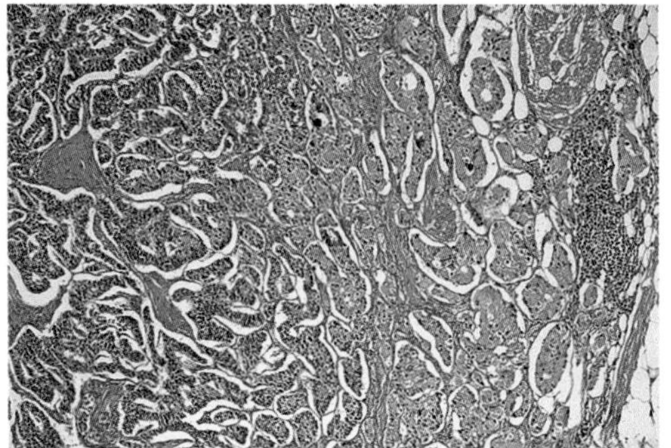

■ **Fig. 7.137** Microscopic view of an appendiceal carcinoid tumor showing insular and acinar growth patterns.

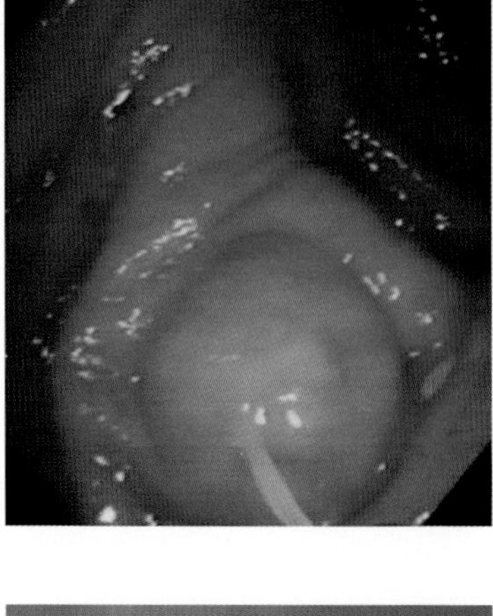

■ **Fig. 7.139** Endoscopic appearance of mucocele of the appendix.

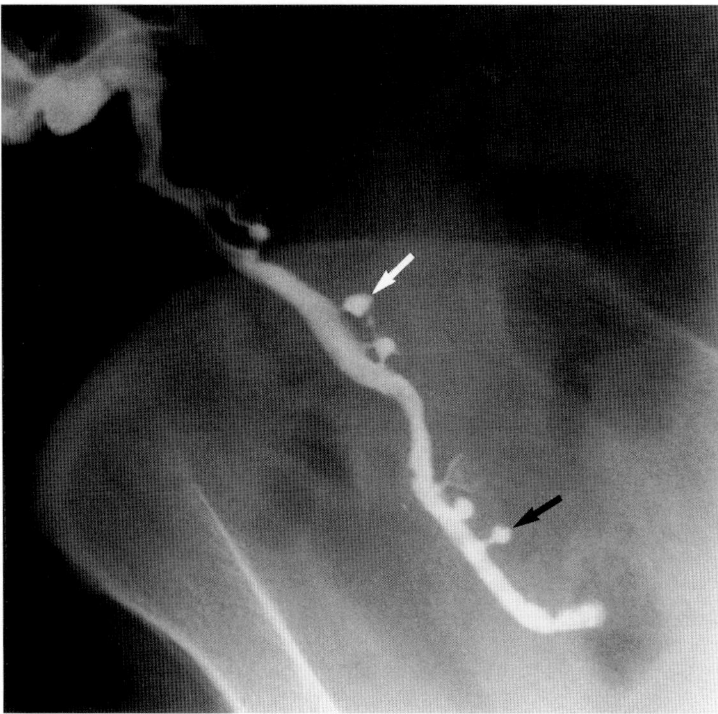

■ **Fig. 7.138** Double-contrast barium enema demonstrating diverticulosis of the appendix. Multiple barium-filled sacs (arrows) protrude from the lumen of the appendix. (Reproduced with permission from reference 6, Fig. 14.4.)

■ **Fig. 7.140** Resected mucocele of the appendix.

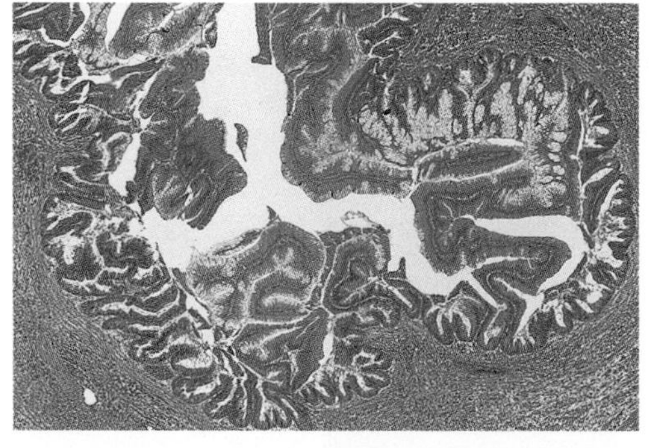

■ **Fig. 7.141** Microscopic view of a circumferential mucin-producing appendiceal adenoma giving rise to a mucocele.

■ **Fig. 7.142** Pseudomyxoma peritoneii associated with mucinous carcinoma of the appendix. Macroscopic appearance of the peritoneum showing confluent involvement by nodular, glistening mucinous deposits.

PSEUDOMYXOMA PERITONEI

This is an uncommon and probably malignant disorder in which the peritoneal cavity becomes filled with mucinous material. This may be in the form of numerous cystic masses or as free-lying mucus. It may follow the rupture of a more-or-less benign lesion such as a mucocele of the appendix (Figs 7.139, 7.140), which may itself be the result of an appendiceal adenoma (Fig. 7.141) or an ovarian cystadenoma, but it may be a feature of a mucus-producing adenocarcinoma of the ovary. Origins alongside primary carcinomas in bowel, urachal cyst, and bile duct have also been described. On histological grounds, it is difficult to determine whether the mucinous material is of benign or malignant origin unless (rarely) frank malignant cells are included (Figs 7.142, 7.143). Since recurrence and invasion frequently occurs whatever the initial histology, it is argued that the disorder almost always indicates spread from a carcinoma even if the primary is never demonstrated.

MELANOSIS COLI

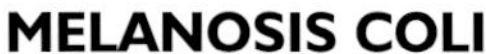

Melanosis coli is a benign condition found in those who habitually use anthracene-containing laxatives. It is characterized by pigmentation of the colonic mucosa, owing to the accumulation of pigment-containing macrophages (Figs 7.144–7.146). These are easily seen histologically (Fig. 7.147). The pigment is not true melanin but more similar to the group of pigments known as lipofuscins. The colon is usually most affected in the proximal parts but the characteristic changes may be recognized sigmoidoscopically in more

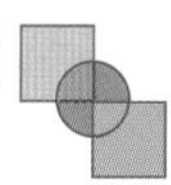

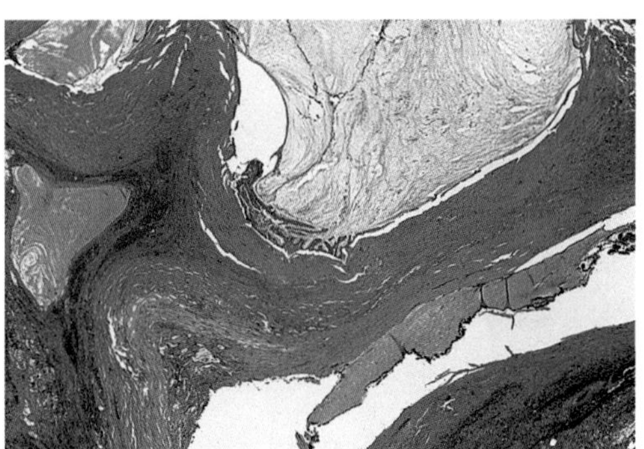

Fig. 7.143 Macroscopic appearance of mucinous carcinoma of the appendix producing pseudomyxoma peritoneii showing strips of malignant epithelium at the edges of massive extra-cellular mucin pools.

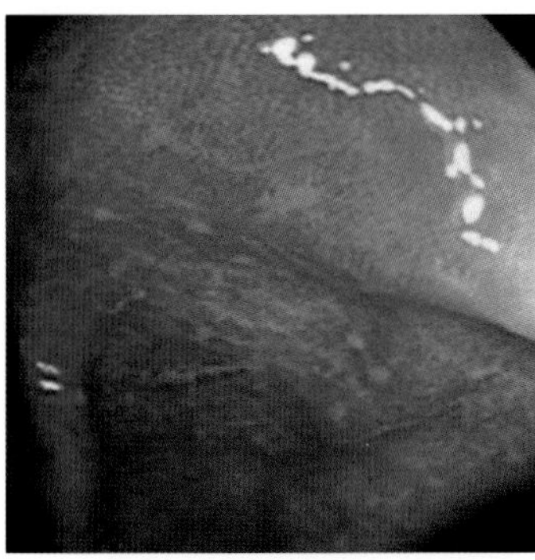

Fig. 7.144 Endoscopic appearance of the brownish discoloration seen in marked melanosis coli.

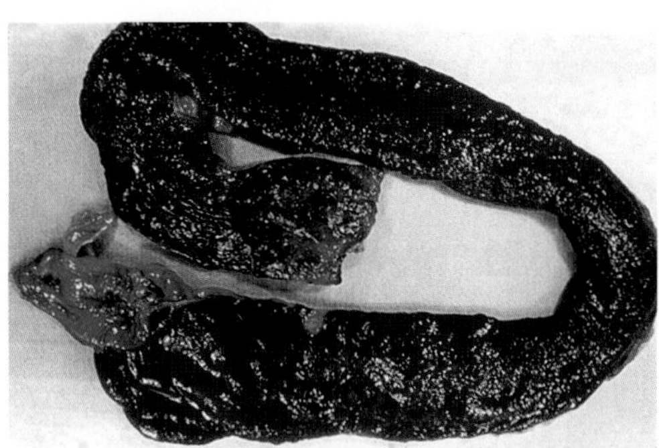

Fig. 7.145 Melanosis coli. Macroscopic appearance of the deeply pigmented mucosal surface in severe melanosis coli.

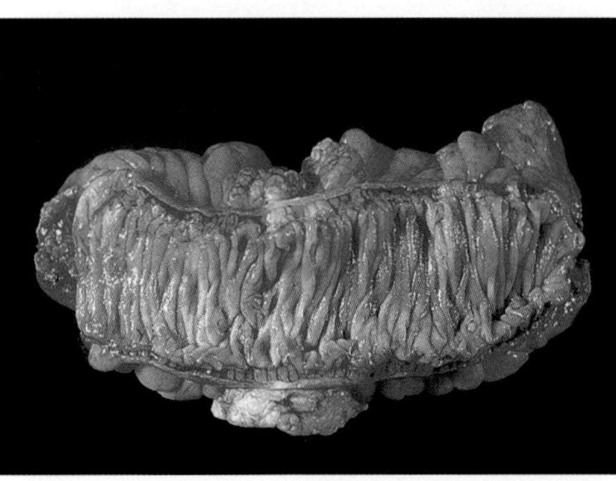

Fig. 7.146 Normal colon. Macroscopic appearance of the normal colonic mucosa for comparison showing the pale pink-tan color.

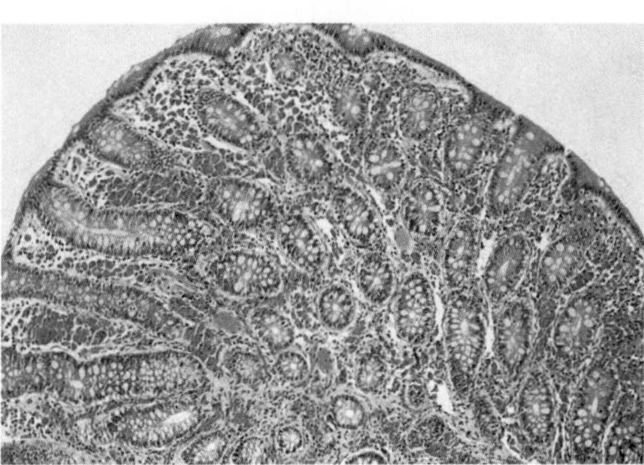

Fig. 7.147 Microscopic view of the mucosa in melanosis coli showing the diagnostic collections of pigmented macrophages in the lamina propria.

advanced cases (Fig. 7.144). The pigmentation does not appear to have any harmful effects and slowly reverses after discontinuing the laxatives. A curious appearance comes from its sparing of co-existent nodules and polyps (Fig. 7.148).

PNEUMATOSIS CYSTOIDES INTESTINALES

In this uncommon disorder, numerous gas-filled cysts are formed within the submucosa and subserosa of the intestine. The cause is unknown but there is a strong association with pyloric obstruction, with chronic obstructive airways disease, and with preceding thoracic surgery. The composition of the gas within the cysts approximates to that of atmospheric air. It has been suggested that gas may track down from the subpleural spaces retroperitoneally along the mesenteric vascular tree to the bowel wall. Pneumatosis has also been described following contrast radiology of the colon and after colonoscopy, and then localized perforation is hypothesized.

Pneumatosis may be an incidental finding on a plain abdominal radiograph (Fig. 7.149), but may be symptomatic, causing cramping lower abdominal discomfort, diarrhea, and, less commonly, tenesmus, rectal bleeding, and mucoid discharge. Cysts can be seen at sigmoidoscopy (Fig. 7.150), and biopsy may result in a loud noise (Fig. 7.151). The diagnosis may also be obvious from barium enema or CT scan (Fig. 7.152). Chilaiditi's sign, in which colonic gas lies between the liver and the diaphragm, may be associated with pneumatosis (Fig. 7.153).

Macroscopically, the bowel has a spongy texture, and the cysts may still be visible in the resected specimen (Fig. 7.154), and microscopy shows giant cells, inflammatory cells, and occasional flat endothelial cells (Figs 7.155, 7.156).

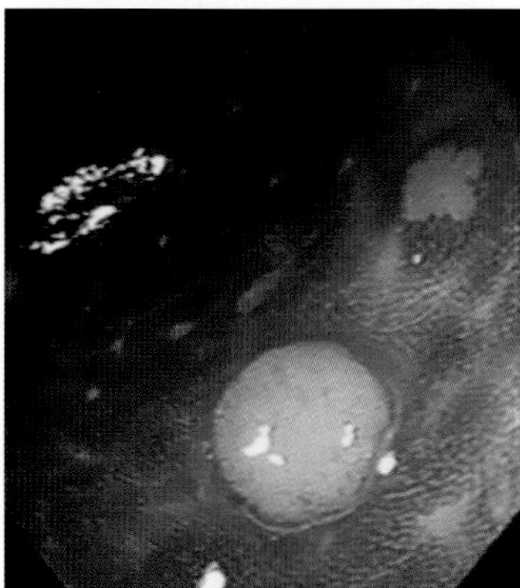

Fig. 7.148 The curious sparing from melanotic changes seen in a patient with a concurrent small adenoma.

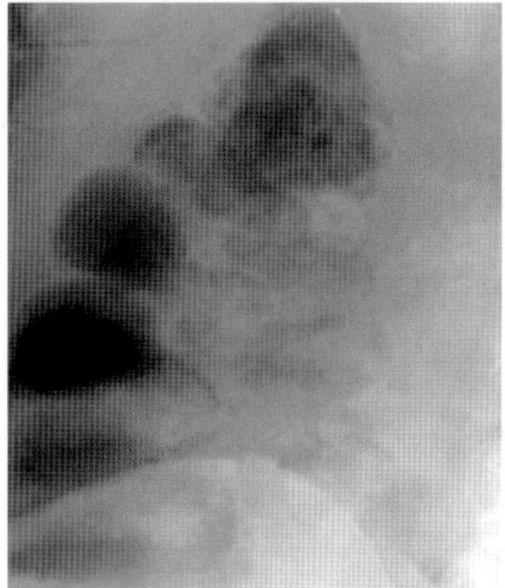

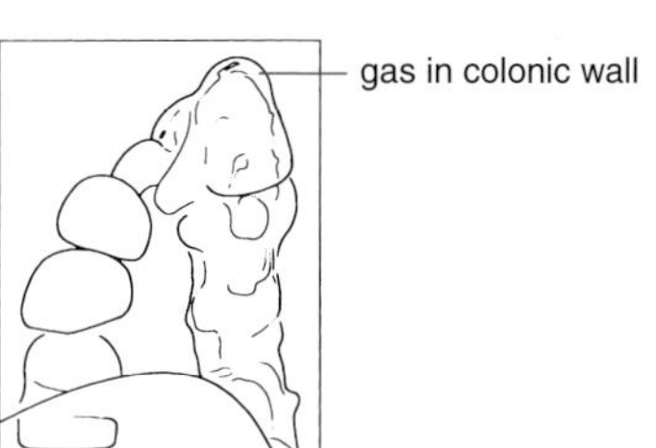

Fig. 7.149 Plain abdominal radiograph showing the appearances of pneumatosis coli. Gas is clearly seen within the colonic wall as well as in the lumen.

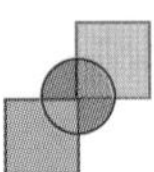

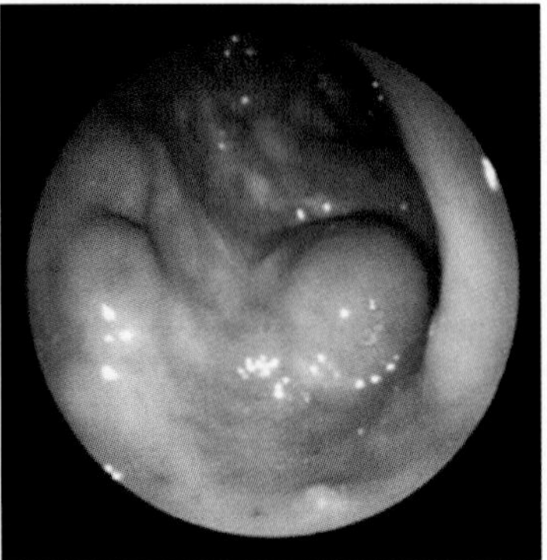

■ **Fig. 7.150** Endoscopic appearance of pneumatosis coli. Gentle probing helps in the distinction from lipomas and other solid lesions.

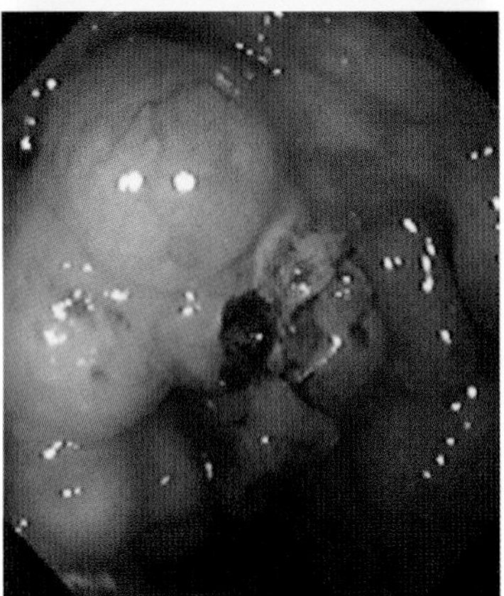

■ **Fig. 7.151** After a generous biopsy sample has been taken (a modest explosion resulting), the inside of the pneumatotic cyst can be clearly seen.

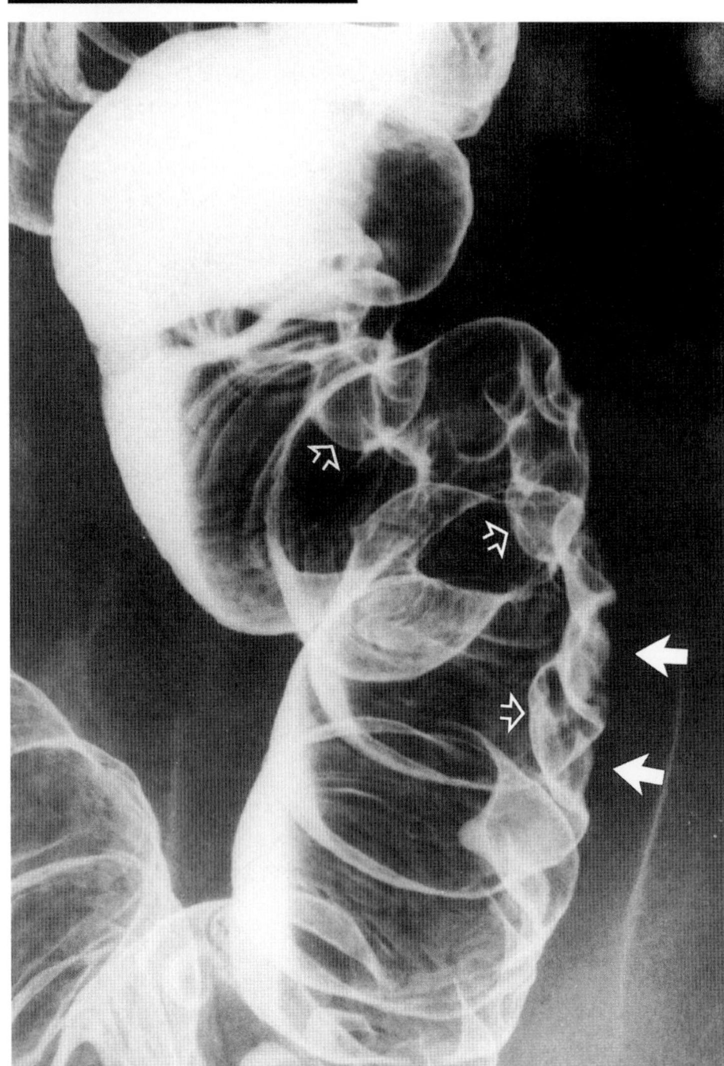

■ **Fig. 7.152** Double-contrast barium enema depicting benign pneumatosis coli. Smooth-surfaced hemispheric elevations of the mucosa (open arrows) are seen in the descending colon. Subtle air-filled spaces are seen in profile (arrows) outside of the luminal contour.

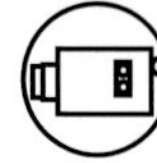

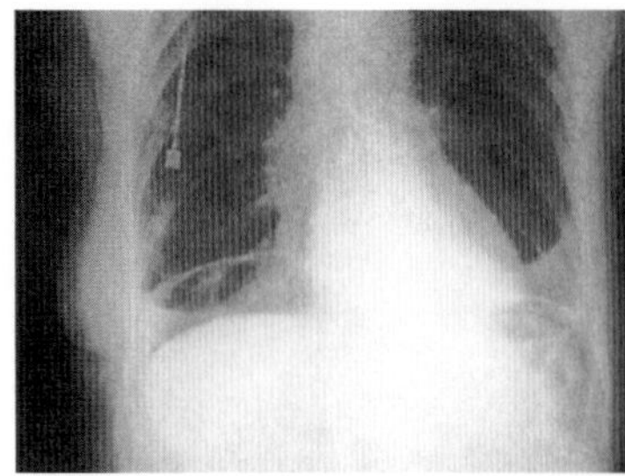

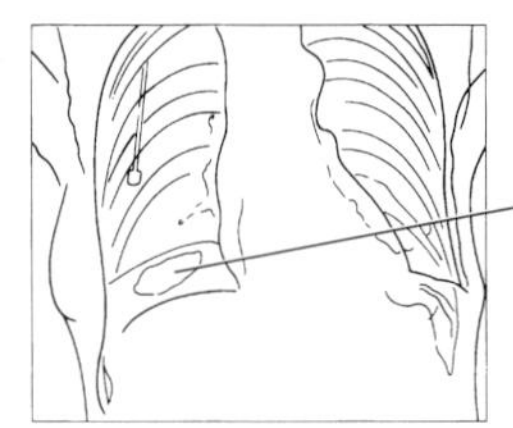

■ **Fig. 7.153** Chest X-ray in Chilaiditi's sign in which pneumatosis coli is suggested by otherwise unexplained colonic gas between the liver and the right hemidiaphragm. (A subclavian venous catheter is also in place.)

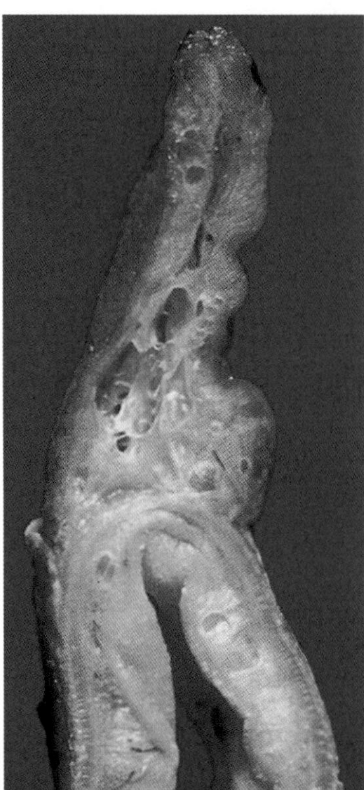

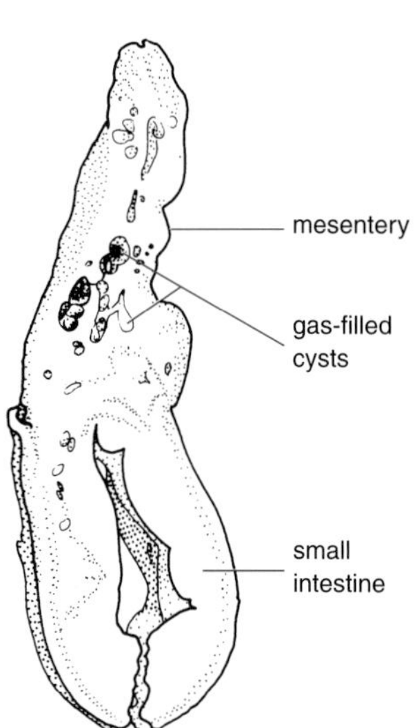

■ **Fig. 7.154** Macroscopic appearance of the cysts in pneumatosis intestinalis.

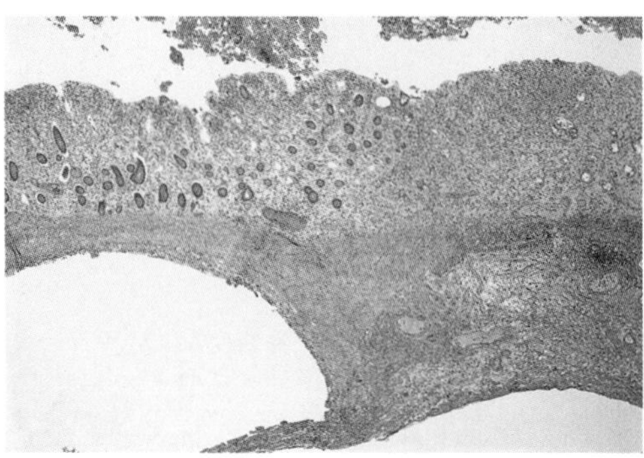

■ **Fig. 7.155** Pneumatosis intestinalis. Microscopic appearance showing large gas-filled cystic spaces in the submucosa.

ENDOMETRIOSIS

The presence of ectopic or extra-uterine endometrial tissue in the bowel may be responsible for cyclical pain and rectal bleeding in women of child-bearing age. The gastrointestinal lesions are generally small, often multiple (Figs 7.157–7.159), but may be invisible at mid cycle. Careful timing of colonoscopy is wise. Very occasionally

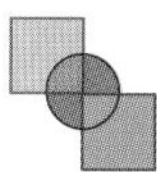

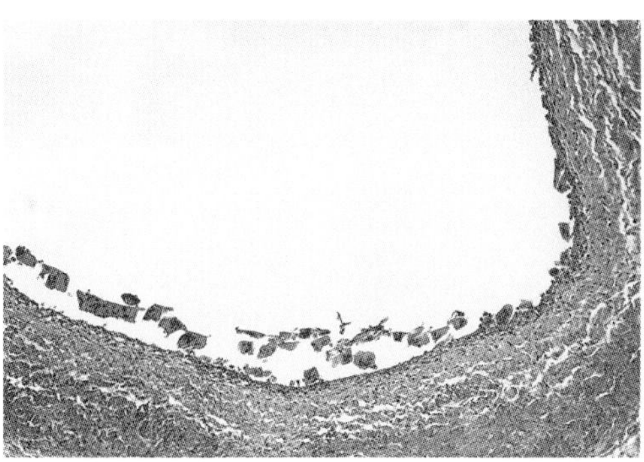

■ **Fig. 7.156** High-magnification view of the edge of a pneumatic submucosal cyst showing a rim of macrophages and foreign body giant cells at the interface between the gas bubble and the stroma.

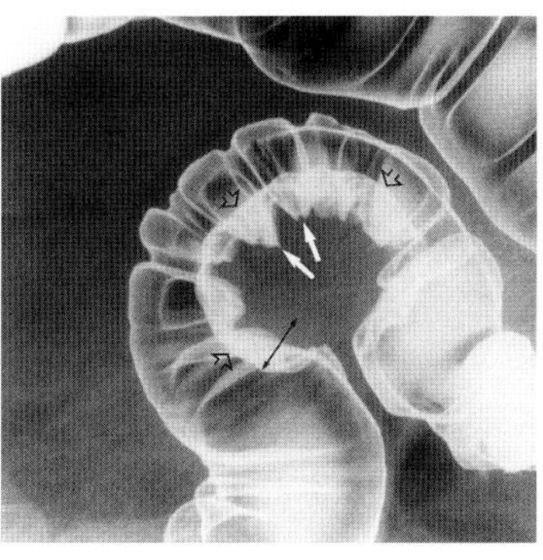

■ **Fig. 7.157** Double-contrast barium enema in a patient with endometrioma. A smooth-surfaced indentation (open arrows) of the inferior border of the sigmoid colon is present. Spiculation of the contour (white arrows) is the result of serosal fibrosis. Muscular hypertrophy causes thickening of the colonic wall (double arrow). (Reproduced with permission from reference 1, Fig. 12.93.)

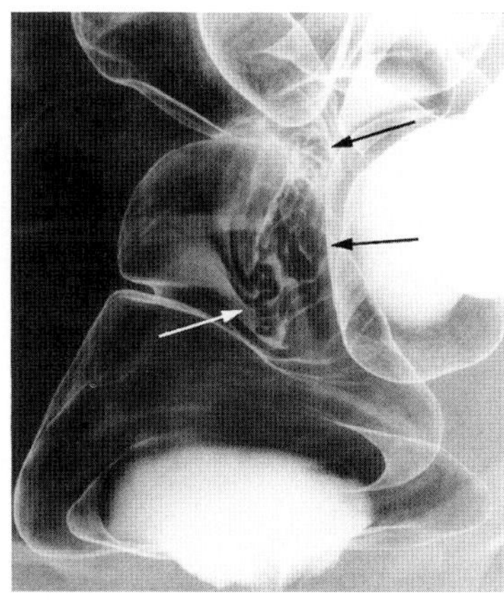

■ **Fig. 7.158** Double-contrast barium enema demonstrating 'pleating' of the mucosa due to endometriosis. The mucosa of the rectosigmoid junction is thrown into smooth, sinuous folds (arrows). (Reproduced with permission from reference 2, Fig. 5.38.)

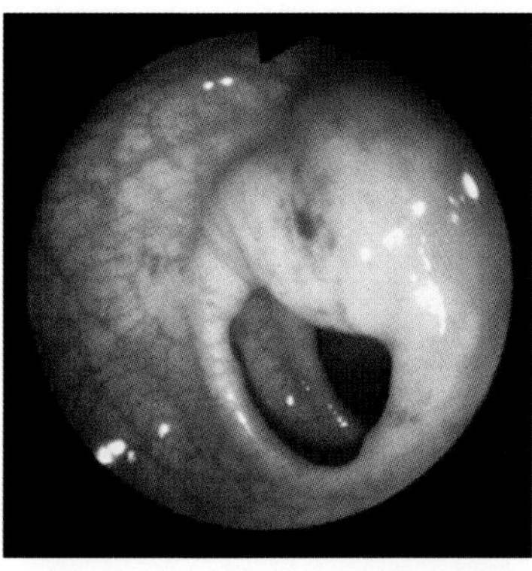

■ **Fig. 7.159** Colonoscopic appearance of one of several endometriosis lesions responsible for cyclical hemorrhage.

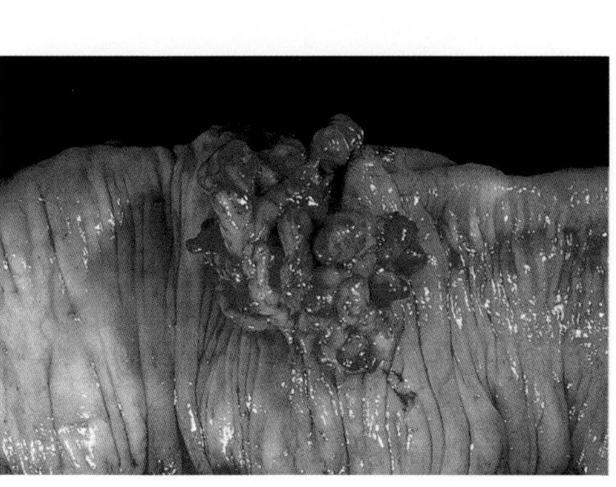

■ **Fig. 7.160** Colonic endometriosis. Segmental resection of colon showing a polypoid endometrioma projecting from the luminal surface.

they grow to sufficient size to cause luminal obstruction. Lesions are usually on the anterior surface of the rectosigmoid (Fig. 7.160), and histological examination is diagnostic (Fig. 7.161).

VASCULAR MALFORMATIONS

The commonest vascular malformation of the colon is angiodysplasia. This is a well-defined clinical and pathological entity, characteristically involving the cecum and/or the ascending colon, and it usually affects patients in the seventh and eighth decades of life. It is occasionally associated with aortic valve disease or chronic obstructive airways disease and may then occur at a younger age. The lesions, which are often multiple, are usually small and flat, and do not generally appear on double-contrast barium enema. The wider availability of colonoscopy confirms, however, that they are not rare, but constitute an important and frequent cause of lower gastrointestinal bleeding (Fig. 7.162). Bleeding may be episodic and dramatic, or low grade and responsible for iron-deficiency anemia. Colonoscopic attempts at therapeutic obliteration by thermal techniques may be followed by early recurrence, probably reflecting the fact that the lesion seen is often only the visible tip of a much broader vascular abnormality deep to the mucosa.

In the acutely bleeding patient, colonoscopy may be difficult; selective angiography will sometimes then show areas of ectatic vasculature, and permit therapeutic embolization. A useful radiological clue comes from the rapid and early filling of the draining vein (Fig. 7.163), as a result of arteriovenous connections present in the lesions. Lesions of less than 3–5 mm in diameter are unlikely to show, however, and resection of presumptively involved bowel is still necessary at times, but even when colonoscopy and angiography have failed to identify a definite causative lesion, they will often guide the surgeon to a less extensive resection. Multiple small lesions are often then identified macroscopically (Fig. 7.164). Histologically, the spectrum ranges from a small number of dilated submucosal veins with only a few thin-walled capillaries in the mucosa, to an obvious cluster of vessels communicating with ectatic capil-

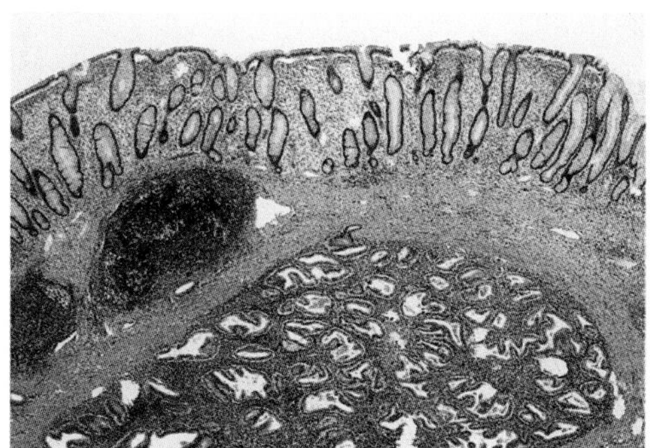

■ **Fig. 7.161** Microscopic view of endometriosis of the colon showing endometrial tissue recognized by the typical dense stroma and serpiginous glands (bottom) extending into the submucosa.

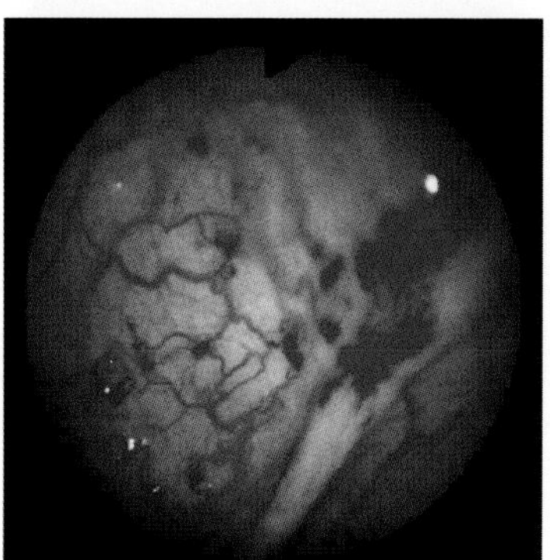

■ **Fig. 7.162** Colonoscopic appearance of angiodysplasia affecting the right colon.

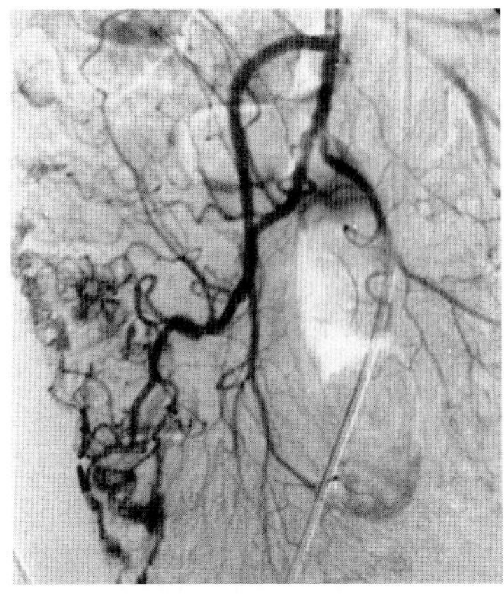

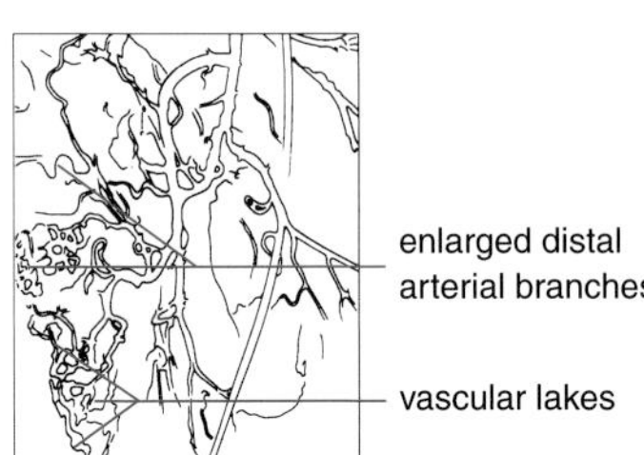

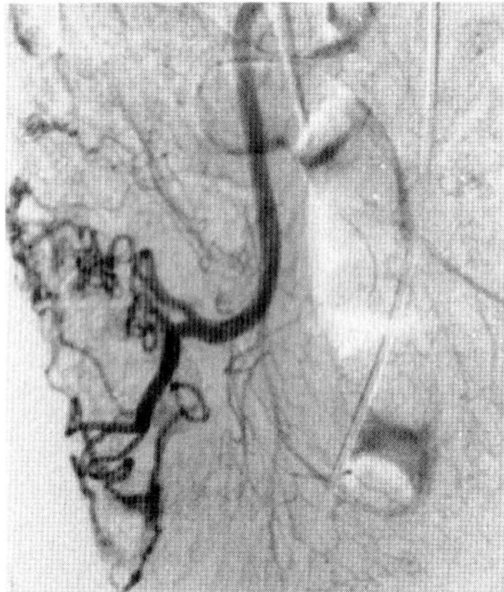

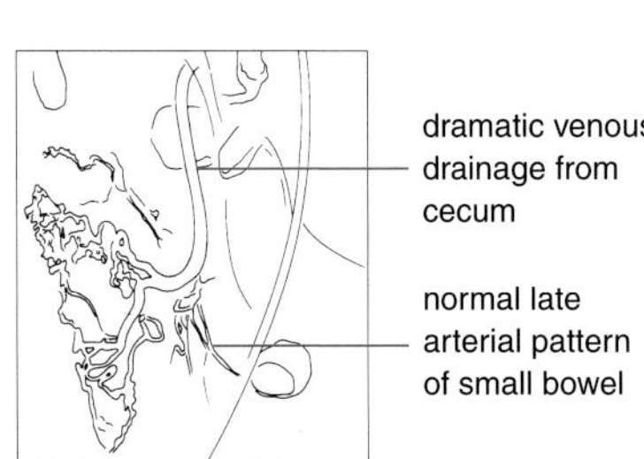

Fig. 7.163 Angiography in angiodysplasia. The early arterial image (a) shows enlargement of the ileocolic artery and of its distal branches supplying the cecum, with vascular lakes and early venous return; the early venous opacification can be seen just below the distal ileocolic artery. The later arterial phase image (b) shows very dramatic venous drainage from the cecum whilst there is still arterial opacification to the small bowel. Courtesy of Dr J.E. Jackson.

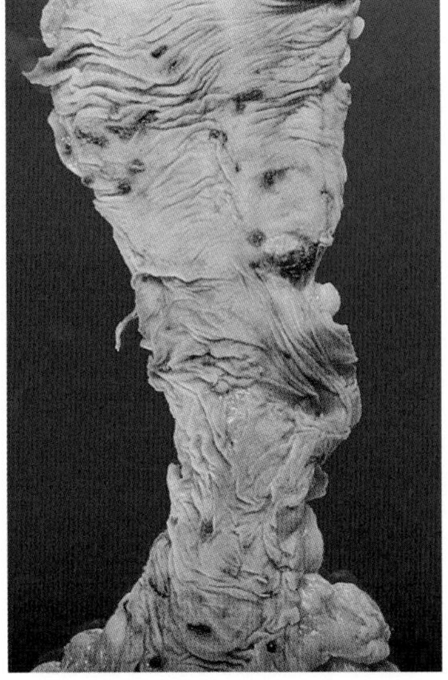

Fig. 7.164 A length of ascending colon in a right hemicolectomy specimen showing multiple angiodysplastic lesions in the mucosa.

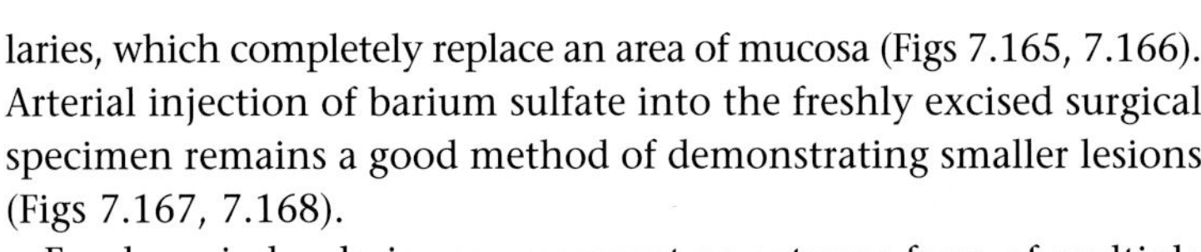

laries, which completely replace an area of mucosa (Figs 7.165, 7.166). Arterial injection of barium sulfate into the freshly excised surgical specimen remains a good method of demonstrating smaller lesions (Figs 7.167, 7.168).

Frank angiodysplasia may represent an extreme form of multiple telangiectasiae, but the genetic background may differ: colonic bleeding may certainly contribute to the clinical picture in Osler–Weber–Rendu syndrome (see Chapters 2, 3, and 4). Colonic

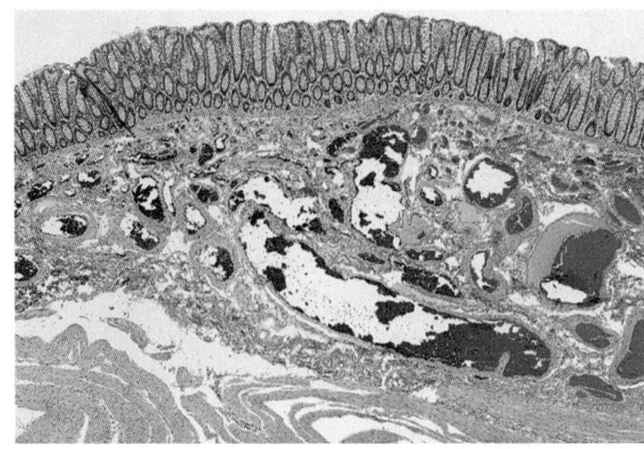

Fig. 7.165 Sporadic vascular ectasia (angiodysplasia) of the right colon. Microscopic view showing a proliferation of congested, ecstatic post-capillary venules and veins in the superficial submucosa.

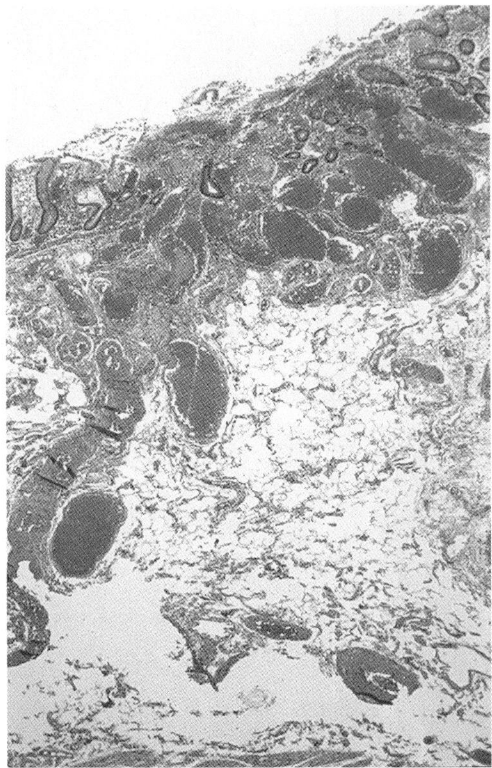

Fig. 7.166 Sporadic vascular ectasia (angiodysplasia) of the right colon. Microscopic view of a mucosal lesion showing extension of the abnormal ecstatic vessels into the lamina propria where they have produced both stromal hemorrhage and bleeding into the lumen.

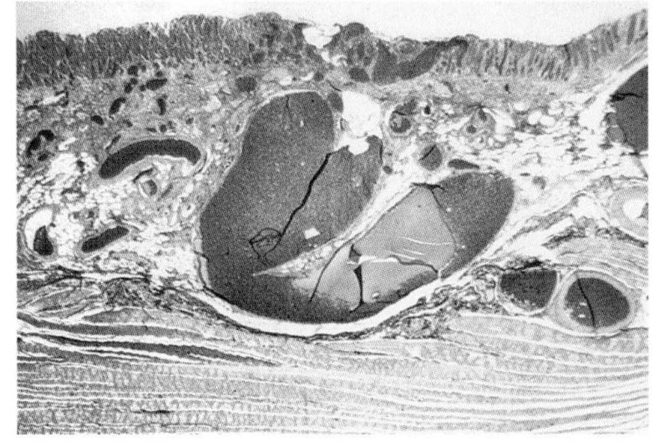

Fig. 7.167 Sporadic vascular ectasia (angiodysplasia) of the right colon. Microscopic view of a submucosal lesion revealed by vascular injection of barium-gelatin in a right colonic resection specimen.

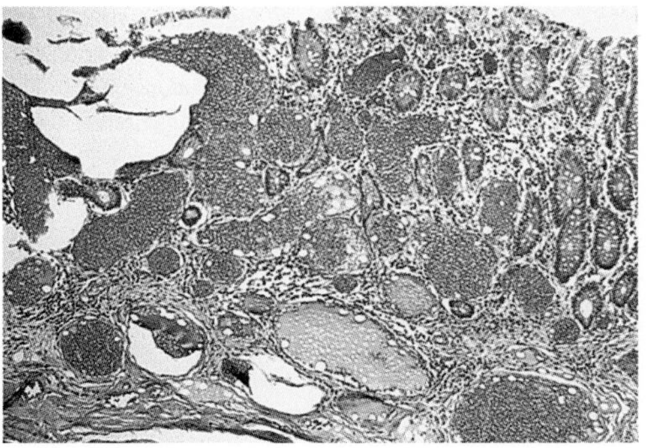

Fig. 7.168 Sporadic vascular ectasia (angiodysplasia) of the right colon. Higher-magnification view of barium-filled ectatic venules and capillaries in the mucosa highlighted by barium injection.

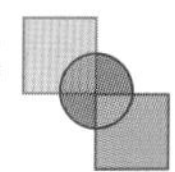

vascular malformations and hemangiomas may cause bleeding as in the Klippel–Trenaunay–Weber syndrome (Fig. 7.169), which also includes cutaneous hemangiomas (Fig. 7.170), varicose veins, and the hypertrophy of the bones and soft tissues of a single limb. Non-syndromic colonic hemangiomas also occur (Fig. 7.171), and colonic varices are often to be found if sought in patients with portal hypertension (Fig. 7.172; see also Chapter 12).

VOLVULUS

A volvulus occurs when a portion of the alimentary tract rotates or twists about itself, and in the colon this usually involves the cecum or the sigmoid. In cecal volvulus, rotation is usually between a particularly mobile cecum and the ascending colon (Figs 7.173, 7.174), which may in turn be associated with malrotation (see Chapter 4). Sigmoid volvulus is more likely when its mesentery is long with a narrow attachment, or when the sigmoid colon is itself abnormally long. Sigmoid volvulus is substantially commoner in populations with a high fiber intake, and tends to affect elderly people. Volvulus is substantially over-represented in patients with the chronic pseudo-obstruction syndromes (see below); while not entirely clear, it is probable that abnormal muscle function predisposes to both conditions. Volvulus of the large bowel presents with intestinal obstruction, which may be acute, recurrent, or chronic. The plain abdominal radiograph, if not diagnostic, is usually highly suggestive (Fig. 7.175). Sigmoid volvulus will sometimes be reduced by performing a contrast study (Fig. 7.176), and usually by the passing of a flatus tube or colonoscope, but the results of endoscopic intervention are less good with cecal volvulus. When conservative measures fail, and when the arterial supply to the gut has been compromised, open reduction with fixation or resection will be necessary (Fig. 7.177).

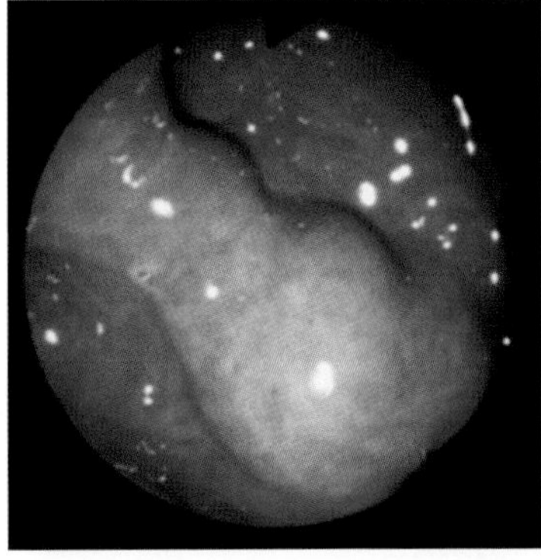

Fig. 7.169 Colonic vascular malformation in a patient with Klippel–Trenaunay–Weber syndrome.

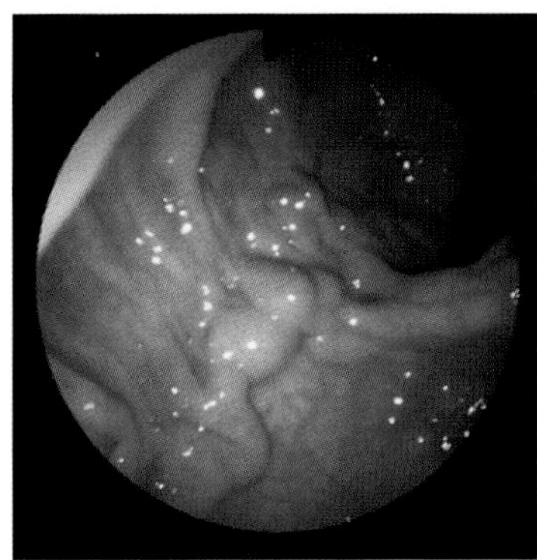

Fig. 7.172 Appearance of colonic varices in a patient with portal hypertension.

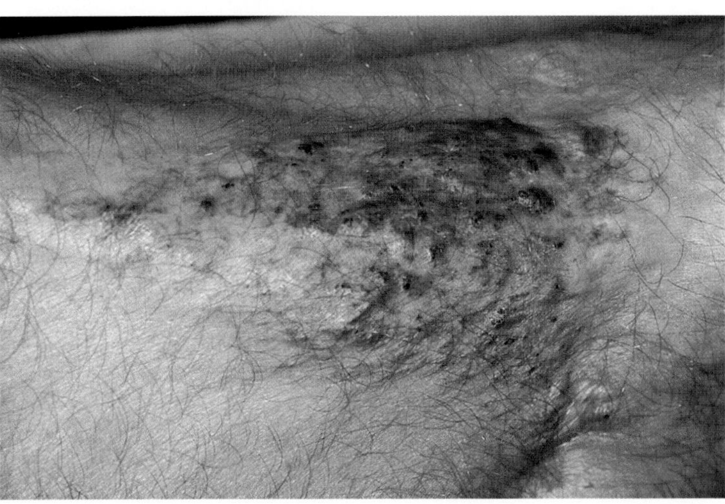

Fig. 7.170 Cutaneous hemangioma affecting the patient shown in Fig. 7.169.

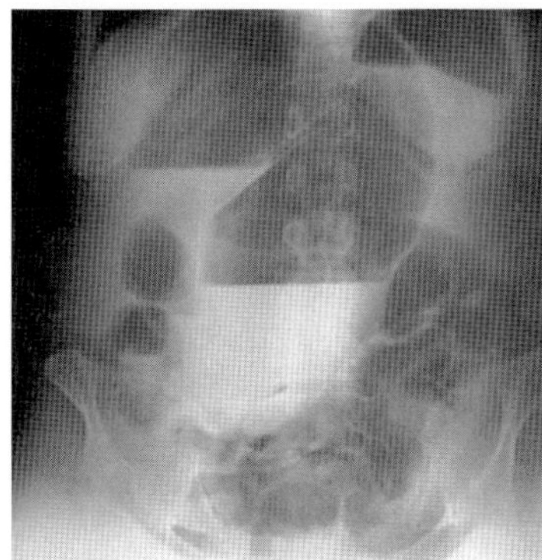

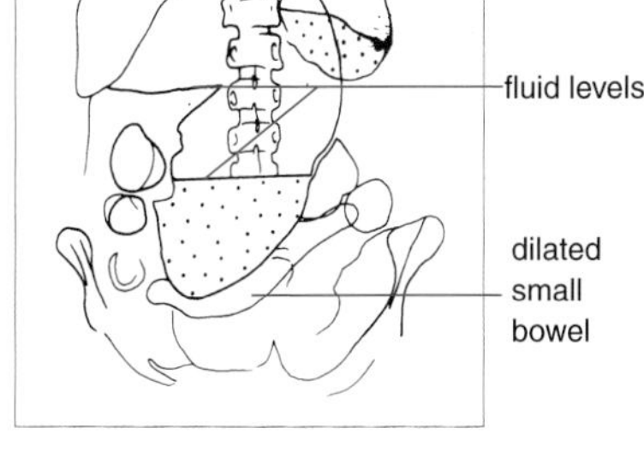

Fig. 7.173 Erect abdominal radiograph in cecal volvulus. There are two large fluid levels in a distended loop of bowel rendering it 'coffee bean' shaped with some gaseous distention in the small bowel. The hilum of the distended loop is formed by the twisted mesentery and points to the right iliac fossa.

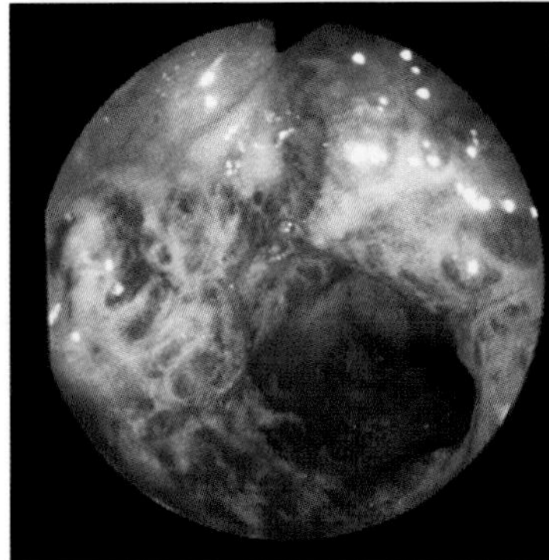

Fig. 7.171 Colonic hemangioma.

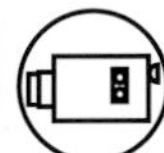

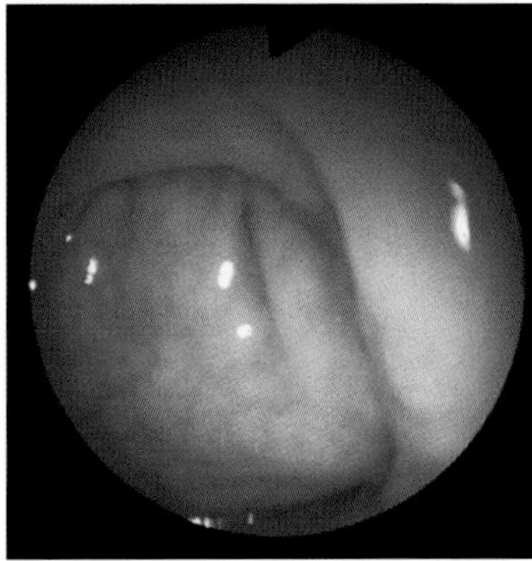

Fig. 7.174 Colonoscopic appearance of the twisted appearance of the bowel in colonic volvulus.

INTUSSUSCEPTION

Intussusception presents with the pain of acute obstruction of the small and large bowel. It is predominantly a disease of childhood and is thought to occur when submucosal aggregates of lymphoid tissue are sufficient to constitute a nidus for peristaltic action; this can then carry the involved section distally, invaginating it into the gut below and thereby causing obstruction. In adults, intussusception is usually provoked by 'peristalsis' of polypoid tumors. Rectal bleeding, which is classically associated with redcurrant stool, is often less typical and may be absent. Diagnosis is often possible from ultrasound scanning (Fig. 7.178), and the intussusception may be reduced by barium enema, which is thus both diagnostic and therapeutic (Fig. 7.179).

HIRSCHSPRUNG'S DISEASE

Hirschsprung's disease results from an absence of the intramural autonomic ganglion cells of the submucosal and myenteric plexuses of the distal bowel, with variable proximal extension into the rectum and colon. In the majority, between 3–10 cm is involved, and only very rarely is the small intestine involved. A hypoganglionic segment is usually found in the transition area between aganglionic and normal bowel. Typically a disease of infants and young children (Fig. 7.180), presentation is also seen amongst older children and adults who will have had lifelong constipation (Fig. 7.181). There is a familial predisposition, and males are more commonly affected than females. Aganglionosis produces functional overactivity such

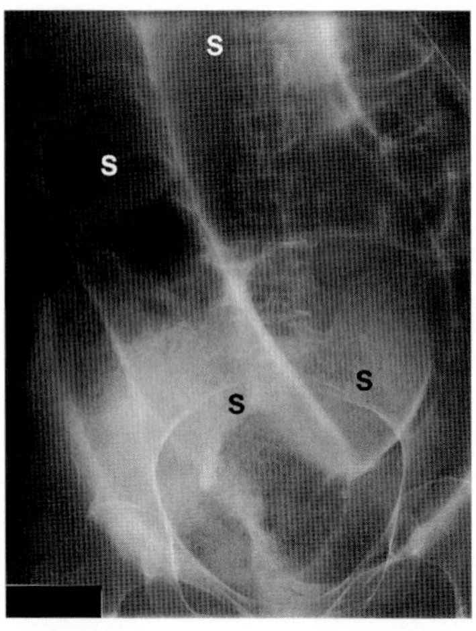

Fig. 7.175 Sigmoid volvulus. Plain radiograph of the abdomen shows two adjacent limbs (S) of a massively dilated sigmoid colon.

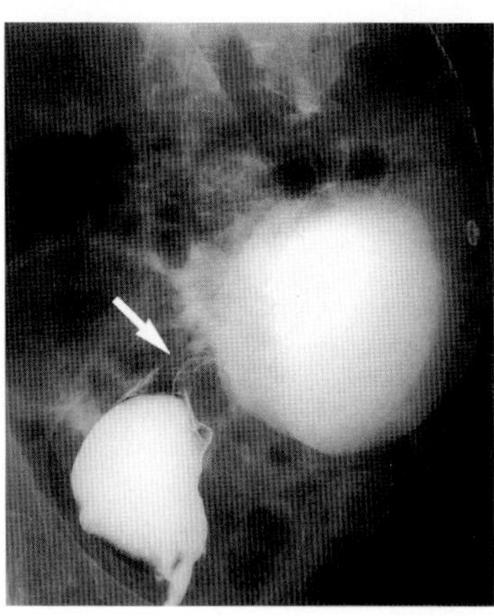

Fig. 7.176 Single-contrast barium enema demonstrates a smooth-surfaced narrowing (arrow). The sigmoid colon proximal to the narrowing is substantially dilated

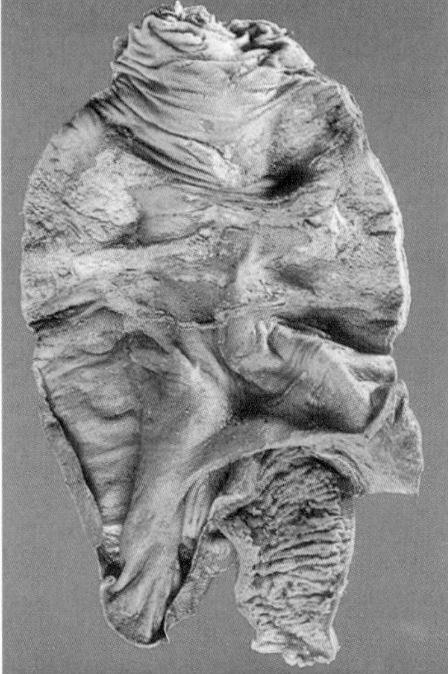

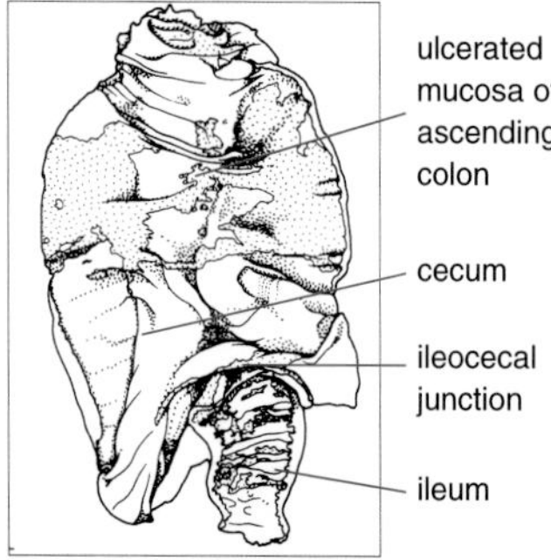

Fig. 7.177 An opened right hemicolectomy specimen following cecal volvulus.

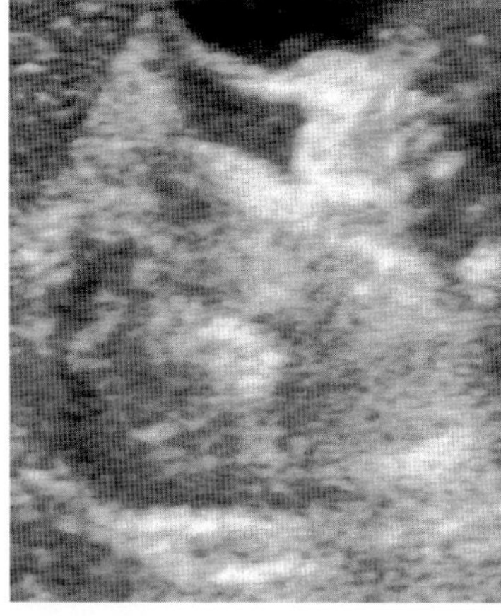

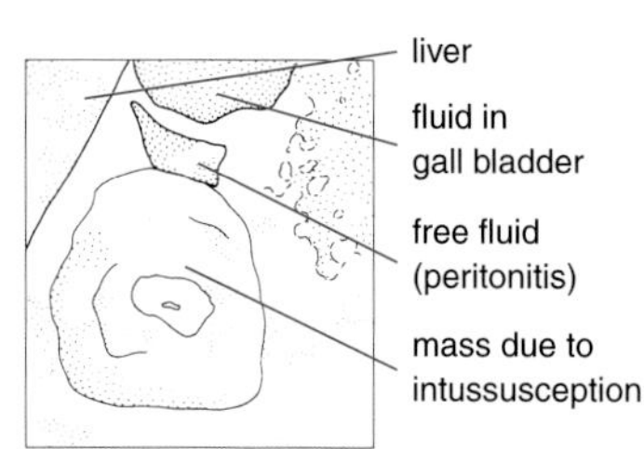

Fig. 7.178 Ultrasound scan in an infant showing a mass formed by the intussusception and a small quantity of free fluid below the gall bladder indicative of secondary peritonitis.

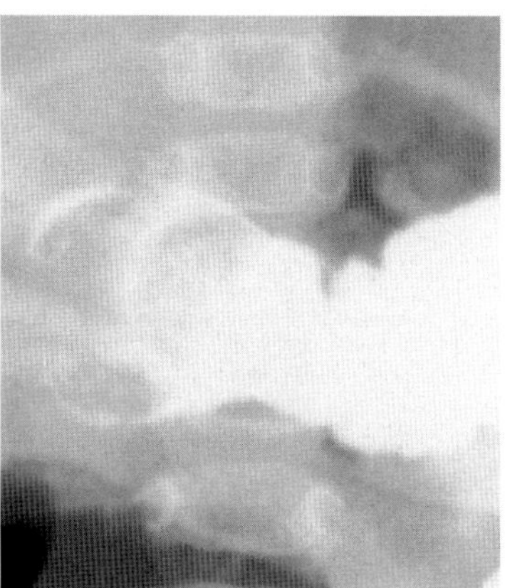

Fig. 7.179 Barium enema in an infant with a colonic intussusception. The examination was of therapeutic as well as diagnostic value.

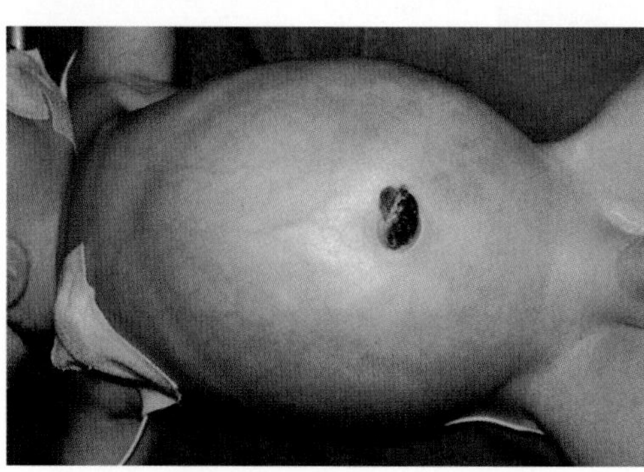

Fig. 7.180 A neonate with Hirschsprung's disease showing the enlarged abdomen. Courtesy of Mr H.H. Nixon.

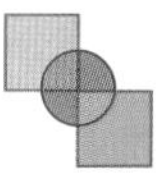

that the internal sphincter is in a state of constant contraction, and – to an extent dependent on the proximal extension – there will also be deficient propulsive motility. Most cases are seen within the first week of life: after a failure to pass meconium, bilious vomiting and abdominal distention engage medical attention (Fig. 7.180). In less dramatic cases, the significance of a mere delay in the passage of meconium followed by constipation and variable degrees of abdominal distention is understandably often missed at first. The stools (when present) are offensive and ribbon like; palpable fecal masses may be felt abdominally, and visible peristalsis may be seen, but soiling is most uncommon.

The diagnosis is often suggested by plain abdominal radiograph showing gaseous distention with no gas in the pelvis (Fig. 7.181). Contrast radiology (preferably with a water-soluble agent) will show a narrowed colorectal segment with proximal dilatation (megacolon) (Fig. 7.182). Manometric studies provide confirmation of the diagnosis by demonstrating the aganglionic segment (Figs 7.183, 7.184) and the failure of the internal sphincter to relax in response to balloon dilatation of the rectum. Delayed diagnosis may permit serious complications, which include intestinal perforation, chronic malnutrition, and failure to thrive. In the mildest cases, chronic constipation, perhaps with stercoral ulceration (Fig. 7.185), may be the only clue. Stercoral ulcer can of course occur in the absence of Hirschsprung's (Fig. 7.186).

Hirschsprung's disease involves both plexuses and, although a full-thickness biopsy is preferable, standard rectal biopsy including submucosa may be adequate for histological diagnosis. The histology confirms the absence of ganglion cells (Fig. 7.187). The presence of abnormal neurons on specific stains is helpful, and fresh tissue demonstrates an excess of acetylcholinesterase. An increase in size and number of positively staining fibers is seen in the mucosa and submucosa. The extent of surgical excision necessary to achieve resolution is determined from multiple biopsies taken from along the rectum and distal colon to define the length of the involved segment.

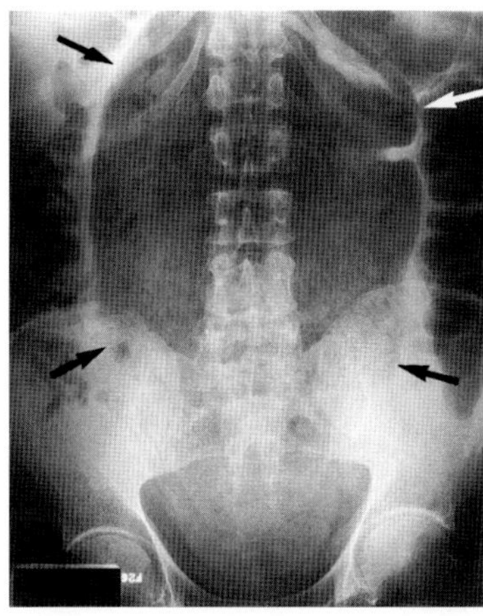

Fig. 7.181 Plain radiograph of the abdomen in adult with newly diagnosed Hirschsprung's disease. The rectum (arrows) is massively dilated.

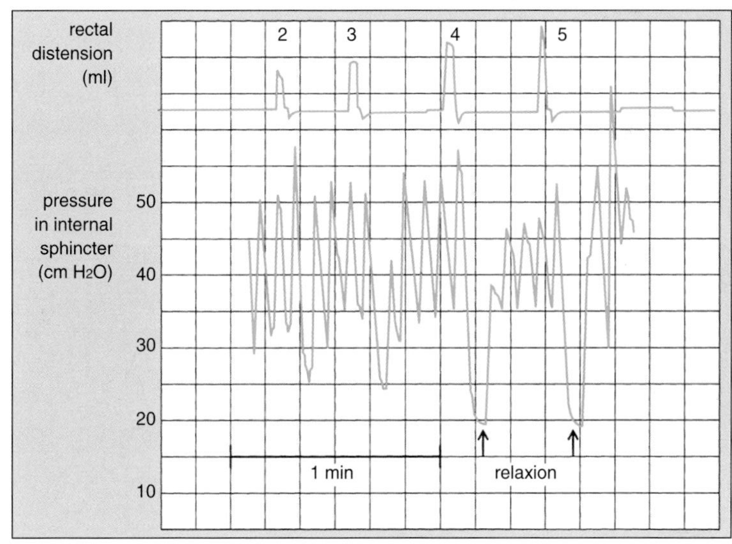

Fig. 7.183 Normal manometric pressure recording in response to rectal distention in an 8-day-old infant. Courtesy of Dr S. Tamate.

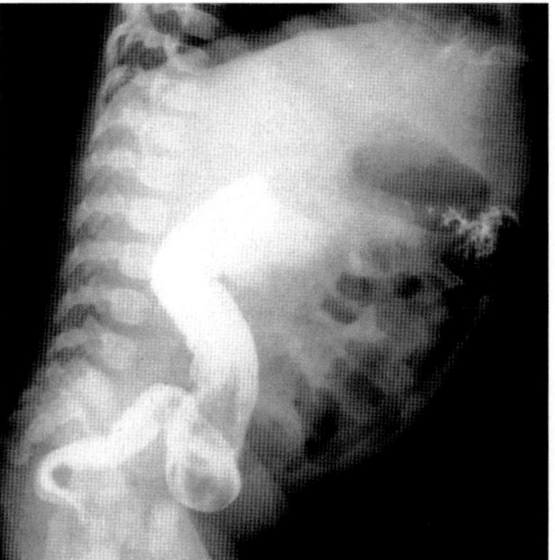

Fig. 7.182 Lateral contrast studies in Hirschsprung's disease. There is a zone of transition from dilated normal bowel to unexpanded aganglionic bowel. Courtesy of Mr H.H. Nixon.

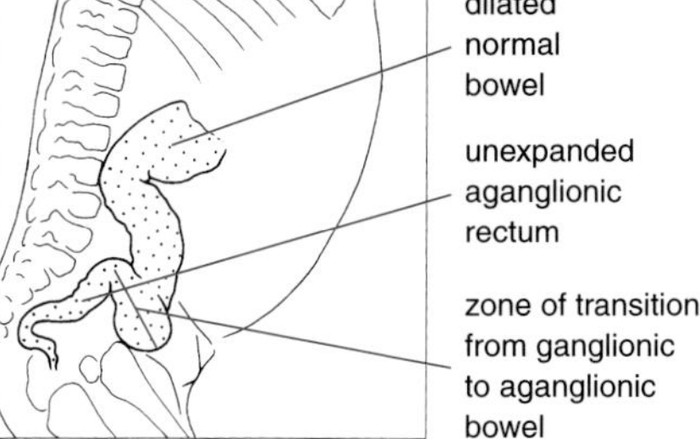

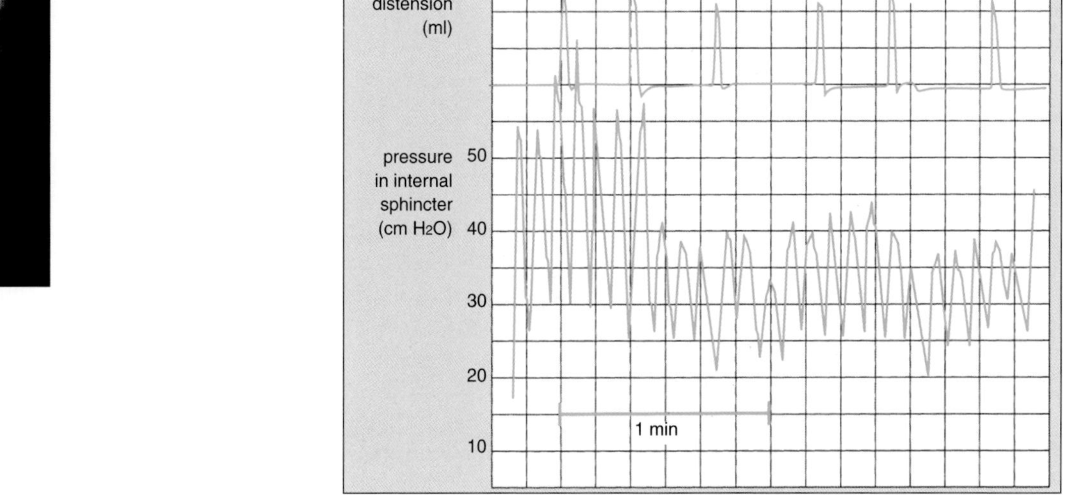

Fig. 7.184 Manometric pressure recordings in Hirschsprung's disease. The failure of internal sphincter relaxation during rectal distention is clearly demonstrated in this 14-day-old child. Courtesy of Dr S. Tamate.

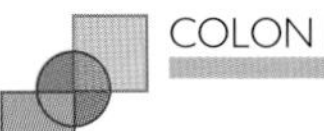

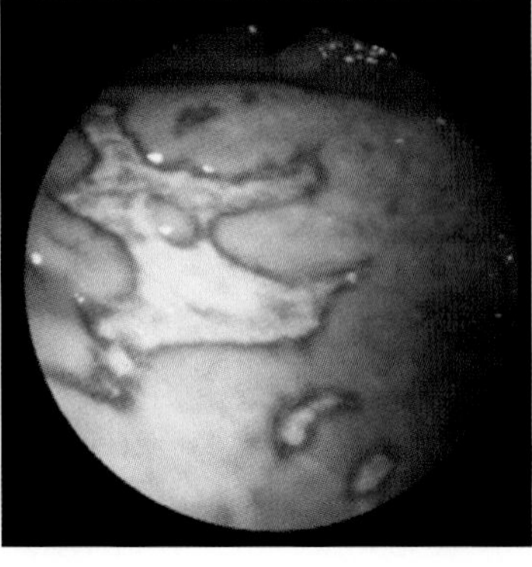

■ **Fig. 7.185** Sigmoidoscopic appearance of marked stercoral ulcers in a patient with Hirschsprung's disease.

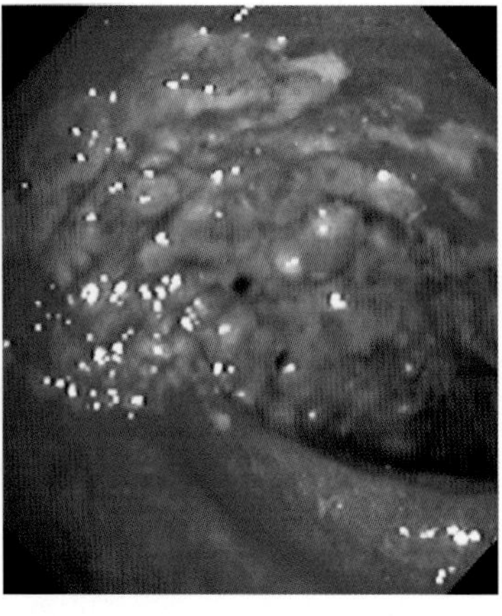

■ **Fig. 7.186** Stercoral ulcer in the lower bowel – in this case associated only with simple constipation.

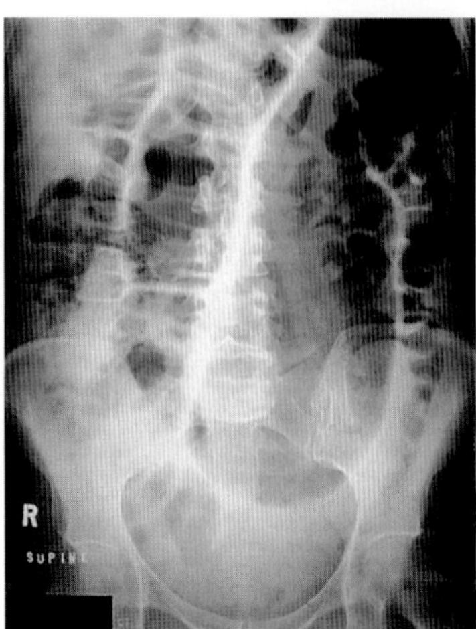

■ **Fig. 7.188** Gross dilatation of the small and large bowel in a patient with acquired megacolon who was found to have globally delayed intestinal transit.

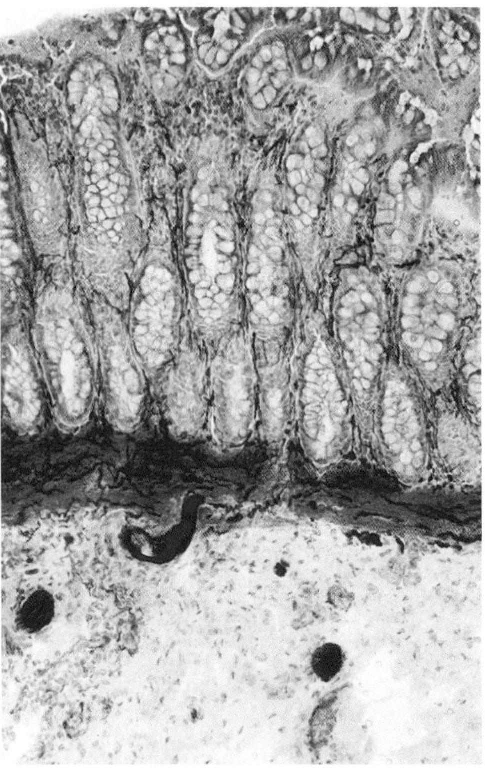

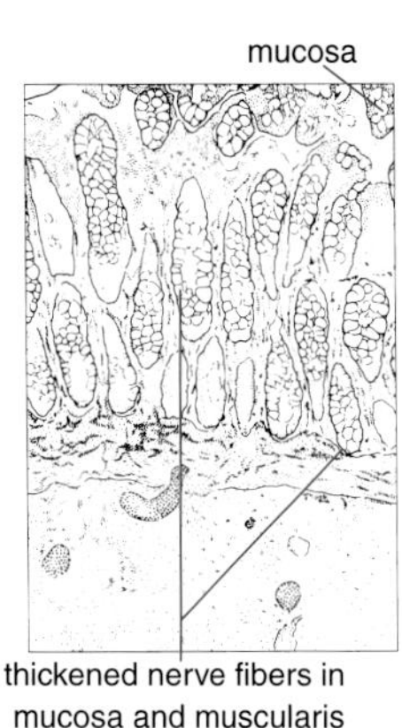

a

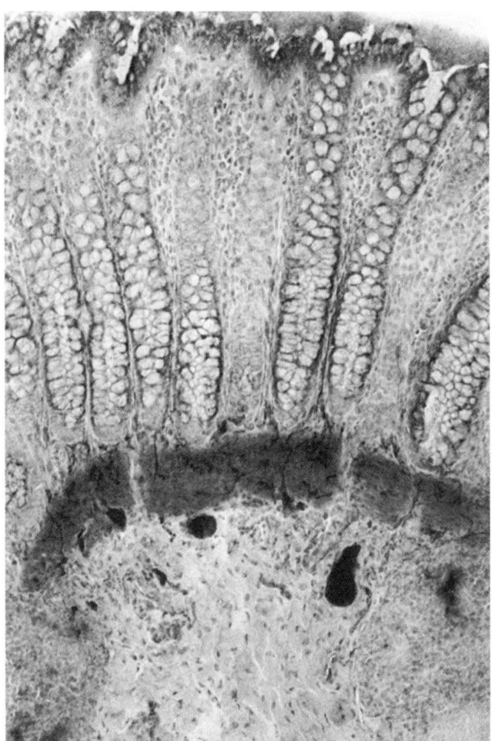

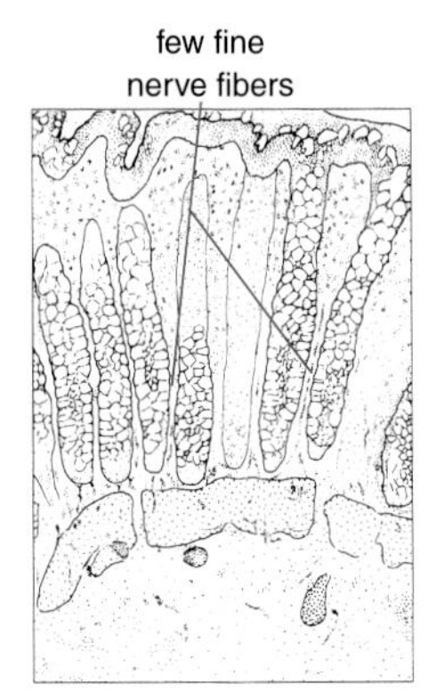

b

■ **Fig. 7.187** Rectal histology in Hirschsprung's disease. These cryostat sections are stained for acetylcholinesterase and contrast the abnormal thickened nerve fibers in the mucosa from a patient with Hirschsprung's (a) with the occasional fine nerve fibers in normal mucosa (b).

PSEUDO-OBSTRUCTION, CHRONIC CONSTIPATION, AND ACQUIRED MEGACOLON

Intestinal pseudo-obstruction is a functional abnormality affecting the entire gastrointestinal tract, but usually responsible mainly for intestinal obstruction in which no demonstrable organic lesion can be shown on plain abdominal radiography, barium studies, or CT scan (Fig. 7.188). There are a number of associated abnormalities, including jejunal diverticulosis and partial malrotation, and it is always wise to demonstrate whether or not there is duodenal dilatation (see Chapter 4). Visceral myopathy can be differentiated from collagenous, and sometimes vacuolated, myopathy of intestinal smooth muscle in a few patients in whom full-thickness biopsies are available (Figs 7.189–7.191); this may be familial.

A primary visceral neuropathy is also occasionally recognized and again may be familial. A variety of neuro-gastrointestinal abnormalities are potentially responsible, but in most patients the cause remains unknown. The association with jejunal diverticula suggests that bacterial overgrowth may be important in some patients and particularly so when diarrhea is a feature (see Chapter 4).

Patients with acquired megarectum and megacolon may have had colonic symptoms since childhood. It is thought that, in most cases, protracted simple constipation is responsible, particularly when in association with mental retardation or psychiatric disorders. Ogilvie's syndrome describes megacolon beginning after a 'crisis'; as obstetric procedures and other abdomino-pelvic trauma are frequently implicated, it is possible that a subtle underlying neuronal injury is to blame. Examination may show fecal soiling, although this is less common with adult-onset disease. The rectum tends to be full of stool: impaction is not unusual. The extent of large bowel dilatation is best confirmed radiologically using a

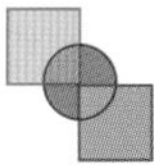

water-soluble contrast medium which does not solidify in the rectum (as may barium) (Fig. 7.192). The examination should be carried out on unprepared bowel, and will then provide an accurate guide to the proximal extent of colonic dilatation and to the rectal diameter. A diameter greater than 6.5 cm at the pelvic brim on a lateral view is considered pathological, as is cecal diameter in excess of 12 cm. Surgery is occasionally necessary (Fig. 7.193).

Intractable constipation is mainly found in young women. When examination is normal and investigations have excluded megacolon, metabolic causes such as hypothyroidism and hypercalcemia, and systemic disorders such as amyloidosis and systemic sclerosis, it is termed severe idiopathic constipation. The rectum is characteristically empty and the condition reflects an underlying motility disturbance. Barium enema is normal, but the slow transit can be documented by the so-called 'shapes' study, in which a single abdominal radiograph is taken 120 hours after ingestion of three sets of radiologically distinguishable markers (ingested at 0, 24, and 48 hours). Normally, at least 80% of markers will have been eliminated by 120 hours (Figs 7.194, 7.195). Some authors believe that the site within the colon at which delayed transit occurs is important in planning management; the results of the simple

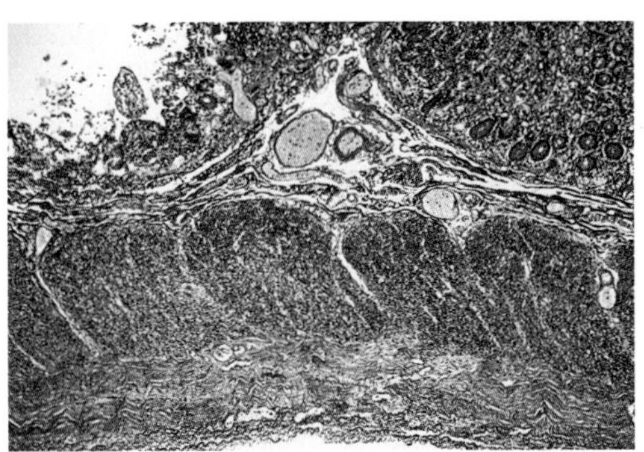

Fig. 7.189 Visceral myopathy. Trichrome-stained microscopic section of the intestinal wall showing the degeneration and fibrous replacement of the outer longitudinal layer of the muscularis propria and the relative sparing of the inner circular layer.

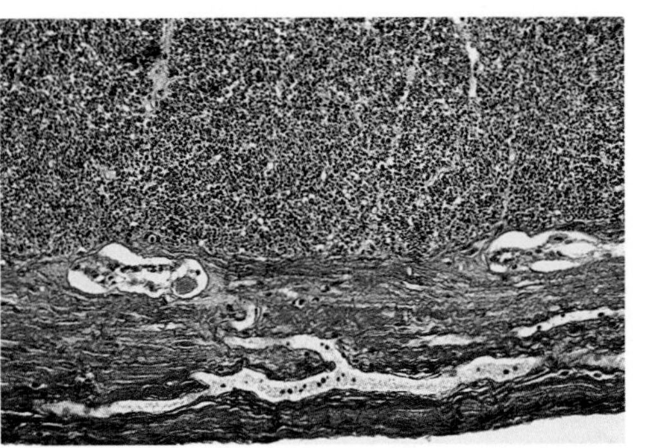

Fig. 7.190 Visceral myopathy. Higher-magnification view showing the characteristic degeneration with myocyte dropout and fibrosis of the outer layer of muscularis propria in the absence of inflammation, vascular disease, or neural abnormalities.

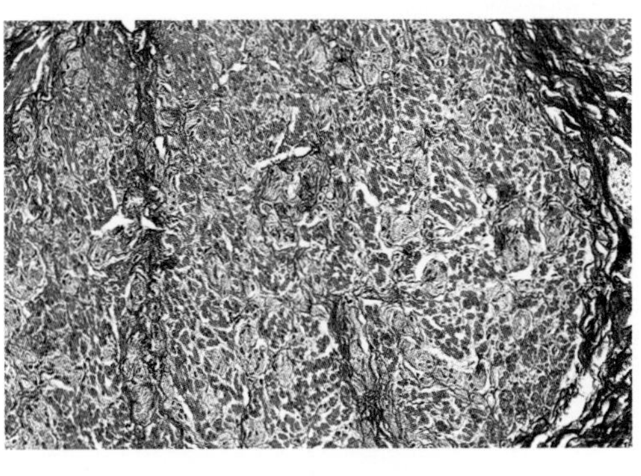

Fig. 7.191 Visceral myopathy. High-magnification view of the degenerating circular layer of the muscularis propria in a trichrome-stained section of the colon showing the characteristic myocyte vacuolization and pericellular fibrosis.

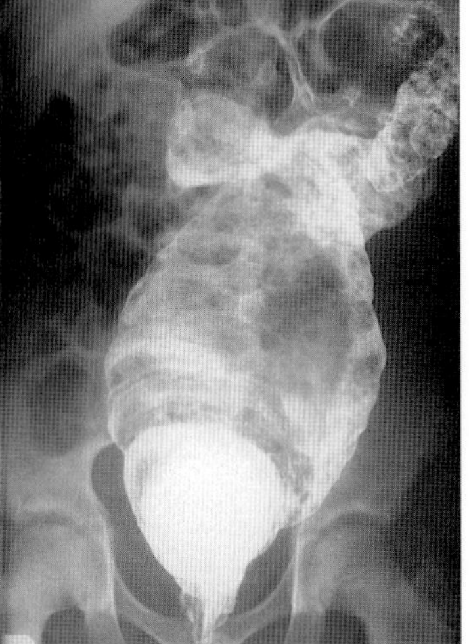

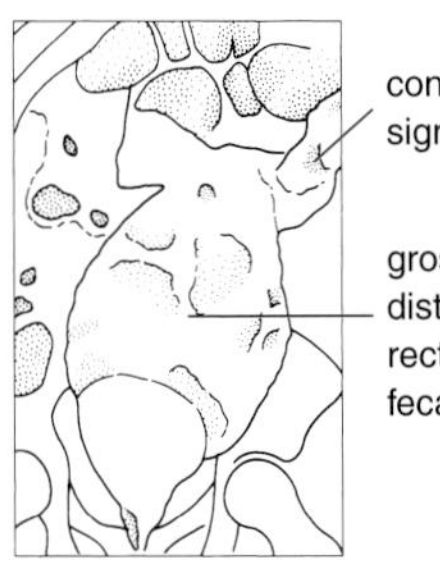

Fig. 7.192 Contrast examination in megarectum. The examination was performed on an unprepared bowel and shows gross distention of the rectum with fecal loading and contrast reaching the sigmoid.

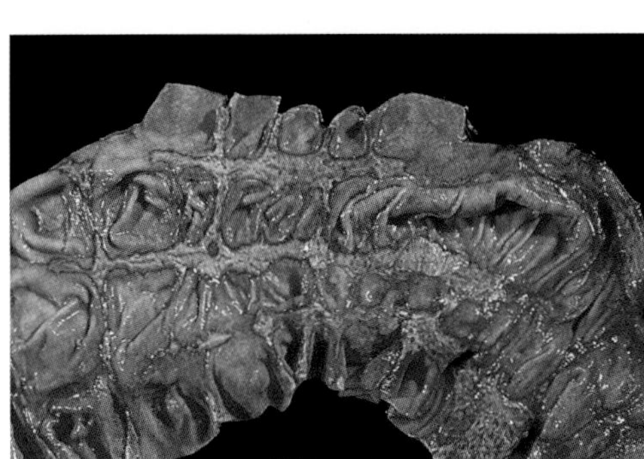

Fig. 7.193 Adynamic colon. Gross appearance of a colon resected for intractable chronic constipation with fecal impaction showing grossly dilated haustra coli and stercoral ulceration of the intervening mucosa.

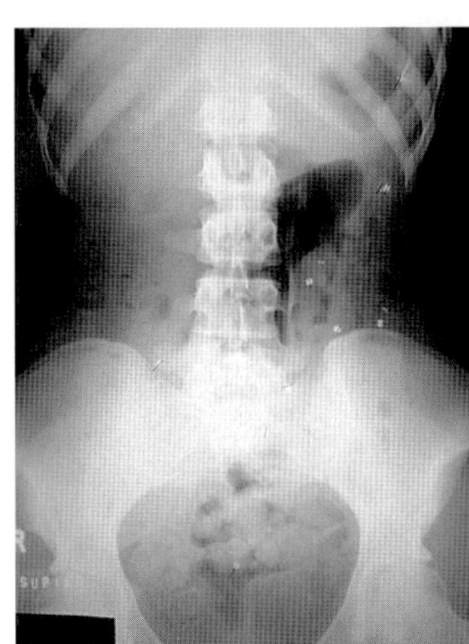

Fig. 7.194 Normal 'shapes' study, with the film taken at 120 hours. Although the patient has considerable fecal loading, the small number of rods and cubes with no rings indicates a normal colonic transit time.

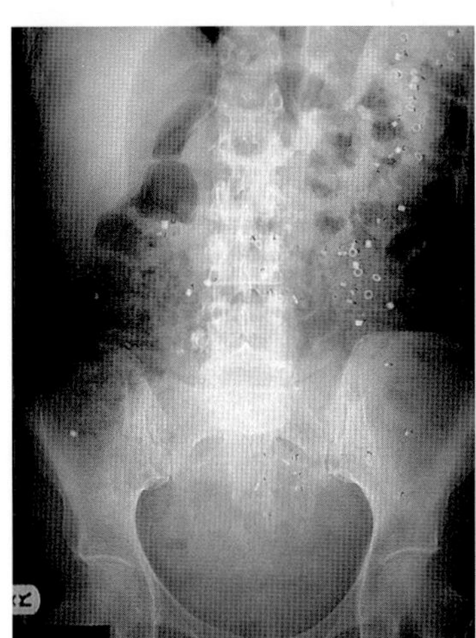

Fig. 7.195 Abnormal 'shapes' study in a woman with generalized slow colonic transit. The ring shapes were administered first, 120 hours before the radiograph. Residual barium is also to be noted within the appendix and sigmoid diverticula, the patient having had an otherwise normal barium enema some days before the 'shapes' study was started.

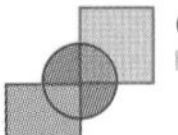

'shapes' study may then be refined by scintigraphic techniques (Fig. 7.196).

Anorectal physiological tests are contributory in excluding myopathy and neuropathy, and also in demonstrating that the act of defecation is impaired by simultaneous contraction of the sphincters and the pelvic floor (see Chapter 8). Biofeedback can then be helpful.

POST-INTERVENTIONAL APPEARANCES AND FOREIGN BODIES

The colonoscopist will not normally be confused by the appearances of a healthy post-operative anastomosis when this is of the simple end-to-end variety (Fig. 7.197), but the two-limbed colo-pouch (Fig. 7.198) or indeed the ileoanal pouch described in Chapter 6 may at first perplex. Ulceration associated with suture material (Fig. 7.199), and diversion colitis seen when the colon is out-of-circuit below a defunctioning stoma (Figs 7.200, 7.201) will be appreciated more readily in the context of the clinical history.

Minor changes are seen immediately after simple mucosal biopsy (Fig. 7.202) and although these normally resolve very quickly indeed, there may still be abnormalities for some days (Fig. 7.203) and perhaps longer still after a 'hot' biopsy of a larger lesion (Fig. 7.204).

Tablets (particularly of the slow-release variety) (Fig. 7.205), and worms (Fig. 7.206) are also sometimes found at colonoscopy.

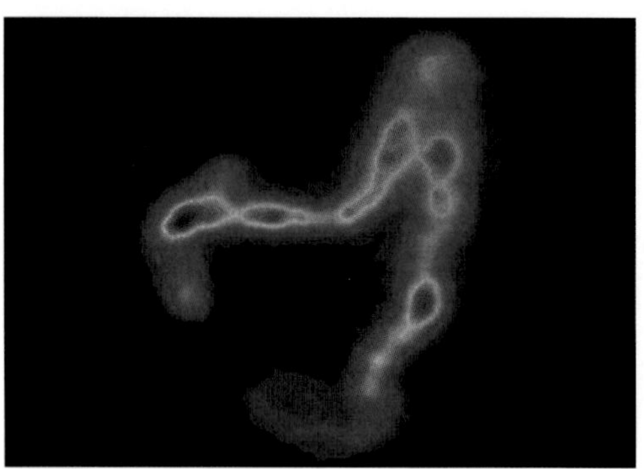

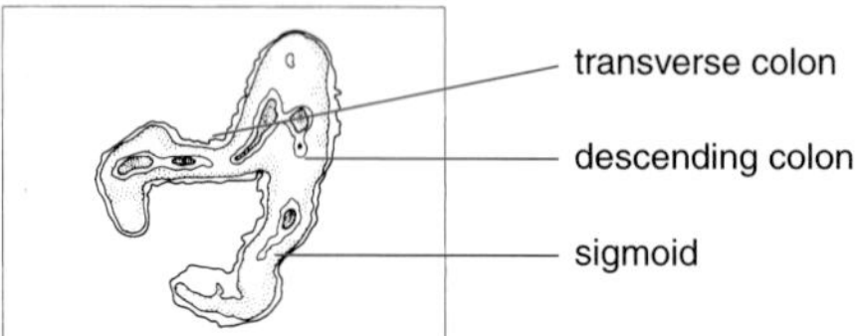

Fig. 7.196 Isotopic study of colonic transit showing the normal appearances at 24 hours. Courtesy of Mr G.T. Morris and Cancer Research UK.

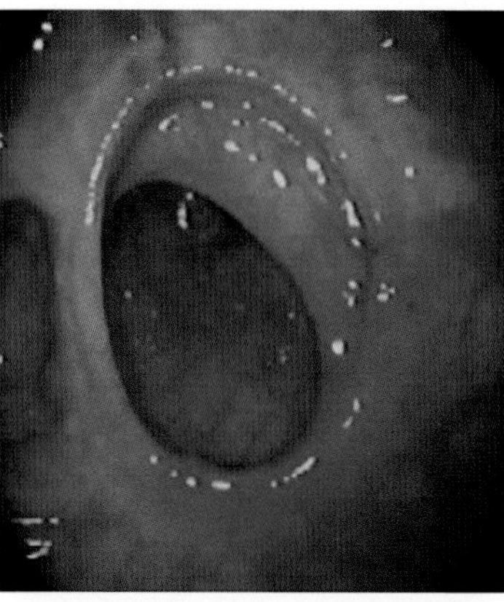

Fig. 7.197 Healthy end-to-end colonic anastomosis seen endoscopically.

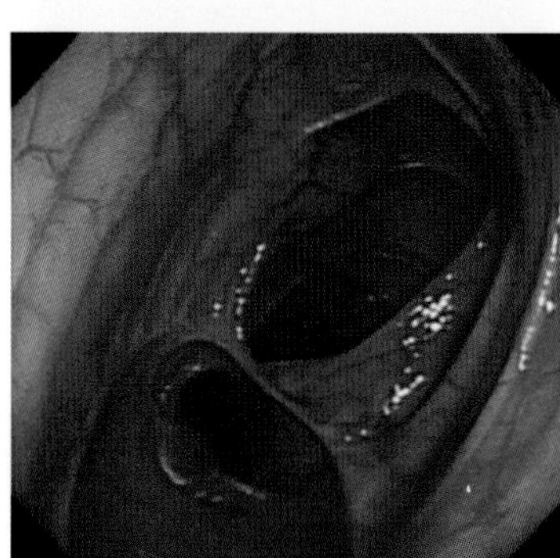

Fig. 7.198 Configuration of healthy coloanal pouch.

REFERENCES

1. Rubesin SE, Laufer I. Tumors of the colon. In: Levine MS, Rubesin SE, Laufer I (eds) Double contrast gastrointestinal radiology, 3rd edn, pp. 357–416. Philadelphia: WB Saunders, 2000, Figs 12.23A, 23B, 62, 91, 93.
2. Rubesin SE, Laufer I. Pictorial glossary of double contrast radiology. In: Gore RM, Levine MS (eds) Textbook of gastrointestinal radiology, 3rd edn, pp. 44–65. Philadelphia: WB Saunders, 2000, Figs 5.9A, 20, 38.

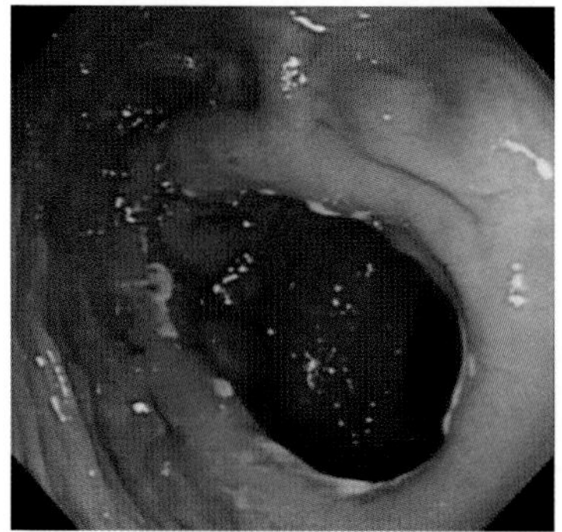

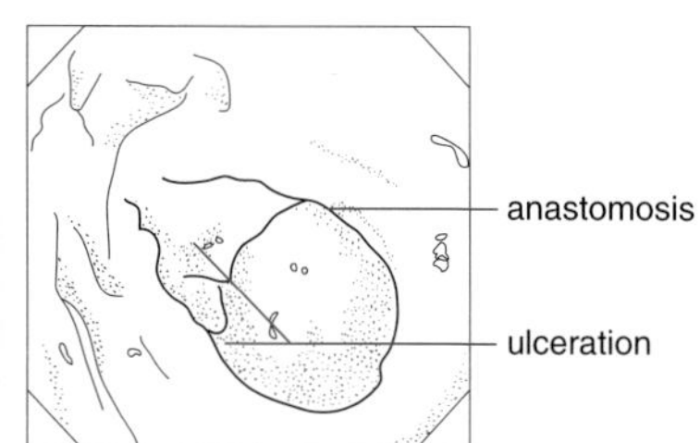

Fig. 7.199 Ulceration at the site of a prior anastomosis after cancer resection. There is no recurrence but benign ulceration associated with the suture material.

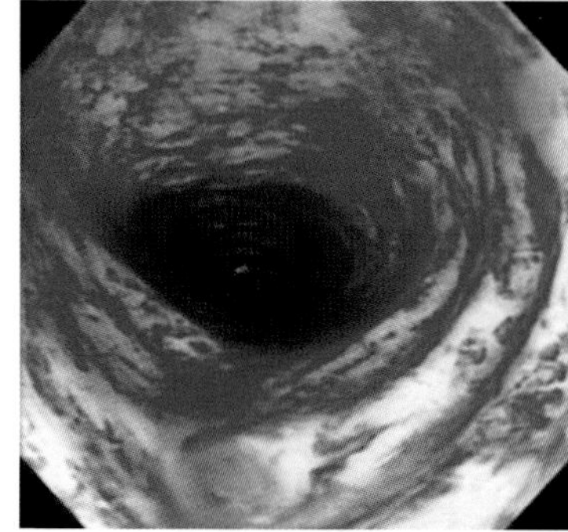

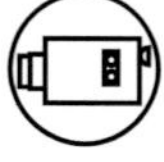

Fig. 7.200 Diversion colitis – non-specific inflammation distal to a defunctioning stoma in a patient with no underlying rectal disease.

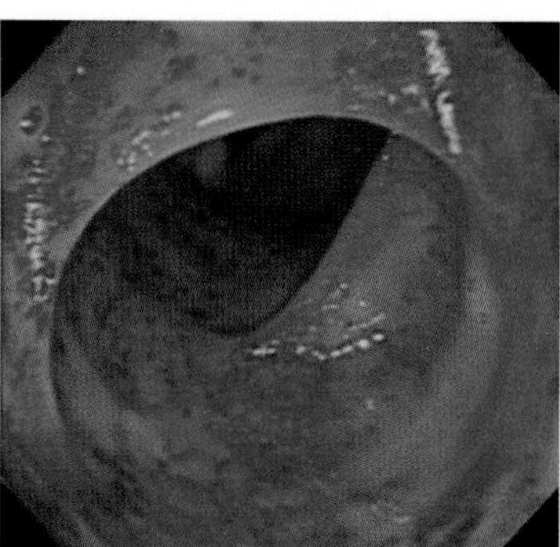

Fig. 7.201 Another view of diversion colitis.

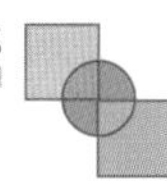

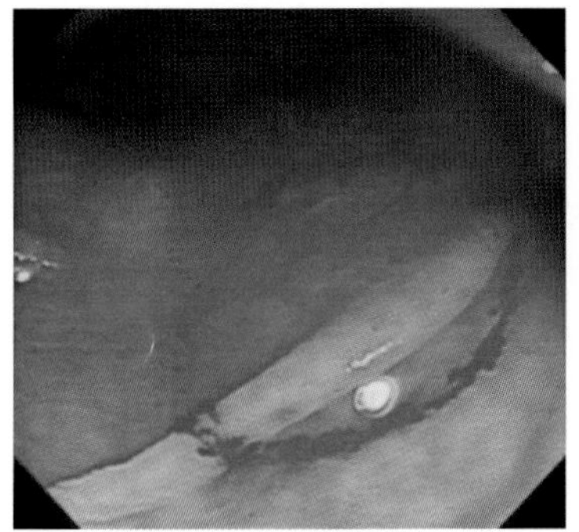

■ **Fig. 7.202** The trivial trauma and bleeding seen immediately after a random mucosal biopsy taken to exclude microscopic colitis in a patient with diarrhea.

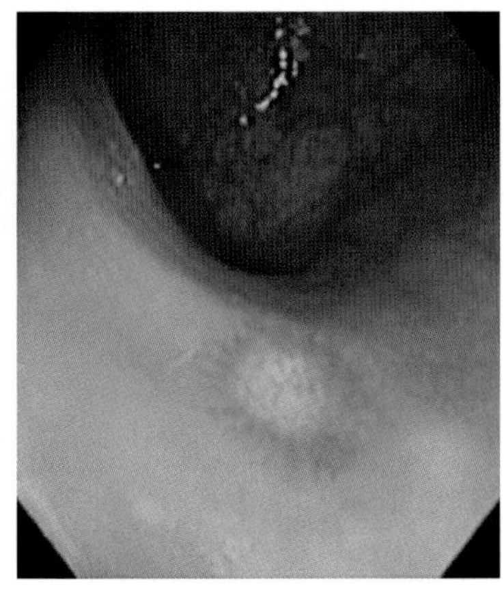

■ **Fig. 7.203** Minor ulceration seen 7 days after biopsies were taken using a rigid sigmoidoscope (and rather larger forceps then would be the case with a flexible instrument).

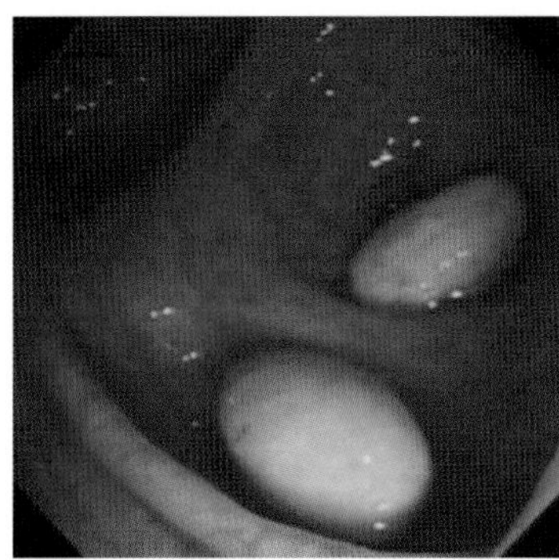

■ **Fig. 7.205** Unfragmented and non-absorbed tablets seen at colonoscopy.

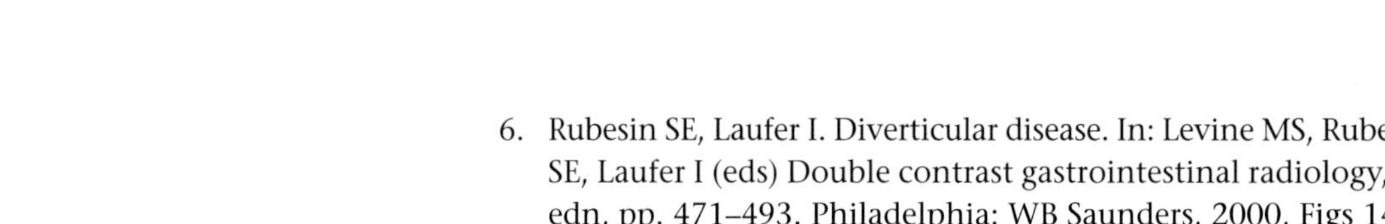

■ **Fig. 7.206** Colonic pinworm observed *in situ* by the endoscopist.

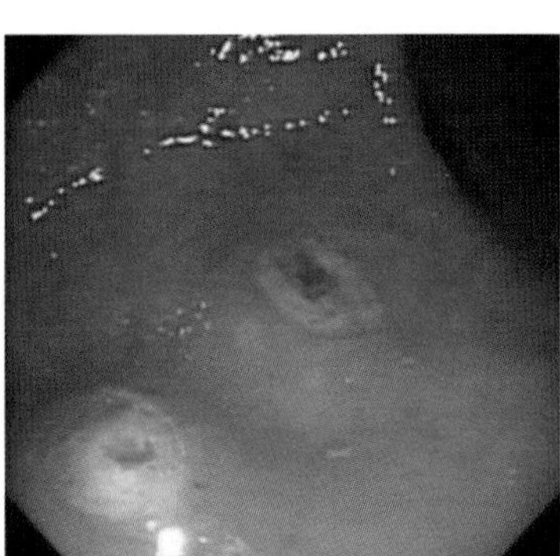

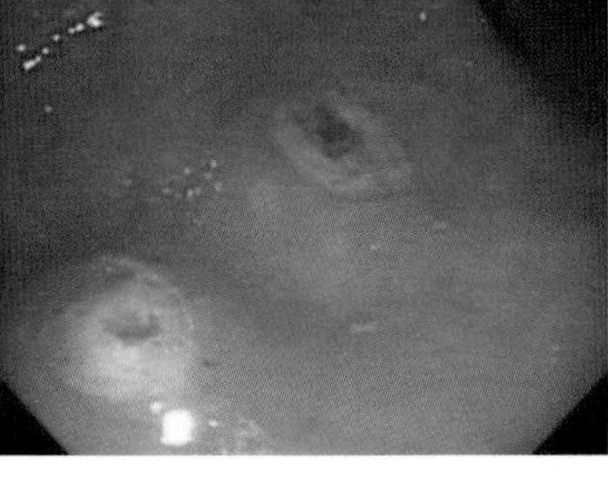

■ **Fig. 7.204** Ulceration at 7 days after hot biopsy to remove what proved to be a small adenomatous polyp.

3. Rubesin SE, Furth EE. Other tumors of the colon. In: Gore RM, Levine MS (eds) Textbook of gastrointestinal radiology, 3rd edn, pp. 1049–1074. Philadelphia: WB Saunders, 2000, Figs 57-3, 13, 14A, 36A and 36B.
4. Rubesin SE, Schnall M. Rectum. In: Gore RM, Levine MS, Laufer I (eds) Textbook of gastrointestinal radiology, 2nd edn, pp. 1261–1309. Philadelphia: WB Saunders, 1994, Figs 68.2, 15.
5. Rubesin SE, Stuzin N, Laufer I. Tumors of the colon. Semin Colon Rectal Surg 1993; 4: 94–111, Figs 11, 12A, 12B, 13.
6. Rubesin SE, Laufer I. Diverticular disease. In: Levine MS, Rubesin SE, Laufer I (eds) Double contrast gastrointestinal radiology, 3rd edn, pp. 471–493. Philadelphia: WB Saunders, 2000, Figs 14.4, 7, 9, 17, 18, 19B, 20, 24, 33.
7. Miller WT, Levine MS, Rubesin SE, *et al*. Bowler hats: a simple principle for differentiating polyps from diverticula. Radiology 1989; 173: 615–617, Figs 2, 3A, 3B.
8. Rubesin SE, *et al*. Carpet lesions of the colon. RadioGraphics 1985; 5: 537–552, Fig. 1.
9. Rubesin SE, Levine MS, Bezzi M, *et al*. Rectal involvement by prostatic carcinoma: radiographic findings. AJR 1989; 152: 53–57, Fig.1B.
10. Dobos N, Rubesin SE. Radiologic imaging modalities in the diagnosis and management of colorectal cancer. Hem/Onc Clin North Am 2002; 16: 875–985, Fig. 2A.

THE ANUS, ANAL CANAL, AND PERIANAL REGION

8

ANATOMY OF THE ANAL CANAL

The anal canal is the terminal 3–4 cm of the large intestine and runs from the anorectal junction to the anus itself. The line of the anal valves, often called the dentate line, is clearly visible, approximately half way along the anal canal. The anal columns extend upwards from this line (Figs 8.1–8.3). The columnar epithelium of the rectum is replaced by mixed columnar and squamous epithelium in the upper anal canal, corresponding to the zone of fusion between the embryological hindgut and the proctodeum. Between the line of the anal valves and the lower border of the internal sphincter, the epithelium is stratified squamous where it may be referred to as the pecten. At the true anal margin, the epithelium becomes hair-bearing skin.

Sphincters

Two sphincters surround the anal canal: the internal sphincter, which is the expanded distal portion of the circular smooth muscle of the large bowel; and the external sphincter, which is derived from the striated muscle of the pelvic floor and becomes continuous with the puborectalis and the levator ani muscles.

Spaces

There are three important spaces in the area. The intersphincteric space contains the terminal fibers of the longitudinal muscle of the gut and the anal intermuscular glands. These anal glands are important in the pathogenesis of abscesses and fistulae. The ischiorectal fossa lies outside the external sphincter, and the supra-levator space is between the rectum and the levator ani muscles.

HEMORRHOIDS

Hemorrhoids are vascular swellings which may involve the internal and external venous plexuses of the anal canal, and be associated with redundancy of the mucosa and/or perianal skin. Internal hemorrhoids arise from the internal venous plexus and are covered by mucosa; external ones come from the external venous plexus below the line of the anal valves and are covered by stratified squamous epithelium and hair-bearing skin (Figs 8.4–8.6). Both types are common and in Western populations approximately 50% of those aged over 50 years will have them to some extent. They are related to engorgement of the venous plexuses (which are the normal anal cushions) and to redundancy of the epithelium. They are characteristically noted during pregnancy, and with persistent straining at stool, and may also be found in association with large pelvic tumors.

Hemorrhoids usually present with the passage of bright red blood, which drips or spurts into the toilet following defecation or is noted on the toilet paper after wiping. Bleeding is almost always self-limited but there may be associated perianal discomfort or pain, prolapse, a mucous discharge and pruritus.

Internal hemorrhoids that do not prolapse are known as first degree, those that prolapse but reduce spontaneously, second degree, and those that require digital reduction, third degree (Fig. 8.7). The three primary hemorrhoidal sites are left lateral, right posterior and right anterior, as illustrated in Fig. 8.7 which shows a patient in the left lateral position who also exhibits the three secondary hemorrhoids (left anterior, left posterior, and right lateral). The internal component is predominantly covered by intestinal columnar

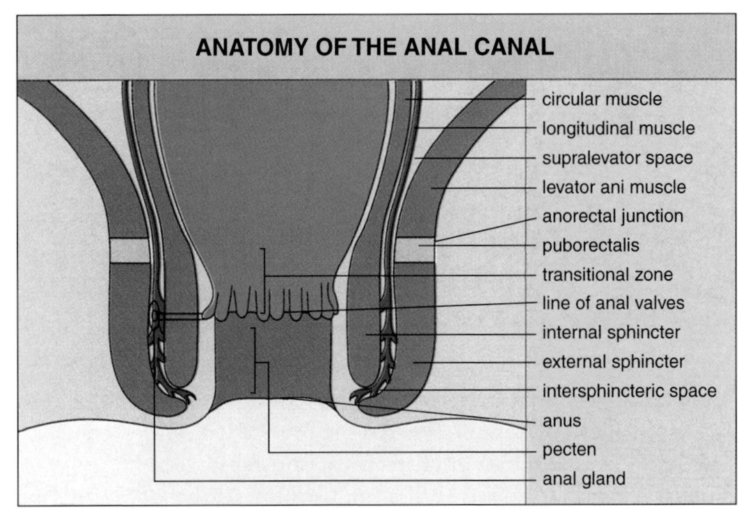

Fig. 8.1 The anatomy of the anal canal.

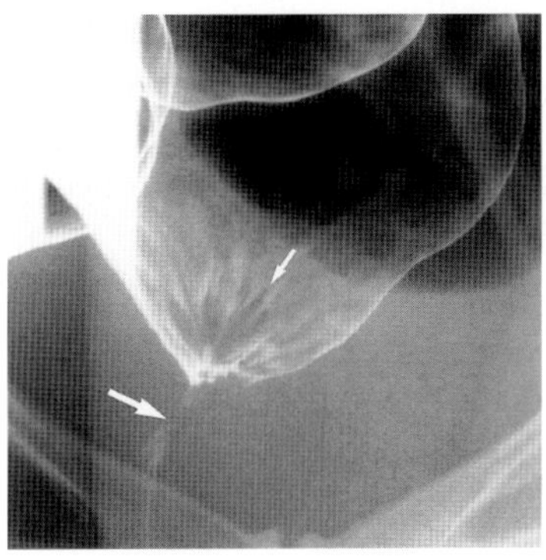

Fig. 8.2 Double-contrast barium enema depicting the location of the anal sphincter. The anal canal (large white arrow) is closed by active contraction of the internal and external anal sphincters. The rectal columns of Morgagni (small arrow identifies one column) are lined by colonic epithelium. (Reproduced with permission from reference 1, Fig. 1.)

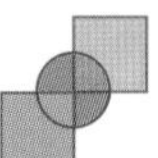

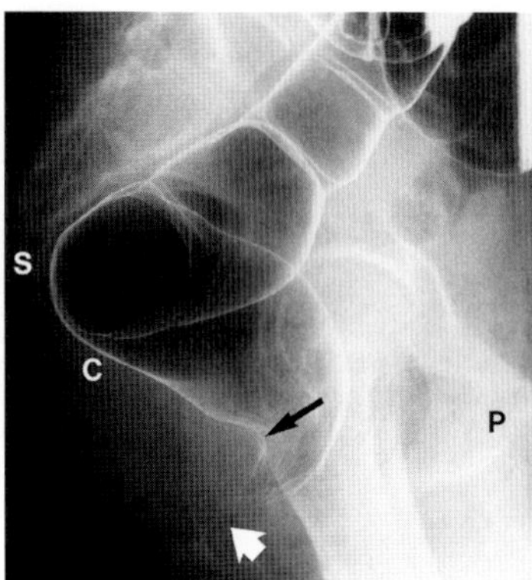

Fig. 8.3 Double-contrast barium enema showing location of anal sphincter. The posterior wall of the rectum abuts the sacrum (S), and coccyx (C). The puborectalis muscle helps support the rectum and is seen as an extrinsic impression (black arrow) on the posterior wall of the rectum. This patient has mild pelvic floor weakness. The anal sphincter (white arrow) is closed. A small amount of barium has spilled onto the perineum. The symphysis pubis is identified (P). (Reproduced with permission from reference 2, Fig. 68.1.)

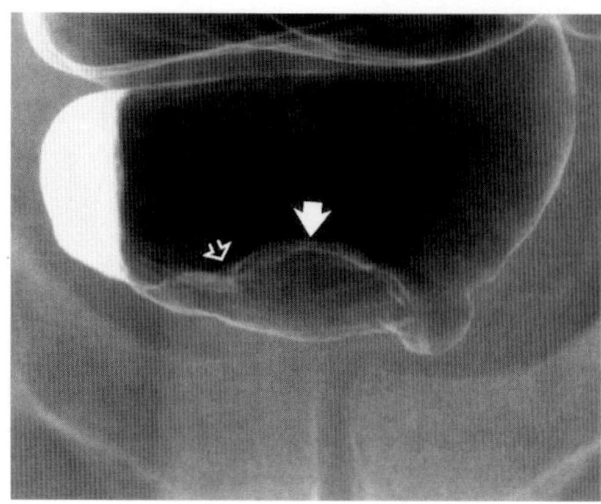

Fig. 8.6 Double-contrast barium enema demonstrating internal hemorrhoids. A large bi-lobed polypoid mass (large arrow) has a focal area of surface ulceration (small arrow). (Reproduced with permission from reference 1, Fig. 5.)

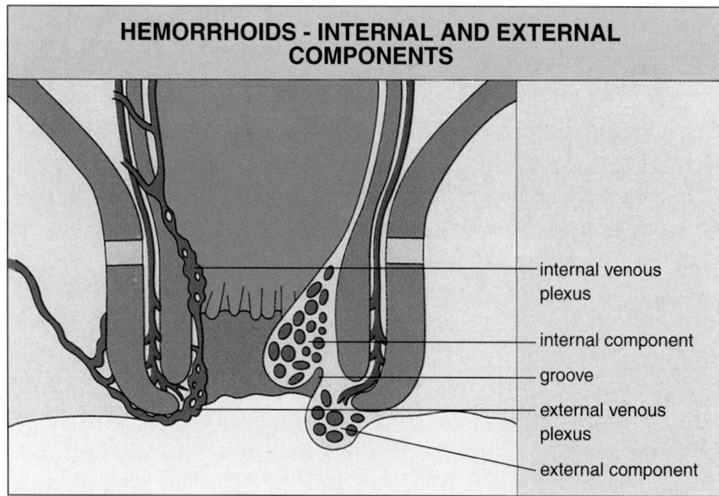

Fig. 8.4 Diagram illustrating the internal and external components of hemorrhoids.

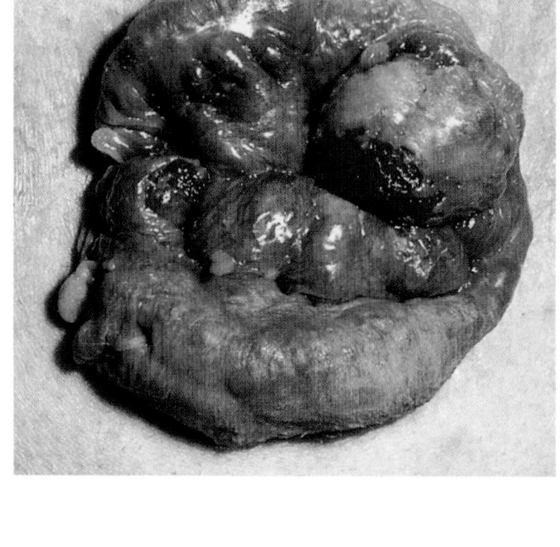

Fig. 8.7 Prolapsed (third degree) hemorrhoids.

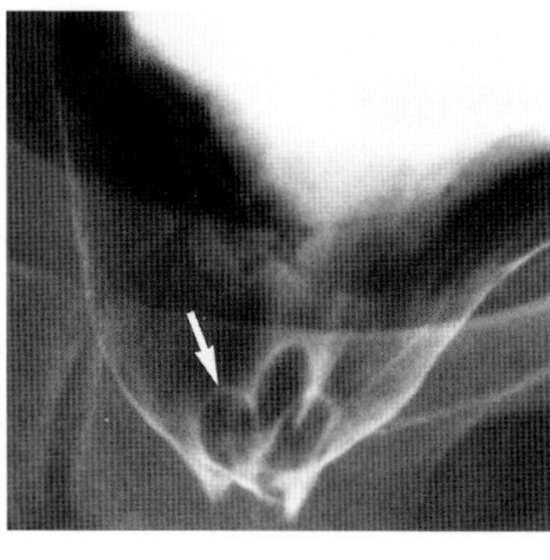

Fig. 8.5 Double-contrast barium enema demonstrating internal hemorrhoids. Three smooth-surfaced polypoid lesions (resembling a bunch of grapes) (arrow) are present at the anorectal junction.

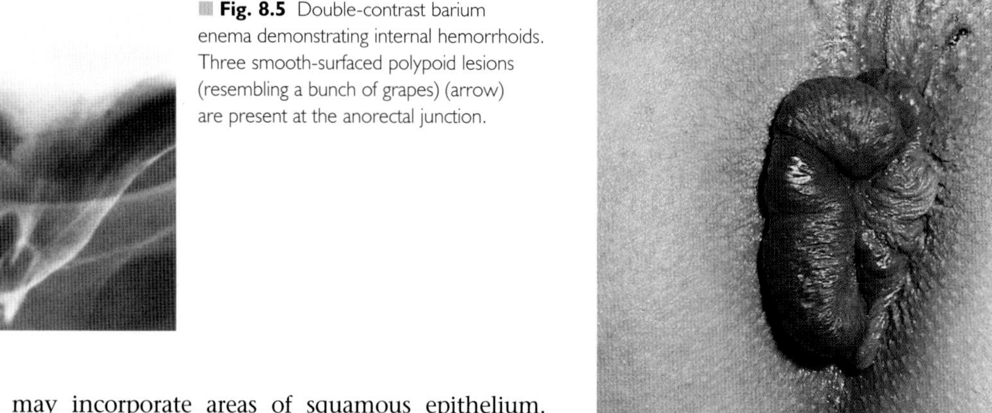

Fig. 8.8 Engorgement of the external hemorrhoidal venous plexus.

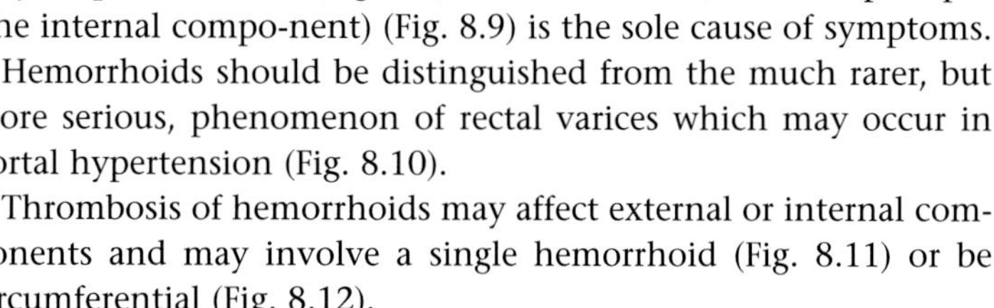

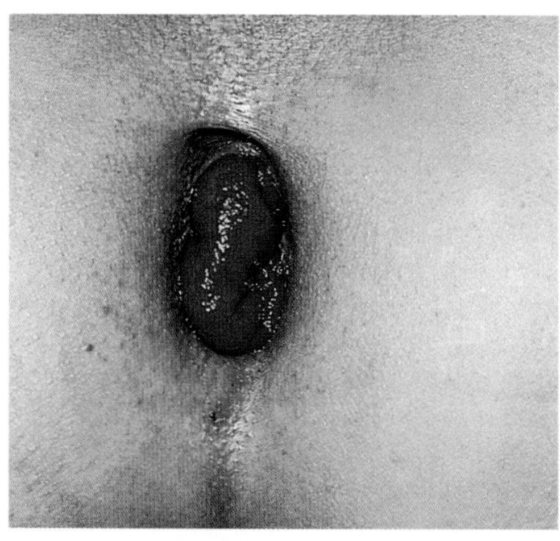

Fig. 8.9 Mucosal prolapse with no external component.

epithelium, but may incorporate areas of squamous epithelium. The colum-nar epithelium may become reddened, and the area of squamous epithelium increased, if prolapse occurs over a prolonged period. This is well demonstrated in the right anterior hemorrhoid in the illustrated patient. The external component may be present alone (Fig. 8.8), while in others, mucosal prolapse (the internal compo-nent) (Fig. 8.9) is the sole cause of symptoms.

Hemorrhoids should be distinguished from the much rarer, but more serious, phenomenon of rectal varices which may occur in portal hypertension (Fig. 8.10).

Thrombosis of hemorrhoids may affect external or internal com-ponents and may involve a single hemorrhoid (Fig. 8.11) or be circumferential (Fig. 8.12).

A small area of involvement of the external plexus is often referred to as a perianal hematoma. However, this is a misnomer (since it is not a bruise) and the preferred term is clotted venous saccule (Fig. 8.13). These are intensely painful and may progress to ulcera-tion (Fig. 8.14) and/or marked hemorrhage.

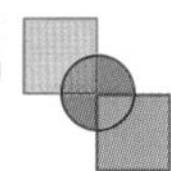

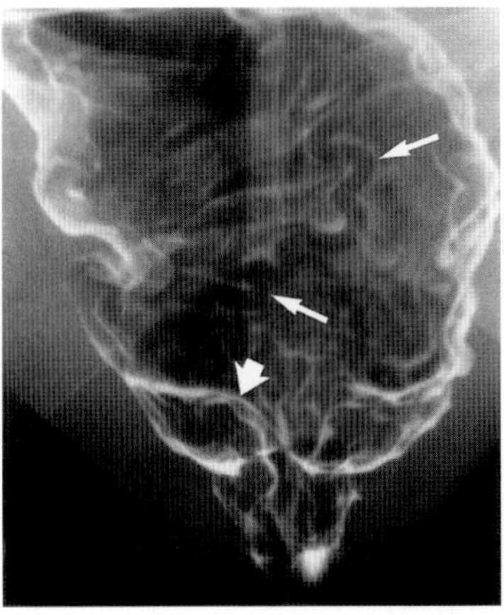

■ **Fig. 8.10** Double-contrast barium enema in patient with portal hypertension demonstrating numerous rectal varices. Varices are seen *en face* (long arrows) and in profile (short arrow) as smooth, surface serpentine folds. (Reproduced with permission from reference 2, Fig. 68.14.)

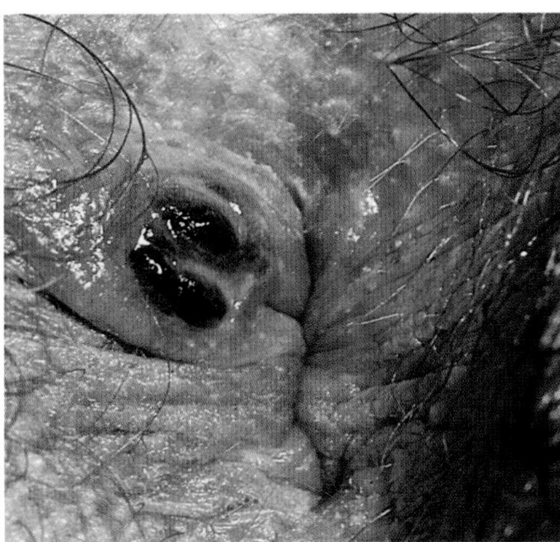

■ **Fig. 8.14** Ulceration of a clotted venous saccule with a visible clot.

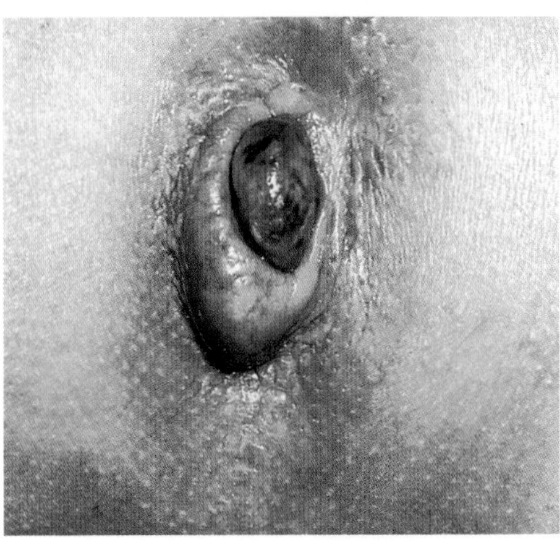

■ **Fig. 8.11** Prolapsed thrombosed right posterior hemorrhoid. The two components are separated by a groove. Reduction is not possible because of the thrombosis and should not be attempted, as this will cause severe pain.

ANAL FISSURE

Anal fissures, the most common anal ulcers, are longitudinal or elliptical defects in the anal canal epithelium which extend for a variable extent from the anal verge towards the line of the anal valves; more than 90% occur in the posterior midline. Many fissures heal spontaneously, but deeper fissures, which often have undermined edges and expose the white circular fibers of the internal sphincter, are more indolent and may be associated with sentinel skin tags or fibrous anal polyps (Figs 8.15, 8.16). Most fissures are tears caused by the combination of unyielding distal anal canal and a tight distal internal sphincter. Affected individuals are usually young or middle-aged adults. The chief symptom is pain, which may be severe and is usually related to defecation, though less severe chronic pain also occurs. Other symptoms include the passage of small amounts of blood or pus, and pruritus ani. Large or multiple fissures, and particularly those away from the midline, should always raise the suspicion of Crohn's disease.

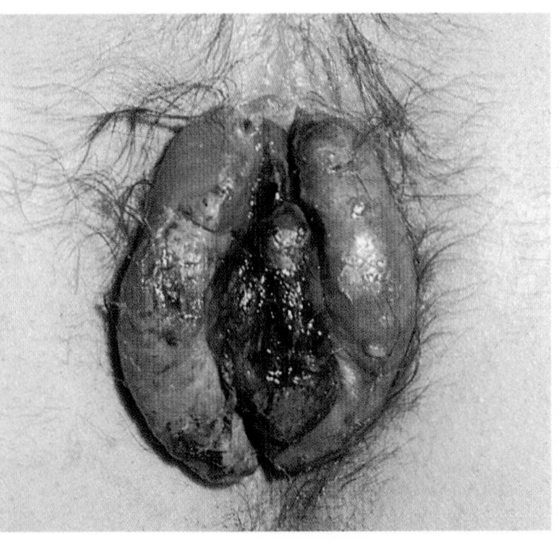

■ **Fig. 8.12** Circumferential thrombosis of both the external and internal plexus, which is prolapsed. The groove between the two components is clearly demonstrated.

CROHN'S DISEASE

Crohn's disease has perianal manifestations in approximately 50% of patients, including about 25% of those with predominantly ileal disease and the great majority of those with rectal disease. The general features of Crohn's disease are considered in Chapters 5 and 6. The perianal disease is characterized by edematous skin tags (Fig. 8.17), bluish discoloration (Fig. 8.18), frank ulceration (Fig. 8.19), and sepsis. The tendency to fistula formation is considered below. Perianal disease also occurs in ulcerative colitis. Perianal ulceration

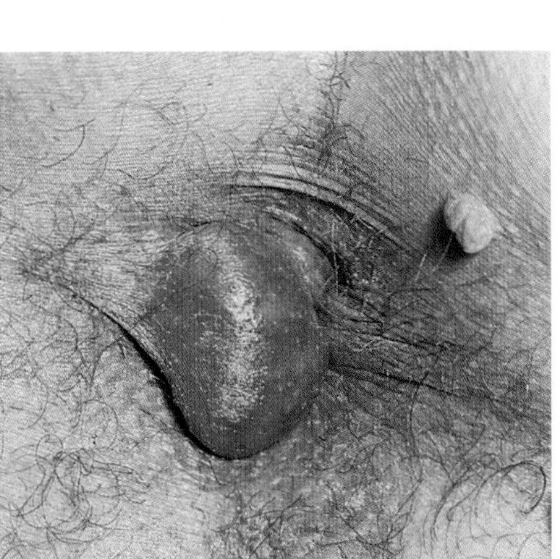

■ **Fig. 8.13** A discrete thrombosis of part of the external venous plexus – a clotted venous saccule.

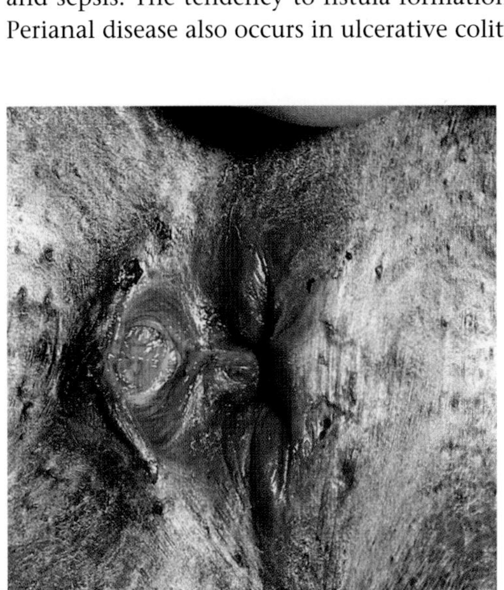

■ **Fig. 8.15** A posterior fissure-in-ano with an associated small sentinel skin tag and enlarged papilla.

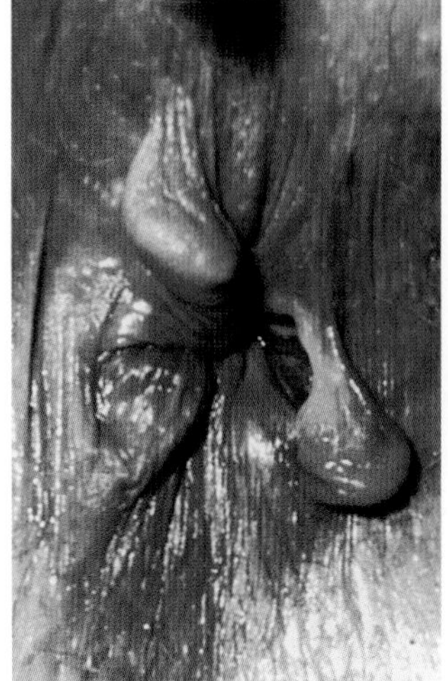
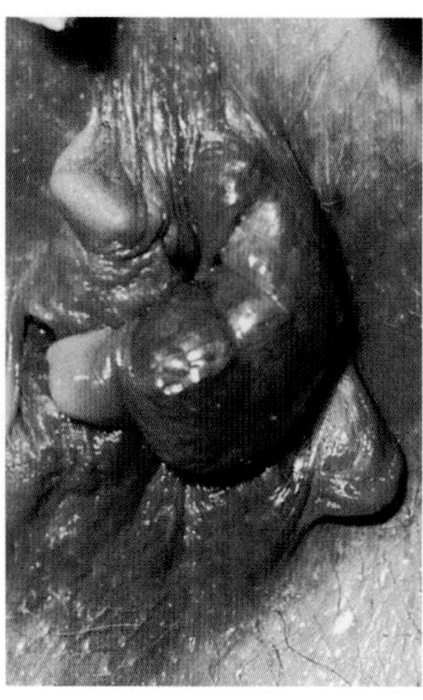

a b

■ **Fig. 8.16** An anterior fissure-in-ano associated with a large sentinel skin tag (a) and the large fibrovascular anal polyp in the same patient (b).

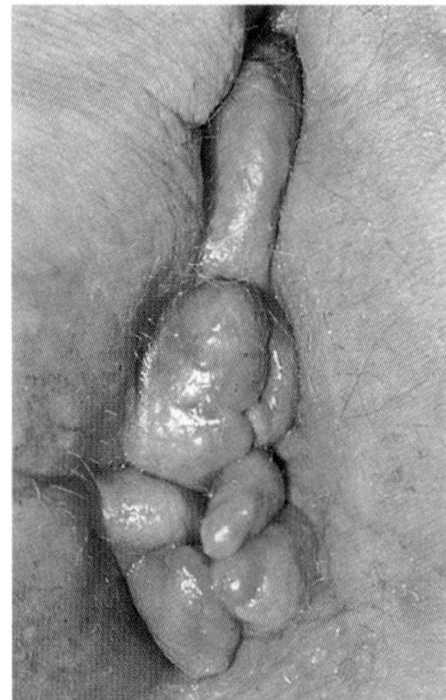

■ **Fig. 8.17** Edematous skin tags in Crohn's disease.

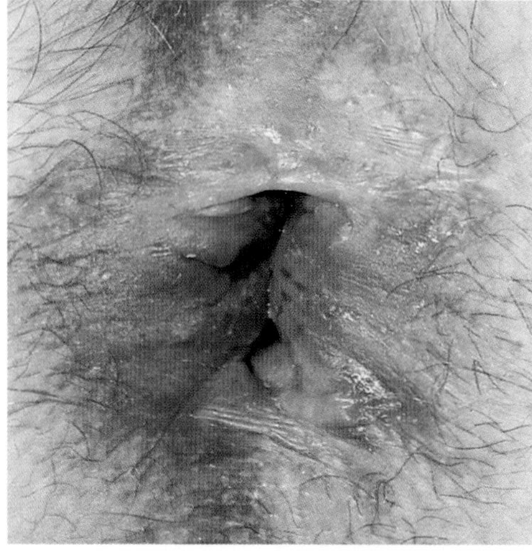

■ **Fig. 8.18** Bluish discoloration of the perianal area in Crohn's disease.

may also be caused by syphilis (see below), tuberculosis, herpes simplex (Fig. 8.20), leukemic states, simple excoriation of the skin, and ulcerating perianal hematoma.

ABSCESSES AND FISTULAE

Abscesses and fistulae in the anal region are different phases of the same disease process, fistula representing the chronic phase of untreated abscess. Most begin as a non-specific infection of the anal glands, which may produce an abscess between the two sphincters – the so-called intersphincteric abscess, but infection may then spread giving rise to what may become a highly complex pattern of sepsis. Spread of infection to the anal margin gives rise to a perianal abscess. Upward spread produces either an intermuscular abscess or a supralevator abscess, depending on whether it is between the two muscle layers of the rectum, or outside the rectum into the supralevator space, respectively (Fig. 8.21). Horizontal spread carries infection back into the anal canal across the internal sphincter, or across the striated muscle into the ischiorectal fossa forming an ischiorectal abscess, which may occur at, below, or above, the level of the anal valves (Fig. 8.22). If the primary track passes through the external sphincter, it is termed trans-sphincteric, but if above the puborectalis, suprasphincteric. Circumferential spread carries infection in the intersphincteric space, supralevator space, or the ischiorectal fossa to the opposite side (Fig. 8.23).

Perianal and ischiorectal abscesses cause throbbing pain and hot, tender, red swellings. A perianal abscess will be seen at the anal margin (Fig. 8.24), while an ischiorectal abscess results in considerable thickening of the ischiorectal fossa. Intersphincteric, intermuscular, and supralevator abscesses are more difficult to diagnose, as there may be no external physical signs. Radiology is occasionally indicated and helpful (Figs 8.25, 8.26).

A fistula is, by definition, an abnormal communication between two epithelial surfaces: in the context of fistula-in-ano, however, either or both of the openings may be closed, or at least not readily apparent, and the communicating track, lined by granulation tissue,

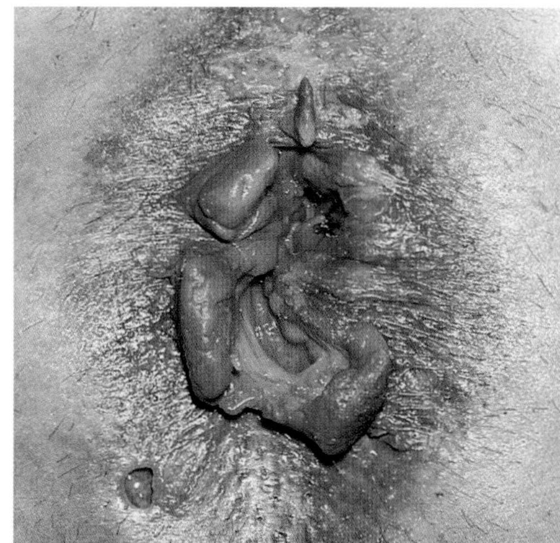

■ **Fig. 8.19** Crohn's disease: edematous skins tags, bluish discoloration, ulceration and sepsis are manifest – there is also a fistula.

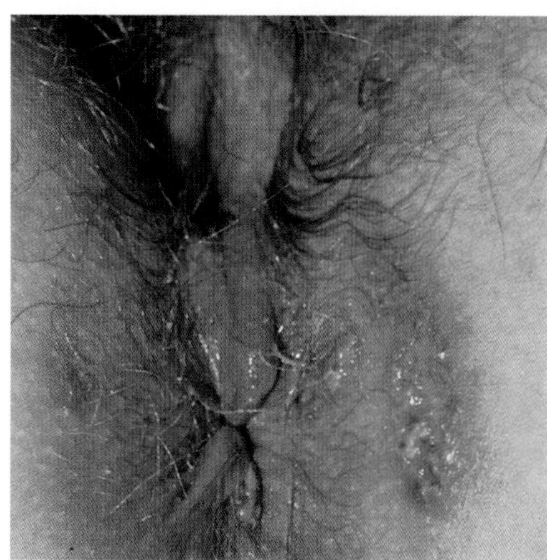

■ **Fig. 8.20** Perianal herpetic vesicles in a patient with severe herpetic proctitis.

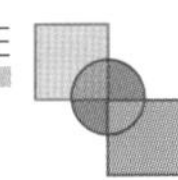

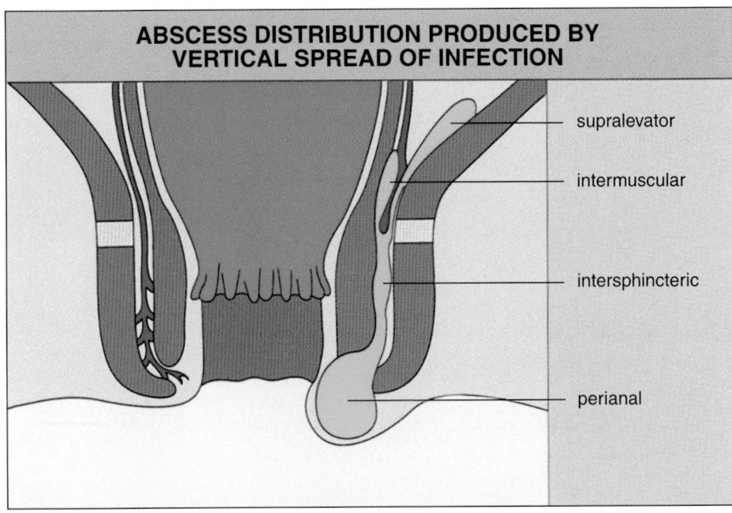

■ **Fig. 8.21** Diagram showing the distribution of abscesses produced by vertical spread of infection.

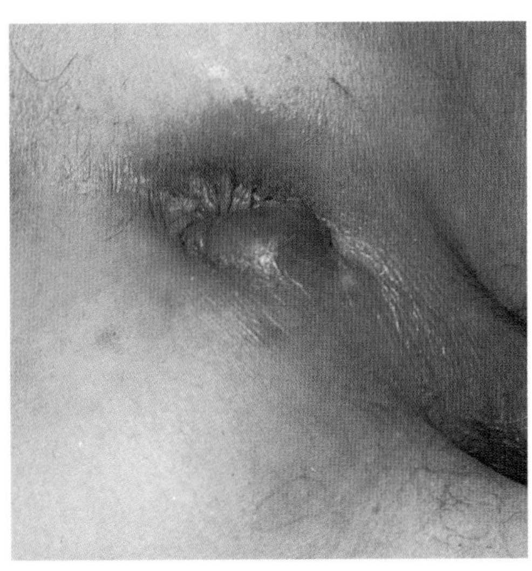

■ **Fig. 8.24** A perianal abscess.

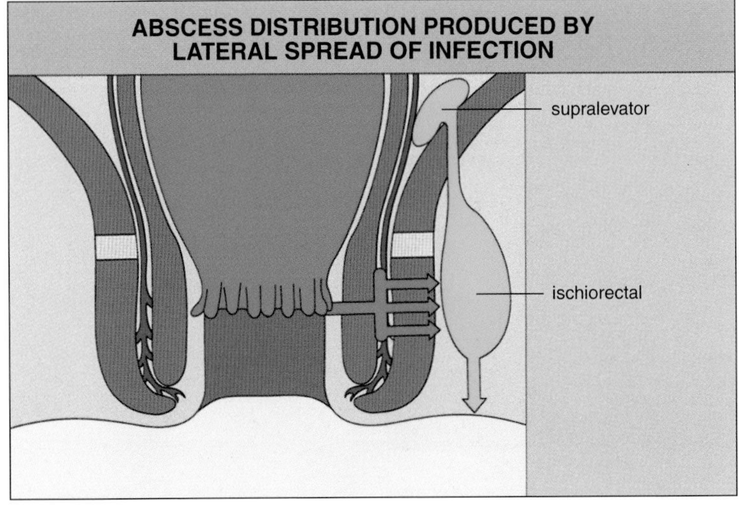

■ **Fig. 8.22** Diagram showing the distribution of abscesses produced by horizontal spread of infection.

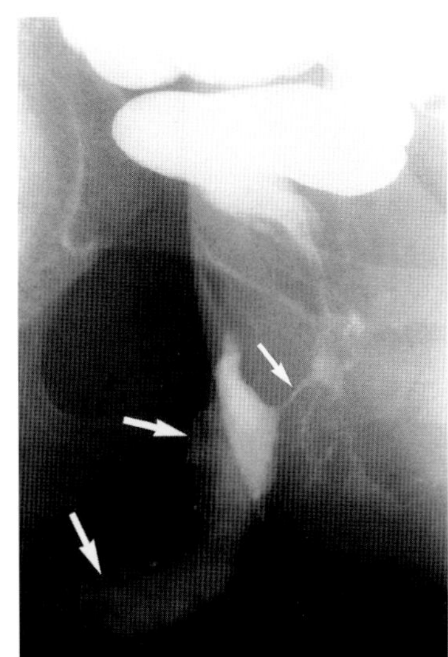

■ **Fig. 8.25** Double-contrast barium enema demonstrating perianal abscess in Crohn's disease. A fistulous track (narrower arrow) courses from the anal canal to fill a tubular perianal abscess (broader arrows). (Reproduced with permission from reference 2, Fig. 68.46.)

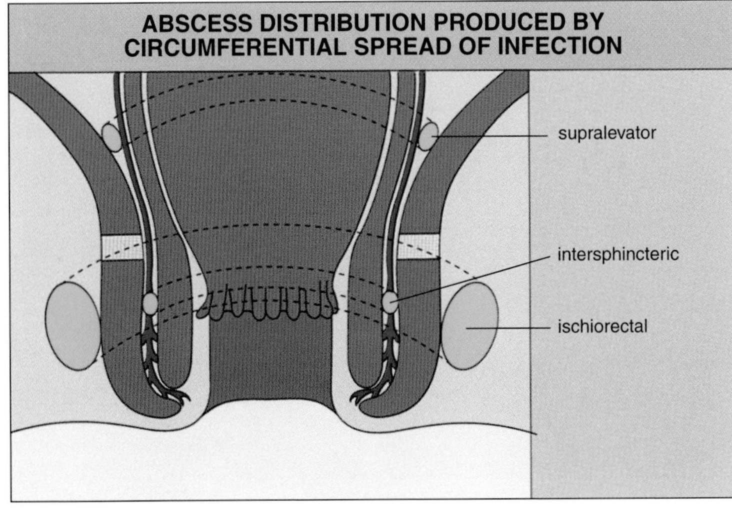

■ **Fig. 8.23** Diagram showing the distribution of abscesses produced by circumferential spread of infection.

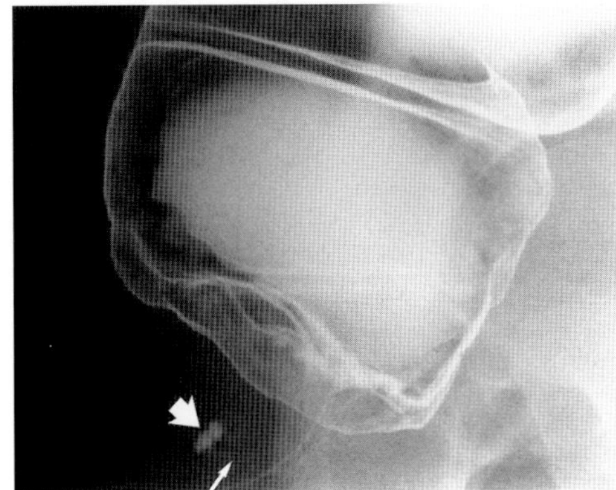

■ **Fig. 8.26** Double-contrast barium enema demonstrating small anal gland abscess. A focal barium collection (large arrow) represents a dilated anal gland at the level of the dentate line. A track of barium (thin arrow) extends from the anal canal to the abscess. (Reproduced with permission from reference 2, Fig. 68.67.)

may be very complex. Although induration is an important physical sign for determining the path of sepsis (Fig. 8.27), diagnostic and therapeutic difficulties often occur. These problems may be ameliorated by MRI scanning, which can often demonstrate the tract and both openings (Fig. 8.28). Fistulae are classified according to the position of the primary track – intersphincteric if it lies between the sphincters (Fig. 8.29), trans-sphincteric when it crosses the external sphincter (Figs 8.28–8.31), and suprasphincteric when it crosses above the puborectalis muscle. Perianal fistulae are a major feature of perianal Crohn's disease (Figs 8.19, 8.32, 8.33), and are usually associated with rectal involvement; only rarely do they represent spread from more proximal bowel disease. Sadly, involvement of the vagina also is quite common (Fig. 8.34).

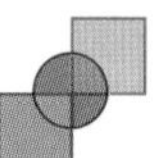

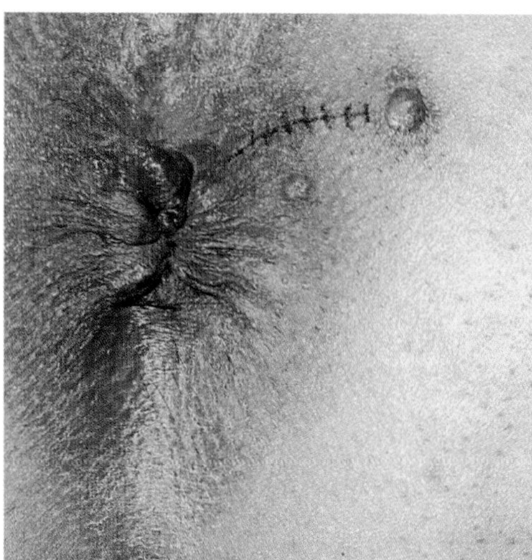

Fig. 8.27 A fistula-in-ano showing the external opening and the course of the indurated track marked in blue.

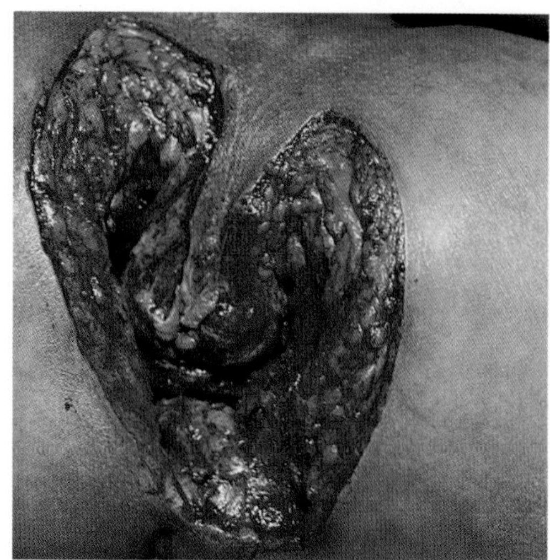

Fig. 8.30 A trans-sphincteric fistula with horseshoe spread of infection to the contralateral ischiorectal fossa; it has been surgically drained.

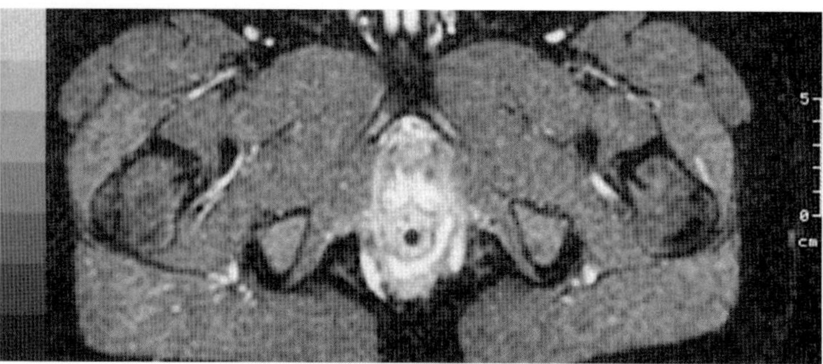

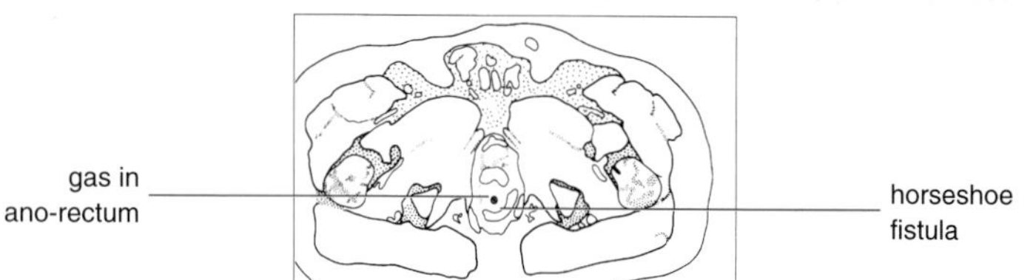

Fig. 8.28 MRI scan illustrating a trans-sphincteric fistula with an inter-sphincteric 'horseshoe'. Courtesy of Mr P. Lunniss.

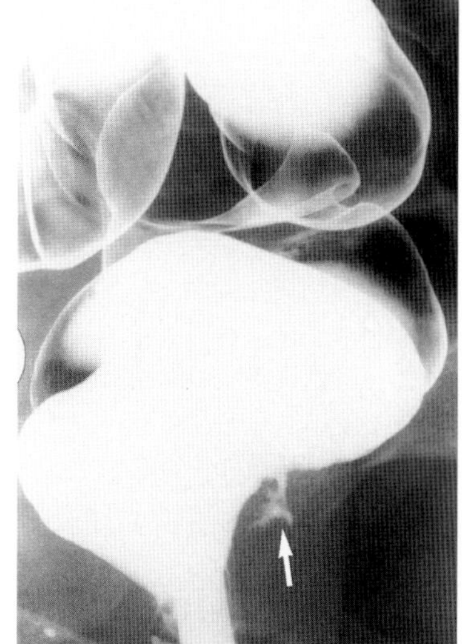

Fig. 8.31 Double-contrast barium enema demonstrating extrasphincteric fistula. An irregular track (arrow) originates from the left lateral wall of the rectum and extends into the perirectal soft tissue. (Reproduced with permission from reference 2, Fig. 68.68; courtesy of S.N. Glick, Philadelphia.)

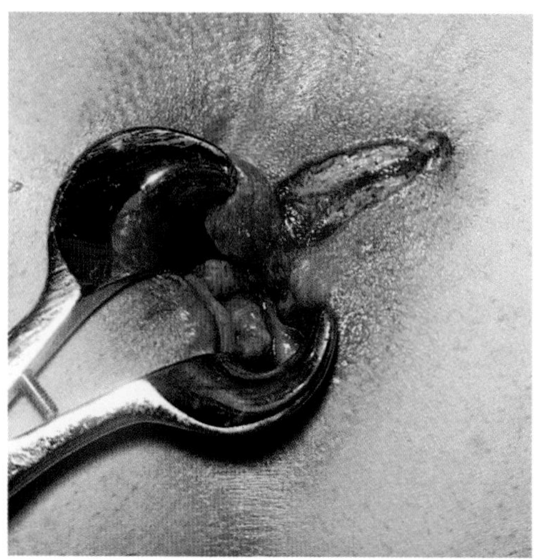

Fig. 8.29 An operating proctoscope inserted into the anal canal of the patient shown in Fig. 8.27 showing the granulation tissue-lined track laid open. This is an intersphincteric fistula with a subcutaneous track.

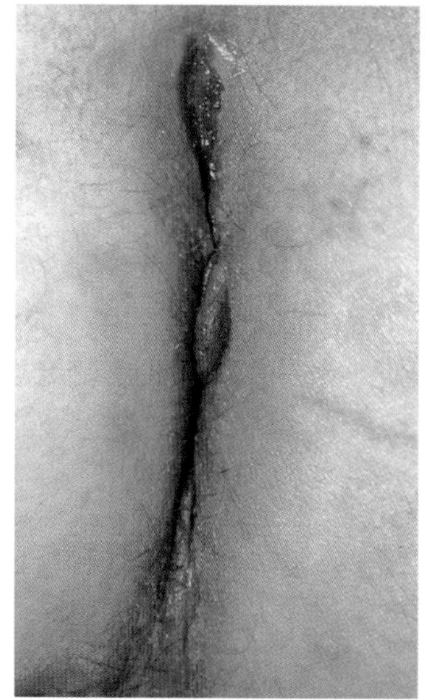

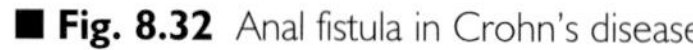

Fig. 8.32 Anal fistula in Crohn's disease.

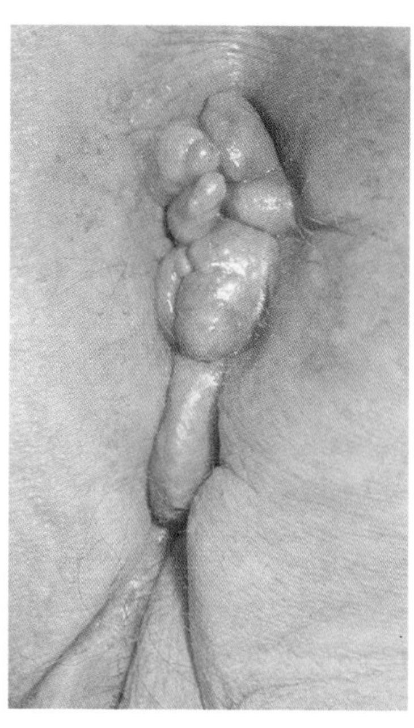

Fig. 8.33 Inflammatory edematous skin tags with severe ulceration and multiple fistulous openings in Crohn's disease.

Pilonidal sinus

Pilonidal sinus is common in young adults (particularly males) and, although sometimes asymptomatic, is a cause of considerable morbidity. It comprises one or more openings in the natal cleft, which have skin-lined edges. The subcutaneous component has a base of granulation tissue and often contains hairs, which may project from the mouth of the sinus (Fig. 8.35). It is thought that pilonidal sinuses follow folliculitis and localized abscess formation within the subcutaneous fat. The relevance of hair is probably secondary, being responsible, once trapped within the sinus, for continued infection and a foreign body reaction (Fig. 8.36).

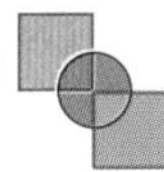

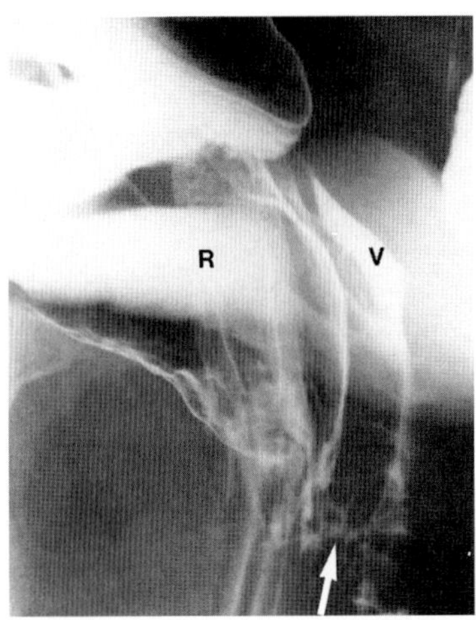

Fig. 8.34 Double-contrast barium enema demonstrating anovaginal fistula in Crohn's disease. Numerous barium-filled tracks (arrow) extend from the distal rectum and proximal anal canal into the distal vagina. The remainder of the vagina (V) is filled retrogradely. Rectum identified by R. (Reproduced with permission from reference 2, Fig. 68.45.)

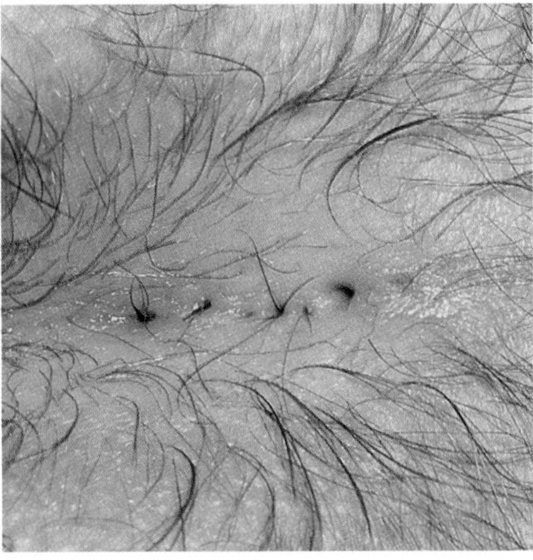

Fig. 8.35 Multiple pilonidal sinus openings in the natal cleft.

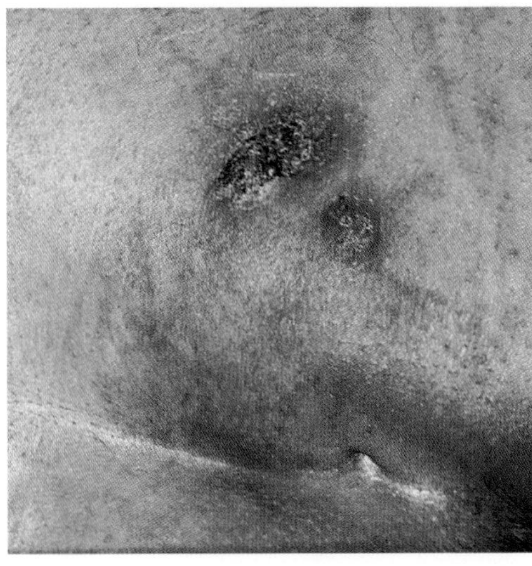

Fig. 8.36 Pilonidal abscess: the site of discharge is clear and the examining finger readily feels induration across the discolored area.

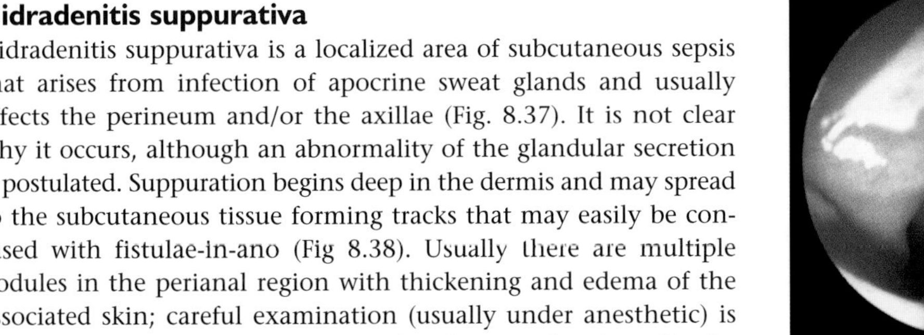

Hidradenitis suppurativa

Hidradenitis suppurativa is a localized area of subcutaneous sepsis that arises from infection of apocrine sweat glands and usually affects the perineum and/or the axillae (Fig. 8.37). It is not clear why it occurs, although an abnormality of the glandular secretion is postulated. Suppuration begins deep in the dermis and may spread to the subcutaneous tissue forming tracks that may easily be confused with fistulae-in-ano (Fig 8.38). Usually there are multiple nodules in the perianal region with thickening and edema of the associated skin; careful examination (usually under anesthetic) is necessary to delineate the disease and to distinguish it from fistula-in-ano (with which there may be an association). Management can be a major problem. It can easily be confused by the inexperienced with the perianal manifestations of Crohn's disease, which is important, as the management of the two conditions is considerably different.

Other forms of sepsis

Abscesses and fistulae may also be associated with tuberculosis, follow appendicitis, or occur in association with diverticular disease: these are all considered elsewhere.

PELVIC FLOOR DISORDERS

The pelvic floor disorders encompass a variety of conditions in which neuromuscular function is disturbed. Difficulty with evacuation, straining at stool, and sensations related to prolapse (of hemorrhoids, rectum or, occasionally, neoplastic masses) are the principal complaints.

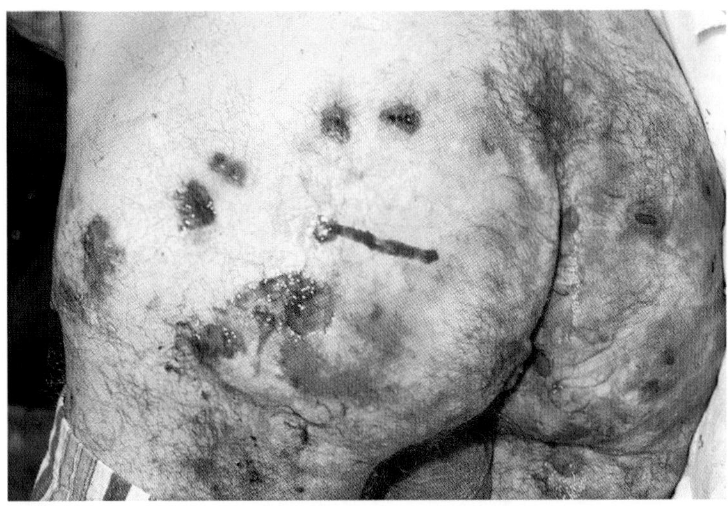

Fig. 8.37 Hidradenitis suppurativa. Multiple discharging sinuses are separated by areas of induration. The terms acne conglobata and watering-can perineum are synonymous.

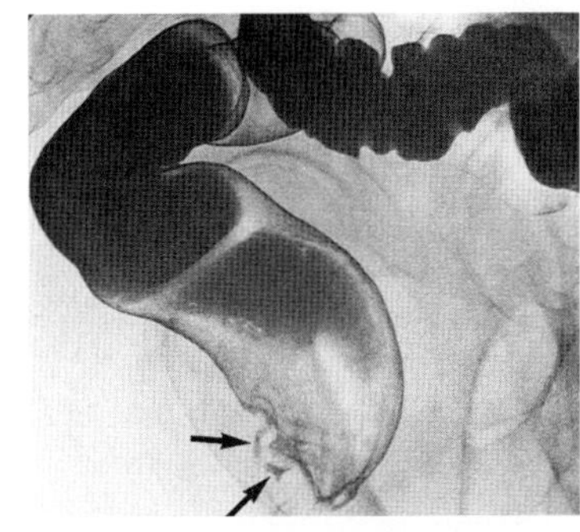

Fig. 8.38 Double-contrast barium enema demonstrating hidradenitis suppurativa. Tracks (arrows) extend from the perineum into the posterior wall of the rectum. (Reproduced with permission from reference 3, Fig. 5.)

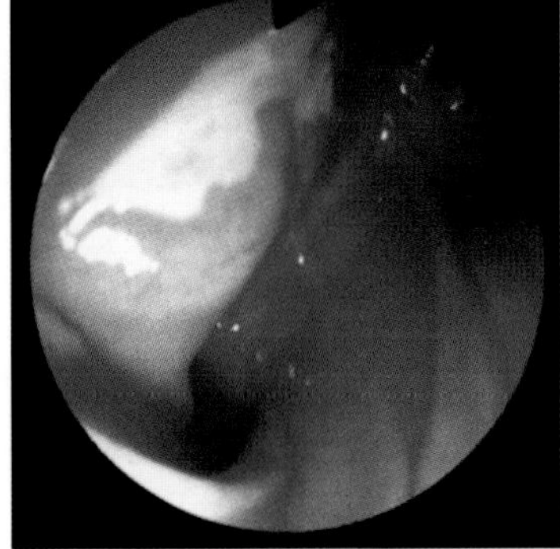

Fig. 8.39 Endoscopic appearance of solitary ulcer syndrome.

Solitary rectal ulcer syndrome (mucosal prolapse syndrome)

The solitary ulcer syndrome is characterized by an indolent, shallow, whitish ulcer surrounded by hyperemic mucosa (Figs 8.39, 8.40) on the anterior wall of the rectum, typically 7–10 cm from the margin. However, the lesions may be circumferential or multiple. There is usually some degree of intussusception of the anterior rectal wall into the anal canal, and its pathogenesis and presentation is the same as that of mucosal prolapse. The ulceration is probably caused by trauma to the mucosa during excessive straining against an actively contracting puborectalis (a muscle that usually relaxes at defecation), and post-inflammatory polyps are commonly seen also (Figs 8.41–8.44). On histological examination the surface epithelium is eroded and there is fibrosis of the lamina propria (Figs 8.44–8.47). Characteristically, muscle fibers extend upwards from the thickened muscularis into the mucosa. There is considerable telangiectasia of superficial capillaries, and submucosal vessels can also be thickened and hyalinized. It is no longer felt that solitary ulcer syndrome arises primarily from self-digitation, but ulceration in the distal rectum may be traumatic (Fig. 8.48), self-induced, or factitious (Fig. 8.49).

Rectal prolapse

Full-thickness rectal prolapse represents an intussusception of the rectum from a point typically some 8 cm above the anus. It may occur at any age but is found most often in elderly nulliparous women (Figs 8.50, 8.51); its cause is unknown.

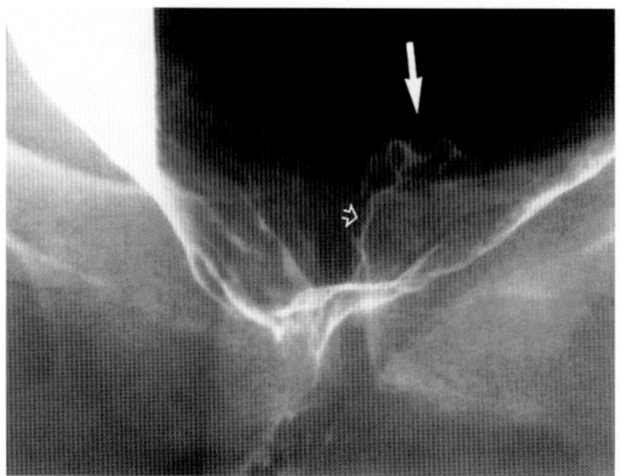

Fig. 8.40 Double-contrast barium enema in chronic mucosal prolapse syndrome (solitary rectal ulcer syndrome). Inflammatory cloacogenic polyp. A 1 cm polypoid lesion (large arrow) is seen associated with a thickened column of Morgagni (open arrow). (Reproduced with permission from reference 1, Fig. 6.)

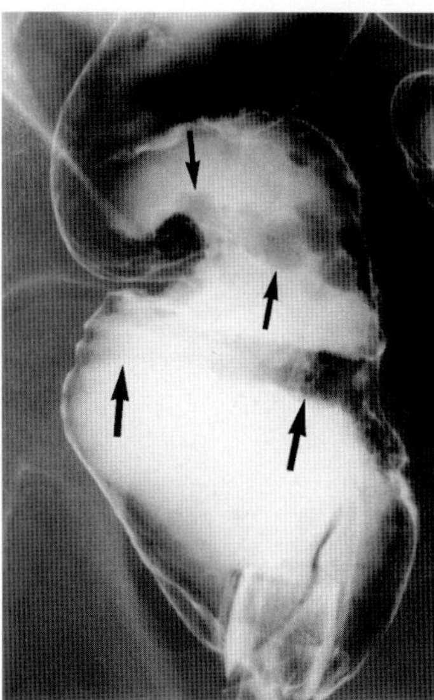

Fig. 8.41 An enlarged, lobulated valve of Houston (long arrows) is seen. The mucosa of the proximal rectum is coarsely lobulated (short arrows). (Reproduced with permission from reference 2, Fig. 68.57.)

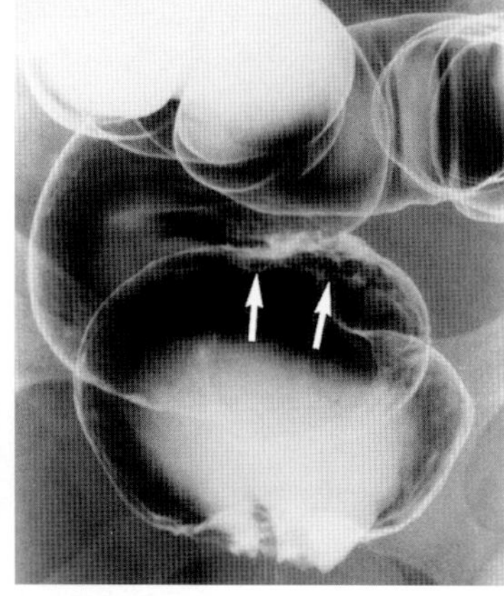

Fig. 8.42 A 2 cm area of focal mucosal nodularity (arrows) is seen in the mid rectum. (Reproduced with permission from reference 4.)

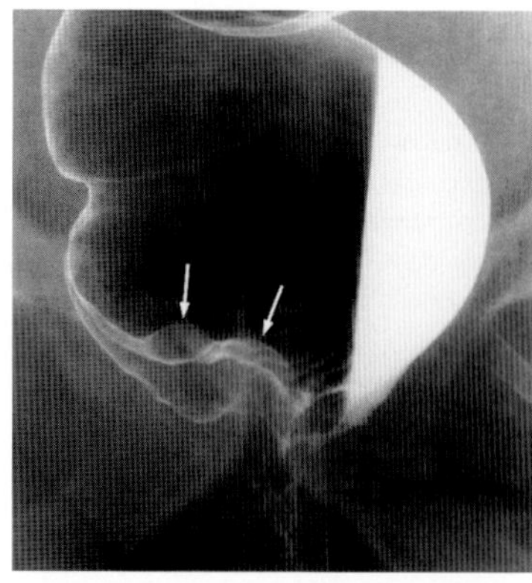

Fig. 8.43 Colitis cystica profunda. A bi-lobed, smooth-surfaced polypoid mass (arrows) arises from the right side of the rectum just proximal to the anorectal junction (Reproduced with permission from reference 2, Fig. 7.)

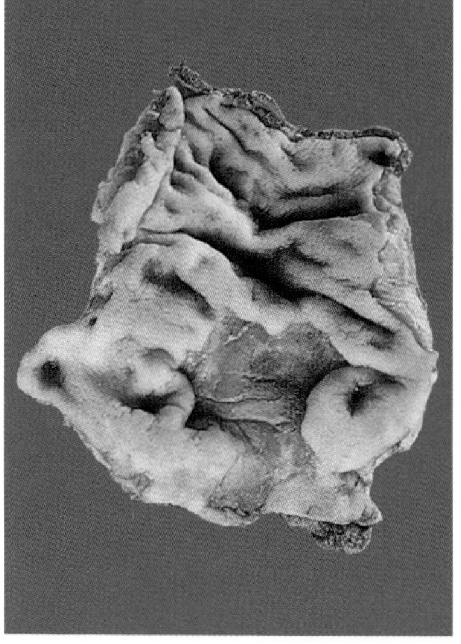

Fig. 8.44 An excised solitary ulcer.

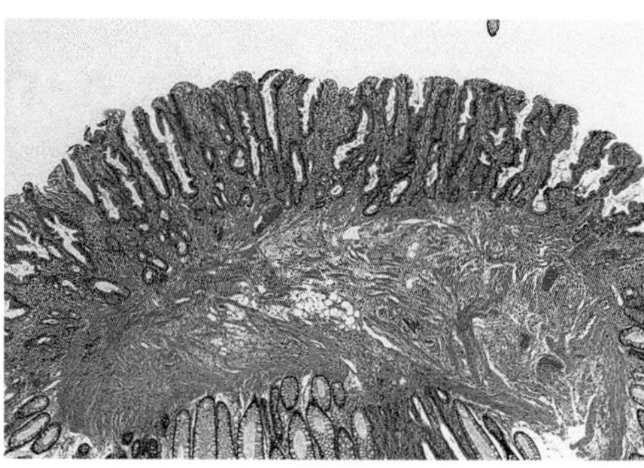

Fig. 8.45 Rectal prolapse. Microscopic view of prolapsed rectal mucosa in the solitary rectal ulcer syndrome showing the irregular shapes of the glands, the reactive, hyperplastic appearance of the epithelium, and the typically dense, eosinophilic stroma (fibromuscular replacement of the lamina propria).

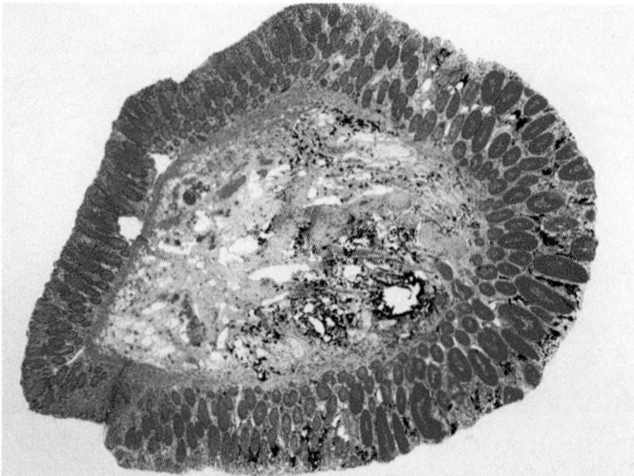

Fig. 8.46 Rectal prolapse. An iron stain shows deep blue-staining deposits of hemosiderin in the mucosa and submucosa, evidence of recent ischemic injury and hemorrhage.

Prolapse is usually associated with generalized laxity of the pelvic floor and defective sphincter function, but it also occurs with conditions in which intra-abdominal pressure is raised, such as cystic fibrosis (see Chapter 9), and should be distinguished from prolapse of an adenoma or other neoplasm (Figs 8.52, 8.53). Marked trau-

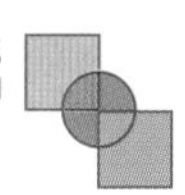

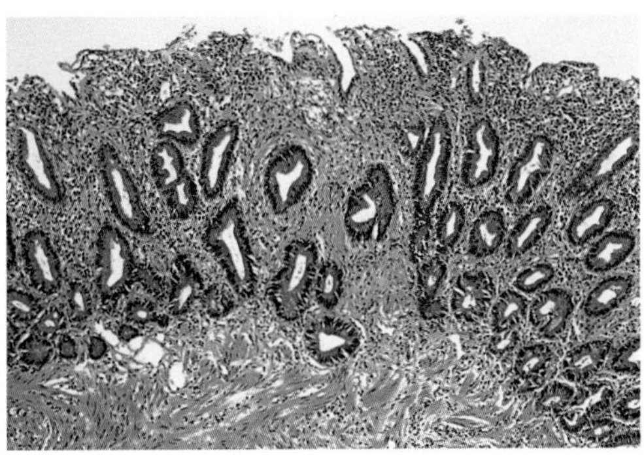

■ **Fig. 8.47** Higher magnification of prolapsed rectal mucosa in the solitary rectal ulcer syndrome, showing the characteristic fibromuscular replacement of the lamina propria. Evidence of ischemic injury includes erosion of the surface, withering of the epithelium in the luminal aspect of the glands, and reparative expansion of the basal proliferative compartment.

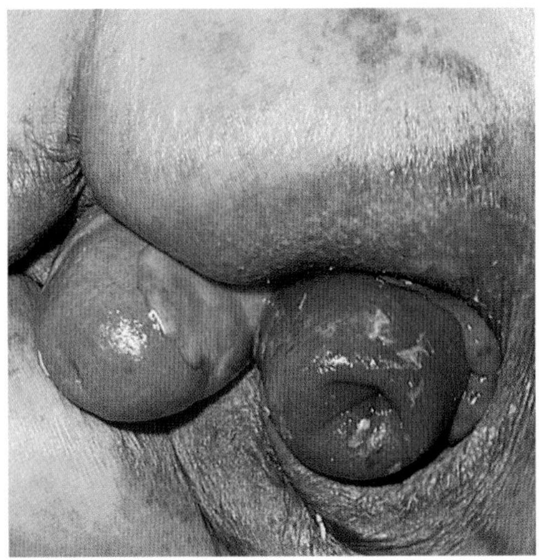

■ **Fig. 8.51** Complete rectal prolapse and complete vaginal procidentia in a nulliparous 95-year-old woman.

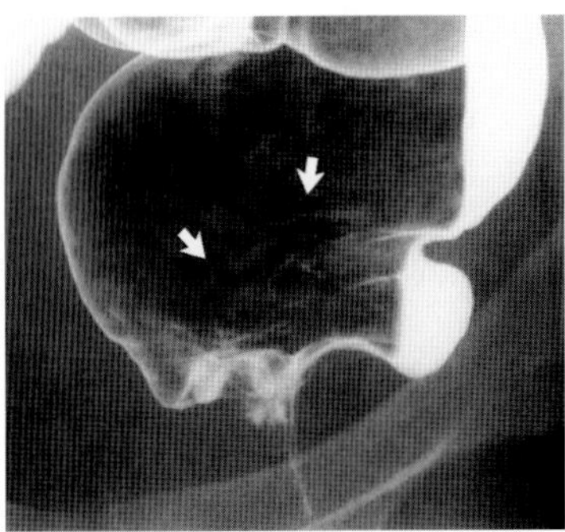

■ **Fig. 8.48** Double-contrast barium enema in patient with traumatic proctitis due to anal intercourse. Fine and coarse mucosal nodularity (arrows) is seen in the distal rectal mucosa. (Reproduced with permission from reference 2, Fig. 68.72.)

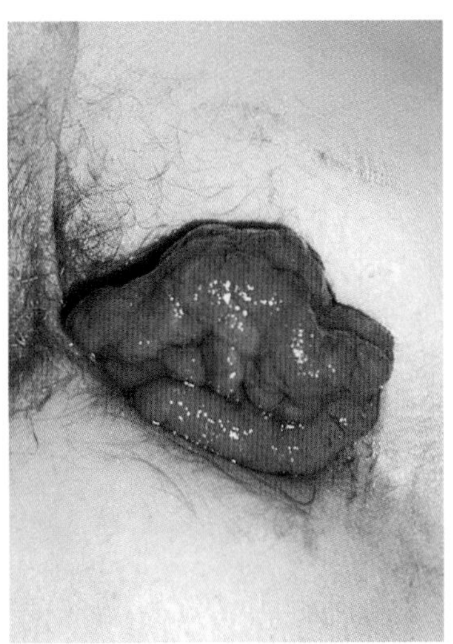

■ **Fig. 8.52** Prolapse of a sessile rectal adenoma in a patient who was found to have three other benign tumors and a sigmoid carcinoma.

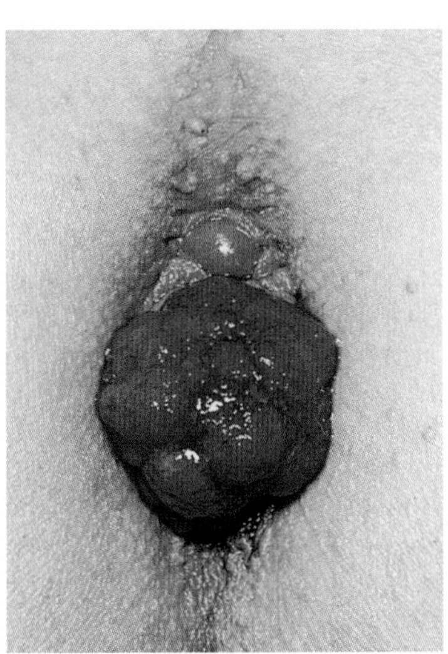

■ **Fig. 8.53** An intussuscepted pedunculated adenoma of the sigmoid colon.

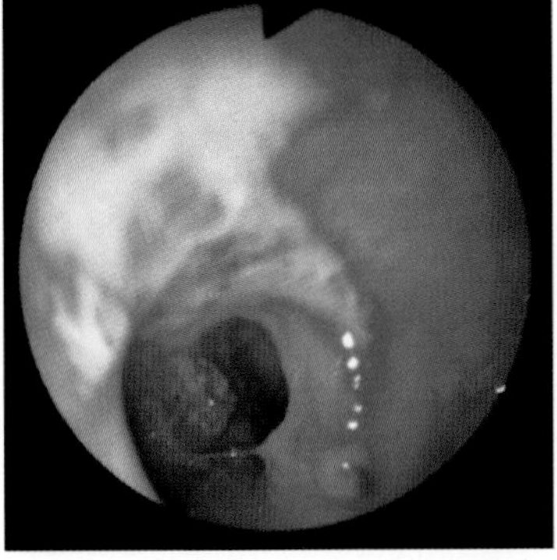

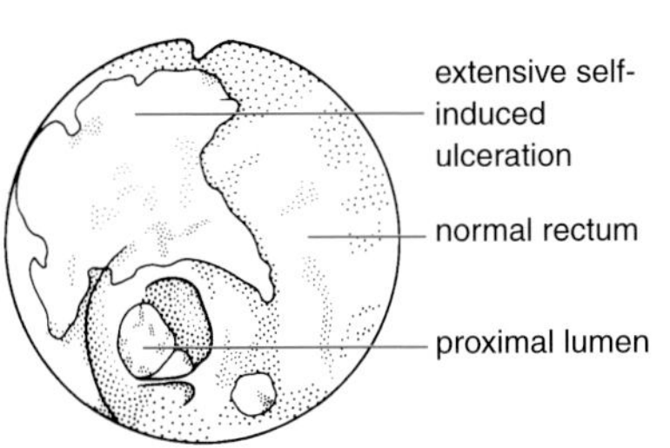

■ **Fig. 8.49** Extensive self-induced ulceration of the rectum.

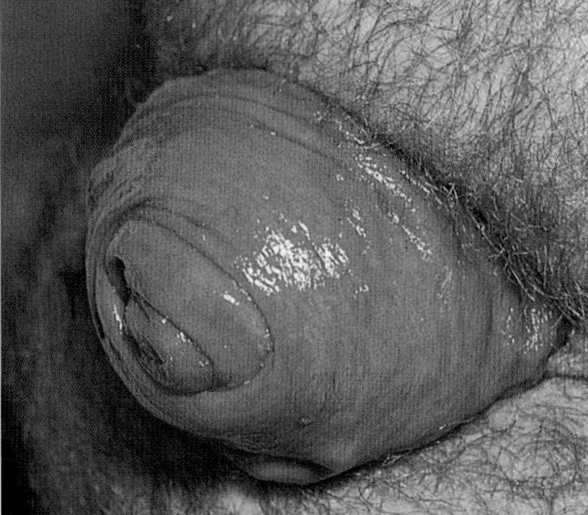

■ **Fig. 8.50** Complete full-thickness rectal prolapse. The mucosa may be reddened and the sphincter is always relaxed.

matic proctitis of the distal rectum may result. This is of course distinct from the less dramatic degrees of solely mucosal prolapse considered above. Straining will reveal the diagnosis when this is not obvious at rest, but it may be necessary for the patient to squat and strain. It is almost always possible to reduce rectal prolapse even when complete.

Descending perineum syndrome

Descent of the pelvic floor on straining (Fig. 8.54) may be present with complete prolapse, but may also occur on its own. Tenesmus, difficulty with evacuation with a need for digitation, and eventual incontinence are associated. Evacuation proctography may be helpful (Figs 8.54–8.58). Failure to relax the puborectalis will be demonstrated – a feature commonly associated with the solitary ulcer syndrome (Figs 8.59, 8.60). In some patients an associated anterior rectocele is found (Fig. 8.55), but the relationship of this to symptoms is far from clear. Small rectoceles are seen in the asymptomatic, and surgical repair is not usually appropriate. Internal prolapse of the anterior rectal wall is significant in disturbed defecation probably only if the wall prolapses before contrast has been passed at defecation proctography. Both rectum and small bowel may intussuscept into the anal canal when the perineal musculature is lax (Figs 8.56, 8.57, 8.61).

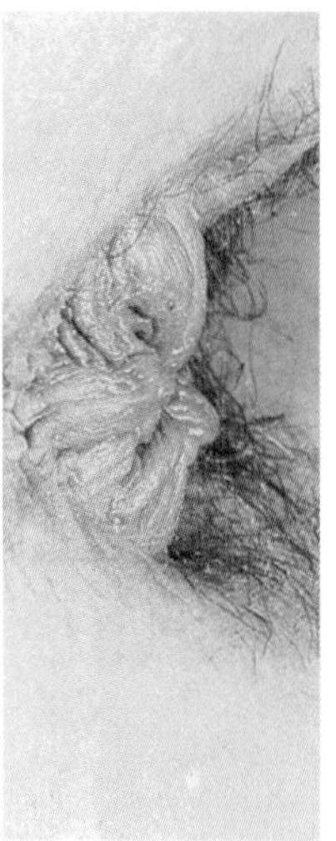

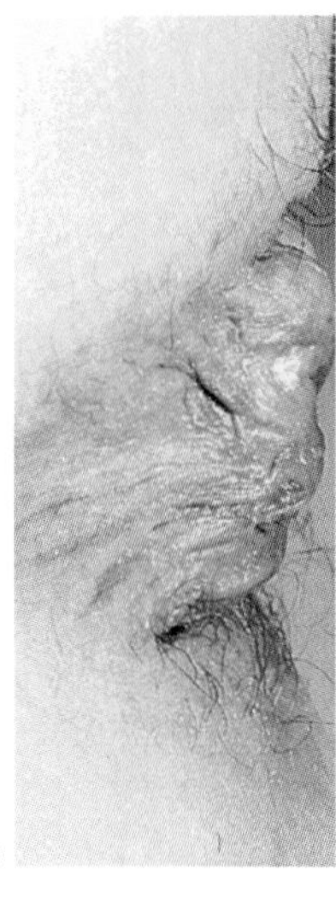

Fig. 8.54 Descending perineum syndrome showing the position of the anus at rest (a) and with straining (b).

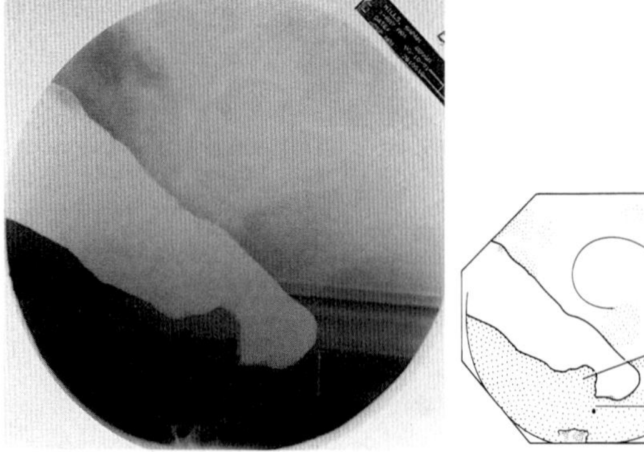

Fig. 8.59 Proctogram illustrating a failure of relaxation of puborectalis at defecation.

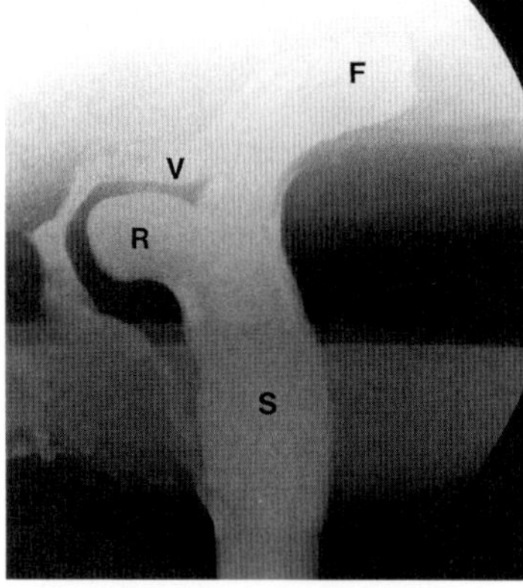

Fig. 8.55 Rectocele and intra-anal intussusception demonstrated during evacuation proctography with patient sitting on a commode and imaged in the right lateral position. Early in defecation the anal sphincter (S) is widely open. A small anterior rectocele (R) has formed and pushes on the vagina (V). F represents the top of the barium paste.

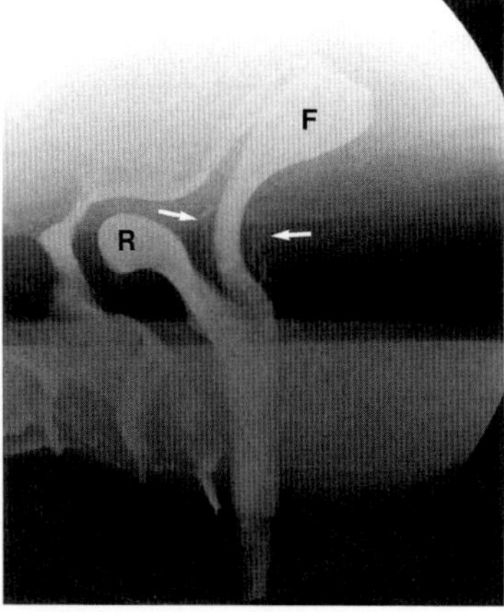

Fig. 8.56 The same patient as in Fig. 8.55. Toward the end of defecation, the rectum is intussuscepting, identified by barium-etched lines (arrows).

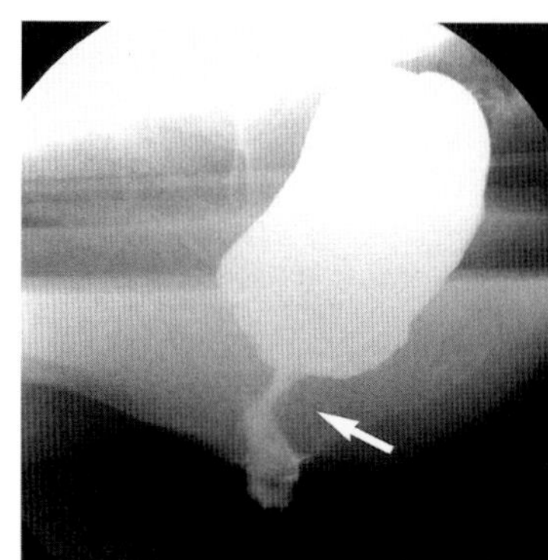

Fig. 8.60 Evacuation proctography demonstrating incomplete opening of the anal sphincter (arrow).

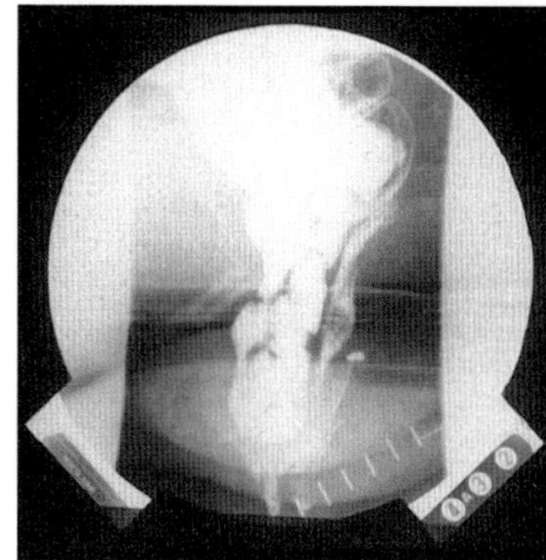

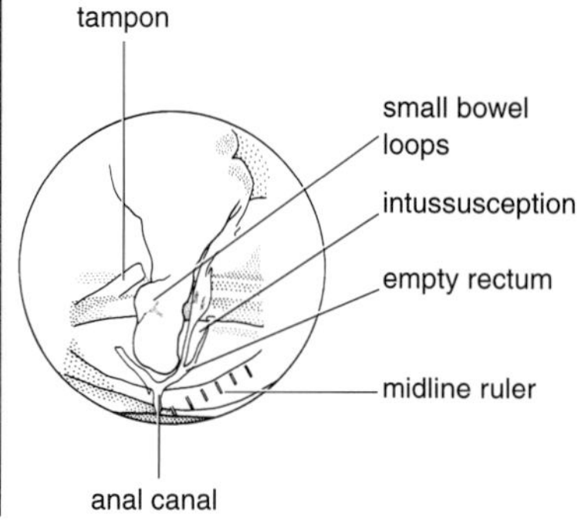

Fig. 8.61 Small bowel loops forming an enterocele with intussusception, shown at proctography.

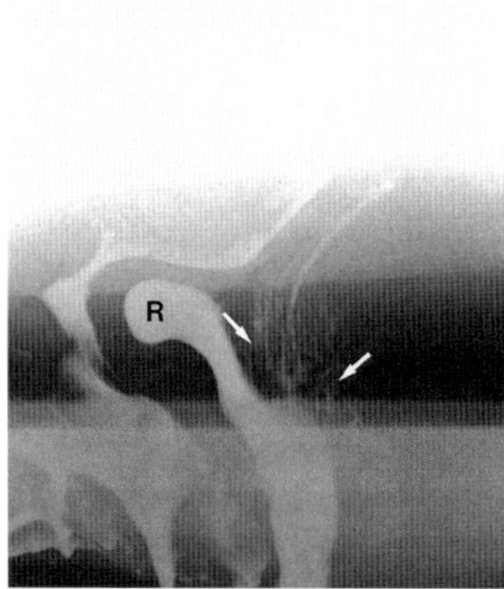

Fig. 8.57 The same patient as in Fig. 8.56. At the end of defecation, the rectum has intussuscepted (arrows) almost toward the edge of the anal canal. The rectocele (R) has incompletely evacuated.

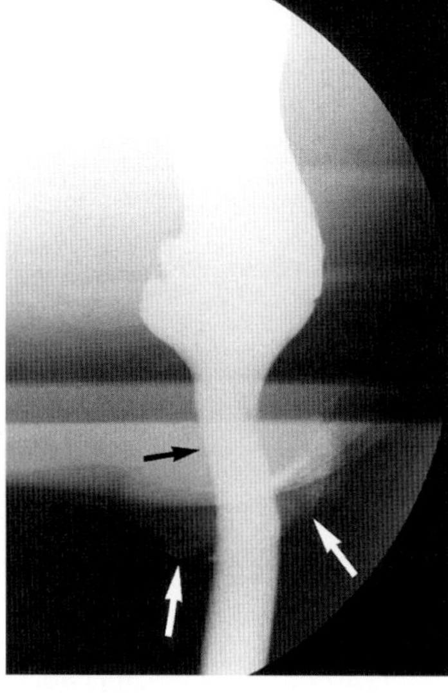

Fig. 8.58 Evacuation proctography demonstrating eversion of anal mucosa. Radiograph obtained during mid evacuation with open anal canal (black arrow). A 4 cm mound of tissue (white arrows) protrudes from the anal canal.

FECAL INCONTINENCE

Fecal incontinence has a number of causes including overt neurological and sphincter injury, but in the majority of cases the causes are more subtle. It may be a late manifestation of injury encountered in childbirth, or result from protracted straining at stool, with or without pathological perineal descent. In each case the cause is traction denervation. Perineal tears during parturition that involve the anal sphincter mechanism are well demonstrated by endoanal ultrasound, which can guide subsequent surgical repair (Figs 8.62, 8.63). Congenital abnormalities are rare, but a variety of obvious neurological disorders (e.g., multiple sclerosis and spinal injuries) are less so. Overflow incontinence remains a problem in the elderly. External and digital examinations are crucial and may provide a diagnosis. If not, ano-rectal manometry, defecating proctography, and endoanal ultrasound then become important tools. Electromyography (EMG) is painful and difficult to standardize and is now rarely used outside a research setting. Manometry will determine whether the anal sphincter tone is normal at rest and with maximal contraction, and what degree of perception/sensation

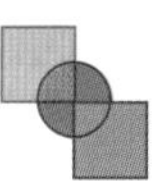

accompanies these. Proctography will assess function of the puborectalis muscle and adequacy of rectal emptying, determine whether there is perineal descent, and show rectoceles, enteroceles and rectal prolapse. Ultra-sound (and endoluminal magnetic resonance imaging) show the degree of muscle integrity. EMG, when performed, can determine whether the innervation of the external sphincter is intact, whether there are re-innervation changes (typical of pelvic neuropathy), and assess pudendal nerve function. Biofeedback is most likely to be helpful when abnormal sensory perception is coupled with normal voluntary sphincter contraction, as with situations of paradoxical contraction. Surgery is unlikely to be successful if there is prolonged motor latency of the pudendal nerve.

SEXUALLY TRANSMITTED DISEASES AFFECTING THE ANORECTUM

Condylomata acuminata

Condylomata acuminata (Fig. 8.64) are viral warts that are usually acquired sexually. They are rarely of serious significance but may be difficult to eradicate, and the possibility of late malignant transformation is not excluded (see anal neoplasia below). Although most often around the opening of the anus, warts may occur in the anal canal and even the lower rectum. Microscopically, there is underlying chronic inflammation, with marked epidermal hyperplasia and many vacuolated cells (Fig. 8.65).

Lymphogranuloma venereum

Lymphogranuloma venereum results from infection with *Chlamydia trachomatis*, and is most prevalent in tropical and sub-tropical climates. It is sexually transmitted and more common in men. The primary lesion is a small painless ulcer or vesicle on the external genitalia that disappears spontaneously within a few days leaving no scar. The secondary stage is manifest as an inguinal or genito-anorectal syndrome. In the inguinal syndrome, the inguinal lymph nodes become enlarged and painful with stretched, discolored overlying skin; these are then known as buboes (Fig. 8.66) and are accompanied by systemic symptoms. Suppuration and the formation of cutaneous sinus tracks may occur. The genito-anorectal syndrome is characterized by a non-specific hemorrhagic proctitis (Figs 8.67–8.69).

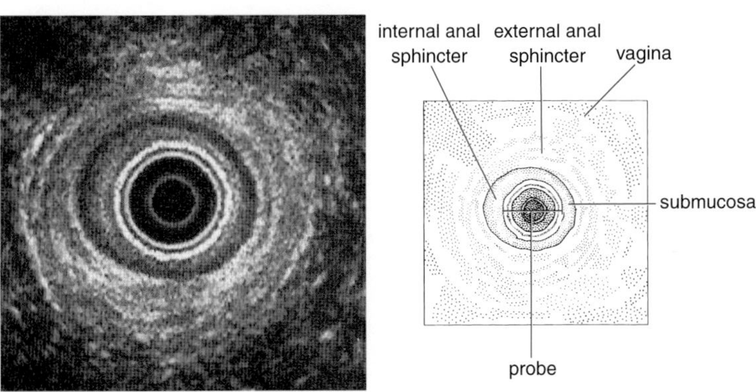

Fig. 8.62 Normal sonographic appearance of the mid-anal canal in a 24-year-old nulliparous woman. The vagina (anterior) is at the top. The internal anal sphincter, the external anal sphincter and the submucosa can be identified. Courtesy of Mr A. Sultan.

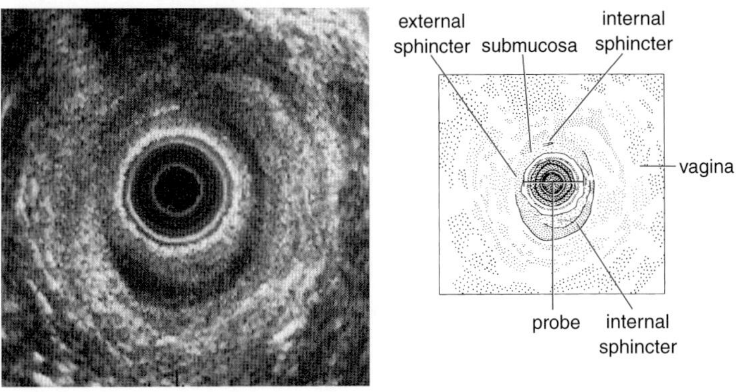

Fig. 8.63 Anal endosonography performed 6 months after delivery in a woman who developed fecal incontinence after a forceps delivery complicated by a third-degree tear. Courtesy of Mr. A. Sultan.

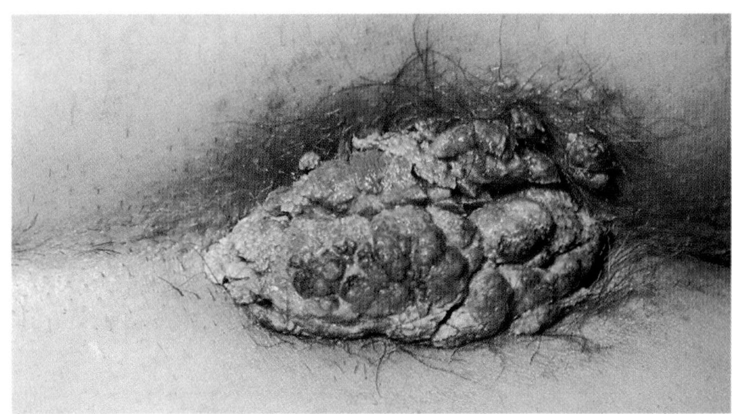

Fig. 8.64 Condylomata acuminata. Although the appearance is of a confluent lesion, it is in fact composed of multiple small warts with normal skin between. The anal canal and lower rectum should be examined to assess the full extent of the problem.

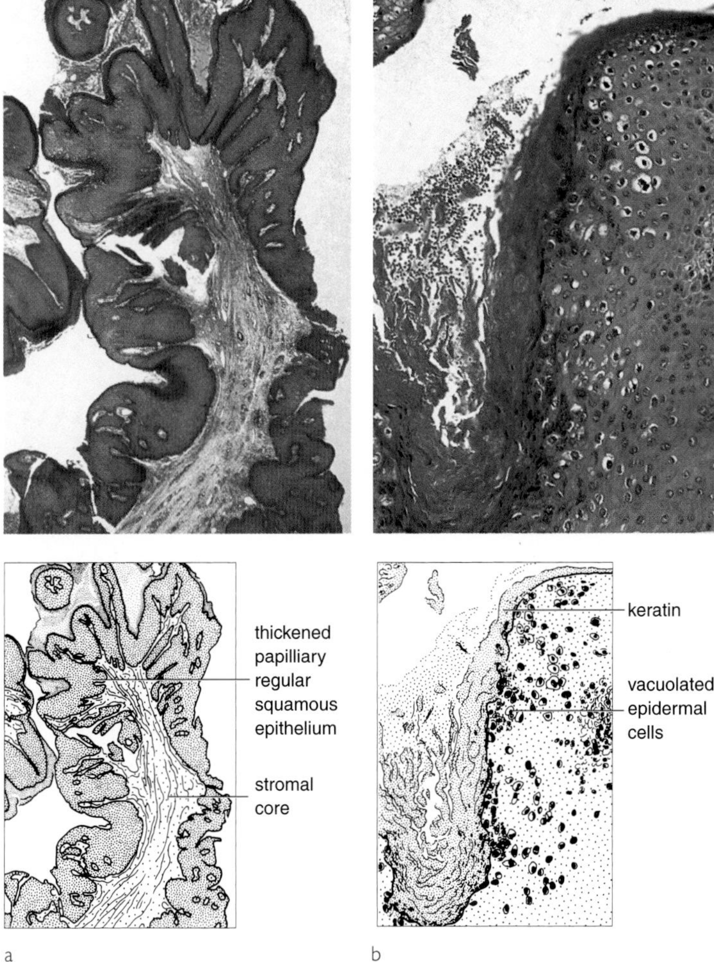

Fig. 8.65 The histology of condylomata acuminata: acanthosis (epithelial hyperplasia) and papillomatosis ((a), H&E stain (x 5)) are accompanied by characteristic cytoplasmic vacuolation ((b) H&E stain (x 120)).

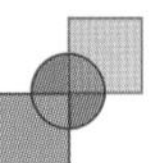

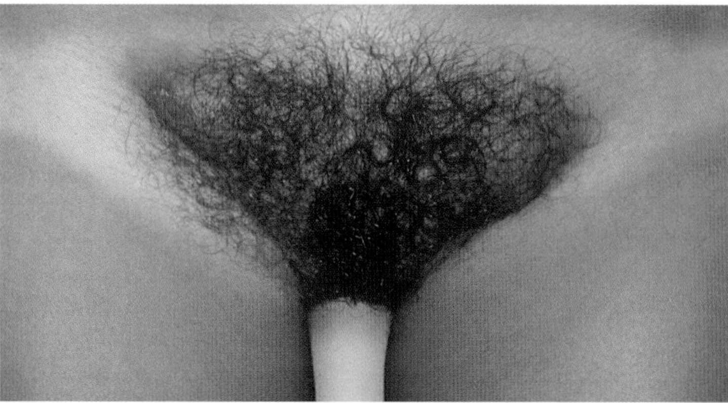

■ **Fig. 8.66** Bilateral buboes in lymphogranuloma venereum. Courtesy of Dr J. Bingham.

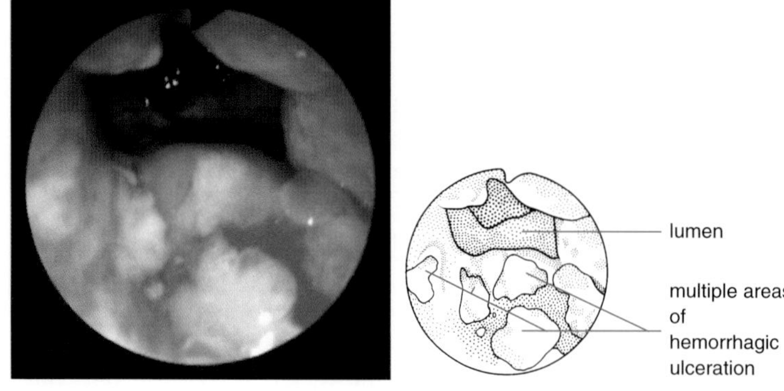

■ **Fig. 8.69** Sigmoidoscopic appearance of the severe proctitis that may occur in lymphogranuloma venereum.

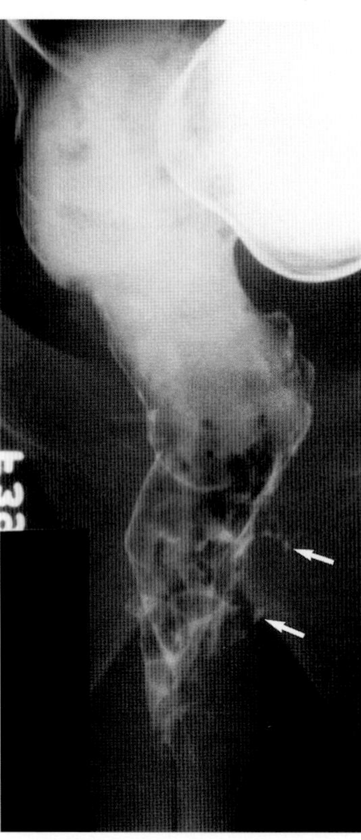

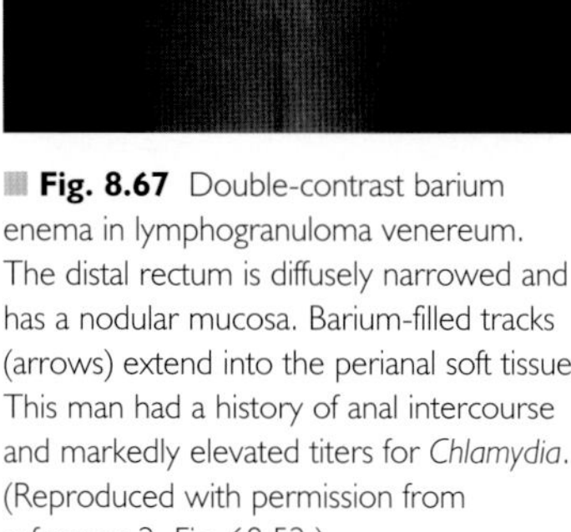

■ **Fig. 8.67** Double-contrast barium enema in lymphogranuloma venereum. The distal rectum is diffusely narrowed and has a nodular mucosa. Barium-filled tracks (arrows) extend into the perianal soft tissue. This man had a history of anal intercourse and markedly elevated titers for *Chlamydia*. (Reproduced with permission from reference 2, Fig. 68.52.)

■ **Fig. 8.68** Double-contrast barium enema in chronic lymphogranuloma venereum. The proximal rectum is diffusely narrowed (arrows). (Reproduced with permission from reference 2, Fig. 68.51.)

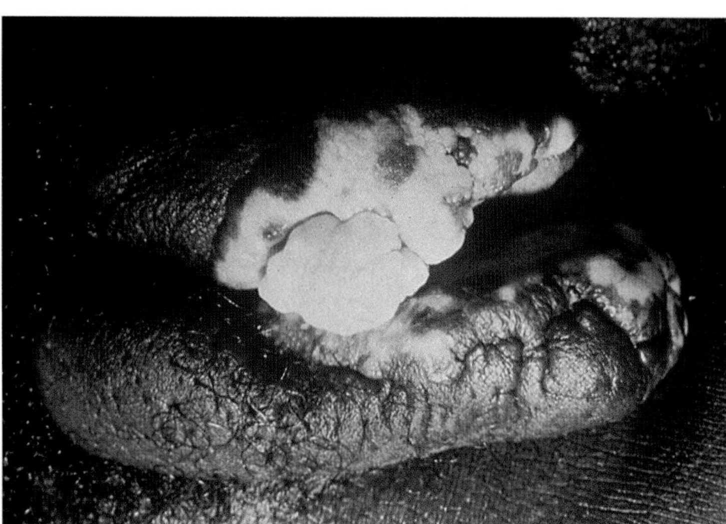

■ **Fig. 8.70** Vulval elephantiasis in lymphogranuloma venereum. Courtesy of Dr J. Bingham.

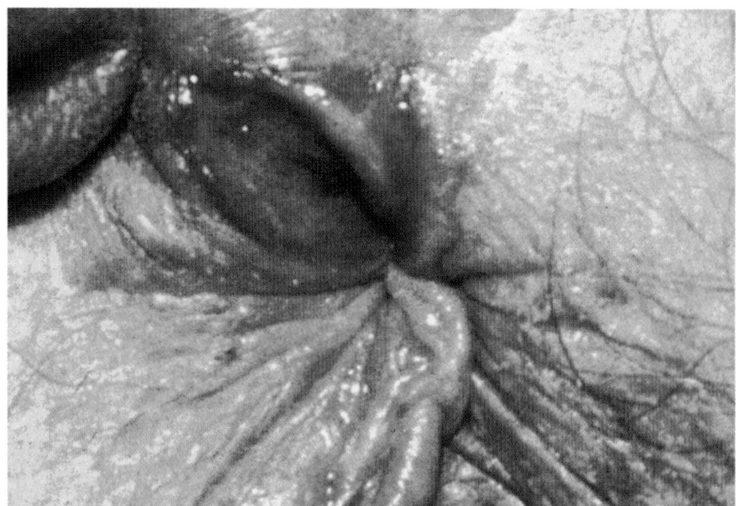

■ **Fig. 8.71** Primary chancre of the anus. Courtesy of Dr J. Bingham.

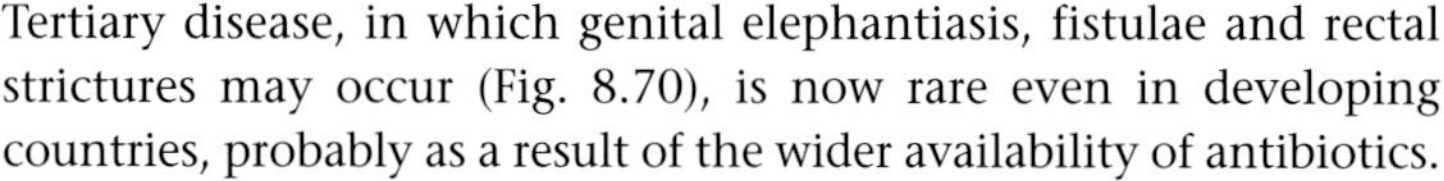

Tertiary disease, in which genital elephantiasis, fistulae and rectal strictures may occur (Fig. 8.70), is now rare even in developing countries, probably as a result of the wider availability of antibiotics.

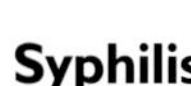

Syphilis

The classical primary syphilitic lesion is the painless ulcer or chancre (Fig. 8.71), but when the anorectum is affected, the lesions may be both painful and tender and are often associated with enlargement of the inguinal nodes. A seropurulent exudate is usual, matting together the hairs around the anus. Nevertheless, chancres heal spontaneously and rectal lesions in particular may be missed completely. The diagnosis is made from the demonstration of *Treponema pallidum* on dark ground illumination of serous fluid from the ulcers (Fig. 8.72)

Secondary syphilis causes condylomata lata. These highly infectious lesions appear as moist, elevated, erythematous papules in the perianal region (Fig. 8.73) and elsewhere. Anorectal syphilis is commoner in male homosexuals.

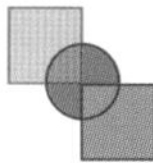

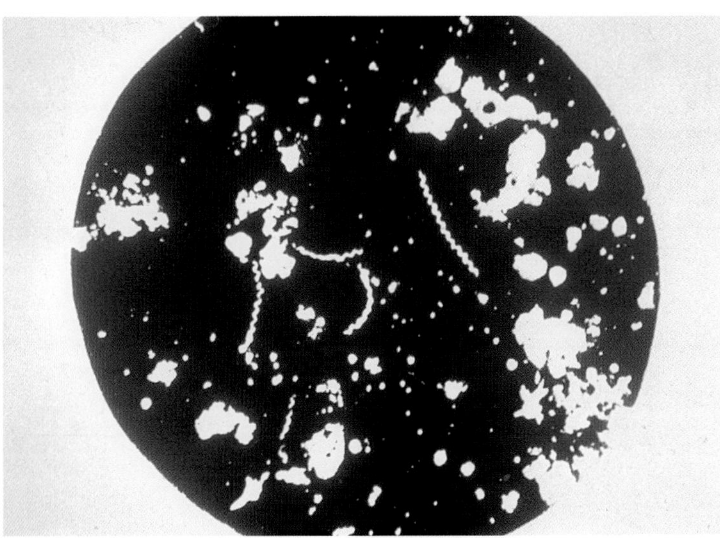

■ **Fig. 8.72** *Treponema pallidum*: dark ground illumination. Courtesy of Dr J. Bingham.

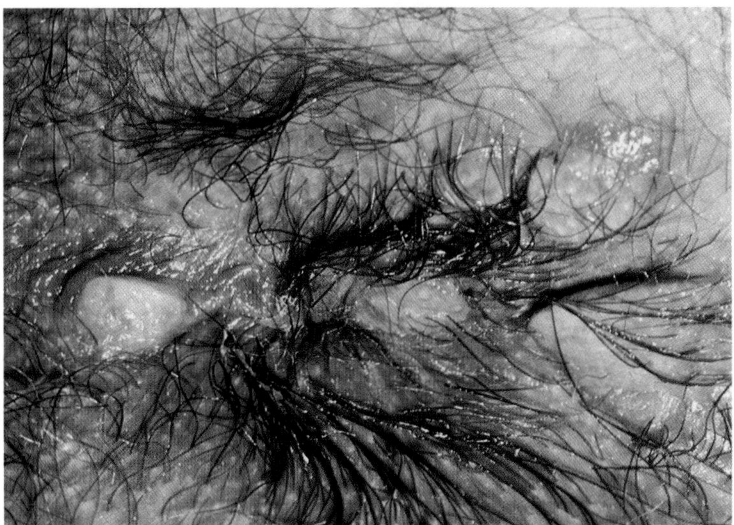

■ **Fig. 8.73** *Condylomata lata*. The flat, fleshy, pink lesions produce a large amount of discharge which mats together the hairs of the perineum. Courtesy of Dr V. Reynolds.

Gonorrhea

Infection of the rectum with *Neisseria gonorrhoea* is common on a worldwide basis. About a third of women with gonorrhea will have rectal involvement, regardless of whether or not anal sex has occurred, in contrast to males in whom rectal involvement is otherwise unusual. The infection is often asymptomatic (as in the urethral carrier state), but there may also be a local inflammatory response. Most such patients describe passage of mucus or muco-pus with the stools, together with rectal discomfort and burning. There may also be bleeding or diarrhea. Sigmoidoscopically, the rectal mucosa is congested, hemorrhagic and friable, with a generalized surface exudate. The organism will only be grown if rectal swabs are immediately placed into an appropriate transport medium and then incubated on highly selective culture media (Fig. 8.74). Rectal biopsy is commonly normal or shows only minimal abnormalities, but in those with a florid proctitis the pattern is similar to that of bacterial dysentery (see Chapter 6).

BENIGN AND PREMALIGNANT CONDITIONS

Viral warts are discussed above, and anal canal adenomas can be considered with rectal adenomas in all crucial particulars (see Chapter 7). Benign polyps of lymphoid origin are also seen (Fig. 8.75). The anal margin shares some of the pathologies seen at other sites of the mucocutaneous junction. In extra-mammary Paget's disease, a reddened, ulcerated, crusting, and scaling lesion is present (Fig. 8.76). Typical Paget's cells are found in the epidermis and may spread down the sweat gland ducts (Figs 8.77–8.79). There is a strong association with adjacent glandular adenexal carcinoma, or regional internal cancer. Keratoacanthoma and Bowen's disease may also be seen.

Malignant neoplasms of the anal canal

Malignancies of the anal canal are appropriately considered separately from those of the anal margin, because of the pattern of spread. Anal canal tumors, which arise above the line of valves in the so-called transitional zone, invade as much as do those of the distal rectum, while tumors of the margin arising from the epithelium up to and including the line of the anal valves behave as skin tumor and spread via the inguinal nodes.

Malignant neoplasms of the anal canal, which are commoner in women, need to be distinguished from adenocarcinomas of the rectum, presenting at the anus (Fig 8.80), since their staging and therapy are clearly different. True anal canal neoplasms are rarer. Pain, pruritus, tenesmus, and bleeding, from ulcerated, indurated lesions with rolled edges are typical (Fig. 8.81). Extensive local invasion is usual by the time of diagnosis (Fig. 8.82), and spread to the inguinal nodes or lymphatics is common, although enlarged inguinal nodes often prove only to be reactive. Despite the apparently obvious distinction from benign lesions such as hemorrhoids (see above), delayed diagnosis still occurs. True tumors arise from the transitional mucosa between the rectal mucosa and the squamous epithelium of the anal margin; most are squamous carcinomas (Fig. 8.83). There may be a histological resemblance to basal cell lesions, and a spectrum from squamous through basal and transitional epithelium to a glandular pattern is recognized (Figs 8.84–8.87). Anal squamous cell carcinoma with a predominantly basaloid differentiation pattern was formerly known as 'cloacogenic carcinoma,' but this

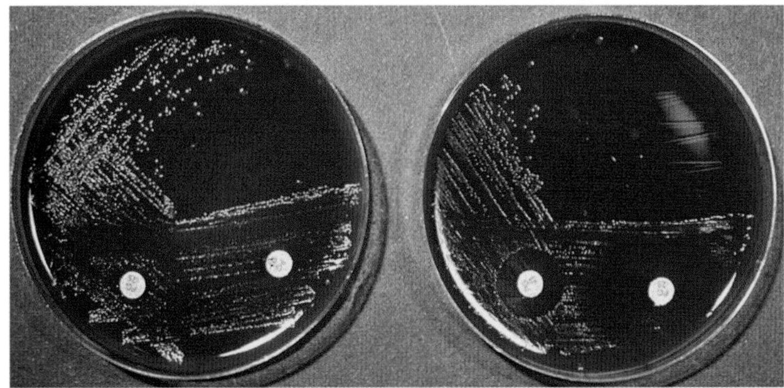

■ **Fig. 8.74** Culture plates of *Neisseria gonorrhoeae*. Antibiotic-impregnated disks demonstrate likely sensitivities. Courtesy of Dr J. Bingham.

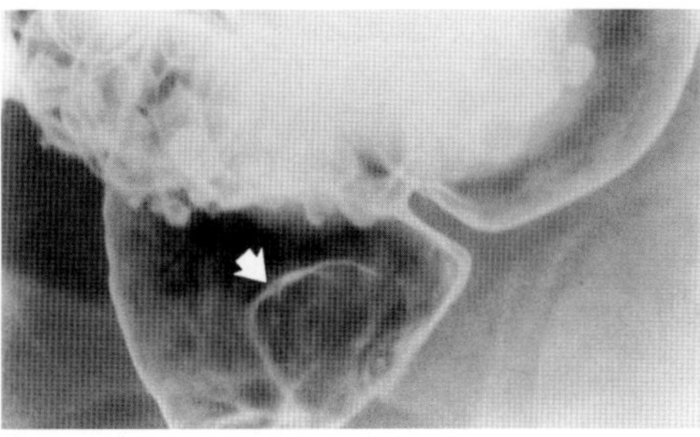

■ **Fig. 8.75** Double-contrast barium enema demonstrating lymphoid polyp just proximal to the anal canal. A finely lobulated polypoid mass (arrow) is seen. (Reproduced with permission from reference 2, Fig. 68.16.)

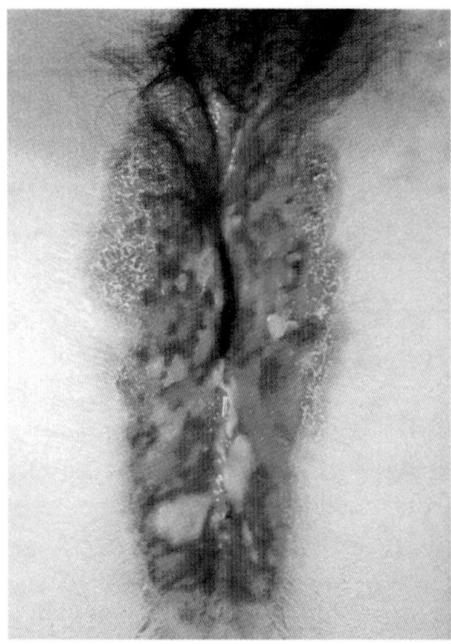

Fig. 8.76 Paget's disease of the perianal skin – abnormal skin in this area should always be biopsied to establish a diagnosis rather than assumed to be harmless eczema or dermatitis.

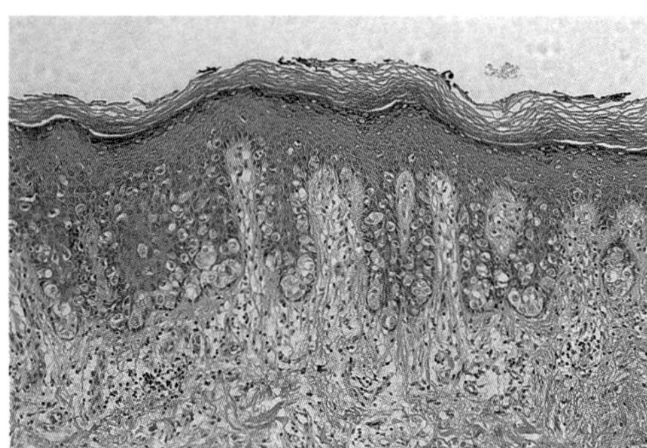

Fig. 8.77 Anal Paget's disease. Perianal skin showing the elongated rete ridges of the epidermis (keratinized squamous epithelium) containing clusters of large pale tumor cells.

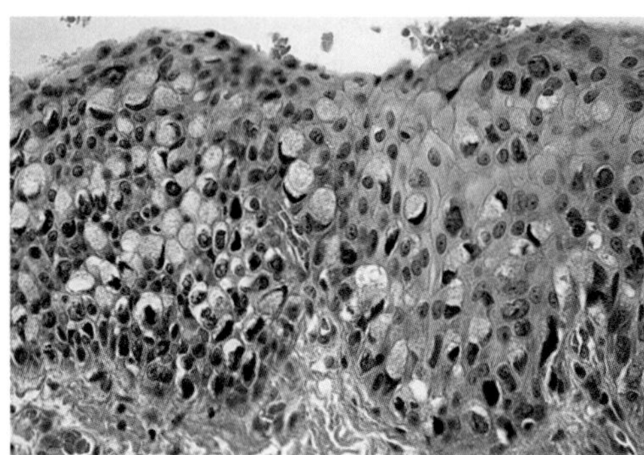

Fig. 8.78 Anal Paget's disease. Mucosa of the anal canal (non-keratinized squamous epithelium) showing numerous mucin-producing tumor cells within the epithelium. The tumor cells have a signet-ring cell morphology with a large pale cytoplasmic mucin vacuole that compresses the nucleus to the cell periphery, giving it a crescent shape.

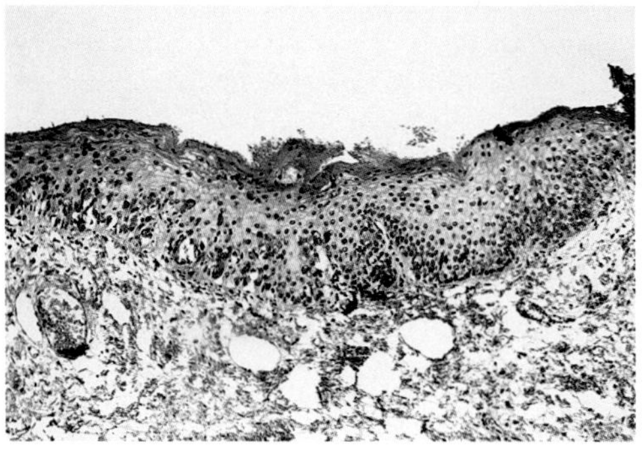

Fig. 8.79 Anal Paget's disease. Immunohistochemical stain for cytokeratin 7, a sensitive method for detecting Paget's cells, showing intense positive staining of the intraepithelial tumor cells.

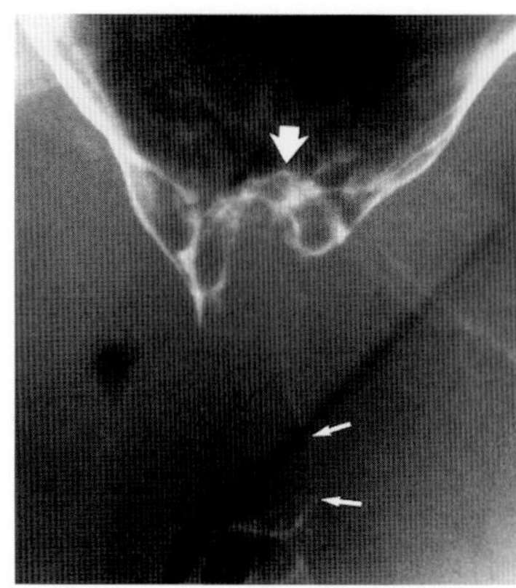

Fig. 8.80 Double-contrast barium enema in rectal adenocarcinoma invading anal canal. A 2 cm polypoid mass (thick arrow) is seen in the distalmost rectum. The anal canal is deformed (small arrows). At surgery the tumor invaded the anal canal and spread into perirectal fat. (Reproduced with permission from reference 1, Fig.11.)

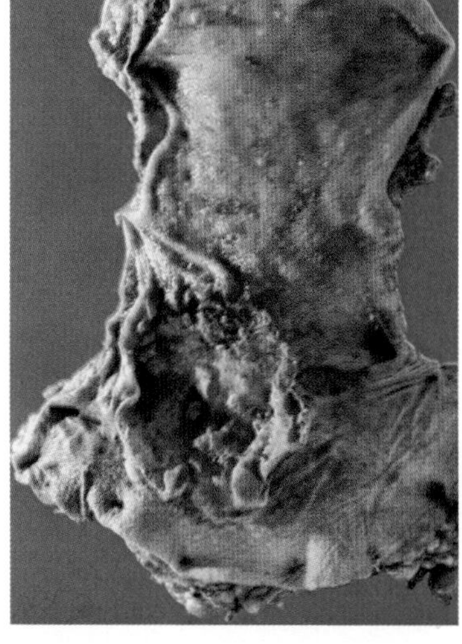

Fig. 8.81 Macroscopic appearance of an ulcerating anal canal carcinoma.

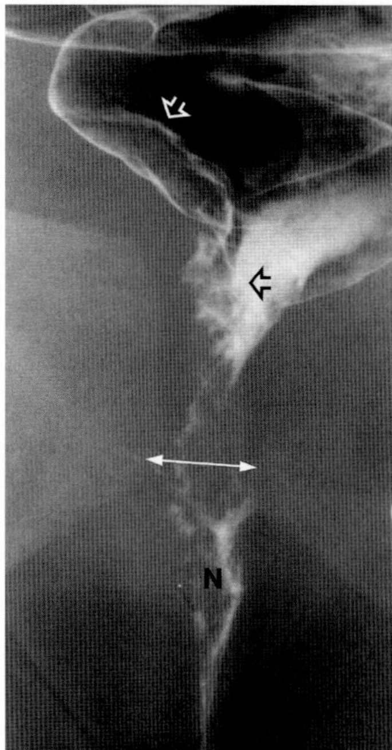

Fig. 8.82 Double-contrast barium enema in a patient with verrucous carcinoma of anal canal invading distal rectum. Nodular tissue (N) is in the perineum at the origin of the anal canal. The anal canal is widened by tumor (double arrow). Infiltrating tumor forms a polypoidal mass (open arrows) in the distal rectum. (Reproduced with permission from reference 1, Fig.13.)

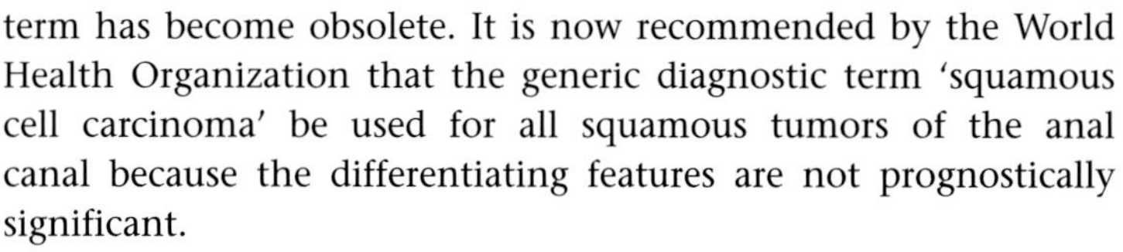

term has become obsolete. It is now recommended by the World Health Organization that the generic diagnostic term 'squamous cell carcinoma' be used for all squamous tumors of the anal canal because the differentiating features are not prognostically significant.

Malignant melanoma has a bluish/black color and a polypoid appearance, and is thus easily mistaken for a thrombosed external hemorrhoid (Figs 8.88, 8.89). The tumor is highly malignant and metastasizes rapidly. The histology is that of melanoma at other sites (Figs 8.90, 8.91).

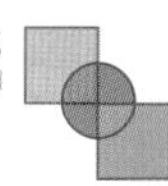

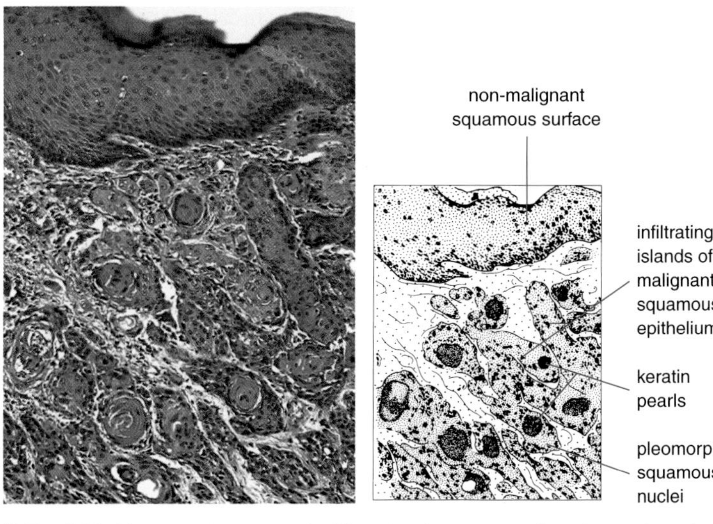

■ **Fig. 8.83** Histology of a moderately differentiated squamous cell carcinoma; irregular islands show keratinization, but there is considerable variation in nuclear size and shape. H&E stain (x 50).

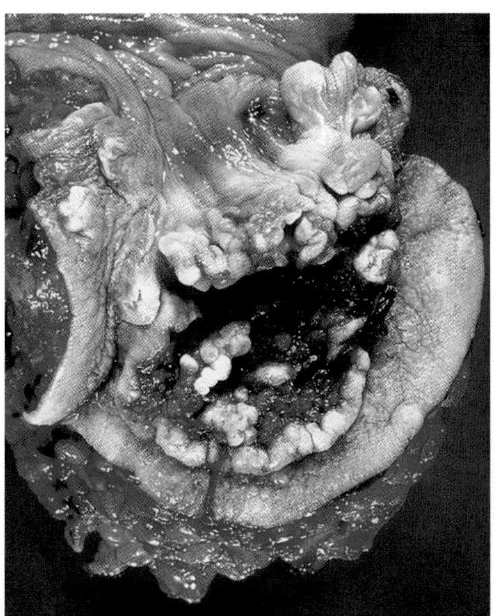

■ **Fig. 8.84** Squamous cell carcinoma of the anal canal. Surgical resection specimen of a squamous cell carcinoma of the anal canal showing a large tan-white ulcerating tumor with raised nodular edges in the anal canal just below the dentate line.

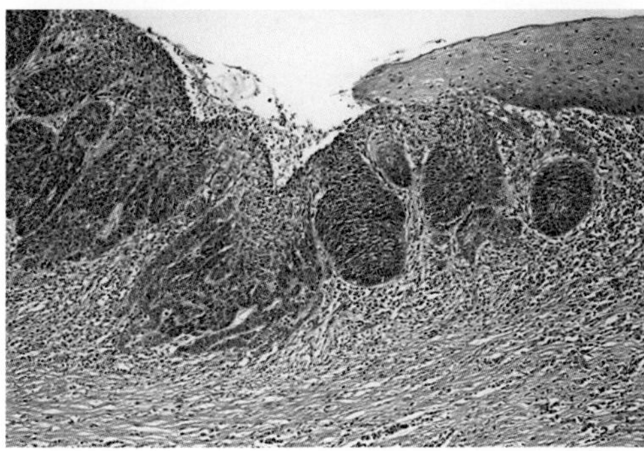

■ **Fig. 8.85** Microscopic view of the periphery of an ulcerating squamous cell carcinoma of the anal canal showing irregular nests of basaloid tumor cells invading the lamina propria and undermining the adjacent anal canal mucosa. Prominent basaloid features and small tumor cell size are related to infection with 'high-risk' human papilloma virus.

Malignant neoplasms of the anal margin

The anal margin is host to squamous (Fig. 8.92) and basal cell carcinomas (Fig. 8.93), with about 80% having the former histology. They are both commoner in males and behave similarly to their counterparts at other sites on the skin. Distinction between a slow-growing verrucous carcinoma and a benign, giant condyloma may be difficult. All lesions should therefore be assessed histologically

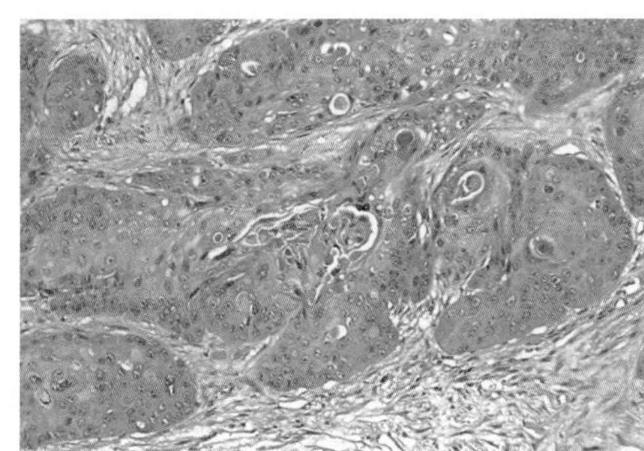

■ **Fig. 8.86** Squamous cell carcinoma of the anal canal. Microscopic view showing a focus of keratinizing tumor with nests of large eosinophilic cells forming numerous keratin 'pearls' (whorls of terminally differentiated cells undergoing apoptosis and producing eosinophilic bodies, some of which show pyknotic nuclei).

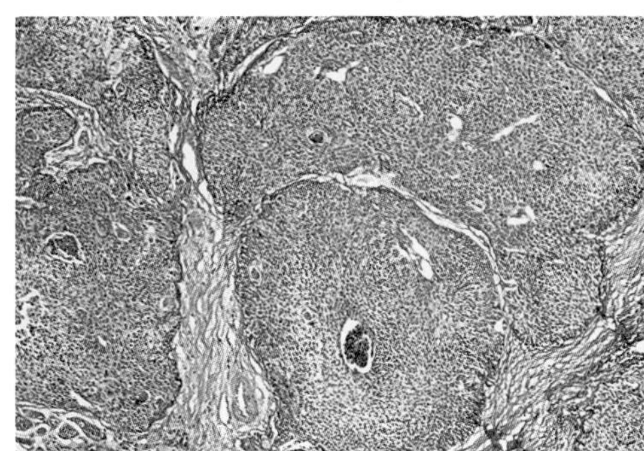

■ **Fig. 8.87** Squamous cell carcinoma of the anal canal. Microscopic view showing a focus of non-keratinizing tumor composed of nests of small tumor cells without peripheral pallisading.

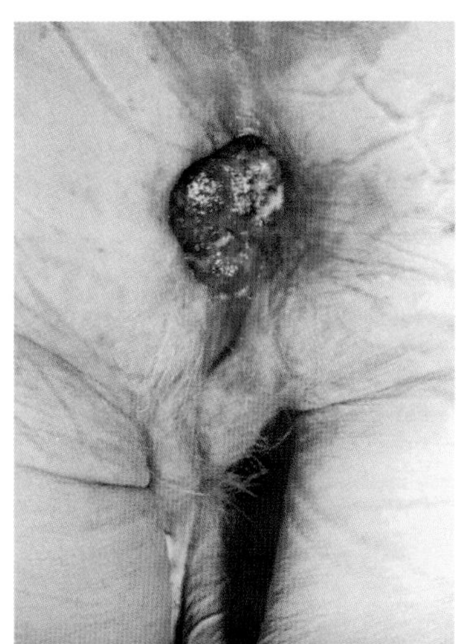

■ **Fig. 8.88** Malignant melanoma of the anal canal.

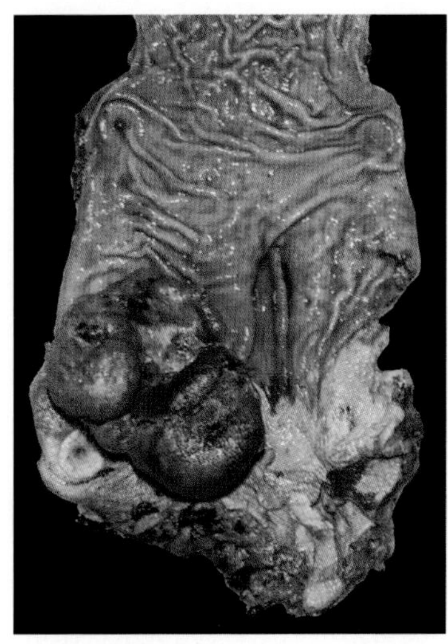

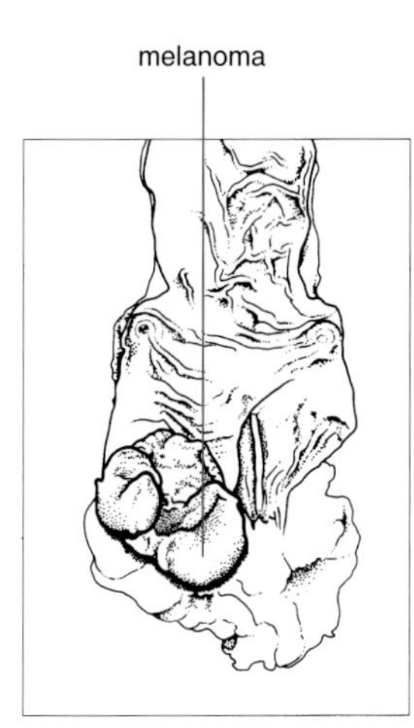

■ **Fig. 8.89** Macroscopic appearance of a polypoid melanoma of the anal canal.

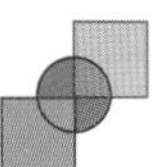

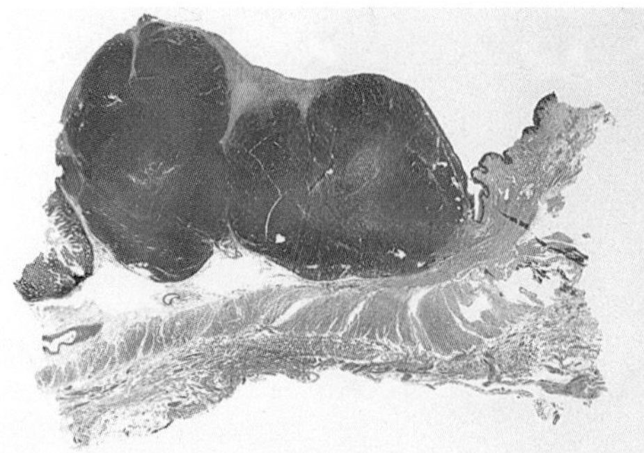

■ **Fig. 8.90** Melanoma of the anal canal. Whole-mount microscopic view showing confluent masses of tumor cells located at the dentate line showing glandular mucosa proximally (left), squamous mucosa distally (right), and ulceration of the mucosa overlying the tumor.

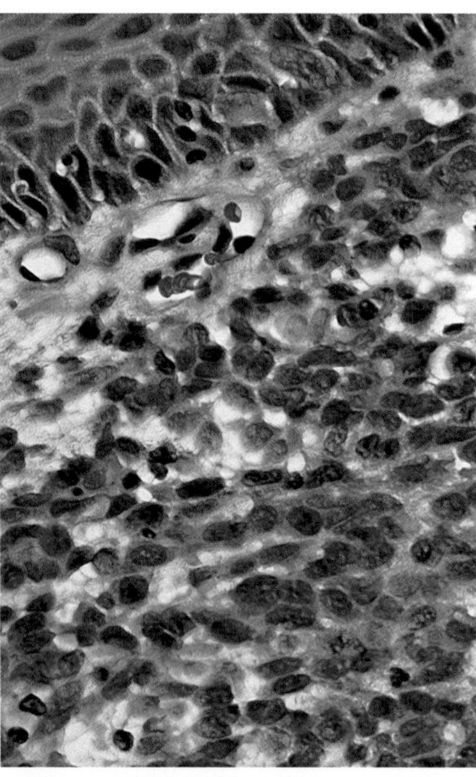

■ **Fig. 8.91** Anal melanoma. High-magnification view showing plump hyperchromatic and pleomorphic tumor cells, some of which show brown melanin pigment in their cytoplasm.

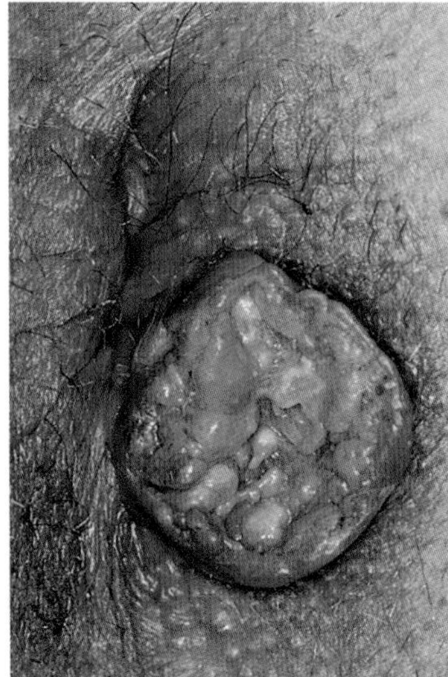

■ **Fig. 8.92** A well-differentiated squamous carcinoma of the anal margin (1 cm in diameter).

(Figs 8.94, 8.95), preferably after excision biopsy. Squamous carcinoma of the anal margin is almost certainly related to human papilloma virus infection. Initial figures in which about half of all squamous tumors at this site had DNA of papilloma virus type 16 and/or 18 within the tumor cell genome have risen to exceed 80% in most recent series. There appears also to be a sequence from prior intra-epithelial neoplasia, analogous to the carcinoma *in situ* recognized in cervical screening. Anal cancers occur at greatly increased frequency in patients with AIDS, and Kaposi's sarcoma may also be seen at this site.

CONGENITAL ANORECTAL ANOMALIES

There are several congenital anorectal anomalies, varying from anal stenosis and imperforate anus through to complete ano-rectal agenesis.

Agenesis accounts for over 75% of anorectal atresias and is often complicated by vaginal, vesical, or urethral fistula (Fig. 8.96). Anal stenosis is usually manifest at birth, with the presence of a small anal aperture containing a dot of meconium (Fig. 8.97). The abdomen may be distended, and defecation – if possible – results in a ribbon-like stool. Fecal impaction and secondary megacolon may occur. During the neonatal period an imperforate anal membrane becomes evident from the failure to pass meconium. A greenish bulging membrane may be visible on examination. The management of anal stenosis and imperforate anal membrane is generally straightforward, with dilatation or simple surgical incision, although subsequent incontinence may occasionally occur. In infants with anorectal agenesis, the most important prognostic and management factor is the site of the abnormality, and whether it is high (supralevator), or low (translevator). The outlook following surgery is good if the

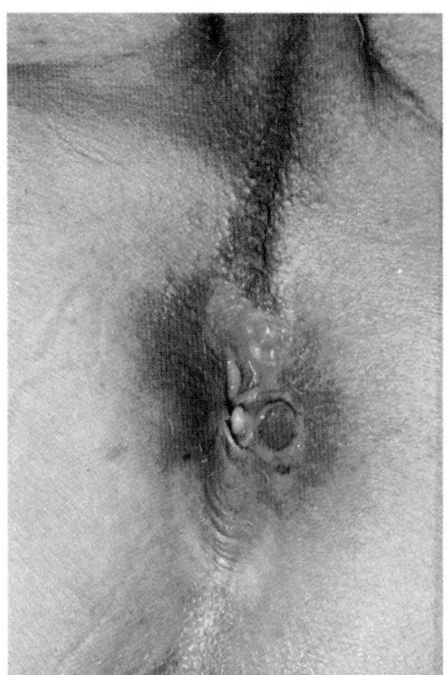

■ **Fig. 8.93** A basal cell carcinoma with a rolled edge.

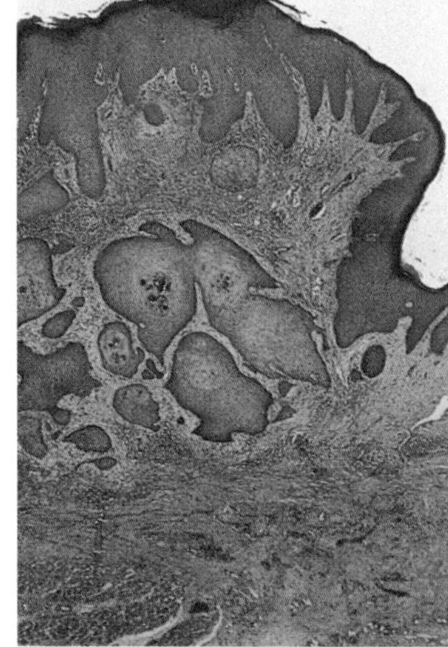

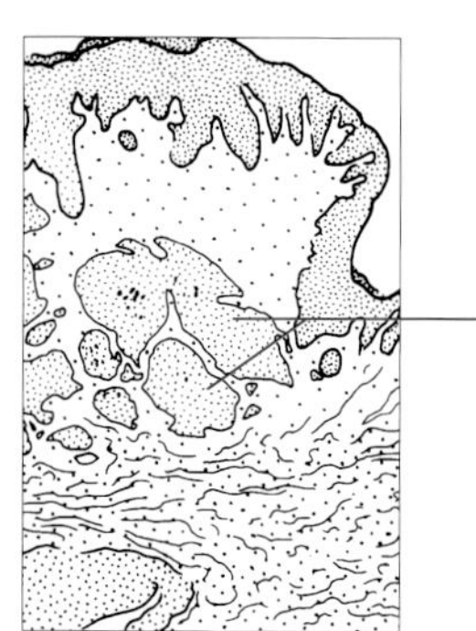

■ **Fig. 8.94** Histology of a well-differentiated squamous cell carcinoma. H&E stain (x 10).

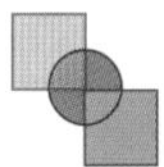

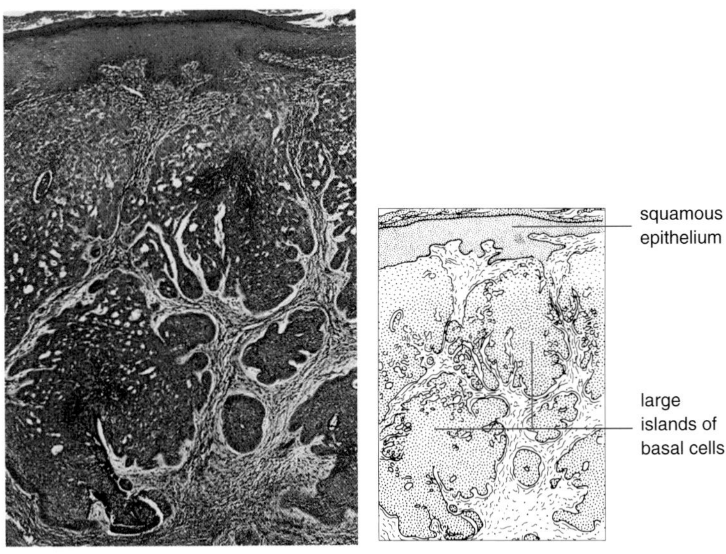

■ **Fig. 8.95** Histology of a basal cell carcinoma in which cystic spaces produce an adenoid appearance. H&E stain (x 20).

LOW AND HIGH ANO-RECTAL AGENESIS

levator ani

normal

covered anus

without fistula

recto-urethral fistula

rectovaginal fistula

■ **Fig. 8.96** Diagrams illustrating low and high ano-rectal agenesis.

bowel has passed through the puborectalis sling during embryological development prior to the development of the abnormalities (Fig. 8.96). However, higher abnormalities (Fig. 8.96), are usually associated with a recto-urethral fistula in the male, or rectovaginal fistula in the female (Fig. 8.96), and necessitate surgical reconstruction. Occasionally there are intact sphincters and normal bowel, but incontinence because the bowel lies anterior to the sphincters (Fig. 8.98).

Radiological examination to determine the site of the abnormality classically relied on an 'invertogram' in which, after the baby was held upside down for a few moments, the air bubble in the distal bowel was related to skeletal markers in the pelvis. Equivalent information is obtained from the prone lateral shoot-through film (Figs 8.99, 8.100). Although this may help to exclude sacral agenesis it is unreliable, and the exact site of the blockage is better determined by running contrast medium into the distal loop of the colon after a colostomy has been performed to relieve the obstruction (Fig. 8.101). CT and, more recently, MRI are sometimes additionally informative (Fig. 8.98). MRI is particularly suited to visualizing anorectal anomalies because of its multiplanar ability and lack of ionizing radiation. In addition to sacral agenesis (Figs 8.98, 8.102), other congenital anomalies such as dermoids (Figs 8.103, 8.104) may be demonstrated.

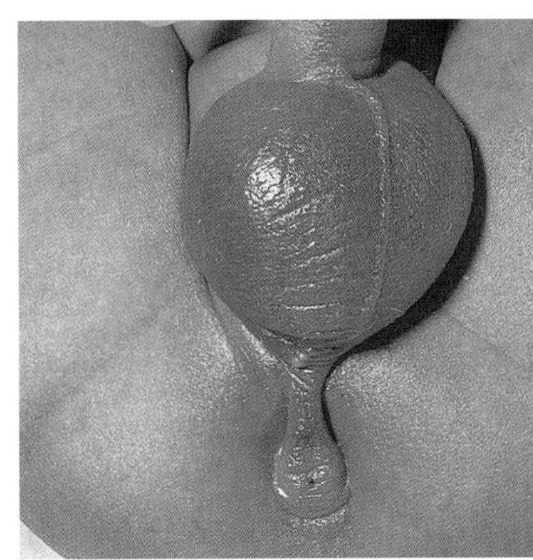

■ **Fig. 8.97** Severe anal stenosis. Courtesy of Miss V. Wright.

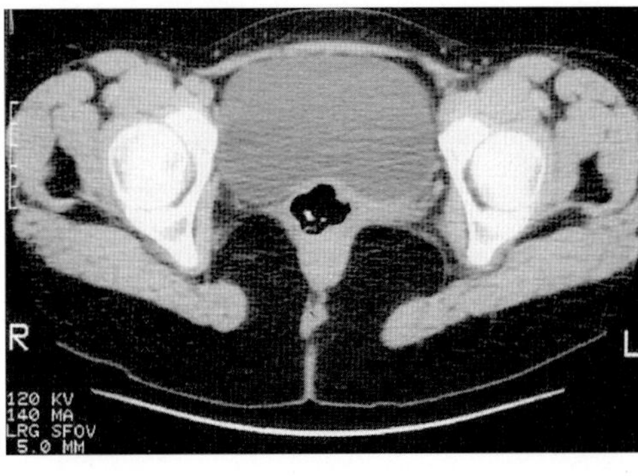

body pelvis and femoral heads

contrast filled bladder

bony pelvis and femoral heads

bowel lumen within anal canal

sphincter muscle posterior to bowel lumen

■ **Fig. 8.98** CT scan of a patient with congenital anterior ectopic anus, in which the bowel lumen is clearly shown lying anterior to the external anal sphincter. The muscle mass could be palpated at rectal examination and surgical re-routing of the bowel through the muscle restored normal continence. Courtesy of Prof R.K.S. Phillips.

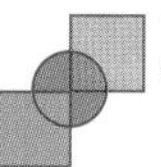

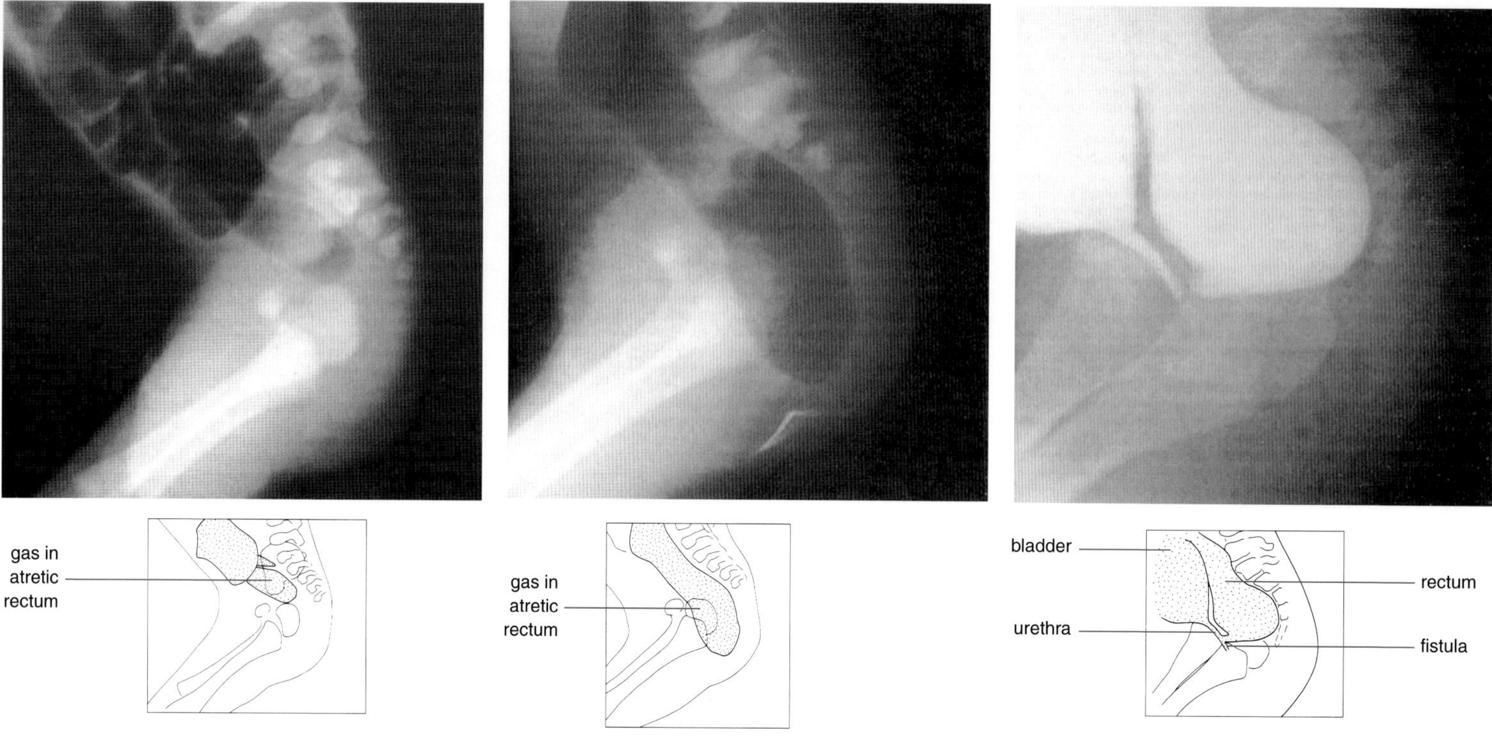

Fig. 8.99 Prone lateral shoot-through film in a neonate showing high ano-rectal agenesis. Courtesy of Dr C. Hall.

Fig. 8.100 Prone lateral shoot-through film in a neonate showing low ano-rectal agenesis. Courtesy of Dr C. Hall.

Fig. 8.101 Distal loopogram showing rectal atresia with a fistula to the posterior urethra in a male neonate. Courtesy of Dr C. Hall.

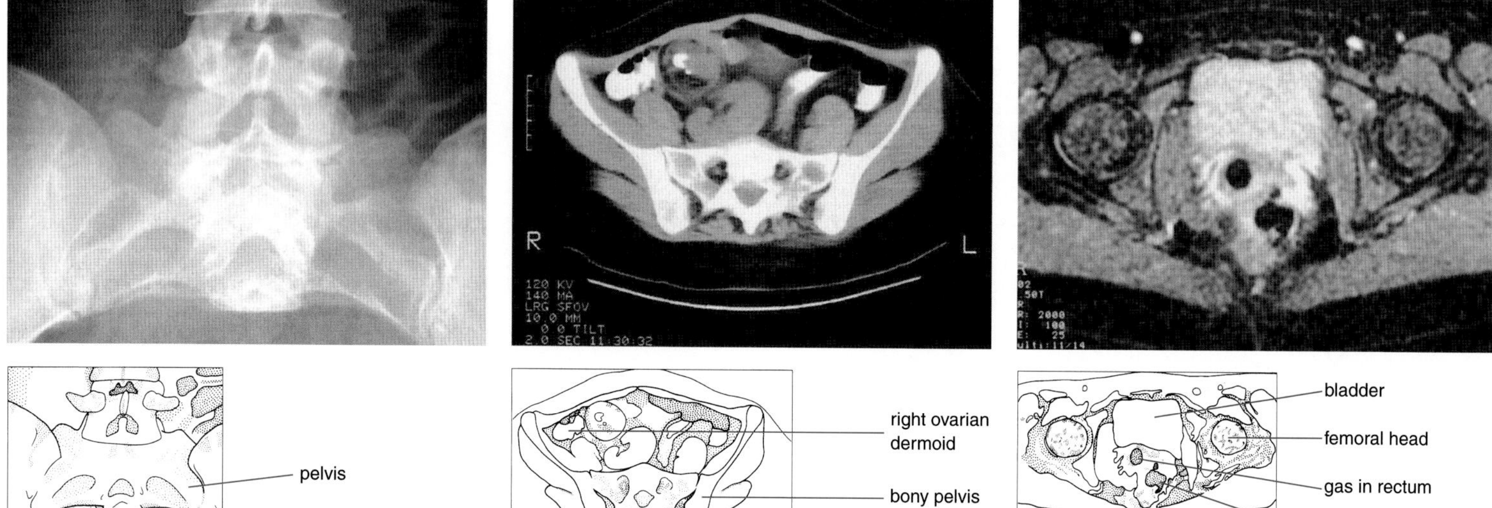

Fig. 8.102 Plain abdominal film in the same patient as in Fig. 8.98 demonstrating associated sacral agenesis. Courtesy of Prof R.K.S. Phillips.

Fig. 8.103 CT scan showing a right ovarian dermoid in the same patient as in Fig. 8.98. Courtesy of Prof R.K.S. Phillips.

Fig. 8.104 MRI scan demonstrating a post-rectal dermoid. Courtesy of Mr P. Lunniss.

REFERENCES

1. Kahn S, Rubesin SE, Levine MS, *et al.* Polypoid lesions at the anorectal junction: barium enema findings. AJR 1993; 161: 339–342, Figs 1, 5, 6, 11, 12.
2. Rubesin SE, Schnall MD. Rectum. In: Gore RM, Levine MS, Laufer I (eds) Textbook of gastrointestinal radiology, pp. 1261–1309. Philadelphia: WB Saunders, 1994, Figs 1, 9, 14, 16, 17, 45, 46, 51B, 52A, 57, 67, 68, 72.
3. Nadgir R, Rubesin SE, Levine MS. On the AJR Viewbox: Perirectal sinus tracks and fistulas caused by hidradenitis suppurativa. AJR 2001; 177: 476–477, Fig. 5.
4. Levine MS, Piccolello ML, Sollenberger LC, *et al.* Solitary rectal ulcer syndrome: a radiologic diagnosis? Gastrointest Radiol 1986; 11: 187–193.
5. Dobos N, Rubesin SE. Radiologic imaging modalities in the diagnosis and management of colorectal cancer. Hem Onc Clin North Am 2002; 16: 875–895, Fig. 7.

THE PANCREAS

9

NORMAL ANATOMY

The pancreas is a lobulated gland which lies retroperitoneally and across the spine, in the posterior part of the upper abdomen (Figs 9.1–9.5). It is 12–15 cm in length; its head and 'uncinate process' lie within the curve of the duodenum, and the tapering body and tail extend to the medial border of the spleen. The splenic vein runs posteriorly to the pancreas, and the splenic artery runs anteriorly and superiorly, while the superior mesenteric artery and vein lie in the angle formed by the head and body of the gland. The superior mesenteric and splenic veins join to form the portal vein at this site.

Histologically, the exocrine pancreas is composed of numerous acini, which consist of pyramidal epithelial cells converging onto a central lumen (Figs 9.6, 9.7). Several acini make up a lobule, and the lumen of each acinus connects with a small duct that drains through the intralobular ducts into larger interlobular ducts. These then drain into the main pancreatic duct, which, together with the common bile duct, enters the duodenum at the ampulla of Vater. The acinar secretions include trypsinogen, chymotrypsinogen, amylase, and lipase, which contribute to intraluminal digestion, and bicarbonate, which alkalinizes the bowel contents.

Distributed within the acinar tissue are small masses of endocrine cells – the islets of Langerhans. These are composed of a variety of cell types including the alpha cells, which produce glucagon; beta cells which produce insulin; delta cells, which produce somatostatin; and other gut hormone-producing cells (Figs 9.8–9.10).

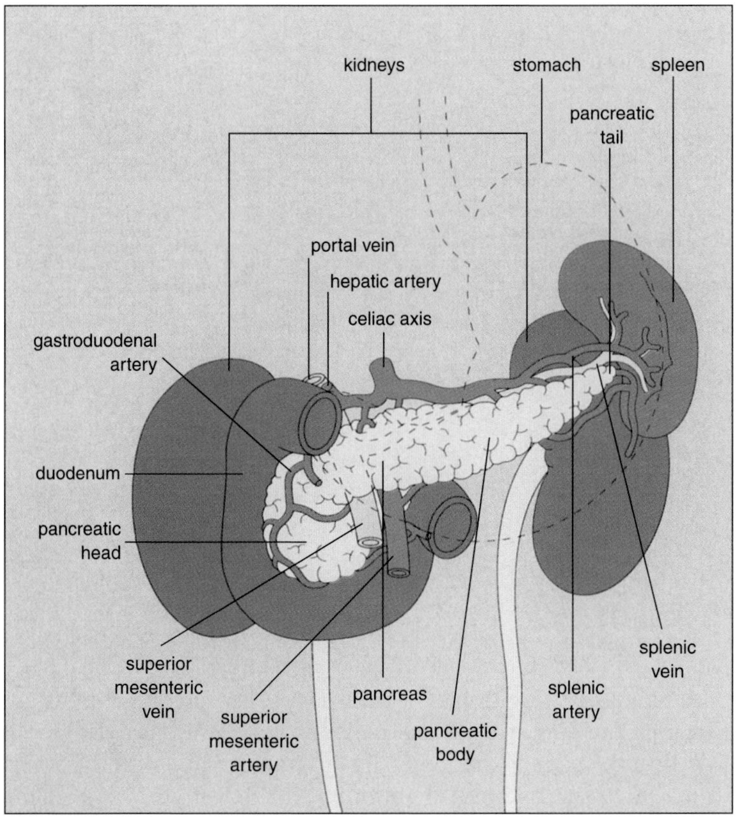

■ **Fig. 9.1** Diagram showing the anatomical relationships of the pancreas with the important vascular structures.

EMBRYOLOGICAL DEVELOPMENT

The pancreas develops from separate ventral and dorsal buds that arise from the junction of the primitive foregut and midgut. The dorsal bud enlarges towards the left, and forms the main bulk of the mature gland. The ventral bud, which is closely associated with the developing common bile duct, is initially carried away from the duodenum; it is brought into apposition with the dorsal system only in the seventh week of intrauterine growth, following its rotation behind the primitive duodenum to lie caudal to the dorsal bud (Fig. 9.11). Both parts of the primitive pancreas contain axial ducts, the dorsal duct arising from the duodenal wall, and the ventral duct from the common bile duct. When they fuse, the ventral duct (of Wirsung) becomes continuous with the dorsal duct (of Santorini) to form the main

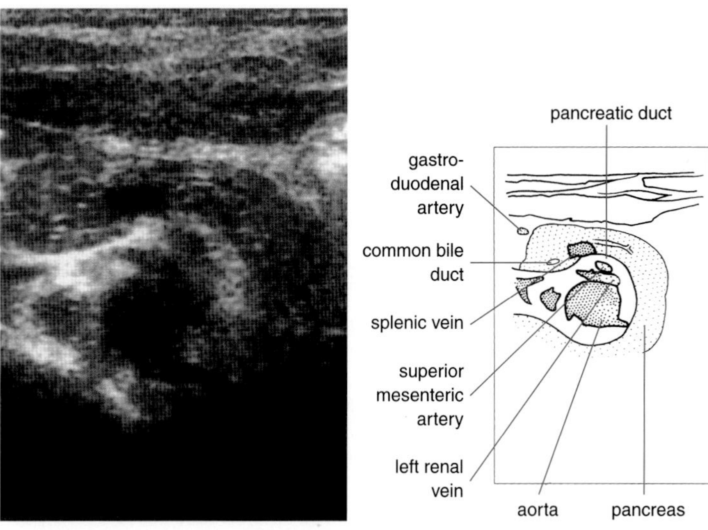

■ **Fig. 9.2** Ultrasound scan appearance of normal pancreas. Courtesy of Prof W. Lees.

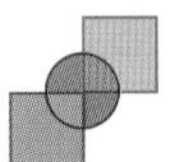

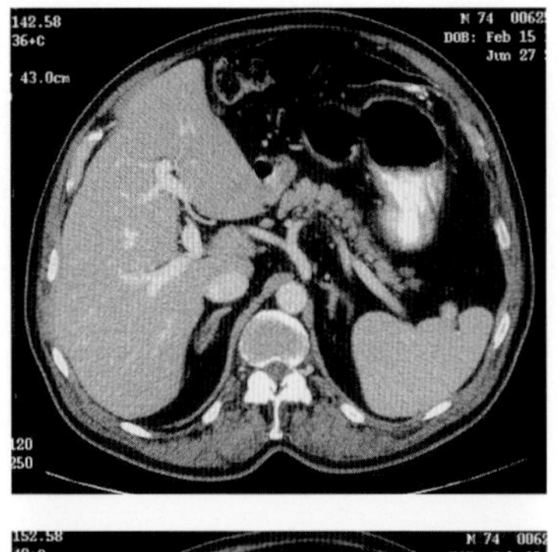

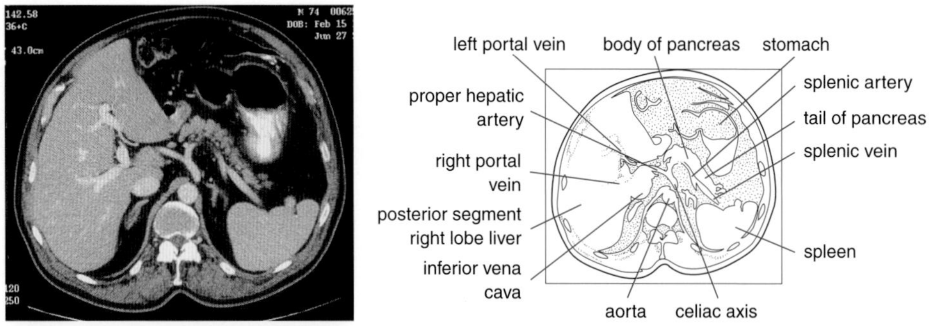

Fig. 9.3 Four images from a CT scan of the abdomen demonstrating the normal pancreas and its anatomical relationships. The pancreas is usually not demonstrated in its entirety on one axial CT image. In this patient, the lobulated acinar structure of the pancreas is evident. Note the relationships of the pancreatic body and tail to the splenic artery, splenic vein, and splenoportal confluence.

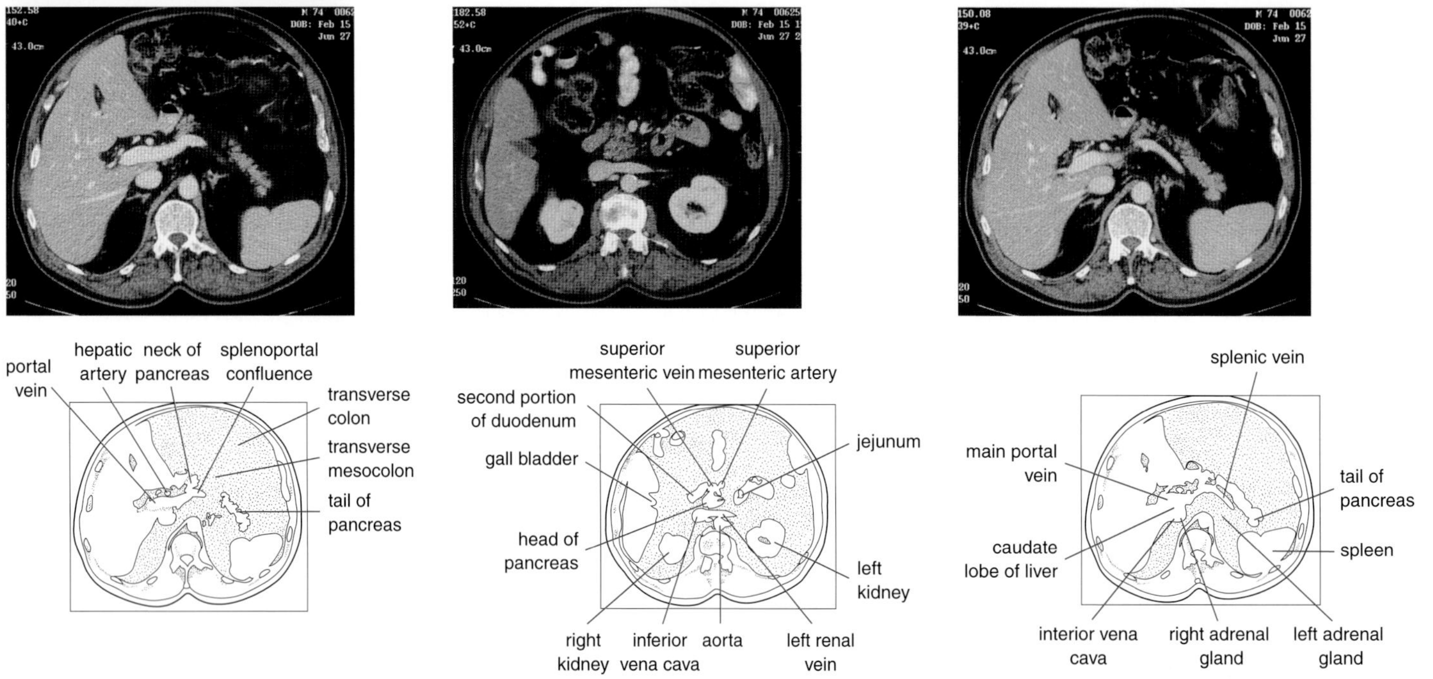

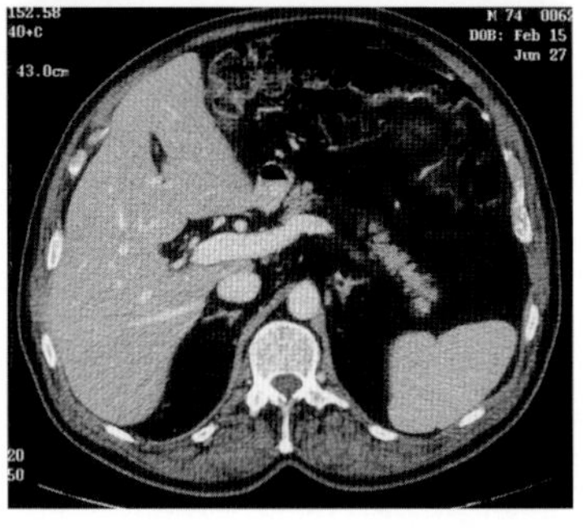

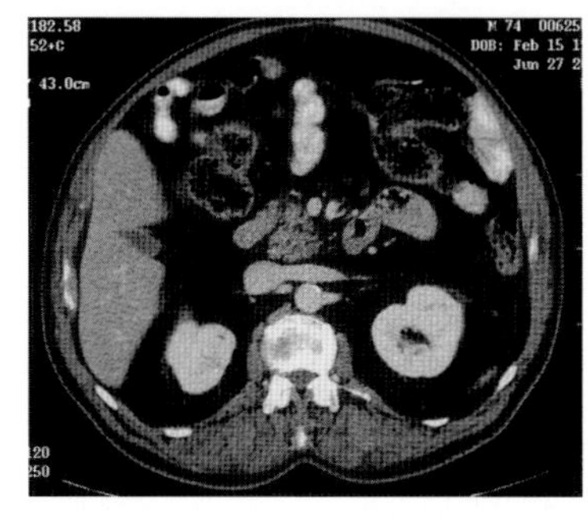

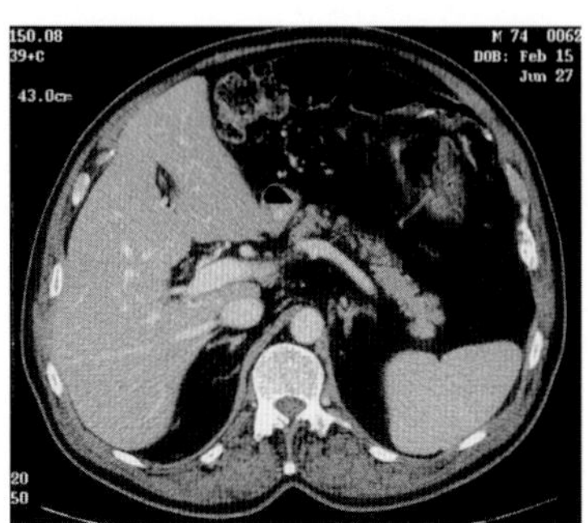

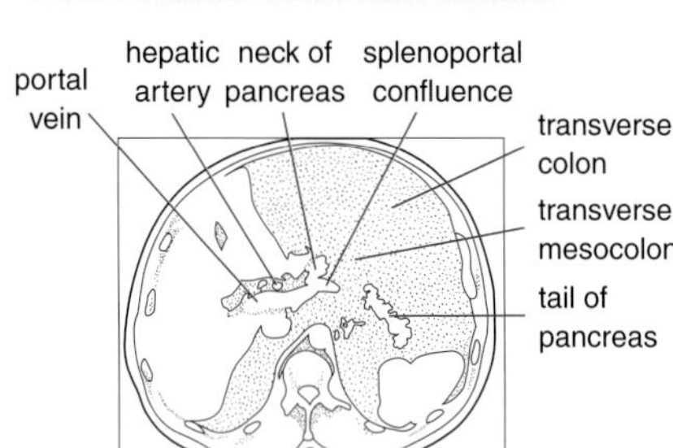

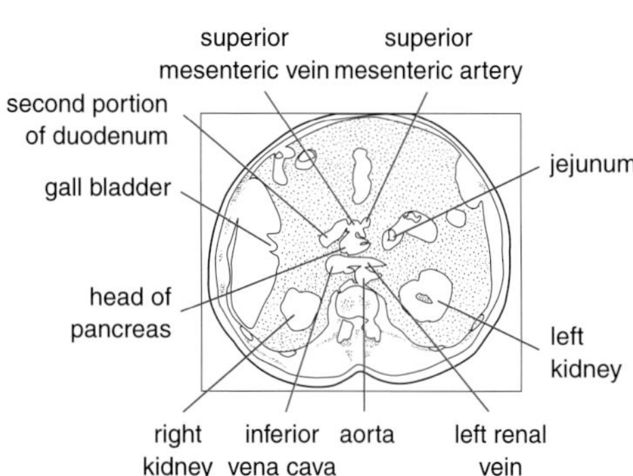

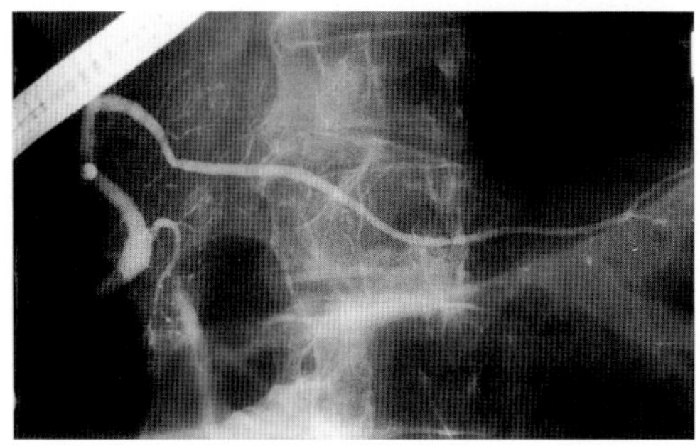

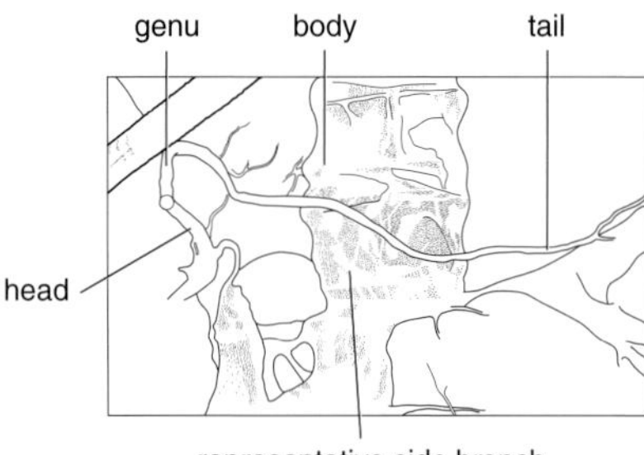

Fig. 9.4 Normal pancreatogram demonstrated at ERCP. In general, the side-branches lie perpendicular to the main pancreatic duct.

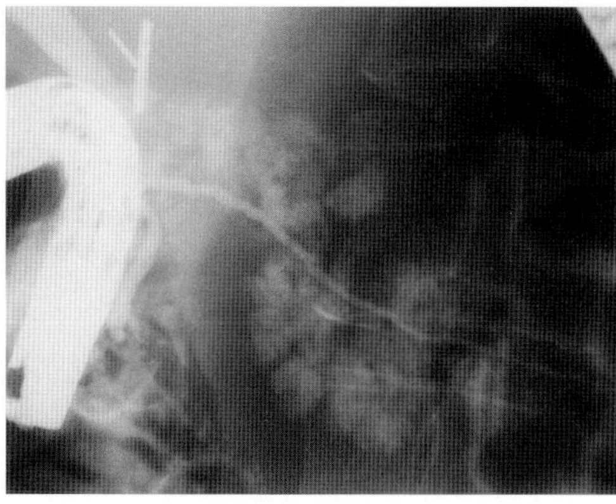

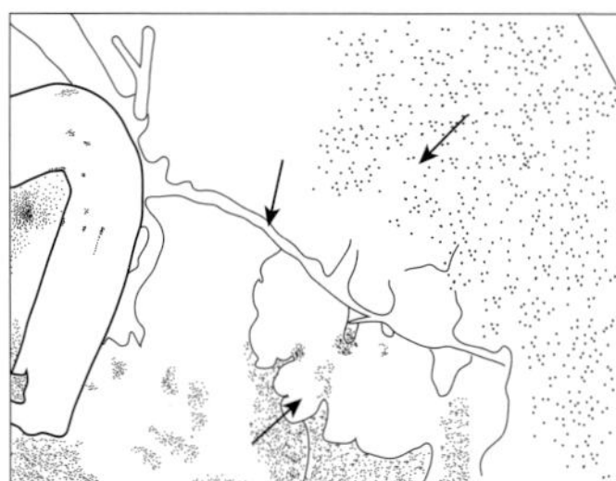

Fig. 9.5 Pancreatic lobules demonstrated during normal pancreatogram. This 'acinarization' of the pancreas implies that this patient is at increased risk for post-ERCP pancreatitis.

pancreatic duct (Fig. 9.11). The common bile duct and pancreatic ducts therefore enter the duodenum at the main papilla (Fig. 9.11), while the portion of the dorsal duct within the head of the pancreas becomes more or less vestigial and enters the duodenum proximally to the main papilla, through a small accessory, or minor papilla (Figs 9.12, 9.13).

Complete failure of the two duct systems to fuse results in a pancreas divisum (Figs 9.14, 9.15). This occurs in about 5% of people and may predispose to pancreatitis (Fig. 9.16). Incomplete fusion, in which the duct of Santorini remains dominant, may also occur. Failure of the body of the ventral bud to rotate in line with the orifice of its duct may give rise to an annular pancreas surrounding the second part of the duodenum (Fig. 9.17). This may be responsible for duodenal obstruction (Fig. 9.18).

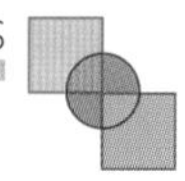

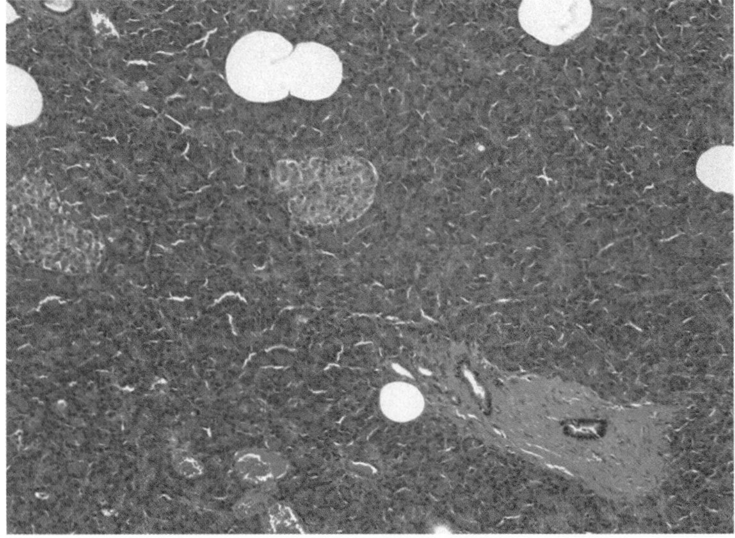

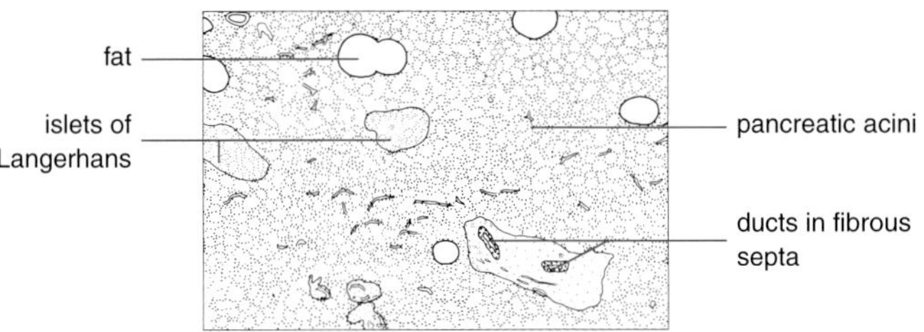

■ **Fig. 9.6** Normal pancreatic histology. The relationship between the exocrine pancreas, the ducts, and the islets of Langerhans is shown. H&E stain (x 75).

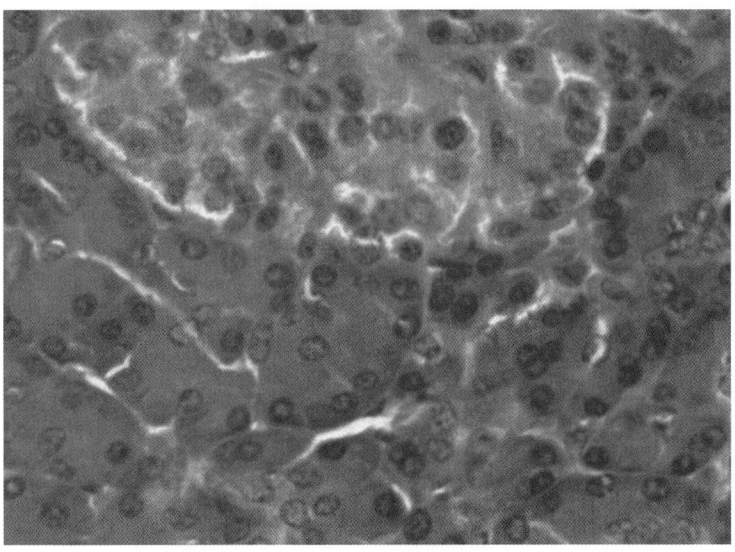

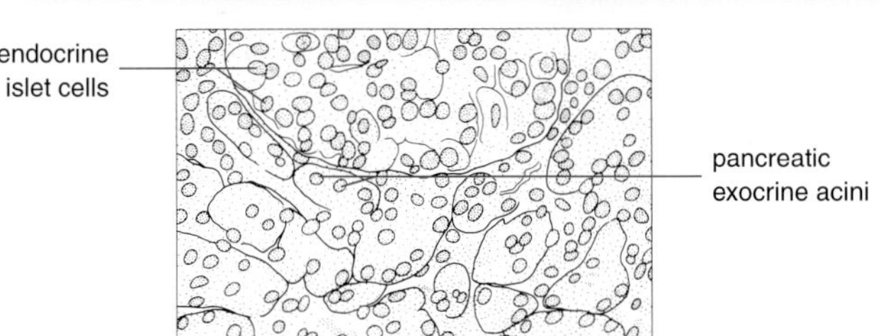

■ **Fig. 9.7** Normal pancreatic histology. H&E stain (x 480).

■ **Fig. 9.8** Immunocytochemical examination of the normal pancreatic islets. Glucagon-like immunoreactivity shown by indirect immunofluorescence method and PAS counterstaining (x 240). Courtesy of Prof J. Polak.

■ **Fig. 9.9** Immunocytochemical examination of the normal pancreatic islets. Somatostatin-like immunoreactivity, peroxidase/antiperoxidase method (x 240). Courtesy of Prof J. Polak.

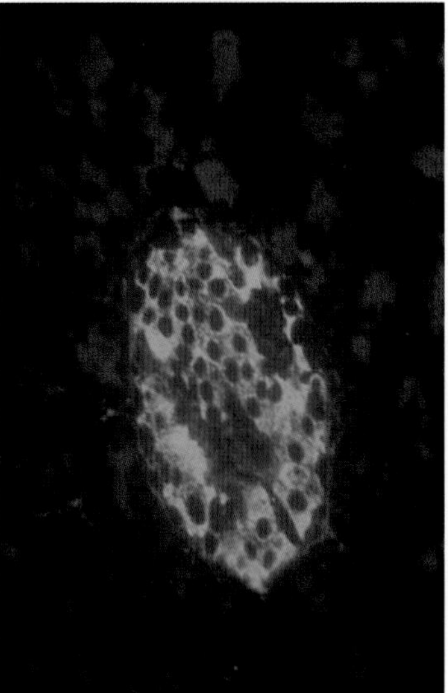

■ **Fig. 9.10** Insulin-like immunoreactivity – indirect immunofluorescence method with PAS counterstaining (x 240). Courtesy of Prof J. Polak.

PANCREATITIS

There are several classifications of pancreatitis, but none is universally accepted. For present purposes, it is convenient to make the distinction between acute and chronic disease.

Acute pancreatitis

In Western populations, acute pancreatitis is most commonly due to gallstones and alcohol. The passage of small gallstones through the ampulla of Vater is particularly likely to trigger an acute episode. Transient obstruction of the pancreatic duct, with or with-

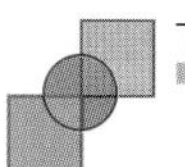

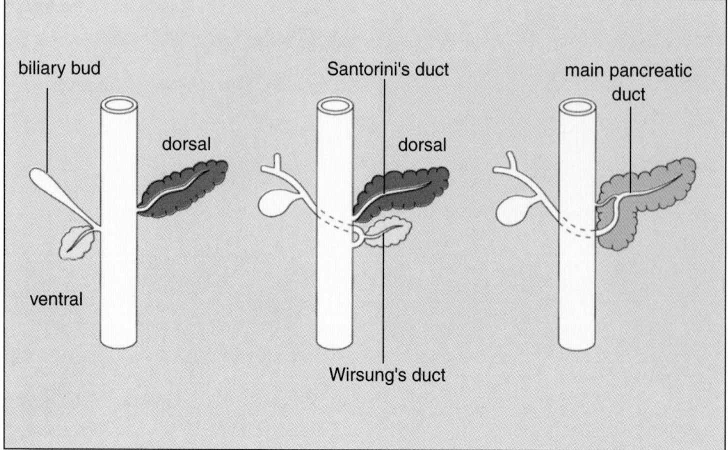

■ **Fig. 9.11** Diagram demonstrating the developmental anatomy of the pancreas.

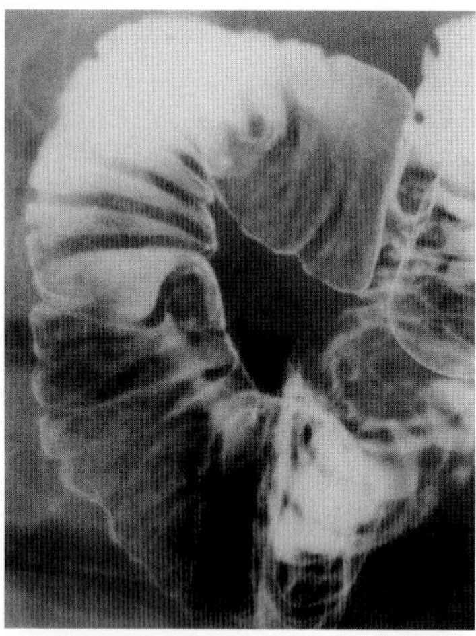

■ **Fig. 9.12** Double-contrast upper GI series showing the major papilla. The folds of Kerckring do not completely encircle the duodenum at the level of the major papilla.

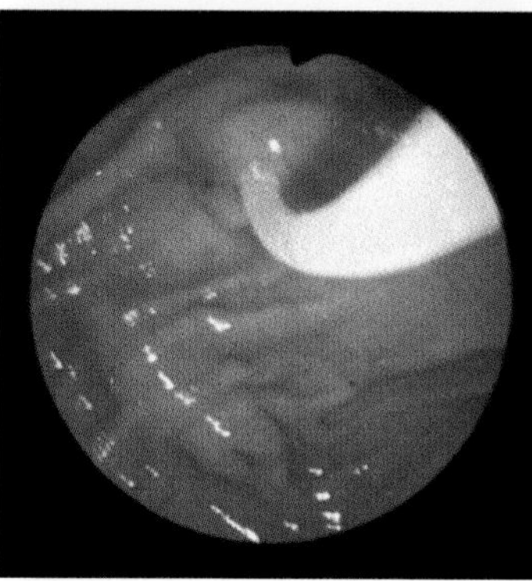

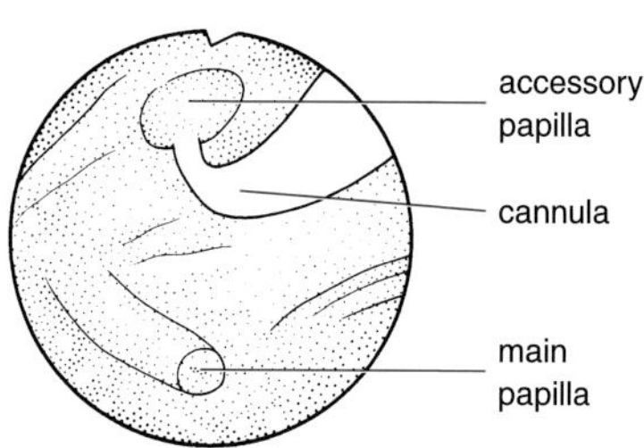

■ **Fig. 9.13** Endoscopic view of the second part of the duodenum showing a cannula within the minor papilla.

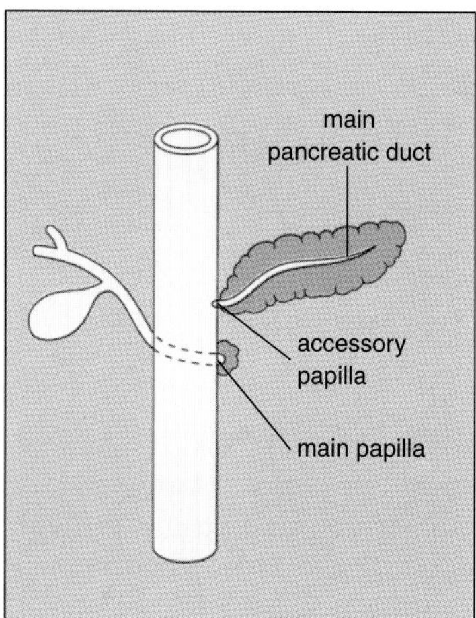

■ **Fig. 9.14** Diagram showing the anatomical arrangement in pancreas divisum.

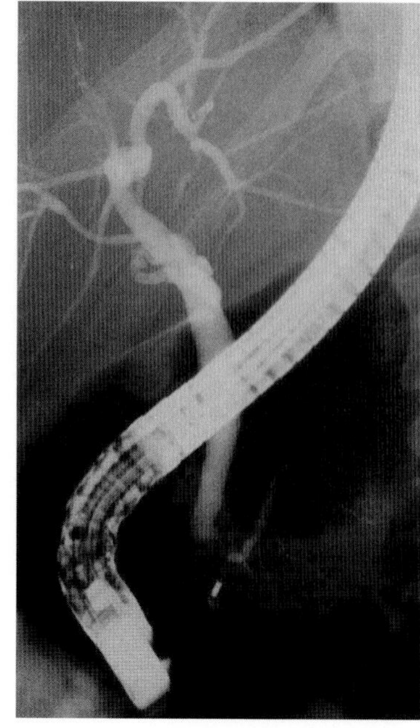

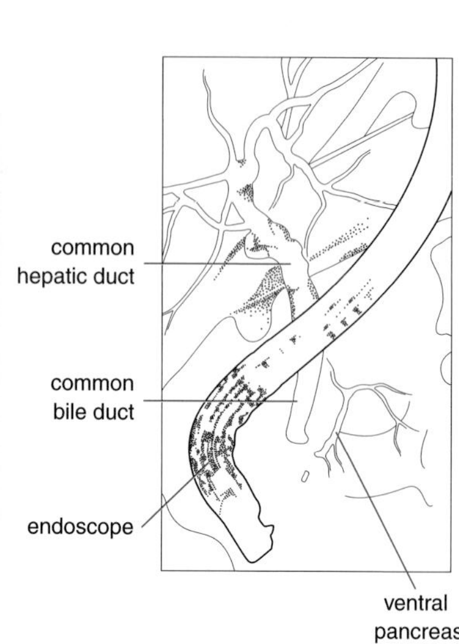

■ **Fig. 9.15** ERCP demonstrating pancreas divisum. The branching system of the ventral pancreas is identified and clearly shows its limitation to the right of the spine. The close relationship of the common bile duct to the ventral pancreas is demonstrated.

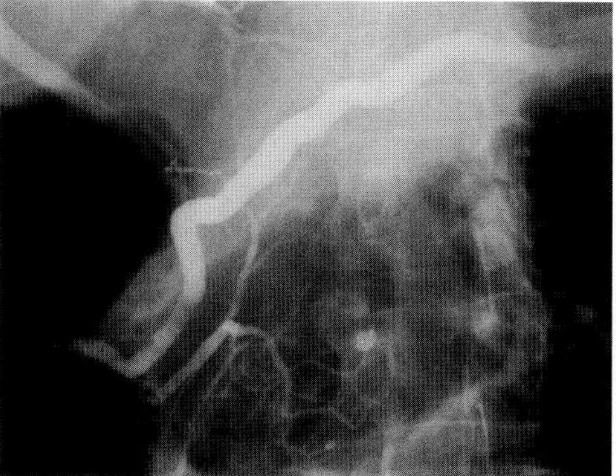

■ **Fig. 9.16** ERCP demonstrating pancreas divisum. The ventral duct of Wirsung and the dorsal duct of Santorini are identified. Changes of chronic pancreatitis are manifested as diffuse dilatation of the dorsal main pancreatic duct.

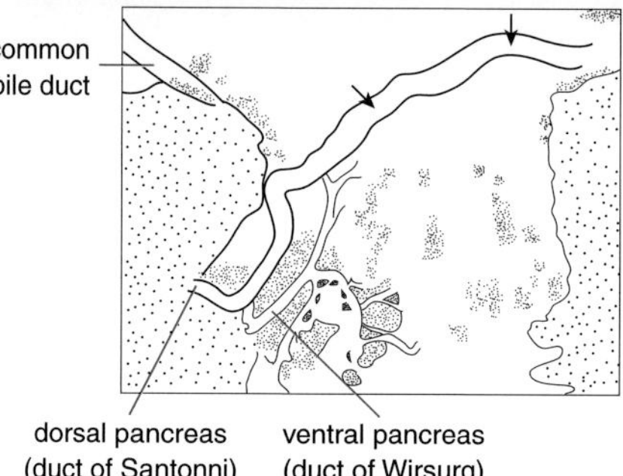

out bile reflux into the duct, is thought to be responsible. Alcohol appears to have a direct toxic effect. Drugs such as azathioprine, infections (e.g. mumps), hypercalcemia, hypertriglyceridemia, and trauma may also be responsible. Pancreatitis also occurs as a complication of cardiac surgery/extracorporeal circulation, and of ERCP.

Acute pancreatitis causes severe abdominal pain, which often radiates to the back. Circulatory collapse may supervene, particularly in hemorrhagic, necrotic pancreatitis. The entrance of blood into fascial plains can cause a blue discoloration of the flanks (Grey–Turner's sign) (Fig. 9.19), or of the periumbilical area (Cullen's sign).

Diagnosis is usually apparent from the clinical features and from a significantly elevated serum amylase or lipase concentration. Ultrasound and CT scanning provide confirmation (Figs 9.20–9.24), but diagnostic peritoneal lavage may help to determine whether

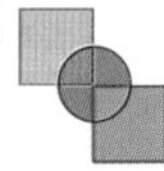

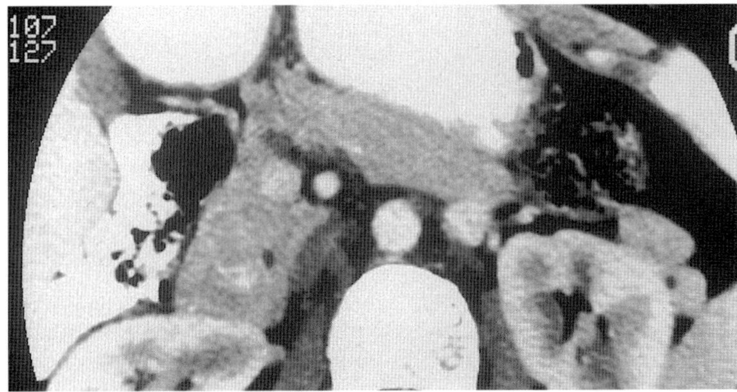

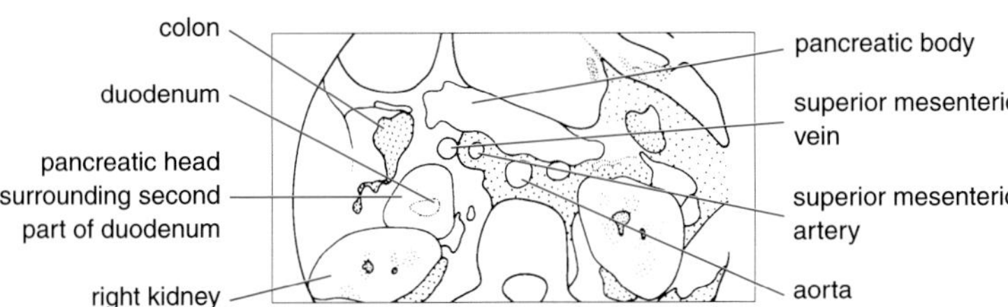

■ **Fig. 9.17** Annular pancreas. CT scan demonstrating the pancreatic head surrounding the second part of the duodenum with the body and tail of the pancreas to the left and anterior to the superior mesenteric vessels.

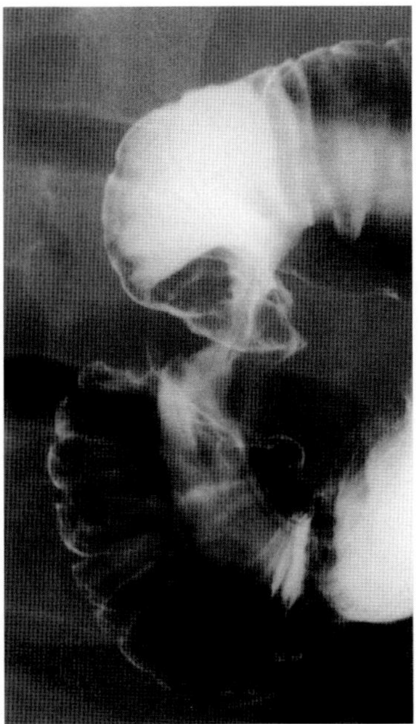

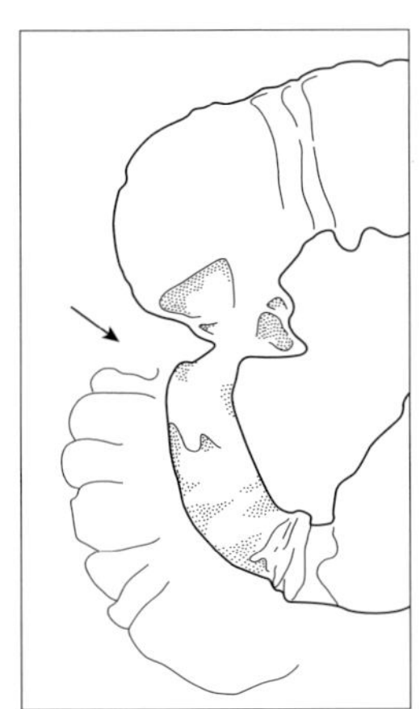

■ **Fig. 9.18** Double-contrast upper GI demonstrating annular pancreas. There is focal circumferential, smooth narrowing of the mid second part of the duodenum. The duodenal folds and mucosa are otherwise normal.

■ **Fig. 9.19** Grey–Turner's sign. Courtesy of Mr C.W. Imrie.

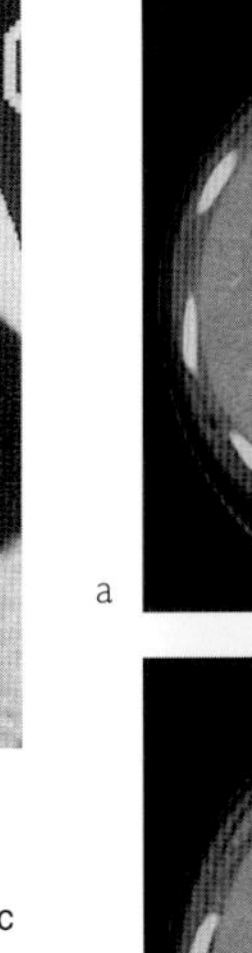

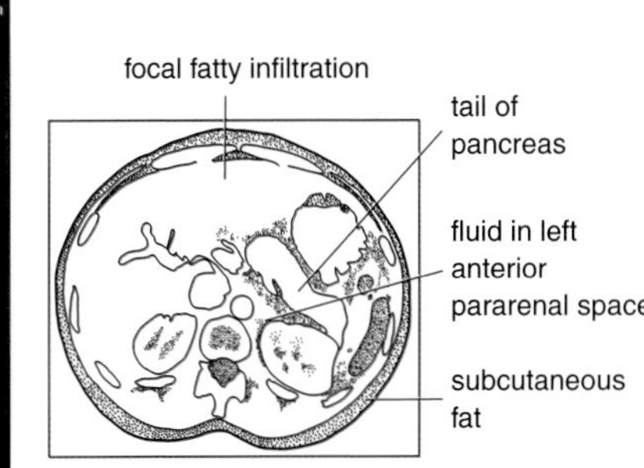

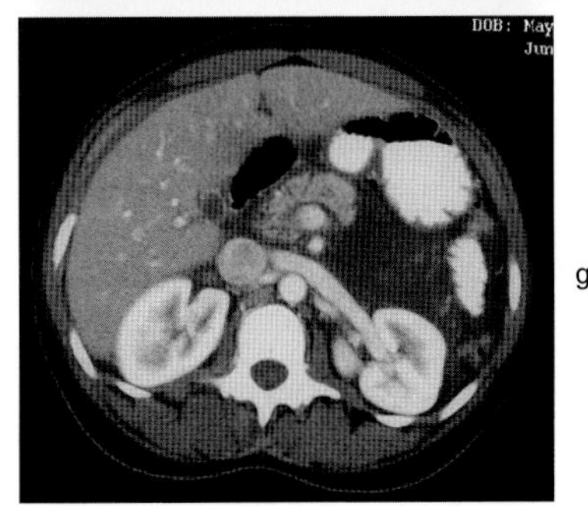

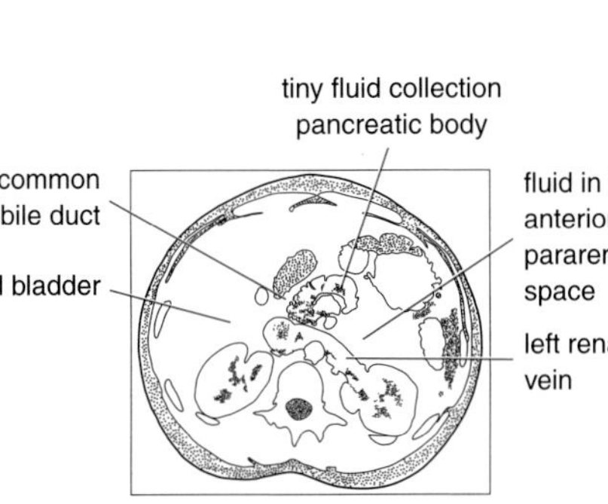

■ **Fig. 9.20** Two images from a CT in a patient with acute pancreatitis. (a) The pancreatic body and tail are enlarged. Fluid tracks into the left anterior pararenal space. Note the difference in attenuation of the fluid in the left anterior pararenal space and the subcutaneous fat. (b) There is a tiny fluid collection in the pancreatic body. Fluid infiltrates the fat of the left anterior pararenal space.

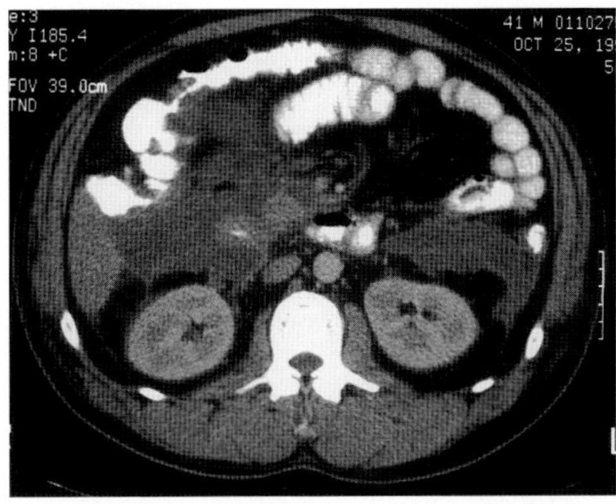

■ **Fig. 9.21** CT demonstrating large fluid collections related to acute pancreatitis. Large fluid collections have spread into the left and right anterior pararenal spaces and the transverse mesocolon. Inflammatory changes related to spread of pancreatic juices are seen in the transverse colon and descending colon.

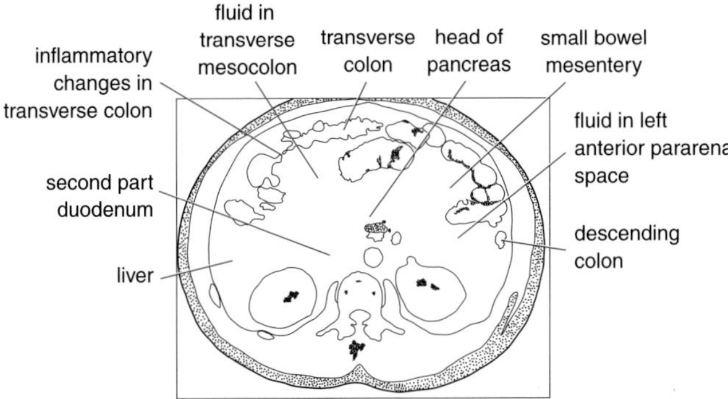

hemorrhagic necrosis, which would warrant laparotomy, is present. In such cases, the subsequent laparotomy demonstrates an edematous, hyperemic gland with fat necrosis (Fig. 9.25), and in the later stages, the pancreas may be necrotic and partially liquefied (Figs 9.22, 9.26, 9.27).

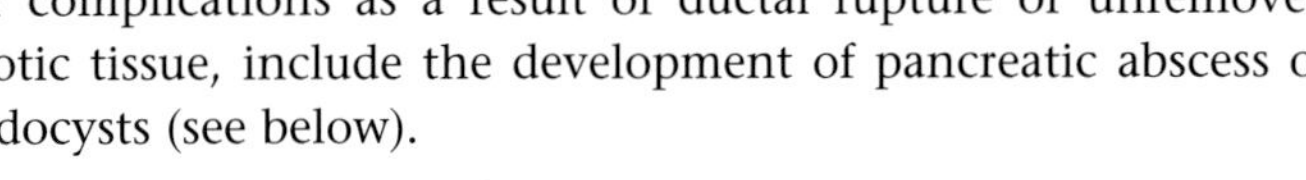

Acute pancreatitis may be complicated by coagulopathy, respiratory and renal failure, encephalopathy, and glucose intolerance. Later complications as a result of ductal rupture or unremoved necrotic tissue, include the development of pancreatic abscess or pseudocysts (see below).

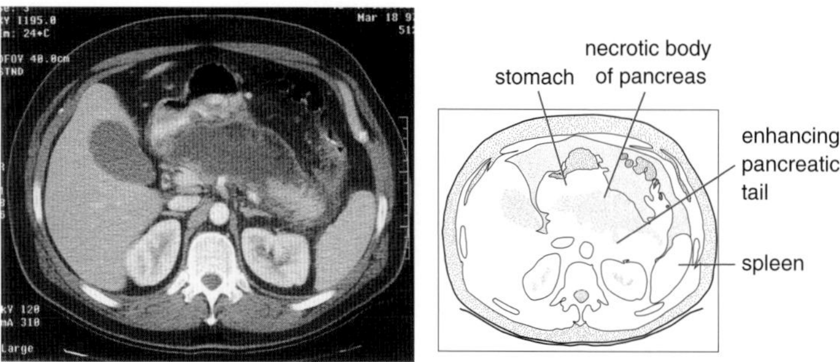

Fig. 9.22 CT demonstrating pancreatic necrosis in a patient with acute pancreatitis. The body and part of the tail of the pancreas are enlarged and of low attenuation. Lack of enhancement of the parenchyma of the pancreatic body and adjacent pancreatic tail indicates pancreatic necrosis. The pancreatic tail adjacent to the spleen enhances with intravenous contrast and is therefore not necrotic.

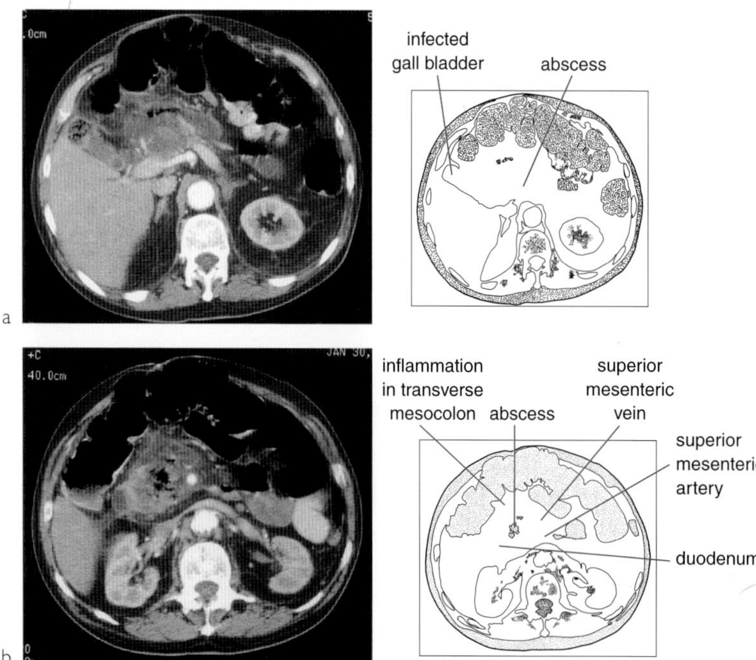

Fig. 9.23 CT demonstrating abscess developing in pancreatic necrosis. (a) The head of pancreas is enlarged and of low attenuation. Bubbles are seen in the anterior portion of the necrotic pancreatic head. Bubbles are also seen in the gall bladder due to retrograde infection spreading up the biliary tree. (b) The infected pancreatic necrosis is manifest by an enlarged head of the pancreas with multiple air bubbles. The inflammatory process has spread to the transverse mesocolon and the medial wall of the duodenum. The superior mesenteric vein is engulfed and partially occluded by the inflammatory process.

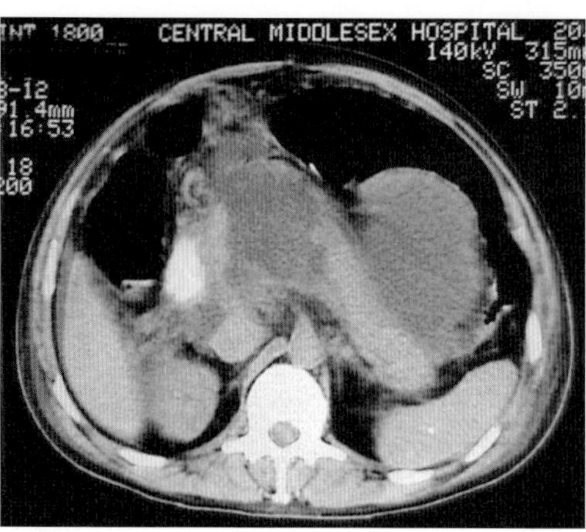

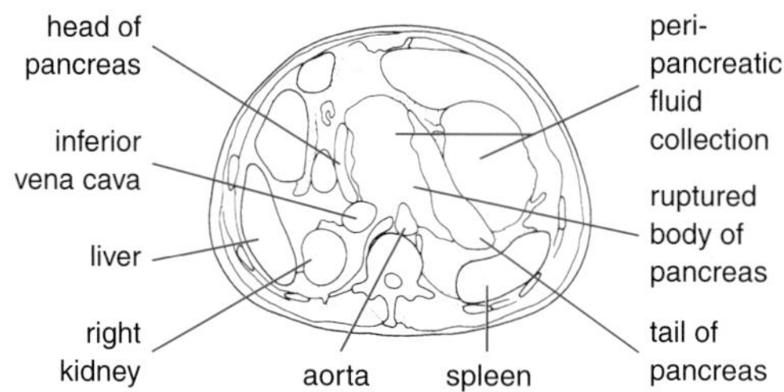

Fig. 9.24 CT scan in traumatic rupture of the pancreas. Typically, the rupture is across the spine, and it is frequently the result of blunt abdominal trauma such as that which occurs in car accidents. The head of the pancreas is seen separately from the tail, with a peripancreatic fluid collection already forming to both sides of the midline.

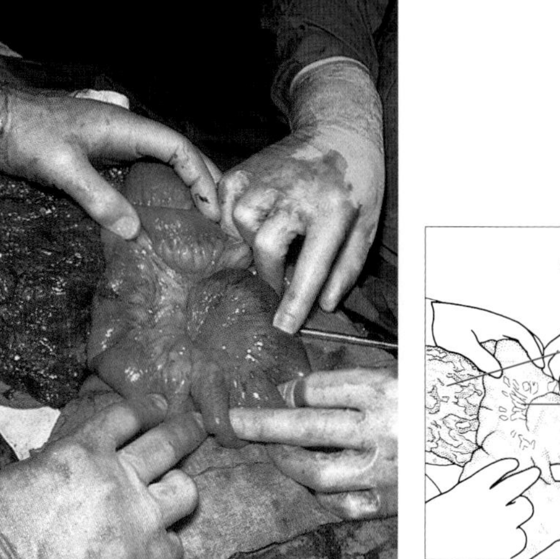

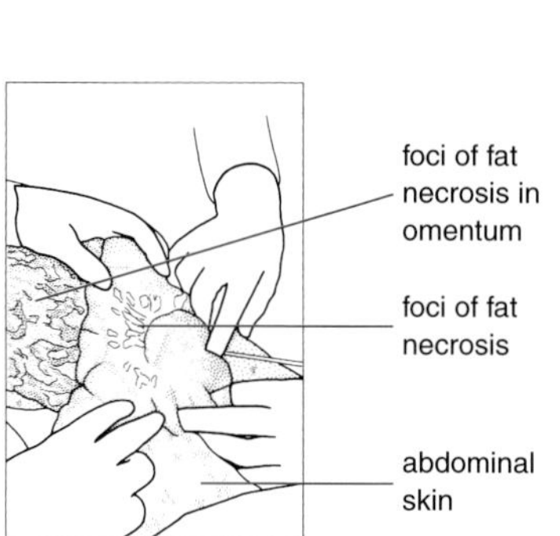

Fig. 9.25 Acute pancreatitis at laparotomy showing extensive small foci of fat necrosis with additional foci in the omentum. Courtesy of Mr C.W. Imrie.

Histologically, the inflammation and destruction are mainly periductular (Fig. 9.28), or perilobular (Fig. 9.29), with relative sparing of the glandular elements. Periductular necrosis is particularly associated with gallstone-related and alcohol-related disease. A perilobular distribution is more common when there has been sustained hypotension. Acute necrotizing pancreatitis produces panlobular necrosis and represents a final common pathway in fatal pancreatitis of any cause (Fig. 9.30). The necrotizing process may spread to the pleura and mediastinum, as well as to the subcutaneous fat, and if the patient survives, these may then become foci for subsequent infection or cysts (see below).

Chronic pancreatitis

Chronic pancreatitis is most commonly the result of alcohol excess, but the other causes of acute pancreatitis are rarely if ever responsible for chronic disease. Protein-calorie malnutrition is implicated in developing countries, and a few rare cases are caused by hereditary pancreatitis (see below). In most series, 10–15% of cases of chronic pancreatitis appear to be idiopathic.

The patient with chronic pancreatitis may be subject to acute exacerbations that share the clinical and pathological features of acute pancreatitis, but even in the absence of superimposed acute episodes, chronic pancreatitis may pose major problems. Although sometimes asymptomatic, it may also be responsible for severe, unremitting upper abdominal pain radiating to the back. Progressive destruction of the pancreatic parenchyma leads to malabsorption, particularly of fat, and ultimately to clinical steatorrhea. The incidence of glucose intolerance is high, but there is relative preservation of the islets, and insulin-requiring diabetes is uncommon. The natural course of chronic pancreatitis is such that pain is a relatively early manifestation and malabsorption relatively late, but either may occur alone. The amylase and lipase levels are usually normal.

Chronic pancreatitis is easily diagnosed from a plain abdominal film if calcification of the gland is present (Fig. 9.31), but a CT scan is the more usual route to prompt diagnosis (Figs 9.31, 9.32). When the site of calcification clearly corresponds to pancreatic topography, there is a very limited differential diagnosis (Fig. 9.33). Diagnosis is otherwise established either from structural changes, demonstrated

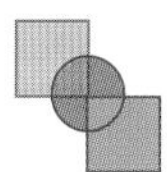

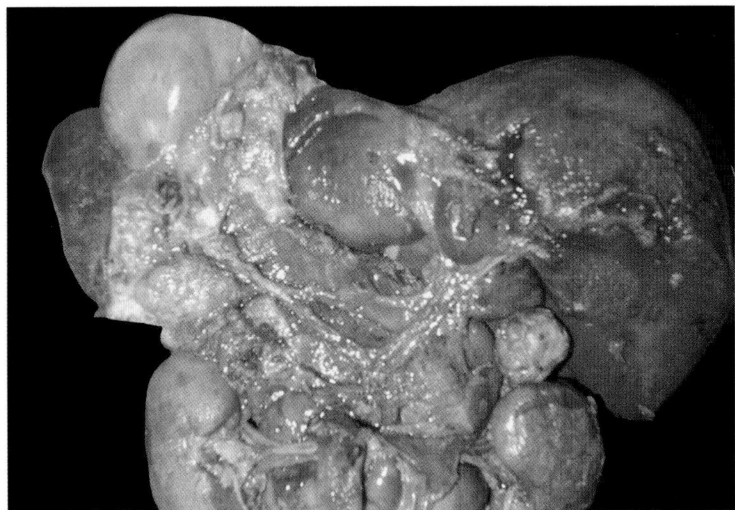

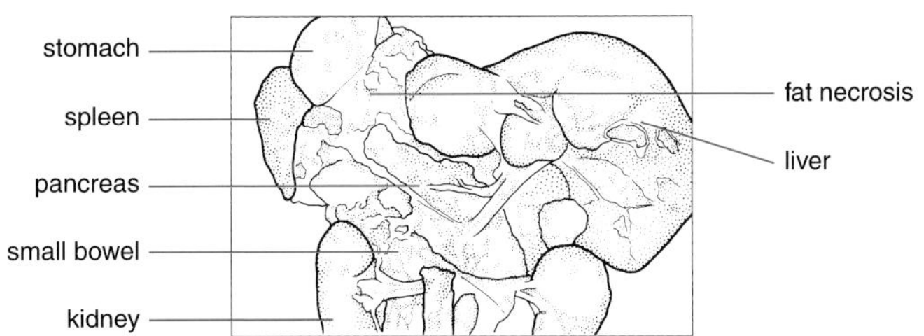

■ **Fig. 9.26** Fatal necrotic acute pancreatitis showing (from behind) massive fat necrosis involving the omentum and the pancreatic tail.

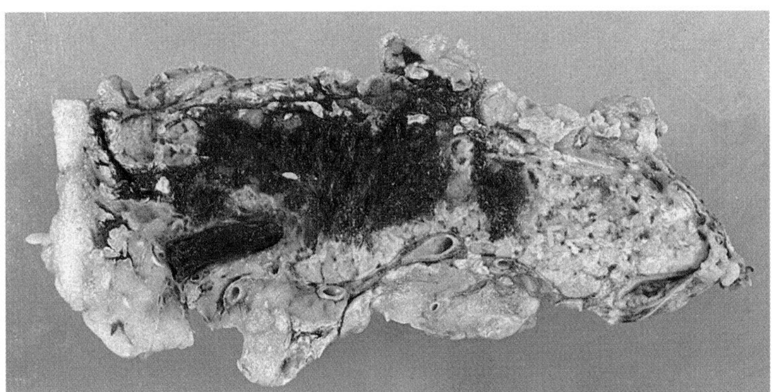

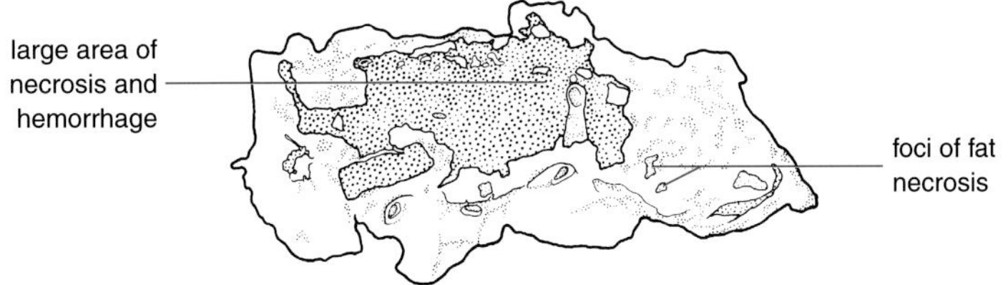

■ **Fig. 9.27** Macroscopic appearance of acute hemorrhagic pancreatitis showing a large area of parenchymal necrosis and hemorrhage. Courtesy of Dr J. Newman.

on imaging, or (less often) from functional abnormalities indicated by the presence of confirmed steatorrhea or the other relatively specific tests of pancreatic function.

The PABA and pancreolauryl tests are indirect, tubeless tests that measure the absorption (and urinary excretion) of a marker dependent for its absorption on cleavage from a carrier molecule. This cleavage is selected to require and depend on adequate pancreatic enzyme availability in the lumen, but the tests are neither especially sensitive nor specific. The best test of function remains the secretin test, which requires intubation of the stomach and duodenum to permit the collection of pancreatic juices in response to intravenous secretin. A variety of enzymes may be studied, but the simplest and most

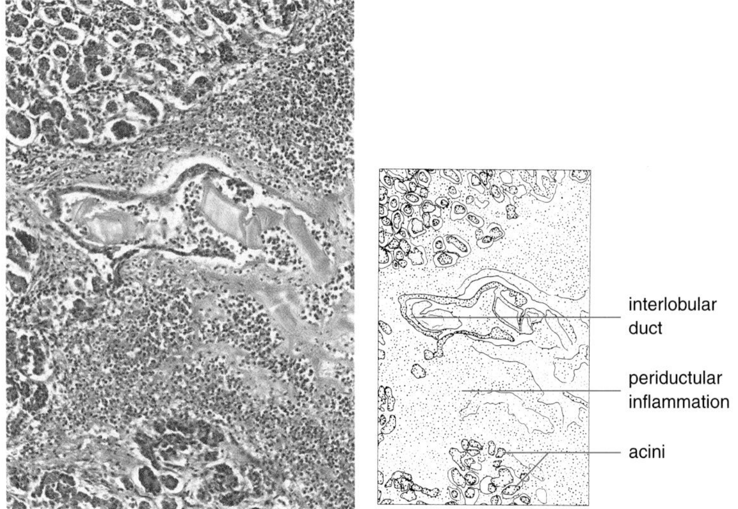

■ **Fig. 9.28** Histological appearance of acute pancreatitis with inflammation around the main duct. H&E stain (x 80). Courtesy of Dr A.K. Foolis.

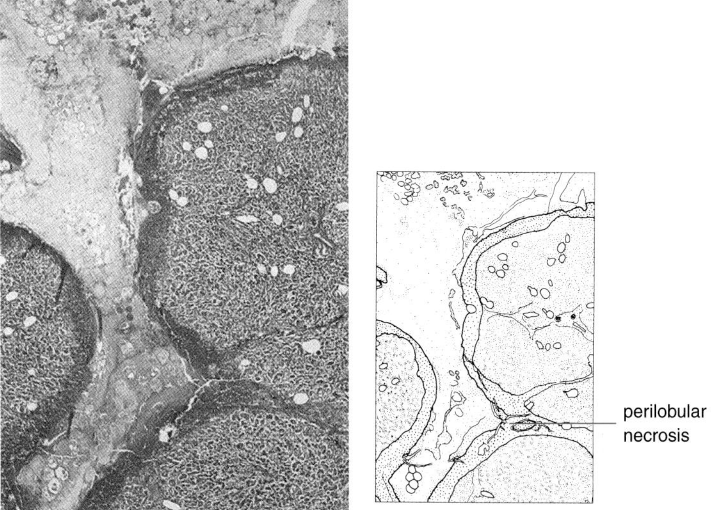

■ **Fig. 9.29** Pancreatitis with inflammation confined to the perimeter of the lobules. H&E stain (x 16). Courtesy of Dr A.K. Foolis.

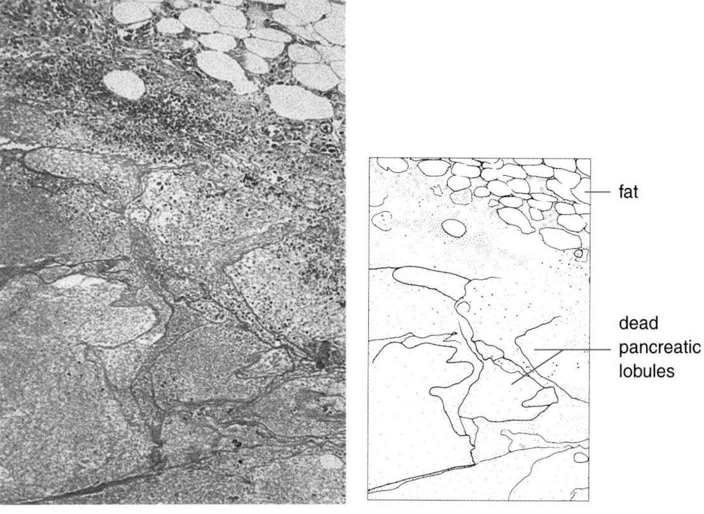

■ **Fig. 9.30** Complete pan-lobular necrosis in severe pancreatitis. H&E stain (x 50).

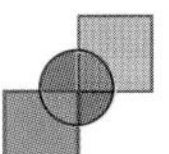

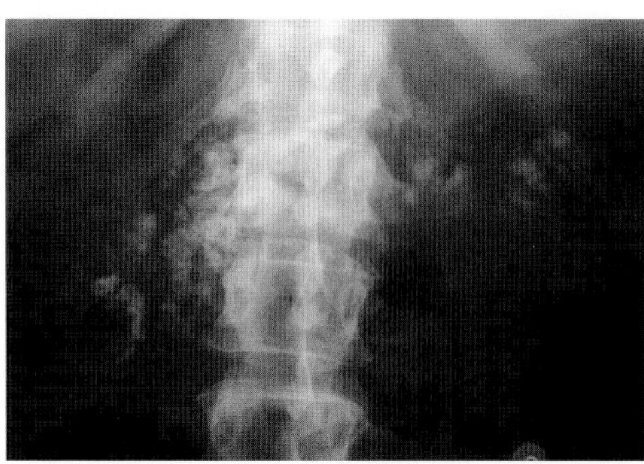

Fig. 9.31 Calcific pancreatitis related to chronic alcohol abuse. Plain radiograph of the abdomen demonstrates coarse lobular calcifications (arrows) throughout the pancreatic ductal system.

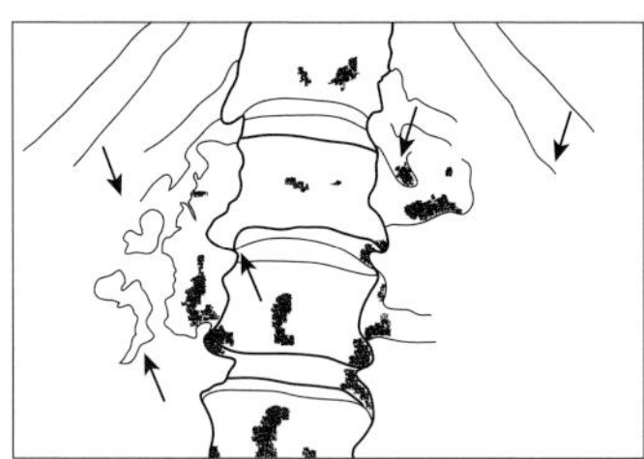

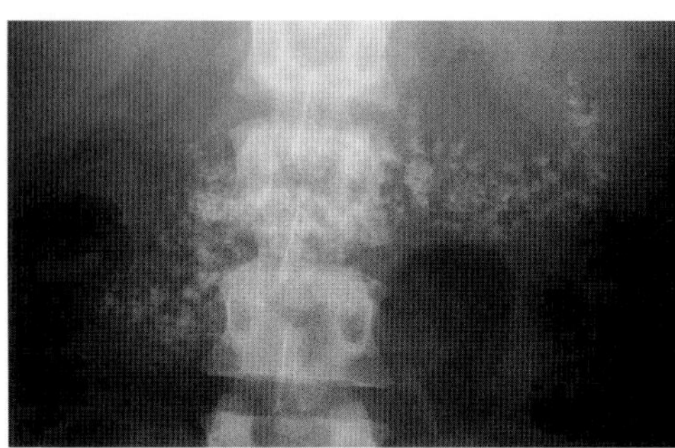

Fig. 9.32 Calcific pancreatitis related to hyperparathyroidism. Plain radiograph of the abdomen shows punctate calcifications in a lobular distribution. Compare the coarse intraductal calcifications due to alcohol abuse in Fig. 9.31 to the fine parenchymal calcifications shown here.

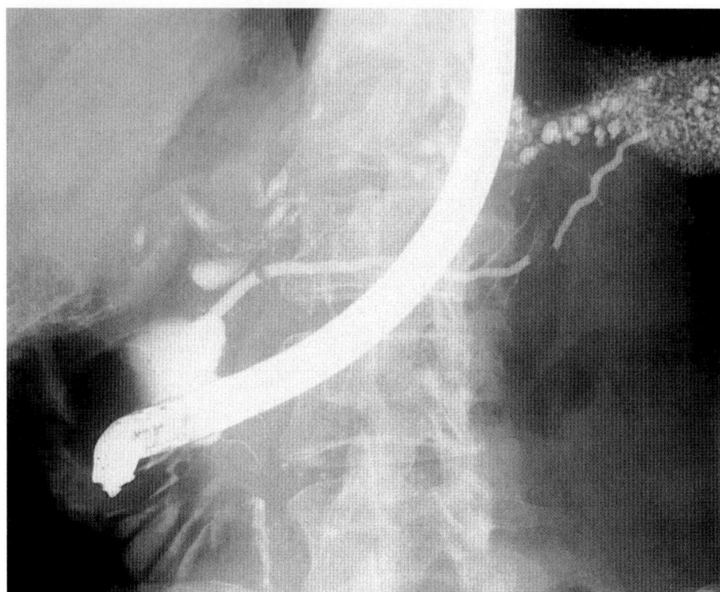

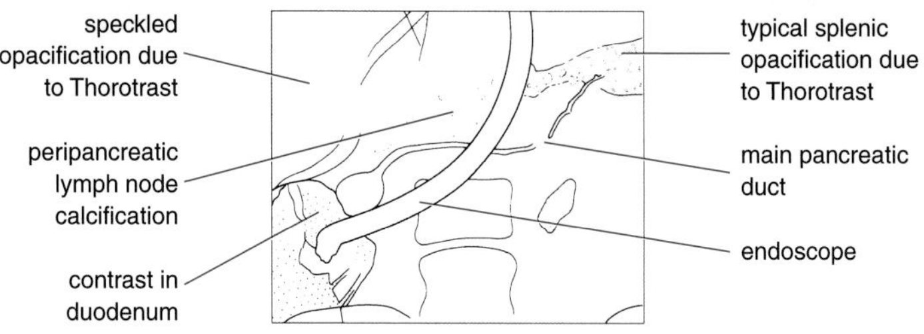

Fig. 9.33 ERCP in a patient given Thorotrast (an α-emitting radiographic contrast agent) many years previously. The agent is typically taken up in the spleen, and it is this splenic opacification that is the pointer to recognition that the other calcification is in lymph nodes and within the hepatic parenchyma rather than in the pancreas (see also Chapter 11). This patient was investigated for suspected chronic pancreatitis before the features were realized.

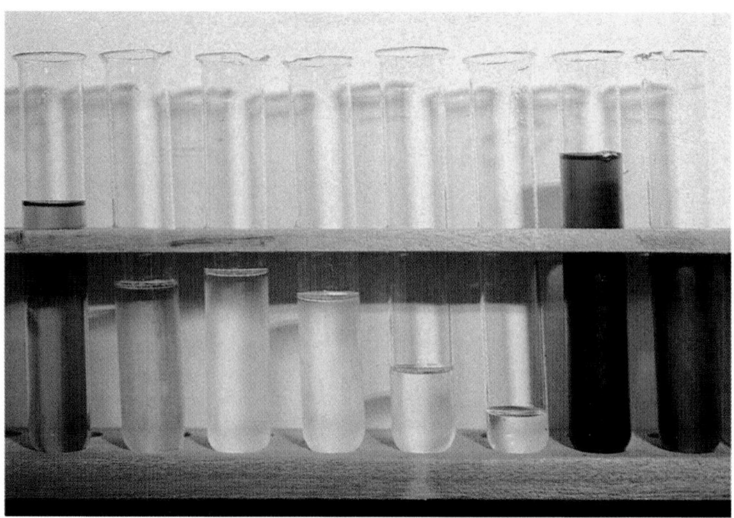

Fig. 9.34 Secretin pancreozymin test. Samples of duodenal juice show progressive clarification as bile is diluted out by pure pancreatic juice following injection of secretin. The two tubes on the right contain heavily bile-stained fluid after a further injection of pancreozymin is given, stimulating bile flow. Courtesy of Dr N. Gilinsky.

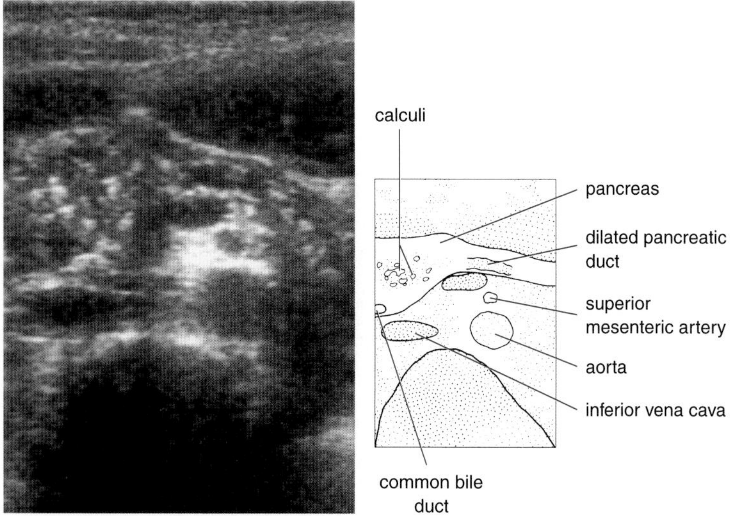

Fig. 9.35 Transabdominal ultrasound showing calcific pancreatitis. Courtesy of Prof W. Lees.

reproducible measure is that of total bicarbonate output which is reduced in chronic pancreatitis (Fig. 9.34).

Structural damage in the absence of overt calcification may be seen on ultrasound scanning or CT (Figs 9.35, 9.36). Barium studies are not normally helpful. Magnetic resonance imaging is informative but not yet as sensitive an investigation for early structural changes as the more invasive endoscopic retrograde pancreatography (ERP). Because the disease is primarily of duct origin, minor changes may be picked up which are too subtle for other forms of imaging and which cause no detectable functional defect (Fig. 9.37). As disease becomes more severe, larger ducts become involved, with eventual destruction and disorganization of the duct system (Figs 9.38, 9.39). The proximity of the distal stomach and duodenum to the pancreas has led to assessment of pancreatic scanning at endoscopic ultrasound (Figs 9.40, 9.41); although resolution is better than from transabdominal probes, the technique remains difficult and uncomfortable for patients and has not become routine. Stones in the pancreatic duct show well also by other forms of imaging (Fig. 9.42).

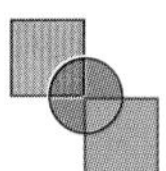

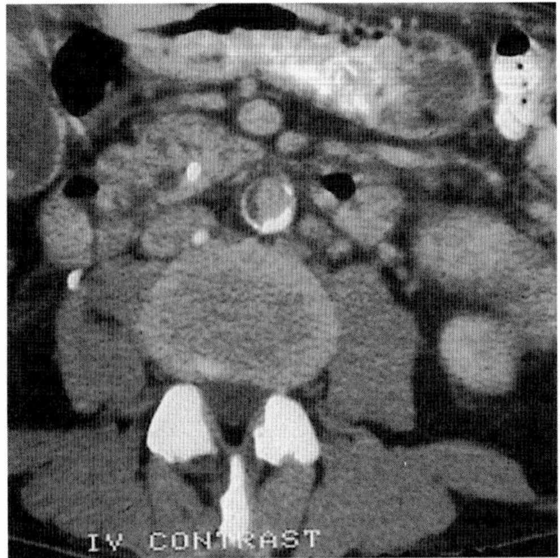

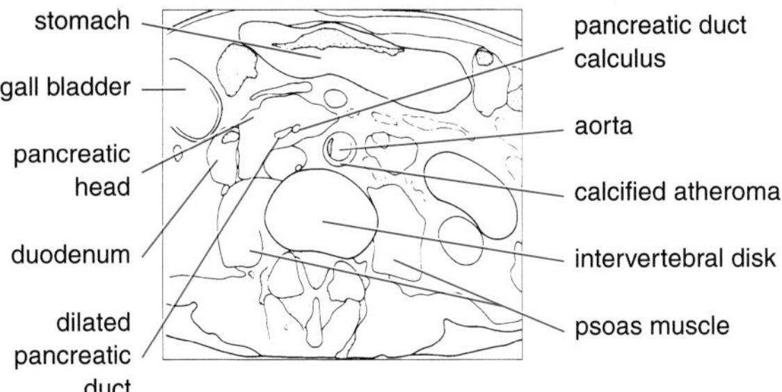

Fig. 9.36 CT scan in calcific pancreatitis affecting the head of the gland.

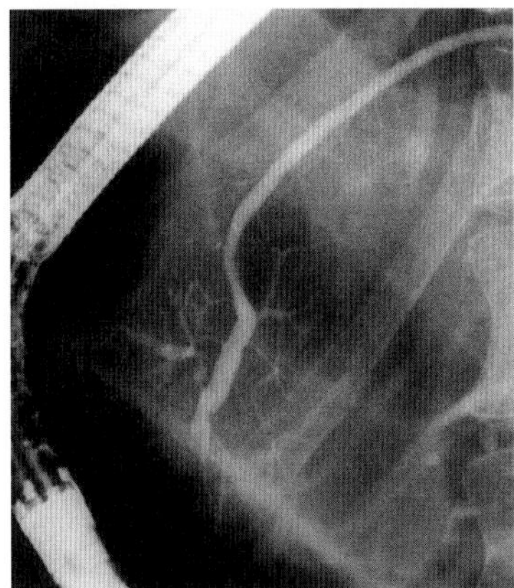

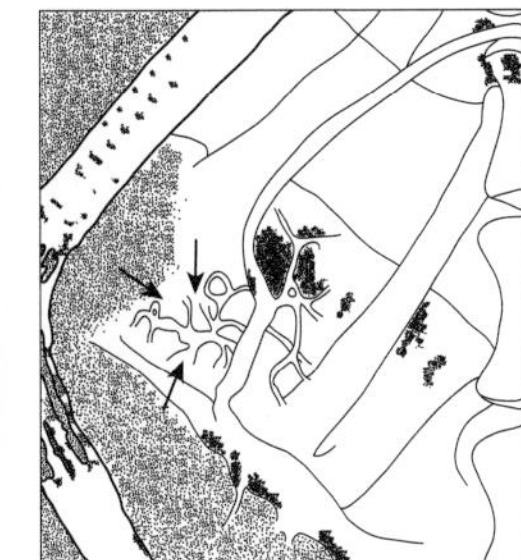

Fig. 9.37 Focal chronic pancreatitis demonstrated at ERCP. The main pancreatic duct is of normal caliber and contour. Focal dilatation and contour irregularity of side branches in the head of the pancreas indicates chronic pancreatitis.

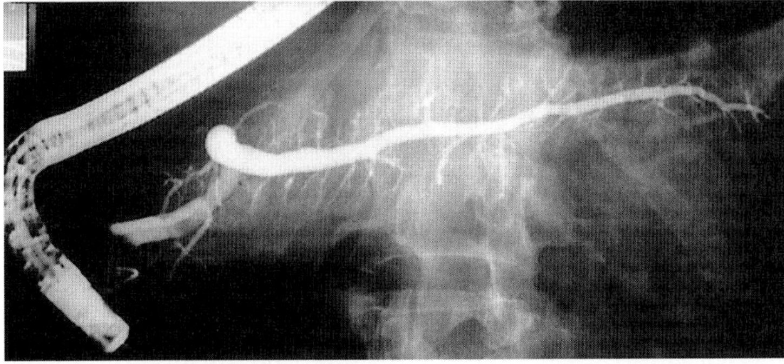

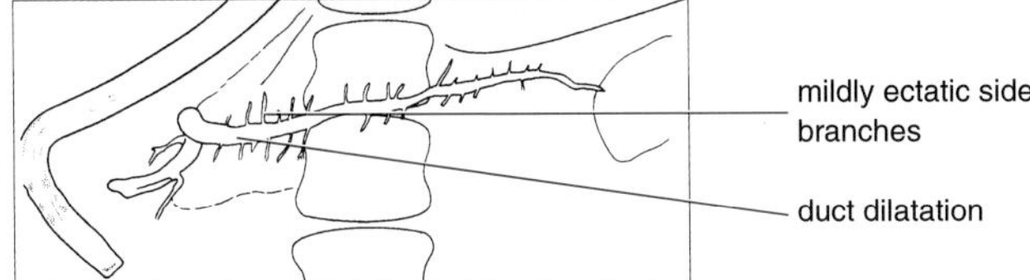

Fig. 9.38 Pancreatogram showing moderate pancreatitis with mild dilatation of the pancreatic duct and mild ectasia of the side branches. Courtesy of Dr D.F. Martin.

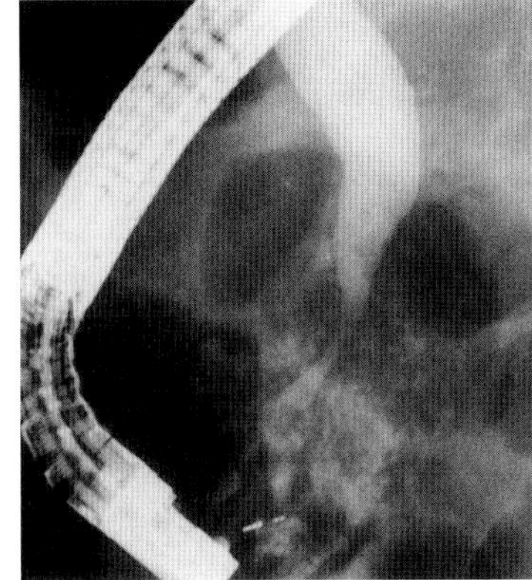

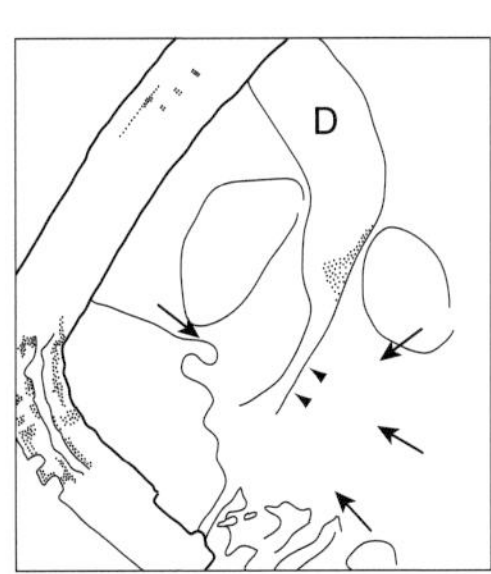

Fig. 9.39 Calcific pancreatitis with common bile duct stricture demonstrated at ERCP. Fine punctate calcifications are seen in the head of the pancreas. The distal common bile duct is mildly and diffusely narrowed. Dilatation of the bile duct proximal to the stricture implies obstruction.

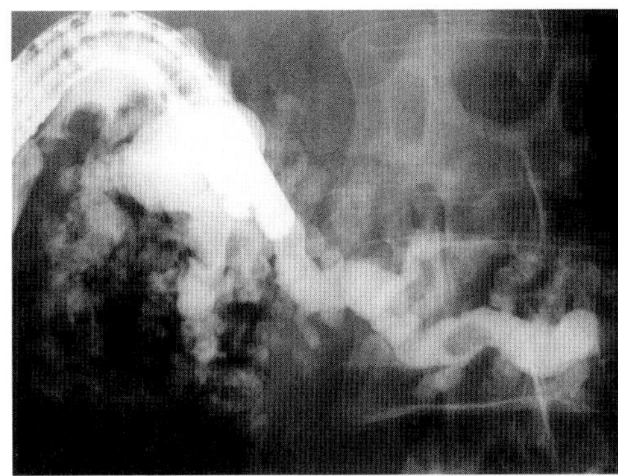

Fig. 9.40 ERCP demonstrating changes of marked chronic pancreatitis. Both the main pancreatic duct and side branches are markedly dilated with irregular, lobular contours. A calculus is manifest as a 6 mm polygonal radiolucency in the contrast filled, dilated main pancreatic duct in the tail of the pancreas.

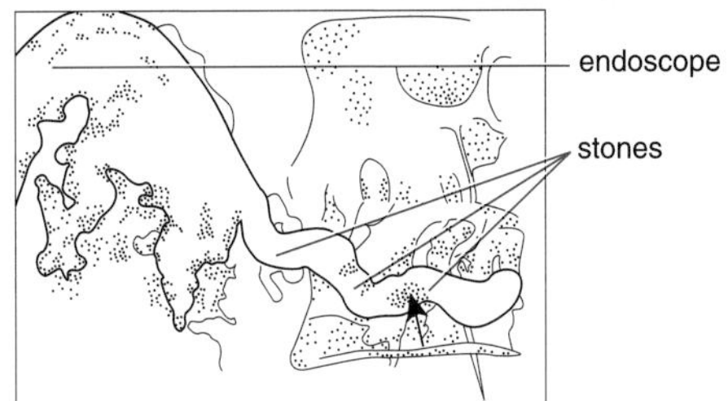

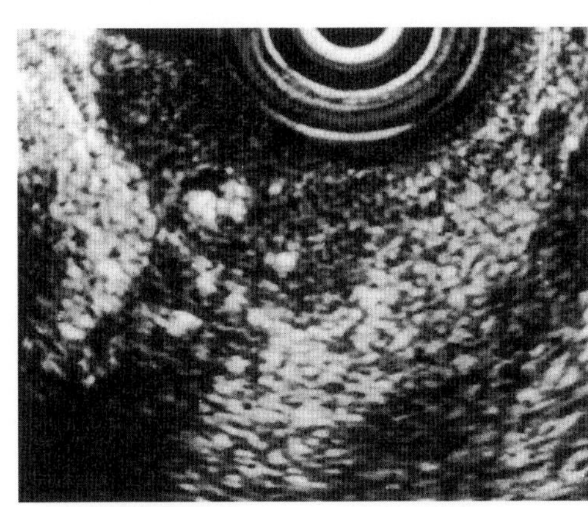

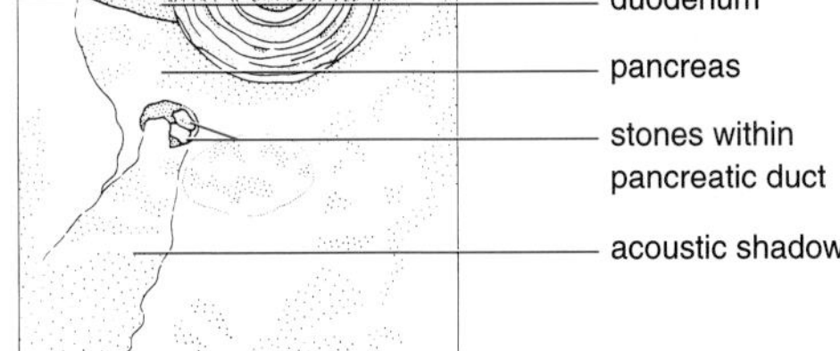

Fig. 9.41 Endoscopic ultrasound scan in chronic pancreatitis showing stones within the pancreatic duct.

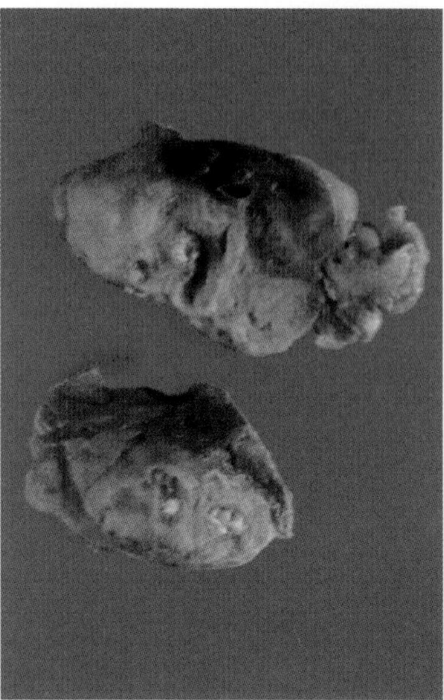

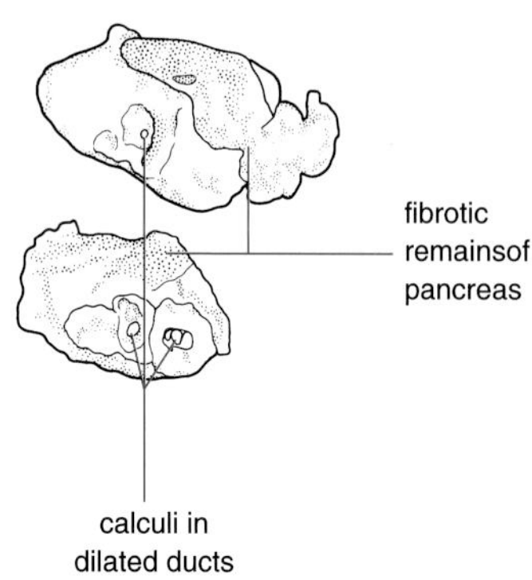

■ **Fig. 9.42** Macroscopic appearance in chronic pancreatitis. The two cross-sections shown were from a patient with severe chronic pancreatitis and demonstrate virtually complete destruction of the pancreatic tissue and the presence of multiple calculi.

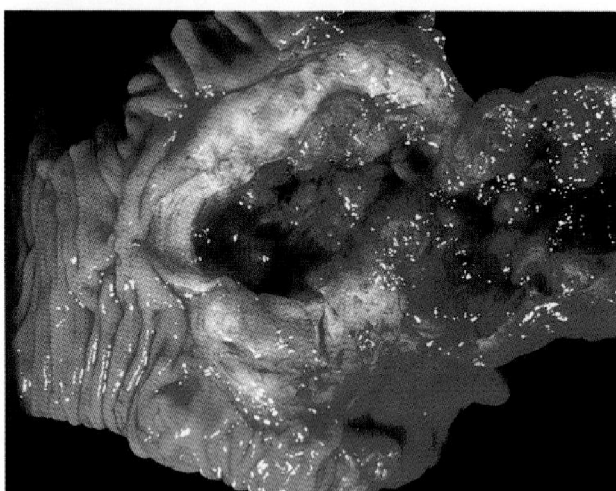

■ **Fig. 9.43** Intraductal papillary-mucinous neoplasm with mucinous ductal ectasia. Pancreatico-duodenectomy specimen with the main pancreatic duct opened longitudinally to reveal an intraductal papillary-mucinous neoplasm that has caused massive ductal dilatation and chronic obstructive pancreatitis of the pancreas. The tumor shows characteristically lush exophytic growth into the ductal lumen and the production of jelly-like masses of extracellular mucin that were seen exuding from the ampulla of Vater at endoscopy.

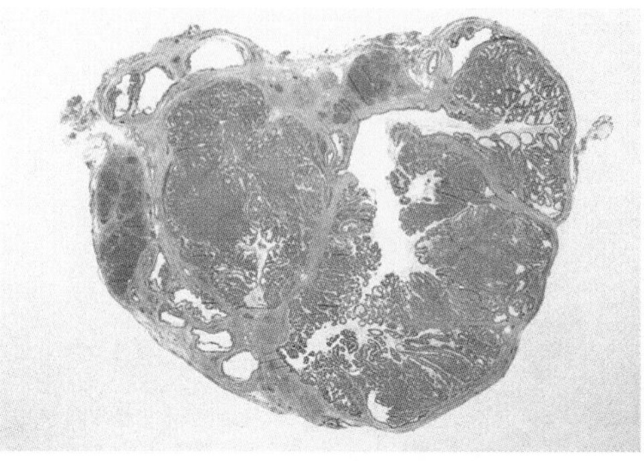

■ **Fig. 9.44** Intraductal papillary-mucinous neoplasm. Whole-mount transverse microscopic section through the head of the pancreas showing massive dilatation of the main pancreatic duct and its major branches, which are all filled with exophytic tumor, and total atrophy and scarring of the surrounding exocrine pancreatic parenchyma.

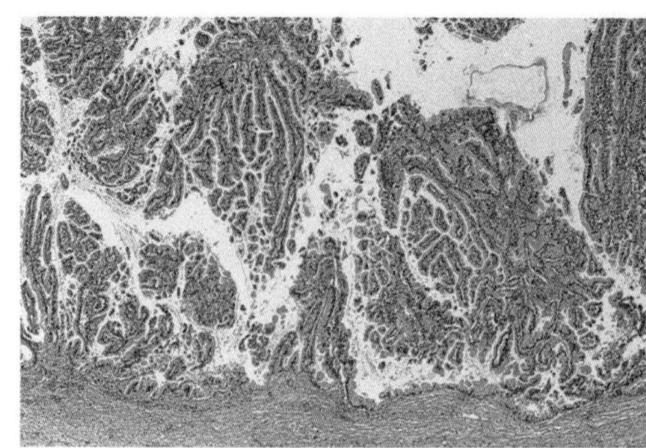

■ **Fig. 9.45** Microscopic appearance of an intraductal papillary-mucinous neoplasm with moderate dysplasia (borderline tumor) showing the villous adenoma-like tumor fronds replacing the normal ductal epithelium and filling the ductal lumen. These tumors tend to grow intraductally for long periods of time before undergoing malignant transformation and stromal invasion.

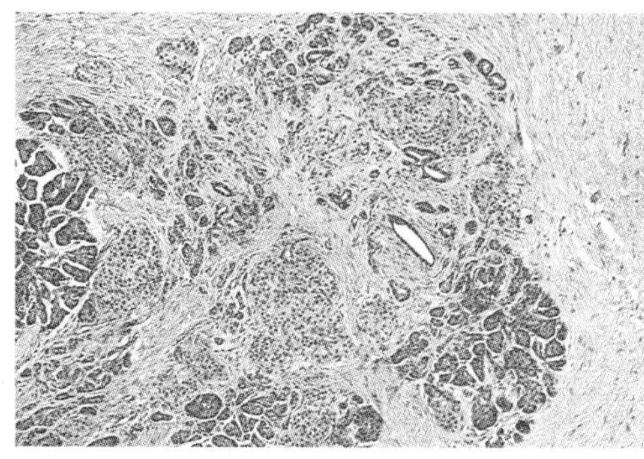

■ **Fig. 9.46** Chronic pancreatitis. Microscopic appearance showing the characteristic dense scarring around and within pancreatic lobules with atrophy of the exocrine pancreas, leaving only ducts and islets amid dense bands of fibrous tissue.

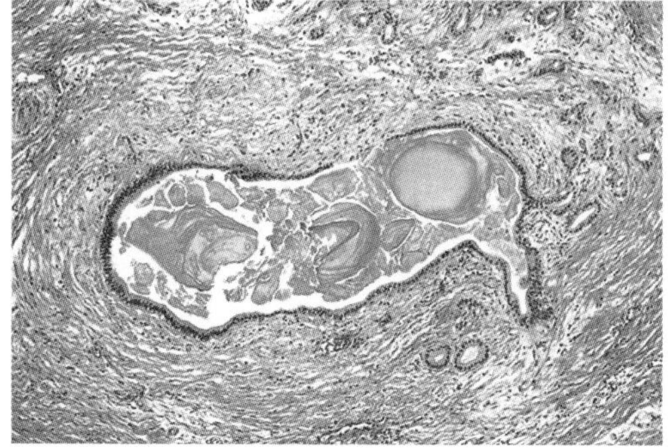

■ **Fig. 9.47** Microscopic view of a dilated duct in chronic pancreatitis that is surrounded by scar tissue and contains concretions of inspissated secretions in the lumen.

Chronic pancreatitis may be focal or generalized. The gland tends to be very firm to the touch, and loses its normal lobulation over the diseased area (Fig. 9.43); there is loss of acinar tissue and its replacement by fibrosis and chronic inflammation. Confusion may arise in the early stages of intraductal neoplasia because of the concurrence of features of pancreatitis (which also exists) (Figs 9.44–9.46). In uncomplicated chronic pancreatitis the islets of Langerhans usually remain intact, and although the ducts remain identifiable, these are usually hyperplastic or otherwise abnormal. Characteristically, the ducts are filled with proteinaceous precipitates (including stone-forming protein), and they become progressively more dilated and cystiform. Finally, the whole gland is replaced by fibrous tissue and associated calcified fat necrosis (Figs 9.47–9.49).

Hereditary pancreatitis and Shwachman's syndrome

Familial pancreatitis was recognized in the 1950s, and several hundred kindreds are now reported. It is probably inherited as an autosomal dominant condition with variable penetrance. The incidence has a bimodal age distribution with peaks at about 10 and 17 years, but the condition may present at any age. Pancreatic calcification often develops in the first decade, but in most respects, the clinical course is similar to that of chronic pancreatitis of other causes (Figs 9.50, 9.51). Children with chronic pancreatitis who do not belong to an affected family usually have a structural abnormality in the pancreas or biliary tree (particularly pancreas divisum or choledochal cyst – see above and Chapter 14).

The association of pancreatic malabsorption, including steatorrhea and failure to thrive, with metaphyseal dysplasia, neutropenia, and other hematological abnormalities, is known as Shwachman's syndrome, and accounts for a high proportion of children presenting with painless pancreatic insufficiency. It is probably inherited as an autosomal recessive condition. With appropriate dietary modification

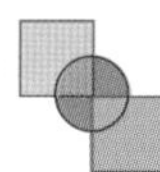

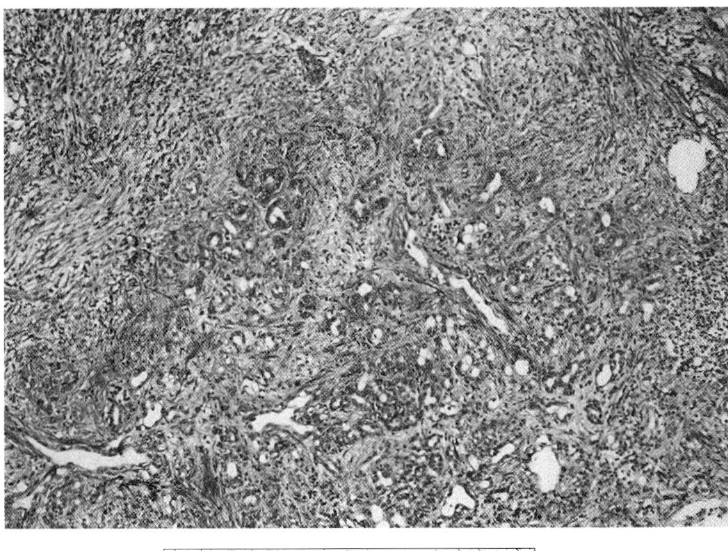

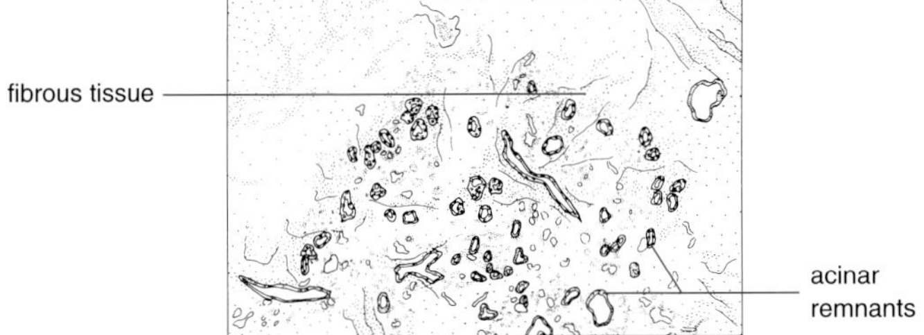

■ **Fig. 9.48** Phosphotungstic acid hematoxylin (PTAH) stain emphasizes the fibrous tissue (rust colored); only scattered pancreatic acini survive (x 75).

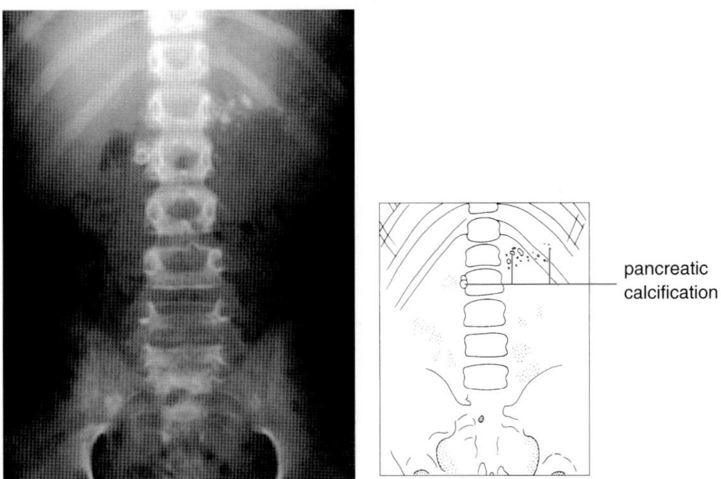

■ **Fig. 9.49** Pancreatic calcification in a child with a strong family history of pancreatitis.

and enzyme supplements, the prognosis is good (see also section on cystic fibrosis below).

Complications of pancreatitis

In addition to pain and malabsorption, edema of the pancreatic head may be responsible for bile duct obstruction and consequent cholestasis. Potential confusion with malignant biliary obstruction exists if the histology for chronic pancreatitis is lacking, but the smooth-bordered tapering of the lower common bile duct should point to the correct interpretation of a benign extrinsic compression (Fig. 9.52).

Pancreatic pseudocyst

Pancreatic pseudocysts are almost always a complication of acute pancreatitis and are unusual in chronic pancreatitis, other than after

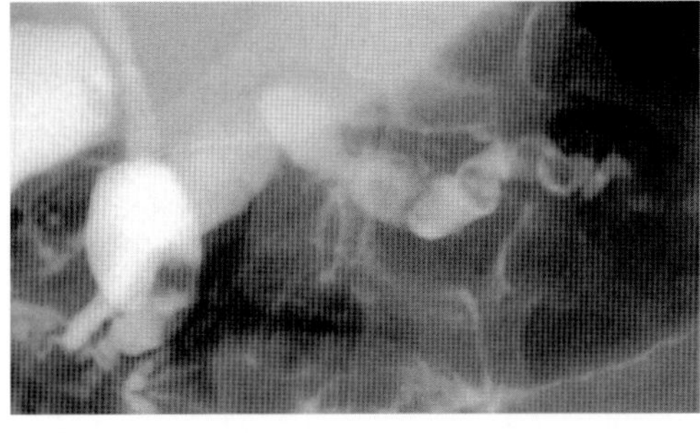

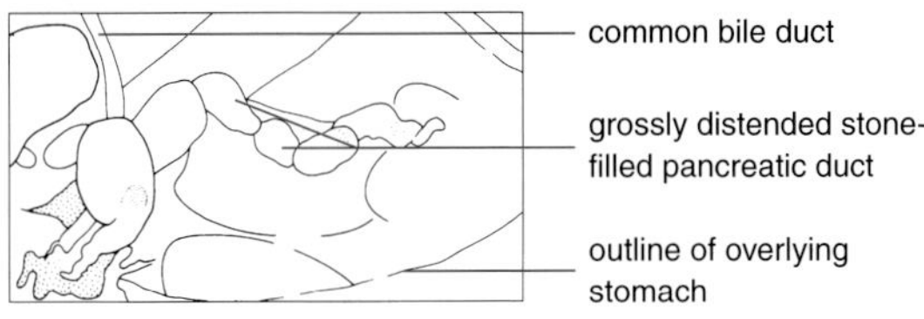

■ **Fig. 9.50** ERCP film of the same patient as in Fig. 9.49 showing the stones and the strictured main pancreatic duct which takes on some of the features of the so-called 'chain-of-lakes.'

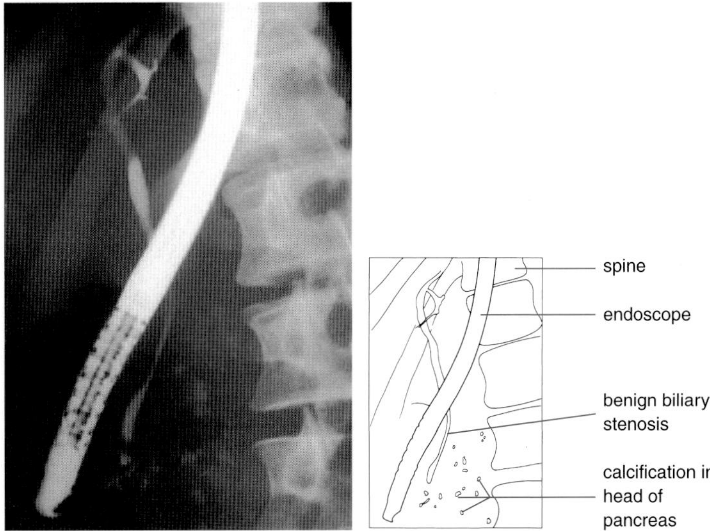

■ **Fig. 9.51** Benign biliary stenosis in calcific chronic pancreatitis. The long smooth narrowing is typical of extrinsic compression.

an attack of acute-on-chronic pancreatitis. Pseudocysts are encapsulated, localized collections of fluid and contain diagnostically useful high concentrations of pancreatic enzymes; they are usually confined to the retroperitoneal areas by a fibrous membrane that is devoid of endothelial lining, and hence they are not true cysts (Fig. 9.53). Although relatively rare outside the peritoneal cavity, pseudocysts may migrate to the mediastinum or pelvis, and associated pleural effusions also occur. Cystic collections may also be the direct result of necrosis during an episode of acute pancreatitis. Since the advent of ultrasound scanning it has been recognized that pseudocysts represent a very common complication of acute pancreatitis (Fig. 9.54), but only rarely does their size warrant intervention. Most lesions with a diameter of 5 cm or less resolve spontaneously. When larger (Fig. 9.55), pseudocysts may cause pain, weight loss, or gastrointestinal obstruction, with or without a palpable mass. ERCP is relatively contraindicated in the presence of cystic disease since it may provoke cyst infection and the subsequent development of abscess formation, but it may be helpful in delineating the limits of disease in pre-intervention assessment (Fig. 9.56). Cysts are usually in communication with the pancreatic duct, although imaging does not always confirm this. Untreated large cysts may become infected spontaneously, and may rupture into the peritoneal cavity or an adjacent

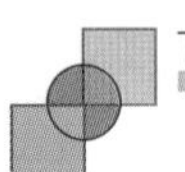

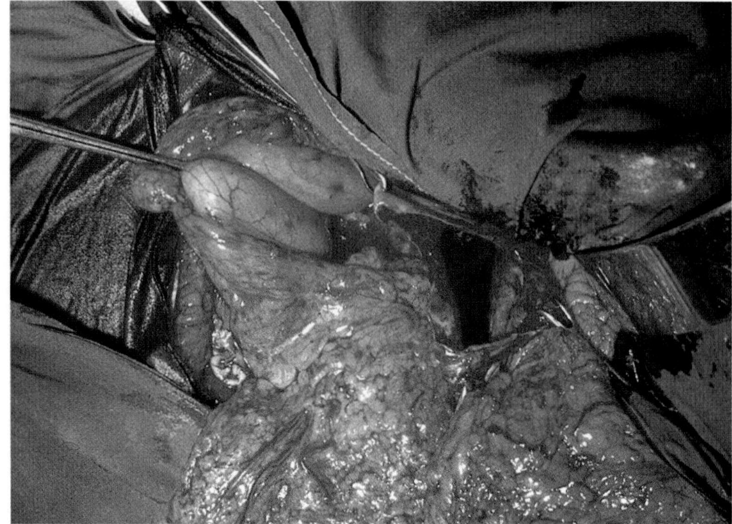

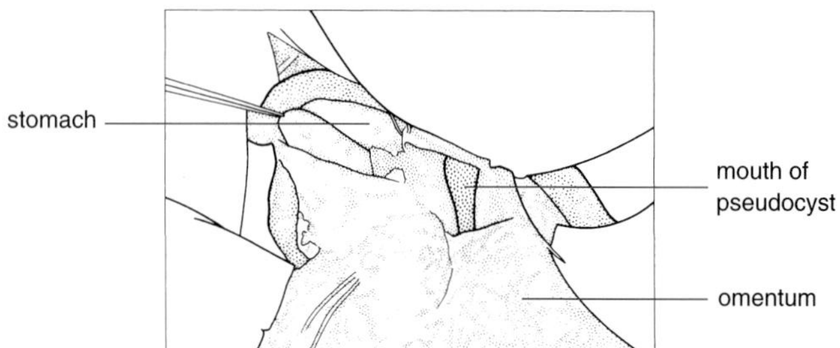

Fig. 9.52 Pancreatic pseudocyst at laparotomy. Courtesy of Mr B. Torrance.

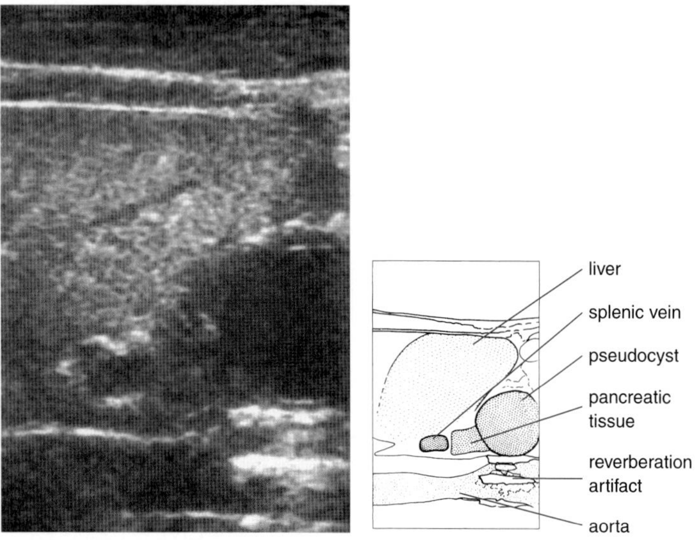

Fig. 9.53 Ultrasound scan (longitudinal section) showing a pancreatic pseudocyst. Courtesy of Prof W. Lees.

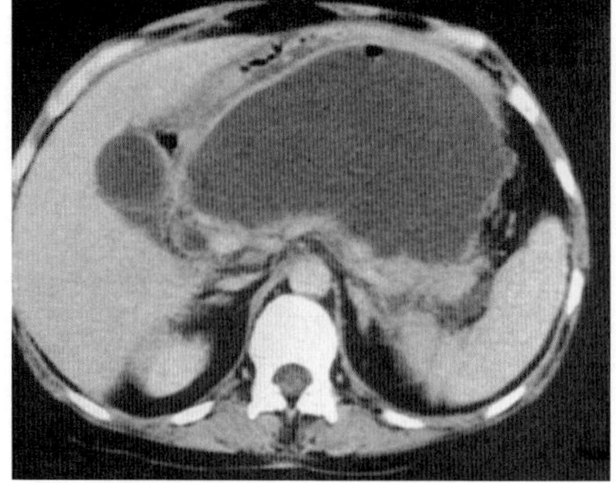

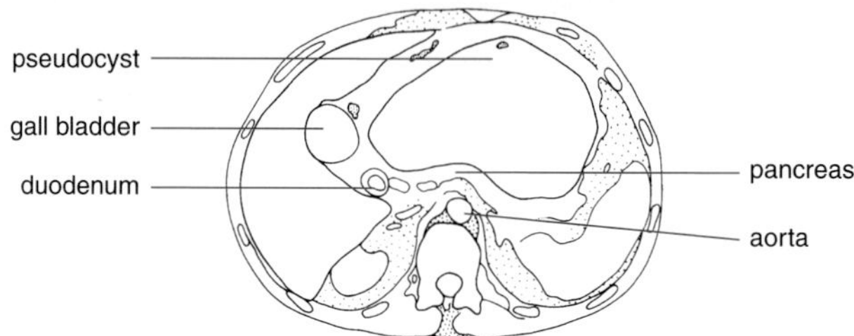

Fig. 9.54 CT scan showing a large pancreatic pseudocyst almost filling the upper abdomen.

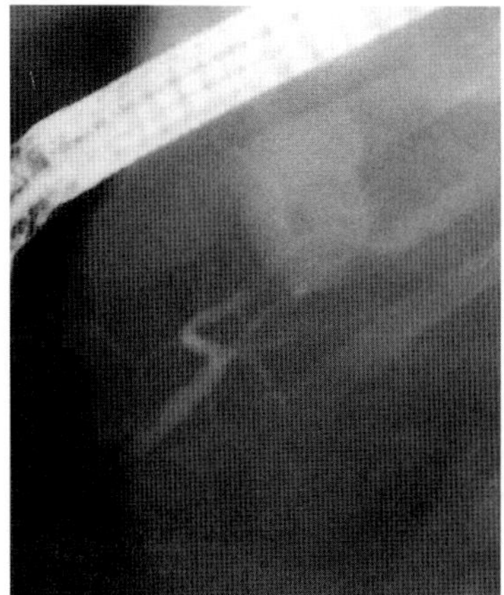

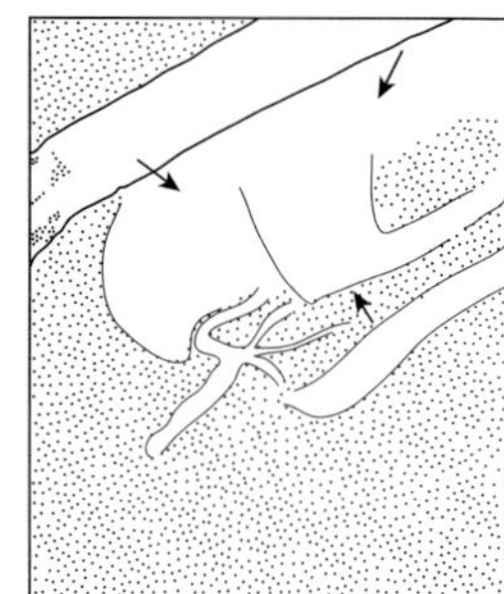

Fig. 9.55 ERCP demonstrating filling of pancreatic pseudocyst after injection of the main pancreatic duct.

viscus; the involvement of major vessels is rare, but devastating if it occurs (Fig. 9.57).

True cysts and cystic neoplasms of the pancreas

True cysts, with an endothelial lining, are usually congenital or dermoid, and are less often a result of widespread hydatid disease (see Chapter 11). They may be single or multilocular and are always separate from the pancreatic duct system. Cystic tumors of the pancreas include serous cystic neoplasms, which are almost always benign (serous cystadenomas) and mucinous cystic neoplasms, which are classified as benign, borderline or malignant (in situ) depending on the degree of epithelial dysplasia present. If any amount of invasive carcinoma if present in a mucinous cystic neoplasm, the entire tumor is classified as a mucinous cyst adenocarcinoma. As a group, cystic tumors are uncommon. They typically cause only vague non-specific abdominal symptoms or are symptomatic and discovered incidently on imaging studies. (Figs 9.58–9.65).

CARCINOMA OF THE PANCREAS

Pancreatic carcinoma has an increasing incidence in Western populations and remains of unknown etiology, although higher incidences in males, in smokers and, to a lesser extent, in those with chronic pancreatitis or diabetes are recognized.

Early symptoms are non-specific, and the diagnosis is often not made until marked weight loss is associated with obstructive jaundice from involvement of the common bile duct (Fig. 9.66). Only rarely is an epigastric mass palpable. Very occasionally, tumors are responsible for apparent acute pancreatitis or a predominantly malabsorptive presentation. Pancreatic carcinoma is particularly associated with an increased tendency to thrombosis (hence Trousseau's description of thrombophlebitis migrans in himself). A pancreatic mass is usually readily shown on ultrasound or CT scanning (Figs 9.67, 9.68). ERCP no longer has a place in diagnosis (Figs 9.69–9.75), but

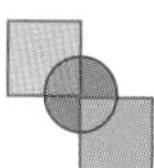

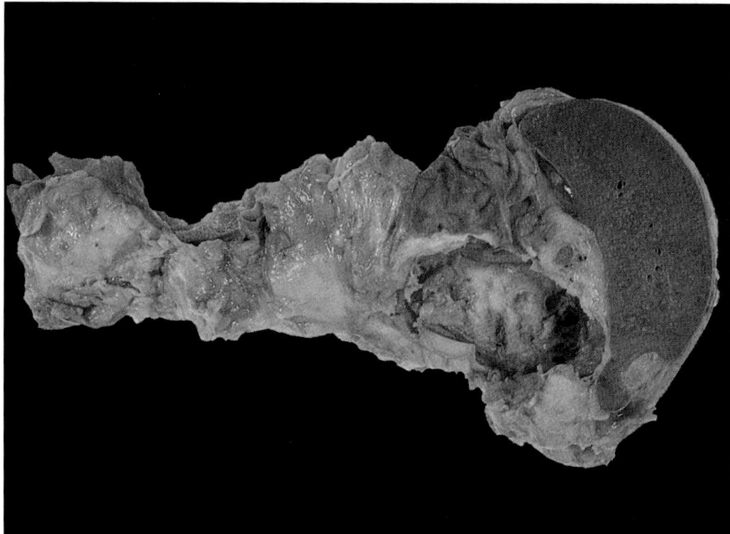

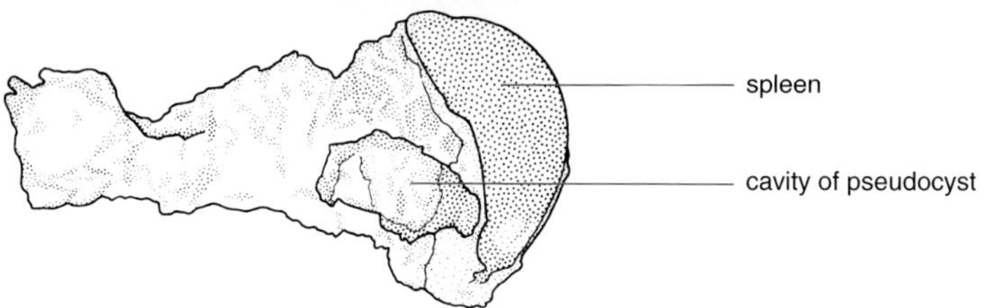

■ **Fig. 9.56** Macroscopic appearance of a pseudocyst in the tail of the pancreas lying adjacent to the spleen. Courtesy of Dr D.W. Day.

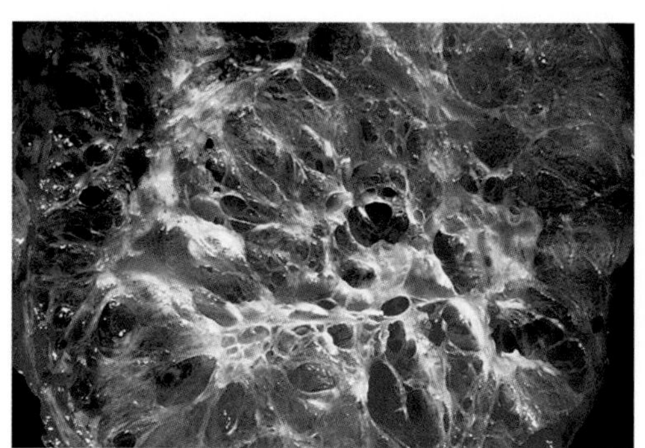

■ **Fig. 9.57** Serous cystadenoma. Surgical resection specimen of a serous cystadenoma of the pancreas showing the typical large size, well-defined borders, and sponge-like macroscopic appearance characterized by myriad small locules with smooth linings and watery contents.

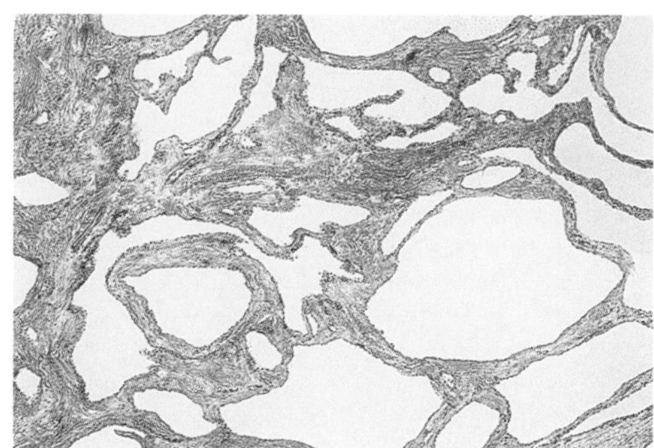

■ **Fig. 9.58** Serous cystadenoma. Microscopic appearance showing the innumerable simple cysts separated by delicate fibrovascular interstices that comprise the tumor.

retains a crucial role in palliative therapy, since most pancreatic tumors are irresectable (Fig. 9.76). Endoscopic ultrasound may be useful, especially if resection is being considered (Fig. 9.77), and most pancreatic surgeons would add to CT (Fig. 9.78), a pre-operative exclusion of vascular encasement or involvement of draining veins by angiography (Figs 9.79, 9.80).

About two thirds of carcinomas occur in the head of the pancreas. Tumors are generally poorly demarcated, grayish hard masses, the cut surface showing variable hemorrhage and necrosis (Figs

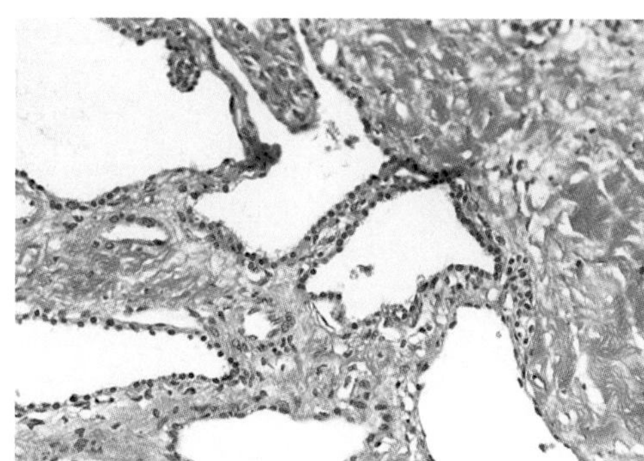

■ **Fig. 9.59** Microscopic appearance of a serous cystadenoma of the pancreas showing the characteristically small, monomorphic epithelial cells with clear, glycogen-rich cytoplasm and no discernible mitotic activity that line the locules.

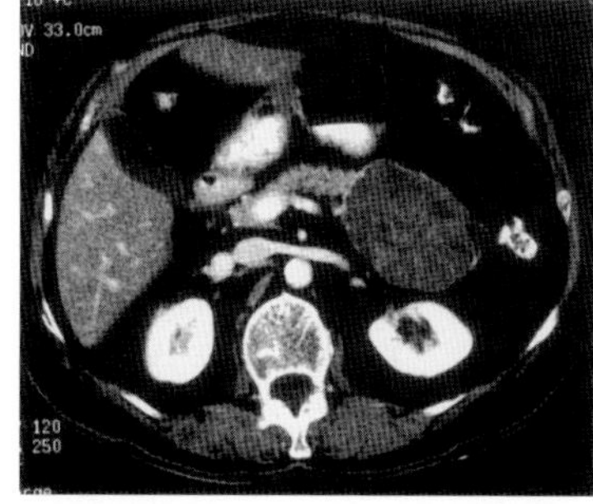

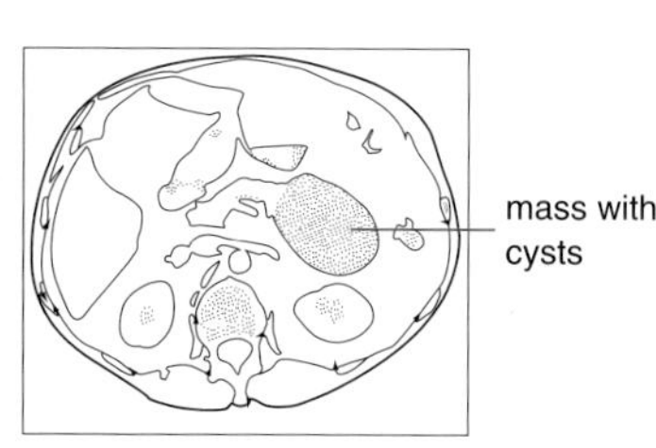

■ **Fig. 9.60** CT demonstrating a microcystic adenoma (serous cystadenoma) of the pancreas. The window level and width are adjusted to bring out tiny 0.5–2 mm cysts in a 4 cm mass in the tail of the pancreas. The normal pancreatic body is identified.

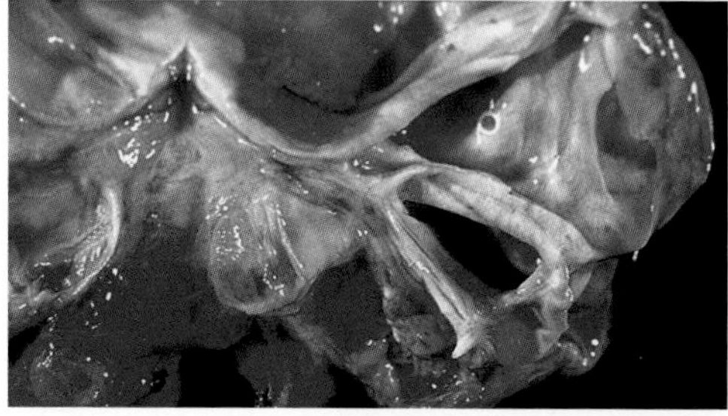

■ **Fig. 9.61** Mucinous cystic neoplasm. Surgical resection specimen showing the typical oligocystic composition, smooth lining, and gelatinous contents.

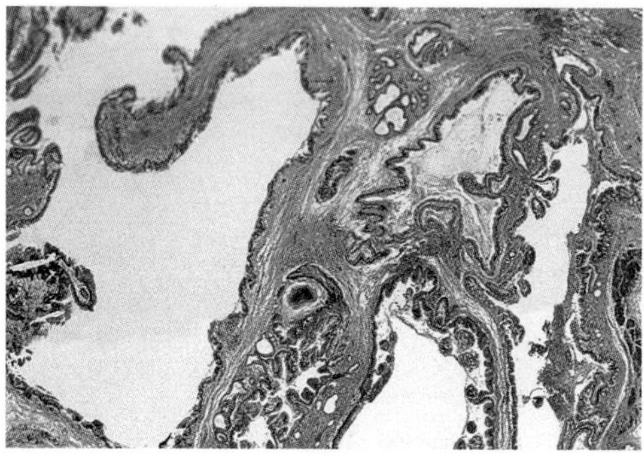

■ **Fig. 9.62** Microscopic appearance of a mucinous cystic neoplasm of the pancreas showing locules lined by a single layer of mucin-producing epithelium lacking significant dysplasia but focally forms small tufts. These tumors are subclassified as benign, borderline, or malignant depending upon the greatest degree of cytological atypia found within the tumor.

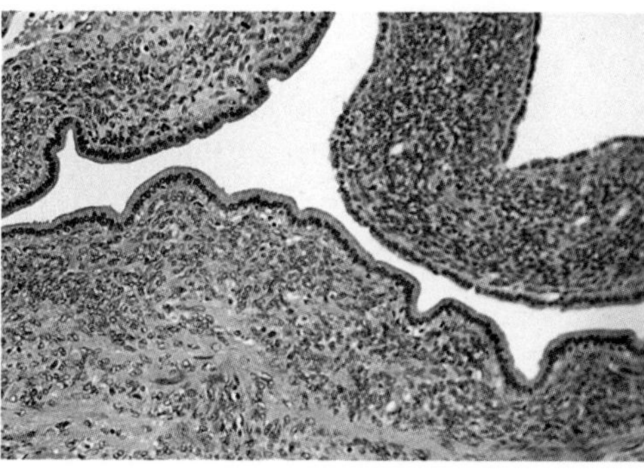

■ **Fig. 9.63** Microscopic view of a mucinous cystic neoplasm showing the uniquely distinctive, highly cellular 'ovarian' stroma that is seen in many tumors in female patients and bears receptors for estrogen and progesterone.

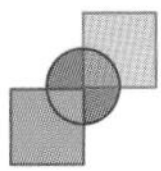

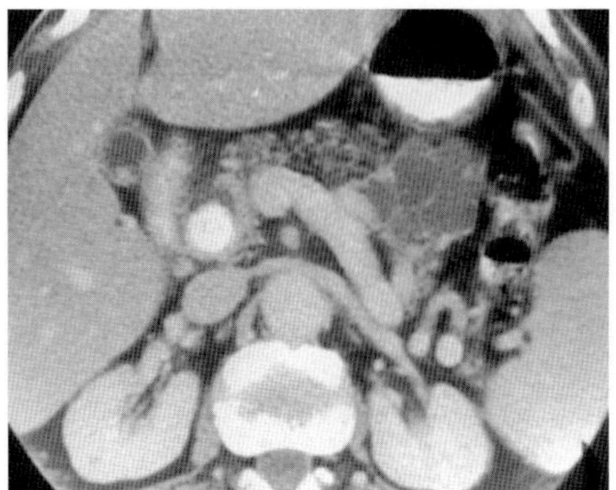

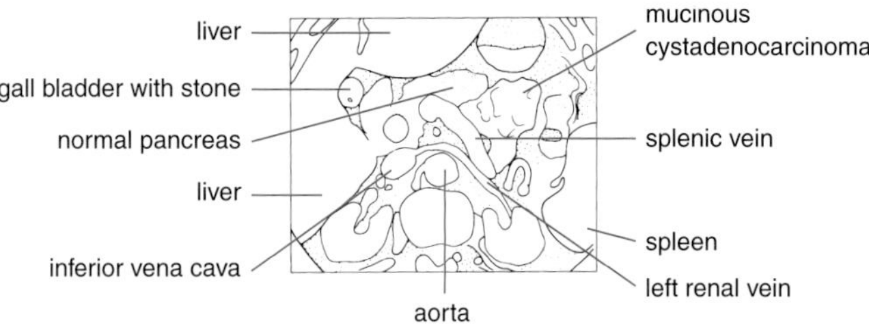

Fig. 9.64 CT scan showing the complex multilocular cystic mass of a mucinous cystadenocarcinoma arising from the tail of the pancreas.

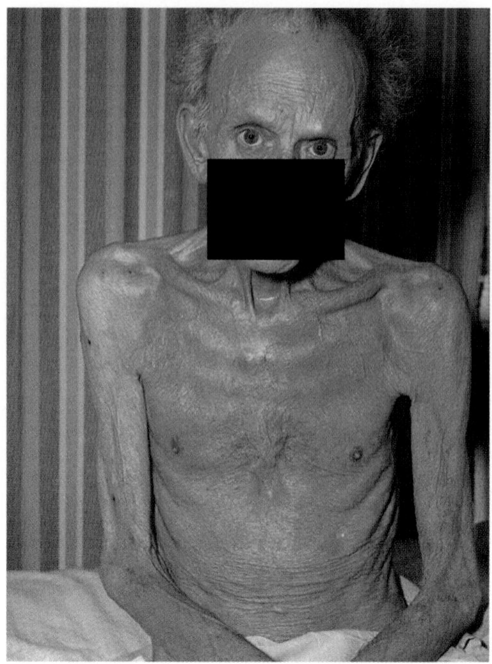

Fig. 9.65 An emaciated jaundiced patient with carcinoma of the pancreas.

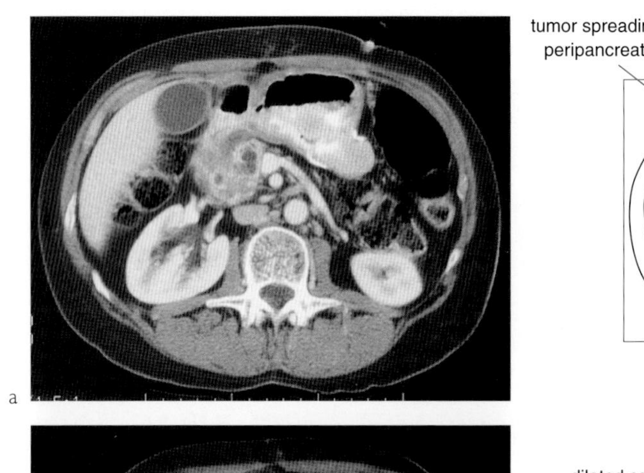

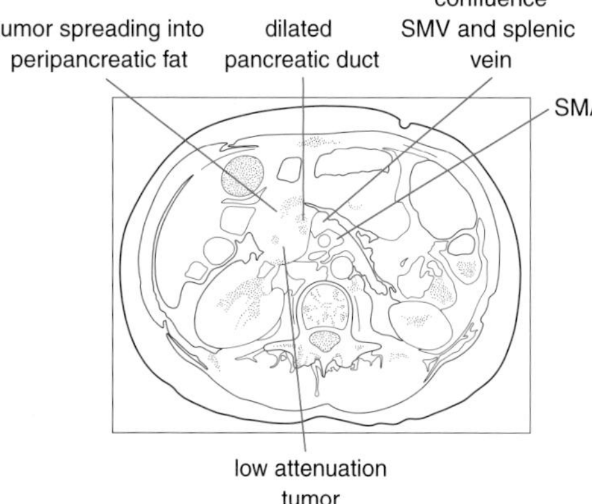

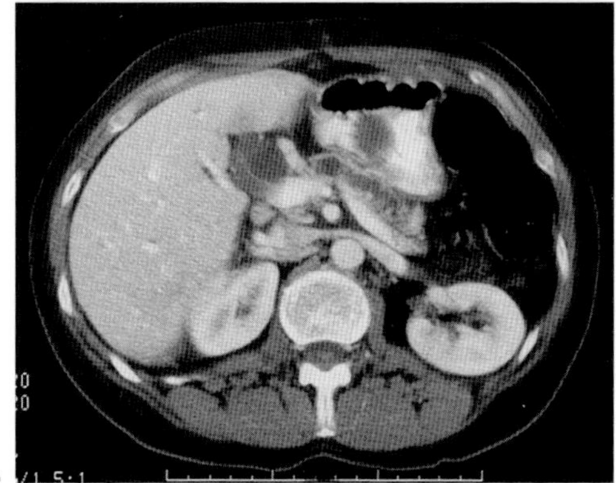

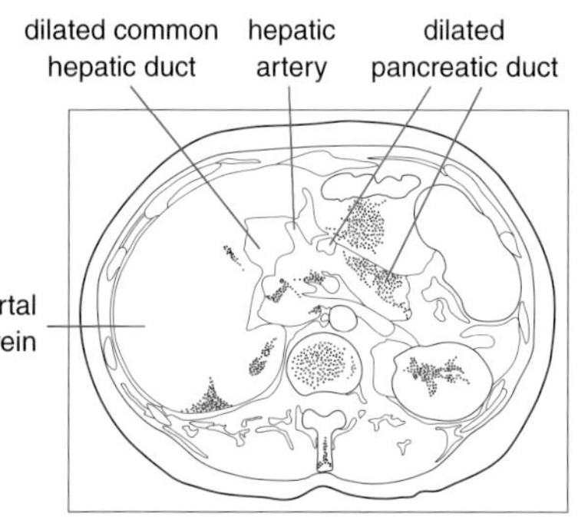

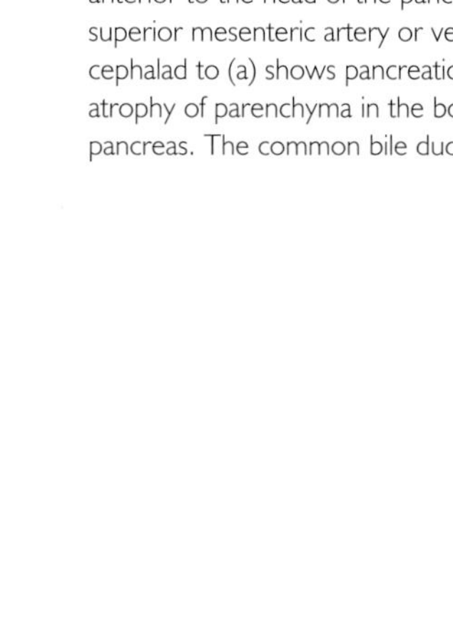

Fig. 9.66 CT demonstrating pancreatic carcinoma with biliary obstruction. (a) The more caudal CT image demonstrates an enlarged head of the pancreas with an irregular area of low attenuation tumor. The main pancreatic duct is dilated. Tumor spreads into the fat anterior to the head of the pancreas. No invasion of the superior mesenteric artery or vein is seen. (b) Image cephalad to (a) shows pancreatic ductal dilatation and atrophy of parenchyma in the body and tail of the pancreas. The common bile duct is mildly dilated.

9.81–9.83). Occlusion of the pancreatic duct with upstream dilatation, and features of chronic pancreatitis, are recognized and contribute to the so-called 'double duct sign' on imaging where both the pancreatic duct and the common bile duct are dilated (Fig. 9.74). By the time of diagnosis, pancreatic carcinoma has usually spread to contiguous structures; unfortunately in most cases jaundice represents invasion, rather than merely compression of the biliary tree.

Confirmation of the diagnosis is achieved in at least 75% of cases, either cytologically with fine-needle aspiration (Fig. 9.84), or histologically with core biopsies guided by ultrasound or CT. Approximately 80% of pancreatic carcinomas are ductal adenocarcinomas, which may be subclassified by degree of differentiation, the presence of mucin, and by the presence or absence of squamous elements or giant cells (Fig. 9.85). Less often, tumors have predominantly acinar characteristics or a major mucinous (colloid) component.

All the variants of pancreatic carcinoma have a poor prognosis, with virtually no survivors to 5 years. Resection may achieve a cure in the occasional patient in whom investigation of pancreatitis reveals apparently incidental early intraductal tumor.

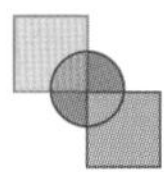

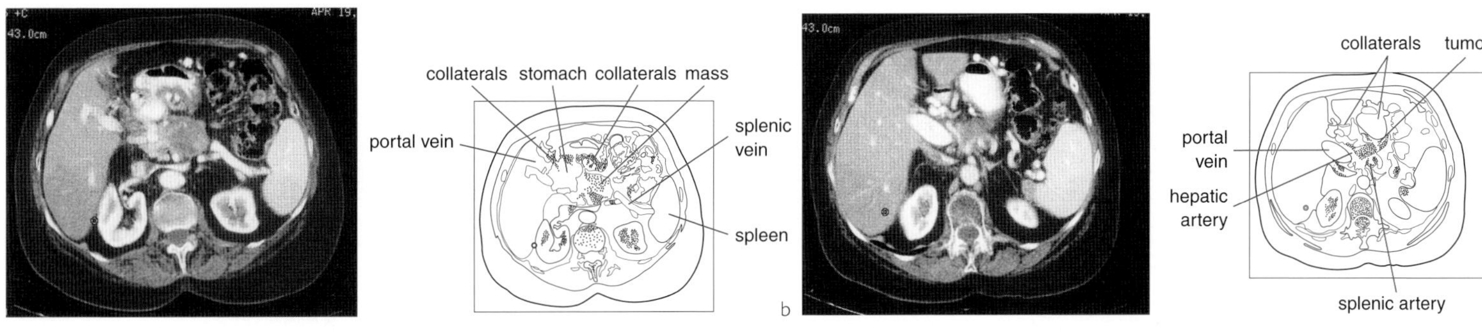

Fig. 9.67 CT demonstrating pancreatic carcinoma with vascular invasion. (a) The more caudal CT image demonstrates an inhomogeneous, low-attenuation mass at the junction of the head and body of the pancreas. The superior mesenteric vein is not seen. Enhancing collateral vessels are indicative of splenic and superior mesenteric venous obstruction. (b) Image cephalad to (a) shows tumor spreading superiorly to encase the splenic artery and hepatic artery. Numerous perigastric and hepatoduodenal ligament collaterals are due to splenic vein and superior mesenteric vein obstruction.

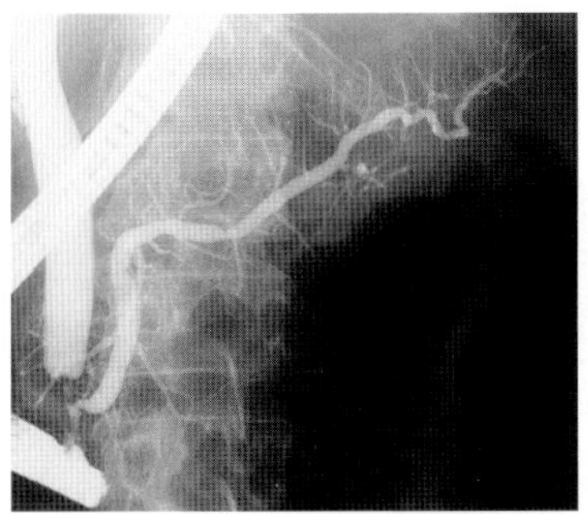

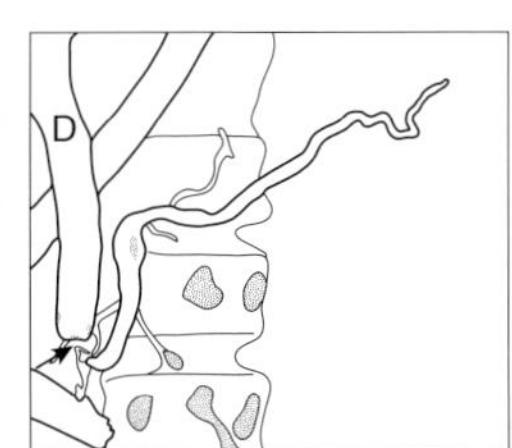

Fig. 9.68 ERCP demonstrating carcinoma in the head of the pancreas obstructing the distal common duct. A focal stricture is seen in the distal common bile duct. The biliary tree proximal to the stricture is dilated. The main pancreatic duct is still normal in this patient.

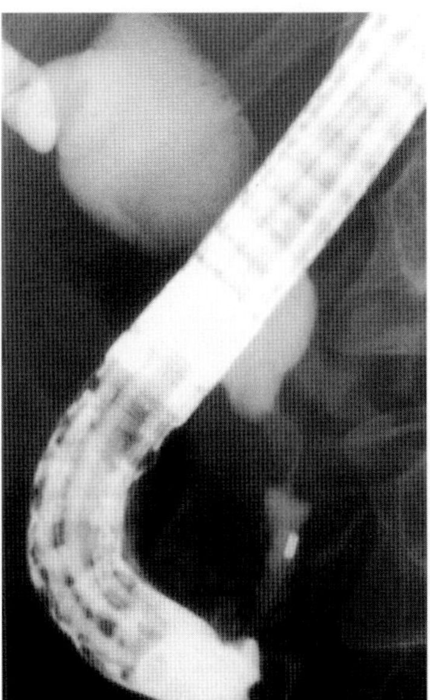

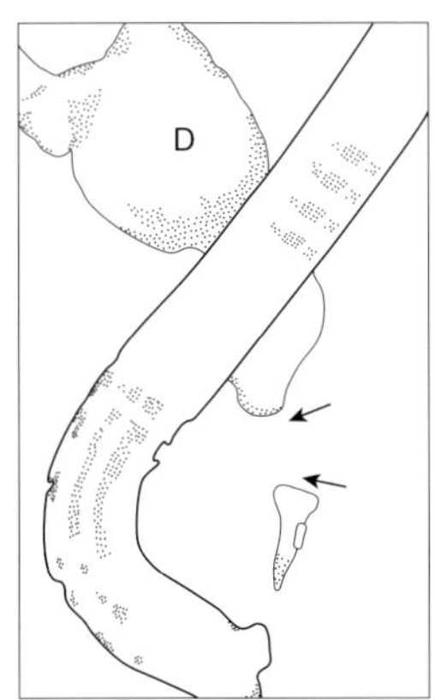

Fig. 9.69 ERCP demonstrating carcinoma in the head of the pancreas obstructing the distal common duct. A focal stricture 18 mm long is seen in the common bile duct. The biliary tree proximal to the stricture is markedly dilated.

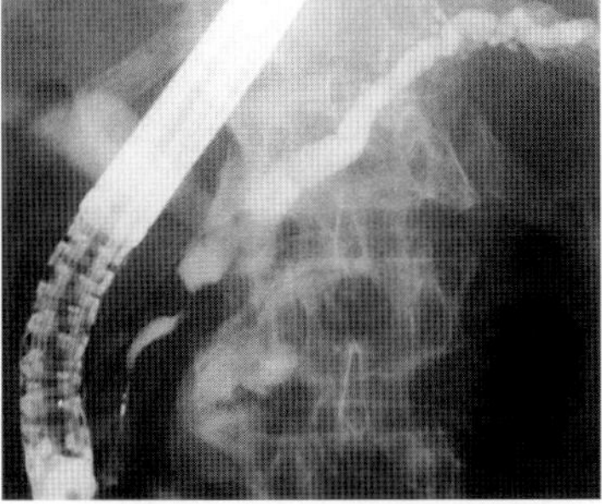

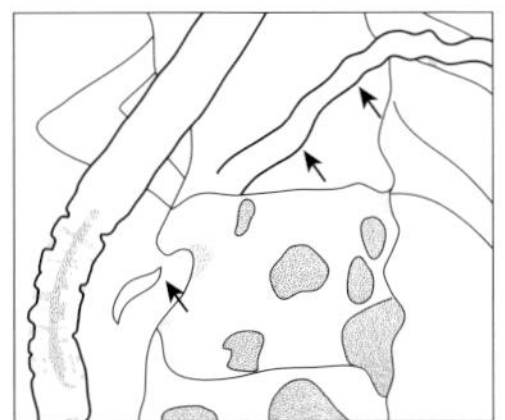

Fig. 9.70 ERCP demonstrating carcinoma in the head of the pancreas obstructing the main pancreatic duct. A short (5 mm) stricture is seen in the head of pancreas. The main pancreatic duct is dilated to the left of the stricture.

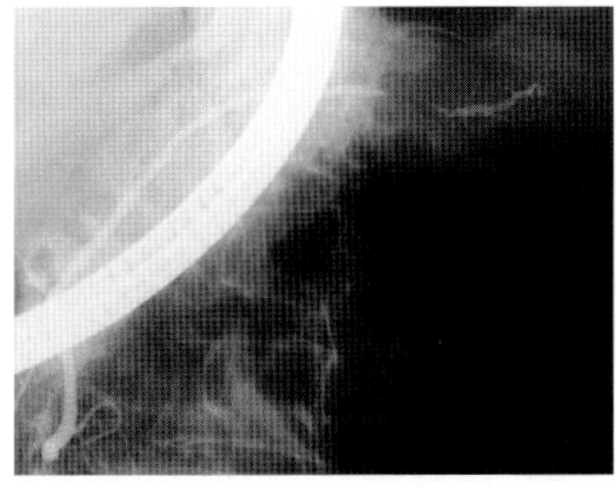

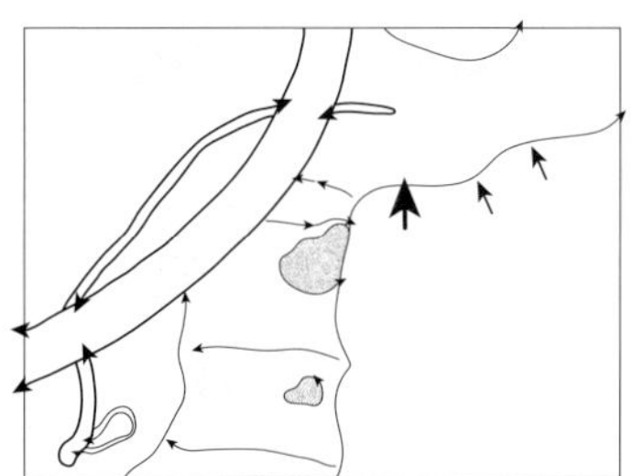

Fig. 9.71 ERCP showing pancreatic carcinoma in the tail of the pancreas. A focal stricture is seen in the tail of the pancreas. The main pancreatic duct and side branches beyond this are dilated.

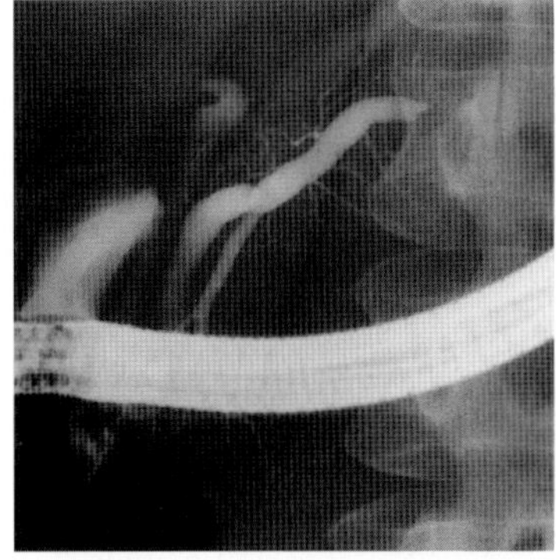

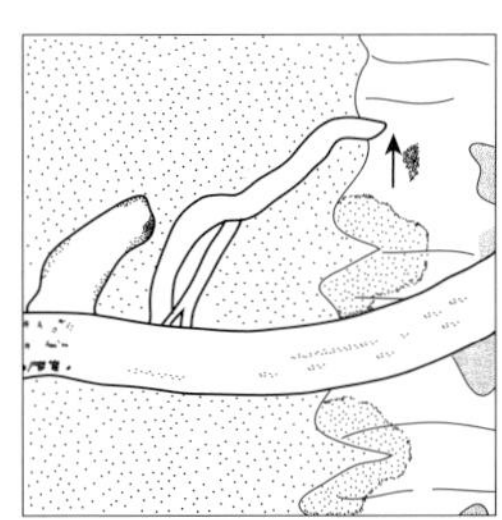

Fig. 9.72 ERCP showing abrupt cut-off of the main pancreatic duct in the body of the pancreas. This radiographic finding is most frequently seen in pancreatic carcinoma, but can be due to pancreatitis or to blunt trauma.

Endocrine pancreatic tumors

Endocrine tumors of the pancreas have excited considerable interest because of their impact on gastrointestinal function: major advances in the understanding of gut endocrinology have been the result. These tumors are almost always small, and present as a result of their hormonal effects, rather than because of an effect on pancreatic exocrine secretion or from mass effects, even when the tumor is malignant. Zollinger–Ellison syndrome – the result of a gastrin-producing adenoma or adenocarcinoma – has been considered already (see Chapters 2 and 3). Adenomas producing vasoactive intestinal peptide are responsible for the Werner–Morrison syndrome of watery diarrhea. The primarily endocrine effects of the insulinoma, and the characteristic dermatological manifestations of glucagonoma, are unlikely to lead to presentation to the gastroenterologist, but it should be remembered that although hypersecretion of one particular hormone generally predominates, hypersecretion to a lesser degree of several gut hormones is usual. Diagnosis is suggested by the clinical manifestations, supported by an assay for the relevant hormone;

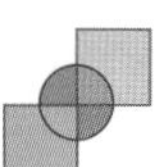

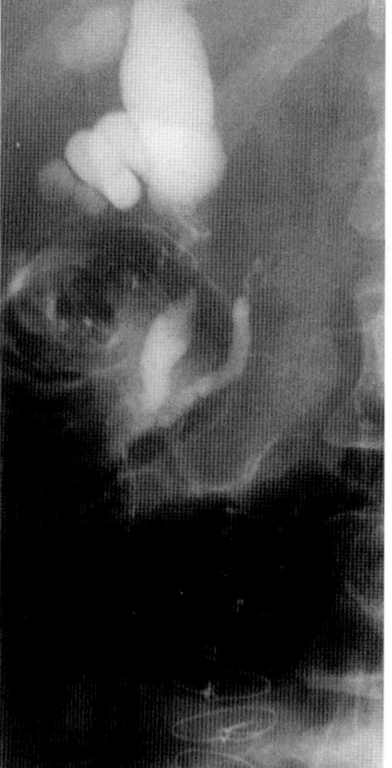

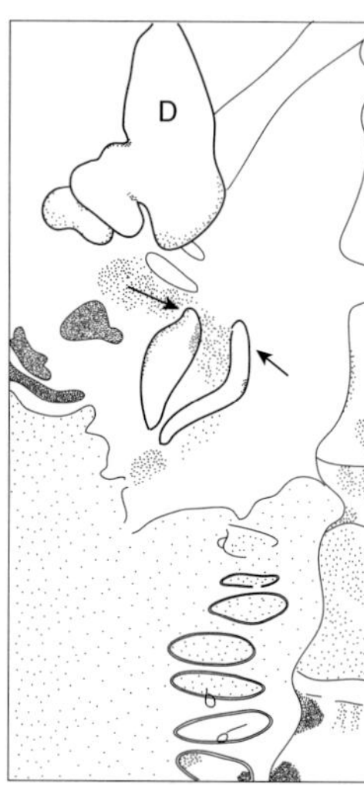

Fig. 9.73 ERCP demonstrating pancreatic carcinoma causing strictures in the pancreatic and bile ducts. Retrograde obstruction to flow of contrast and a stricture are seen in the main pancreatic duct in the head of the pancreas. Adjacent to this stricture, there is a stricture in the common bile duct. The common hepatic duct proximal to the stricture is dilated implying obstruction. This is the so-called 'double duct sign,' most frequently seen in patients with pancreatic carcinoma.

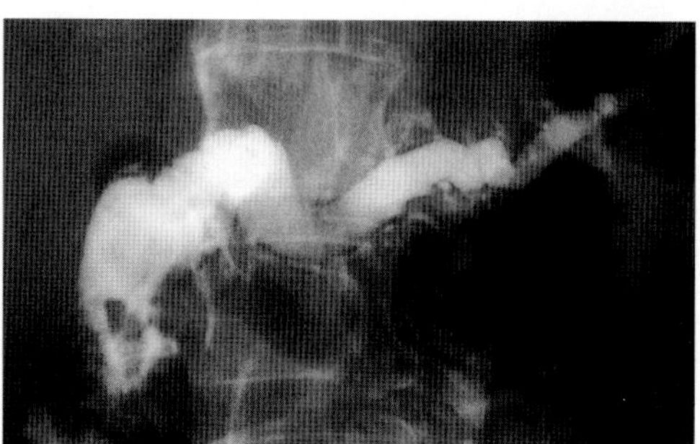

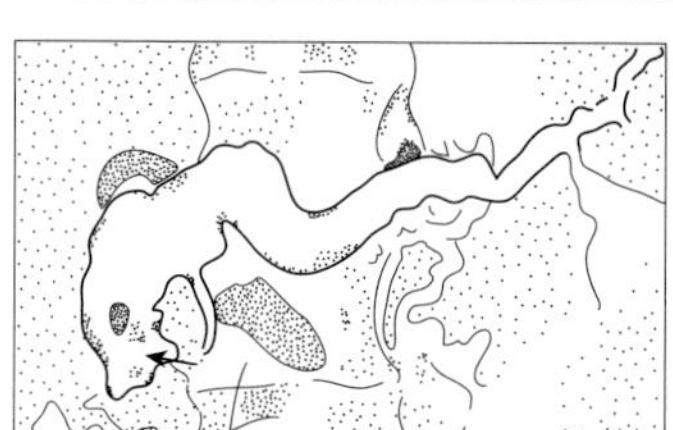

Fig. 9.74 ERCP in a patient with an intraductal papillary mucinous neoplasm (IPMT). The main pancreatic duct is diffusely and markedly dilated. Side branches are dilated.
A polypoid radiolucent filling defect is seen in the contrast column in the head of the pancreas, representing a papillary component of the tumor. At endoscopy, mucin poured out of a bulging papilla of Vater. This tumor was previously termed 'mucinous duct ectasia.'

localization requires careful imaging, endoscopic ultrasound having a particular role in identifying these small lesions (Figs 9.86–9.89). Selective arteriography may be helpful but selective venous sampling is now rarely performed.

PERI-AMPULLARY CARCINOMA

Peri-ampullary carcinomas are not strictly of pancreatic origin, but their clinical presentation and endoscopic appearances render consideration here appropriate. In distinction from pancreatic carcinoma, prompt diagnosis is often valuable, as resection may well be possible and of long-term therapeutic benefit. Obstructive jaundice is the usual presenting feature, and ultrasound (especially endoscopic) or a CT scan may demonstrate the causative lesion (Fig. 9.90). At ERCP, the endoscopic appearance is immediately suggestive of a malignant tumor at the ampulla (Fig. 9.91), and when contrast is introduced the absence of extension along the pancreatic duct or bile duct helps in the distinction from an infiltrating pancreatic carcinoma or (more rarely) downwards extension of a cholangiocarcinoma which may otherwise be responsible for similar endoscopic appearances (see Chapter 14). Biopsies, taken at endoscopy or ERCP, should confirm the diagnosis and further reduce the potential confusion with a spreading pancreatic or bile duct tumor. Ampullary neoplasms usually only invade locally (Figs 9.92, 9.93).

The usual histological pattern is of moderately well-differentiated adenocarcinoma. Softer papillary tumors of the ampulla may resemble colonic villous adenoma (see Chapter 7) but are almost always malignant. There can be difficulty in assessment of ampullary histology given the interlacing of normal periductular glands with the adjacent smooth muscle; the histologist is helped by a careful description of the endoscopic findings and well-orientated biopsy samples, to be sure that invasive tumor is recognized but also that florid benign cases are not overcalled as examples of infiltrating tumor.

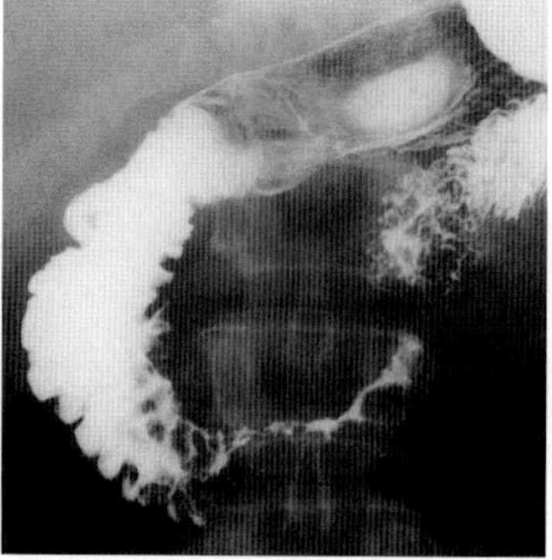

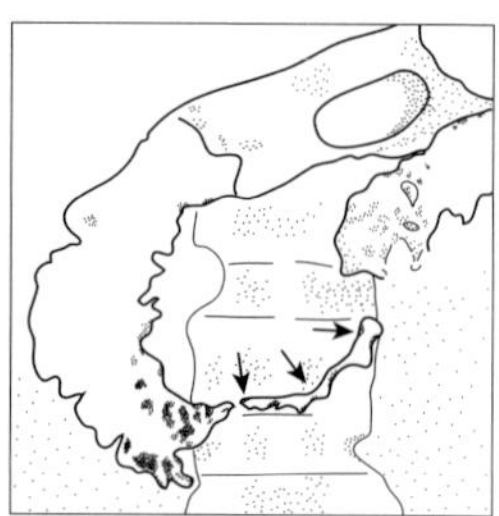

Fig. 9.75 Double-contrast upper GI study showing pancreatic carcinoma invading the third and fourth portions of the duodenum. There is diffuse narrowing of the distal duodenum with thick, nodular mucosal folds. Upper endoscopy had been 'negative' in this patient with vomiting.

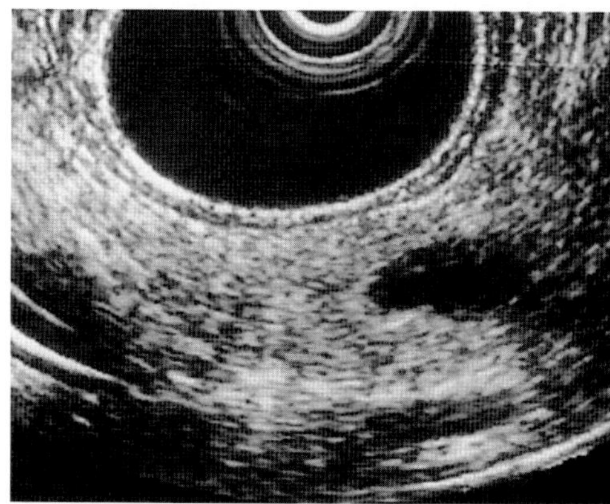

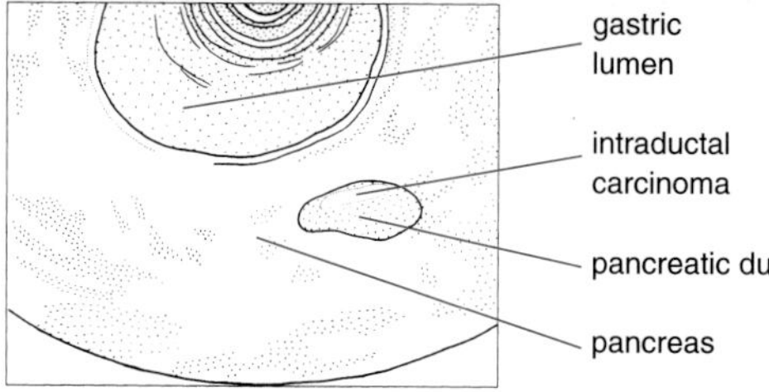

Fig. 9.76 Endoscopic ultrasound appearance of an early intraductal pancreatic carcinoma, which was not demonstrable at conventional ultrasound or CT scanning.

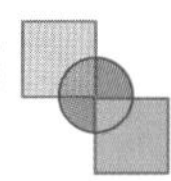

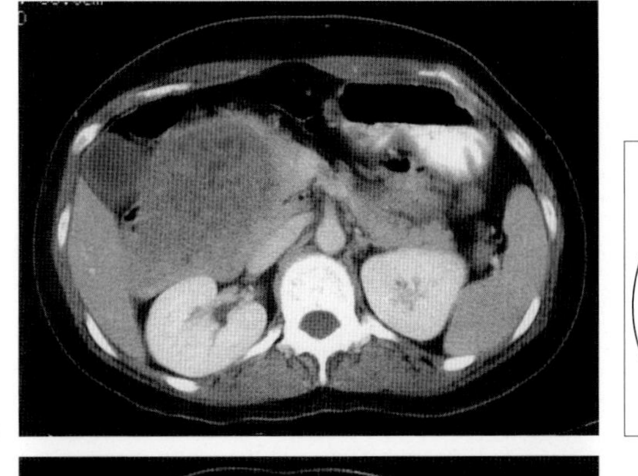

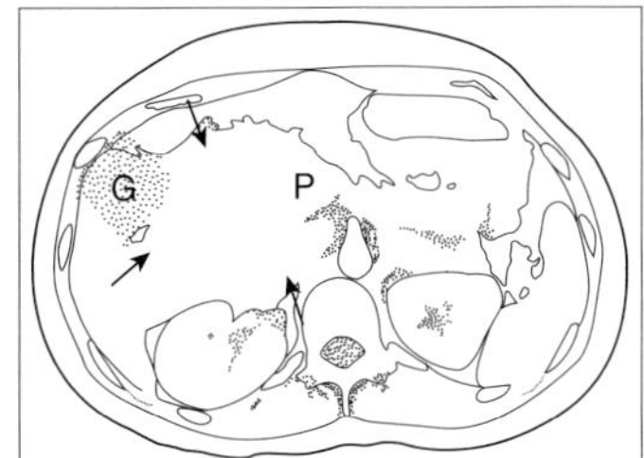

a

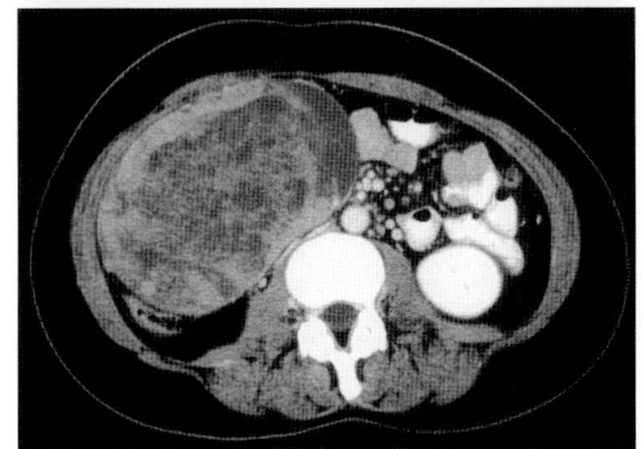

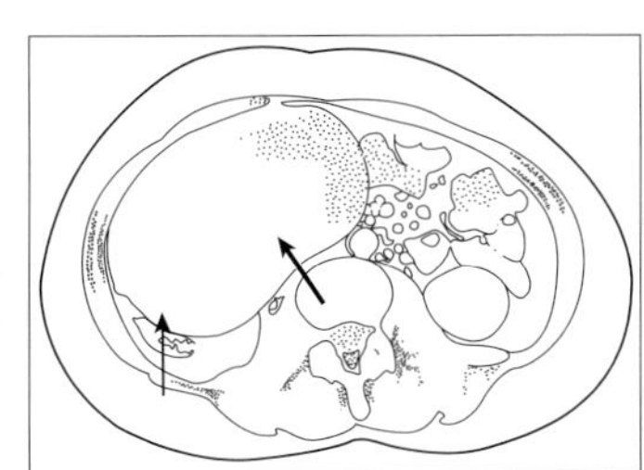

b

■ **Fig. 9.77** CT demonstrating a solid and papillary epithelial neoplasm (SPEN). (a) A huge heterogeneous mass arises in the head of the pancreas. (b) A more caudal image is photographed at window width and levels to increase 'contrast.' There are a few areas of increased attenuation representing hemorrhage, and numerous areas of low attenuation due to tumor necrosis.

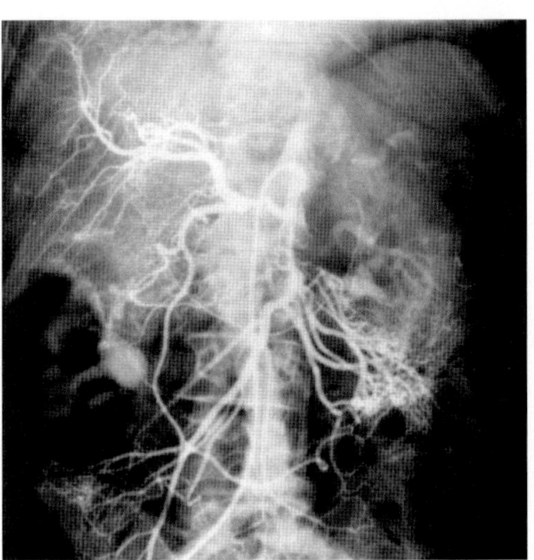

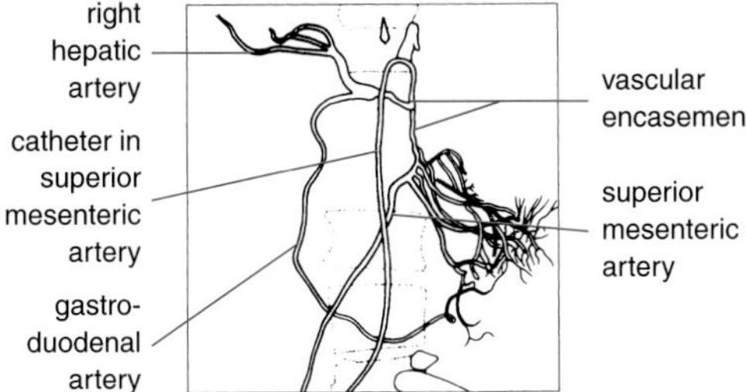

■ **Fig. 9.78** Angiogram demonstrating vascular encasement in a patient with pancreatic carcinoma.

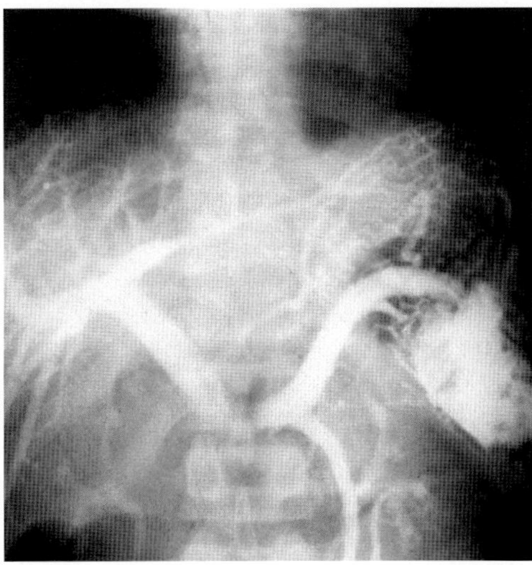

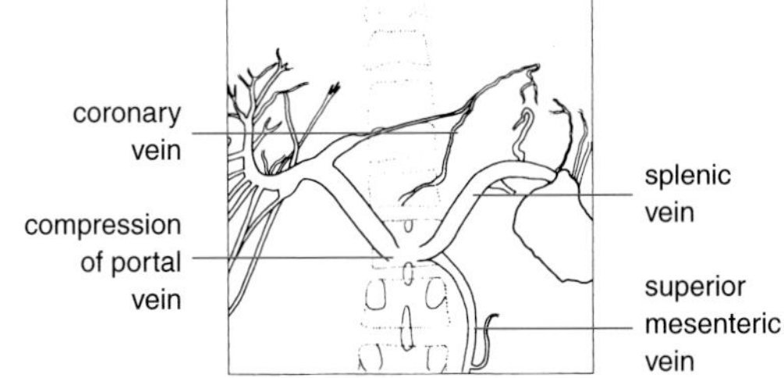

■ **Fig. 9.79** Splenoportogram demonstrating portal vein compression caused by a carcinoma in the head of the pancreas.

CYSTIC FIBROSIS

The gene defect for this, the commonest disease of autosomal recessive inheritance, is the so-called cystic fibrosis transmembrane conductance regulator (CFTR). Apart from its obvious importance in the disease, it has broader implications in gastroenterology since the gene product is one of two well-characterized epithelial cell chloride channels. There is evidence that heterozygotes for CFTR are protected against acute diarrheal illness such as cholera, and this presumably accounts for the evolutionary persistence of the gene.

Cystic fibrosis is most often diagnosed in childhood from respiratory symptoms, but presentation with intestinal obstruction may occur in the neonatal period, inspissated meconium having caused meconium ileus (Fig. 9.94). This results from diminished intestinal secretion of mucus, and consequently increased viscosity of the meconium. A water-soluble contrast enema (for example gastrografin) is both diagnostic and therapeutic (Fig. 9.95). Meconium ileus-equivalent, which may be responsible for intestinal obstruction in those with cystic fibrosis at any age, has a similar pathogenesis and responds in the same way to contrast enemas.

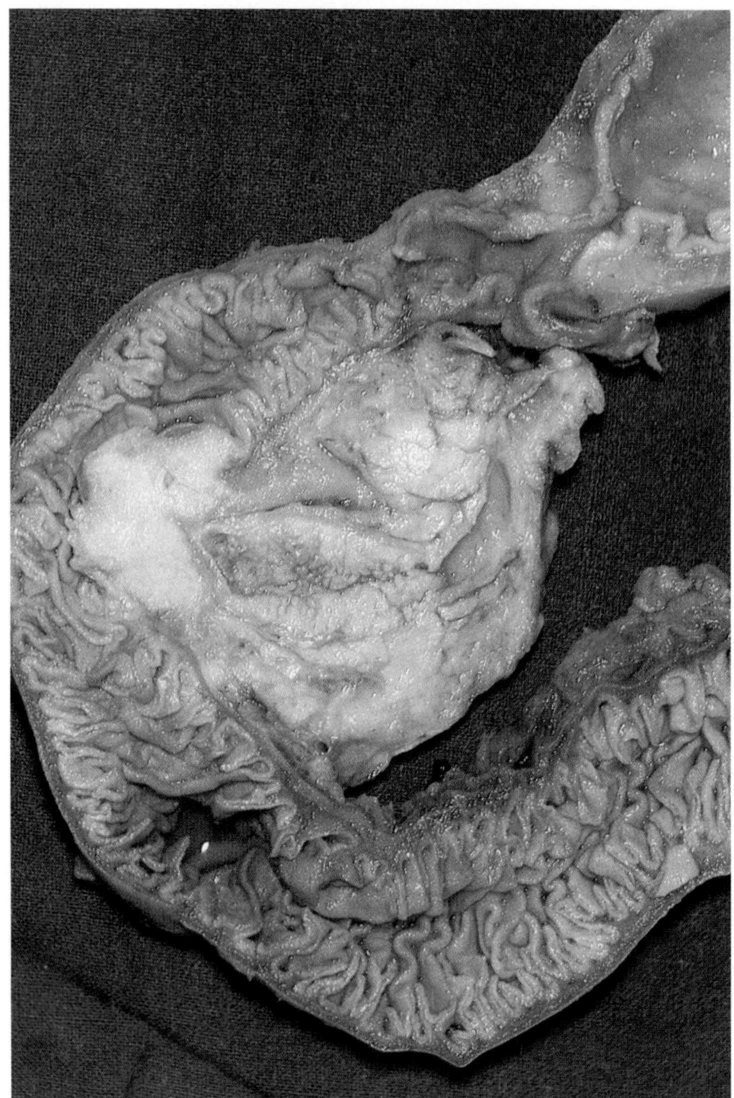

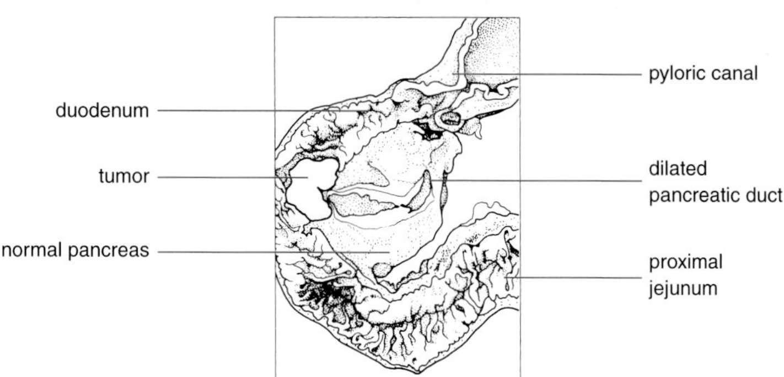

■ Fig. 9.80 Macroscopic appearance of a carcinoma invading the head of the pancreas, infiltrating the duodenum, and destroying the pancreatic duct. Courtesy of Mr M. Knight.

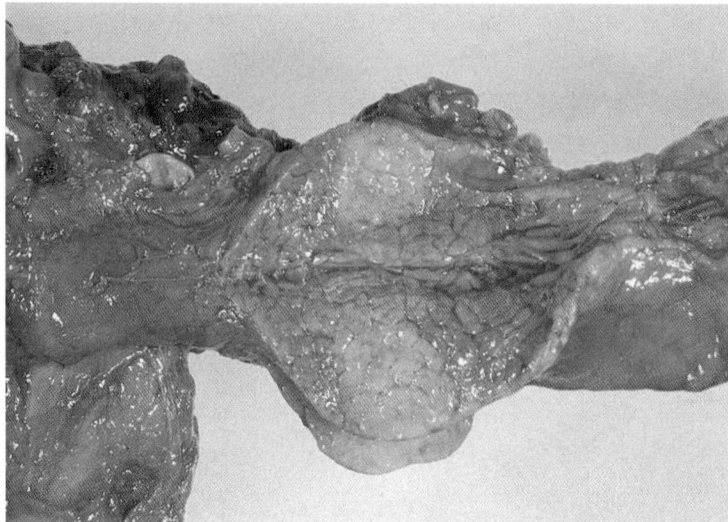

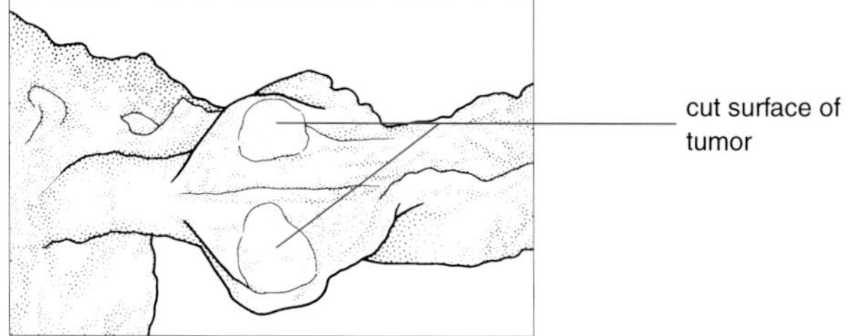

■ Fig. 9.81 Macroscopic appearance of a carcinoma of the body of the pancreas. Courtesy of Dr J. Newman.

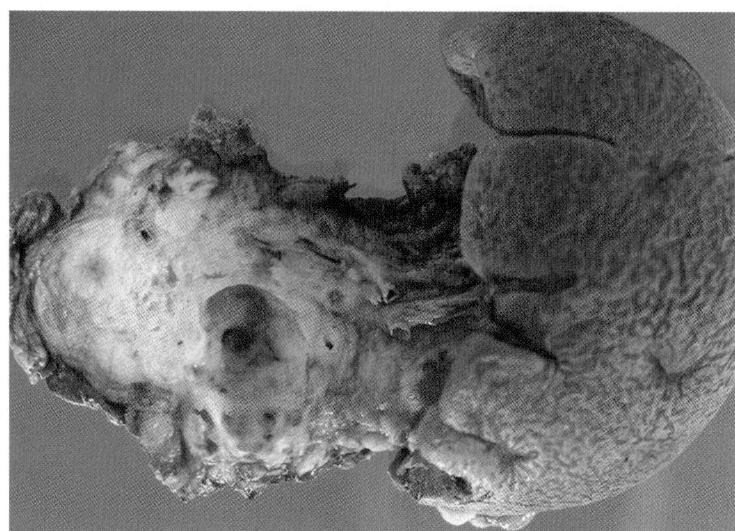

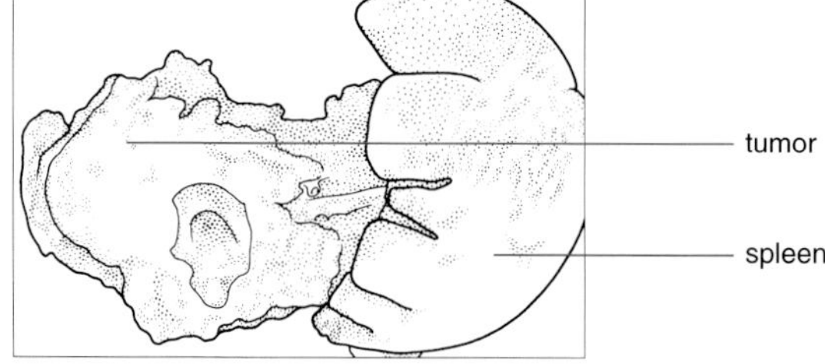

■ Fig. 9.82 Macroscopic appearance of a carcinoma of the pancreatic tail.

As respiratory management steadily improves – including successful pulmonary transplantation – and death in childhood becomes unusual, the relative importance of gastrointestinal manifestations increases. Failure to thrive despite a large appetite and effective treatment of bronchopulmonary sepsis may be overcome by supplementary enteral nutrition; the use of an endoscopically placed percutaneous gastrostomy tube is then particularly helpful (e.g. in facilitating overnight tube feeding in addition to normal daytime eating). Other gastroenterological problems include steatorrhea from pancreatic malabsorption, hemorrhagic diathesis from vitamin K deficiency, and abdominal wall herniae or rectal prolapse (Fig. 9.96) as a result of chronic cough and increased abdominal pressure (see also Chapter 8).

Chronic pancreatitis is mainly the result of blockage of the duct system by tenacious secretions, with duct dilatation and subsequent destruction of exocrine tissue: fibrosis gradually replaces the

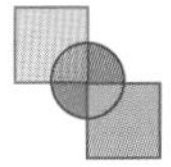

gland (Figs 9.97, 9.98). As in other forms of chronic pancreatitis, there is relative preservation of the islets.

Hepatic manifestations of cystic fibrosis are relatively late (i.e. not usual before the late teens) and therefore used to be considered rare, but this is no longer the case. A form of cirrhosis is increasingly recognized, and examination of the biliary tree at CT or ERCP shows features indistinguishable from those of primary sclerosing cholangitis (Fig. 9.99). Pancreatic carcinoma is seen in patients with cystic fibrosis at a younger age and at a higher incidence than in control groups.

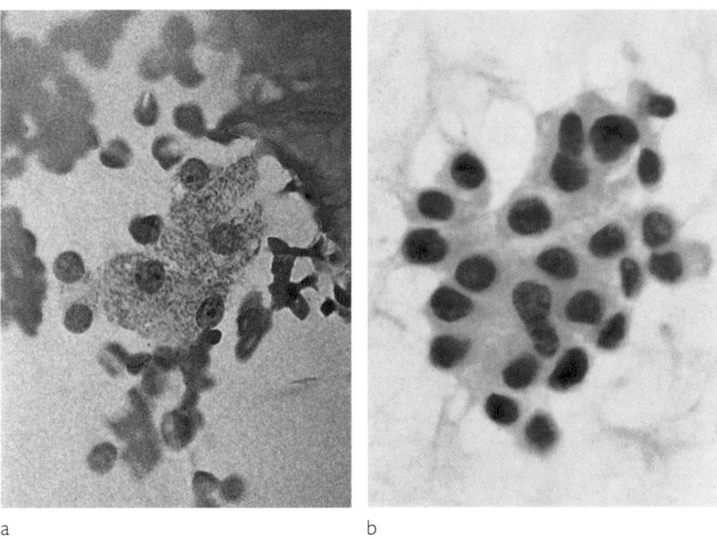

Fig. 9.83 Pancreatic cytology contrasting benign (a) and malignant (b) exocrine cells. The latter possess the usual characteristics of malignant cells with increased nuclear to cytoplasmic ratio, and hyperchromatic nuclei. Papanicolau stain (x 400). Courtesy of Dr E.A. Hudson.

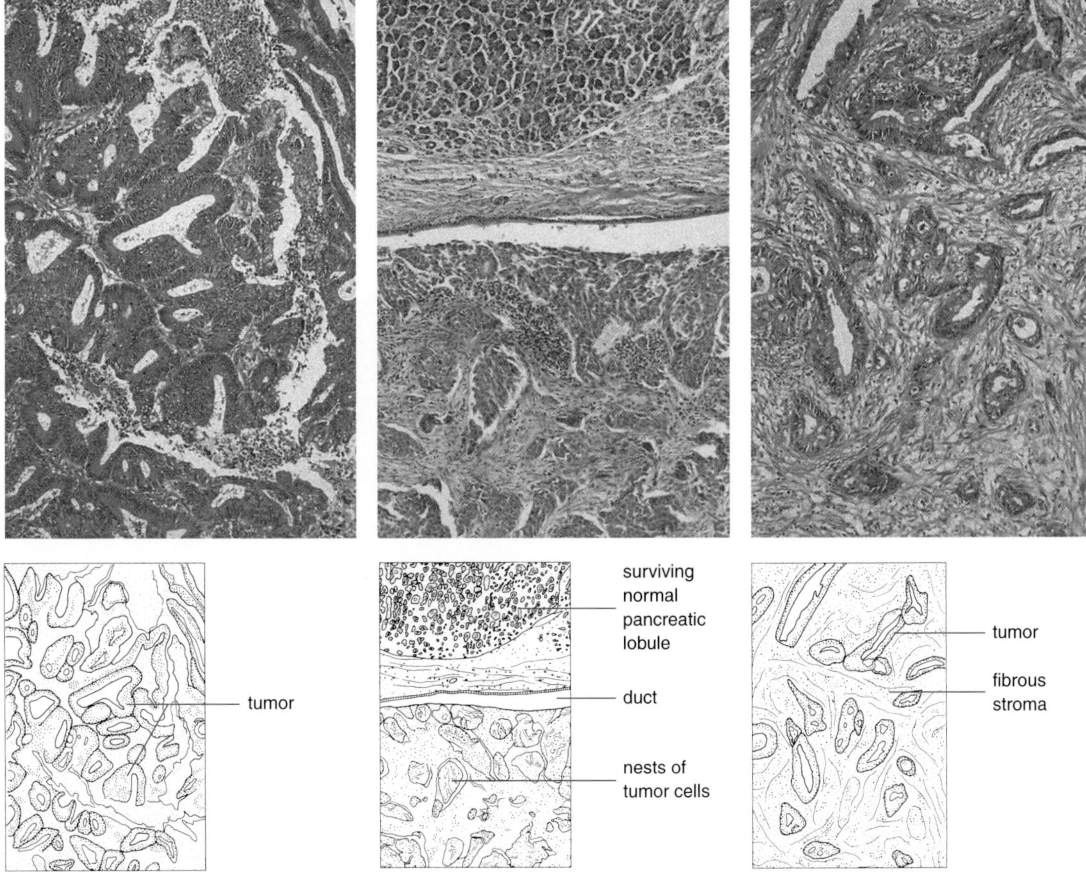

Fig. 9.84 Histological patterns of pancreatic carcinoma. A typical well-differentiated tumor (a), a moderately differentiated lesion with nests of cells producing a squamoid configuration (b), and an adenocarcinoma with a dense fibrous stroma (c). When fibrous stroma predominates, the results of fine needle aspiration are least able to discriminate from chronic pancreatitis. H&E stain (x 50).

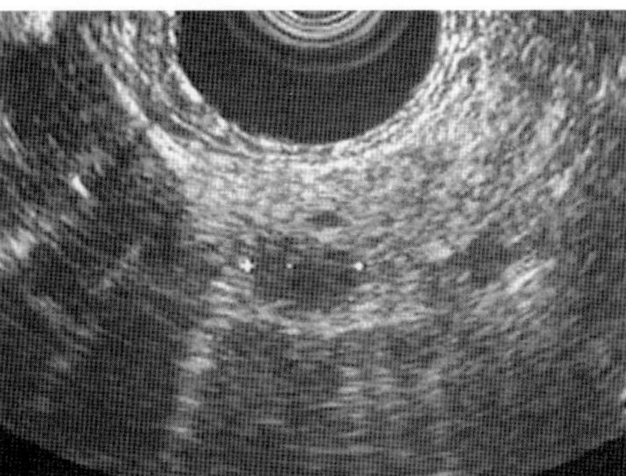

Fig. 9.85 Endoscopic ultrasound scan in a patient with a functional gut hormone-secreting tumor. The insulinoma lies just below the (normal) pancreatic duct in this scan.

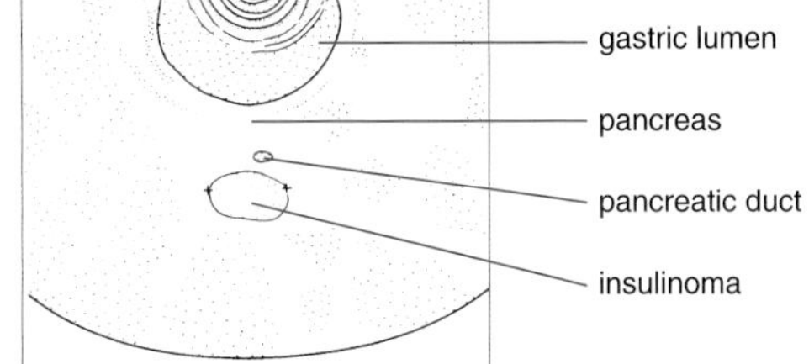

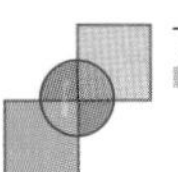

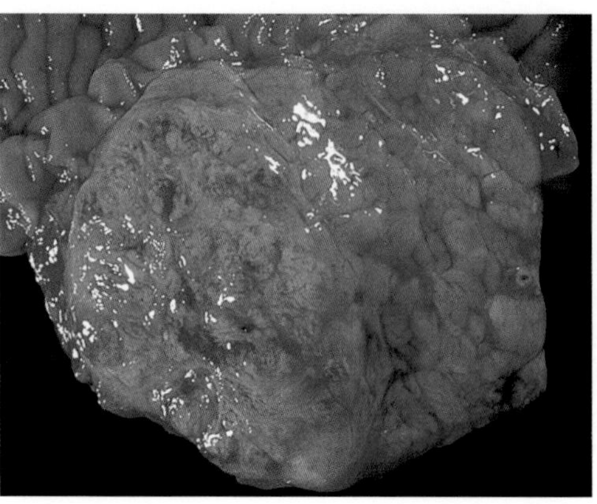

■ **Fig. 9.86** Pancreatic endocrine tumor. Surgical resection specimen showing the typically well circumscribed borders and tan, lobulated cut surface of this tumor type.

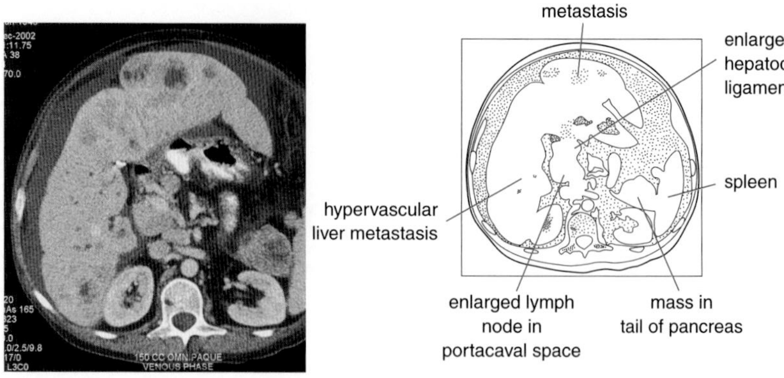

■ **Fig. 9.88** CT demonstrating islet cell tumor with liver and lymph node metastases. A mixed attenuation mass is seen in the tail of the pancreas. Metastases to portacaval and hepatogastric ligament lymph nodes are present. Numerous liver metastases are seen, some hypervascular, some predominantly hypovascular.

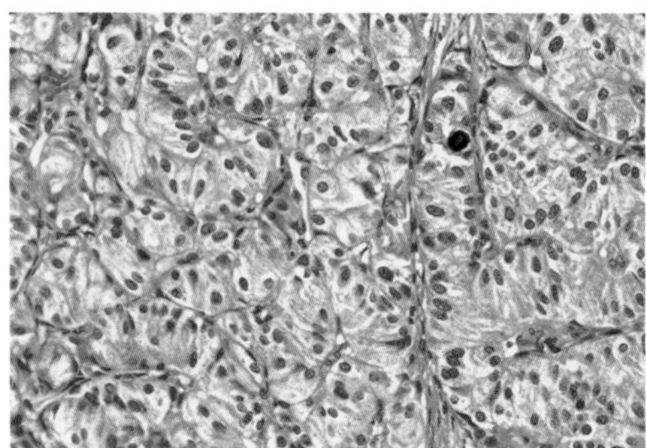

■ **Fig. 9.87** Pancreatic endocrine tumor. Microscopic view of an insulinoma showing monomorphic tumor cells with central nuclei and clear cytoplasm arranged in compact pseudoacinar groups.

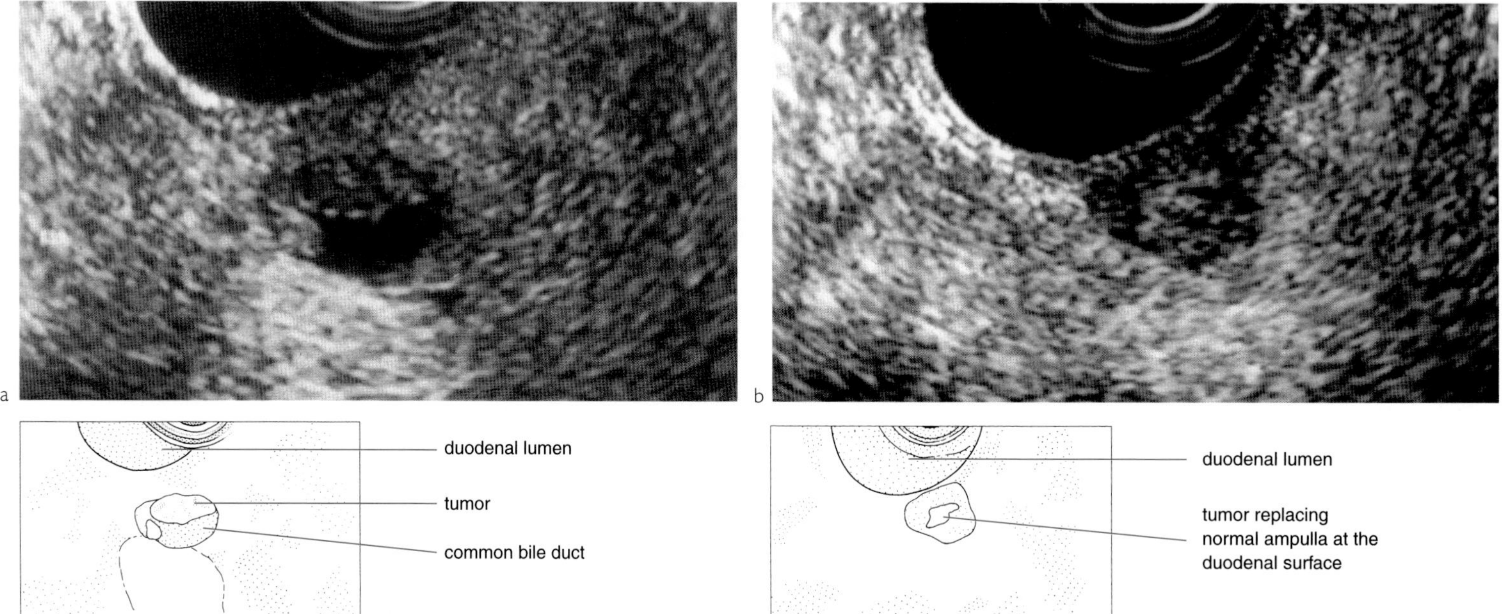

■ **Fig. 9.89** Endoscopic ultrasound in a patient with an ampullary carcinoma. In (a) the tumor mass is seen in the low common bile duct; scan (b) reveals its true nature as an ampullary lesion with origins at the duodenal level.

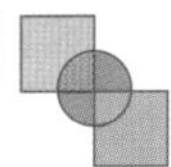

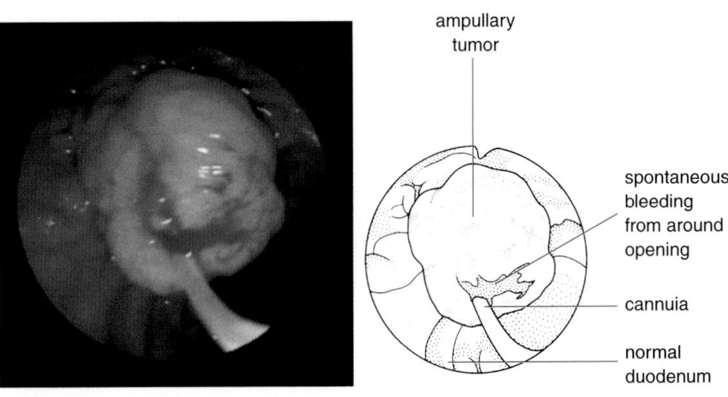

■ **Fig. 9.90** Endoscopic appearance of an ampullary carcinoma; the rather pale mucosa and spontaneous hemorrhage are characteristic. A diagnostic cannula is inserted into the duct system.

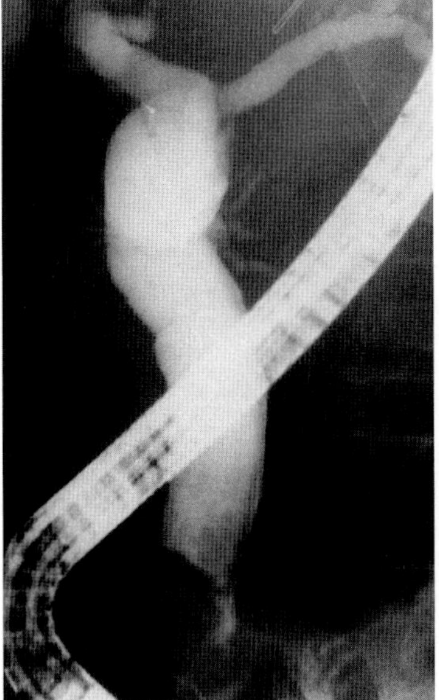

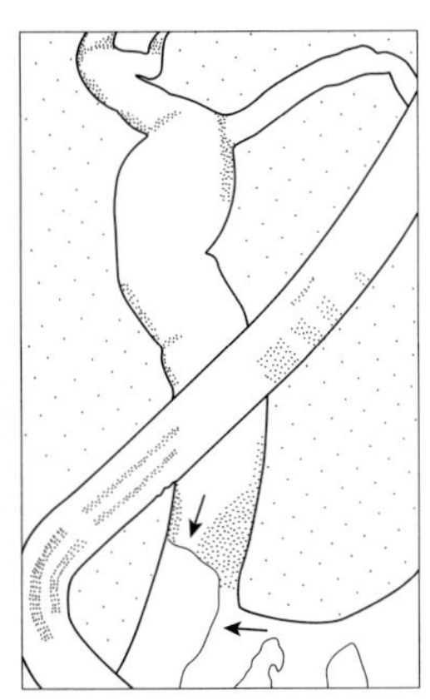

■ **Fig. 9.91** ERCP in patient with carcinoma of the papilla of Vater invading and obstructing the distal common bile duct. A 1.8 cm lobulated mass protrudes into the lumen of the distal-most common bile duct. The biliary tree is diffusely dilated.

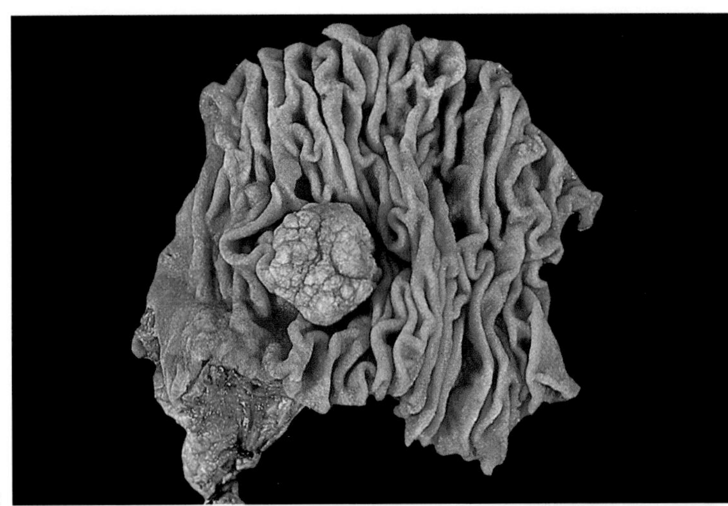

a

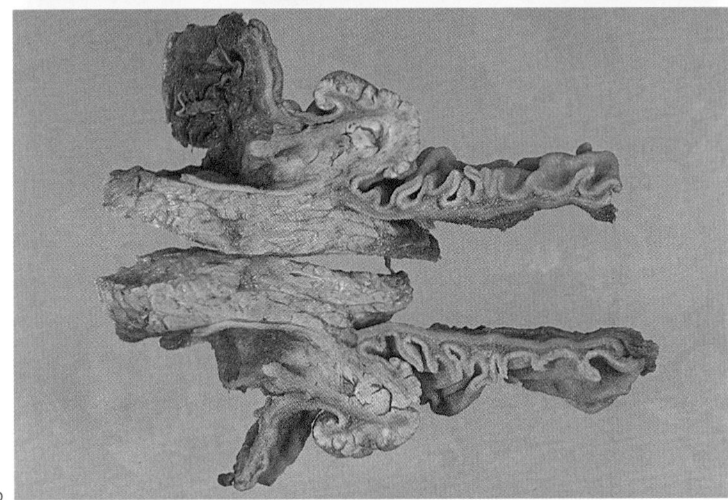

b

■ **Fig. 9.92** The luminal aspect (a), and the cut surface (b), of a carcinoma of the ampulla of Vater. The carcinoma has not invaded pancreatic tissue. Courtesy of Dr J. Newman.

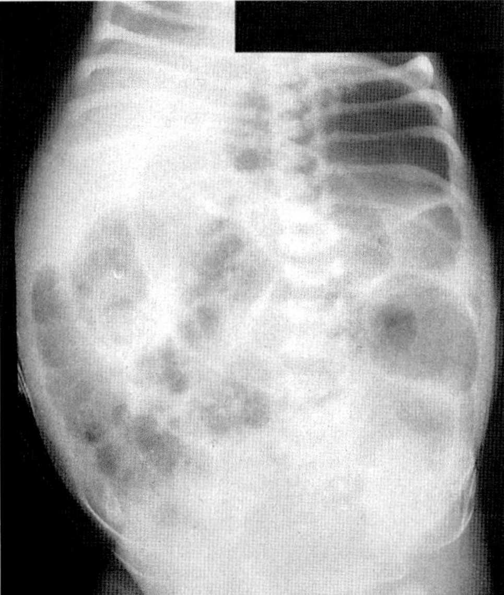

■ **Fig. 9.93** Plain abdominal film in a neonate with meconium ileus. Obvious small bowel dilatation is accompanied by the presence of air on both sides of the bowel wall indicative of perforation.

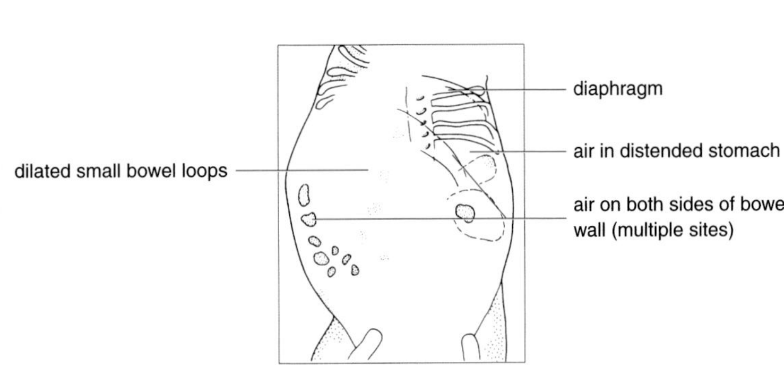

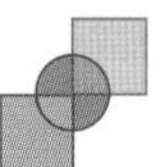

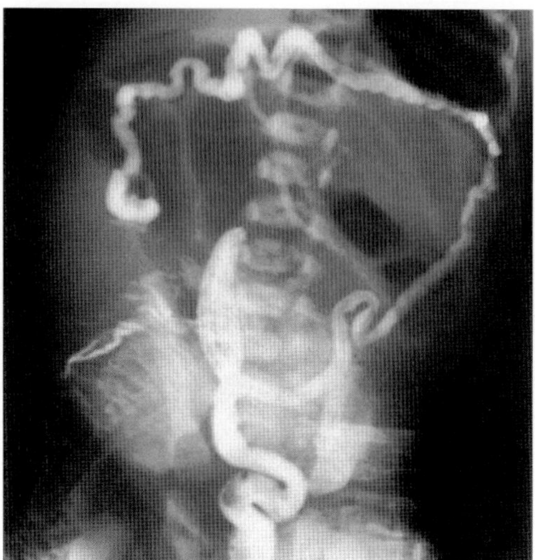

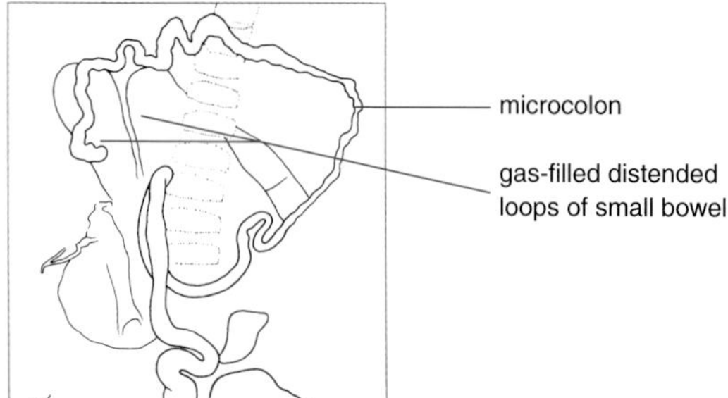

Fig. 9.94 Meconium ileus. Water-soluble contrast enema outlines a microcolon secondary to distal small bowel obstruction from inspissated meconium. Gas-filled distended loops of small bowel are seen proximal to distal obstruction.

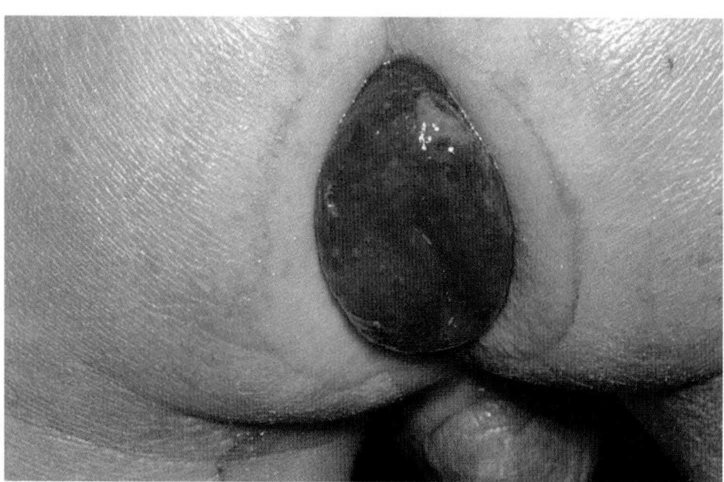

Fig. 9.95 Rectal prolapse in a child with cystic fibrosis. Courtesy of Dr J.A. Dodge.

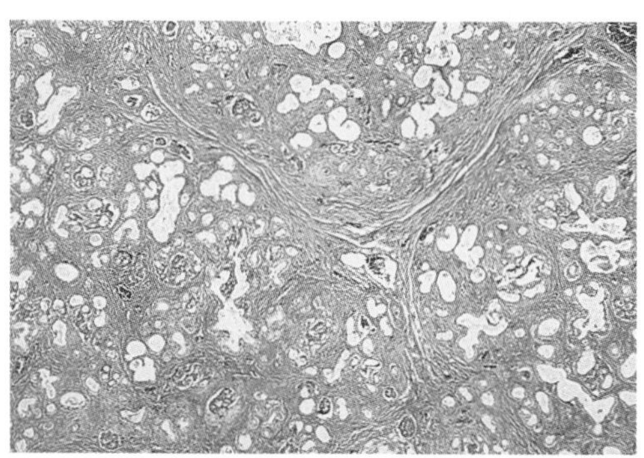

Fig. 9.96 Cystic fibrosis. Microscopic appearance showing cystic ductal dilatation and panlobular fibrosis throughout the pancreas.

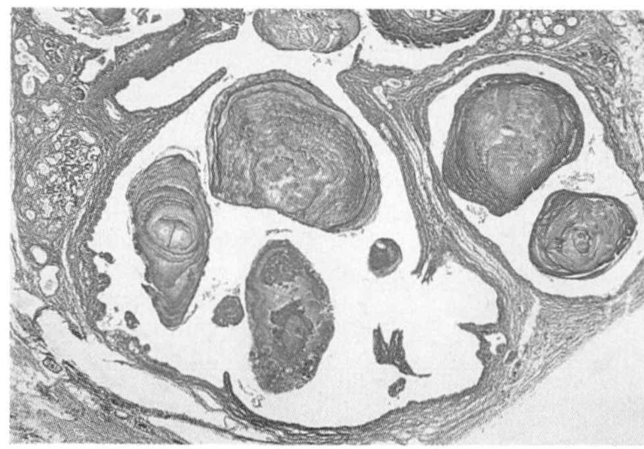

Fig. 9.97 Cystic fibrosis. High-magnification view of a dilated pancreatic duct containing numerous lamellar concretions in cystic fibrosis of the pancreas.

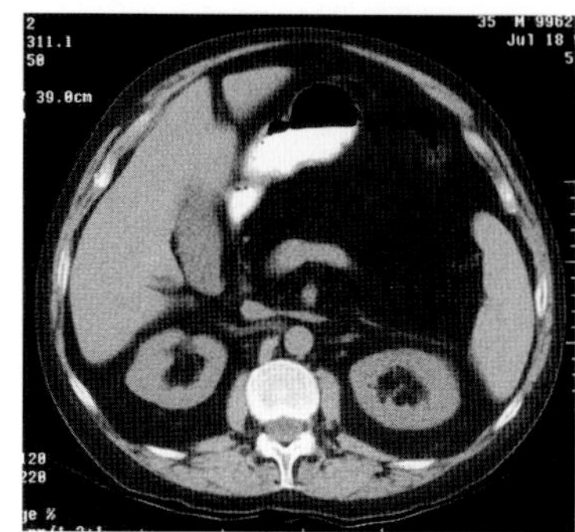

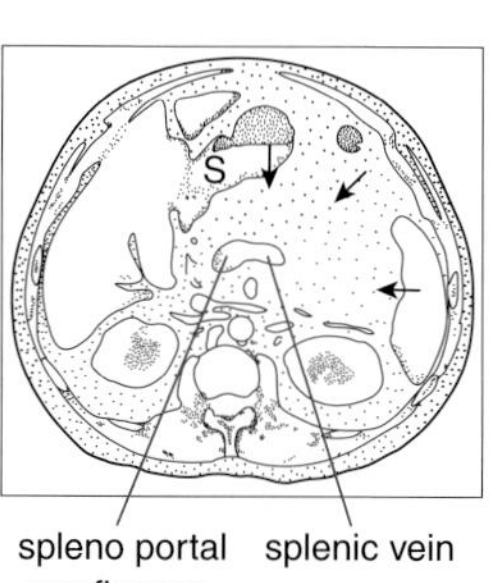

Fig. 9.98 CT demonstrating fatty replacement and enlargement of the pancreas in cystic fibrosis. No normal pancreatic parenchyma is seen anterior to the splenoportal confluence and splenic vein. Instead, the pancreas is enlarged and replaced by fat. Extrinsic impression of the posterior wall of the stomach can be discerned immediately anterior to the pancreas.

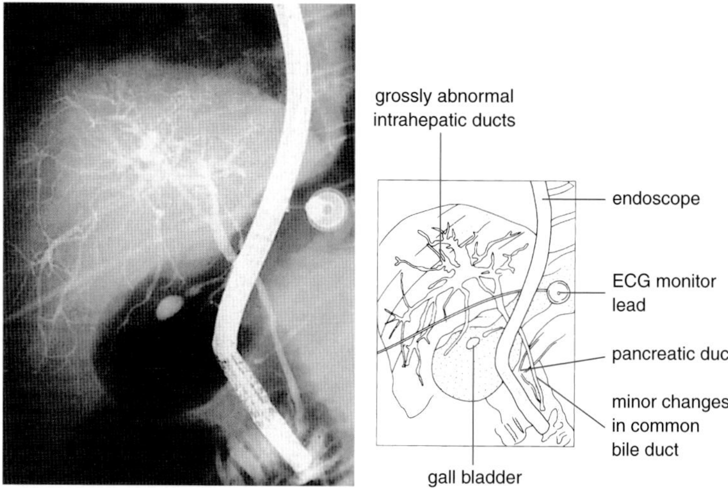

Fig. 9.99 ERCP cholangiogram in cystic fibrosis showing the changes similar to those of primary sclerosing cholangitis. Note the presence of an electrocardiogram electrode – exquisite attention to cardiorespiratory status during relatively invasive endoscopy in cystic fibrosis patients is essential. Courtesy of Dr S. Williams.

THE NORMAL LIVER AND BILIARY TREE AND JAUNDICE

10

The liver is the largest organ in the body, weighing 1200–1500 grams in the adult, and it comprises approximately 2% of the total adult body weight. It is relatively larger in infancy, accounting for about 5% of the birth weight. Its anatomy can be described both in terms of its surface markings (morphological anatomy), and in functional terms.

The upper border of the liver normally reaches the fourth right intercostal space anteriorly, while the lower border extends down to and approximately parallel with the right costal margin. The surface of the liver is divided into lobes, the left separated from the much larger right lobe by the embryological falciform ligament. Below and behind this ligament, the liver is further divided into the small quadrate and caudate lobes (Figs 10.1–10.7).

BLOOD SUPPLY

The liver has a dual blood supply: it receives about 70% of its blood from the portal vein (Fig. 10.8), and the remainder from the hepatic artery. Branches of the hepatic vein are responsible for draining blood from the liver to the inferior vena cava, and it is the complex inter-relationship between these various vessels that forms the basis of the functional anatomy of the liver (Figs 10.8, 10.9). It effectively divides the organ into eight segments, and this is of importance from a surgical point of view, as segmentectomy is frequently preferable to lobectomy as a surgical procedure. Segment 1 (the caudate lobe) is, in effect, an autonomous segment, since it is supplied by both right and left branches of the portal vein as well as the hepatic artery, while its hepatic venous drainage is directly into the inferior vena cava. The significance of this is illustrated in the Budd–Chiari syndrome, where thrombosis of the main hepatic vein results in the entire hepatic venous outflow passing through the caudate lobe which, consequently undergoes gross hypertrophy (Fig. 10.10).

The liver is often visible on a plain abdominal radiograph (Fig. 10.11): an inferior extension of the right lobe towards the right iliac fossa is a common variant – the so-called Riedel's lobe (Fig. 10.12).

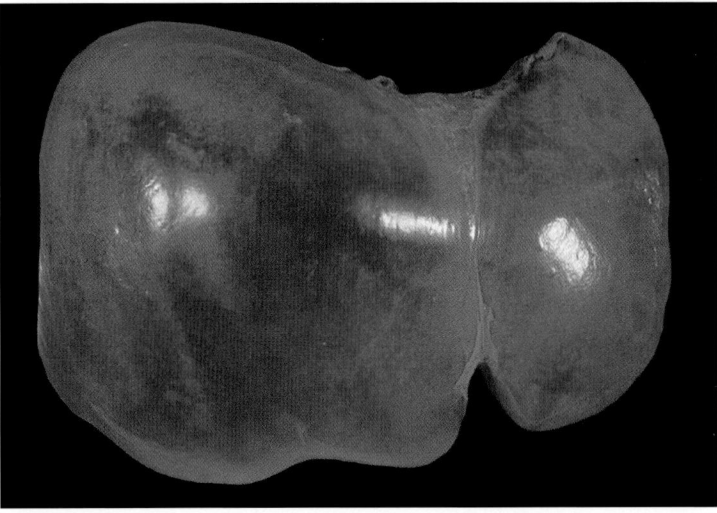

Fig. 10.2 Normal liver: anterior view. Courtesy of Prof B. Portmann.

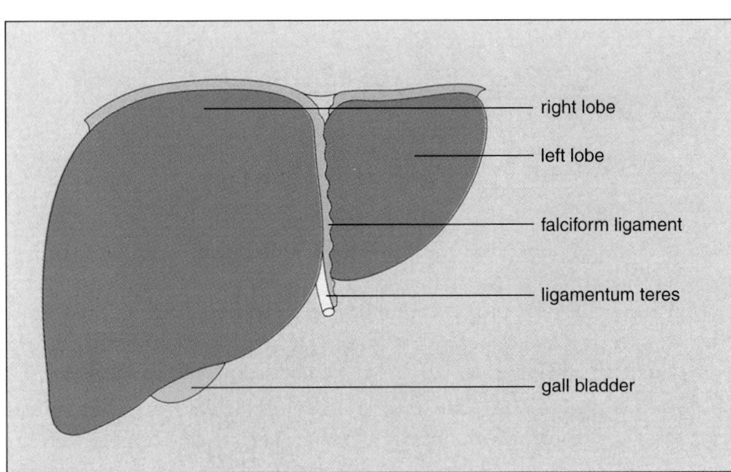

Fig. 10.1 Diagram showing the anterior view of the liver.

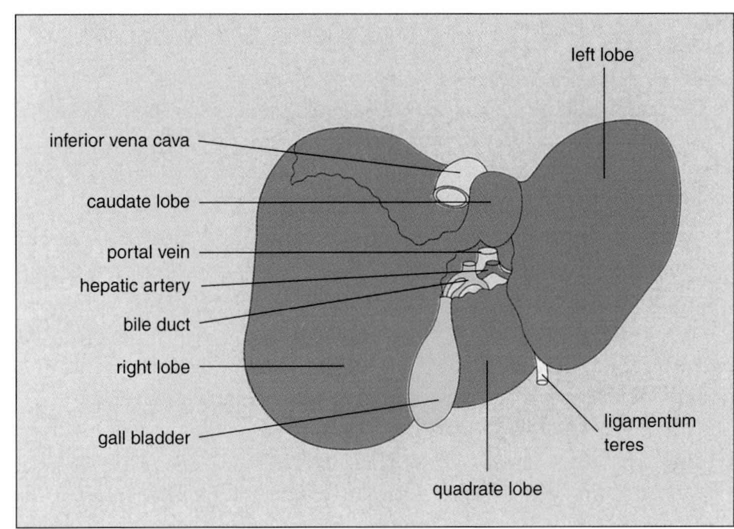

Fig. 10.3 Diagram showing the inferior and posterior aspects of the liver.

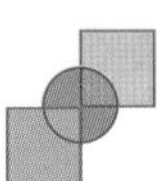

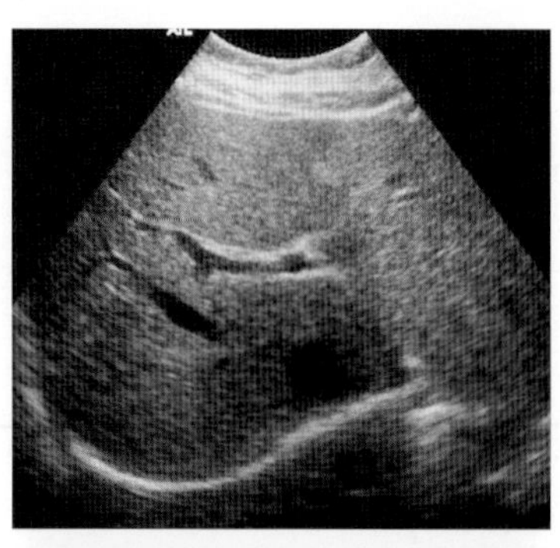

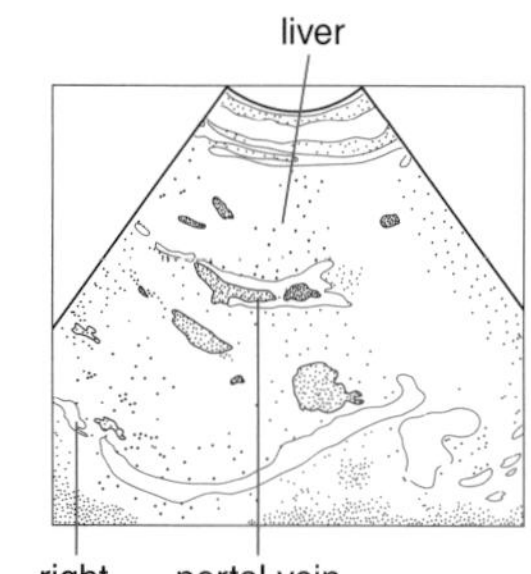

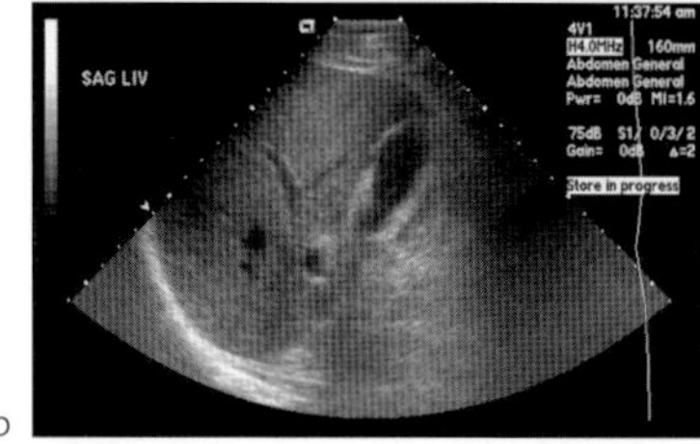

■ **Fig. 10.4** (a) Ultrasound of normal liver. Transverse view of the liver demonstrates the echogenicity of the hepatic parenchyma, the right hemidiaphragm and the portal vein. (Courtesy of Dr Jill E. Langer.) (b) Sagittal scanning is complementary.

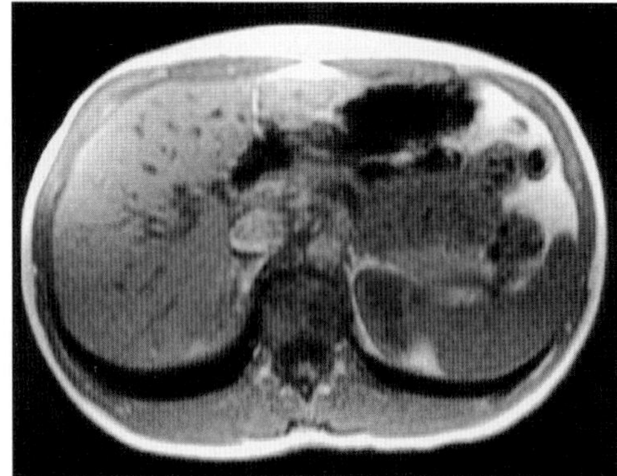

■ **Fig. 10.5** T_1-weighted MRI scan through normal liver. Courtesy of Dr Drew Torigian.

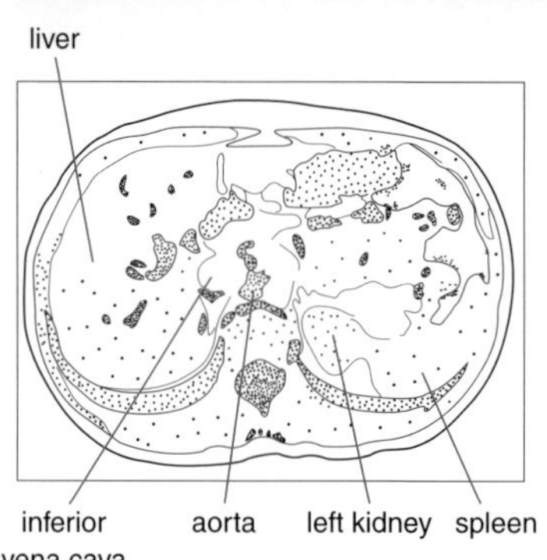

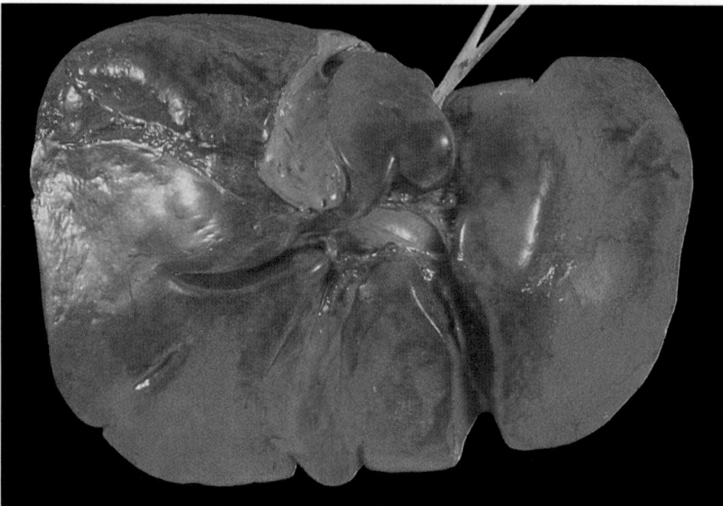

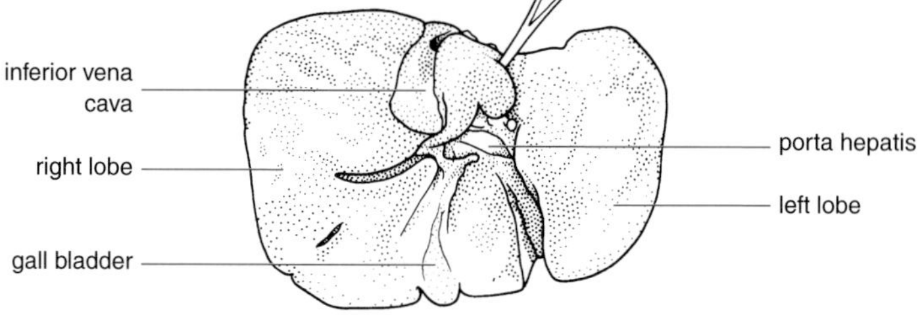

■ **Fig. 10.6** Normal liver: inferior and posterior view. Courtesy of Prof B. Portmann.

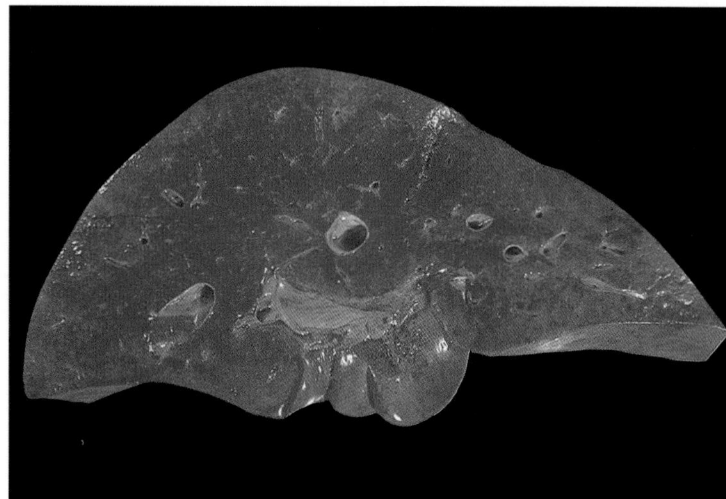

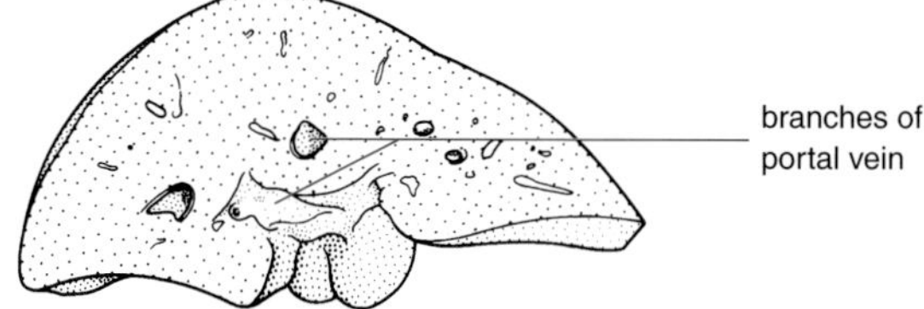

■ **Fig. 10.7** Slice of a normal liver. Courtesy of Prof B. Portmann.

The main bile ducts draining the left and right lobes join at the porta hepatis to form the common hepatic duct which, at a variable distance, is joined by the cystic duct to become the common bile duct (Figs 10.13, 10.14). This passes down along the edge of the lesser omentum behind the first part of the duodenum and the head of the pancreas, and enters the medial wall of the duodenum with the main pancreatic duct (duct of Santorini) in the papilla of Vater (see Chapter 9). The two ducts may join together to form an ampulla within the papilla (see Fig. 10.32), or the bile duct may first join the pancreatic duct up to 1 cm proximal to the orifice (Figs 10.14, 10.15). Oral cholecystography is no longer used to visualize the gall bladder, having been replaced by ultrasonography (Fig. 10.16). The biliary system is demonstrable by endoscopic retrograde cholangiography (ERC) (Fig. 10.17), or, more safely but less clearly, by magnetic resonance imaging (Fig. 10.18). Direct injection into the liver for percutaneous transhepatic cholangiography should no longer be necessary for diagnostic purposes.

The hepatic artery, portal vein and common hepatic duct are found in close proximity in the porta hepatis (Fig. 10.19). The hepatic artery is normally a branch of the celiac axis, whereas the gall bladder derives its blood supply from the cystic artery (Fig. 10.20); anatomical variations in these blood vessels are common. The portal vein is formed behind the head of the pancreas by the junction of the splenic and superior mesenteric veins. It may be opacified by several routes.

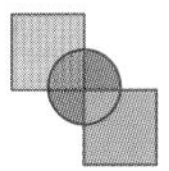

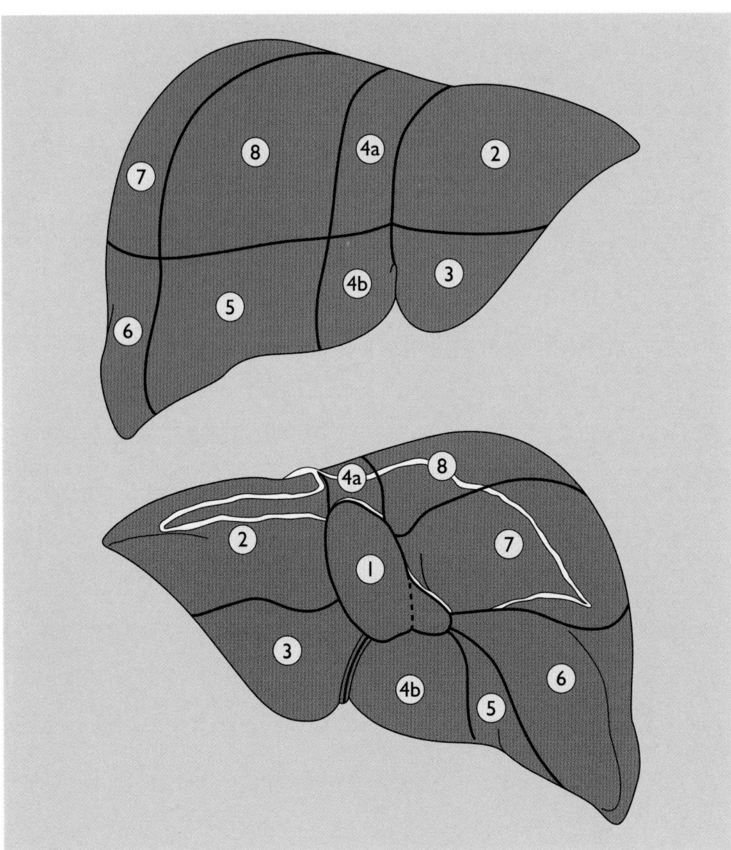

■ **Fig. 10.8** Anterior and posterior views of the liver showing the distribution of the eight segments. Note that segment I is the caudate lobe. Courtesy of the website of the GI Unit at Johns Hopkins.

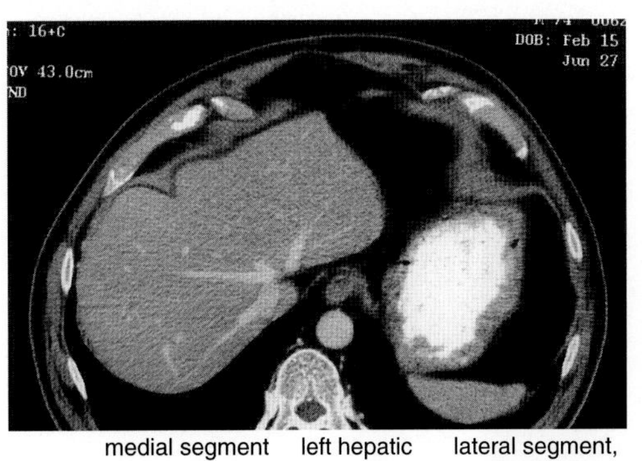

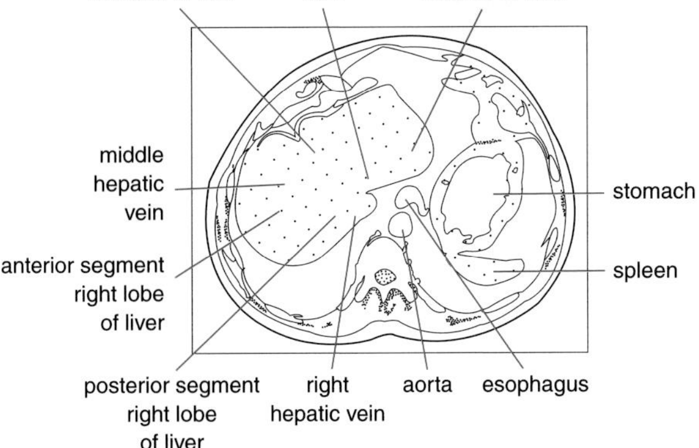

■ **Fig. 10.9** CT of liver. Axial image through the dome of the liver demonstrates the hepatic veins dividing the hepatic parenchyma into segments. The posterior segment of the right lobe of the liver is barely visible at this level, as the bulk of this segment lies inferior to the anterior segment of the right lobe.

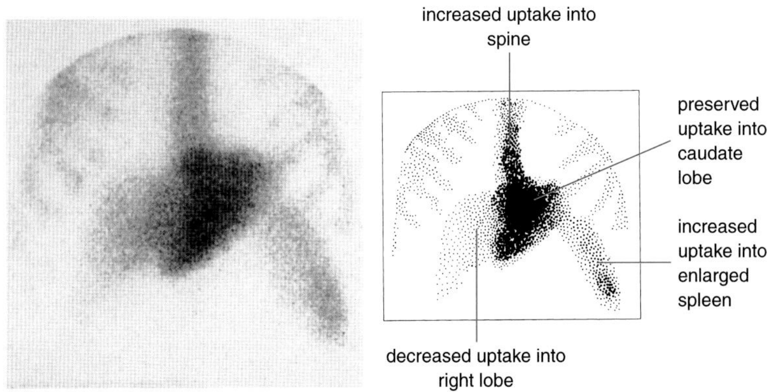

■ **Fig. 10.10** Technetium scintiscan in Budd–Chiari syndrome showing reduced uptake of colloid by the liver, with preserved caudate lobe, and increased uptake by the spleen and bones.

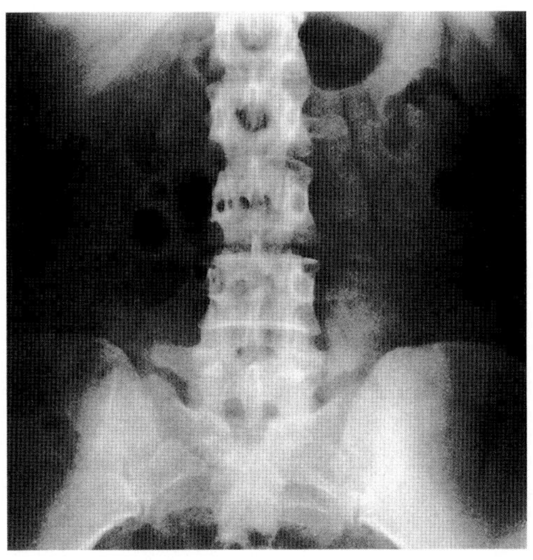

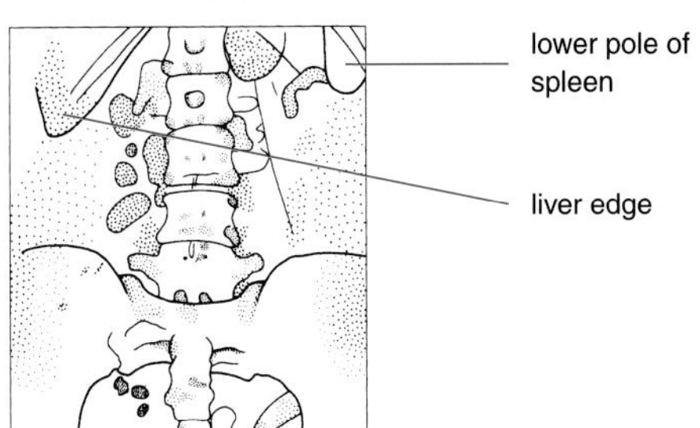

■ **Fig. 10.11** Plain abdominal radiograph showing the liver.

Direct percutaneous injection into the splenic pulp (splenic venography) used to be widely utilized but is now a rare investigation even when the spleen is enlarged and there is evidence of portal hypertension (Fig. 10.21). In infants in whom the umbilical vein is still patent, this can be cannulated directly and contrast material injected into the left portal venous system. More often now selective angiography is used, demonstrating the portal venous system by catheterization of the splenic artery and visualization of the venous return phase after the contrast material has passed through the spleen (Fig. 10.22). The image quality may be unsatisfactory in patients with portal hypertension because of hemodilution of the contrast agent, and this is improved using the technique of digital subtraction angiography (Fig. 10.23). Hepatic veins can be cannulated directly after passing a catheter transvenously through the right side of the heart; both radiological visualization and venous pressure measurement then become possible. For the latter the free hepatic venous pressure is first recorded and then the catheter is pushed gently into the parenchyma. A balloon at its tip is inflated, and measurement of this pressure (the wedged hepatic venous pressure) approximates to the portal venous pressure, and allows the hepatic venous pressure gradient to be calculated (Fig. 10.24). Such catheters are most easily introduced via the right internal jugular vein, as the direction of approach is then more or less a straight line. Essentially the same technique is used for access in transvenous biopsy of the liver.

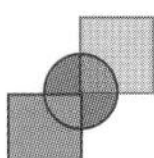

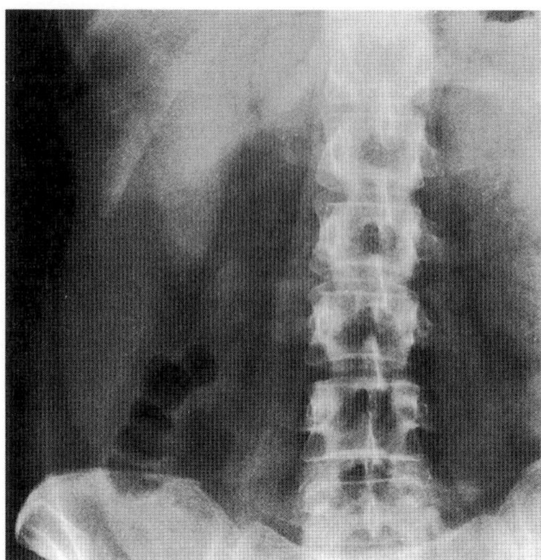

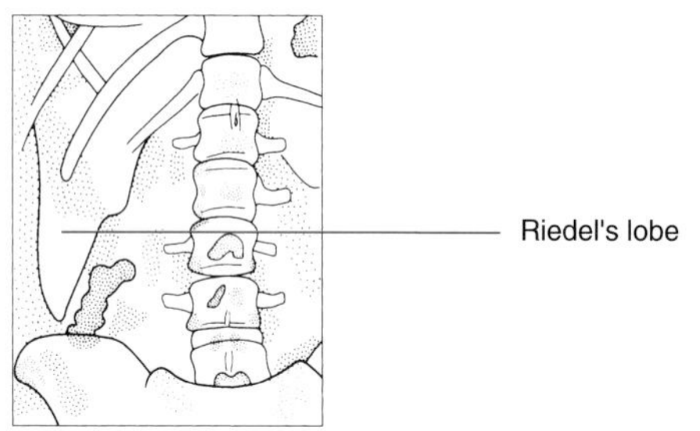

Fig. 10.12 Normal abdominal radiograph showing a Riedel's 'lobe' in the right hypochondrium.

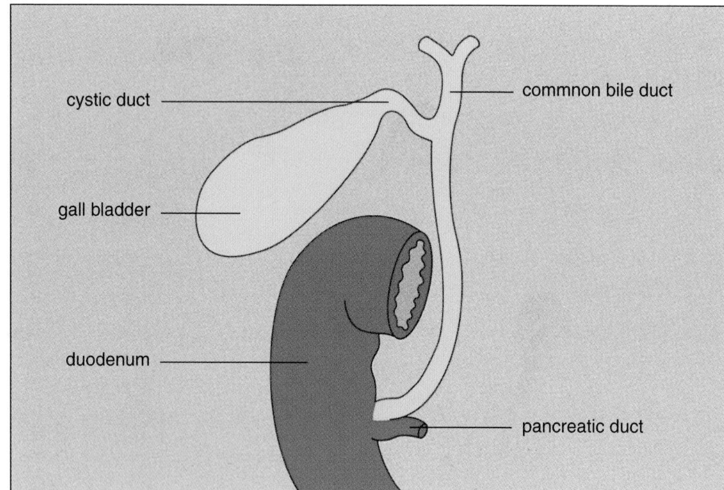

Fig. 10.13 Diagram showing the normal biliary tract.

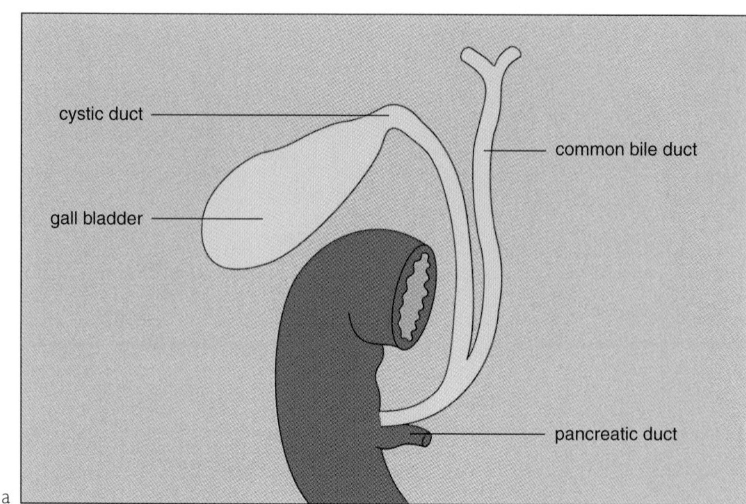

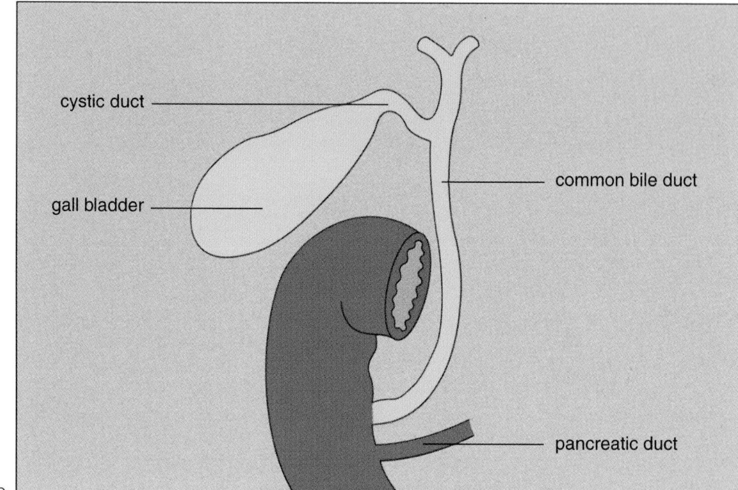

Fig. 10.14 Diagram showing common variants of the biliary tree anatomy. (a) The long cystic duct entering the common hepatic duct within the head of the pancreas. (b) Common bile duct and pancreatic ducts enter the duodenum separately.

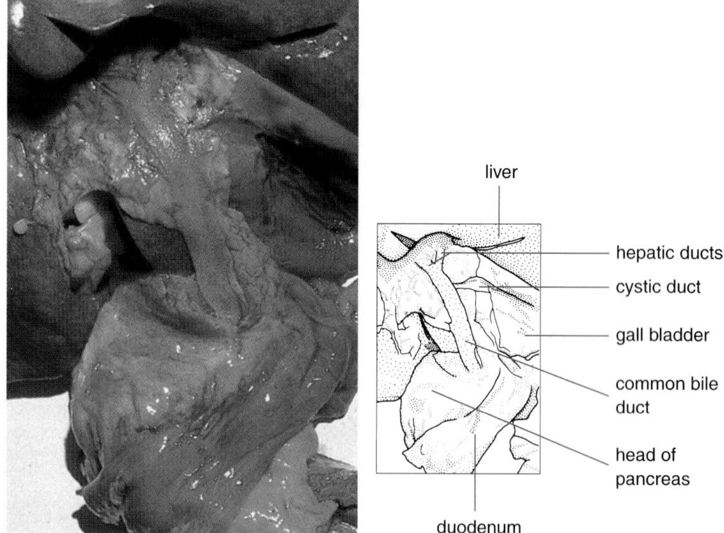

Fig. 10.15 Autopsy specimen showing the relationship of the hepatic, common bile, and cystic ducts from behind (thus the right of the image is also the right of the cadaver).

Ultrasound examination of the normal liver shows its size and consistency, filling defects, and often the anatomy of the biliary tree and portal vein (Figs 10.25, 10.26). The liver parenchyma and surrounding tissues can also be demonstrated by computerized tomography (CT scanning) (Fig. 10.27).

Magnetic resonance cholangio-pancreatiography (MRCP) utilizes long T_1 and T_2 relaxation time of fluids. Fluids exhibit very low signals (dark) on T_1-weighted images and high (bright) signal on T_2-weighted images (Figs 10.28, 10.29a). For MRCP, heavily T_2-weighted images are used to obtain cholangiogram and pancreatogram. Sensitivity and specificity of MRCP varies with the technique and indication. When the clinical index of suspicion is very low, MRCP is the preferred diagnostic modality. However, ERCP is preferable when there is a very high likelihood of intervention. Moreover, peri-ampullary lesions are often missed because of the artifacts caused by air in the duodenum. In addition, MRC is not sufficiently sensitive to detect early bile duct lesions such as subtle lesions often seen in PSC. TESLA scan is another modality, rarely used, that can visualize bile ducts (Fig. 10.29b).

Liver lesions are better characterized using CT or MRI. Using contrast agents and taking images in both arterial and venous phase,

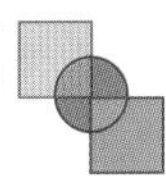

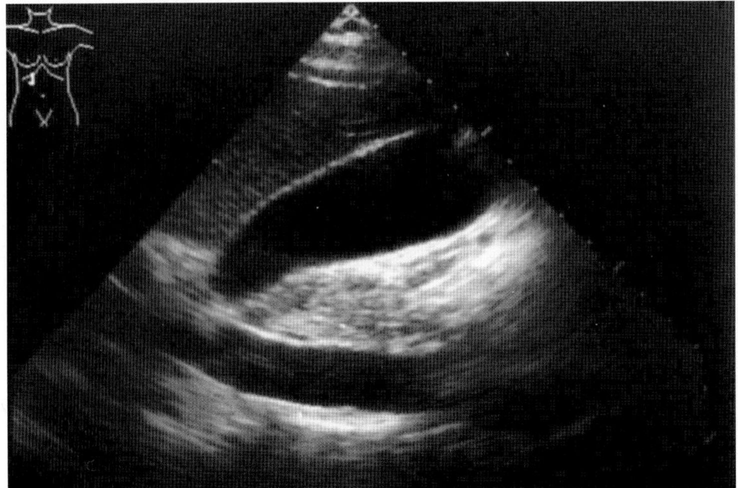

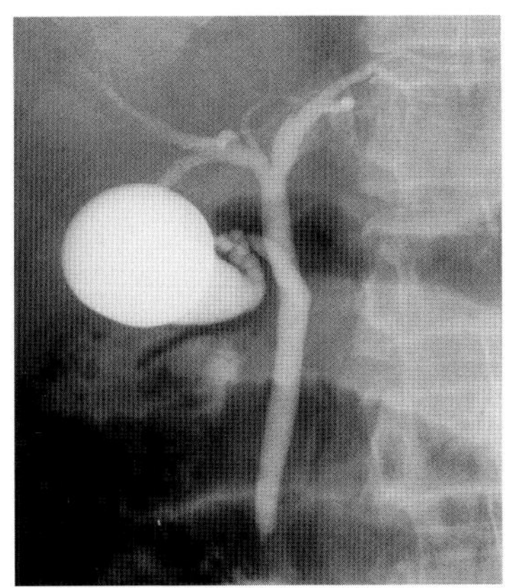

Fig 10.17 Biliary anatomy demonstrated by endoscopic retrograde cholangiography.

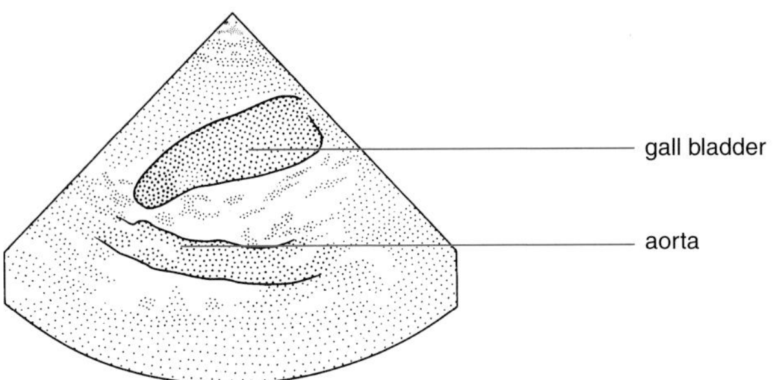

Fig. 10.16 Ultrasound showing normal gall bladder. Courtesy of Dr M.C. Collins.

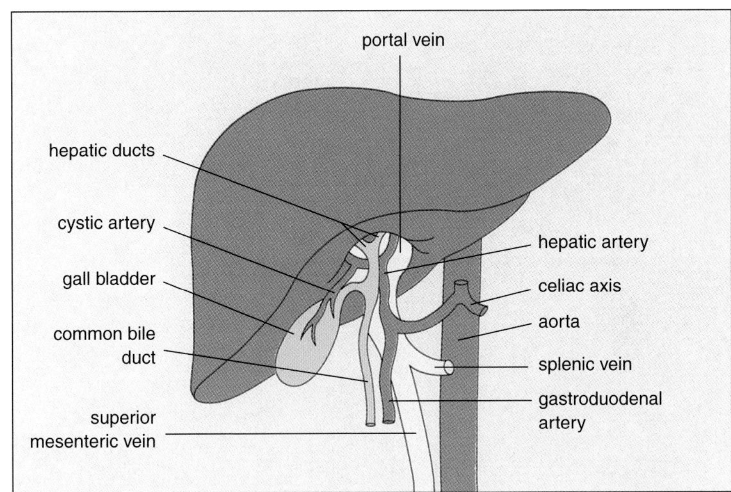

Fig. 10.19 Diagram showing the blood supply of the liver.

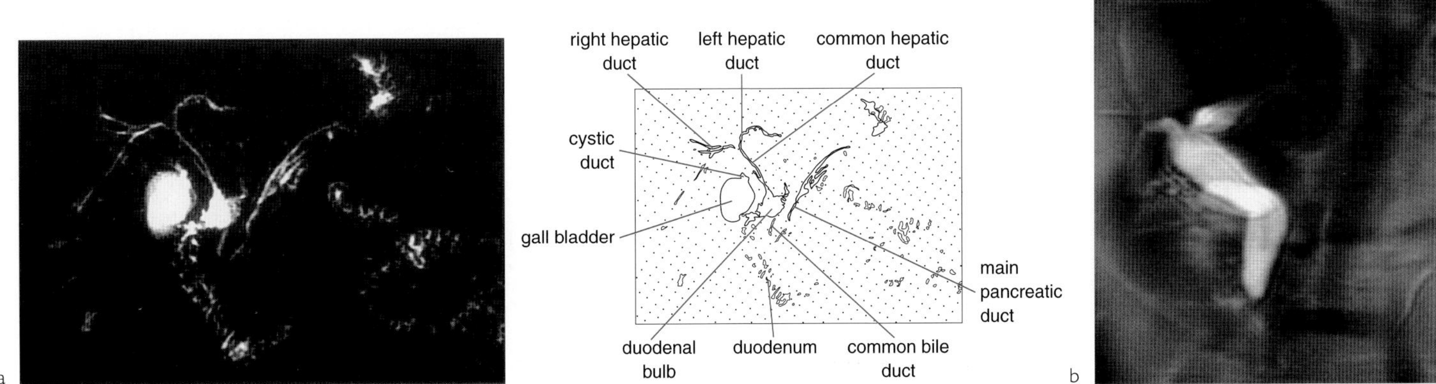

Fig. 10.18 (a) Normal biliary anatomy demonstrated by magnetic resonance cholangiopancreatography (MRCP). Courtesy of Dr Drew Torigian. (b) MRC showing a low insertion of the bile duct. Courtesy of Dr Ihab Kamel.

it has been possible better to diagnose both benign and malignant lesions within the liver. 3D-CT scans and MRA also could be used to delineate vascular anatomy. In addition, biliary cancers can be staged further with either MRC and TESLA scans. CT or MRI could be used as a single modality to visualize the tumors, delineate vascular anatomy and characterize the extent of biliary involvement.

Radio-isotope scanning of the liver, in which technetium-labeled colloid is injected intravenously and its concentration in the hepatic reticulo-endothelial (Kupffer) cells studied, is now much less often used (Fig. 10.30a). HIDA scan may be used to diagnose sphincter of Oddi or gallbladder dysfunction, and rarely to detect bile leak (Fig. 10.30b). Laparoscopy is not often performed primarily for hepatic imaging, but shows the inferior surface of the liver very clearly (Fig. 10.31) and permits access for biopsy under direct vision.

FUNCTIONAL ANATOMY

Within the liver, the hepatic artery and portal vein come together with the bile ducts and lymphatics. The branches of all these vessels extend into the liver until, in the final portal tracts, they interdigitate with the first tributaries of the hepatic veins (central lobular veins). Microscopically, there is a cylinder of tissue roughly 1 mm in diameter around each central vein.

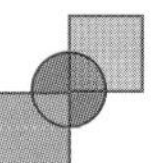

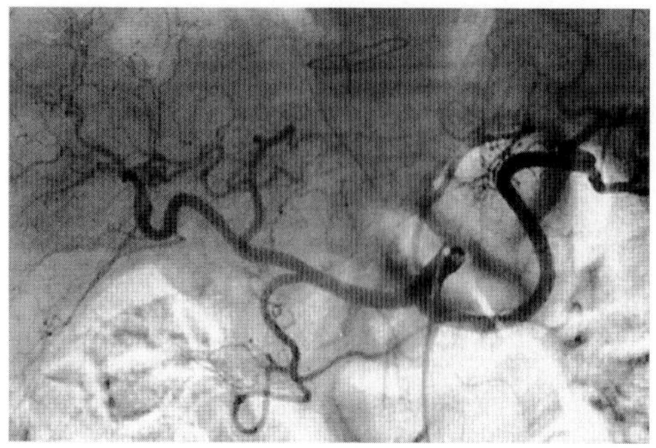

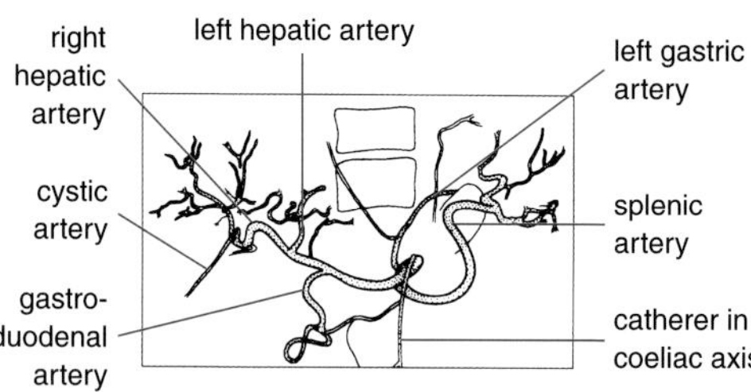

Fig. 10.20 Normal celiac axis.

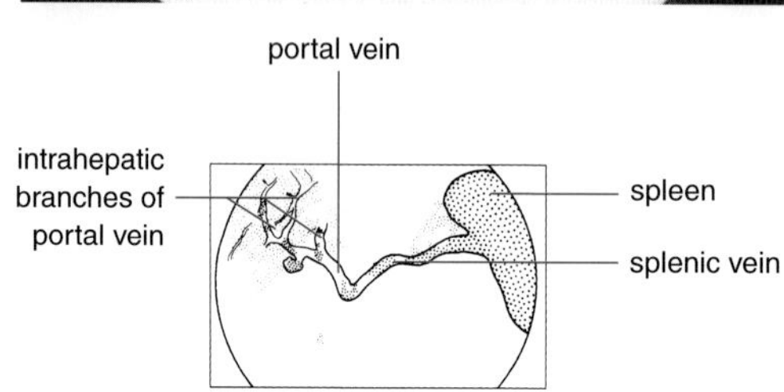

Fig. 10.23 Digital subtraction angiogram.

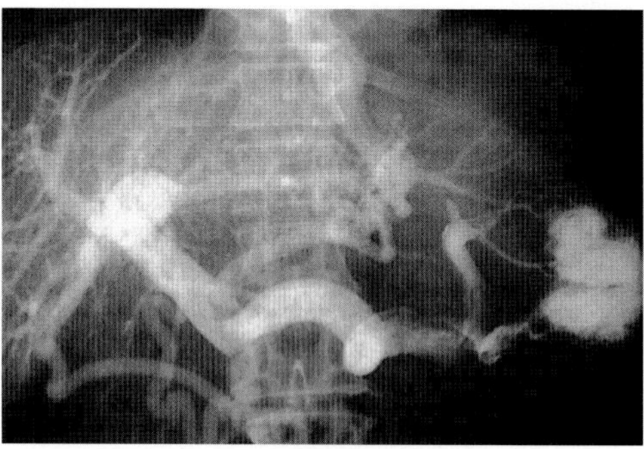

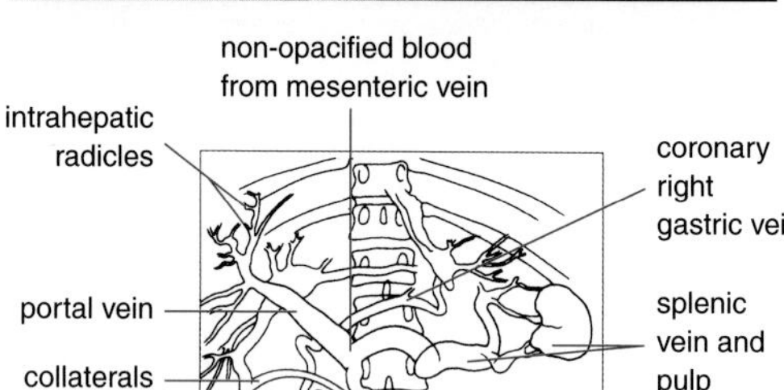

Fig. 10.21 Percutaneous splenic venogram showing anatomy in cirrhosis.

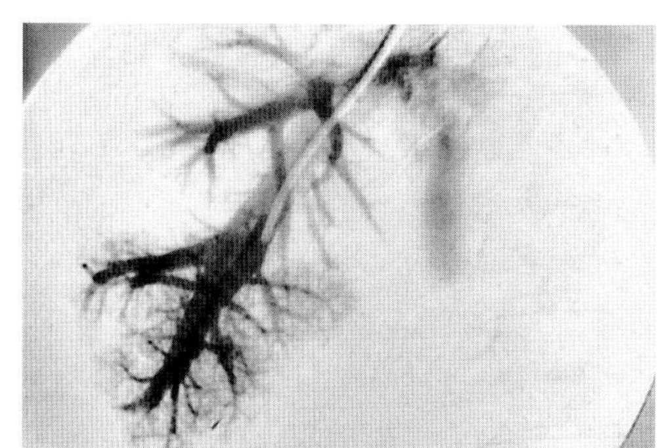

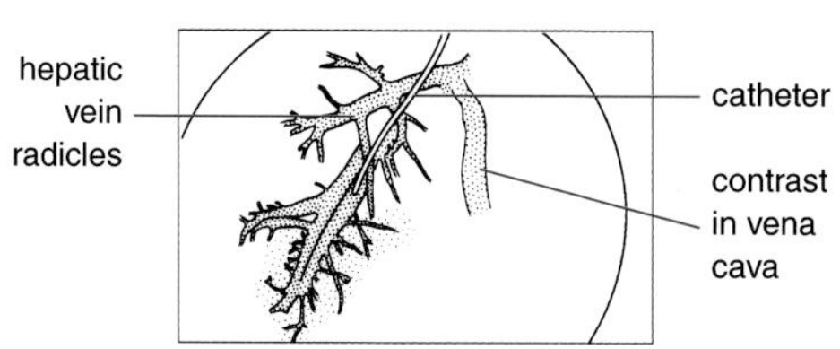

Fig. 10.24 Normal hepatic venogram. Courtesy of Prof A. Hemingway.

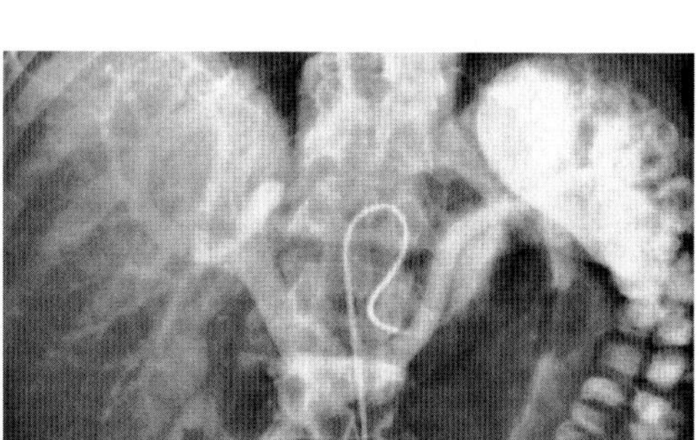

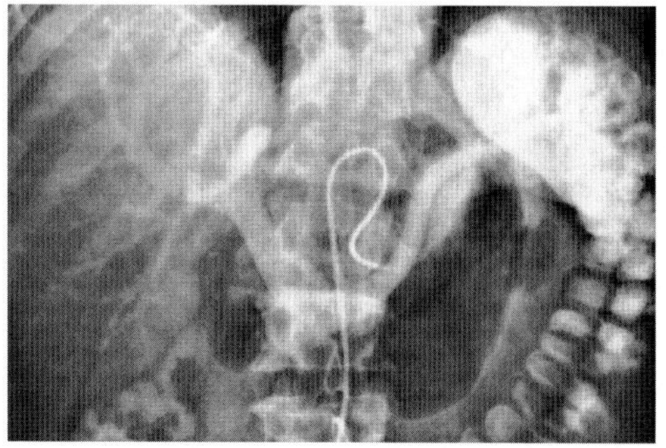

Fig. 10.22 Normal arterial splenic venogram. Courtesy of Prof A. Hemingway.

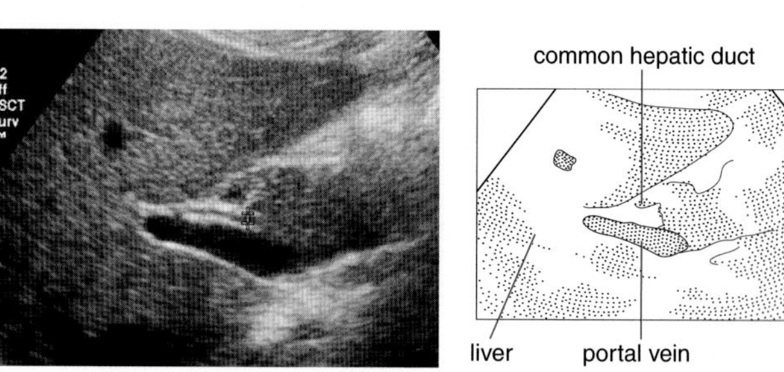

Fig. 10.25 Ultrasound of normal liver demonstrates the relationship of the common hepatic duct (between calipers) to the portal vein. Courtesy of Dr Jill E. Langer.

It has been conventional to consider the normal histology in relation to a lobule, with a central efferent vein and radiating plates of hepatocytes leading to the portal tracts at the periphery (Figs 10.32, 10.33). An alternative (and preferable) approach is to consider the acinus as the primary functional unit of the liver (Fig. 10.34). A portal tract, which contains distal branches of the hepatic artery, bile duct, and branches of the portal vein, lymphatics and connective tissue, is thus surrounded by a limiting plate of hepatocytes (Fig. 10.35). The acinar concept is important in understanding the pathophysiology of the liver, as there is then a natural

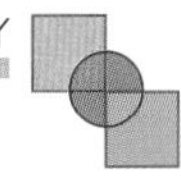

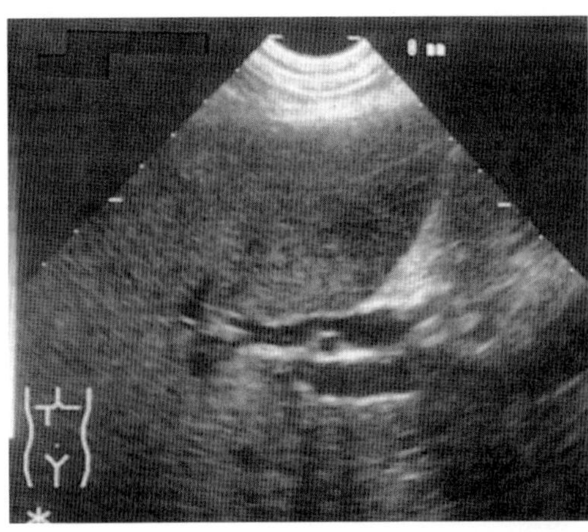

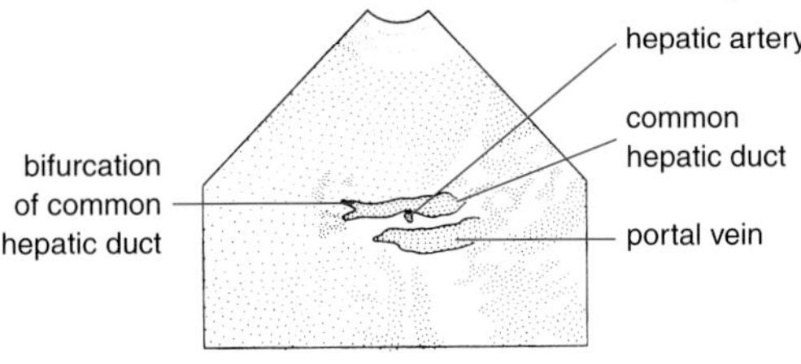

Fig. 10.26 Ultrasound showing the structures in the porta hepatis. Note the hepatic artery between the common hepatic duct (dilated) and the portal vein. Courtesy of Dr M.C. Collins.

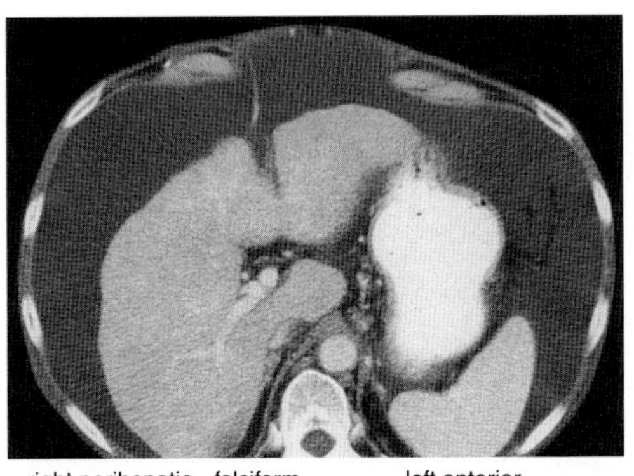

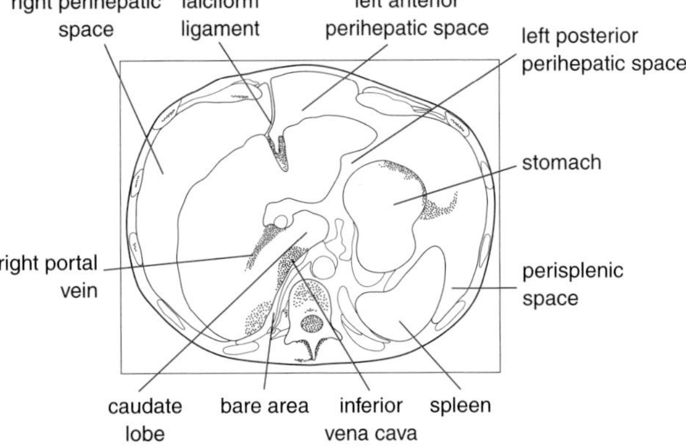

Fig. 10.27 CT demonstrates the perihepatic spaces filled with ascites in a patient with cirrhosis. The falciform ligament divides the potential space surrounding the liver into the right and left perihepatic spaces. The liver is suspended from the bare area by the coronary and triangular ligaments. Note the difference in the fat attenuation of the bare area attenuation of d.

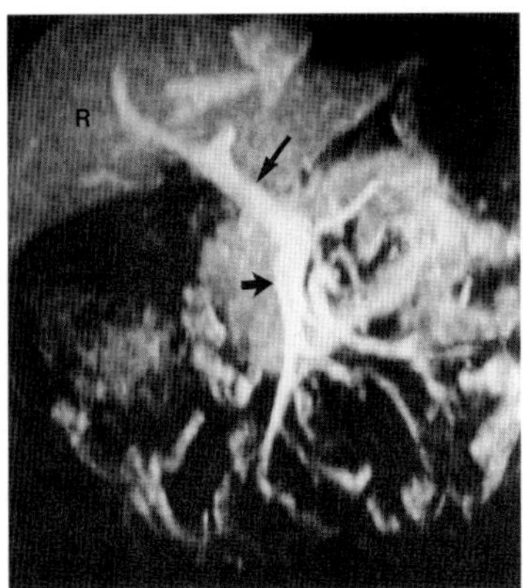

Fig. 10.28 MRI demonstrating normal portal venous system. The superior mesenteric vein (short arrow) and its major branches are seen. The portal vein (long arrow) extends into the liver. The right lobe of the liver (R) is identified. Courtesy of Dr Drew Torigian.

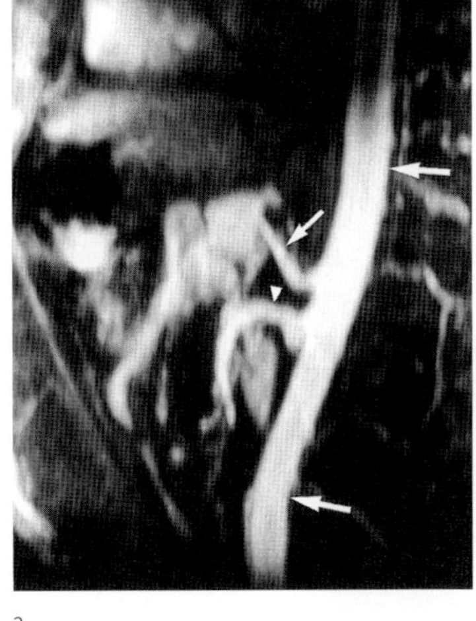

a

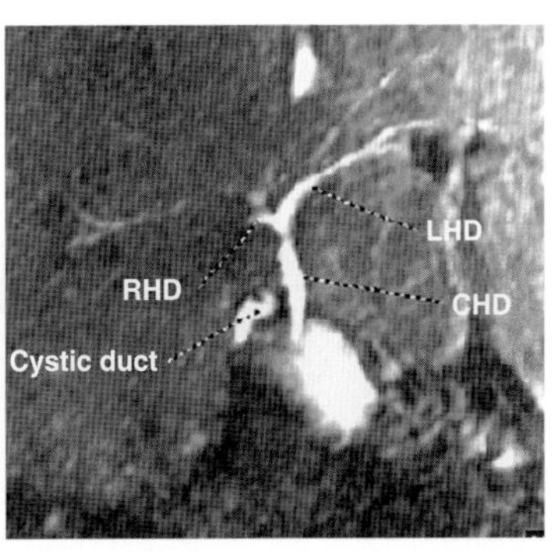

b

Fig 10.29 (a) MRI in the mid-sagittal plane demonstrates aorta (long arrows), celiac axis (short arrow) and root of superior mesenteric artery (arrowhead). Courtesy of Dr Drew Torigian. (b) TESLA scanning is also a non-invasive way to show biliary anatomy. Courtesy of Dr Ihab Kamel.

division of the liver into zones (Rappaport zones 1–3), which reflect a progressive reduction in oxygen supply from the portal tract to the central vein. Thus, zone 3 is the area most susceptible to tissue damage, and this is where necrosis tends to occur in response to severe liver injury.

Within the portal tract, both large and small bile ducts are found; these are termed septal and interlobular respectively. These bile ducts communicate with the bile canaliculi of the lobular parenchyma through the ductules and canals of Hering. Small numbers of macrophages and lymphocytes occur normally within the portal tracts, but the presence of plasma cells and polymorphonuclear cells is abnormal.

The lobular parenchyma comprises the central vein and the plates of hepatocytes (Fig. 10.36). Between the plates of hepatocytes are the sinusoids, which are lined by endothelial cells. The endothelial cells and hepatocytes are separated by the space of Disse, which in viable tissue is visible only by electron microscopy (Fig. 10.37). In addition to endothelial cells, there are two other major types of sinusoidal cells. Kupffer cells are derived from the mononuclear-phagocyte system and are the major scavenger cells of the liver (Fig. 10.38). The Ito, or hepatic stellate, cells also lie within the space of Disse. They were thought to function mainly as fat storage cells (e.g. for excess vitamin A and other fat-soluble vitamins) (Fig. 10.39), but it is now clear that they have other and more important roles. They become actively contractile when the liver is exposed to injury, such as that from ischemia, and this contractility is thought to have a major impact on the integrity of the sinusoidal microcirculation. They are also the primary cell type responsible for matrix deposition in liver fibrosis, during which they undergo a process of differentiation into fibrogenic myofibroblasts, in which they are major targets for the fibrogenic agent, transforming growth factor-beta.

The hepatocytes are regular polygonal cells with round nuclei and well-defined nucleoli. They normally contain glycogen, often some lipofuscin ('wear and tear' pigment), and occasional fatty vacuoles (Fig. 10.40). Each hepatocyte has an intercellular surface, surfaces that abut the sinusoids and space of Disse, and a canalicular surface. The bile canaliculi run between the liver cells (Fig. 10.41), forming a network converging towards the bile ducts within the portal tracts.

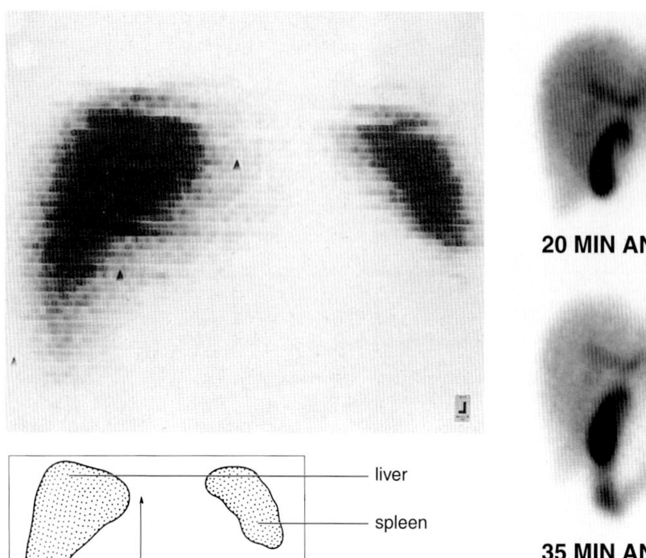

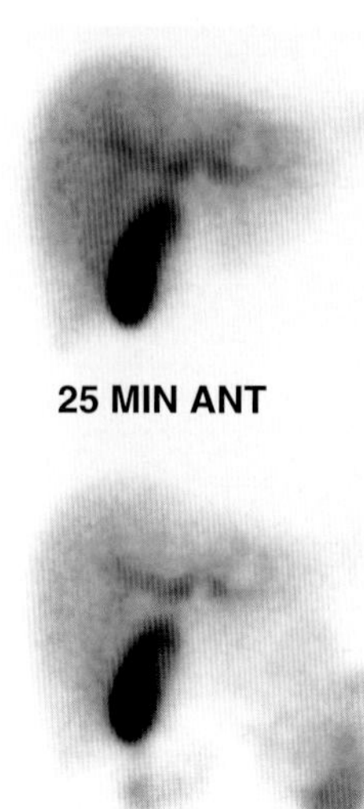

Fig. 10.30 (a) Normal ^{99m}Tc tin colloid scan of the liver and spleen. (b) HIDA scan showing normal uptake and excretion into the bile duct; this can be combined with cholecystokinin stimulation to assess gall bladder or sphincter of Oddi dysfunction. Courtesy of Dr Ihab Kamel.

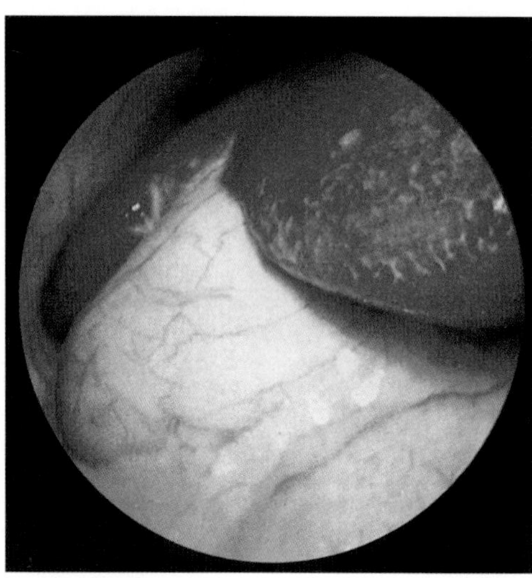

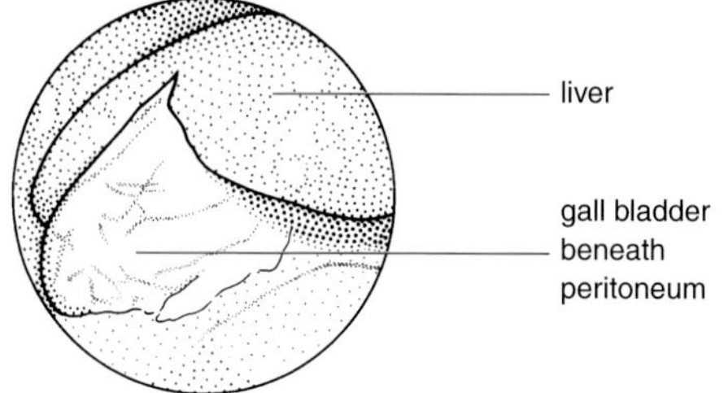

Fig. 10.31 Normal laparoscopic appearance of the liver.

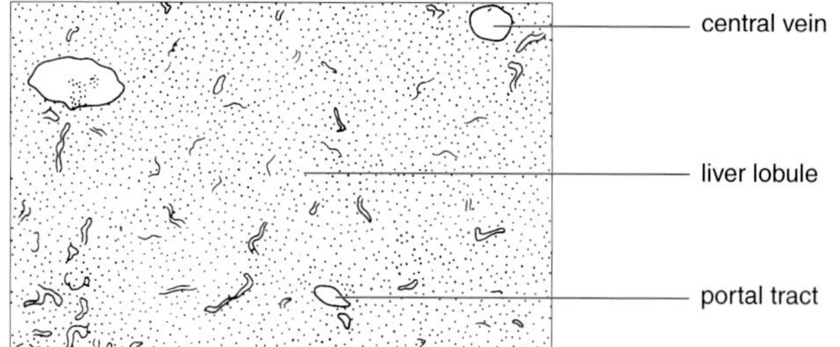

Fig. 10.32 Normal adult liver section showing the radiating plates of liver cells between the portal tracts and central veins. H&E stain (x 75).

JAUNDICE

Jaundice, or icterus, is the yellow coloration first of the sclera and later of the skin caused by an excess of bilirubin pigment (Fig. 10.42). This hyperbilirubinemia may be conjugated or unconjugated (Fig. 10.43). Clinically, conjugated and unconjugated hyperbilirubinemia are usually distinguishable by examining the urine. The unconjugated form of bilirubin is not filtered by the kidney, and so the urine is of a normal color – hence the old term acholuric jaundice.

Unconjugated bilirubinemia

Bilirubin appears in the blood following the breakdown of red cells, and unconjugated hyperbilirubinemia occurs when the rate of bilirubin production exceeds the ability of the liver to eliminate the pigment. This may be caused by excessive hemolysis (as in hemolytic anemia) or by defects in hepatic bilirubin metabolism. This is seen transiently in healthy newborn infants as 'physiological' jaundice.

Hepatic glucuronidation is required for the efficient biliary excretion of bilirubin. In the hereditary condition of Gilbert's syndrome

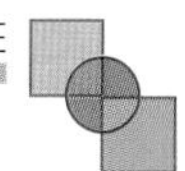

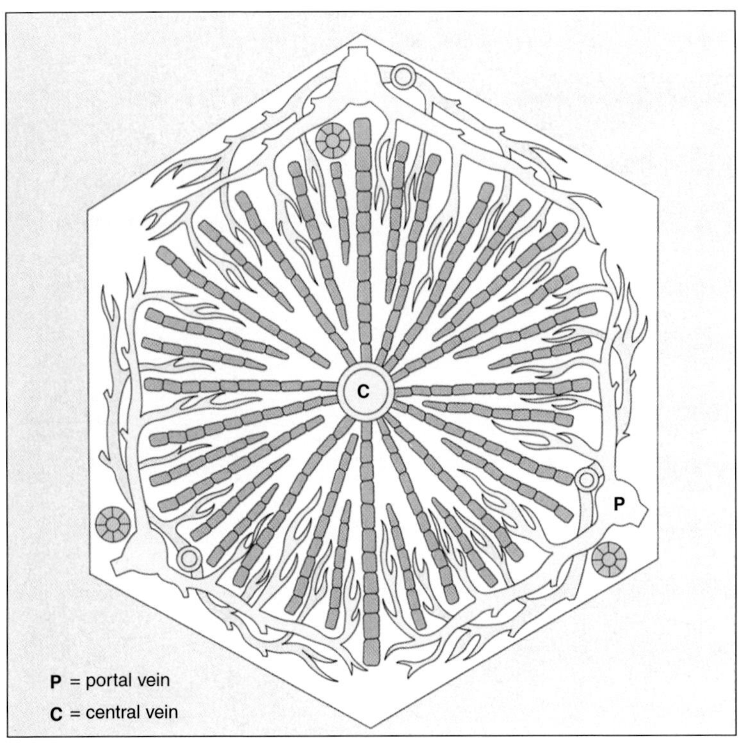

■ **Fig. 10.33** Diagrammatic representation of the acinus.

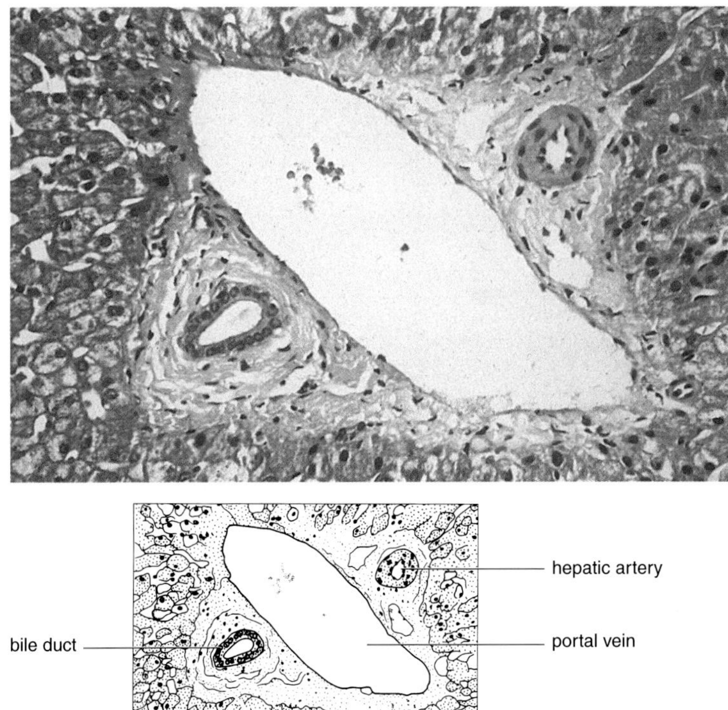

■ **Fig. 10.35** Normal liver section showing the constituents of the portal tract. H&E stain (x 175). Courtesy of Prof B. Portmann.

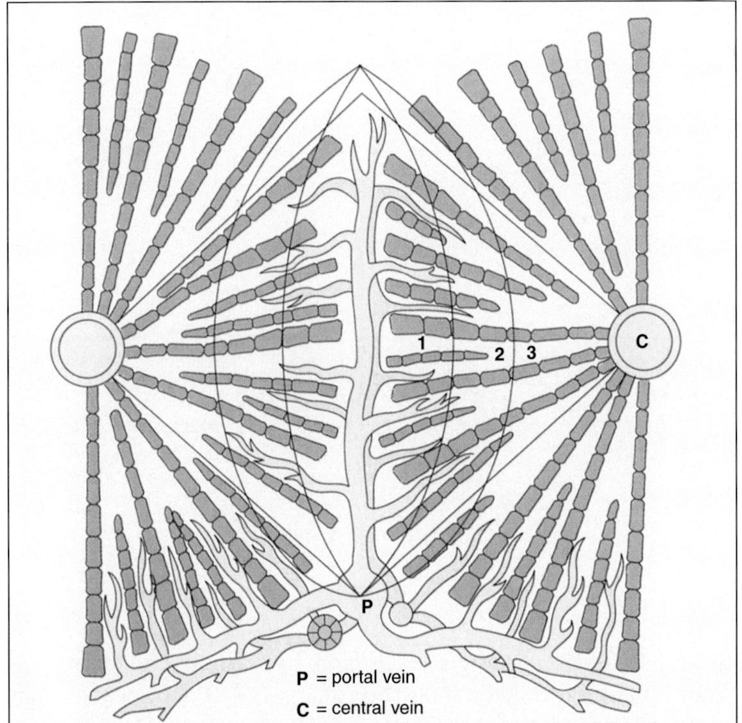

■ **Fig. 10.34** Diagrammatic representation of the lobule, in which the portal vein is perceived to be at the periphery rather than at the center of the structural unit. Blood flows from the portal space towards the central vein. Relative hypoxia in zone 3 (compared with zones 1 and 2) means that this zone is most susceptible to injury.

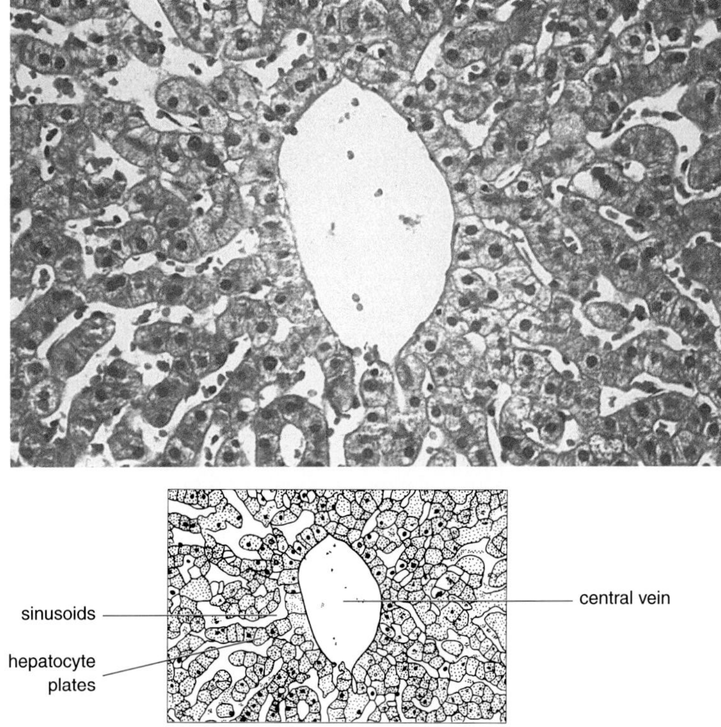

■ **Fig. 10.36** Normal liver section showing the central vein. H&E stain (x 175). Courtesy of Prof B. Portmann.

levels of UDP glucuronosyl transferase are reduced to about 30% of normal as a result of one of a series of mutations in the UDP-glucuronosyl transferase 1 promoter gene. A mild unconjugated hyperbilirubinemia is seen which is greater when fasting and maximal at times of additional stress such as with intercurrent illness.

None of the above is associated with any histological abnormality in the liver, apart from the accumulation of small amounts of pigment in the parenchymal cells. Very rarely the glucuronosyl transferase may be completely absent, and in this case a severe unconjugated hyperbilirubinemia develops (Crigler–Najjar disease).

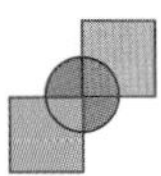

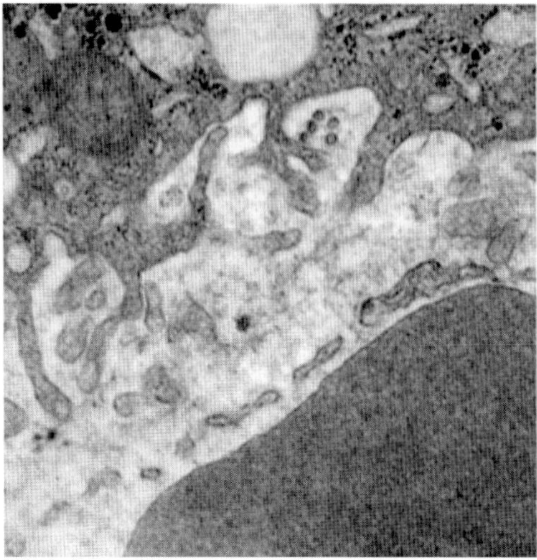

■ **Fig. 10.37** Electron micrograph showing the space of Disse. This is the space between the sinusoidal cytoplasm and the hepatocytes (x 50 000). Courtesy of Prof J.C.E. Underwood.

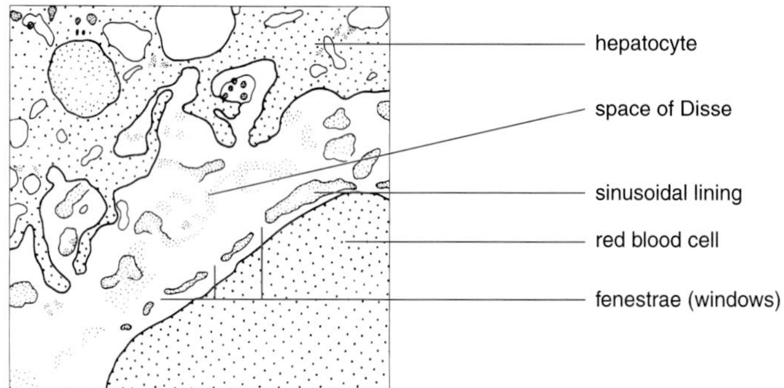

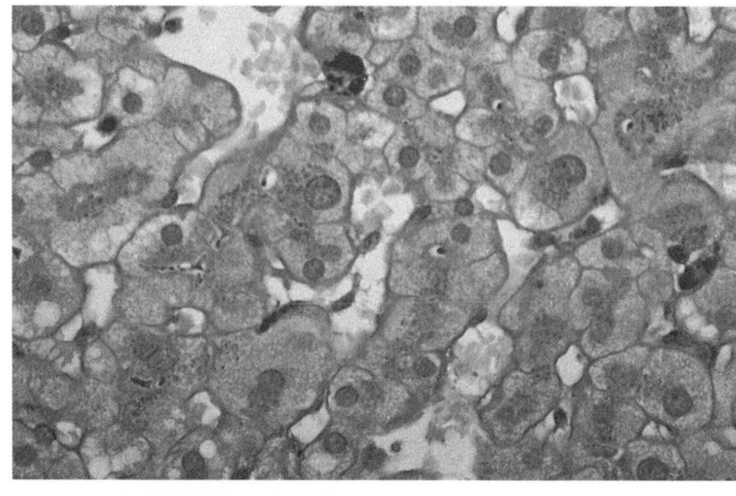

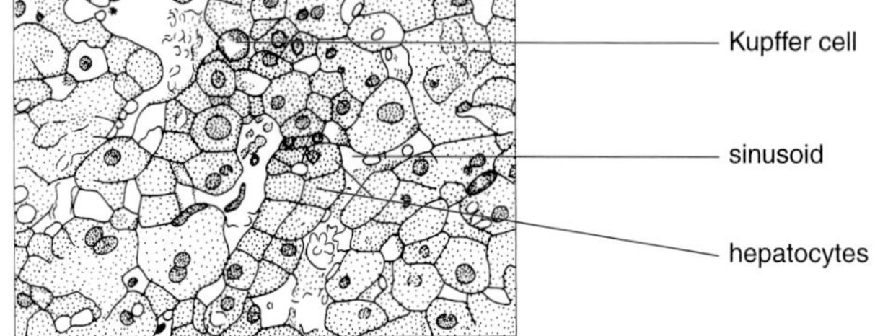

■ **Fig. 10.38** Normal liver cell plates with PAS-positive Kupffer cells in the sinusoids. PAS stain (x 450).

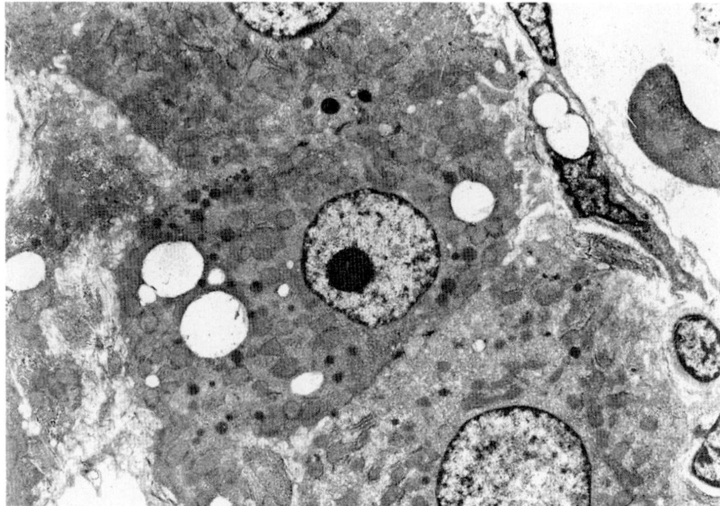

■ **Fig. 10.39** Electron micrograph of a normal hepatocyte showing its relationship to the adjacent sinusoid (x 3000).

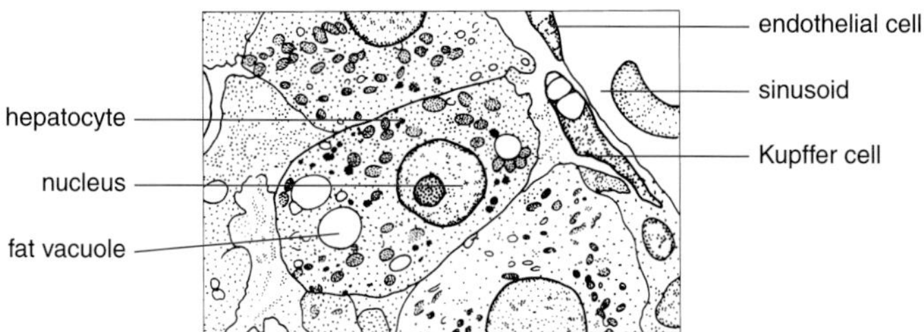

Conjugated hyperbilirubinemia and cholestasis

Conjugated hyperbilirubinemia occurs when there is obstruction to the flow of bile, either within the liver (intrahepatic cholestasis), or at any level in the biliary tree. Failure to excrete bile pigments into the intestinal lumen results in the feces being pale in color; instead the conjugated bilirubin is excreted by the kidneys, giving rise to dark urine (Fig. 10.44). Ultrasonography provides the simplest method of distinguishing between intra- and extrahepatic obstruction, because the bile ducts are dilated in the latter (Fig. 10.45), but excellent views with minimal invasiveness comes also from CT scanning (Fig. 10.46). Cholestasis is frequently accompanied by pruritus and hence by scratch marks on the skin (Fig. 10.47), as well as being associated with generalized pigmentation in more advanced cases (Fig. 10.48). Prolonged cholestasis leads to secondary hypercholesterolemia, and in turn to cholesterol deposition around the eyes (xanthelasmata; Fig. 10.49), or elsewhere in the body (xanthomata; Figs 10.48, 10.50).

Bile is easily recognizable in liver sections by its green/brown color, although within hepatocytes it may resemble lipofuscin (Fig. 10.51). Intra- and extrahepatic cholestasis typically have very different histological appearances. Centrilobular cholestasis with relatively little liver cell damage is an early feature of extrahepatic obstruction. Later the hepatocytes degenerate and groups of necrotic cells can then be seen in periportal zones, forming bile infarcts. The most striking changes are seen in the portal tracts, which dilate due to edema. Inflammatory cells (mainly neutrophils) are seen, especially around the bile ducts (Fig. 10.52). Proliferation of small ducts at the periphery of the portal tracts is a characteristic feature. Bile can leak out of the

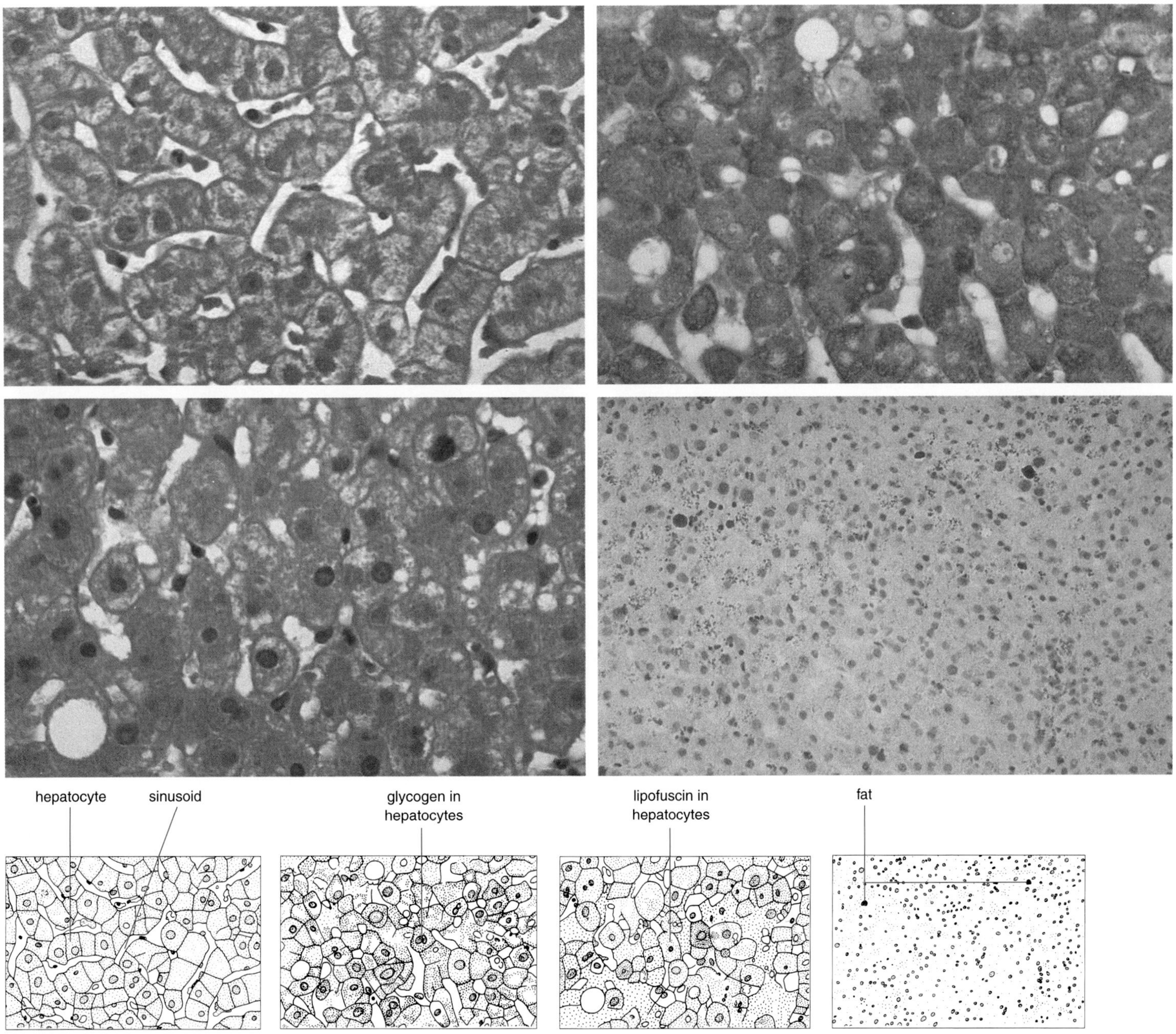

hepatocyte
sinusoid
glycogen in hepatocytes
lipofuscin in hepatocytes
fat

■ **Fig. 10.40** Normal liver section (upper left, H&E stain (x 450)) and sections stained for glycogen (upper right, PAS stain (x 450)), lipofuscin (lower left, H&E stain (x 450)), and fat (lower right, staining with oil red-O (x 175)). Upper left is courtesy of Prof B. Portmann.

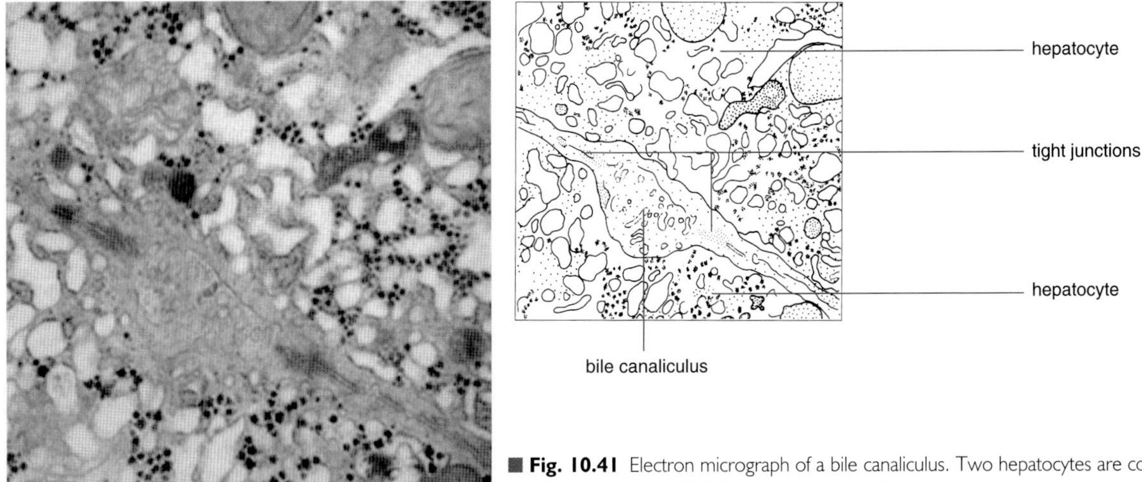

■ **Fig. 10.41** Electron micrograph of a bile canaliculus. Two hepatocytes are connected by 'tight junctions' between which lies the canaliculus (x 30 000). Courtesy of Prof J.C.E. Underwood.

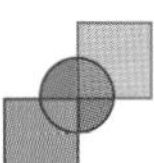

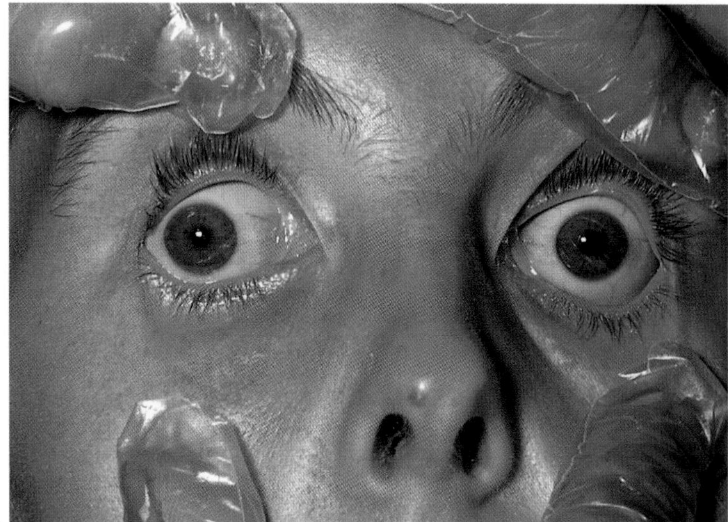

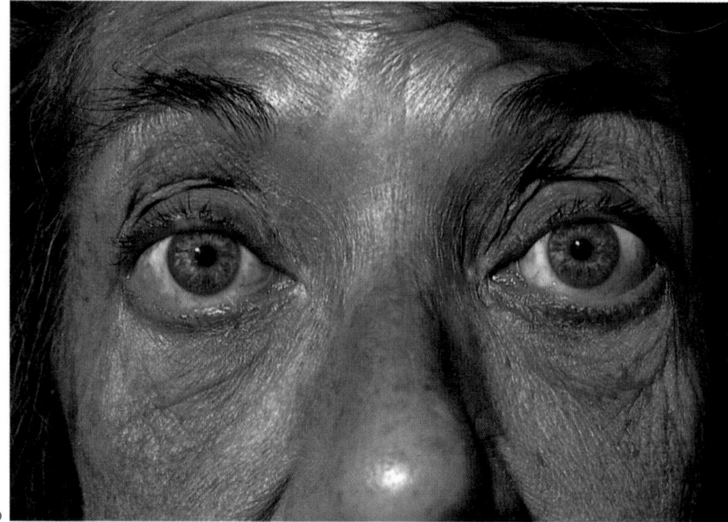

■ **Fig. 10.42** Facial appearance of two patients with jaundice. Acute hepatitis (a), and primary biliary cirrhosis ((b) – note the pigmentation in addition to the jaundice).

HYPERBILIRUBINEMIA		
	Unconjugated	
pre-hepatic	hemolytic anemia hemoglobinopathies systemic infections	
hepatic	Gilbert's syndrome neonatal jaundice	
	Conjugated	
intrahepatic	hepatitic	viral drugs alcohol
extrahepatic	cirrhosis gall stones carcinoma pancreatitis	 pancreas bile ducts ampulla
non-cholestatic	Dubin-Johnson syndrome	

■ **Fig. 10.43** Classification of hyperbilirubinemia.

RBC
bilirubin (300mg/day)
bilirubin/albumin (unconjugated)
conjugated
bilirubin
diglucuronide
unconjugated
conjugated
bilirubin
conjugated
fecal
stercobilinogen

■ **Fig. 10.44** Diagram showing the metabolism of bilirubin.

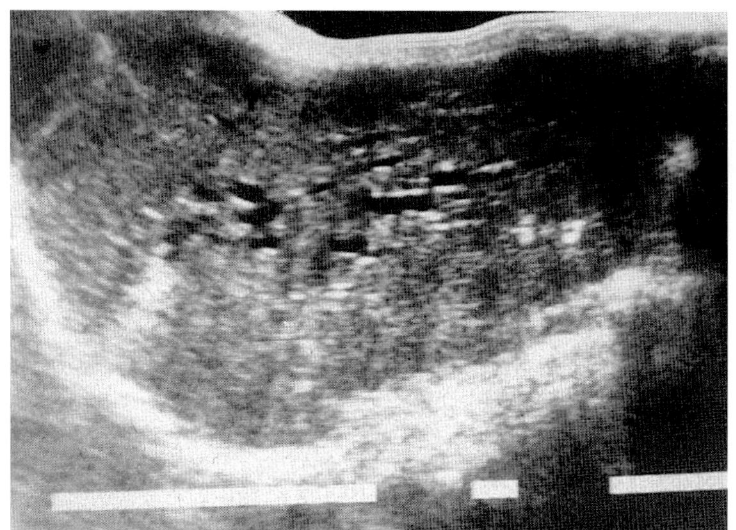

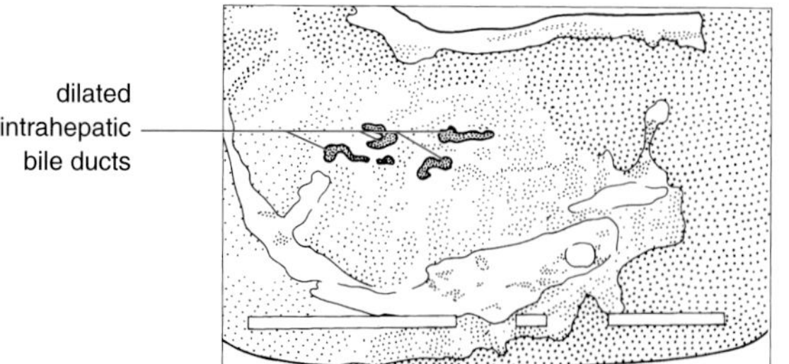

■ **Fig. 10.45** Ultrasound showing a large calculus in the extrahepatic biliary tree. Dilated bile ducts can be seen to the left. Courtesy of Dr M.C. Collins.

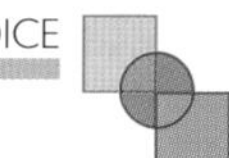

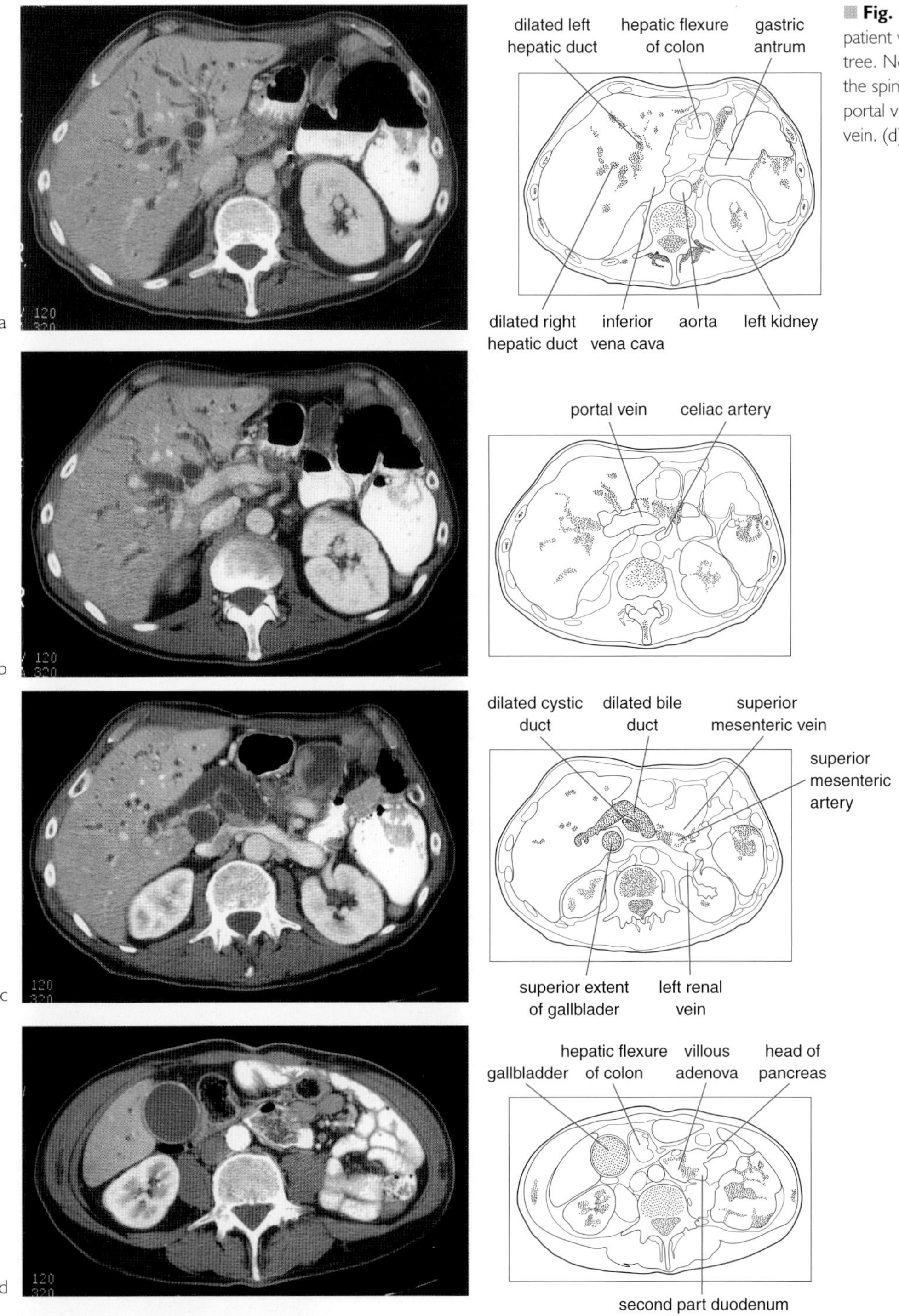

Fig. 10.46 Cross-sectional biliary anatomy demonstrated by CT in patient with villous adenoma of the papilla of Vater obstructing the biliary tree. Note that the pancreas and duodenum are deviated to the left of the spine. (a) Image through upper liver. (b) Image through level of main portal vein. (c) Image through level of common bile duct and left renal vein. (d) Image through level of lower portion head of pancreas.

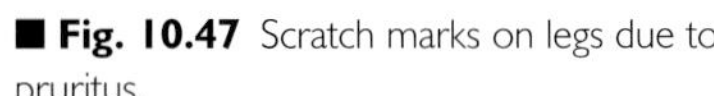

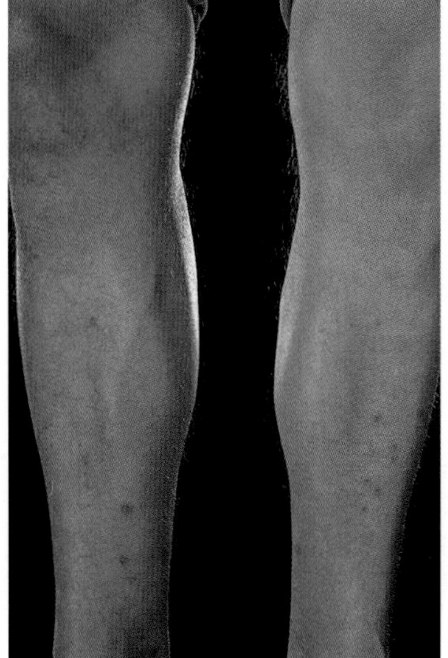

Fig. 10.47 Scratch marks on legs due to pruritus.

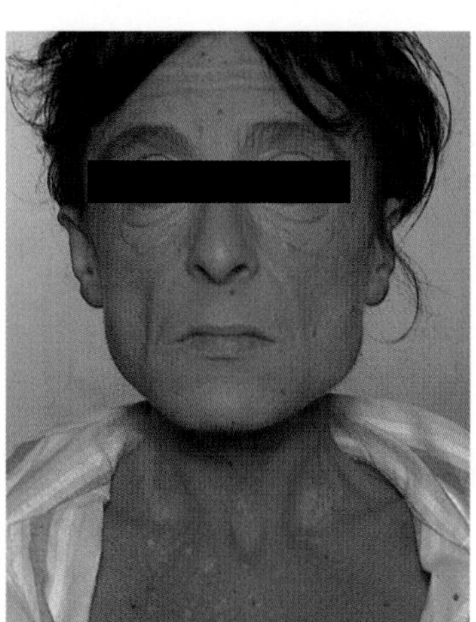

Fig. 10.48 Cutaneous pigmentation and xanthomata in chronic cholestasis.

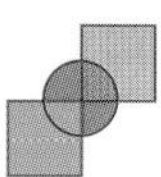

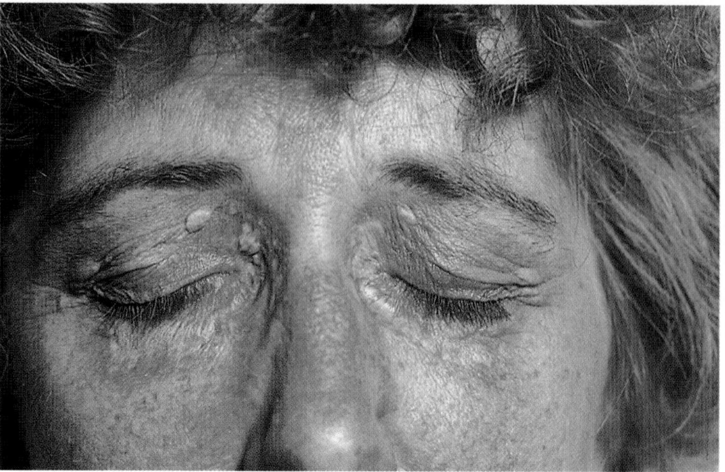

■ **Fig. 10.49** Periorbital xanthelasmata in a patient with early (pre-icteric) primary biliary cirrhosis.

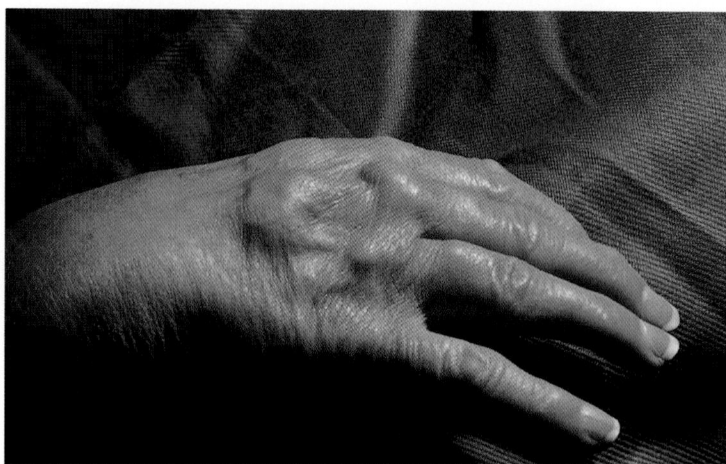

■ **Fig. 10.50** Subcutaneous xanthomas on the dorsum of the hand in a patient with primary biliary cirrhosis.

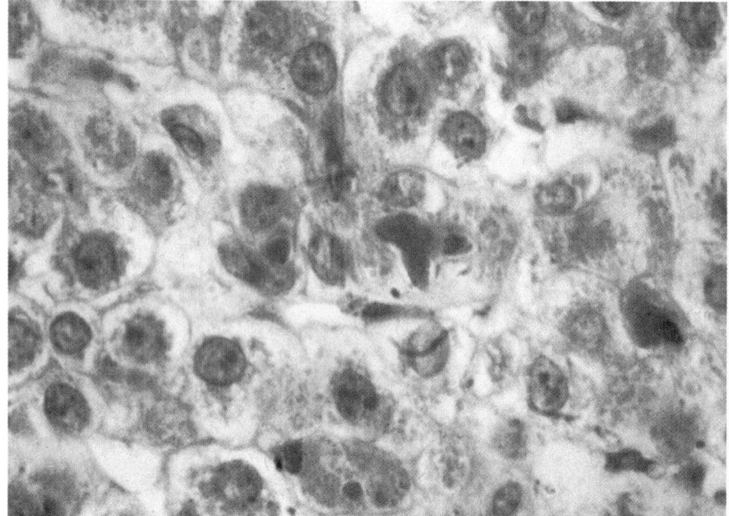

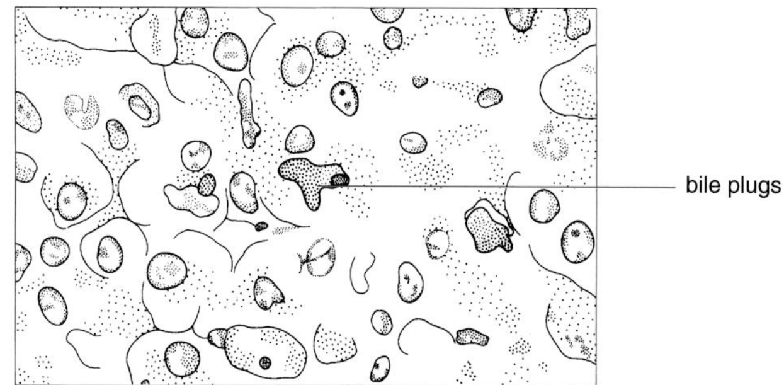

■ **Fig. 10.51** Liver section in cholestasis showing a bile plug. H&E stain. Courtesy of Prof J.C.E. Underwood.

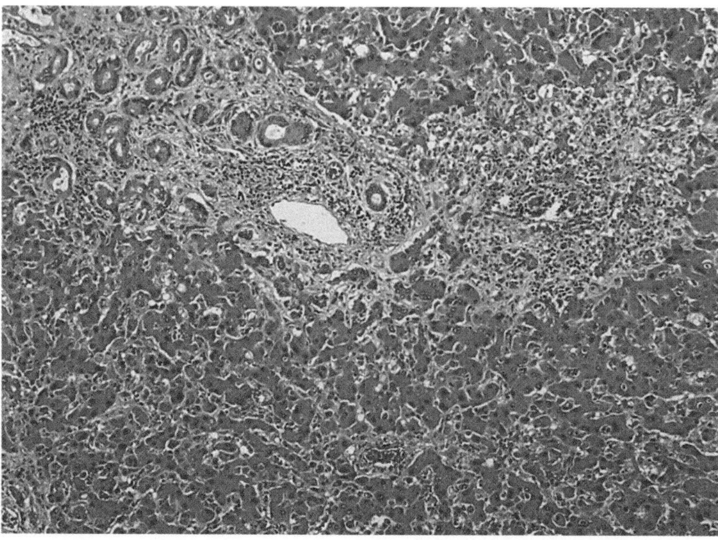

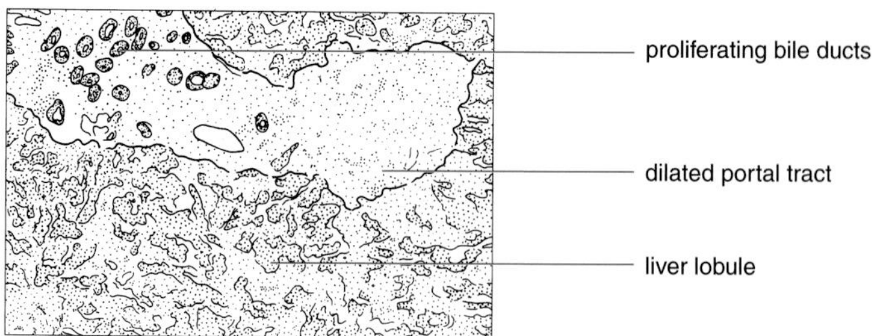

■ **Fig. 10.52** Liver section showing inflammatory cells in a portal tract and proliferation of small ductules. H&E stain (x 75).

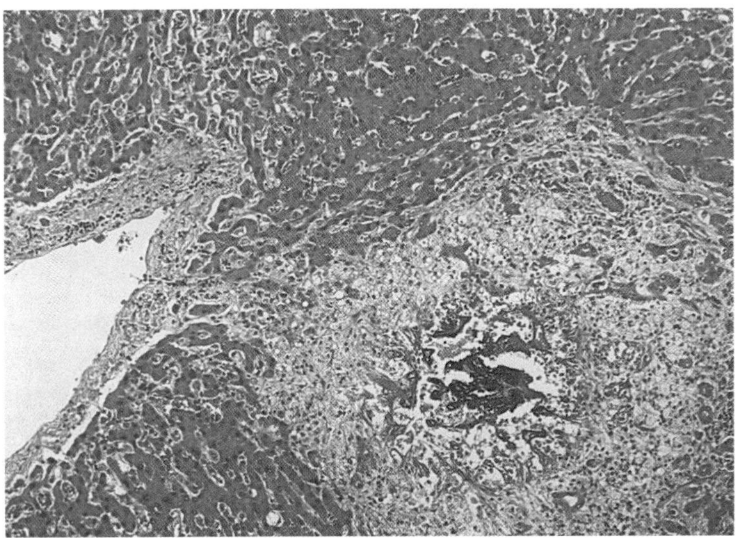

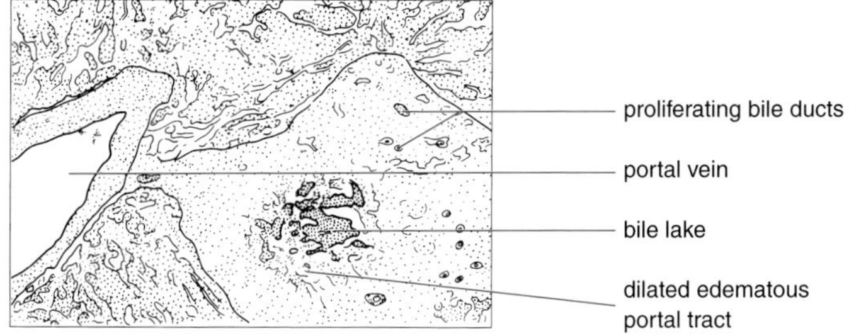

■ **Fig. 10.53** Liver section showing a bile 'lake' at the site of a damaged duct, with extravasation of bile into the adjacent portal connective tissue. H&E stain (x 75).

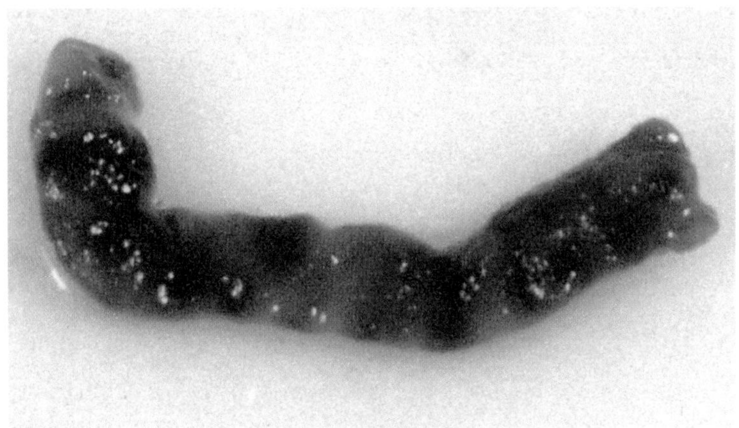

■ **Fig. 10.54** A needle liver biopsy specimen in Dubin–Johnson syndrome.

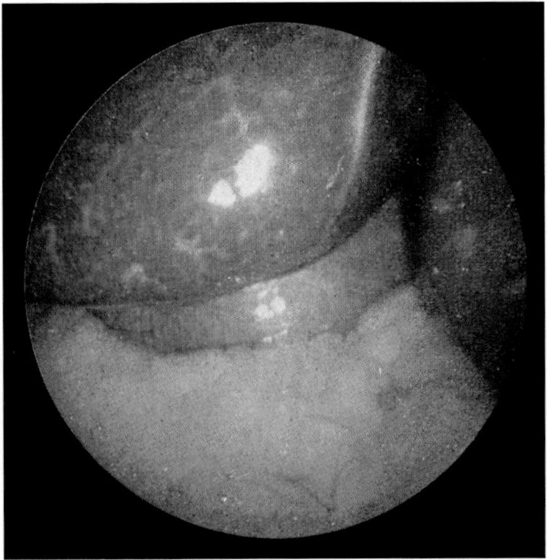

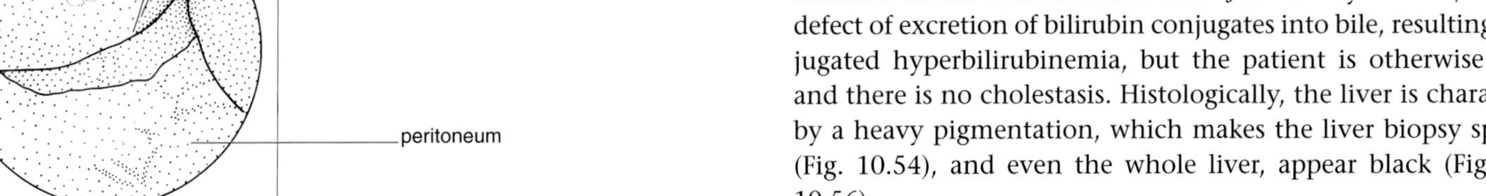

■ **Fig. 10.55** Laparoscopic appearance of the liver in Dubin–Johnson syndrome.

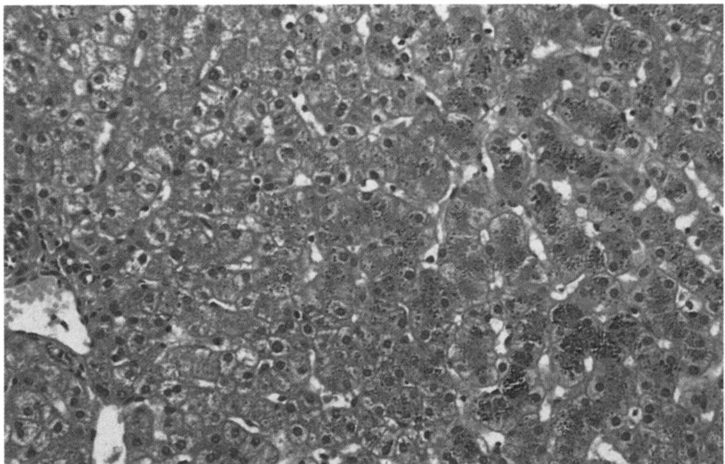

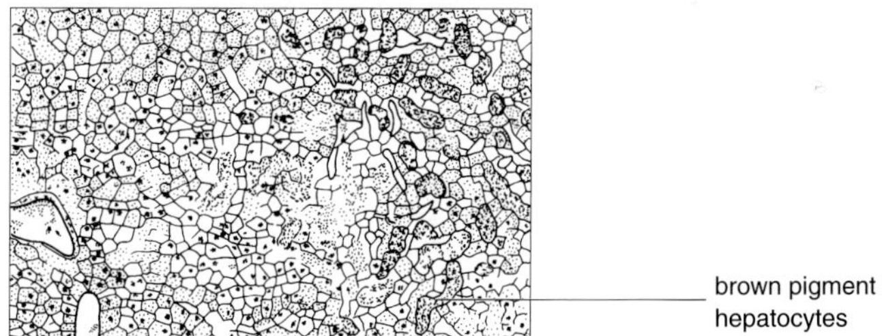

■ **Fig. 10.56** Liver section in Dubin–Johnson syndrome showing pigment-laden hepatocytes. H&E stain (x 175).

ducts to form extracellular bile 'lakes' (Fig. 10.53), and, although rare, this is pathognomonic of large duct obstruction. If unrelieved, chronic obstruction ultimately leads to fibrosis and secondary biliary cirrhosis.

The histopathology in intrahepatic cholestasis depends upon the etiology of the liver damage. Cholestasis commonly accompanies hepatocellular jaundice, such as in viral hepatitis, even if it is not the predominant feature. This will be considered separately in later sections. In the rare familial Dubin–Johnson syndrome, there is a defect of excretion of bilirubin conjugates into bile, resulting in conjugated hyperbilirubinemia, but the patient is otherwise normal and there is no cholestasis. Histologically, the liver is characterized by a heavy pigmentation, which makes the liver biopsy specimen (Fig. 10.54), and even the whole liver, appear black (Figs 10.55, 10.56).

HEPATITIS AND INFECTIONS OF THE LIVER

11

HEPATOTROPIC VIRUSES

The liver may be involved in many viremias, but certain viruses are classified as being hepatotropic because of their predilection for this organ (Table 11.1). To date, five such viruses have been positively identified (hepatitis A to hepatitis E), and there is increasing evidence to suggest the existence of other hepatitis viruses. Most cases of viral hepatitis are subclinical and hence undiagnosed.

Hepatitis A (Fig. 11.1) is an RNA virus which is responsible for an acute short-lived illness with a very low mortality and no long-term sequelae. In contrast, hepatitis B (HBV) (Fig. 11.2) is a DNA virus which tends to cause a more severe acute illness, other than in small children, and may give rise to a chronic carrier state that is accompanied by the persistence of the virus in the blood, and progression to chronic hepatitis and cirrhosis.

Hepatitis C (HCV) is an RNA virus that, like HBV is transmitted parenterally, and is a common cause of chronic liver disease, affecting about 200 million people worldwide. It appears that the virus is approximately 30–60 nm in diameter (Fig. 11.3). The genome of HCV is a single-stranded RNA and the molecular structure of HCV is shown in Figure 11.4. The structural and non-structural proteins

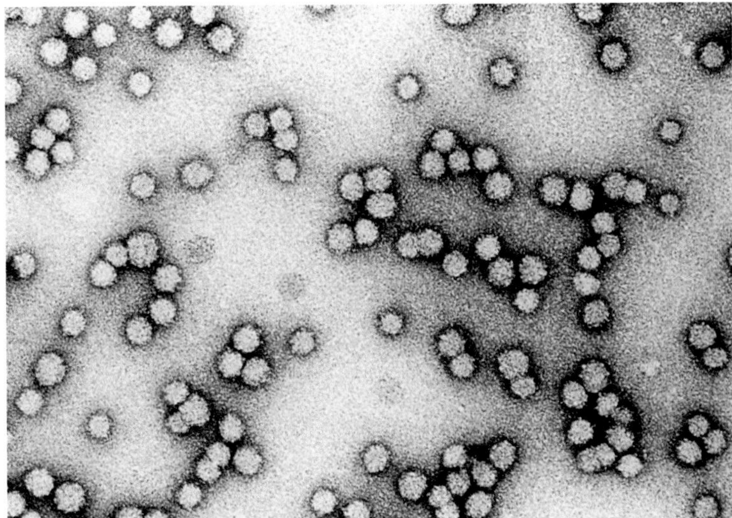

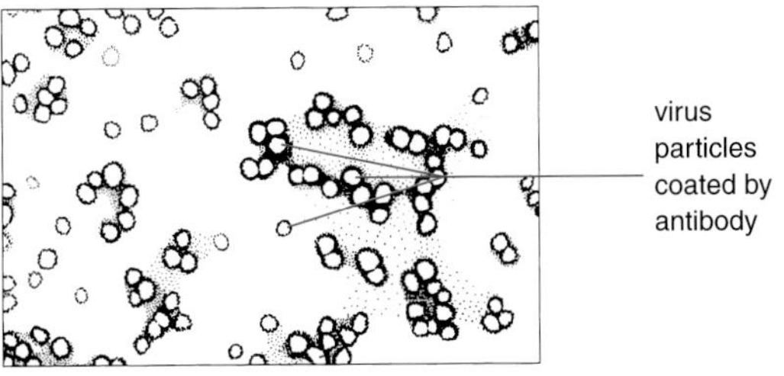

■ **Fig. 11.1** Electron micrograph showing hepatitis A virus particles (27–32 nm diameter) with antibody coating their surfaces.

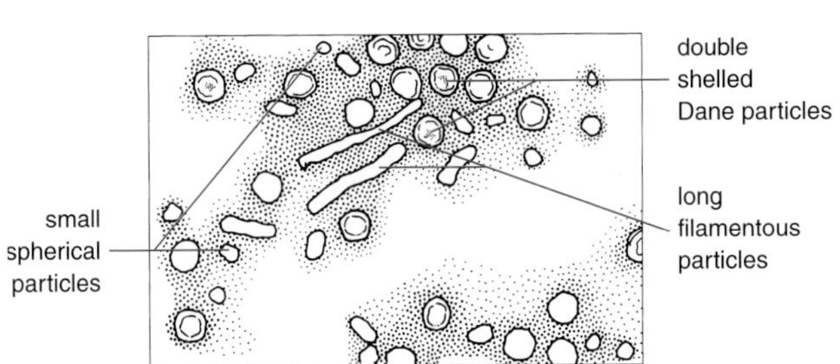

■ **Fig. 11.2** Electron micrograph of hepatitis B virus. The slide includes: small 28 nm spherical particles (HBsAg); larger 42 nm spherical, double shelled Dane particles; long filamentous particles.

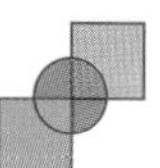

are encoded at the 5′ and 3′ ends of the open reading frame. Untrans-lated regions (UTR) flank both 5′ and 3′ ends and UTR is required for the translation of proteins and replication of the virus.

Hepatitis D (delta antigen) is a small RNA virus which in itself is non-pathogenic but, when occurring in association with HBV, renders the liver disease more severe, more likely both to run a fulminant course and to be progressive.

An enterically transmitted virus associated with large water-borne epidemics throughout Asia, Africa, and Latin America has been termed hepatitis E (Fig. 11.5). This usually causes a benign self-limiting illness like hepatitis A, although it causes a high mortality in pregnant women.

The different types of acute hepatitis cannot be distinguished clinically, and their distinction depends upon serological tests. Similarly, reliable histological differentiation between them cannot be made in most cases. The classical histological appearance in uncomplicated, acute (lobular) hepatitis is of liver cell damage and necrosis in the centrilobular area (Fig. 11.6). The hepatocytes show ballooning degeneration and degenerate acidophil bodies. Kupffer cells are active and engulf degraded liver cells (Fig. 11.7). These changes are accompanied by an inflammatory infiltrate within the lobules which is predominantly lymphocytic with some plasma cells. Mild edema in the portal tract, together with mononuclear cells and some macrophages, is usually found. Bile duct proliferation is minimal. The degree of cholestasis is variable, but occasionally in patients who are deeply jaundiced, the changes in the portal tract may mimic those seen in extrahepatic obstruction (see Chapter 10). As the lobular inflammation subsides, the centrilobular collapse of reticulin becomes more apparent (Fig. 11.8), thus giving the appearance of architectural distortion, but these changes are transient. Inflammation of the portal tracts persists for long periods, and this may result in the formation of fibrous septa between portal tracts.

In more severe cases of acute hepatitis, there is bridging necrosis between central veins and portal tracts (subacute hepatic necrosis; Fig. 11.9). The portal tracts at this stage are enlarged; there may be bile duct proliferation and neutrophil infiltration, which may also be confused with extrahepatic obstruction. The boundary between the hepatic lobule and portal tract (limiting plate) is usually preserved, but disruption tends to be associated with the development of chronic hepatitis (see below). Subacute hepatic necrosis may progress to liver failure and death, although full recovery is possible. A more acute and severe hepatitis may lead to fulminant hepatic failure, in which few viable parenchymal cells remain and the liver is shrunken and yellow (acute yellow atrophy; Fig. 11.10).

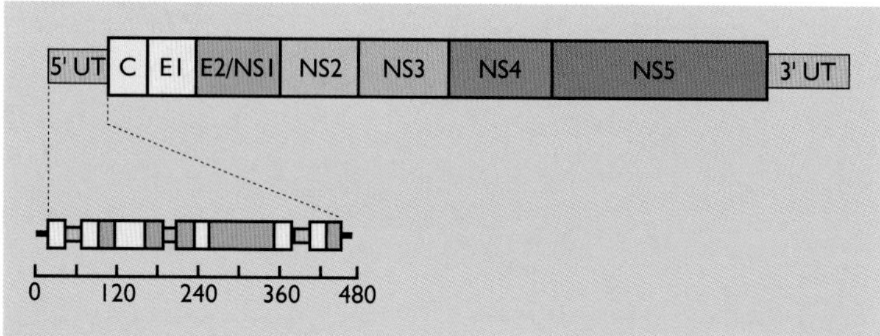

Fig. 11.3 Schematic diagram of hepatitis C virus showing structural and non-structural components together with some of the antigens currently used in antibody testing.

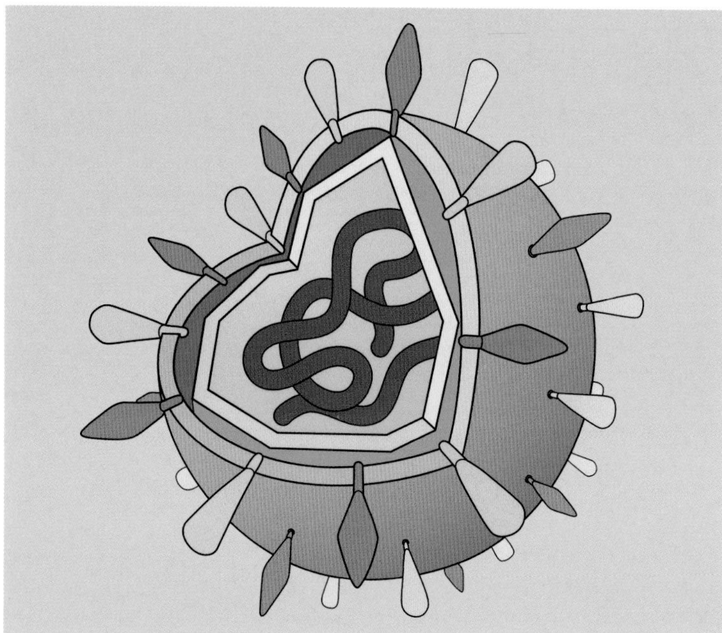

Fig. 11.4 The hepatitis C virion.

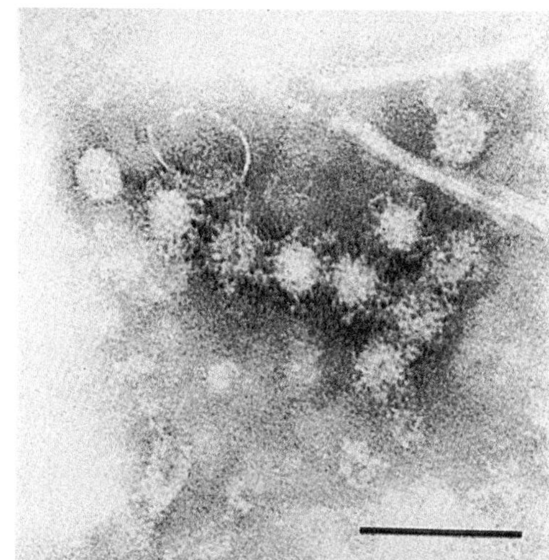

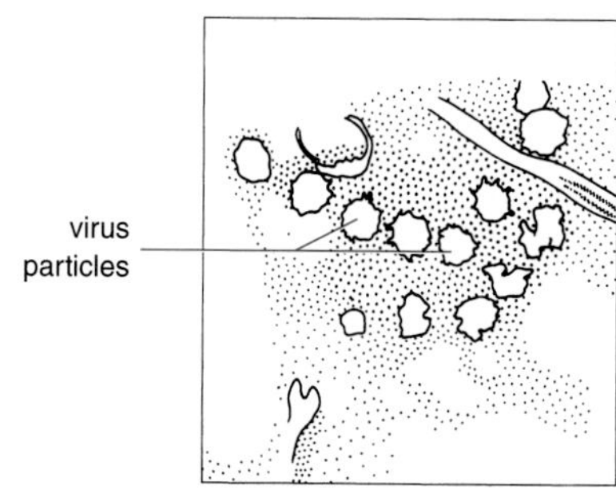

Fig. 11.5 Electron micrograph of hepatitis E virus particles (bar = 100 nm).

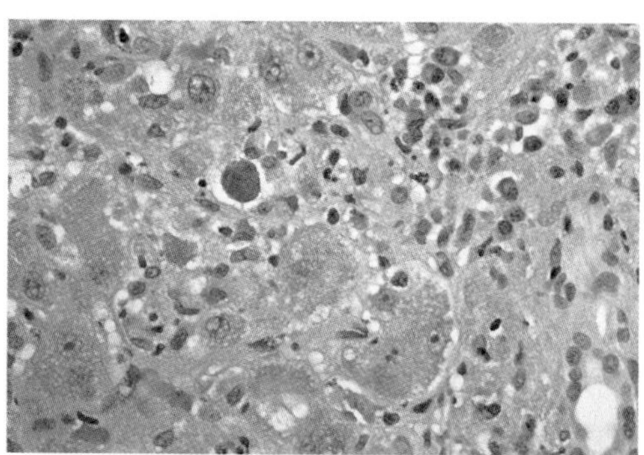

Fig. 11.6 Acute hepatitis. Microscopic view of acute lobular hepatitis showing parenchymal infiltration by inflammatory and immune cells, disarray and vacuolization of hepatocytes, and focal hepatocyte apoptosis (single cell necrosis seen as a dense eosinophilic body (Councilman body) containing karyorrhectic nuclear fragments).

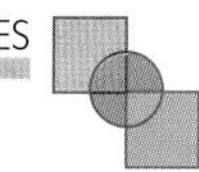

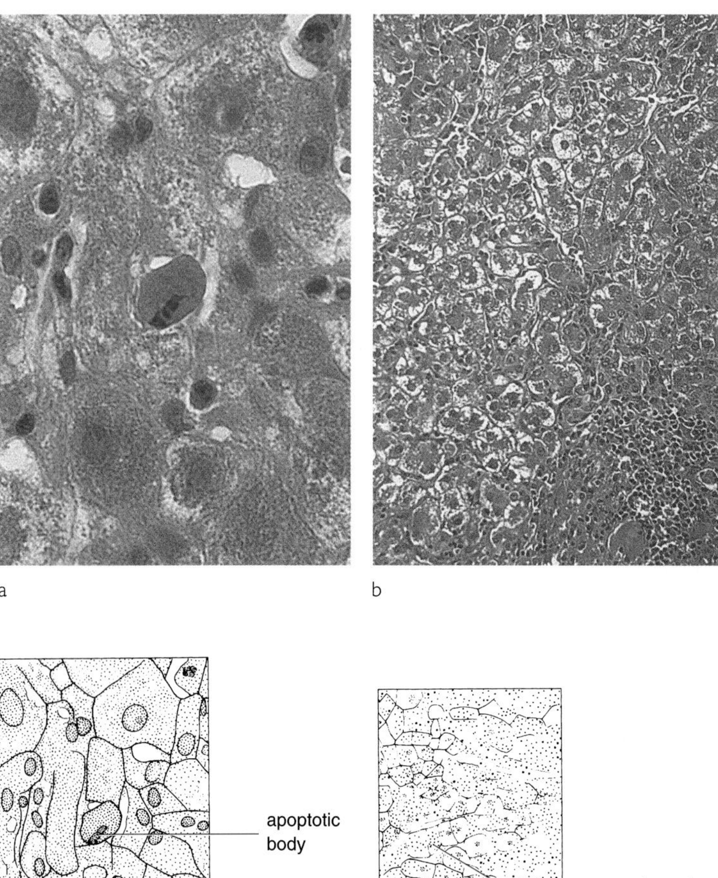

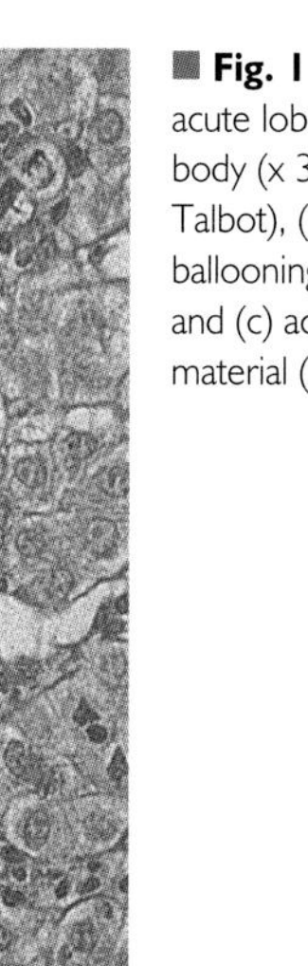

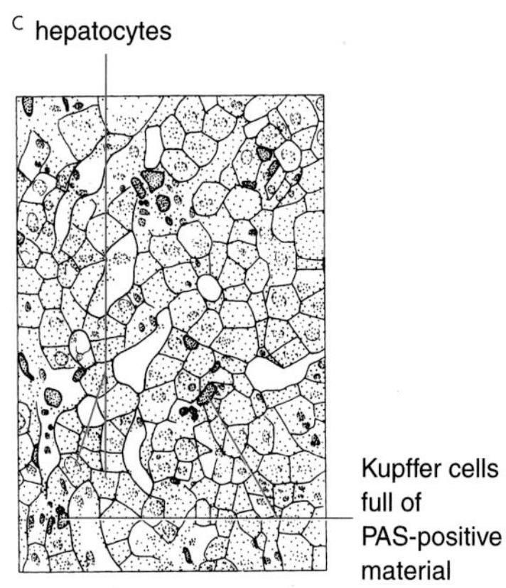

■ **Fig. 11.7** (a) Histological appearance in acute lobular hepatitis showing an apoptotic body (x 320, H&E stain) (Courtesy of Prof I. Talbot), (b) enlarged hepatocytes due to ballooning degeneration (x 125, H&E stain), and (c) active Kupffer cells full of PAS-positive material (x 320, PAS stain).

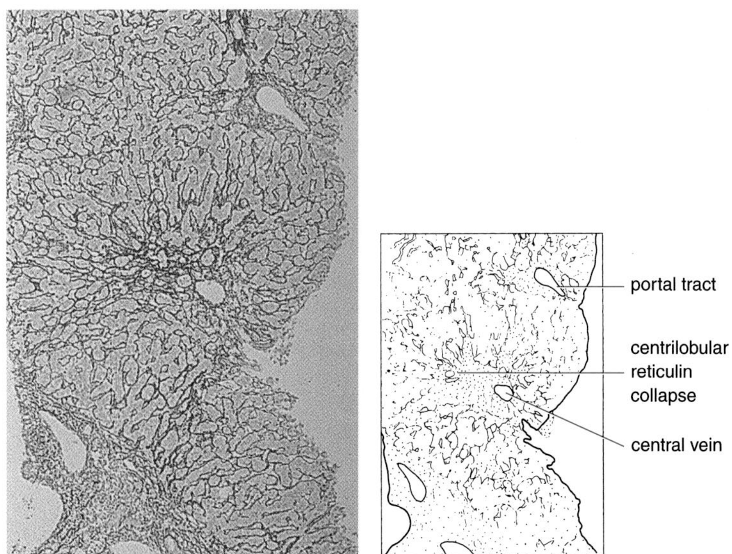

■ **Fig. 11.8** Histology in acute lobular hepatitis showing centrilobular reticulin collapse. Reticulin stain (x 50).

Acute viral hepatitis secondary to HBV and HCV infection often leads to chronic inflammation. The main histological changes are seen in the portal tracts, which contain large numbers of lymphocytes and plasma cells. Adjacent tracts may link up (Fig. 11.11).

In some cases, the etiology of the hepatitis can be discerned histologically. HBV can be recognized in liver cells by their 'ground glass' appearance, and by special stains such as orcein. Alternatively, an anti-HBV antibody, incorporating immunofluorescence or horse-radish peroxidase techniques, can be used (Figs 11.12–11.14). Hepatitis C infection is characterized by specific histological features of microvesicular fat and lymphocyte infiltration of the sinusoids (Fig. 11.15).

SYSTEMIC VIRUSES

Many other viruses may damage the liver (see Table 11.1), although the primary site of infection is usually extrahepatic. During infection with the Epstein–Barr virus, although jaundice is unusual, elevated transaminases are found in the majority of cases. Liver damage is usually mild, consisting of an infiltrate of atypical mononuclear cells in sinusoids and small foci of necrosis (Fig. 11.16). Herpes simplex (herpes virus type 1) may invade the liver in infants and immunocompromised adults. Foci of coagulative necrosis with little surrounding inflammation are characteristic (Fig. 11.17). A similar histological pattern is found with varicella zoster (chicken pox) infection (Fig. 11.18).

In cytomegalovirus infection the liver damage is variable. Liver cells are swollen and have nuclear inclusions surrounded by a halo, giving an 'owl's eye' appearance (Fig. 11.19).

Two severe tropical viral hepatitides are yellow fever in South America and Central Africa, and Lassa fever in Central Africa. These can be accompanied by widespread systemic features such as renal failure and skin hemorrhage. In fatal yellow fever, the liver is yellow and soft, and classically the necrosis is 'mid-zonal' (Fig. 11.20). Eosinophilic nuclear inclusions (Torres bodies) may be detected.

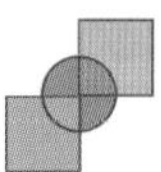

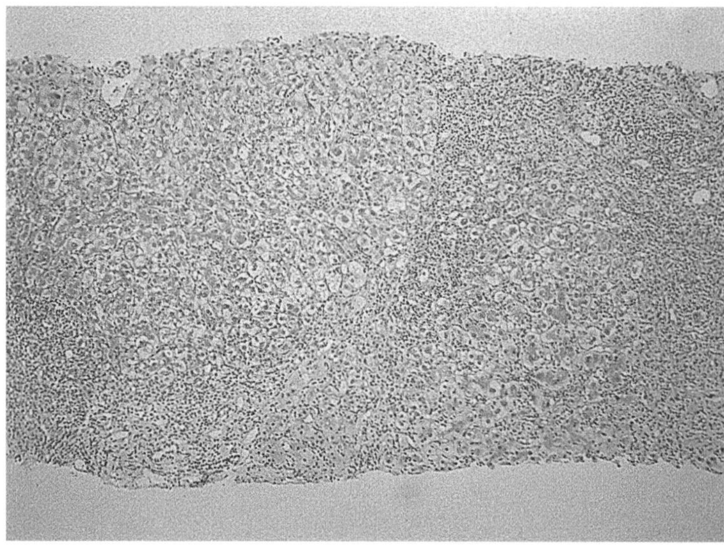

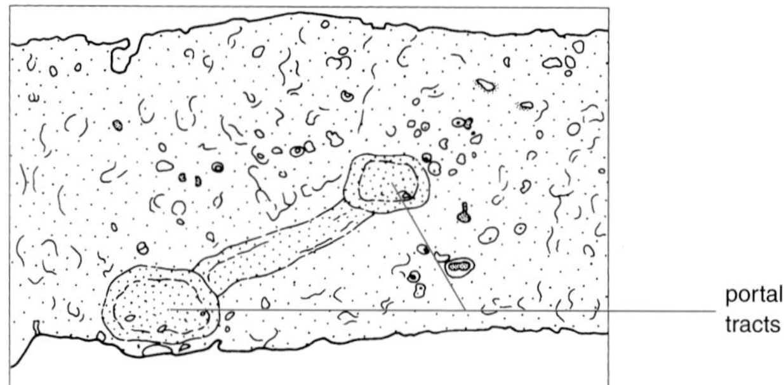

■ **Fig. 11.9** Histological appearance of subacute hepatic necrosis showing bridging necrosis between portal tracts. (H&E stain).

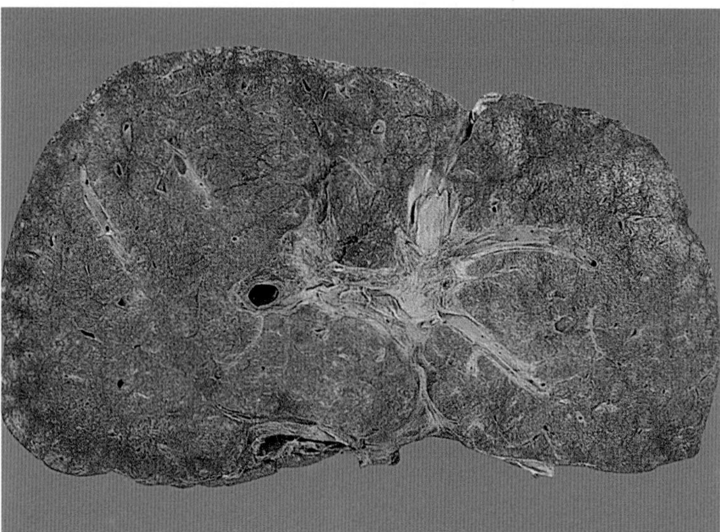

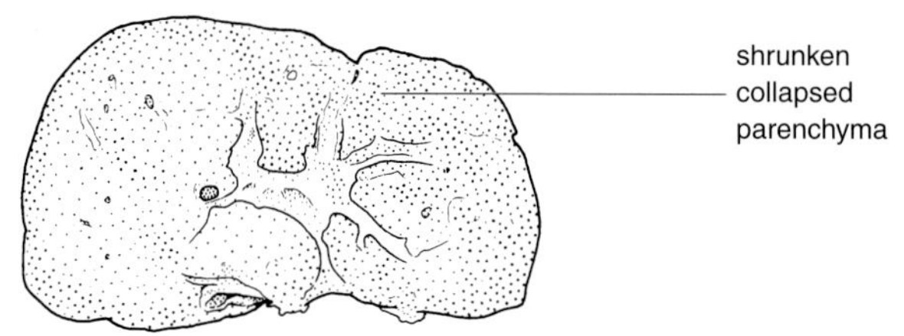

■ **Fig. 11.10** Autopsy liver from a patient who died with acute submassive viral hepatitis. Courtesy of Prof I. Talbot.

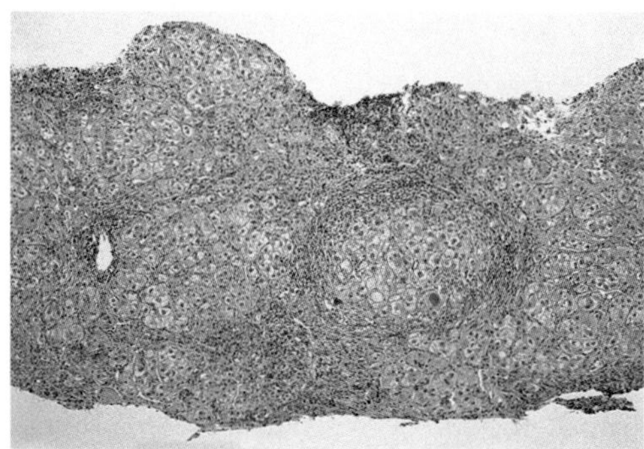

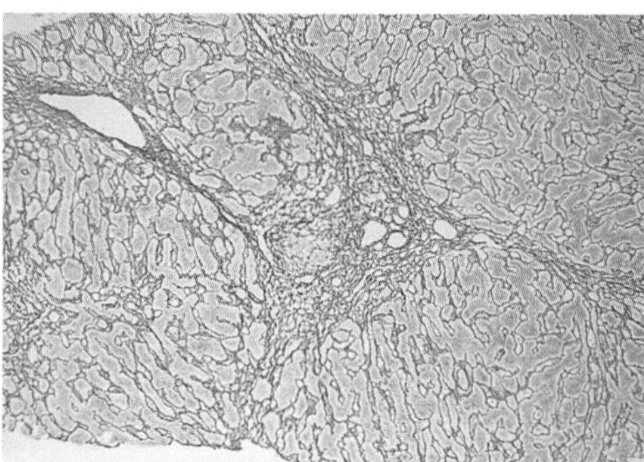

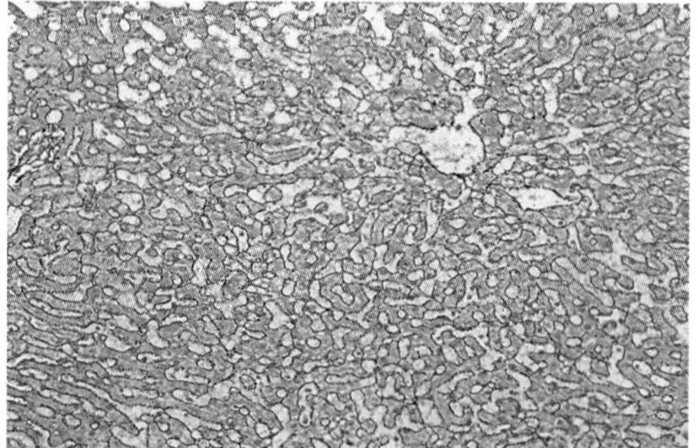

■ **Fig. 11.11** Massive hepatic necrosis. Microscopic appearance of a fatal case of drug-related massive hepatic necrosis showing pale portal–portal zones of parenchymal necrosis and stromal collapse separating foci of viable hepatocyte within residual lobules.

BACTERIAL HEPATITIS

Minor histological changes and abnormalities of liver biochemical tests occur during bacterial septicemia. In leptospirosis, particularly if it is caused by *Leptospira icterohaemorrhagica* (Weil's disease), there can be severe renal and liver damage together with cutaneous hemorrhage. Deep jaundice is a common feature, but the histological changes in the liver are usually mild and non-specific.

Tuberculosis involves the liver more often than is clinically apparent; the most characteristic feature on liver biopsy is the presence of granulomas that are typically caseating (Fig. 11.21), but small non-caseating lesions indistinguishable from sarcoid may be present. In tuberculosis such granulomas tend to be found within the lobules, but acid-fast bacilli are rarely identifiable. Brucellosis is another granulomatous condition, in which small collections of lymphocytes, plasma cells and a few histiocytes are commonly seen. The presence of granulomas within the liver biopsy is very non-specific as they are found in a wide range of conditions, including infectious diseases, drugs, and lymphoma (Fig. 11.22). Congenital

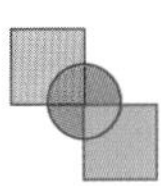

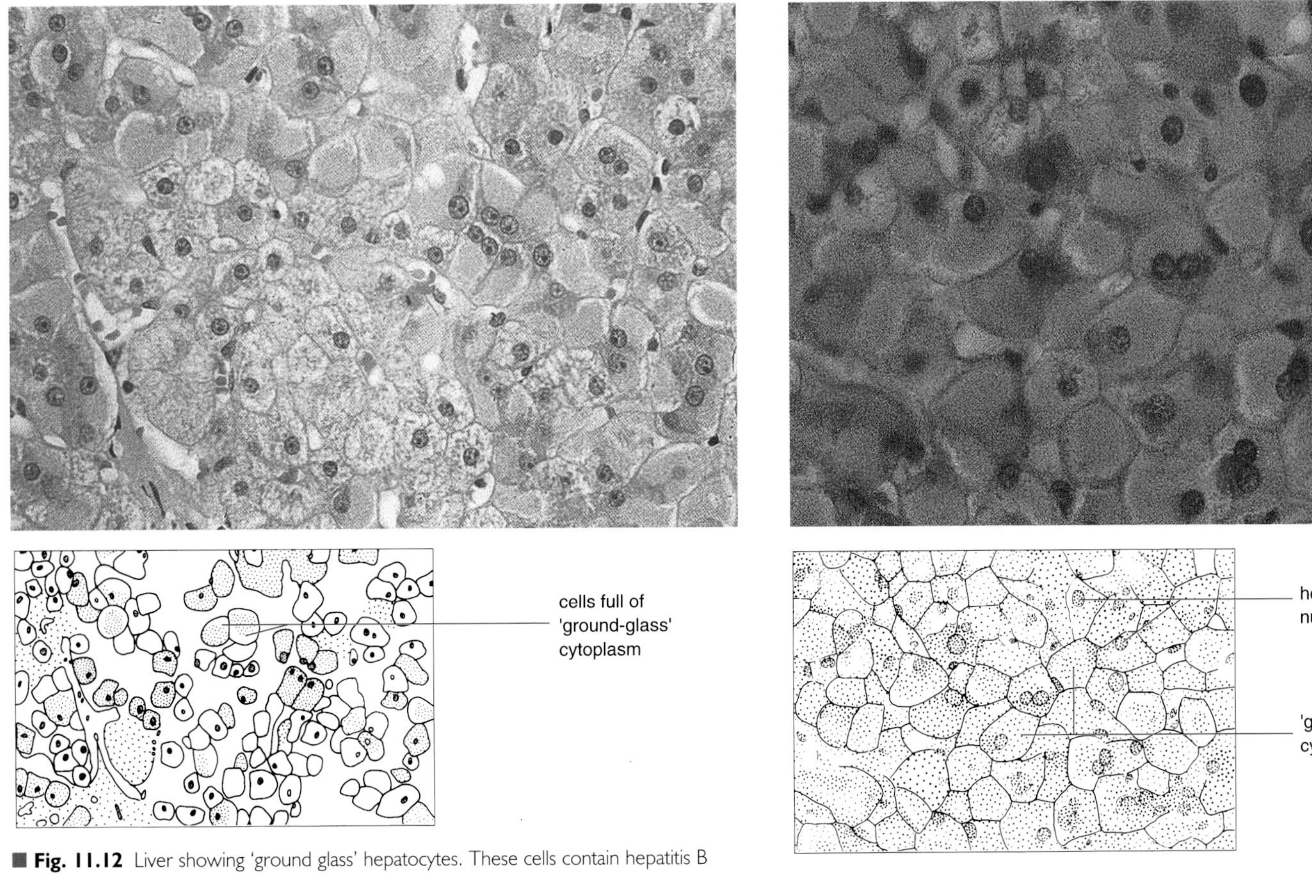

■ **Fig. 11.12** Liver showing 'ground glass' hepatocytes. These cells contain hepatitis B antigen. H&E stain.

■ **Fig. 11.13** 'Ground glass' hepatocytes. These cells are rich in hepatitis B surface antigen. H&E stain (x 460).

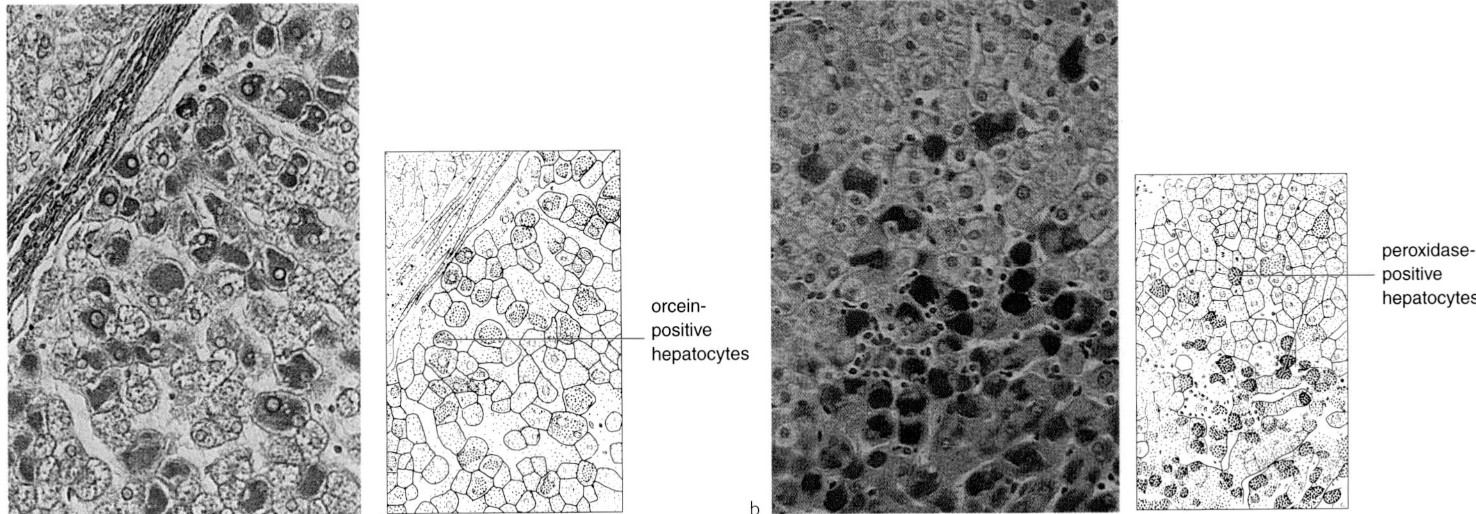

■ **Fig. 11.14** 'Ground glass' hepatocytes demonstrated using orcein ((a), courtesy of Prof I. Talbot) and immunoperoxidase ((b), courtesy of Dr D.R. Davies) with anti-hepatitis B antibody (x 240).

syphilis is characterized by the presence of spirochetes within the liver, and diffuse fibrosis (Fig. 11.23). This may even progress to a true pericellular cirrhosis. Granulomatous hepatitis is a common feature of secondary syphilis. Granulomas may also be present in the tertiary stages, but the classical lesion is the syphilitic gumma (Fig. 11.24). This is a necrotic nodule surrounded by granulation tissue that produces deep scars (hepar lobatum) as it heals, with the development of fibrosis.

OTHER INFECTIOUS HEPATITIDES AND SYSTEMIC MYCOSIS

In Q fever, liver damage may vary from small, discrete foci to extensive necrosis. A characteristic feature is the presence of lipogranulomatous-like lesions with eosinophilic material surrounding the central vacuole (Fig. 11.25). The liver is rarely primarily involved by fungal infections but can frequently suffer from hemato-

Viruses causing Acute Hepatitis	
Hepatotropic viruses	
hepatitis A (HAV)	hepatitis D (delta)
hepatitis B (HBV)	hepatitis E (enterically transmitted hepatitis)
hepatitis C (HCV)	? hepatitis F/G
Systemic viruses	
Epstein–Barr virus	Marburg virus
cytomegalovirus	rubella
varicella	flavivirus (causing yellow fever)
herpes simplex types 1/2	zoonotic arenavirus (causing Lassa fever)
paramyxoviruses	
coxsackievirus	

Table 11.1 Viruses that can cause acute hepatitis.

genous spread. A liver biopsy speci-men often aids diagnosis since it may involve the recognition of the individual fungal organism within the organ (Figs 11.26, 11.27) (see also Liver abscess below).

AIDS AND THE LIVER

Human immunodeficiency virus (HIV) infection is associated with a high prevalence of liver abnormalities. Hepatitis B and C infections are commonly found in such patients since many AIDS sufferers are hemophiliacs or drug addicts who are at high risk for infection by these hepatotropic viruses. Most liver abnormalities are due to the invasion of the organ by a variety of opportunistic organisms (Figs 11.28–11.31).

HIV cholangiopathy

Biliary tract abnormalities are sometimes seen in advanced AIDS. The common presentation is with cholestatic liver tests or with right upper quadrant pain. The two most common findings are

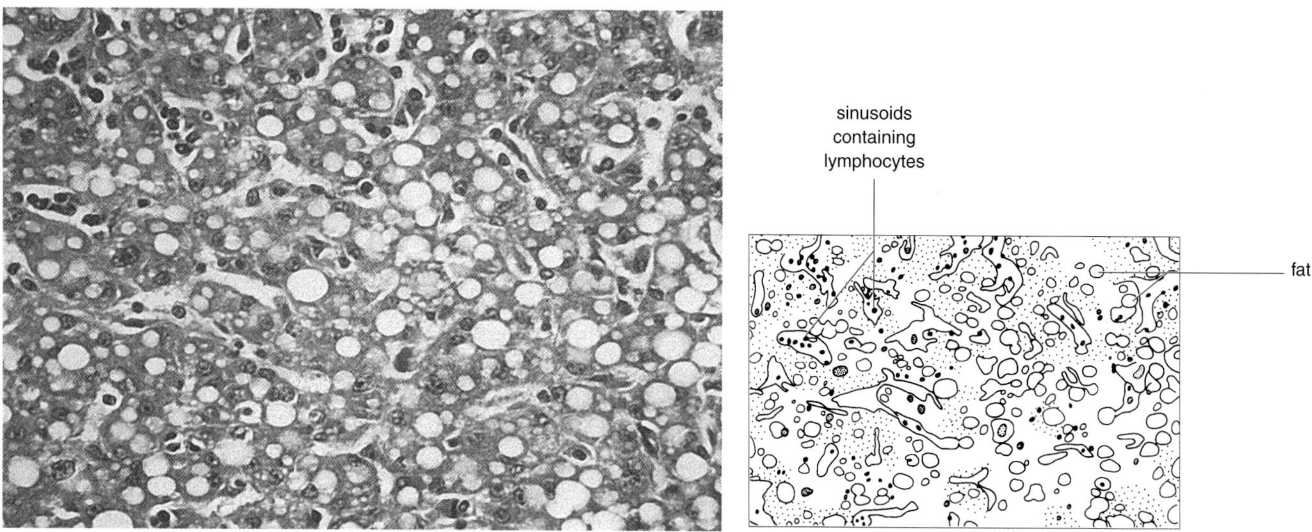

■ **Fig. 11.15** Hepatitis C infection, showing lymphocytic infiltrate of sinusoids and microvesicular fat. H&E stain. Courtesy of Prof J.C.E. Underwood.

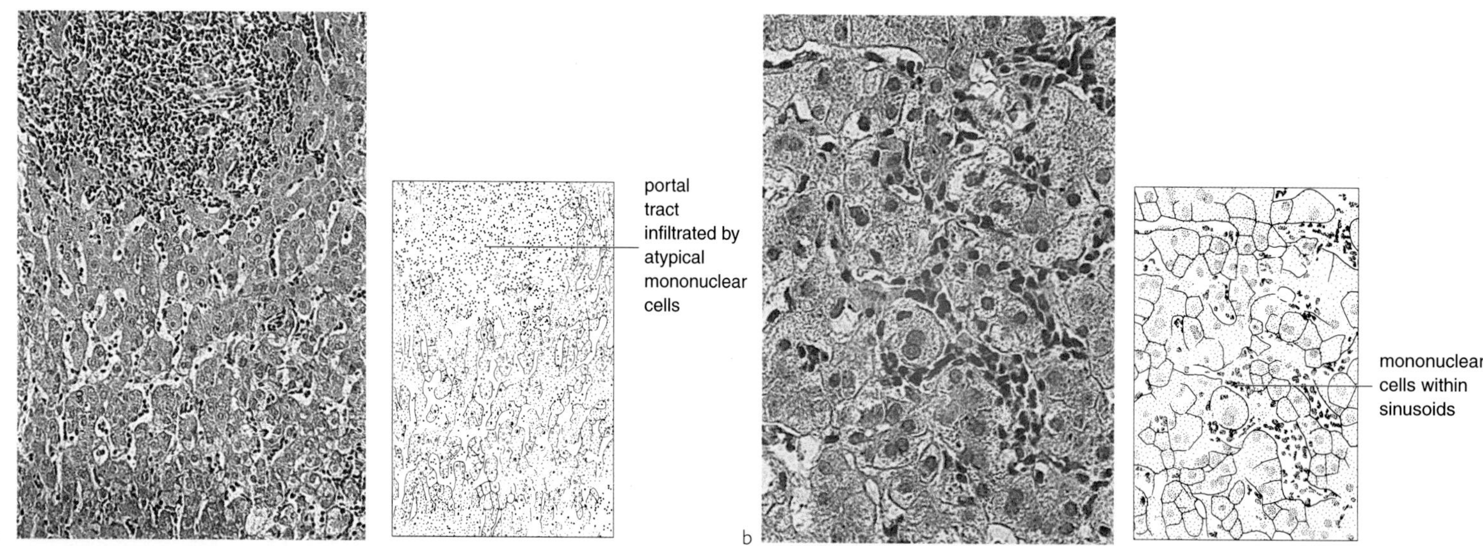

■ **Fig. 11.16** Liver histology in infectious mononucleosis showing a portal tract infiltrated by atypical mononuclear cells ((a), x 70, courtesy of Prof I. Talbot) and mononuclear cells extending into the sinusoids ((b), x 320). H&E stain.

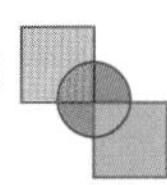

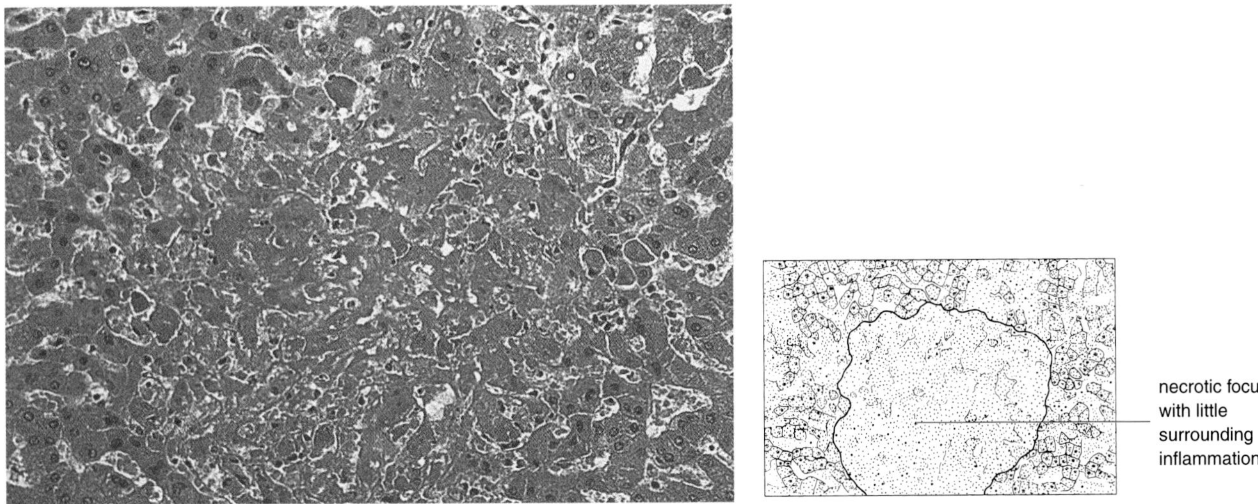

■ **Fig. 11.17** Liver histology in herpes simplex showing a necrotic focus with little surrounding inflammation. H&E stain (x 180).

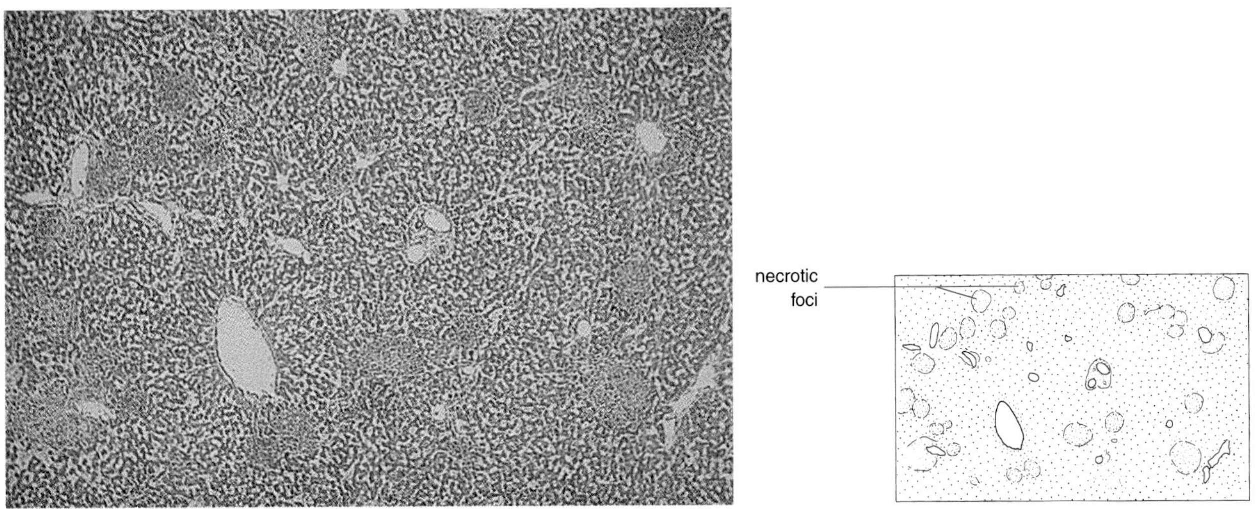

■ **Fig. 11.18** Liver histology in chicken pox showing necrotic foci. H&E stain (x 30). Courtesy of Prof I. Talbot.

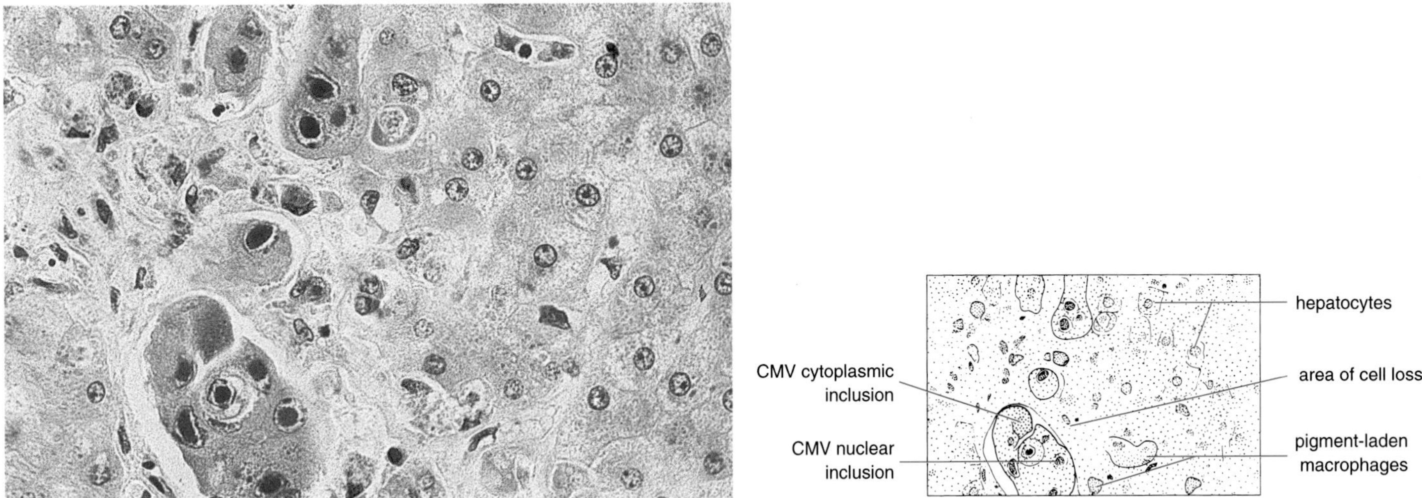

■ **Fig. 11.19** Liver histology showing cytomegalovirus inclusions. H&E stain (x 460). Courtesy of Prof B. Portmann.

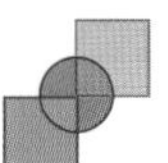

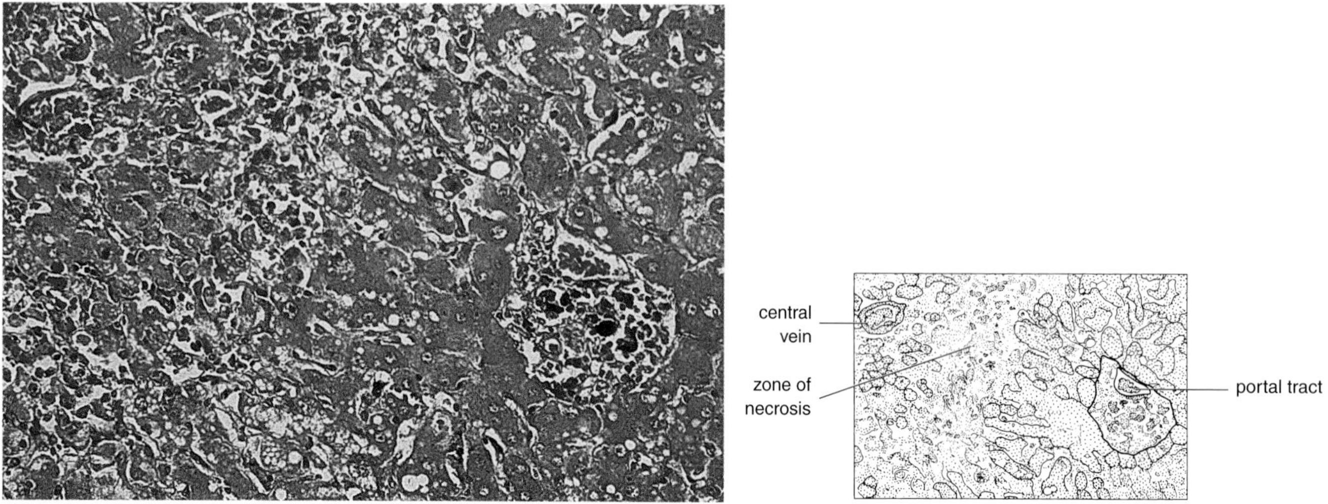

■ **Fig. 11.20** Liver histology in yellow fever showing the characteristic mid-zonal necrosis between central vein and portal tract. Masson trichrome stain (x 180).

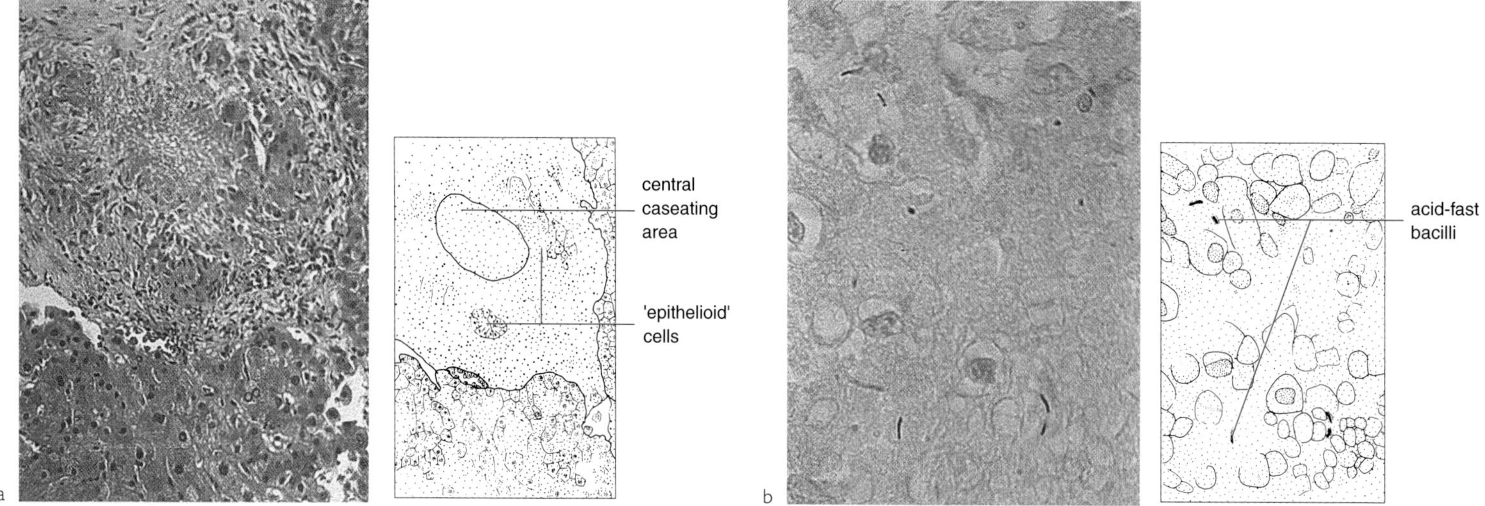

■ **Fig. 11.21** Liver histology in tuberculosis showing a caseating granuloma ((a), H&E stain, x 125), and acid-fast bacilli ((b), Ziehl–Neelsen stain, x 800, courtesy of Prof I. Talbot).

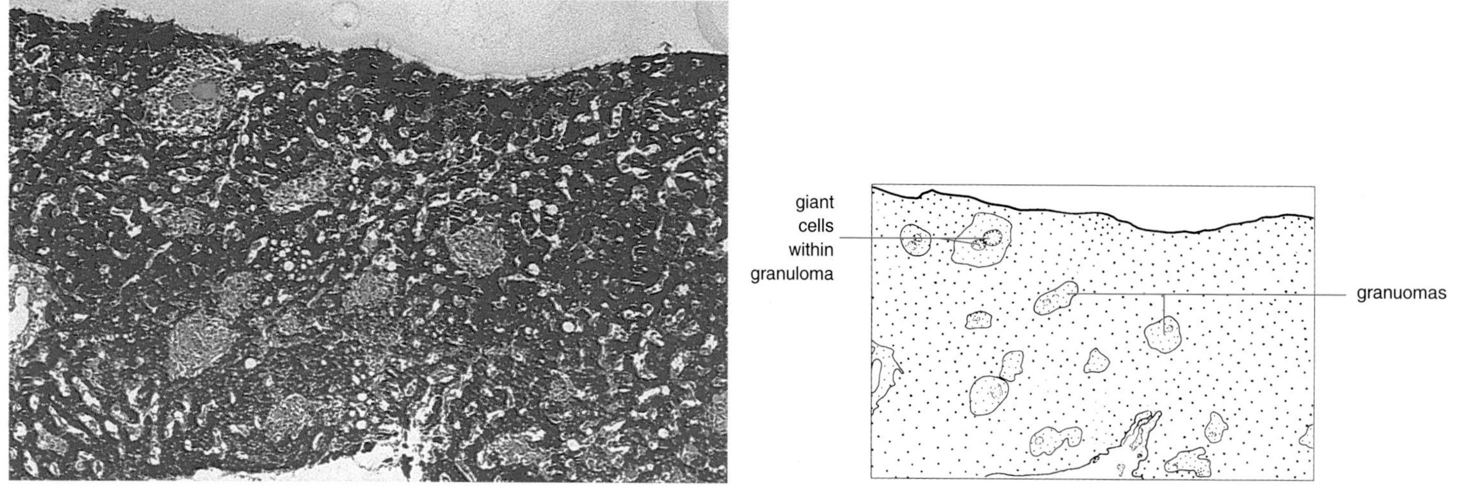

■ **Fig. 11.22** Granulomatous hepatitis found during the investigation of a pyrexia. PAS stain (x 180).

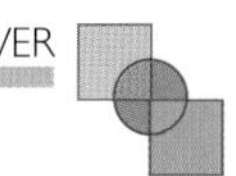

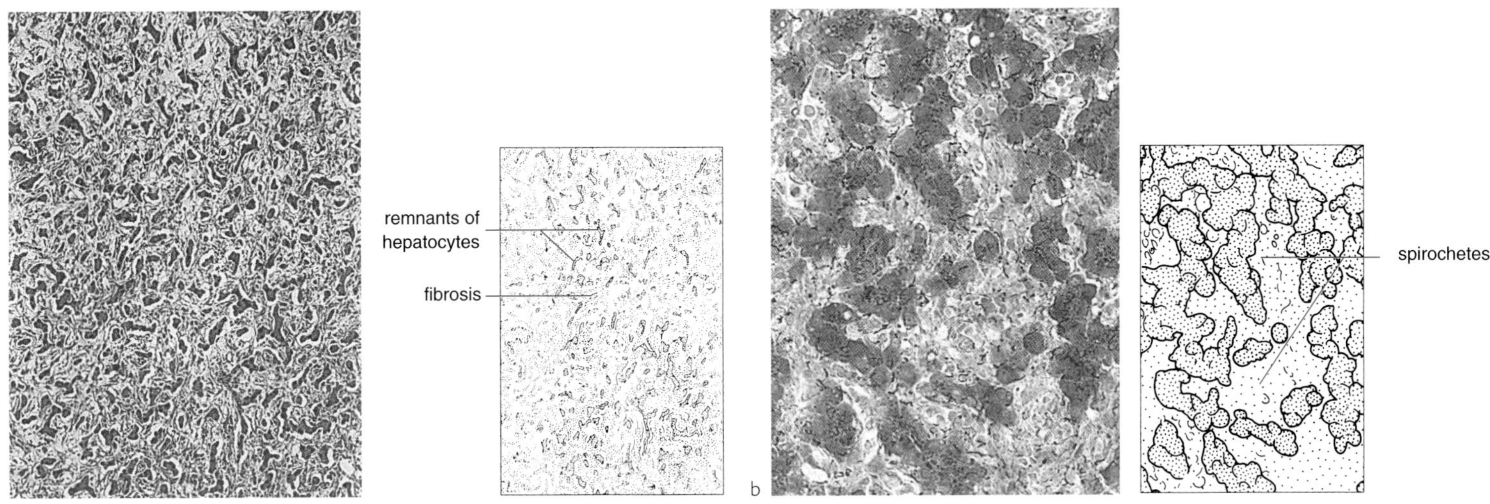

■ **Fig. 11.23** Liver histology in congenital syphilis showing diffuse pericellular fibrosis ((a), H&E stain, x 160), and spirochetes ((b), Levaditi stain, x 600). Courtesy of Prof I. Talbot.

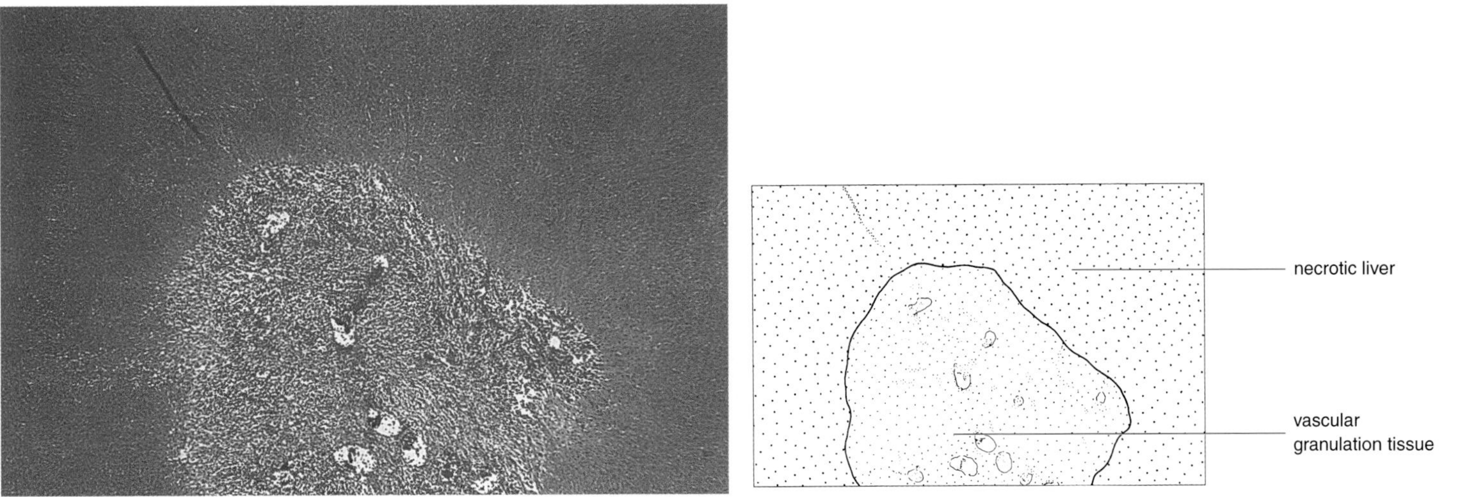

■ **Fig. 11.24** Liver histology in tertiary syphilis showing a gumma. H&E stain (x 70). Courtesy of Prof I. Talbot.

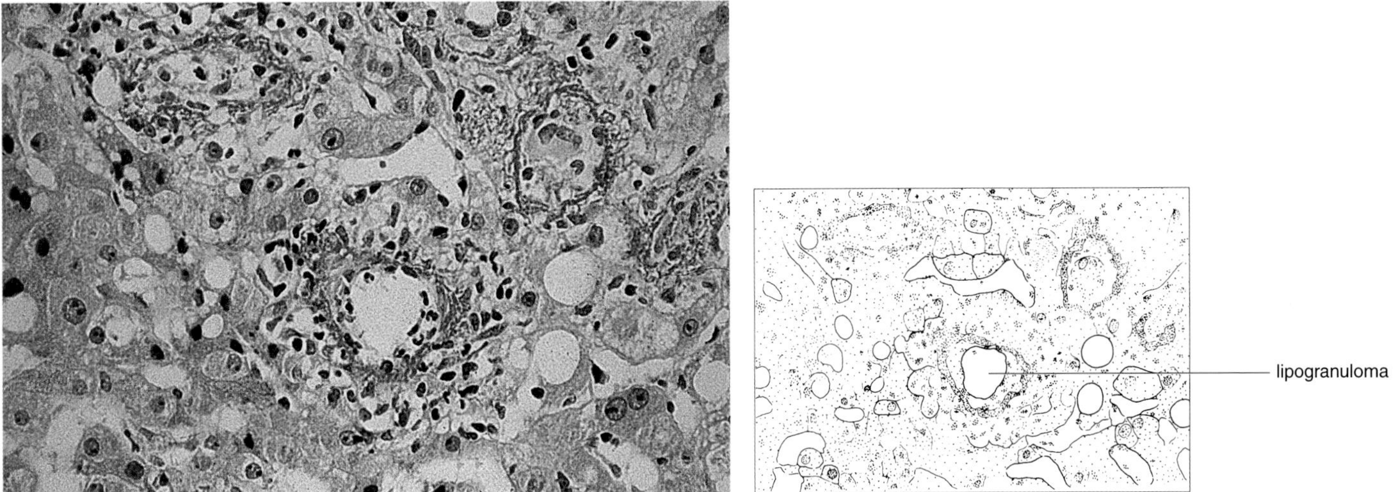

■ **Fig. 11.25** Liver histology in Q fever showing the characteristic lipogranulomatous-like lesion: a granuloma with a central vacuole and a red 'fibrinoid' rim. Martius scarlet blue stain (x 460). Courtesy of Prof P. Scheuer

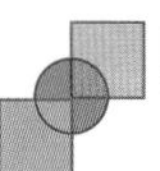

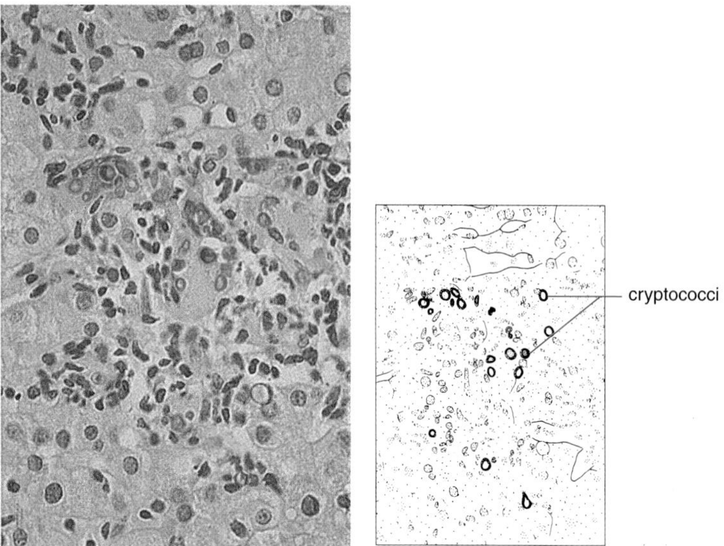

■ **Fig. 11.26** Liver histology showing cryptococci staining blue with alcian blue stain (x 320).

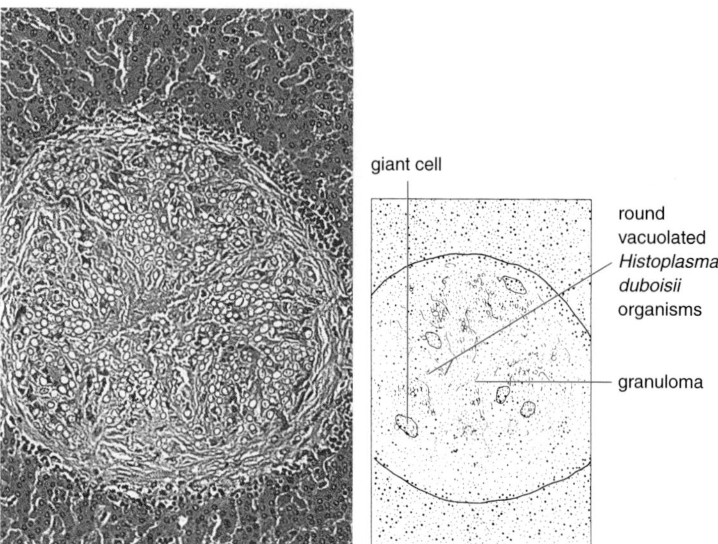

■ **Fig. 11.27** A hepatic granuloma in histoplasmosis. H&E stain (x 125).

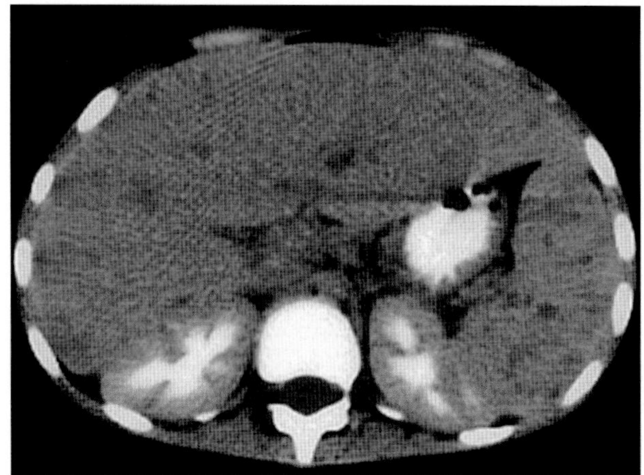

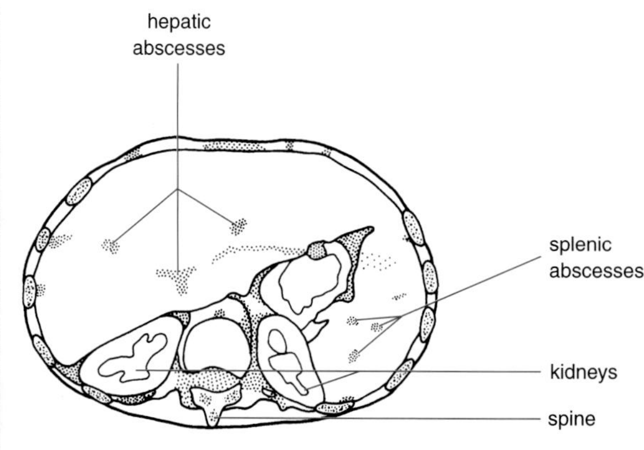

■ **Fig. 11.28** CT scan showing multiple hepatic fungal abscesses in a patient with AIDS. Note also the multiple abscesses in the spleen. Courtesy of Dr R.A. Nakielny.

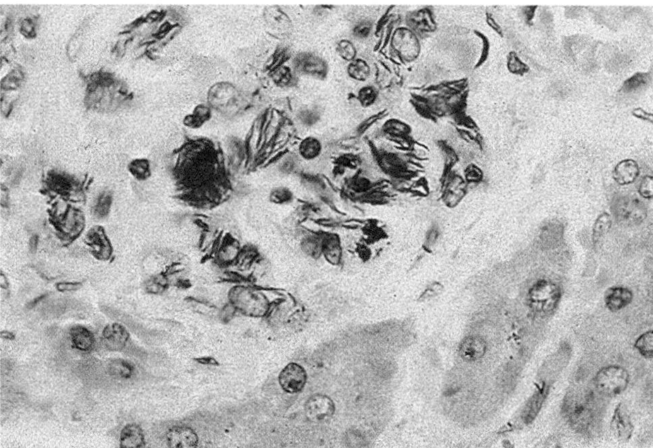

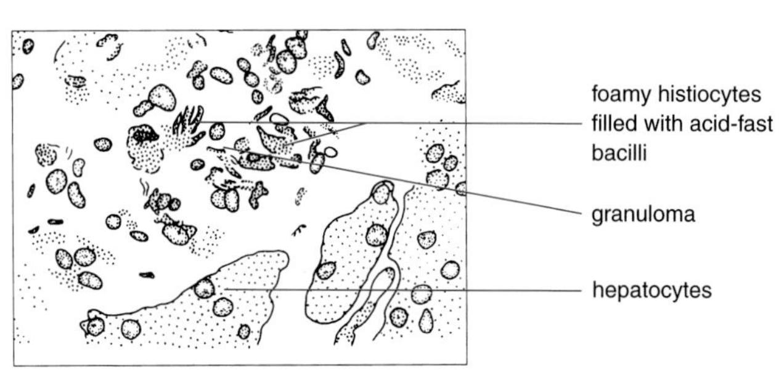

■ **Fig. 11.29** Liver biopsy showing foamy histiocytes in a hepatic granuloma filled with *Mycobacterium avium-intracellulare*. Kinyoun's stain.

dilated bile ducts, presumably from papillary stenoses (Fig. 11.32), or a sclerosing cholangitis-like picture with irregularity of bile ducts (Fig. 11.33). However unlike PSC, even in those with a sclerosing cholangitis-like picture, the ducts are marginally dilated.

ALCOHOLIC HEPATITIS

Acute alcohol abuse produces two distinct histological patterns in the liver. Fatty infiltration or steatosis is a universal response to alcoholic binges, when fat globules accumulate in parenchymal cells due to impaired metabolism of triglycerides by the hepatocytes. In severe cases, this leads to extensive involvement of the entire lobule (Figs 11.34, 11.35). Steatosis is predominantly centrilobular and mid-zonal (Fig. 11.36). Large cytoplasmic vacuoles may also distort the cell and compress the sinusoids (Fig. 11.37); these appear empty on many stains but their fatty nature is apparent from fat staining (Fig. 11.38). This appearance is distinct from the microvesicular fatty changes of the fatty liver of pregnancy

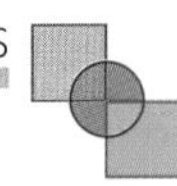

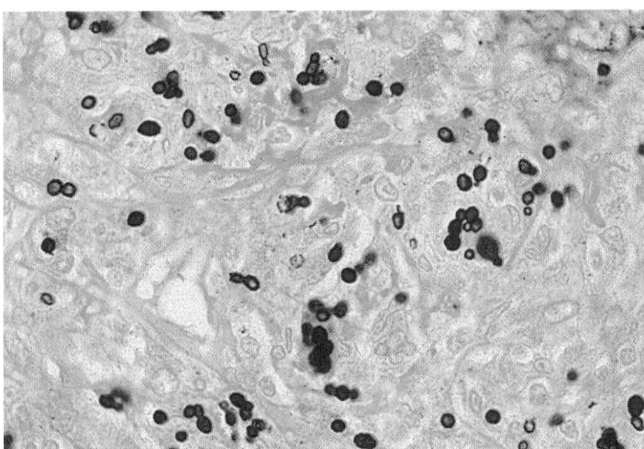

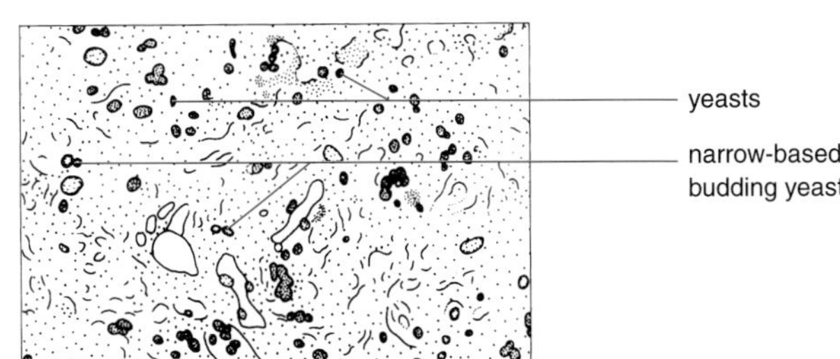

■ **Fig. 11.30** Liver biopsy of a patient with AIDS showing infiltration with yeasts. Grocott's methanamine silver stain.

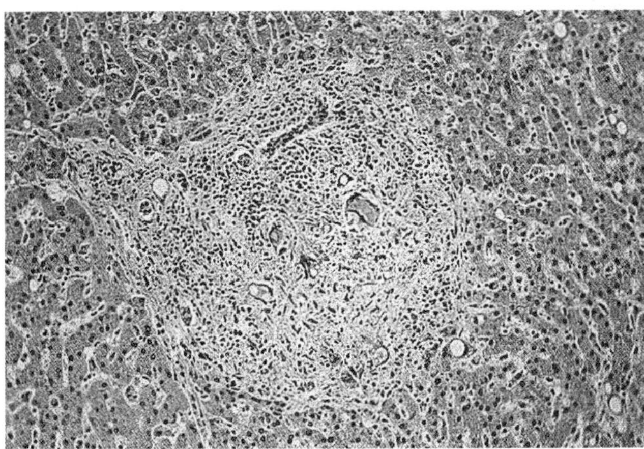

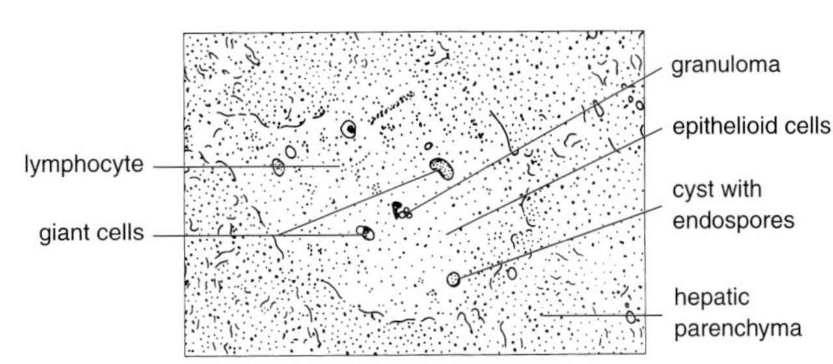

■ **Fig. 11.31** Granulomatous infiltration of the liver due to coccidioidomycosis showing numerous cysts, some containing distinguishable endospores.

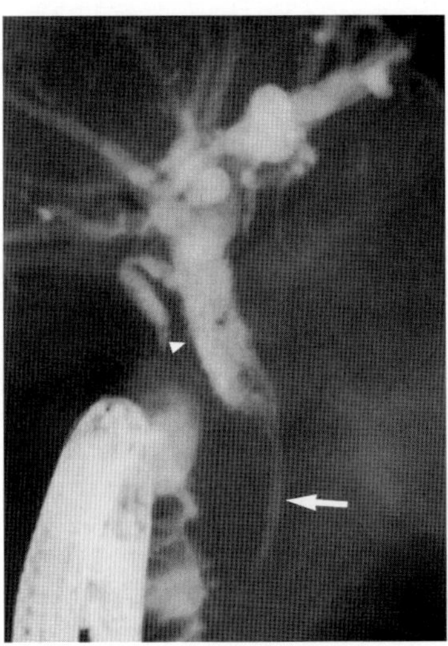

■ **Fig. 11.32** Endoscopic retrograde cholangiogram demonstrating AIDS-related cholangitis. A long tapered stricture (arrow) is seen in the common bile duct. The contour of the common hepatic duct (arrowhead) is irregular. Debris fills the lumen of the common hepatic duct.

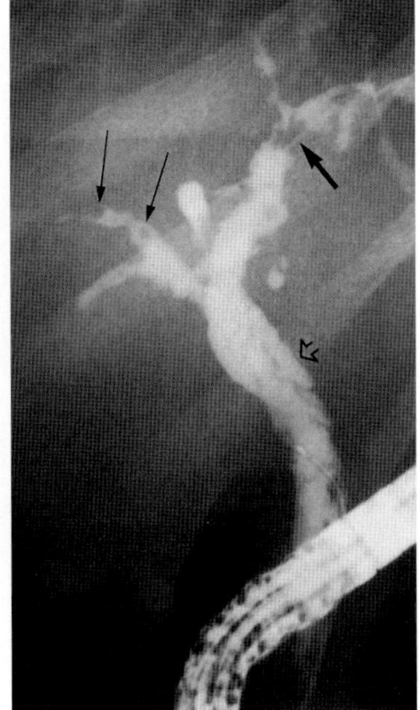

■ **Fig. 11.33** Endoscopic retrograde cholangiogram demonstrating AIDS-related cholangitis. The contour of the intrahepatic biliary tree is irregular. A focal stricture is seen in branches to the left lobe (thick arrow). Small calculi are present in a duct to the right lobe (thin arrows). Strands of mucus are seen in the common hepatic duct (open arrow).

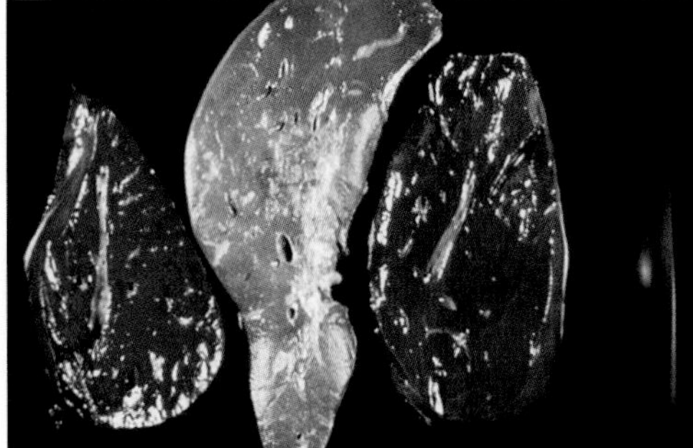

■ **Fig. 11.34** Liver: steatosis (middle), hemochromatosis, and normal. The typical yellow macroscopic appearance of steatotic liver (middle) contrasted with the brown liver of hemochromatosis (left) and red-pink normal liver (right) to show the marked difference in color.

(Fig. 11.39). In addition to fatty infiltration, in some individuals alcoholic steatotic hepatitis develops in which there is focal necrosis of liver cells with clusters of neutrophils and Mallory's hyaline (Figs 11.40, 11.41). Mallory's hyaline is a clumped inclusion of eosinophilic material within a swollen hepatocyte. It is not exclusive to alcoholic liver disease, occurring in many other conditions, such as primary biliary cirrhosis and Wilson's disease, but its presence in association with fat and neutrophil infiltration is virtually diagnostic of alcohol abuse. Clinically, alcoholic hepatitis may resemble acute viral hepatitis, with jaundice, fever, tender hepatomegaly and elevated serum transaminases, but the two lesions are histologically entirely different.

Continued or recurrent alcoholic hepatitis eventually leads to fibrosis and cirrhosis. The fibrosis may be pericellular around centrilobular hepatocytes (Fig. 11.42) or present as stellate extensions

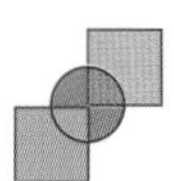

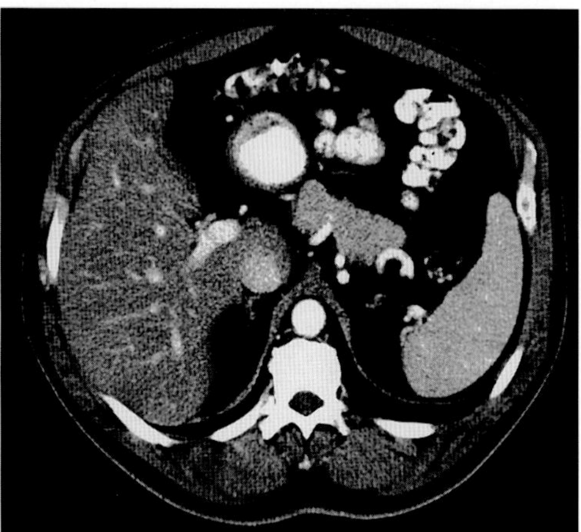

Fig. 11.35 CT demonstrating steatosis of the liver. Hepatic parenchyma is usually of slightly less attenuation (less than 25 Hounsfield units) than the spleen on scans obtained during the portal venous phase. In this patient, the hepatic parenchyma is of much lower attenuation (60 Hounsfield units 'darker') than the spleen. Given differences in attenuation depending on the amount of contrast/blood flow to liver or spleen, however, it is better to assess for steatosis on a non-contrast CT scan, where liver parenchyma should be 10 Hounsfield units or less than splenic parenchyma.

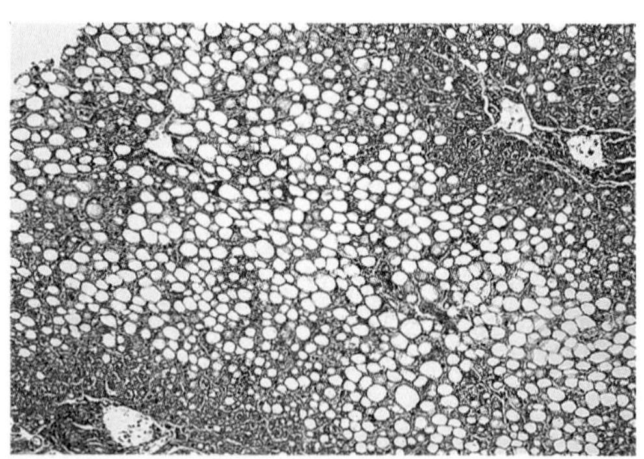

Fig. 11.36 Macrovesicular steatosis. Microscopic appearance of alcohol-induced macrovesicular fatty change in a trichrome-stained section that accentuates the location of portal tracts (blue-stained collagenous stroma) and shows the predominantly centrilobular to midzonal distribution of the steatosis.

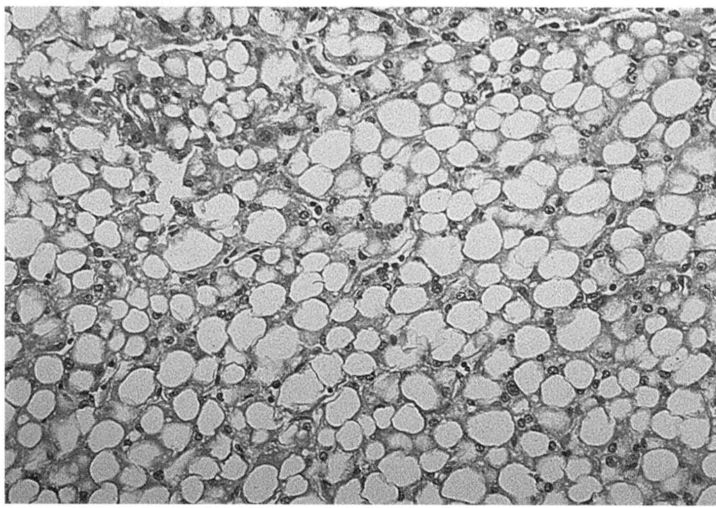

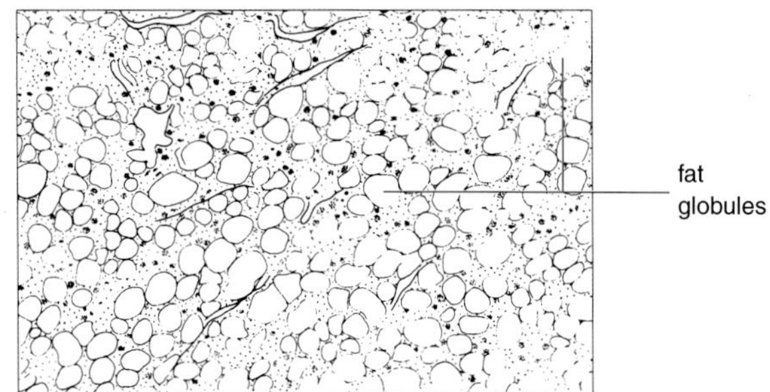

Fig. 11.37 Macrovesicular steatosis. Microscopic appearance of macrovesicular fatty change showing the characteristic single large cytoplasmic vacuoles of fat that distort the hepatocytes, displacing their nuclei to the cell periphery, and compress sinusoidal spaces. H&E stain (x 180). Courtesy of Prof I. Talbot.

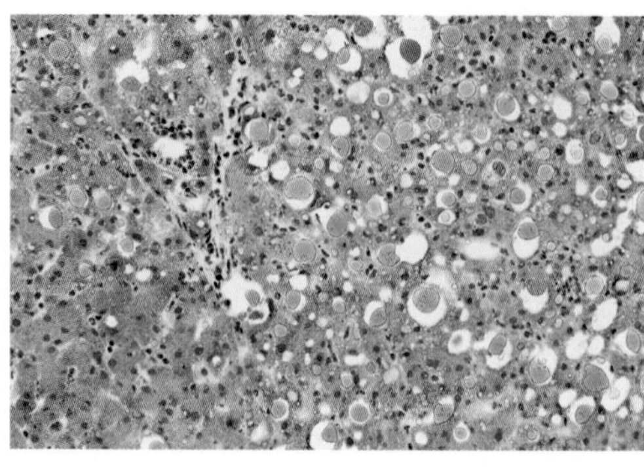

Fig. 11.38 Macrovesicular steatosis. An oil red O stain of a frozen section of fatty liver showing the orange-red staining of the neutral lipid within the cytoplasmic vacuoles, which, on permanent sections appear clear due to dissolution of the fat by organic solvents during specimen processing.

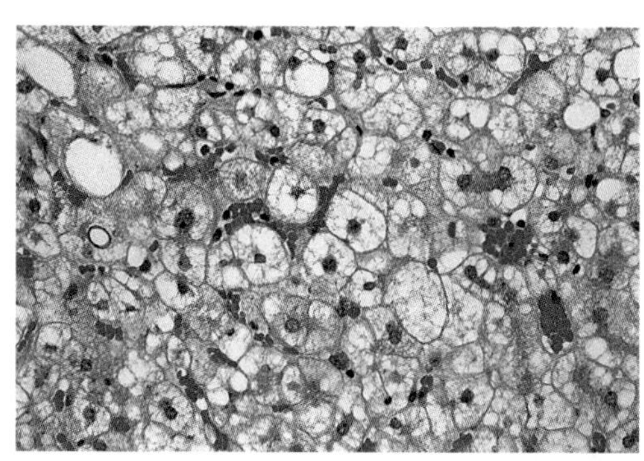

Fig. 11.39 Microvesicular steatosis. Microscopic view of microvesicular fatty change on fatty liver of pregnancy illustrating the myriad small vacuoles of cytoplasmic lipid that indent and scallop the hepatocyte nuclei in contrast to the appearance of macrovesicular fat.

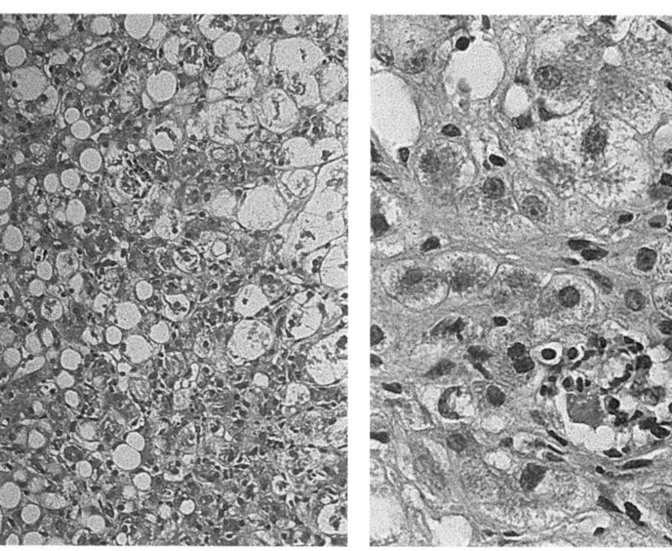

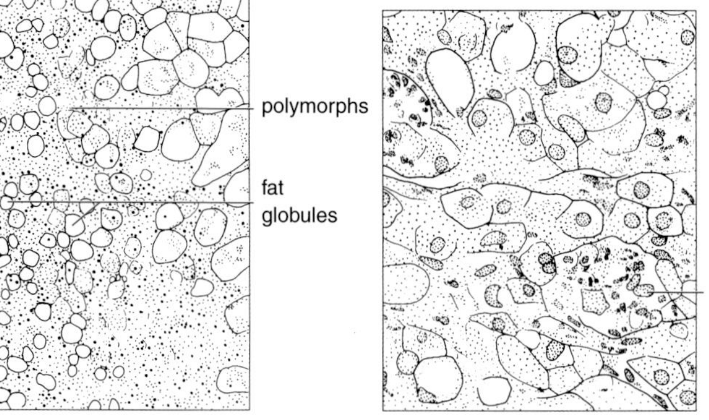

Fig. 11.40 Steatotic hepatitis. Microscopic appearance of steatosis hepatitis caused by alcohol showing the four characteristic features: macrovesicular fatty change, ballooning of hepatocytes, neutrophilic inflammatory infiltrates, and Mallory's hyaline in injured hepatocytes. Classic 'string of pearls' rimming of the nucleus by Mallory's hyaline droplets is seen in the ballooned hepatocyte in the center of the field (x100 (left, x320 (right)).

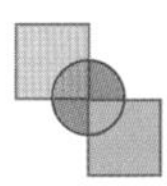

from portal tracts (Fig. 11.43). Another characteristic is 'central sclerosing hyaline necrosis' in which the fibrosis surrounds central veins and radiates around hepatocytes (Fig. 11.44). Pericentral vein fibrosis, in which the fibrosis is initially limited to a rim surrounding the central vein (Fig. 11.45), is another well-recognized histological pattern. All these lesions ultimately progress to alcoholic cirrhosis, which is typically micronodular and discussed in Chapter 12. Alcoholic liver disease is often complicated by the accumulation of iron, leading to hemosiderosis (Fig. 11.46).

DRUG-INDUCED HEPATITIS

The list of drugs and toxins that can damage the liver is almost endless, and it is now recognized that their effects may mimic almost any form of acute or chronic histological pattern. A selection of the recognized hepatic injuries associated with drugs is shown in Table 11.2. There are relatively few poisons that have a predictable dose-related effect on the liver (Table 11.3), and the majority produce unpredictable non-dose-related idiosyncratic effects. In predictable liver injury, zonal necrosis is usual, and this is the typical lesion seen in the liver following paracetamol/acetaminofen overdose (Fig. 11.47). Such reactions are usually acute and self-limiting, resulting either in death following massive necrosis, or full recovery.

The most common types of idiosyncratic liver injury are both clinically and histologically identical to acute viral hepatitis. Halothane hepatitis, following repeated exposure to this anesthetic agent, is now rare but remains an examplar of drug-related hepatitis (Fig. 11.48). Cholestasis is also commonly encountered,

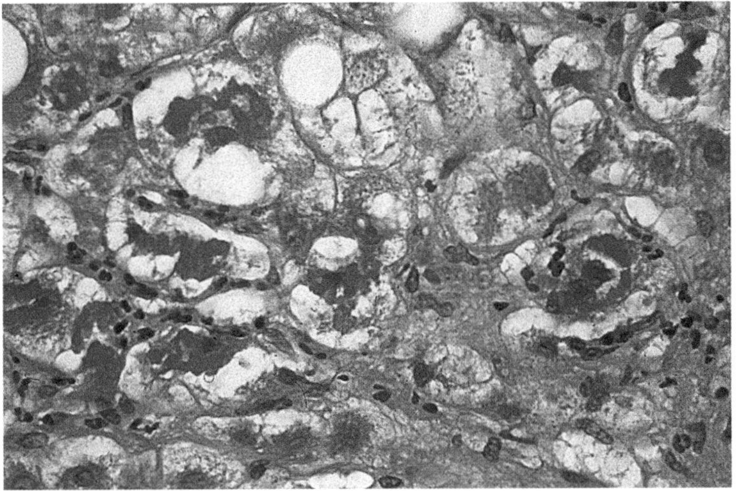

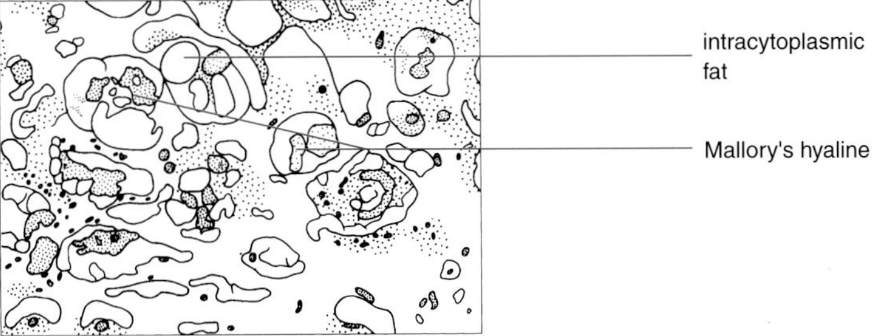

■ **Fig. 11.41** Steatotic hepatitis. High-magnification microscopic appearance of Mallory's hyaline in steatotic hepatitis showing the deeply eosinophilic condensations of intermediate filaments (cytokeratins) that occur in injured, ballooned hepatocytes. H&E stain. Courtesy of Prof J.C.E. Underwood.

Histological Spectrum of Drug-Induced Liver Damage	
Histology	**Drug**
fatty liver	tetracycline/sodium valproate
granulomas	phenytoin/sulphonamides
acute hepatitis	halothane/monoamine oxidase inhibitors
cholestasis	chlorpromazine/oral contraceptives
phospholipidosis	amiodarone
alcoholic hepatitis	perhexilene maleate
peliosis	corticosteroids
Budd–Chiari	senecio alkaloids/azathioprine/mercaptopurine
chronic active hepatitis	methyldopa
noncirrhotic portal hypertension	arsenicals
adenoma	oral contraceptives
hepatocellular carcinoma	anabolic steroids
angiosarcoma	vinyl chloride

Table 11.2 Histological spectrum of drug-induced liver damage.

Predictable Hepatotoxins
paracetamol
carbon tetrachloride
benzene/phenol derivatives
yellow phosphorus
amanitin (from mushrooms)

Table 11.3 Dose-related hepatotoxins.

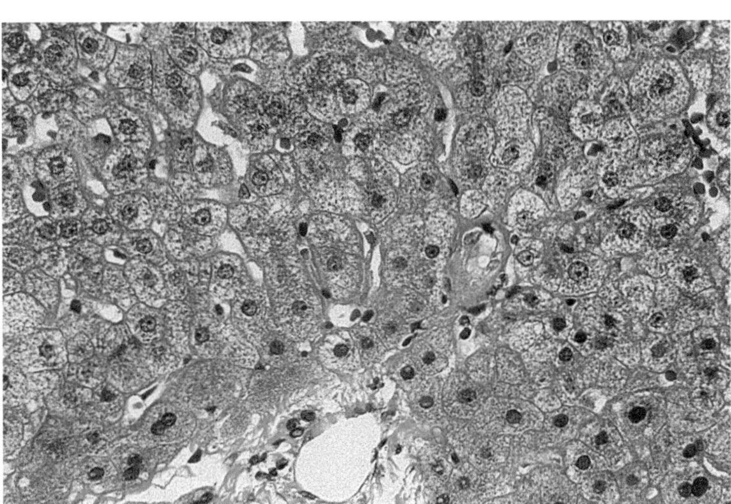

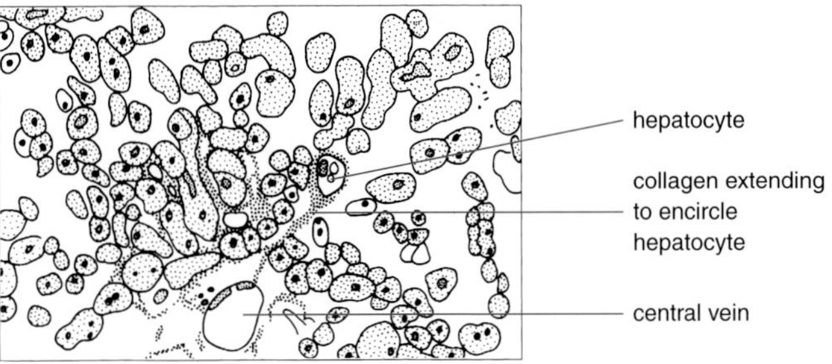

■ **Fig. 11.42** Liver histology showing pericellular fibrosis secondary to chronic alcohol abuse. Collagen stains green. Masson trichrome stain. Courtesy of Prof J.C.E. Underwood.

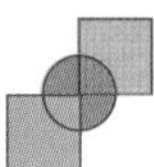

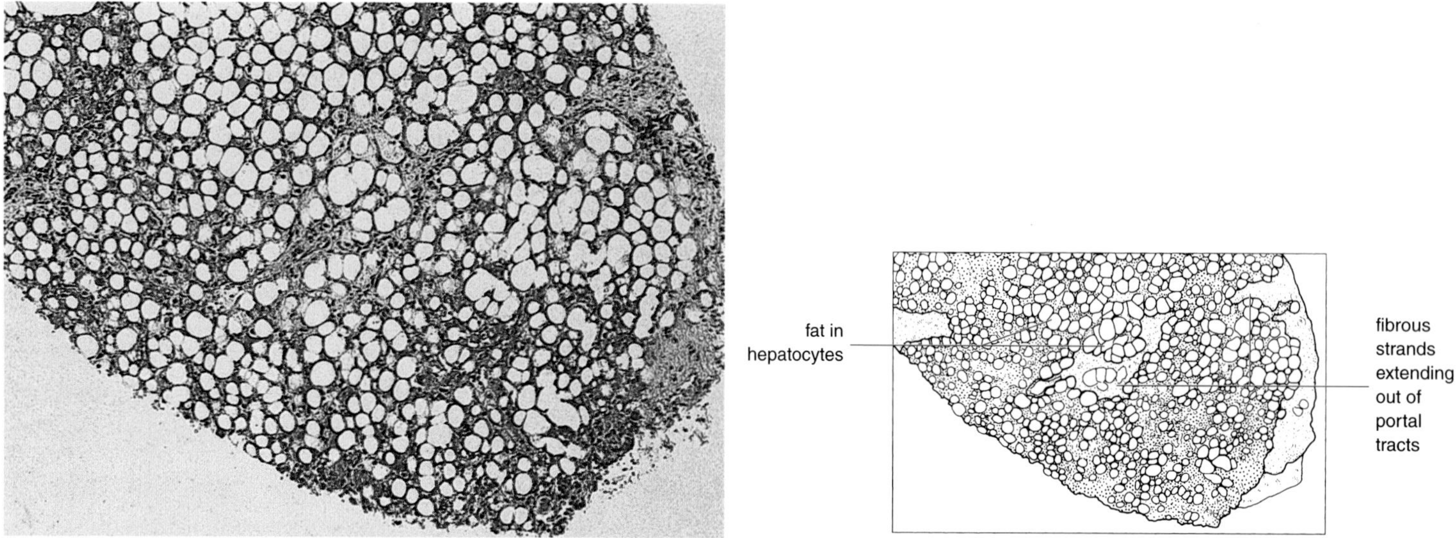

■ **Fig. 11.43** Liver histology showing early fibrosis with extensions from portal tracts and severe fatty change. Masson trichrome stain (x 180). Courtesy of Prof I. Talbot.

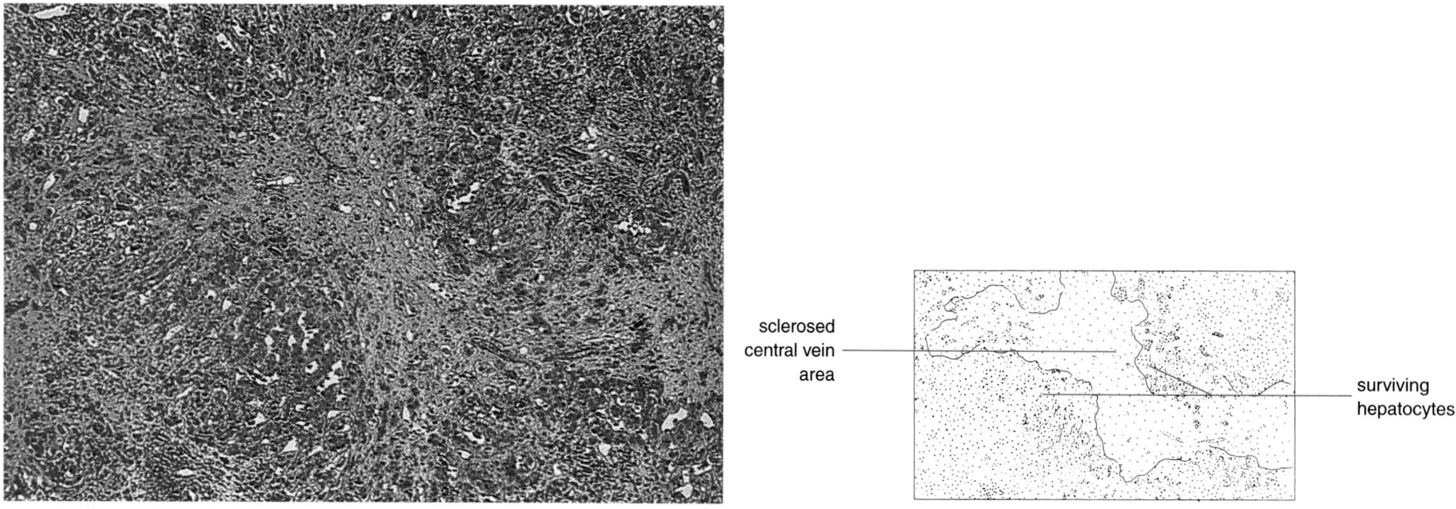

■ **Fig. 11.44** Liver histology in alcoholic central sclerosis showing hyaline necrosis. H&E stain (x 120). Courtesy of Prof I. Talbot.

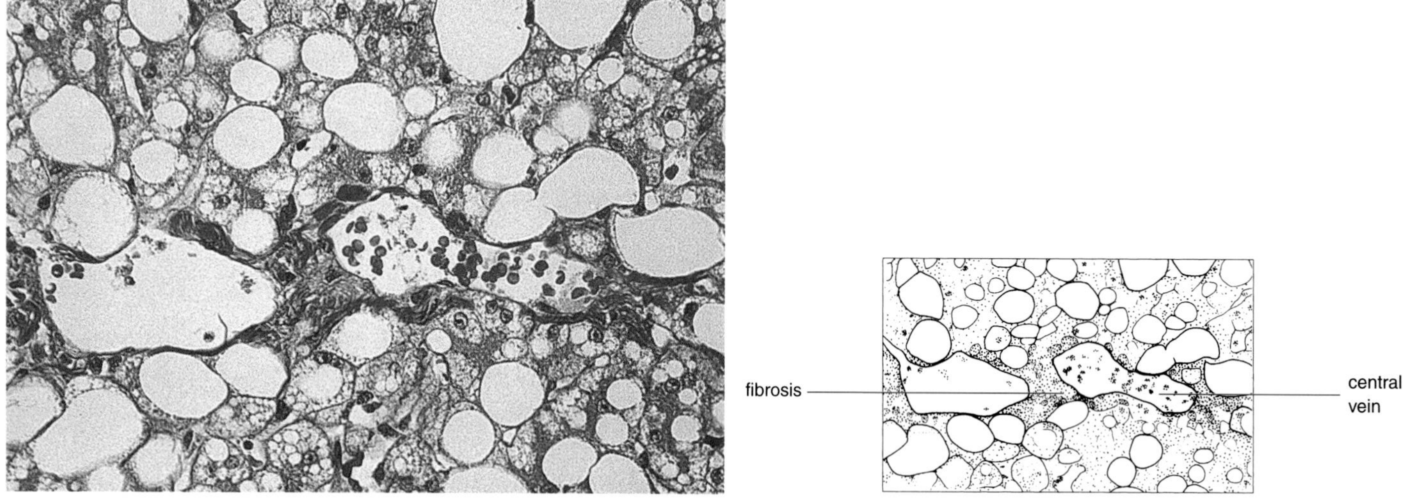

■ **Fig. 11.45** Liver histology in an alcoholic showing central vein fibrosis. Masson trichrome stain (x 180). Courtesy of Prof P. Scheuer.

where the typical lesion is that of bile stasis which must be distinguished from bile duct obstruction. The presence of eosinophils in the liver biopsy suggests a drug etiology, but this is by no means diagnostic (Fig. 11.49). The chronic sequelae of long-term drug prescriptions are often much more serious, since severe irreversible liver damage may have developed by the time any signs or symptoms are apparent. The now rarely used antihypertensive, methyldopa, may induce a chronic aggressive hepatitis accompanied by high-titer autoantibodies, thereby mimicking lupoid hepatitis. Oral contraceptive administration may result in cholestasis after an

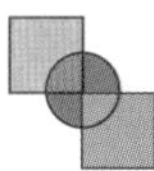

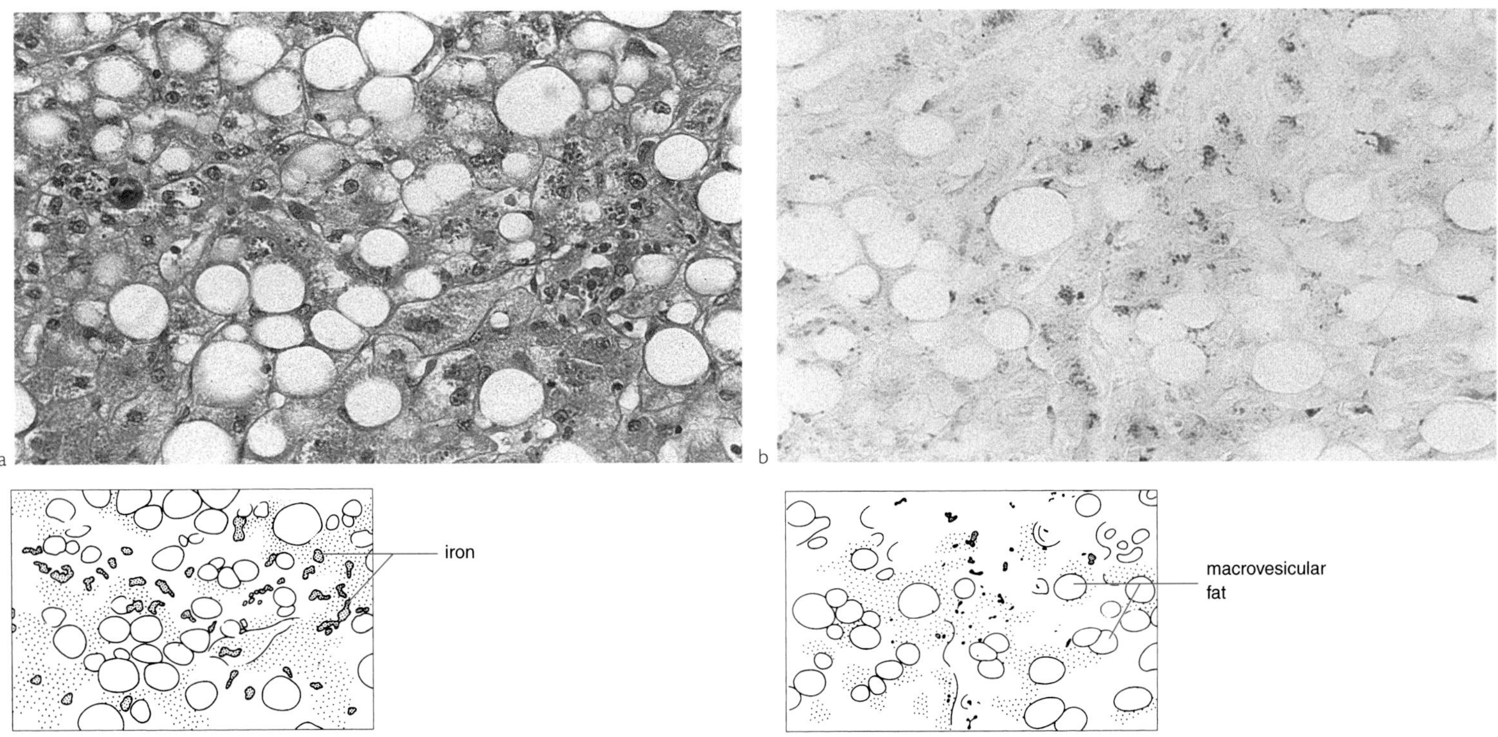

■ **Fig. 11.46** Alcoholic fatty liver with iron overload. H&E stain shows fat and iron (a). The iron is stained specifically using Perls' stain (b). Courtesy of Prof J.C.E. Underwood.

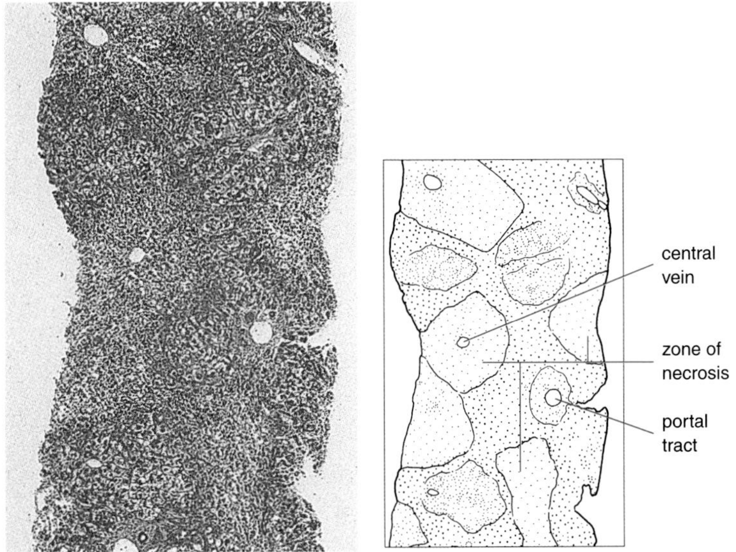

■ **Fig. 11.47** Liver histology showing centrilobular necrosis following paracetamol overdose. H&E stain (x 80). Courtesy of Prof I. Talbot.

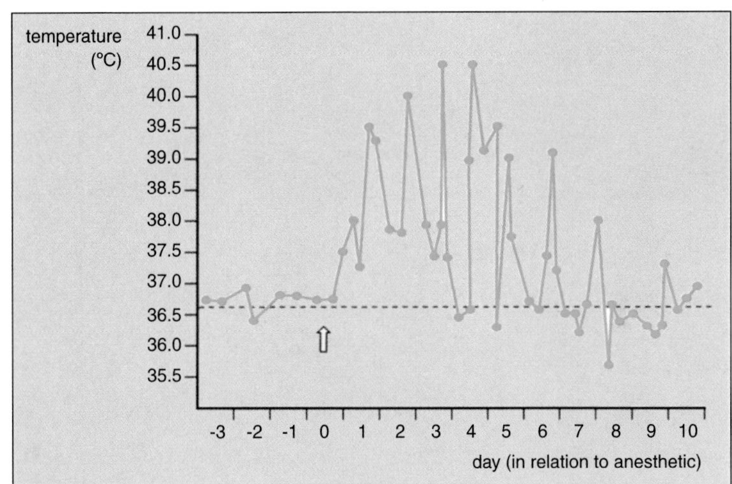

■ **Fig. 11.48** Temperature chart of a 38-year-old woman with a fractured femur receiving halothane for the second time in 3 weeks. No infective cause was found for the post-operative fever and rigors, which were accompanied by the development of typical hepatitic features. Fever is a characteristic of many drug-related hepatitides.

interval of a few months, while regular use over several years can lead to hepatic adenomas (Figs 11.50, 11.51). Hepatocellular carcinoma rarely complicates oral contraceptive use but is more commonly found as a consequence of anabolic steroid use (Fig. 11.52).

In many cases, the mechanism whereby liver damage is induced is poorly understood, but it frequently depends upon characteristics of the individual's rate and type of hepatic metabolism. Two particular drug-related effects on the liver involve benoxaprofen (Fig. 11.53) and thorotrast (Fig. 11.54). Benoxaprofen, a non-steroidal anti-inflammatory drug, was withdrawn because of severe cholestasis which resulted from bile duct accumulation of its insoluble glucuronide metabolite. Thorotrast, used widely during the 1940s as an intravenous contrast material, was selectively taken up by the hepatic and splenic reticuloendothelial system, where thorium proved to be carcinogenic by virtue of its alpha ray emission and extremely long half life (see Fig. 11.54 and Chapter 9).

NEONATAL HEPATITIS

Jaundice within the first 2 weeks of life may be caused by a hepatitis of viral or unknown etiology and characterized by the presence of giant cells (Figs 11.55, 11.56). These cells are grossly enlarged and may contain up to 30 nuclei. The liver architecture is often distorted, with connective tissue septae extending irregularly into the

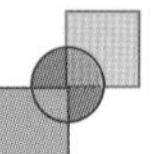

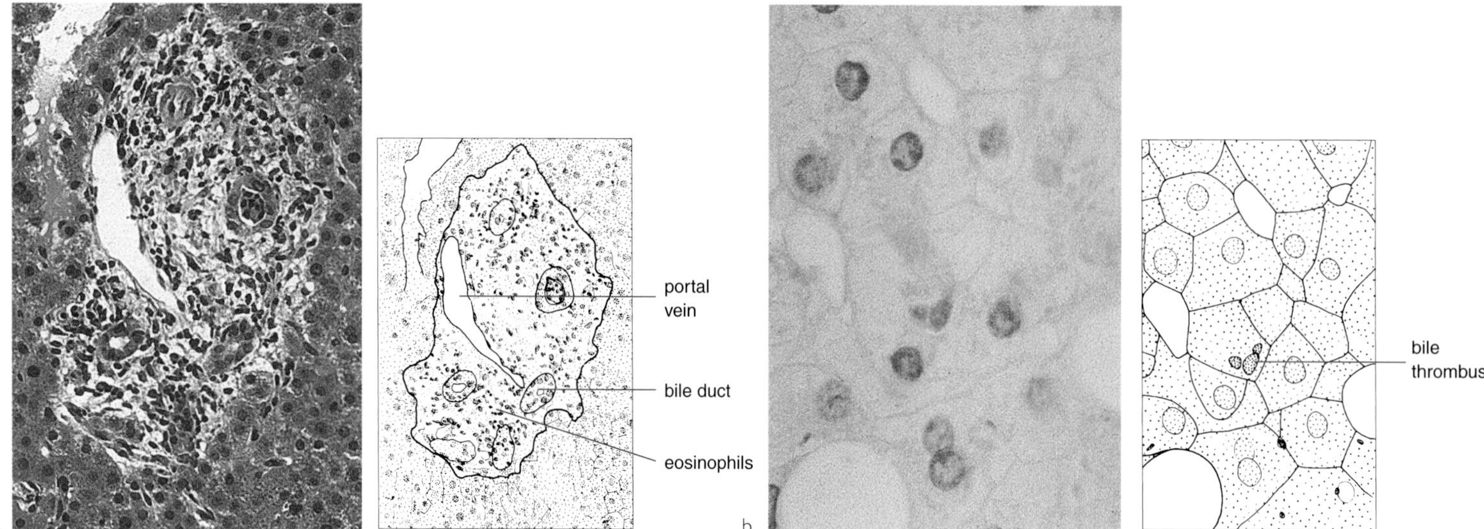

Fig. 11.49 Histology in chlorpromazine jaundice showing eosinophils infiltrating the portal tract ((a), H&E stain, x 350) and cholestasis without any liver damage or inflammation ((b), hematoxylin & van Gieson stain, x 400). Courtesy of Prof I. Talbot.

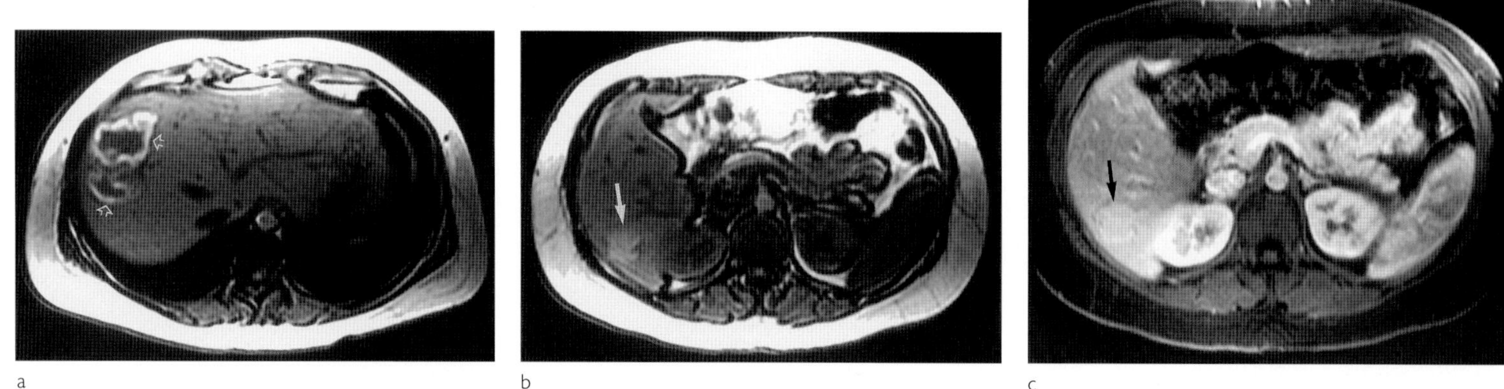

Fig. 11.50 Sub-acute bleed in a hepatic adenoma in 24-year-old woman on oral contraceptives. (a) Out of phase T_1-weighted MR image demonstrates a lobulated ring of high signal surrounding a heterogeneous lobulated mass (arrows) spanning the anterior segment of the right lobe and the medial segment of the left lobe of the liver. The rim of high signal is hemosiderin. The true size of the adenoma underlying the area of hemorrhage is difficult to determine. (b) Out of phase T_1-weighted MR image through the tip of the liver shows a lobulated mass (arrow) of increased signal in the posterior segment of the right lobe. (c) T_1-weighted image during after intravenous injection of Omniscan (gadodiamide, Nycomed, Princeton, NJ) demonstrates enhancement of the mass (arrow) in the tip of the liver. This second lesion also proved to be an adenoma. Courtesy of Drew Torigian, M.D., Philadelphia.

parenchyma. Multinucleate giant cells can also be seen in hepatitis in older children and young adults, as well as in neonates, and it is likely that giant cell transformation is a non-specific response by a young liver to a variety of stimuli.

CHRONIC HEPATITIS

Chronic hepatitis is arbitrarily defined as any acute inflammatory process of the liver persisting for more than 6 months. The etiology of chronic hepatitis is varied and includes alcoholic liver disease, primary biliary cirrhosis, drug-induced liver damage, Wilson's disease, α_1-antitrypsin deficiency, sclerosing cholangitis, and hemochromatosis. Autoimmune chronic active hepatitis (otherwise known as lupoid hepatitis) is a disorder which characteristically occurs in women and is associated with hyperglobulinemia, numerous systemic disorders, the presence of serum autoantibodies (antinuclear antibody and/or anti-smooth muscle antibody) and responsiveness to immuno-suppressive therapy.

The most common occurrence of chronic hepatitis is as a sequel to acute viral hepatitis, particularly hepatitis B or C. Figure 11.57 illustrates the possible different outcomes of acute viral hepatitis. About 5% of patients with acute HBV infection develop chronic hepatitis, but the figure is nearer 30% for acute HCV. Subclinical anicteric hepatitis is more likely to lead to chronic disease than are classical acute icteric cases. HBV is a worldwide problem, but marked geographical variations in its prevalence are found (Fig. 11.58). HCV is particularly common in Japan and the Mediterranean countries, as well as in Egypt where, sadly, a bilharzial eradication program with non-sterile injections led to many HCV infections.

The main histological forms of chronic hepatitis are chronic persistent hepatitis (CPH) and chronic aggressive hepatitis (CAH). These can only be distinguished by histological means, and the importance of this distinction relates to prognosis. CPH is usually a benign, non-progressive or self-limiting condition, in contrast to CAH, which has a high rate of progression to cirrhosis. The term chronic aggressive hepatitis is a histopathological description and is to be preferred to chronic active hepatitis, or active chronic hepatitis, in order to avoid confusion with lupoid hepatitis or chronic hepatitis or other non-viral etiologies. Generally accepted scoring systems for the classification of viral hepatitis have now been agreed (Table 11.4).

CPH is characterized by an inflammatory infiltrate, which is confined to the portal tract (Fig. 11.59). The infiltrate consists mainly of mononuclear cells and some plasma cells. Short fibrous septae

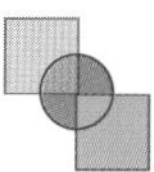

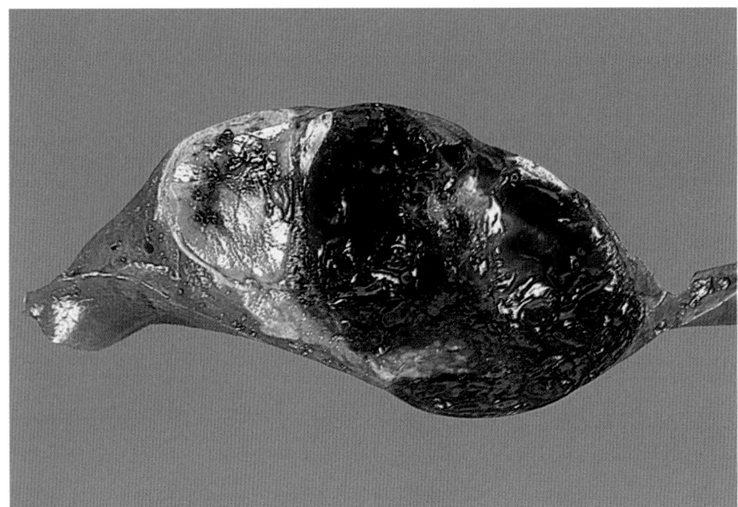

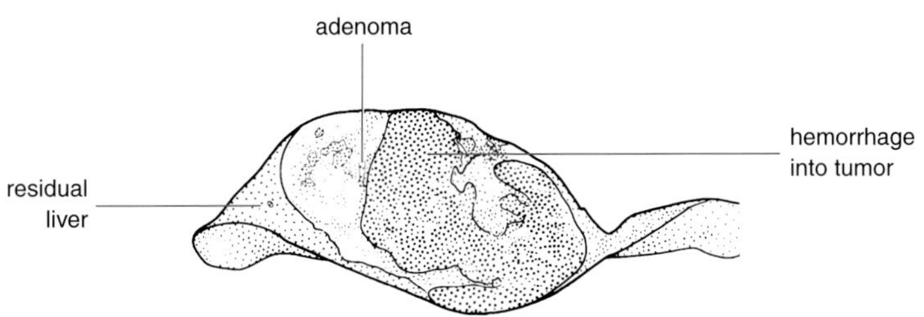

■ **Fig. 11.51** A hepatic adenoma from a patient taking an oral contraceptive. Courtesy of Prof B. Portmann.

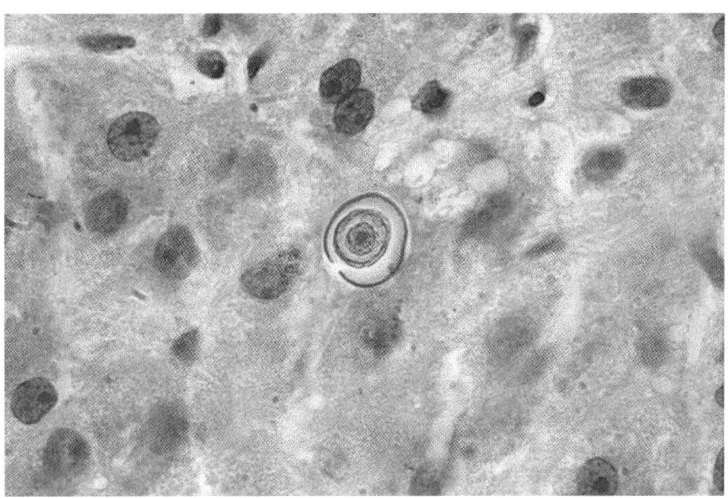

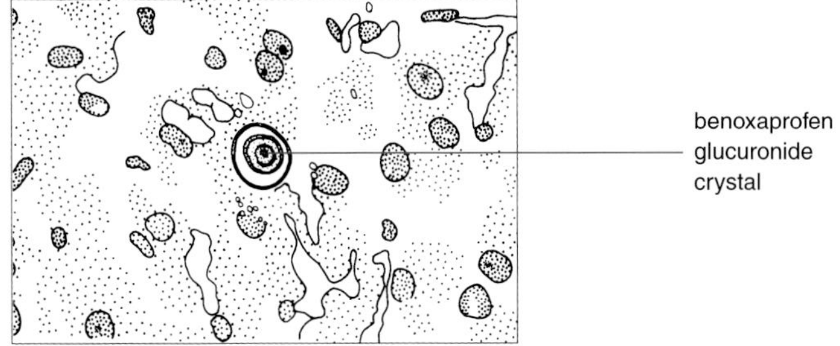

■ **Fig. 11.53** Liver biopsy of a 60-year-old man with cholestatic jaundice who had been prescribed benoxaprofen for 6 months for rheumatoid arthritis. The jaundice was caused by the presence of insoluble crystals of benoxaprofen glucuronide between hepatocytes. H&E stain.

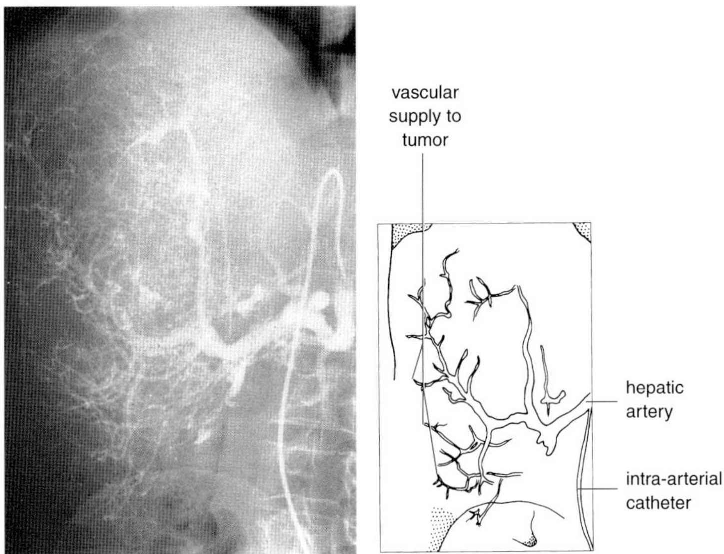

■ **Fig. 11.52** Hepatic arteriogram of a 29-year-old man showing a huge vascular mass due to hepatocellular carcinoma. The patient had been receiving the anabolic steroid oxymethalone for 5 years as treatment for aplastic anemia.

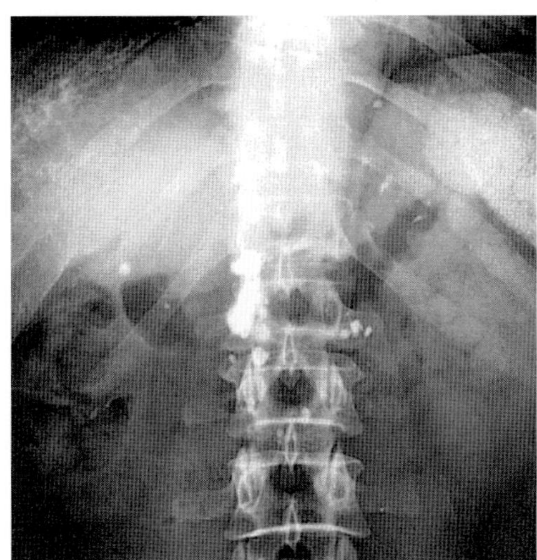

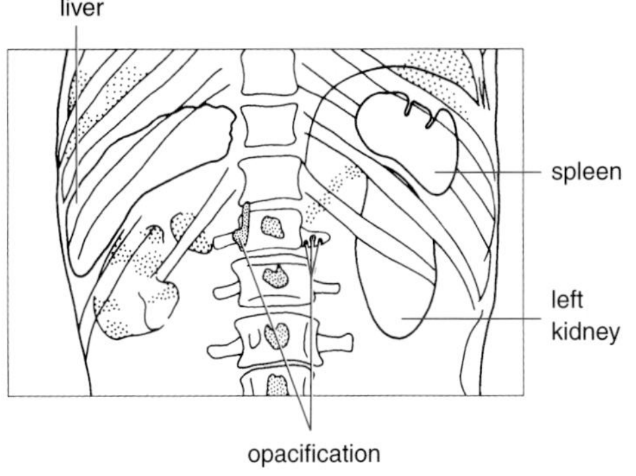

■ **Fig. 11.54** Plain abdominal X-ray showing the deposition of contrast material in the liver and spleen 30 years after the injection of thorotrast for carotid angiography. Note the opacification in the upper abdominal lymph nodes.

may extend outwards, but the hepatic lobule remains intact apart from minor non-specific inflammatory changes.

In CAH the changes are not confined to the portal tract, and the inflammatory cells spill out across the limiting plate into the adjacent parenchyma (Fig. 11.60). Local hepatocytes become surrounded and destroyed, leading to piecemeal necrosis or interface hepatitis. Subsequently, bridging occurs, with fibrous septae that link adjacent portal tracts as well as central veins to portal tracts (Fig. 11.61). This ultimately may progress to cirrhosis.

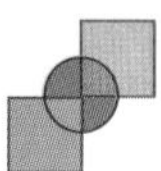

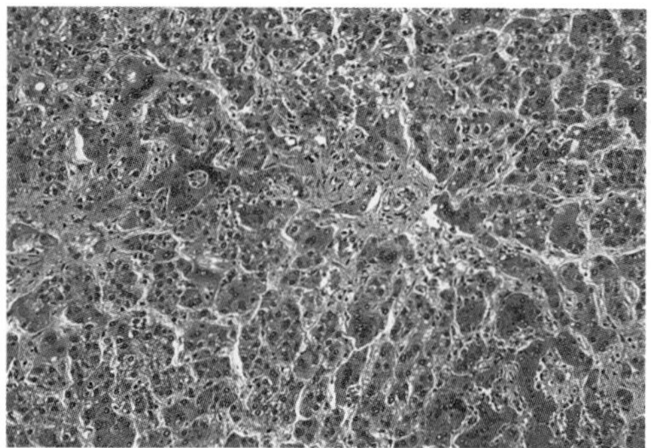

■ **Fig. 11.55** Giant cell hepatitis. Microscopic appearance of neonatal giant cell hepatitis caused in this case by rubeola infection showing edema, panlobular inflammatory infiltration, and marked disarray of cords with the formation of numerous syncytial hepatocytes (giant cells).

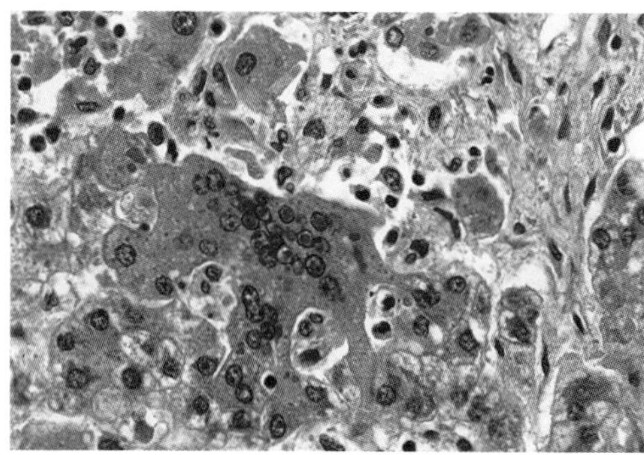

■ **Fig. 11.56** Giant cell hepatitis. High-magnification appearance of a hepatocyte giant cell in measles hepatitis showing the typical glassy eosinophilic intranuclear inclusions of rubeola virus infection.

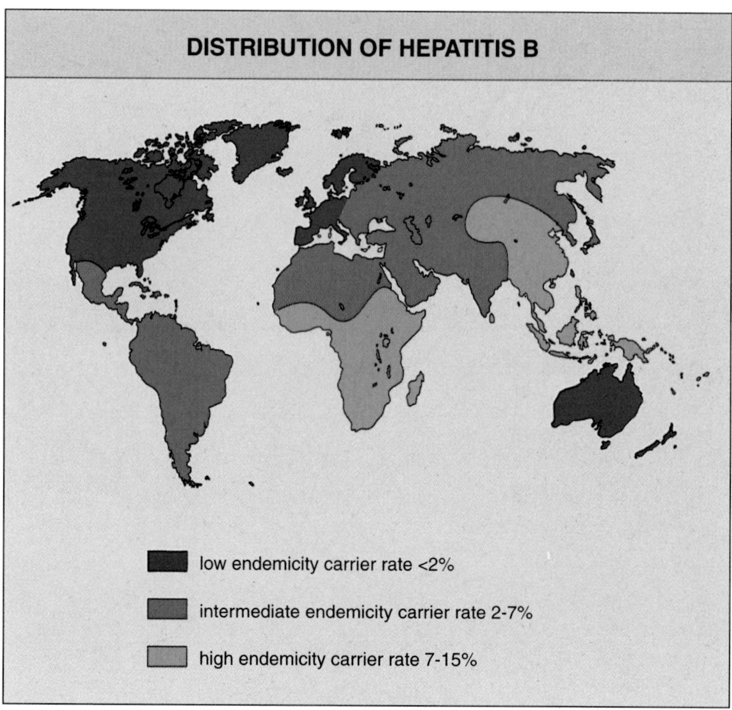

■ **Fig. 11.58** The worldwide distribution of hepatitis B.

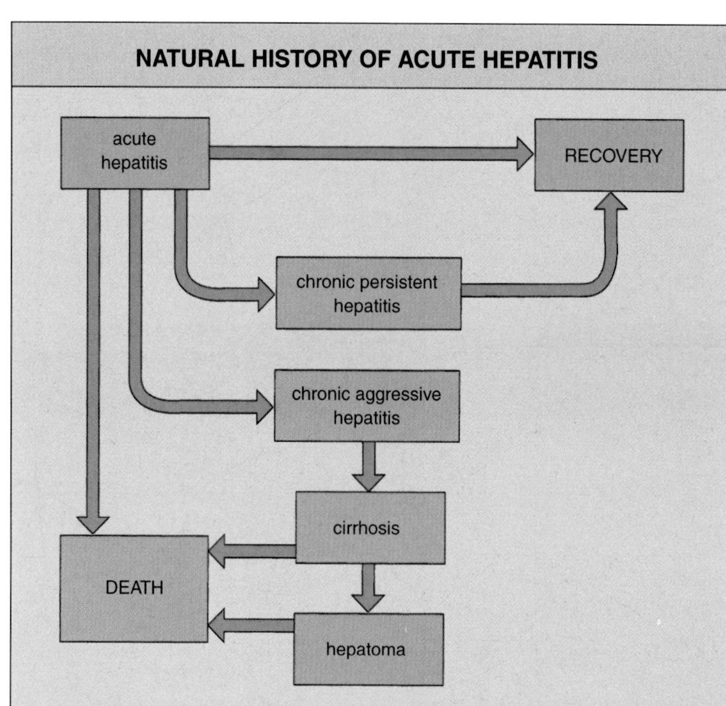

■ **Fig. 11.57** The natural history of acute hepatitis.

LOBULAR ACTIVITY	
Grade	**Histological features**
0	No inflammation or necrosis
1	Inflammation but no necrosis
2	Focal necrosis and acidophil bodies
3	Severe focal cell damage
4	Damage includes bridging necrosis
PORTAL/PERIPORTAL (SEPTAL) ACTIVITY	
Grade	**Histological features**
0	No or minimal inflammation
1	Portal inflammation (chronic persistent hepatitis)
2	Mild piecemeal necrosis (mild chronic active hepatitis)
3	Moderate piecemeal necrosis (moderate chronic active hepatitis)
4	Severe piecemeal necrosis (severe chronic active hepatitis)
FIBROSIS	
Stage	**Histological features**
0	No fibrosis
1	Enlarged, fibrotic portal tracts
2	Fibrous septa with intact architecture
3	Bridging fibrosis with architectural distortion
4	Probable or definite cirrhosis

Table 11.4 Microscopic scoring of chronic viral hepatitis.

A third type of chronic hepatitis is chronic lobular hepatitis in which the histological pattern resembles acute viral hepatitis (see Fig. 11.7); this carries an excellent prognosis.

Until recently chronic active hepatitis was considered to be an uncommon but recognized complication of inflammatory bowel disease. A wide range of histological abnormalities is seen, ranging from pericholangitis (Fig. 11.62) through to chronic aggressive hepatitis and cirrhosis. Recent advances, however, have shown these to be histological manifestations of primary sclerosing cholangitis, where both intra- and extrahepatic ducts may be involved (Fig. 11.63).

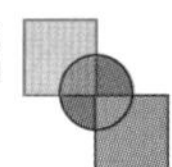

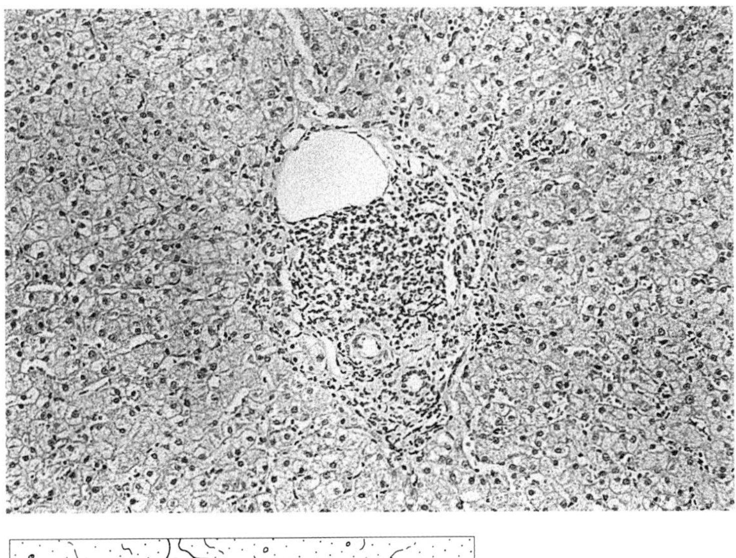

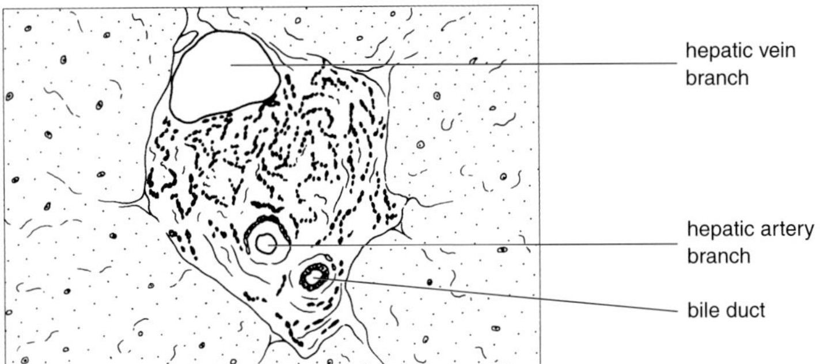

■ **Fig. 11.59** Chronic persistent hepatitis. Inflammatory cells are confined to the portal tract. H&E stain. Courtesy of Prof J.C.E. Underwood.

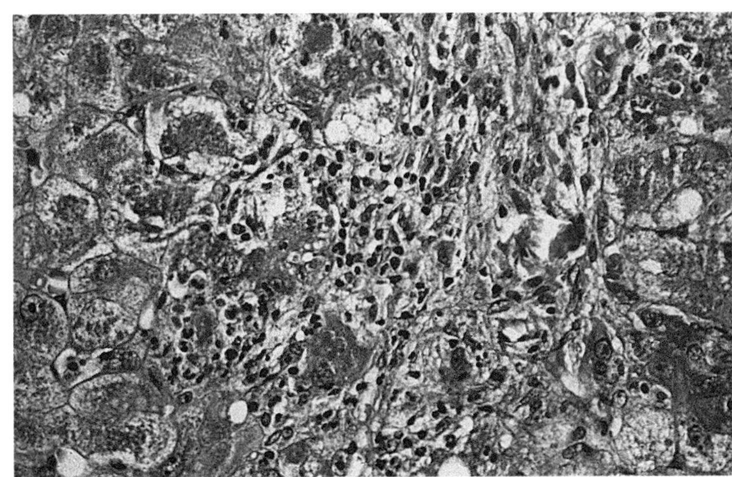

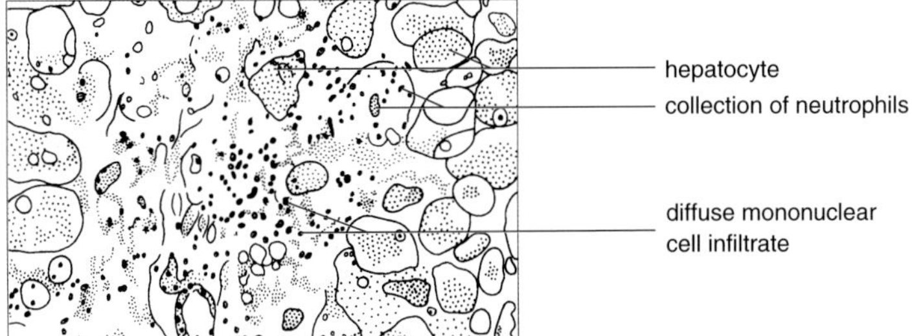

■ **Fig. 11.60** Liver biopsy of chronic aggressive hepatitis. The inflammatory infiltrate is not confined to the portal tract and 'spills over' into the liver parenchyma. H&E stain. Courtesy of Prof J.C.E. Underwood.

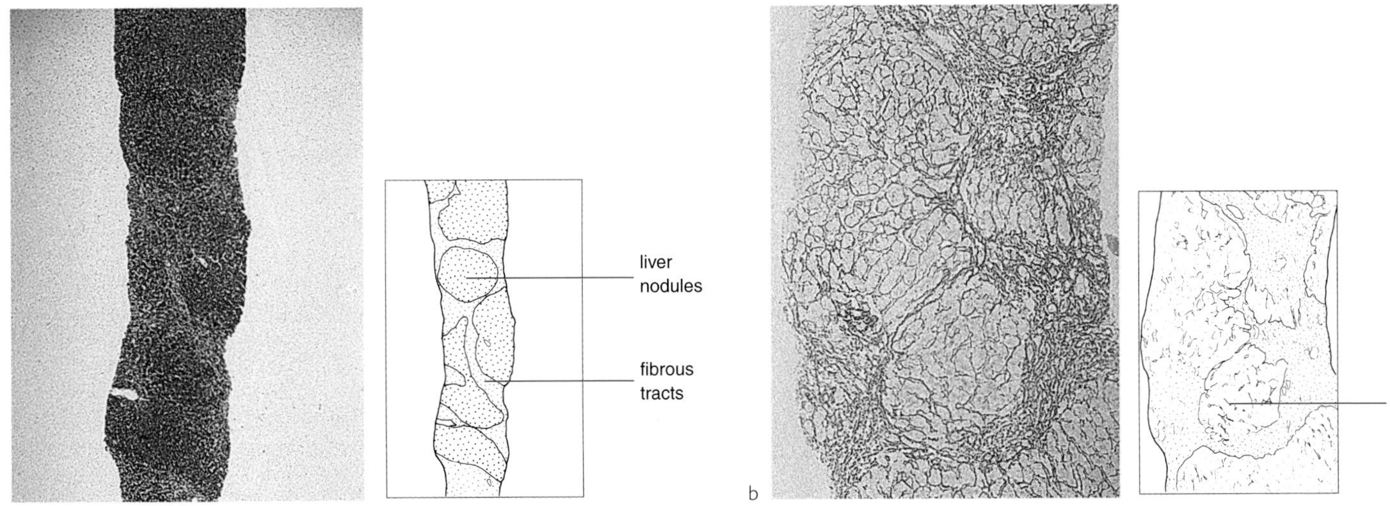

■ **Fig. 11.61** Histology in severe chronic aggressive hepatitis bordering on cirrhosis showing the fibrous dissection of normal architecture and isolated liver nodules ((a), Masson trichrome stain, x 20) and expanded fibrotic portal tracts isolating nodules of liver parenchyma ((b), reticulin stain, x 50).

LIVER ABSCESSES

Localized infections within the liver causing macroscopic areas of liver cell necrosis, namely abscesses, are uncommon. Liver abscesses can be caused by bacteria, fungi, or ameba. In Western countries, bacterial (pyogenic) abscesses are seen more commonly, while in less developed countries amebic abscess which follows invasion of the bowel wall by the protozoan *Entamoeba histolytica* predominates.

Pyogenic abscesses may be caused by complications of gall stones and cholangitis, result from intra-abdominal sepsis, or be idiopathic. Microaerophilic or anaerobic organisms are being increasingly isolated as causes of such abscesses. Fever, rigors, malaise, jaundice, and right hypochondrial pain are typical features, and the liver is usually large and tender. External drainage may be required. The CT scan of one affected patient shows a multiloculated abscess that was resected because of (unsubstantiated) concerns about malignancy (Figs 11.64–11.66). Liver abscess may also complicate abscess formation at other sites (Fig. 11.67), and where foreign bodies have been left behind (Fig. 11.68).

Fungal abscess is seen in immunosuppressed subjects or more often as a superinfection. The abscess may appear as a single, large, fluid-filled cyst with debris (Fig. 11.69) or as multiple lesions (Fig. 11.70).

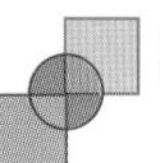

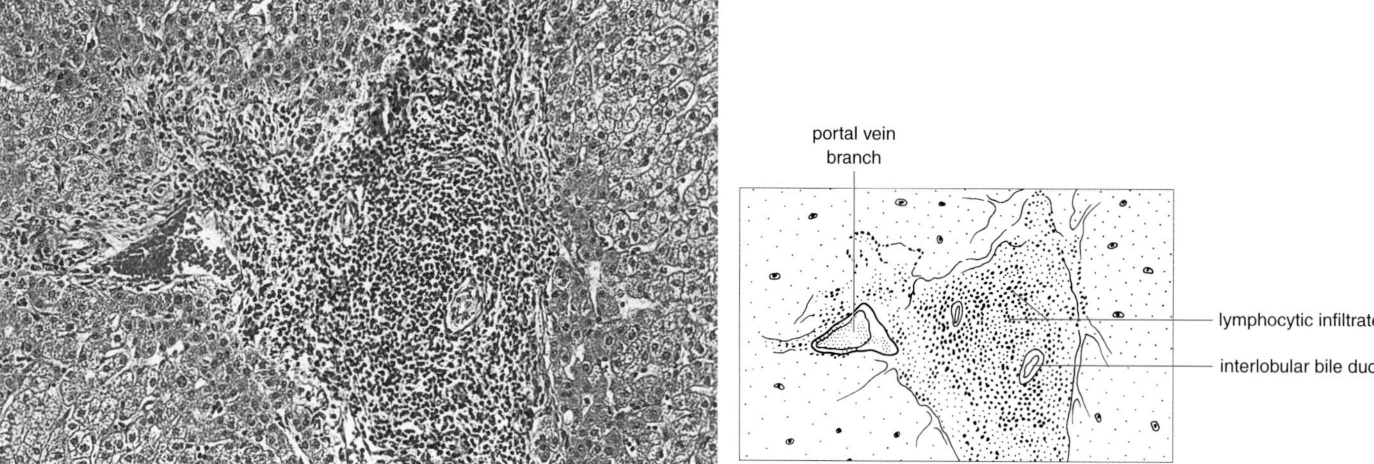

Fig. 11.62 Liver biopsy showing pericholangitis in a patient with ulcerative colitis. There is a heavy inflammatory infiltrate surrounding the bile duct. H&E stain. Courtesy of Prof J.C.E. Underwood.

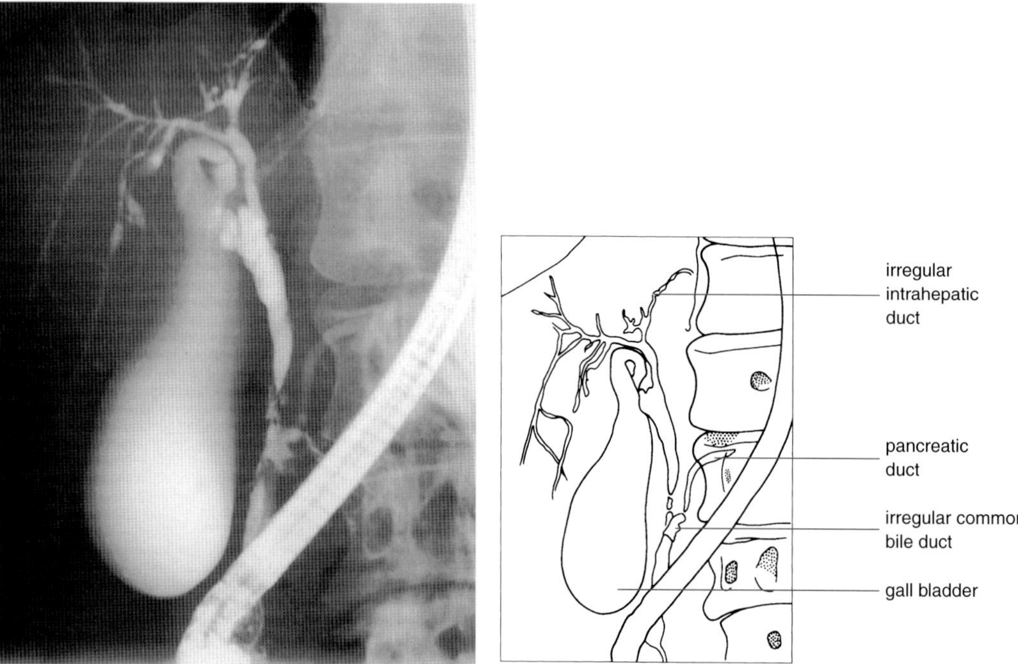

Fig. 11.63 Endoscopic retrograde cholangiopancreatogram showing primary sclerosing cholangitis in a 40-year-old man with ulcerative colitis. Note the irregularities in the common bile duct and in the left intrahepatic ducts.

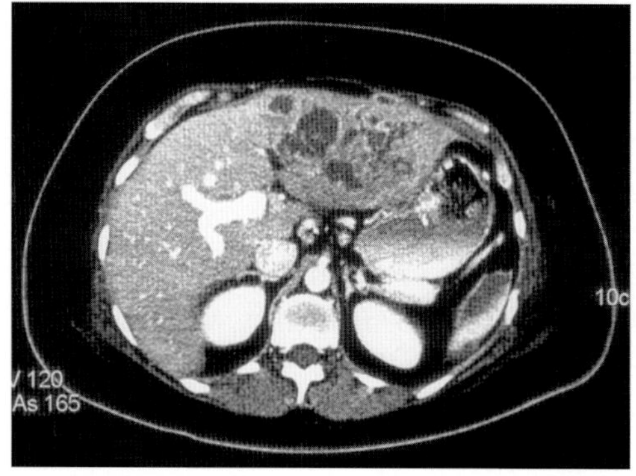

Fig. 11.64 CT scan showing suspicious lesion in the left lobe. Courtesy of Dr Richard Schulick, MD.

Abscesses may rupture into adjacent abdominal organs, the lung or the pericardium, but pulmonary problems also arise when a right pleural effusion occurs as a reaction to the sub-diaphragmatic pathology. If the abscess penetrates the diaphragm there may be spontaneous discharge into the bronchial tree (Fig. 11.71).

Abscesses may be detected by ultrasound or CT scanning (Figs 11.72, 11.73), and these techniques are also useful in enabling directed needle aspiration.

Histologically a pyogenic abscess shows a central area of pus with a rim of acute inflammatory cells and eventually a fibrous capsule. Amebic 'pus' is sometimes pink and has been likened to anchovy sauce (Fig. 11.74). In amebiasis there is little host reaction and the abscess contains necrotic liver cells rather than pus, with a rim of compressed liver cells (Fig. 11.75).

PARASITIC INFECTIONS OF THE LIVER

Hydatid disease

Ingestion of eggs of the dog tapeworm *Echinococcus granulosus* may cause hydatid disease. Man and sheep ingest the cysts in food contaminated by canine feces. The cysts dissolve in the stomach and the liberated ovum penetrates the intestinal wall. Dogs eat the viscera of dead infected sheep, and hence the cycle is maintained, but man is a so-called futile intermediate host (Fig. 11.76).

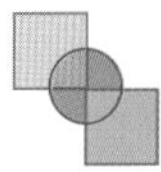

The embryos leave the bowel in portal blood and most are filtered off by the liver where they cause slowly expanding double-layered cysts full of infectious scolices (Figs 11.77, 11.78). The cysts may harmlessly die, when they can be seen on plain abdominal radiographs if the wall is calcified (Fig. 11.79).

Symptoms of hydatid cysts depend on the location of the cyst. Large cysts may present as masses (Fig. 11.80), or with hepatomegaly. Hydatid disease may appear as a single cyst (Fig. 11.81) or multi-

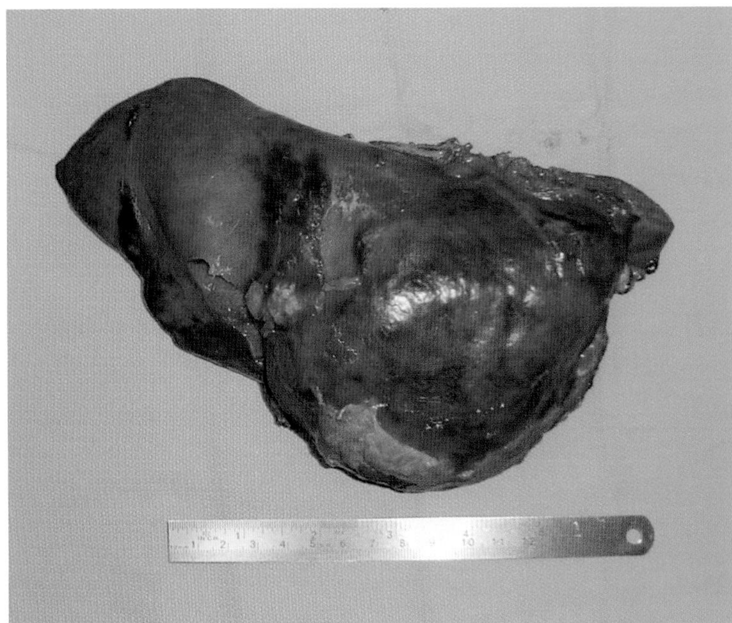

Fig. 11.65 At laparotomy of the same patient as in Fig. 11.68 the solely infective nature of the problem became clear. Courtesy of Dr Richard Schulick, MD.

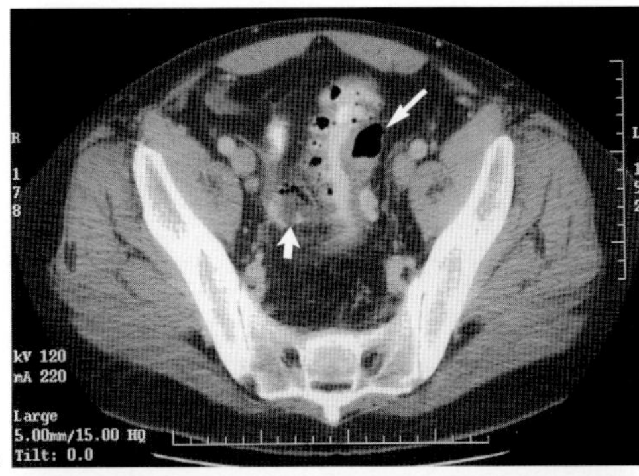

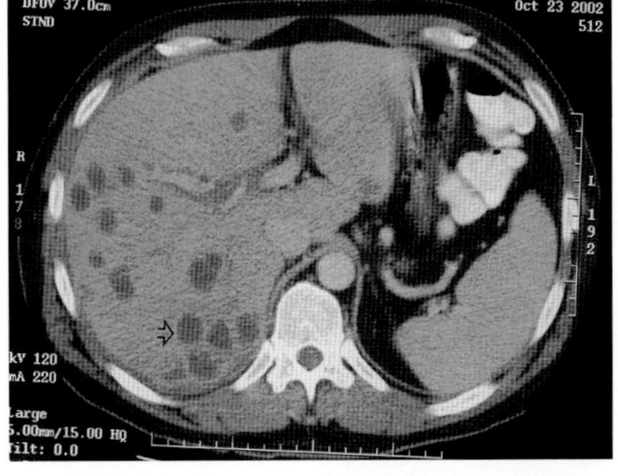

Fig. 11.67 Liver abscesses in patient with smoldering diverticulitis. (a) CT through pelvis showing diverticulosis and two pericolic abscesses. A 3 cm mass with an air–fluid level (long arrow) and a 2.5 cm round area with contrast, air bubbles and soft tissue debris (short arrow) abut the sigmoid colon. (b) CT demonstrating 16 small abscesses predominantly in the posterior segment of the right lobe of the liver. Numerous small low attenuation masses are seen (representative abscess identified by arrow).

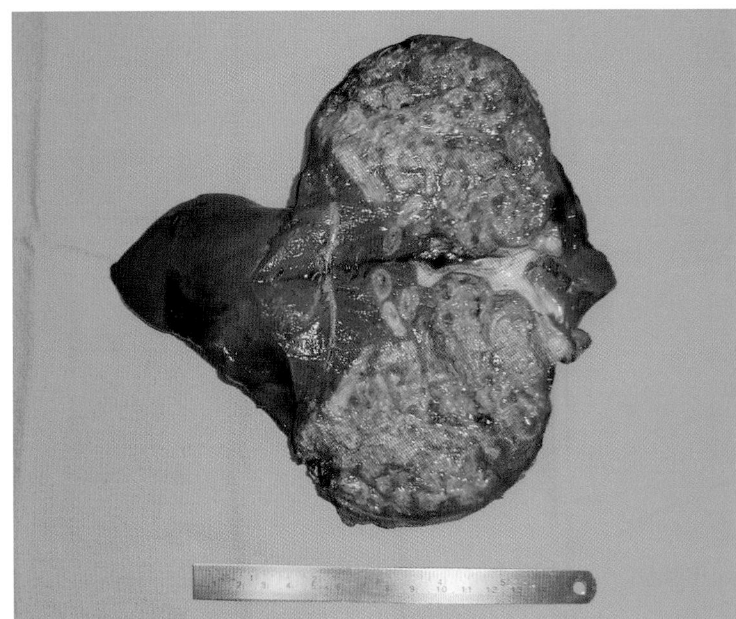

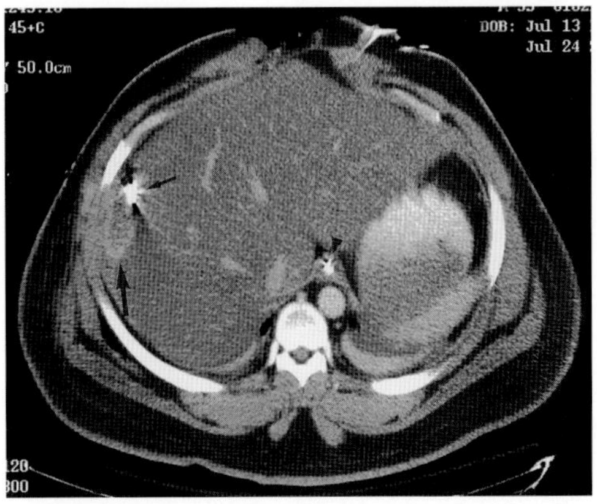

Fig. 11.66 Resection of the lobe was, however, necessary. Courtesy of Dr Richard Schulick, MD.

Fig. 11.68 Liver abscess related to laparotomy pad left in subcapsular region. An ovoid area of increased attenuation (long arrow) is seen. The area of very high attenuation (short arrow) is due to the radio-opaque marker manufactured into the pad.

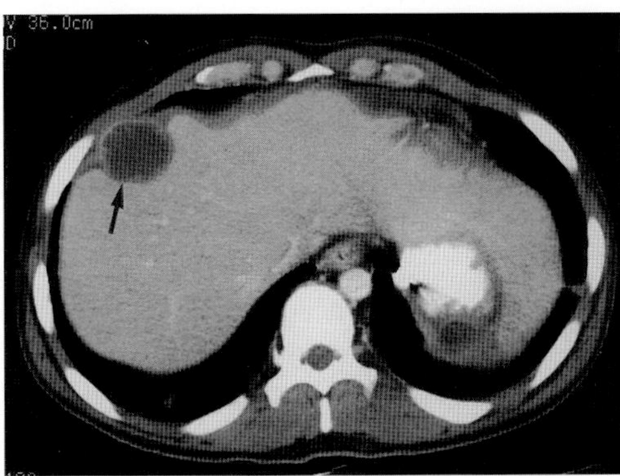

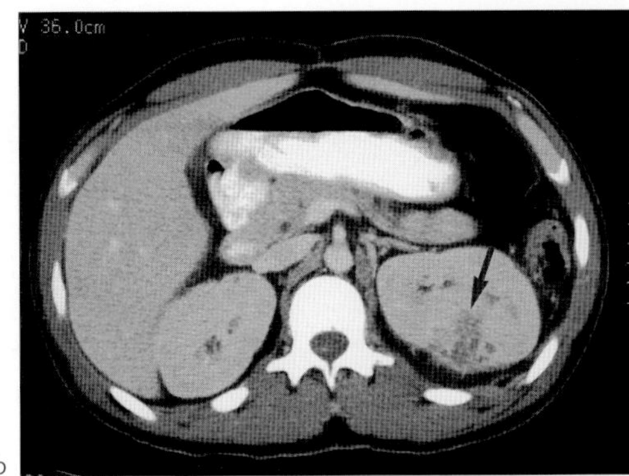

Fig. 11.69 Liver and renal abscesses in a patient with disseminated aspergillosis. (a) CT demonstrates a 3.5 cm mass (arrow) with a thick rim in the subcapsular portion of the medial segment of the left lobe. (b) CT demonstrates an ill-defined low-attenuation wedge-shaped mass (arrow) in the posterior mid left kidney.

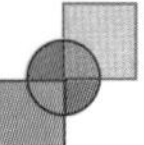

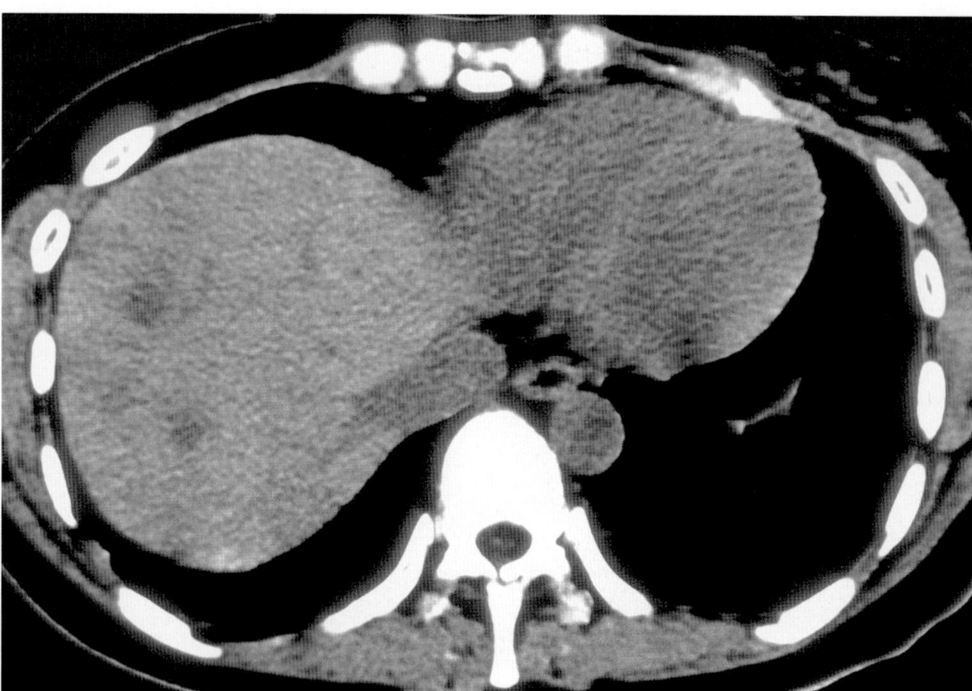

Fig. 11.70 Multiple fungal liver abscesses seen on CT.

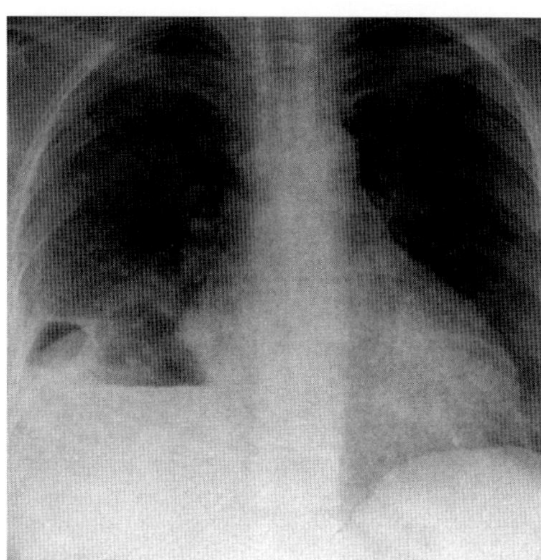

Fig. 11.71 Chest radiograph showing air–fluid level within a loculated liver abscess, secondary to abscess rupture and bronchial communication.

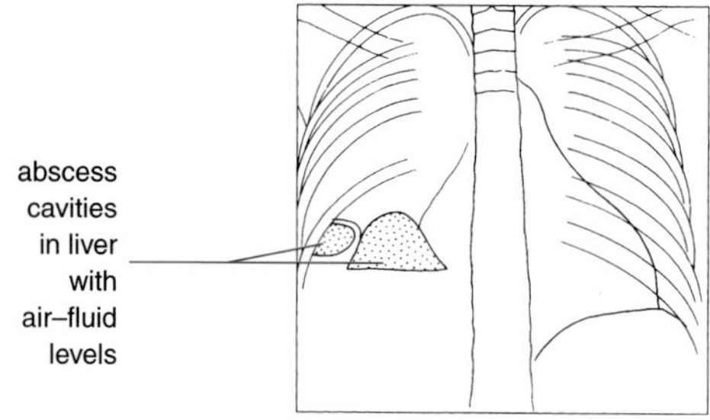

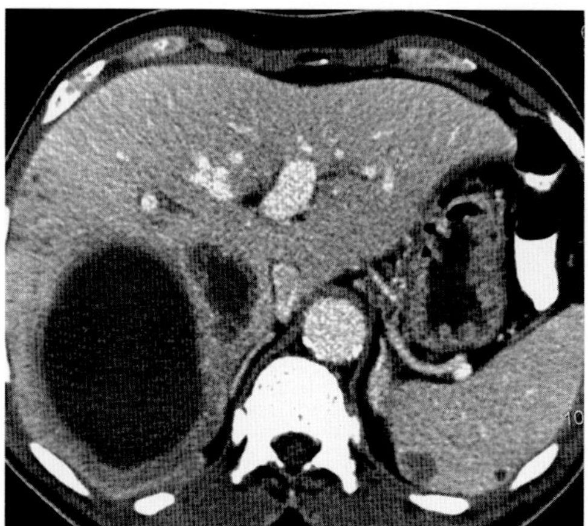

Fig. 11.72 Large pyogenic abscess in the right lobe of the liver.

loculated cysts (Fig. 11.82) on ultrasound, CT, or MRI. Compression of the biliary tree, or rupture into it (see Fig. 11.86), causes jaundice, and there can be secondary infection, or rupture into the abdomen, causing peritonitis if the cysts lie on the surface of the liver (Figs 11.83, 11.84).

Symptomatic cysts may be treated by surgery, but it is important not to spill the contents into the peritoneal cavity. Aspiration of the contents and instillation of cysticidal agents is done prior to surgical removal of the cyst wall or resection.

Schistosomiasis

The cercaria of *Schistosoma mansoni* or *S. japonicum* penetrate the skin and develop into adult worms in the portal veins, where they lay their eggs. These are carried back into the portal tracts, where they stimulate fibrosis and eventually obstruct the portal venous supply to the liver and cause portal hypertension. Hepatosplenomegaly is prominent, but liver function is preserved. Histologically, in the acute infection, the portal tracts are inflamed with prominent eosinophils. Kupffer cells are active and there is focal hepa-

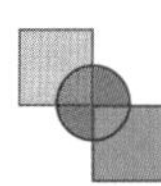

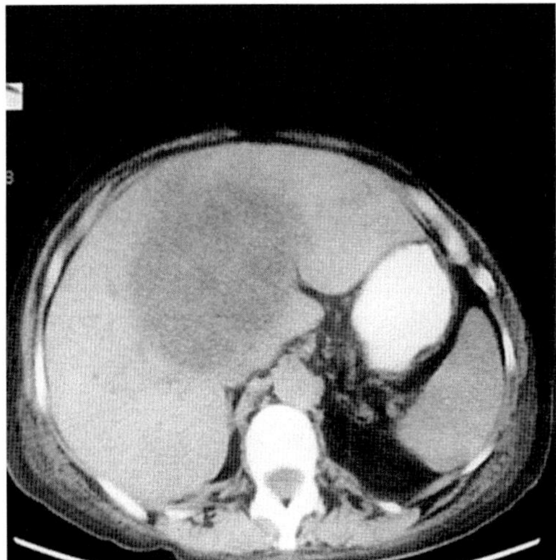

Fig. 11.73 CT scan of the liver showing a single, large multiloculated abscess. Courtesy of Dr R.A. Nakielny.

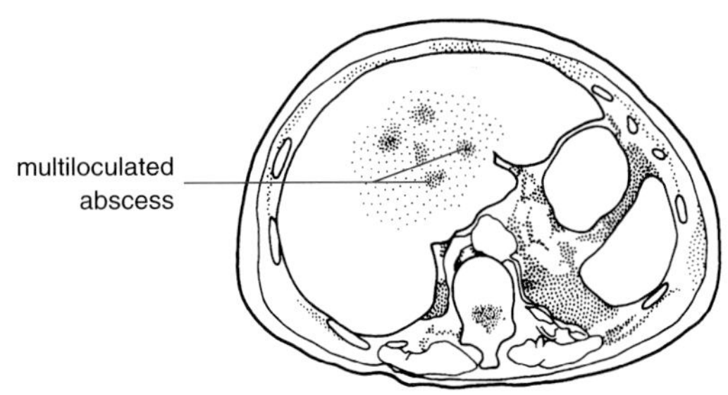

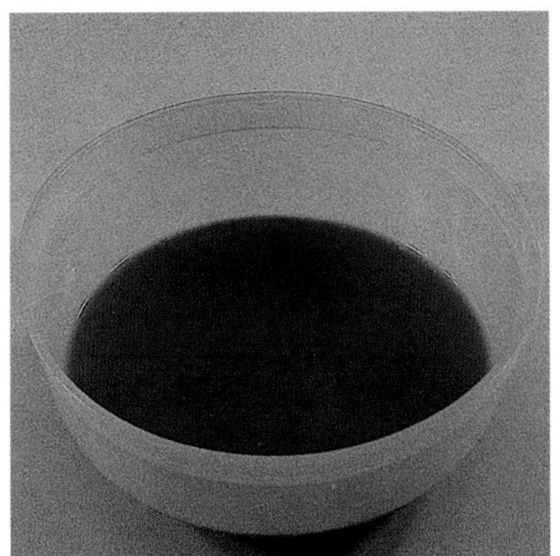

Fig. 11.74 Aspirated contents of an amebic abscess.

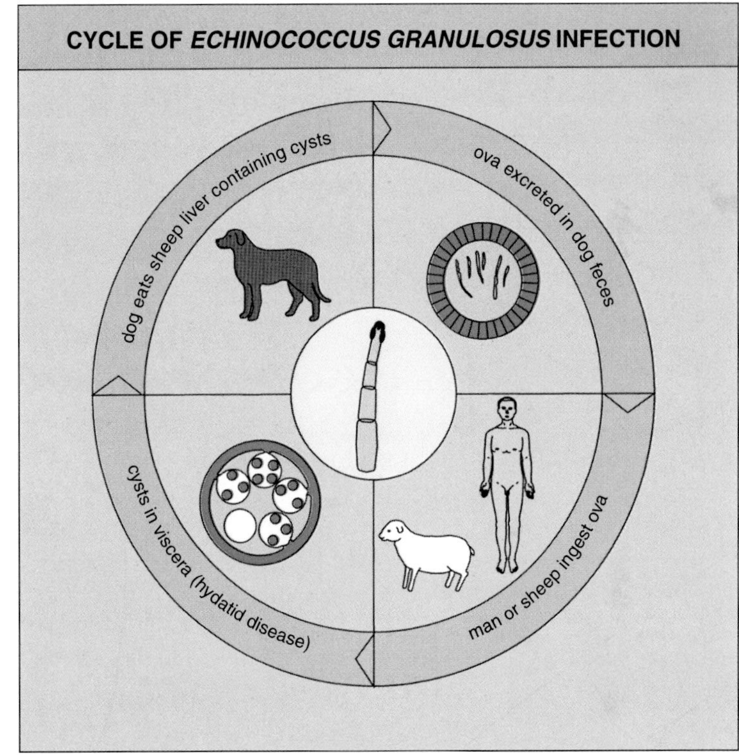

Fig. 11.76 The cycle of *Echinococcus granulosus* infection.

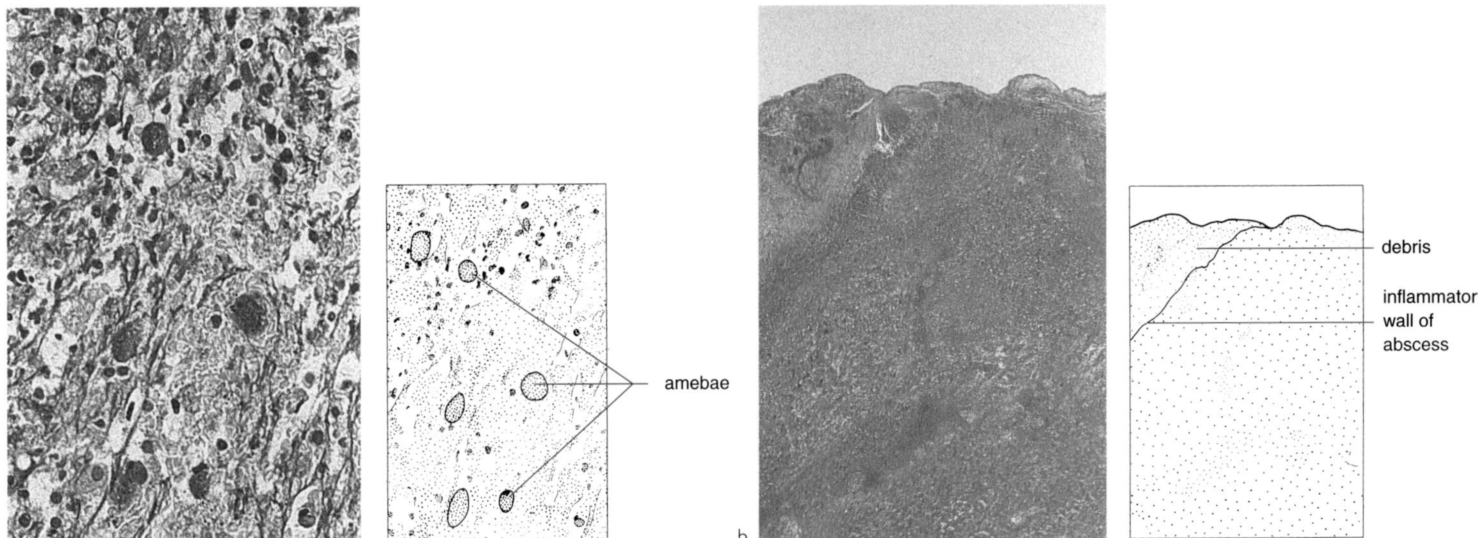

Fig. 11.75 Liver histology showing an amebic abscess and amebae in the wall of the abscess (x 20 (b), x 320 (a), H&E stain).

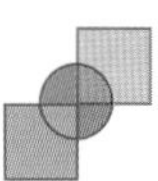

titis. Granulomas are not usually found, in contrast to the chronic progressive variety in which they develop around the ova (Fig. 11.85). In suspected cases where a granuloma is detected, serial sections of the liver biopsy may identify ova.

Malaria

Following a mosquito's bite, malarial sporozoites reach the liver where they develop into schizonts within parenchymal cells. The schizonts contain thousands of merozoites that are released into the blood. In the acute attack of *Plasmodium falciparum* the sinusoids are congested and filled with parasitized erythrocytes. The Kupffer cells are active and there may be mild centrilobular hepatic necrosis. In the non-immune patient, there is florid Kupffer cell hyperplasia. These Kupffer cells contain malarial dark brown

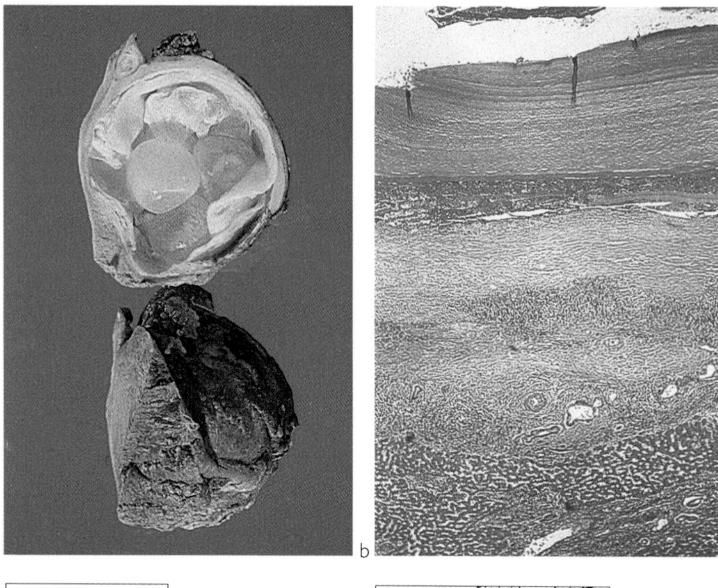

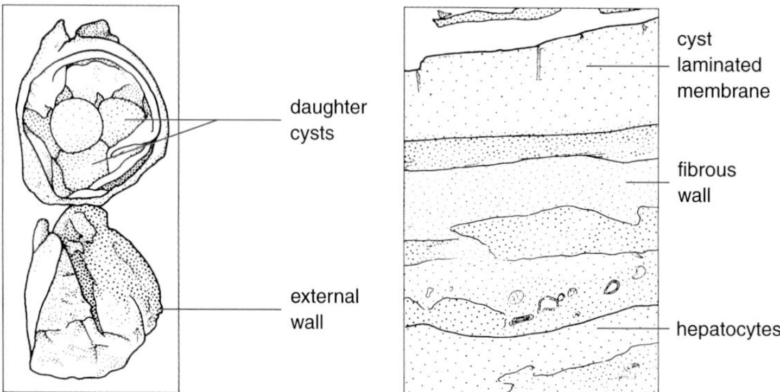

Fig. 11.77 An echinococcal cyst showing daughter cysts, resected from the liver (a), and histology showing the layers of an hydatid cyst ((b), H&E stain, x 20).

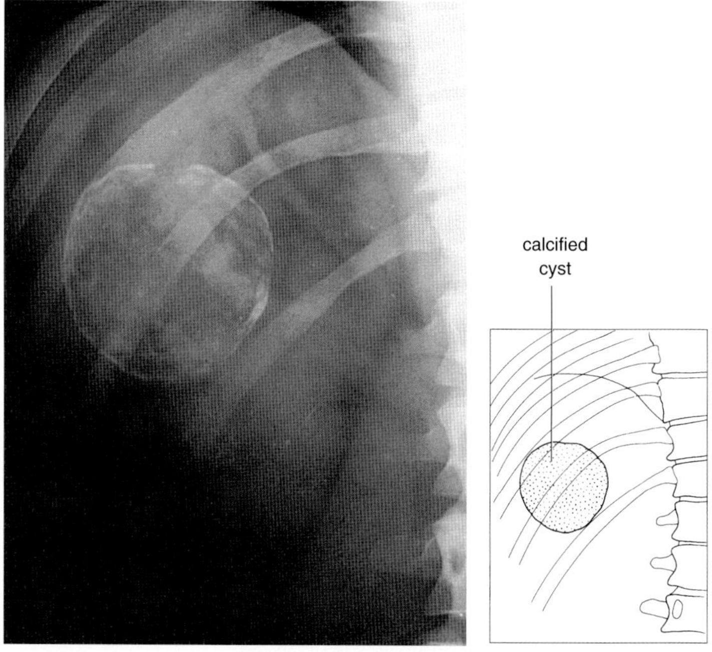

Fig. 11.79 Abdominal radiograph showing a calcified hydatid cyst in the liver.

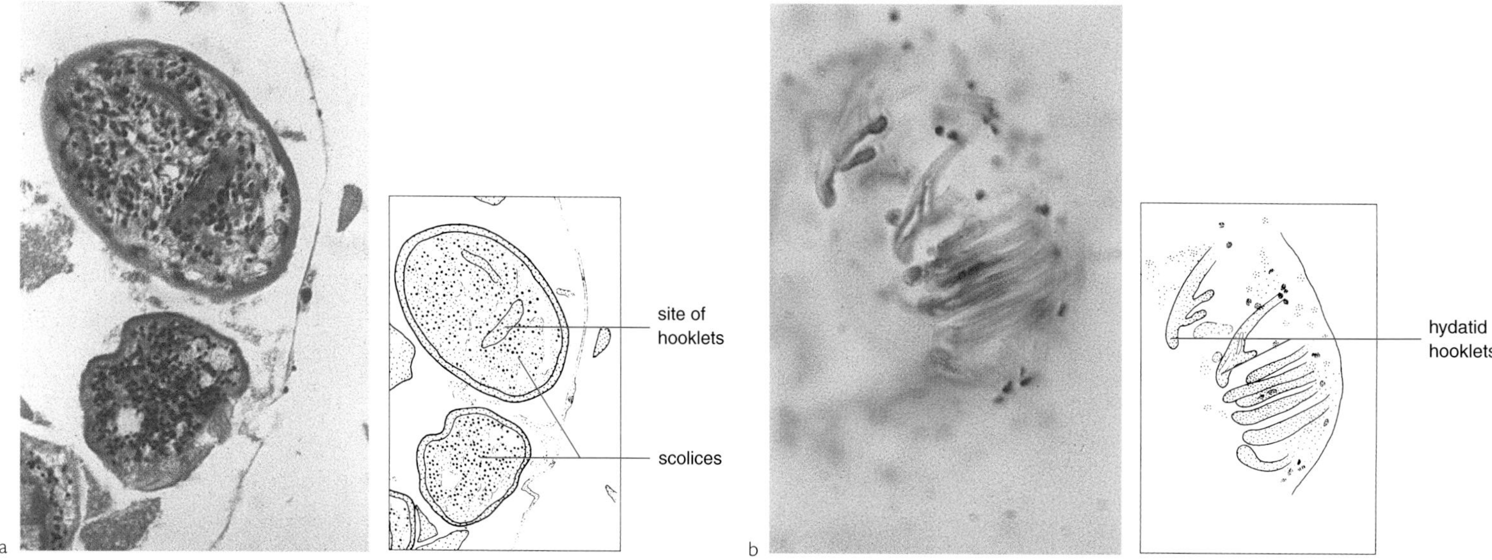

Fig. 11.78 Scolices of *E. granulosus* ((a), H&E stain, x 400), and the hooklets at a higher magnification ((b), Ziehl–Neelsen stain, x 800).

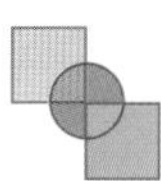

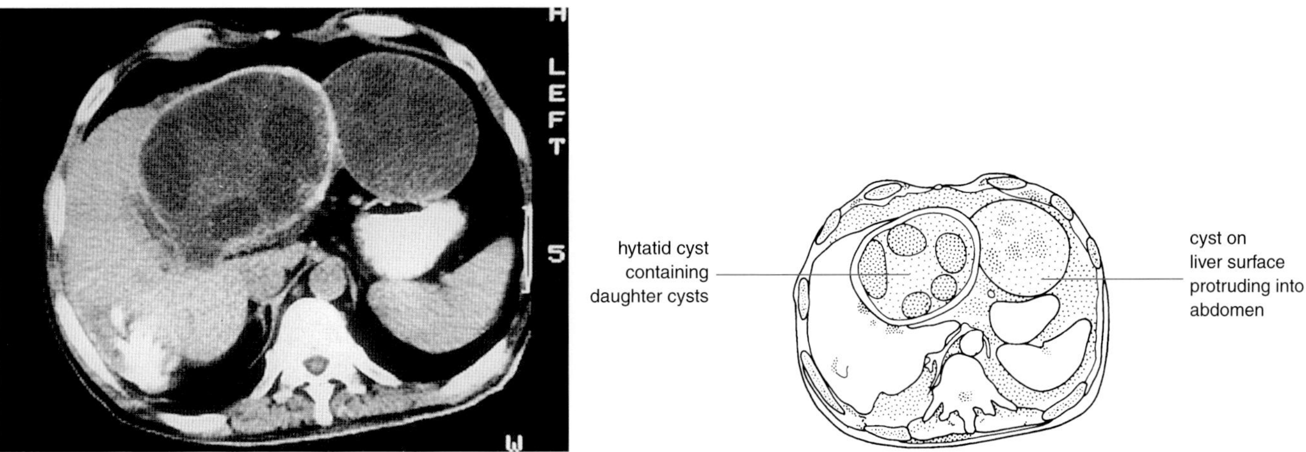

Fig. 11.80 CT scan of the liver showing a large cyst in the left lobe containing several daughter cysts. In addition there is a cyst on the liver surface protruding into the abdomen.

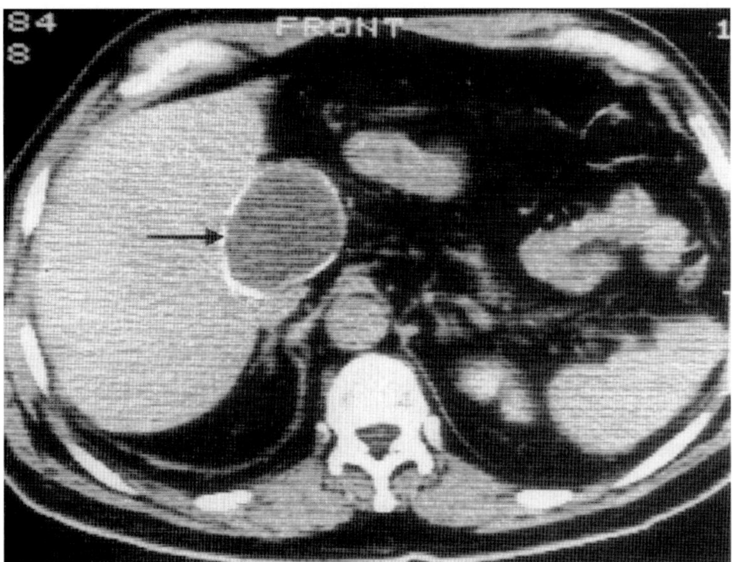

Fig. 11.81 CT showing single hydatid cyst protruding from the liver surface.

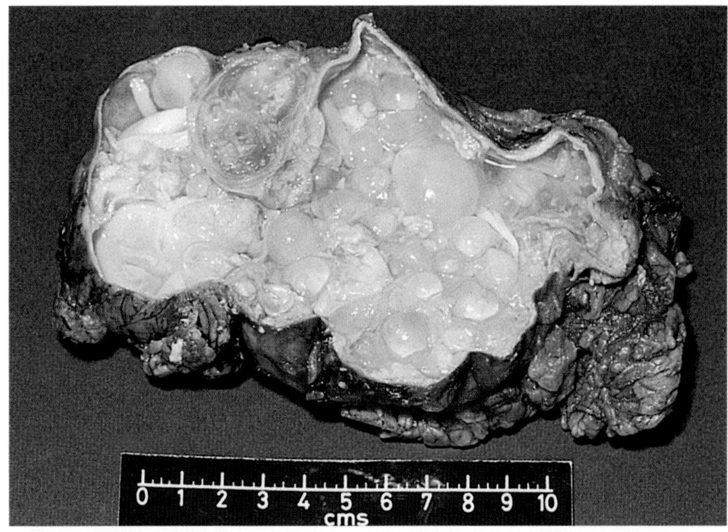

Fig. 11.84 Resected hydatid cyst of the liver containing numerous daughter cysts. Note the adherent omentum.

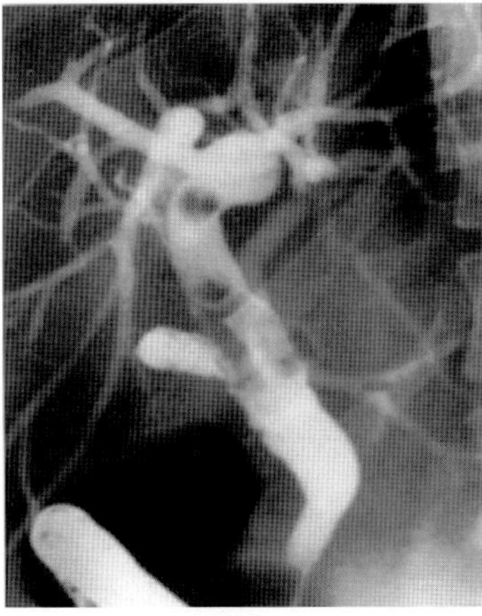

Fig. 11.82 ERCP of ruptured hydatid.

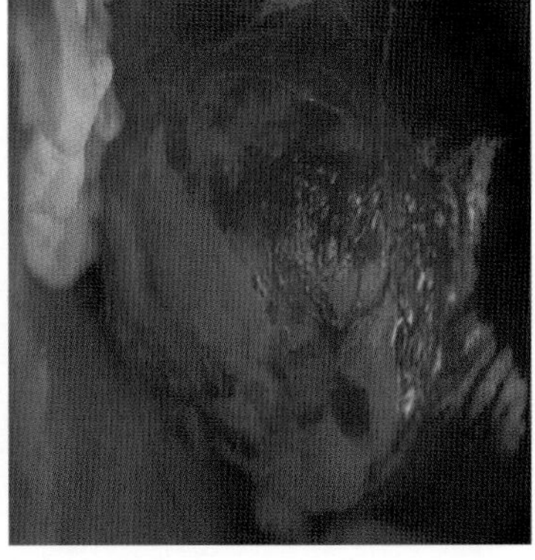

Fig. 11.83 Hydatid cyst surface seen at surgery.

pigment (hemozoin) (Fig. 11.86). It resembles schistosomal and formalin pigments. As immunity develops, the pigment disappears from the sinusoids but remains in the portal tract areas.

In endemic malarious areas, tropical splenomegaly syndrome develops, probably due to an abnormal immune response to malarial antigens. Non-specific sinusoidal lymphocytosis is found in the liver.

Leishmaniasis

In visceral leishmaniasis, or kala-azar, the trypanosomes invade reticuloendothelial cells in the liver and other organs. Clinically there is usually substantial splenomegaly, and histologically the trypanosomes are seen as the Leishman–Donovan bodies within the Kupffer cells and macrophages (Fig. 11.87).

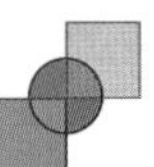

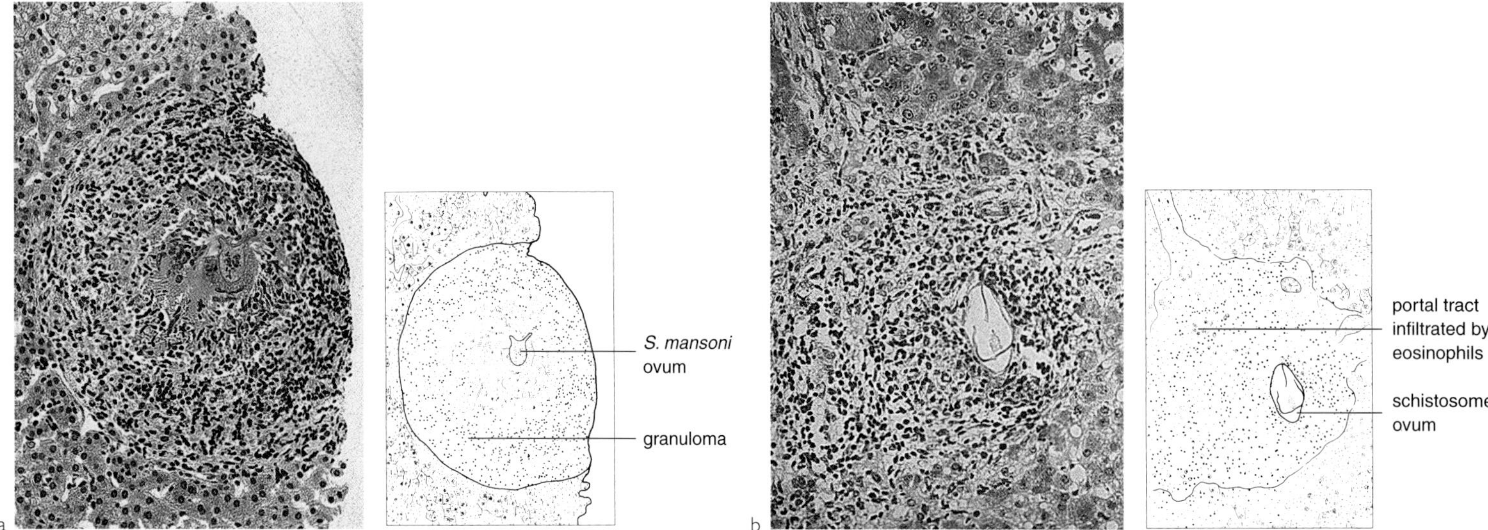

■ **Fig. 11.85** (a) Chronic schistosomal liver disease with portal fibrosis. Post-mortem specimen from patient with chronic hepatic schistosomiasis showing the grossly lobulated liver produced by broad portal scars that transect the hepatic parenchyma and produce a segmented macroscopic architecture. H&E stain (x 200). Courtesy of Prof I. Talbot. (b) Chronic schistosomal liver disease with portal fibrosis. Microscopic appearance of chronic hepatic schistosomal infection characterized by marked portal scarring showing the expansion of the portal areas by dense fibrosis that produces portal hypertension without true cirrhosis. When transected longitudinally, a scarred portal branch has the appearance of the stem of a clay pipe ('pipe-stem fibrosis'). H&E stain (x 200). Courtesy of Prof I. Talbot.

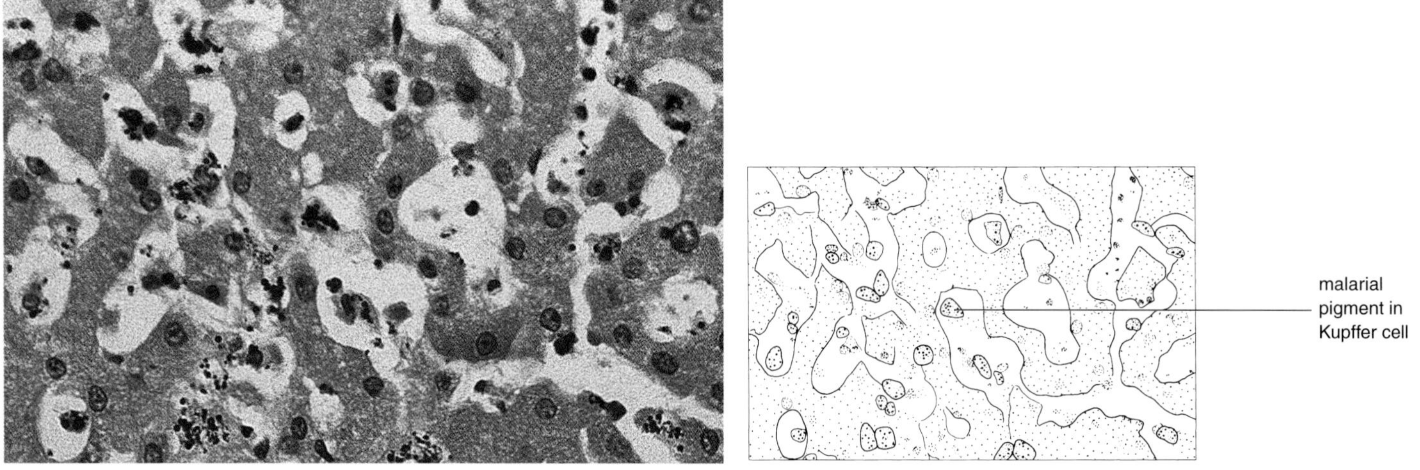

■ **Fig. 11.86** Liver histology in malaria showing Kupffer cells containing malarial pigment. H&E stain (x 450).

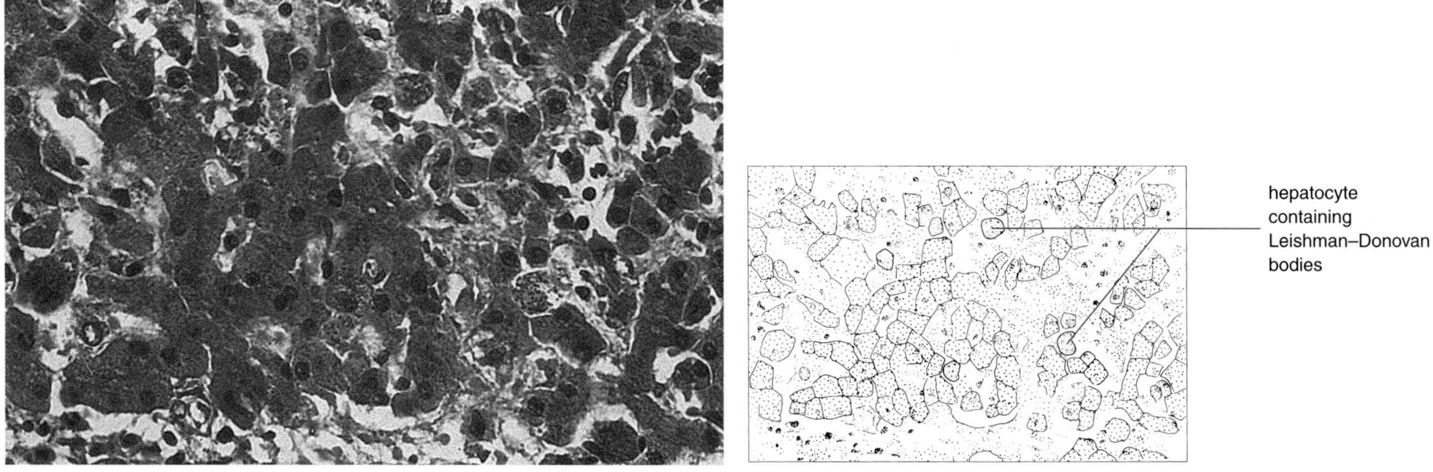

■ **Fig. 11.87** Liver histology in kala-azar showing Leishman–Donovan bodies in the hepatocytes. H&E stain (x 1100). Courtesy of Prof I. Talbot.

FIBROSIS, CIRRHOSIS, AND PORTAL HYPERTENSION

12

The word cirrhosis is derived from the Greek *kirros* meaning tawny, as this is often the color of the cirrhotic liver. Cirrhosis is defined as diffuse fibrosis involving the whole organ with the formation of nodules. It is the diffuse involvement which distinguishes the process from fibrosis or scarring, although post-necrotic scarring may progress to cirrhosis. Liver biopsy is the most sensitive tool to diagnose cirrhosis, but about 10% of cirrhosis would be missed on simple needle biopsy alone. Traditionally cirrhosis is classified morphologically into macronodular and micronodular types, the nodule in the micronodular variety being 3 mm or less in diameter (Figs 12.1, 12.2). In practice, however, this is a somewhat artificial distinction, since in many patients both macronodular and micronodular changes can be found in the same liver, and there is often a tendency for progressively larger nodules to develop as cirrhosis becomes more established. Alcoholic cirrhosis is typically micronodular.

The major types of cirrhosis according to etiology are shown in Table 12.1. Macroscopically the cirrhotic liver may be large, normal in size, or small and shrunken. In micronodular cirrhosis no recognizable normal architecture survives, the nodules being devoid of central veins and portal tracts (Fig. 12.3). In contrast, areas of normal architecture can survive within the dissecting fibrous bands in macronodular cirrhosis (Fig. 12.4). This may result in sampling errors in needle biopsies of the liver; the tendency of specimens from cirrhotic livers to fragment is a further feature which may complicate the diagnosis. Active cirrhosis is characterized by the presence of inflammatory cells and piecemeal necrosis, but variable amounts of cholestasis, iron, and fat may be found according to the etiology of the liver disease (see Chapter 11). As cirrhosis progresses, activity tends to subside, and in end-stage liver disease it is often impossible to distinguish between the consequences of different etiologies.

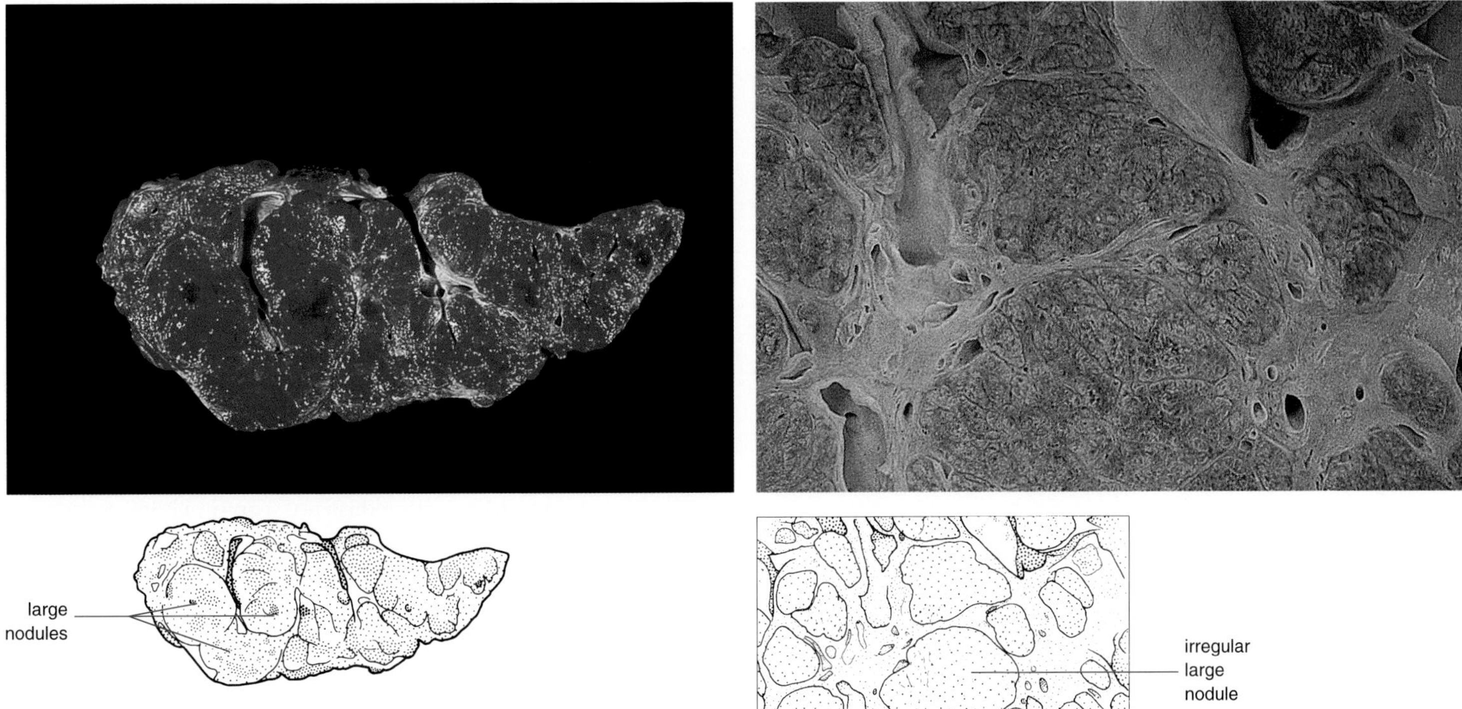

Fig. 12.1 Gross appearance of the liver of a patient with macronodular cirrhosis.

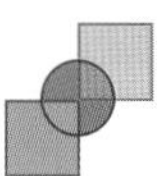

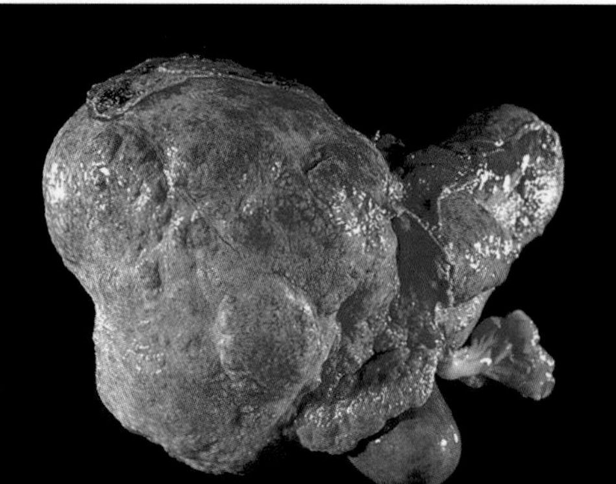

a

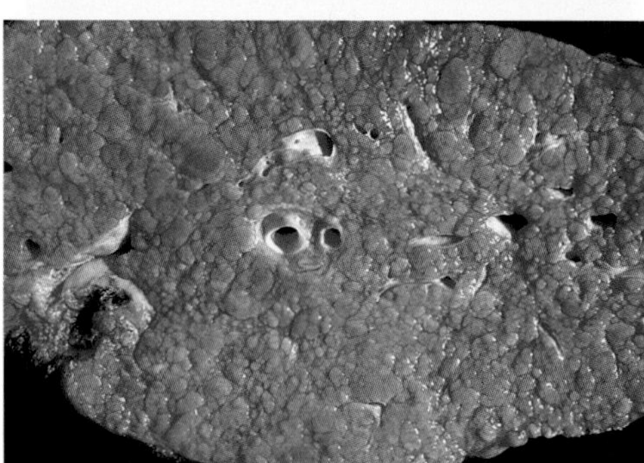

b

Fig. 12.2 (a) Micronodular cirrhosis. Hepatectomy (explant) specimen from a liver transplant patient showing the overall distortion of the liver contour produced by scarring, and the granular surface reflecting the myriad small regenerative nodules of the cirrhotic parenchyma. (b) Cut surface of the liver in micronodular cirrhosis showing the diffuse replacement of the normally smooth parenchyma by innumerable small regenerative nodules of relatively uniform size, each encircled by slender fibrotic bands. The nodules have a yellow color reflecting the on-going steatosis of the hepatocytes.

Etiology of Cirrhosis	
Viral hepatitis	
HBV	hepatitis B
HCV	hepatitis C
Toxins	
alcohol	alcoholic cirrhosis
iron	hemochromatosis
copper	Wilson's disease
methyldopa arsenic	drug-induced cirrhosis
Cholestasis	
small ducts	Caroli's syndrome
	primary biliary cirrhosis
large ducts	secondary biliary cirrhosis
small/large ducts	sclerosing cholangitis
Venous obstruction	
small veins	veno-occlusive disease
large veins	Budd–Chiari syndrome
	congenital web lesion
	cardiac cirrhosis
Others	
autoimmune	lupoid hepatitis
non alcoholic fatty liver disease (NAFLO)	cryptogenic cirrhosis

Table. 12.3 Etiology of cirrhosis.

A number of cutaneous features (stigmata) may develop in a patient with cirrhosis, and these are important as they aid clinical recognition of chronic liver disease. Palmar erythema ('liver palms'; Fig. 12.5), involves the thenar and hypothenar eminences whilst sparing the center of the palm. This is a reflection of a hyperdynamic circulation and is not specific to cirrhosis. Bright red telangiectases of the face are characteristic of the alcoholic ('paper money' skin; Fig. 12.6), as is parotid enlargement. Another classical feature of chronic liver disease is the presence of spider naevi (Fig. 12.7), which are red arterioles with fine radiating branches. These are only found on the arms and upper trunk (in the drainage area of the superior vena cava).

Leuconychia (white nail syndrome), is a feature of defective protein metabolism, which is often found in association with chronic liver disease (Fig. 12.8). Clubbing of the fingers (Fig. 12.9) is an uncommon but recognized complication of chronic liver disease. Rarely it may be associated with cyanosis due to intrapulmonary shunting (Fig. 12.10). Dupuytren's contracture (Fig. 12.11) has been linked with alcoholic cirrhosis, but it is commonly seen in other conditions and also in an entirely benign familial form. Bruising at venepuncture sites and purpura occur when advanced liver disease has led to coagulation abnormalities (Fig. 12.12). Generalized pigmentation of the skin is more characteristic of primary biliary cirrhosis (Fig. 12.13), and hemochromatosis (Fig. 12.14). Arthralgia and arthritis occur in autoimmune chronic active hepatitis and primary biliary cirrhosis, while in hemochromatosis, chondrocalcinosis and erosive arthritis are recognized features (Figs 12.15, 12.16). Loss of body and pubic hair (especially of the male escutcheon), and testicular atrophy reflect the hormonal changes of cirrhosis. A pathognomonic feature of Wilson's disease is the deposition of copper on the cornea (Kayser–Fleischer ring; Fig. 12.17).

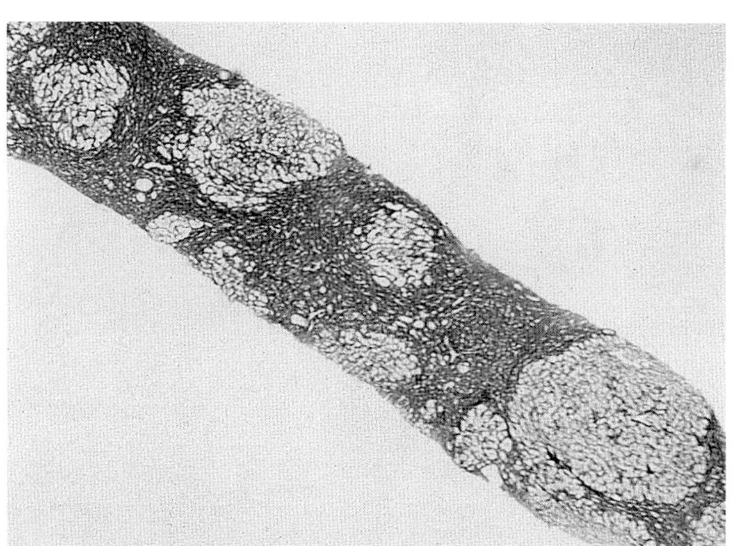

Fig. 12.3 Histology of micronodular cirrhosis showing distortion of liver architecture by fibrous tissue. Reticulin stain.

Peripheral edema and ascites may be the presenting symptoms of cirrhosis, and careful inspection of the abdomen often reveals dilated abdominal veins which carry blood in a radial direction (as distinct from the inferior to superior route of the dilated collaterals when the inferior vena cava is blocked) (Fig. 12.18). Umbilical varices forming a frank caput medusa are seen much less frequently (Figs 12.19, 12.20). Spontaneous bacterial peritonitis is a major complication of ascites, which is often rapidly fatal unless treated promptly. It is diagnosed by the finding of large numbers of leukocytes in the ascitic fluid (more than 250/mm^3; Fig. 12.21), and the condition should be suspected in any patient with ascites who deteriorates without obvious reason. Behavioral disturbances (encephalopathy) are a further clinical manifestation of cirrhosis and are sometimes accompanied by typical EEG features (Fig. 12.22).

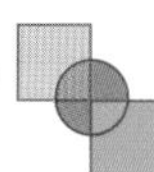

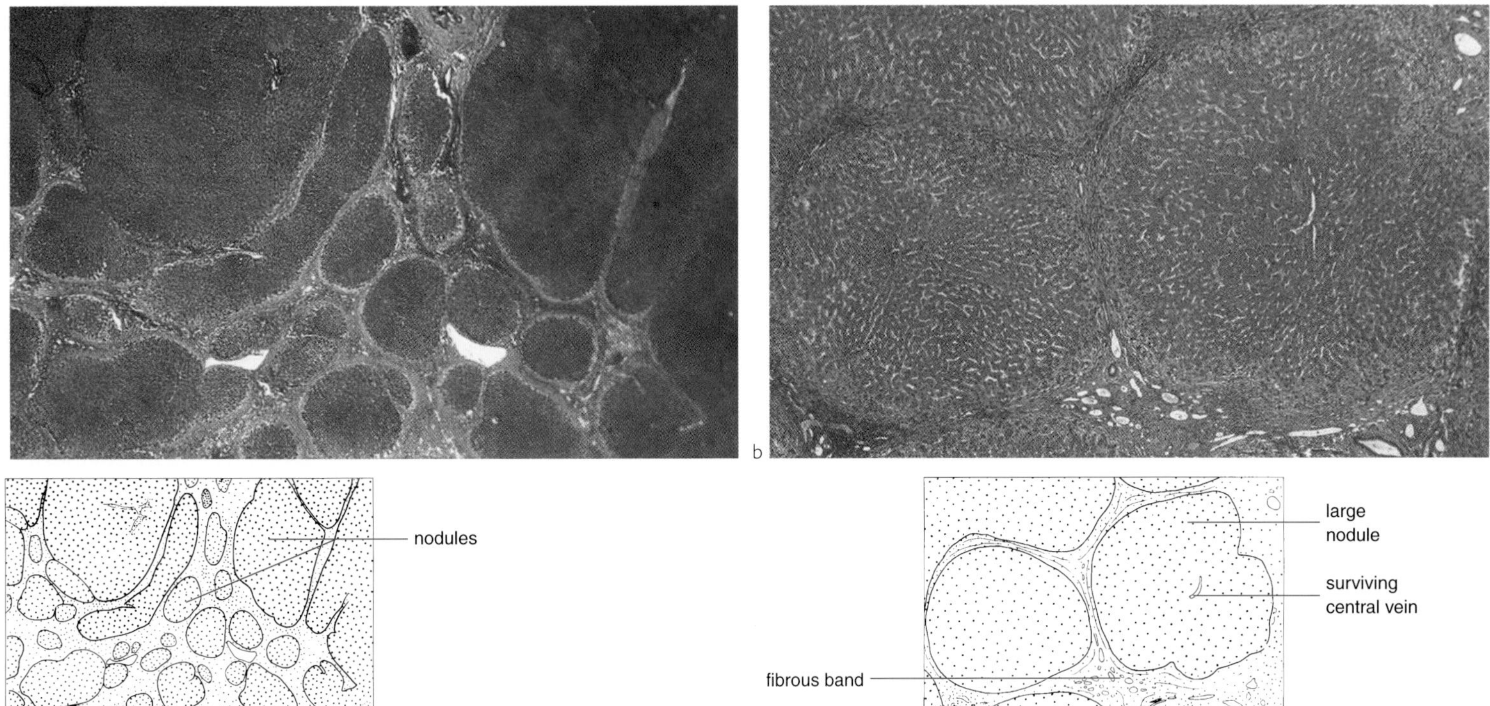

■ **Fig. 12.4** Appearance of the liver in cryptogenic macronodular cirrhosis. The overall architecture is destroyed, but the nodules are large enough to contain some residual normal features ((a), Masson trichrome stain x 12; (b), trichrome staining at a higher magnification; H&E stain, x 30).

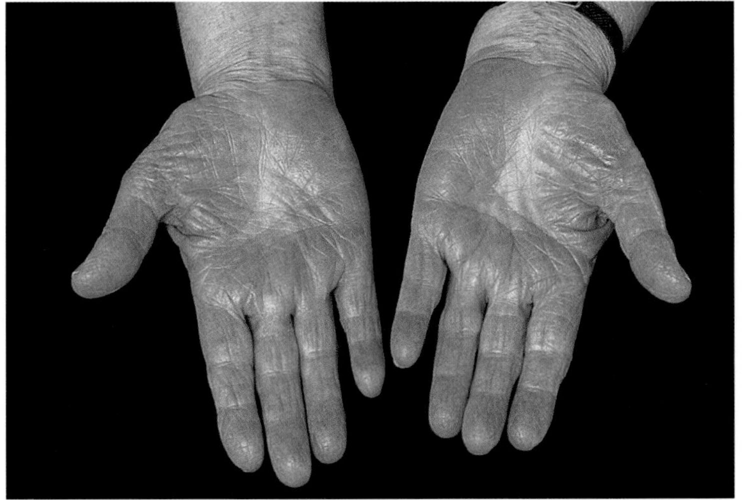

■ **Fig. 12.5** Palmar erythema (liver palms). Gross reddening of the thenar and hypothenar eminences and fingers with sparing of the center of the palm.

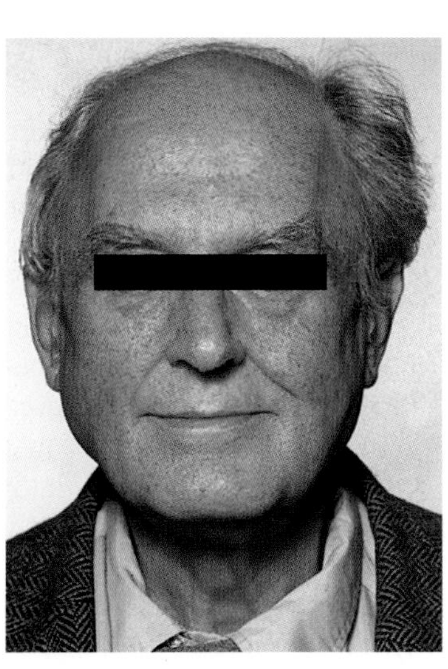

■ **Fig. 12.6** Parotid enlargement, facial telangiectases ('paper money' skin) and the cheerful appearance of the alcoholic.

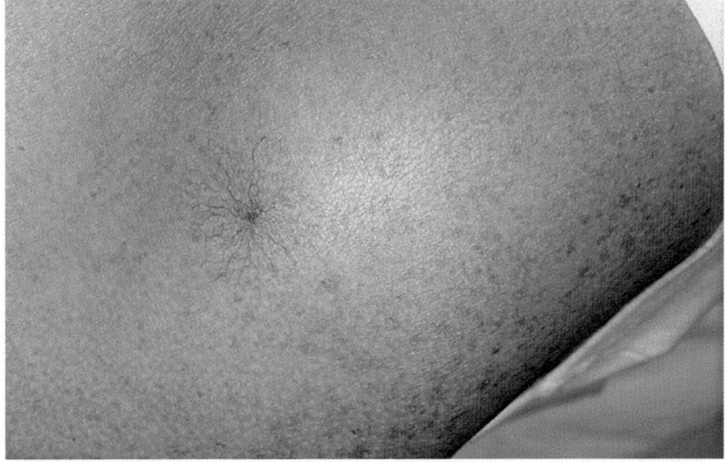

■ **Fig. 12.7** A typical spider naevus, with a central arteriole and fine radiating vessels.

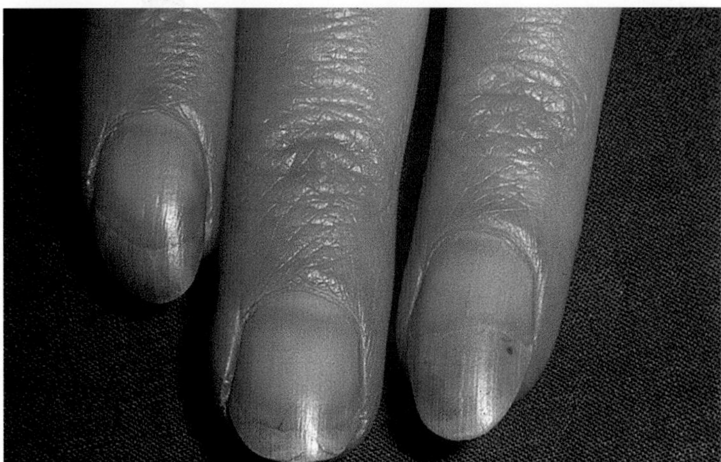

■ **Fig. 12.8** The fingernails of a patient with autoimmune chronic active hepatitis. The patient presented with acute decompensation which responded to steroid therapy. Following control of the hepatitis, the normal nail at the base reflects improved protein synthesis.

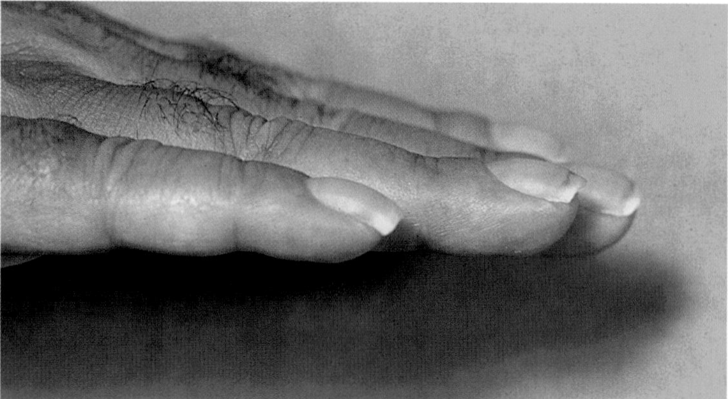

■ **Fig. 12.9** Finger clubbing associated with primary biliary cirrhosis.

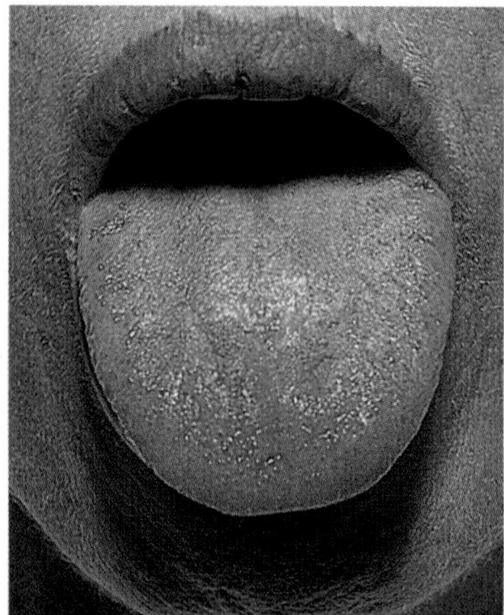

■ **Fig. 12.10** Central cyanosis of mucous membranes in alcoholic cirrhosis.

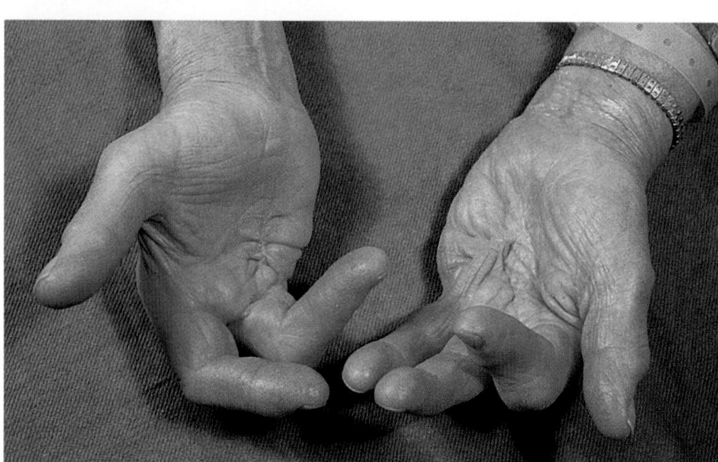

■ **Fig. 12.11** Gross Dupuytren's contracture in a patient with alcoholic liver disease. Note the contractures on the palms as well as the fingers, together with the amputations performed because of earlier deformities.

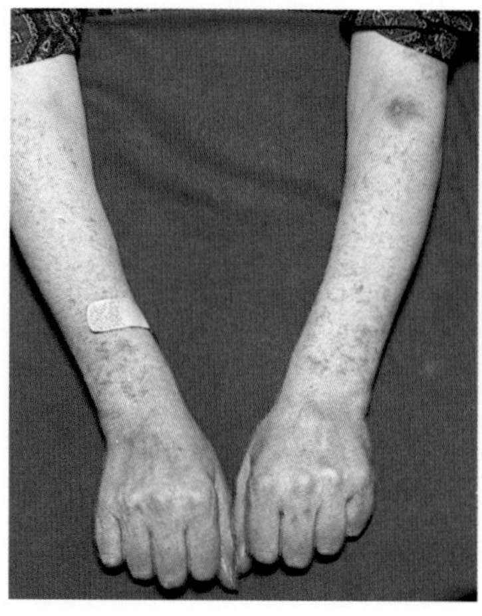

■ **Fig. 12.12** Bruising and telangiectases in alcoholic cirrhosis.

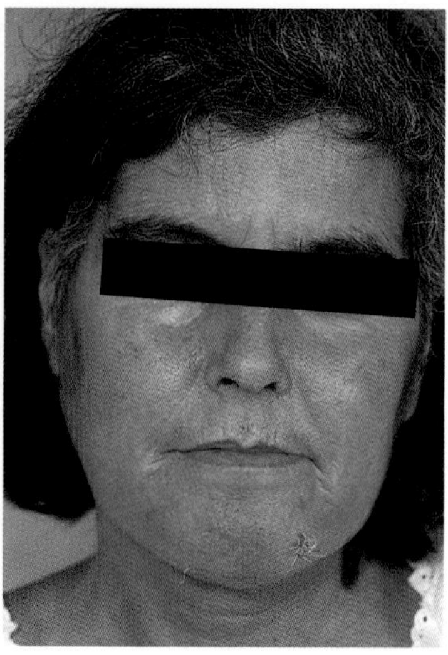

■ **Fig. 12.13** Facial pigmentation associated with primary biliary cirrhosis.

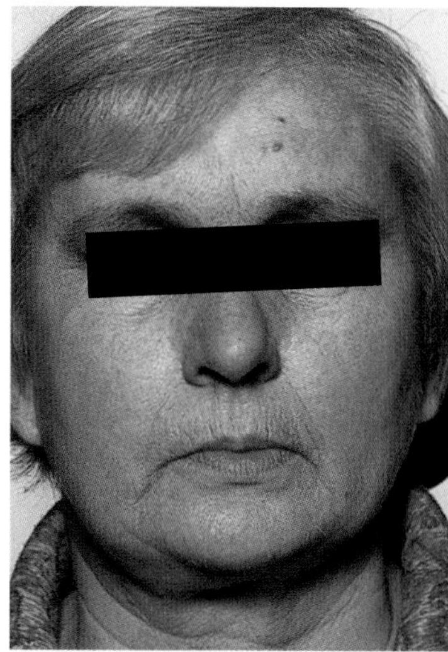

■ **Fig. 12.14** Facial pigmentation in hemochromatosis.

Attenuation of the intrahepatic bile ducts occurs in cirrhosis, and this can be demonstrated by retrograde cholangiography (Fig. 12.23), but this invasive technique is not warranted for diagnostic purposes alone. Ultrasound is a valuable diagnostic tool in portal hypertension. In addition to the coarse parenchymal texture of the liver, it may demonstrate both the presence of ascites and an irregular outline to the liver (Fig. 12.24), but absence of these features by no means excludes the diagnosis.

CT scan or MRI could be used to diagnose advanced cirrhosis, but early cirrhosis (Fig. 12.25a) can be missed on these scans too. Rarely, CT scan may also give an indication of the etiology of liver disease as in hemochromatosis (Fig. 12.25b). MRA and 3D-CT scans could be used to assess patency of hepatic vessels and these scans also may give an indication of the severity of portal hypertension (Figs 12.26, 12.27).

Esophageal varices can be demonstrated by barium swallow (Fig. 12.28) and by CT scanning (Fig. 12.29a–c), but fiber-optic endoscopy is the preferred means of examination, since this can be used to ascertain whether or not varices are bleeding.

Esophageal varices are seen in a third of patients with cirrhosis and bleeding from varices (Fig. 12.30) accounts for a third of deaths in patients with cirrhosis (Fig. 12.31). The size, color, red signs, and hepatic venous wedge pressure gradient are the best predictors of bleeding. The varices could be classified as F0 (none), F1 (small, non-tortuous), F2 (<50% radius, tortuous), and F3 (>50% radius) based on Japanese Association of Portal Hypertension grading (Figs 12.32–12.34). Red color signs including cherry red spots (Fig. 12.35), vale signs (Figs 12.36, 12.37) and hematocystic spots (Fig. 12.38) are highly indicative of imminent bleeding.

Other vascular abnormalities in the gastrointestinal tract may also complicate portal hypertension. Varices are seen in the stomach in 5–15% of patients with cirrhosis (Figs 12.39, 12.40a–c). Large, isolated fundal varices, without esophageal varices, should raise the suspicion of splenic vein thrombosis (Fig. 12.39).

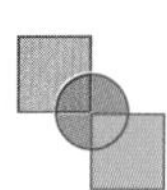

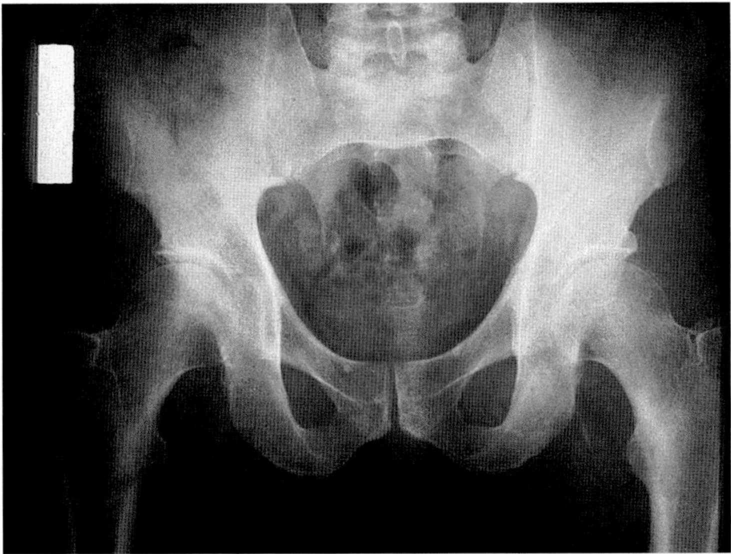

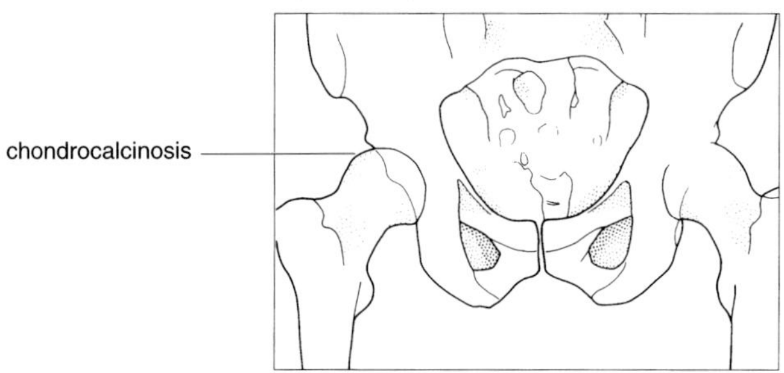

Fig. 12.15 Pelvic X-ray of a patient with primary hemochromatosis showing marked chondrocalcinosis in both hip joints. Courtesy of Dr R.S. Amos.

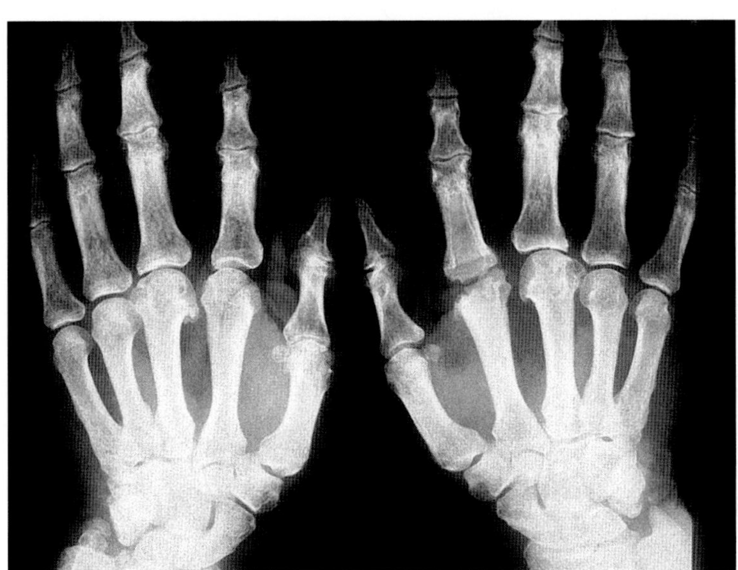

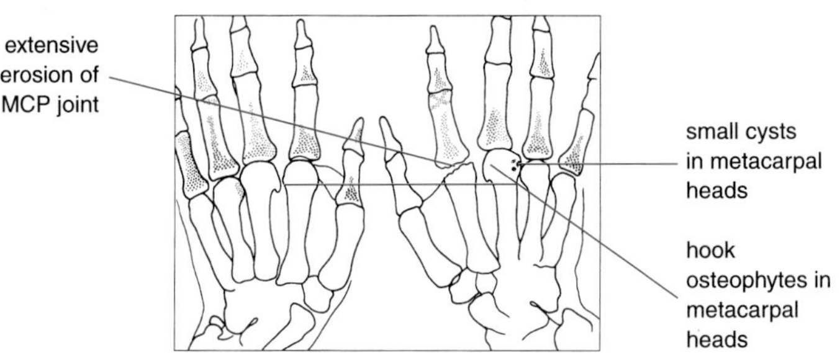

Fig. 12.16 Hand X-rays of a patient with primary hemochromatosis showing typical hook osteophytes and cystic lesions in the metacarpal bones. The erosive changes in the metacarpophalangeal joint of the right index finger are the result of previous surgery. Courtesy of Dr R.S. Amos.

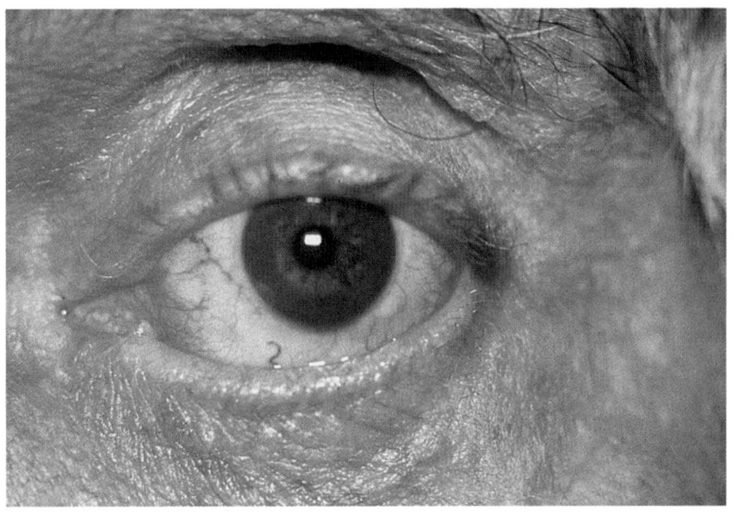

Fig. 12.17 Kayser–Fleischer ring in Wilson's disease. In gross cases such as this the ring of copper is circumferential, while in early cases it is confined to crescents at 12 o'clock and 6 o'clock.

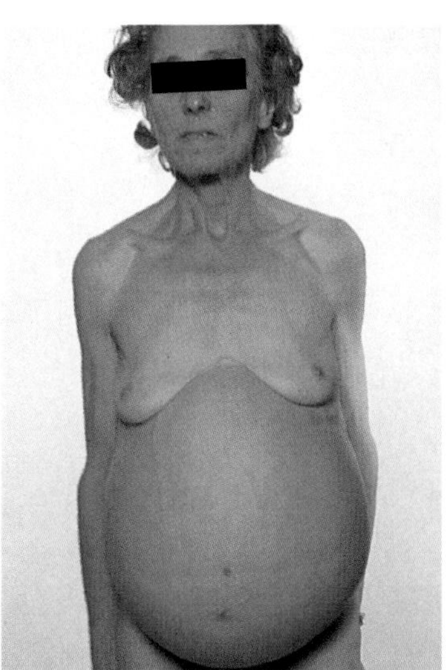

Fig. 12.18 Ascites secondary to portal hypertension. Note the dilated collateral vein running up the right side of the abdomen.

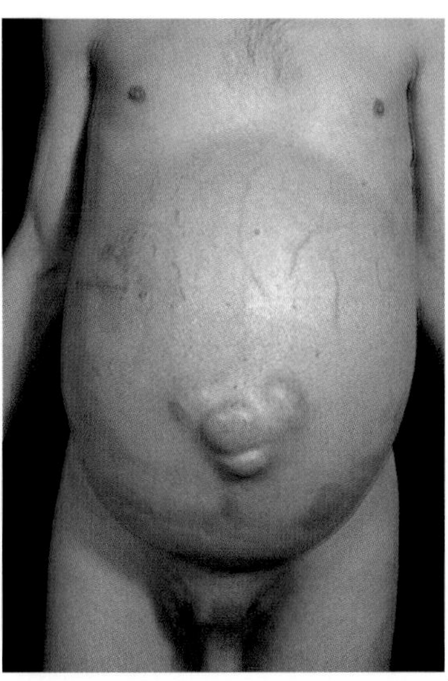

Fig. 12.19 Ascites in a patient with alcoholic cirrhosis showing: distended abdomen; dilated superficial collateral veins; hemorrhagic scratch marks due to pruritus and coagulopathy; umbilical varices; plaster in left iliac fossa indicating diagnostic paracentesis.

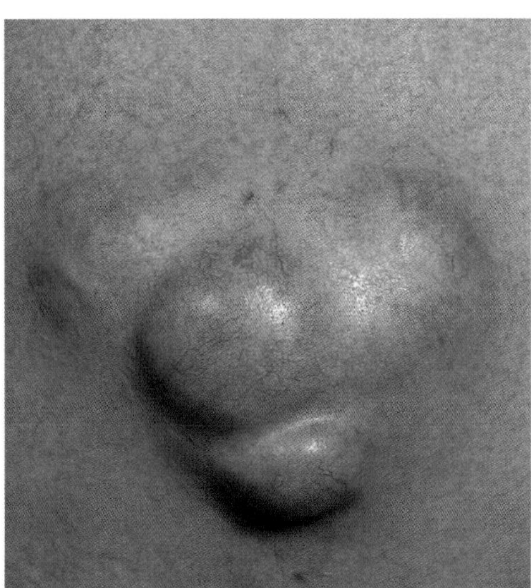

Fig. 12.20 Close-up of umbilical varices. A venous hum was audible over the veins (Cruveilher–Baumgarten murmur).

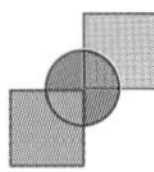

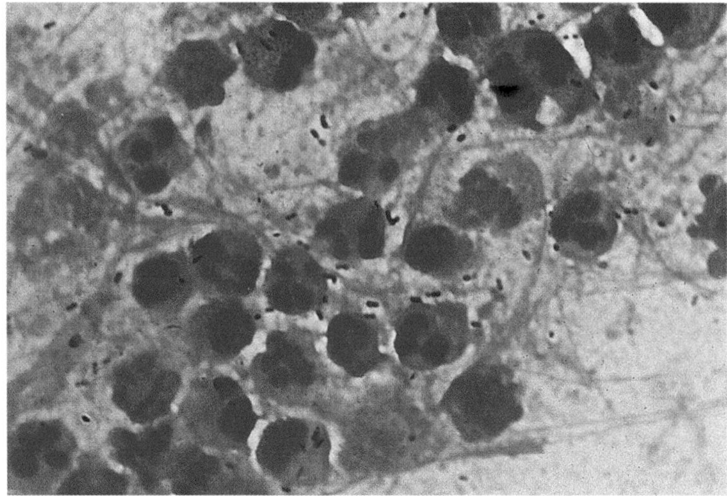

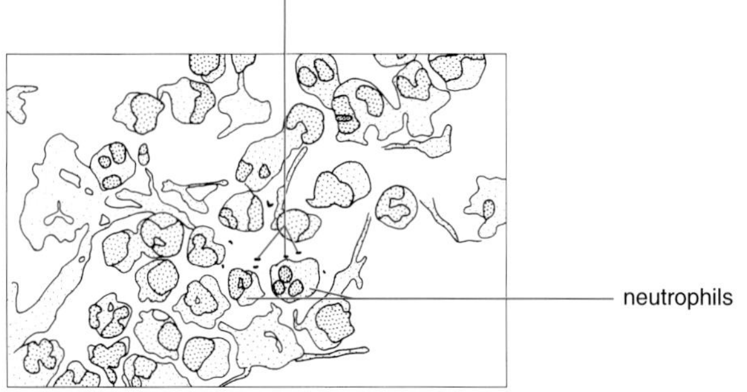

■ **Fig. 12.21** Gram stain of ascitic fluid in spontaneous bacterial peritonitis showing neutrophils and Gram-positive pneumococci.

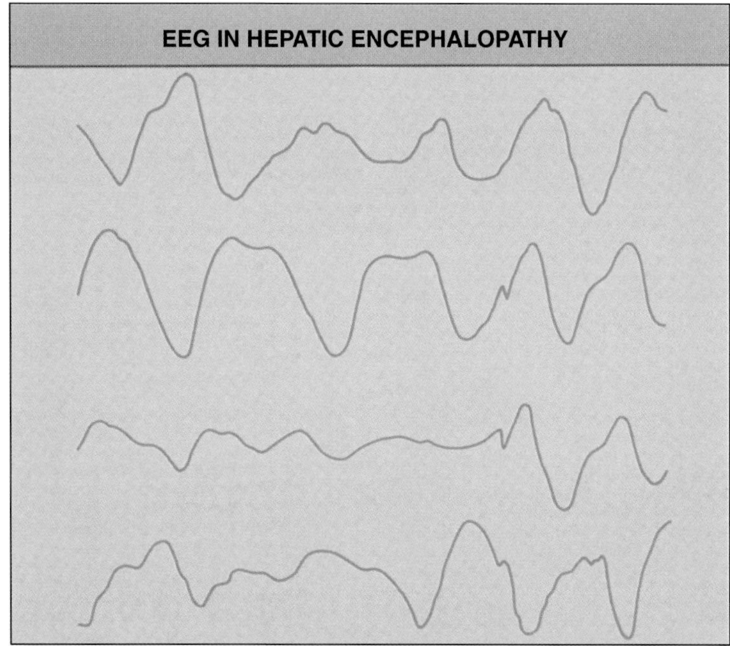

■ **Fig. 12.22** EEG tracing of hepatic encephalopathy. This shows characteristic triphasic electrical activity predominantly over the frontal regions.

Patients with portal hypertension also may develop rectal varices that may appear as an isolated tortuous varix (Fig. 12.41) or as multiple varices (Fig. 12.42), but these are only infrequently the cause of major lower GI bleeding (Fig. 12.43). More proximal true colonic varices are very rare indeed. Anal varices (Fig. 12.44) should not be confused with hemorrhoids (see Chapter 8).

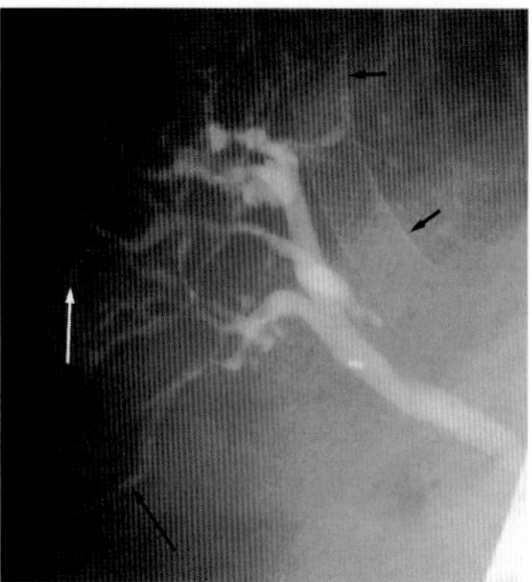

■ **Fig. 12.23** Endoscopic retrograde cholangiogram in a patient with cirrhosis treated by a TIPSS procedure. The peripheral bile ducts have a 'squiggly' contour (white arrow) related to scarring and shrinkage of the liver. The liver is small. A wallstent (short black arrows) bridging the hepatic and portal venous systems is present.

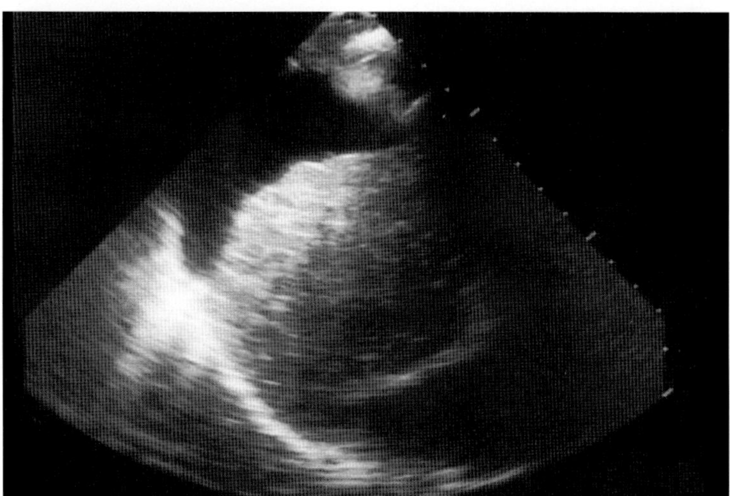

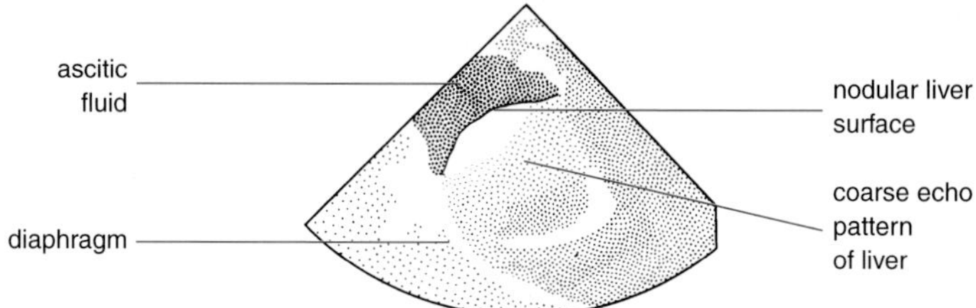

■ **Fig. 12.24** Ultrasonogram of a patient with ascites and cirrhosis. The dark area is the ascitic fluid and the irregular outline of the cirrhotic liver is readily visible. Courtesy of Dr M.C. Collins.

Portal hypertensive gastropathy (PHG) is an increasingly recognized entity, which is commonly found in patients with portal hypertension in whom it will be found in 40–80%. PHG may be classified as mild (Fig. 12.45), moderate (Fig. 12.46), or severe (Fig. 12.47). Mild gastropathy is an asymptomatic clinical observation, but severe changes are associated with a high incidence of hemorrhage.

Less often, patients with portal hypertension may also have gastric antral vascular ectasia (GAVE) (Fig. 12.48). Although these appearances are also seen in the absence of portal hypertension it is not known whether this is a distinct entity or a variant of portal hypertensive gastropathy when seen in patients who do have portal hypertension. Changes similar to PHG are also occasionally seen in other parts of the gastrointestinal system including the colon (Fig. 12.49).

Although macroscopically resembling inflammatory gastritis, portal hypertensive gastropathy is histologically quite different, with dilated mucosal and submucosal vessels and no significant inflammatory infiltrate (Fig. 12.50).

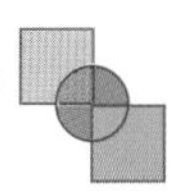

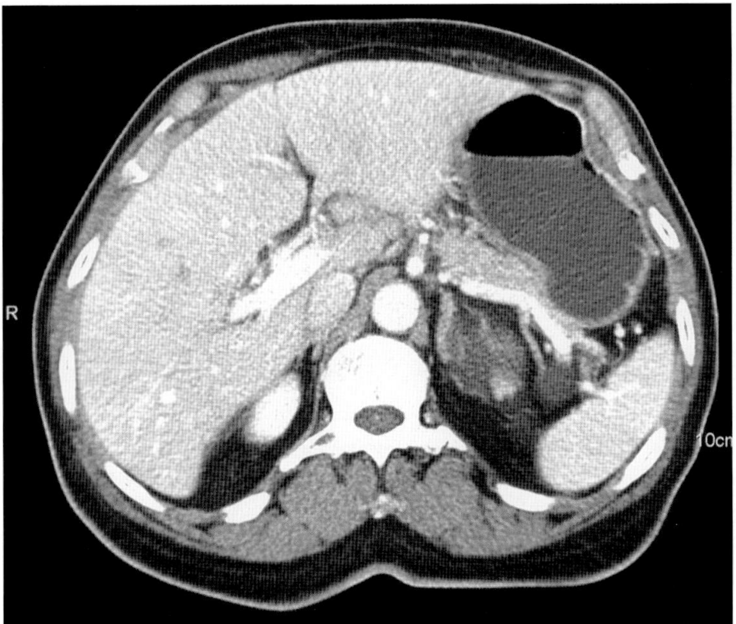

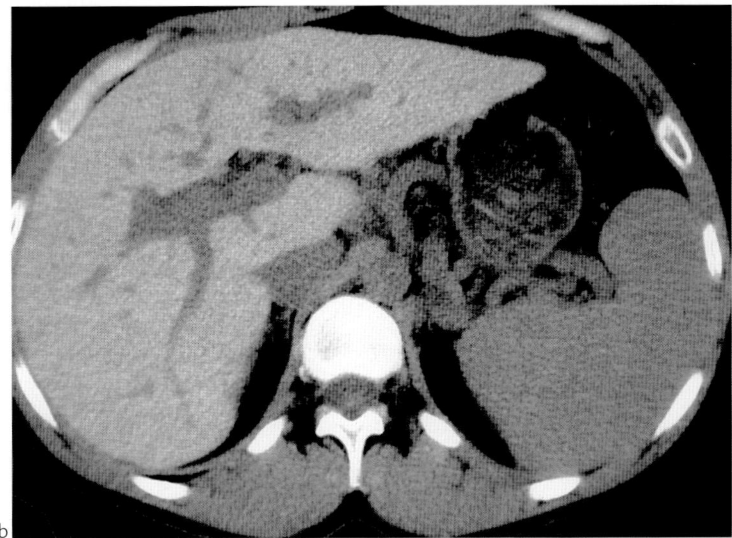

■ **Fig. 12.25** (a) CT scan indicating the earliest features of cirrhosis as judged from a slightly small liver with a disordered parenchymal pattern; the diagnosis was confirmed histologically. (b) CT scan showing the contrast distinctions that permit a radiological working diagnosis of hemochromatosis (which was again confirmed histologically); note in particular the relative density of the liver and spleen as compared to the differential in Fig 12.25a.

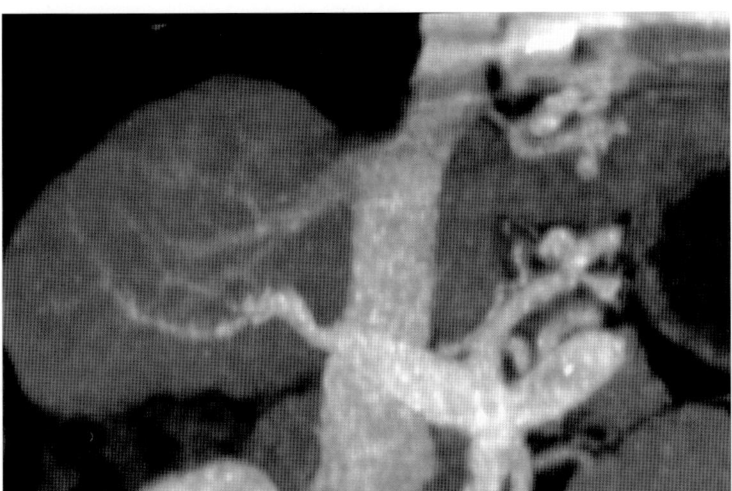

■ **Fig. 12.26** MR angiography showing portal hypertension with collaterals. The shrunken liver and collateral circulation is obvious.

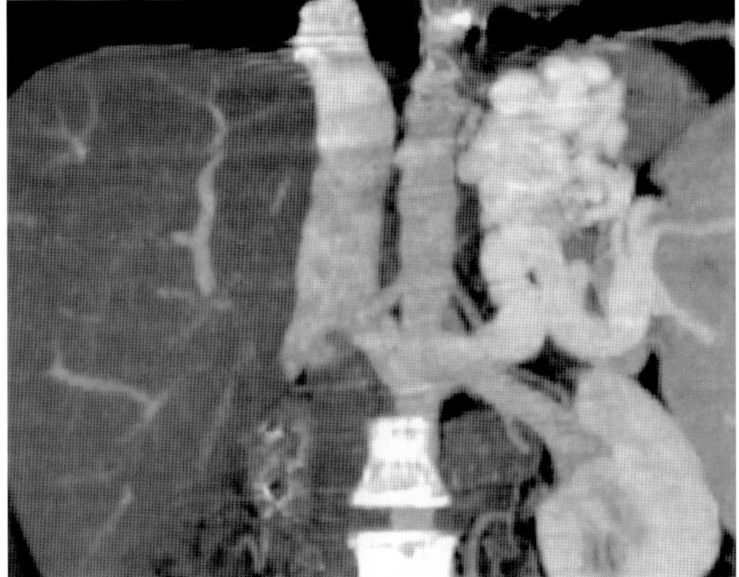

■ **Fig. 12.27** MR of another patient with portal hypertension and collaterals in whom huge varices are apparent.

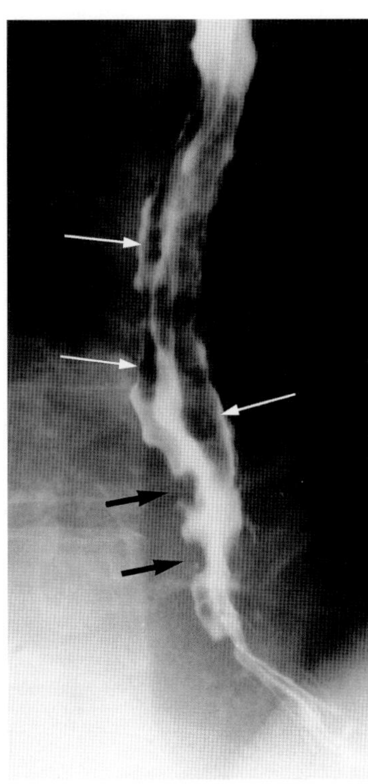

■ **Fig. 12.28** Single-contrast esophagram demonstrating esophageal varices. Smooth, coarsely lobulated folds are seen both *en-face* (white arrows) and in profile (black arrows) in the distal esophagus.

Several techniques are available for investigating the dilated portal venous system in portal hypertension. CT scanning may reveal dilated para-esophageal or parasplenic veins, and intervascular shunts, as well as confirming the presence of ascites (Figs 12.51, 12.52). CT scanning can also be helpful in the demonstration of changes that are not due to cirrhosis such as the 'pseudo-cirrhosis' that is occasionally seen with metastases and their treatment (Figs 12.53a, b). There must be some degree of additional caution when using contrast media in patients with advanced liver disease since these are known to pose a significant risk of provoking hepatorenal syndrome.

Ultrasound is useful in assessing the size of the portal vein, while Doppler ultrasonography can identify both the patency and direc-

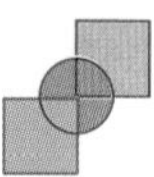

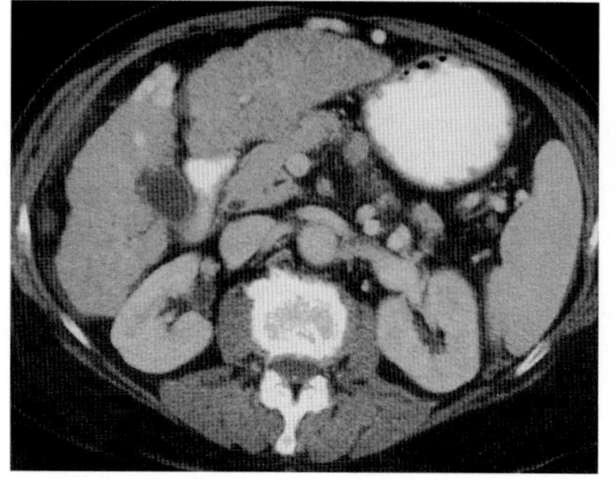

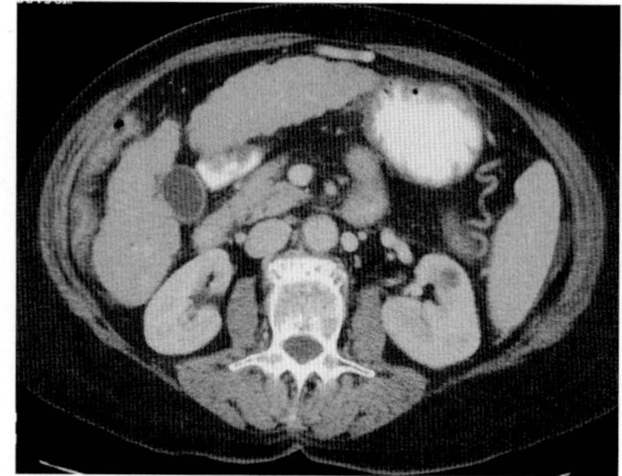

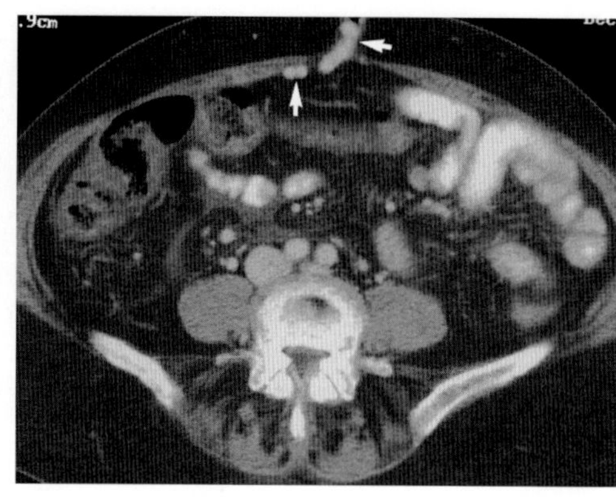

a

b

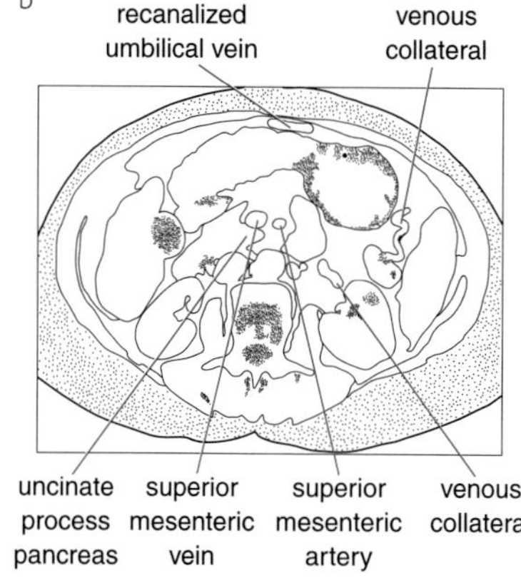

c

■ **Fig. 12.29** (a–c) CT demonstrating moderately severe cirrhosis with a small lobulated liver, with the presence of varices and a recanalized umbilical vein (arrows in (c)).

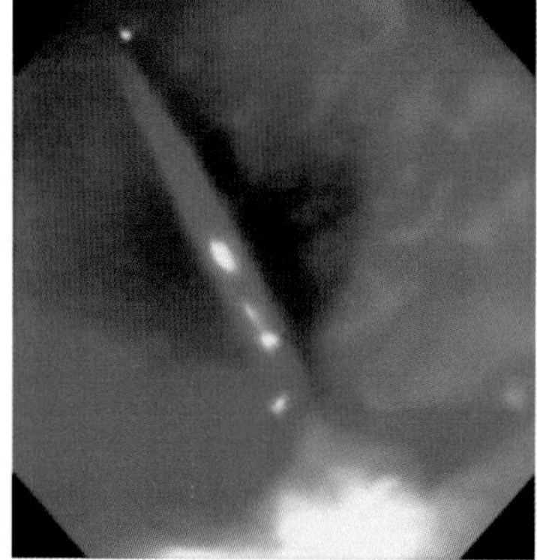

■ **Fig. 12.30** Endoscopic appearance of an actively bleeding varix.

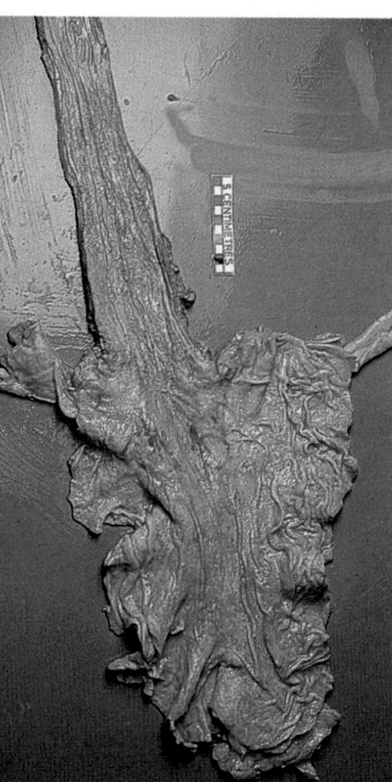

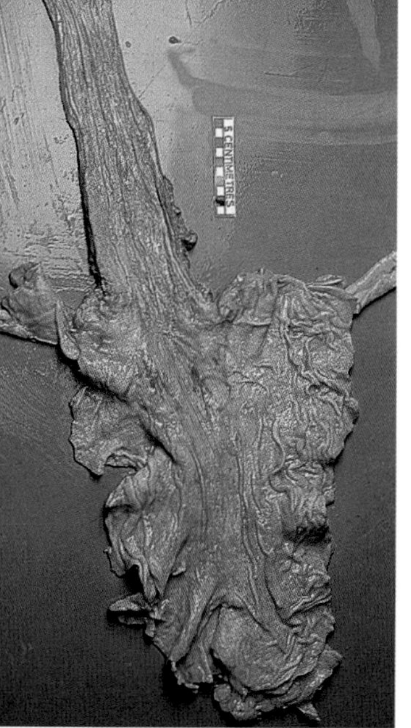

■ **Fig. 12.31** Autopsy view of esophageal varices.

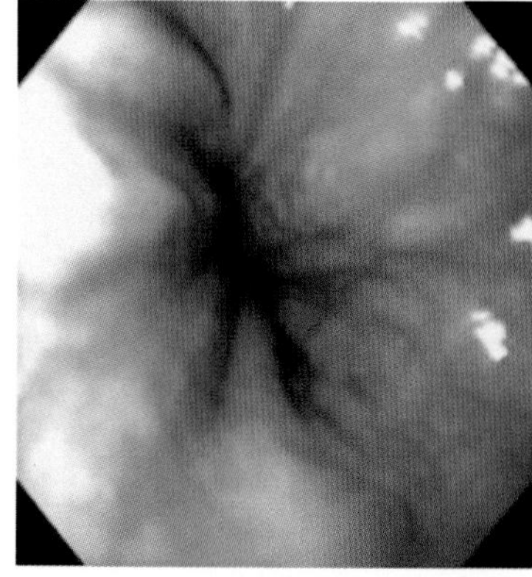

■ **Fig. 12.32** Early small (F1) varices.

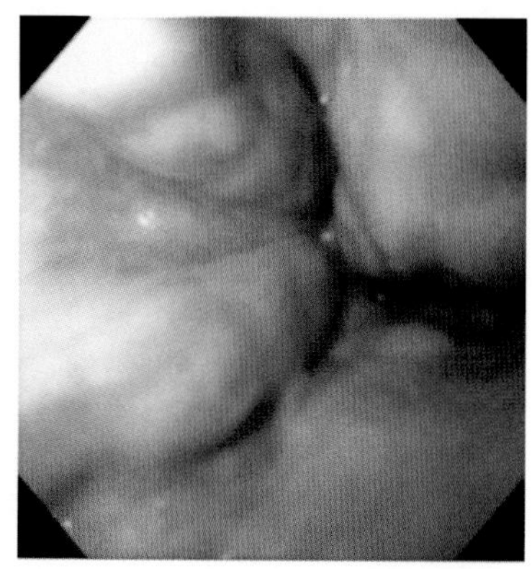

■ **Fig. 12.33** Larger tortuous (F2) varices.

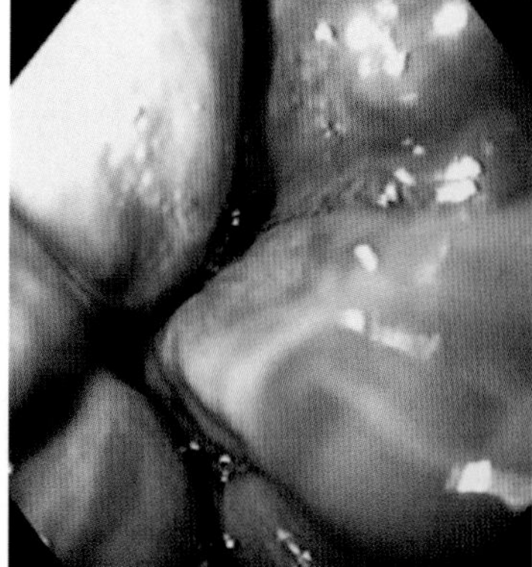

■ **Fig. 12.34** Major (F3) varices encompassing more than 50% of the radius of the esophagus which have the highest risk of bleeding.

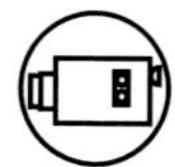

tion of portal venous blood flow (Figs 12.54, 12.55). Delineation of the venous collaterals can be achieved by percutaneous splenic venography but this hazardous technique is now rarely performed (Fig. 12.56). Injection of contrast material into the splenic or superior mesenteric artery, followed by late venous phase pictures, is less satisfactory in portal hypertension, due to the dilution of the contrast material, but it can still be useful in identifying venous abnormalities (Fig. 12.57).

Radioisotopic scintigraphy using labeled technetium sulfur colloid in cirrhosis shows diversion of the colloid away from the liver with increased uptake in the spleen and bone marrow (Fig. 12.58). Its use has declined considerably in recent years with the advent of ultrasound and CT scanning.

The mottled irregular liver surface of cirrhosis is readily demonstrable on laparoscopy (Figs 12.59, 12.60). This technique is widely used in certain countries, and enables a confident diagnosis of cirrhosis to be made when needle biopsy samples may be equivocal or inadequate.

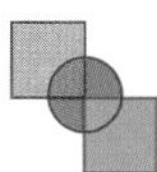

PRIMARY BILIARY CIRRHOSIS

The pathological changes of primary biliary cirrhosis are commonly divided into four stages. Stage one is the florid duct lesion. The septal and large interlobular bile ducts are damaged, but smaller portal tracts are normal. Affected ducts have atypical epithelium that may be disrupted. An infiltrate of lymphocytes and plasma cells occurs in the portal tracts adjacent to the ducts (Fig. 12.61). The lymphocytes can form follicles, and granulomas occur within the portal tracts (Fig. 12.62). The hepatic lobule shows minimal abnormality at this stage.

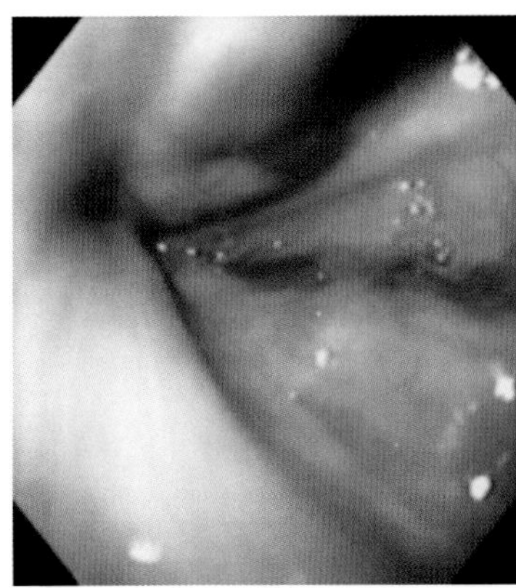

Fig. 12.37 Another example of the vale sign.

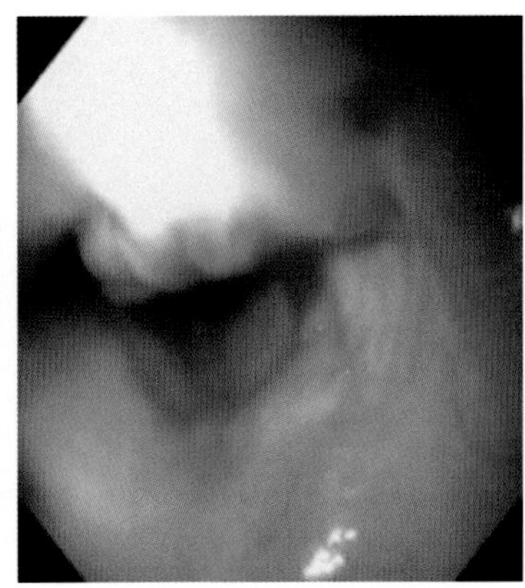

Fig. 12.38 The hematocystic spot but with a very high risk of bleeding.

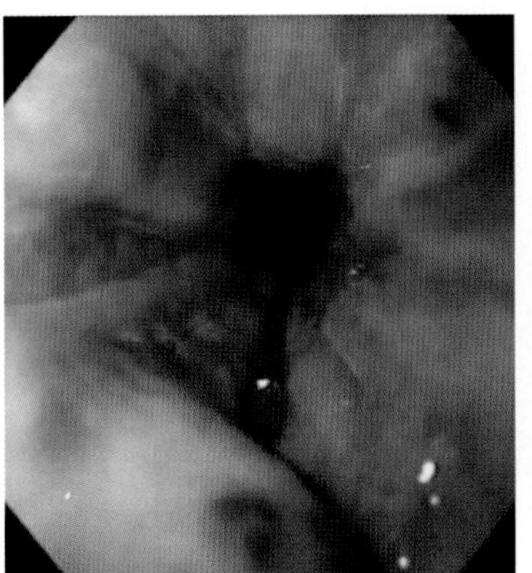

Fig. 12.35 Cherry red spots associated with varices.

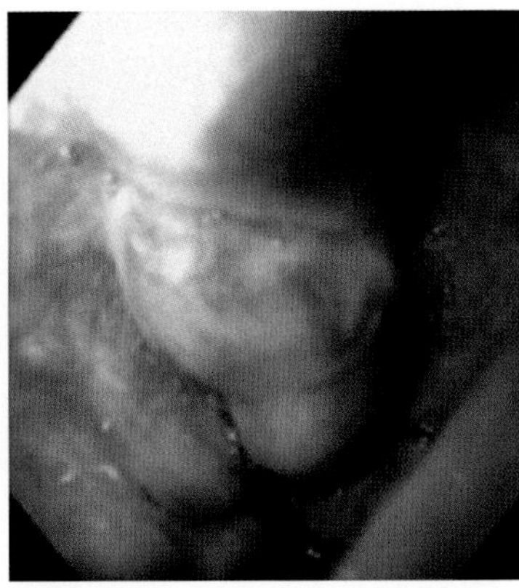

Fig. 12.36 The so-called vale signs of conformational change associated with high risk of variceal bleeding.

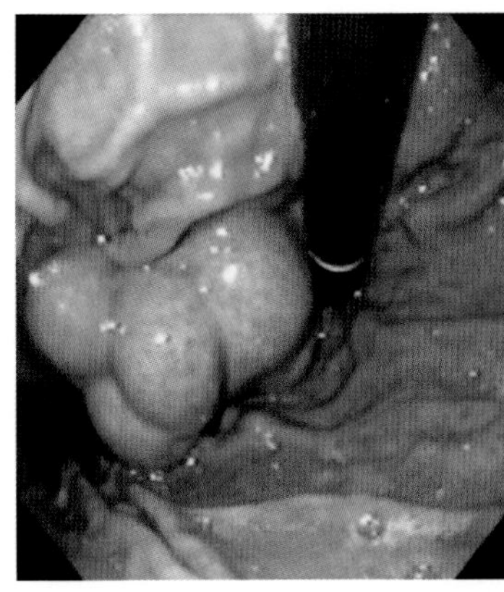

Fig. 12.39 Endoscopic view of large fundal varices. In this case the cause was splenic vein thrombosis and there were no esophageal varices.

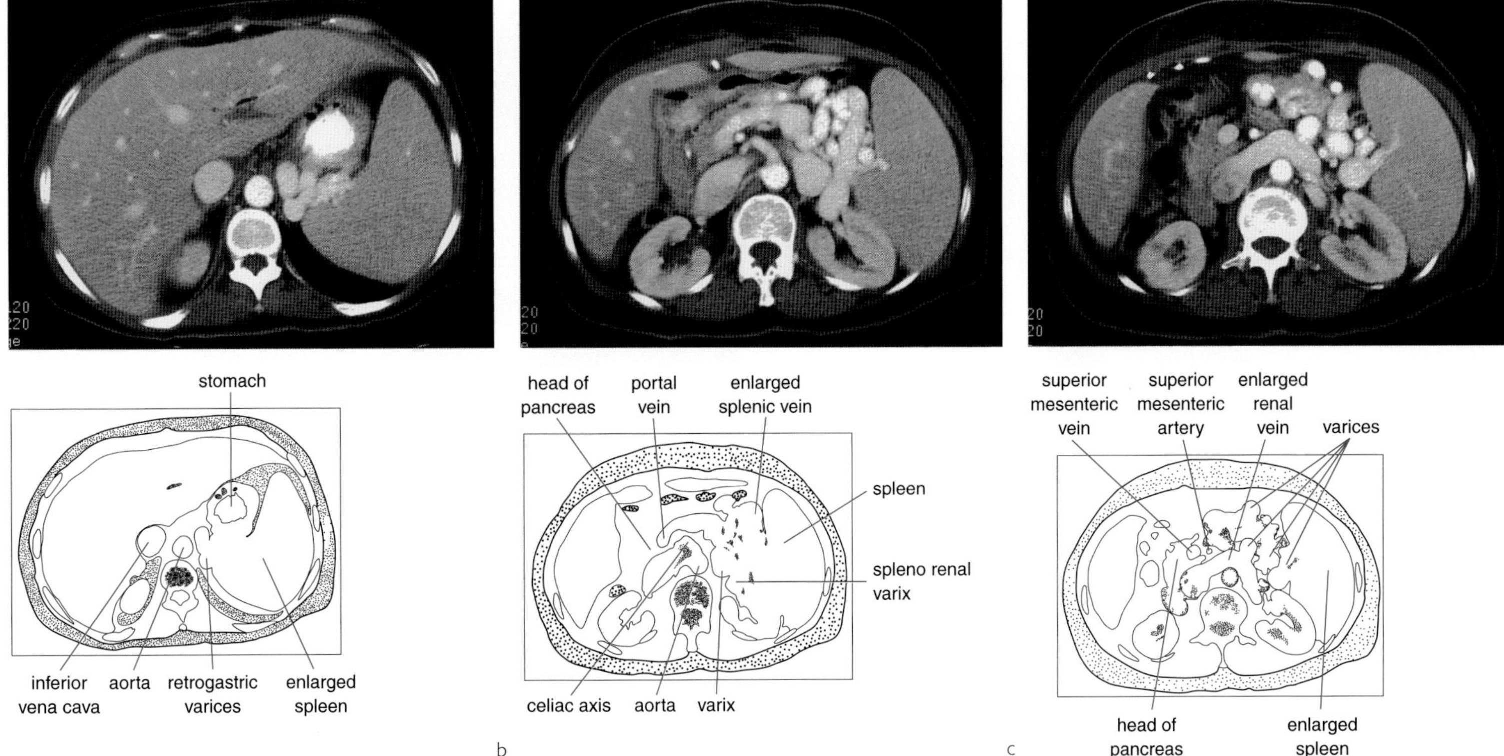

Fig. 12.40 (a–c) CT scan demonstrating perigastric varices. The CT demonstrates a relatively normal-appearing liver in a patient with mild cirrhosis. There is, however, moderate splenomegaly and numerous varices in the perigastric (a) and splenic hilar (b, c) regions. A spontaneous splenorenal shunt is present resulting in a dilated left renal vein.

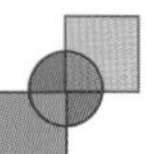

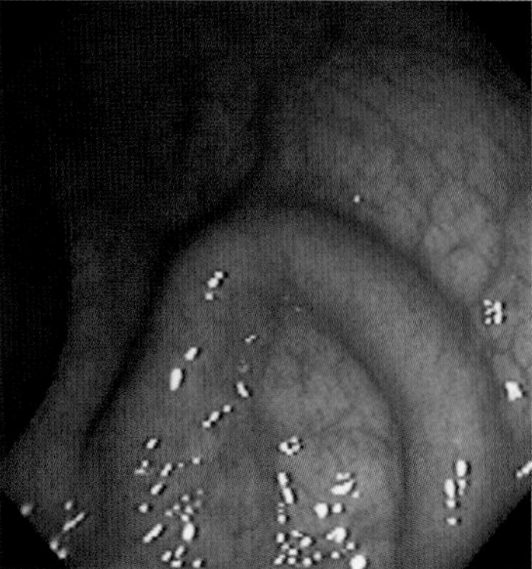

■ **Fig. 12.41** Rectal varices, appearing here as an isolated tortuous varix.

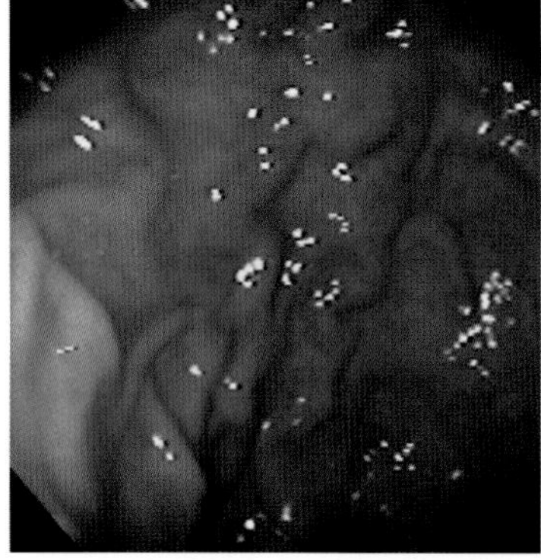

■ **Fig. 12.42** Multiple rectal varices.

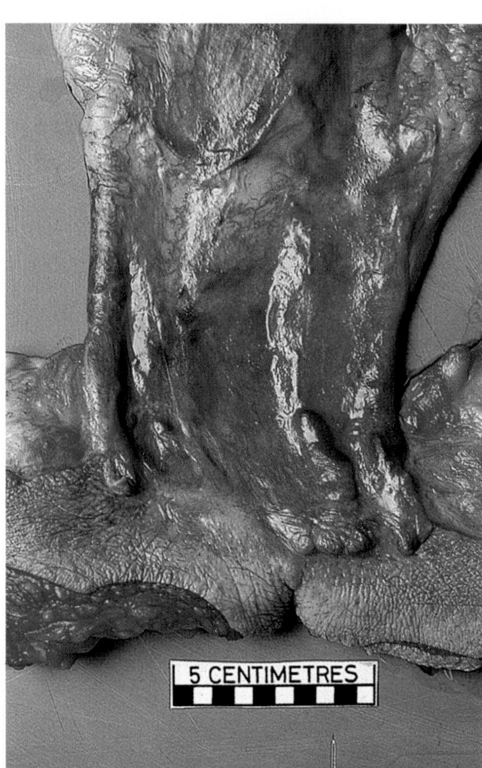

■ **Fig. 12.43** Post-mortem demonstration of rectal varices.

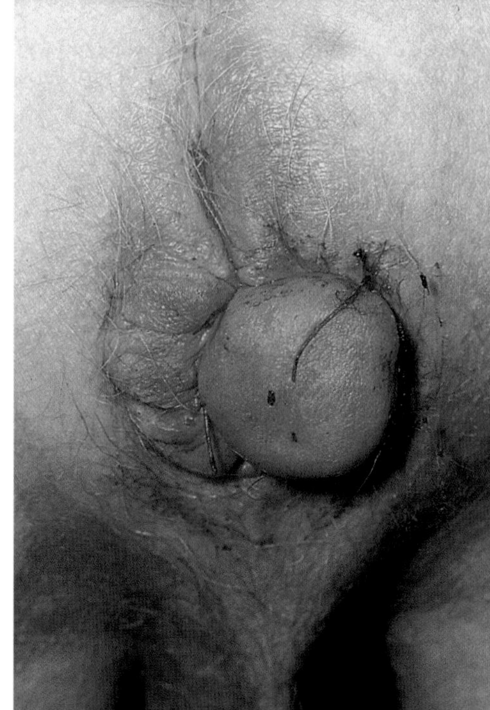

■ **Fig. 12.44** External view of anal varices.

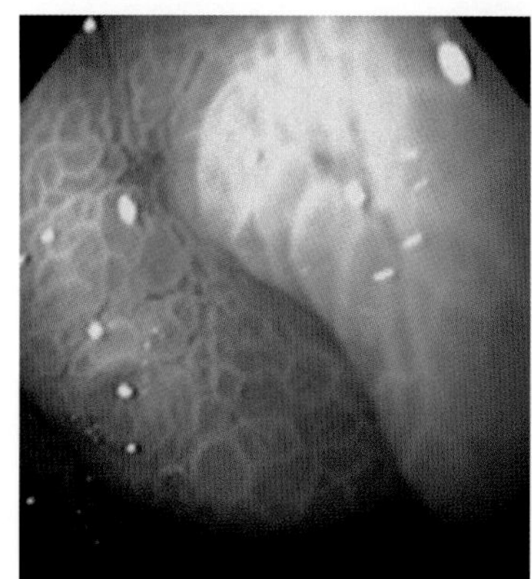

■ **Fig. 12.45** The earliest endoscopic features of mild portal hypertensive gastropathy.

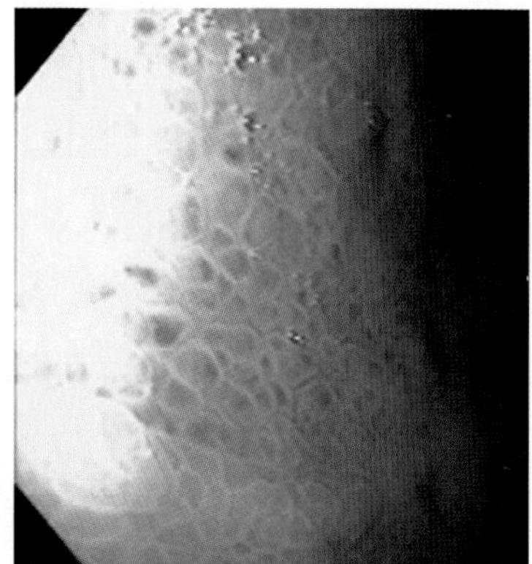

■ **Fig. 12.46** Moderate portal hypertensive gastropathy.

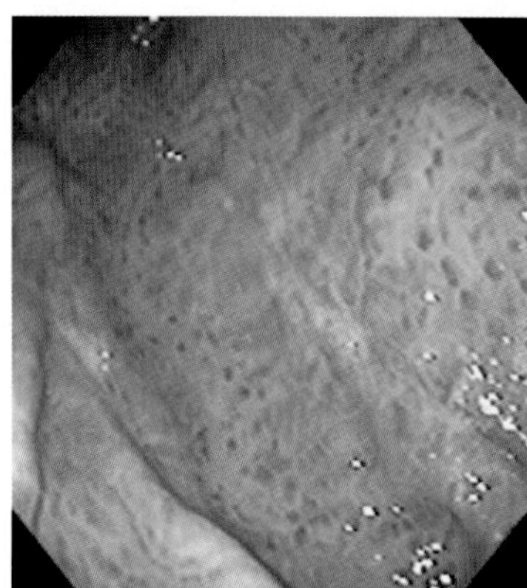

■ **Fig. 12.47** Severe portal hypertensive gastropathy.

In the second stage, that of duct proliferation, the periductal inflammation regresses and the number of bile ducts diminishes. However, there is proliferation of atypical peripheral ductules in the portal tracts. The limiting plate between tract and lobule now becomes involved in the inflammatory process, with piecemeal necrosis. Cholestasis also occurs and is often periportal. With greater lobular inflammation and piecemeal necrosis, the picture is hard to distinguish from chronic aggressive hepatitis. The lymphoid aggregates within the portal tract marking the sites of former bile ducts (Fig. 12.63) are the diagnostic feature. The third and fourth stages represent scarring and cirrhosis (Fig. 12.64) with extension of fibrosis outward from the tracts. Accumulation of copper in periportal and periseptal hepatocytes is a frequent finding; this

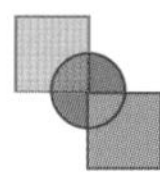

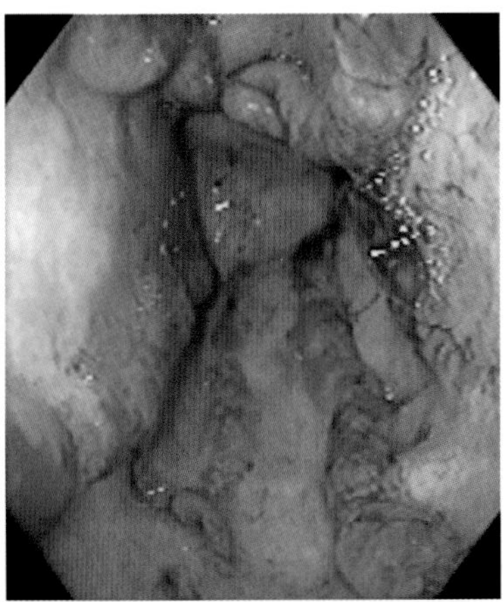

Fig. 12.48 Gastric antral vascular ectasia.

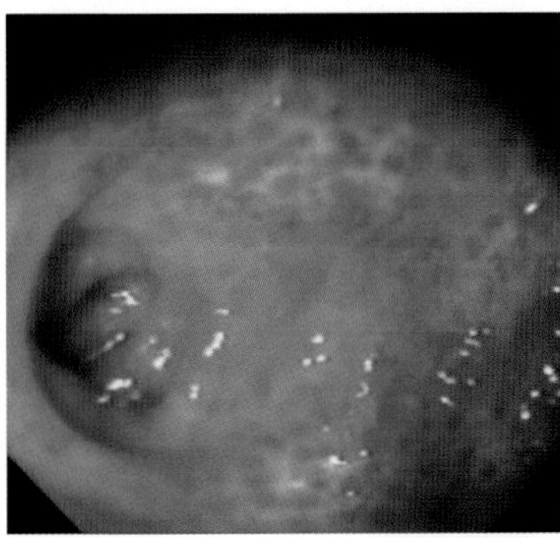

Fig. 12.49 Vascular changes which have been termed the colonic equivalent of portal hypertensive gastropathy.

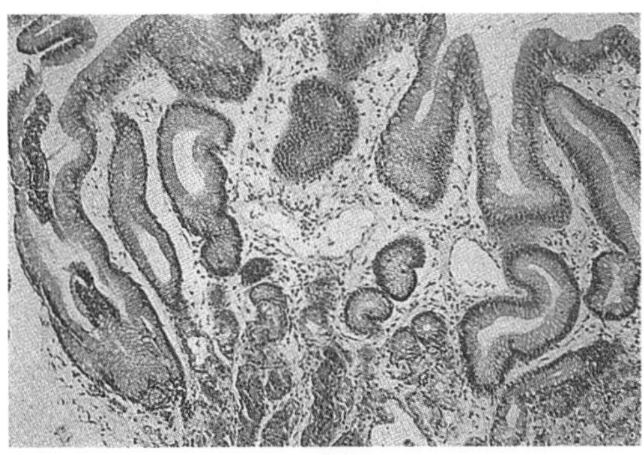

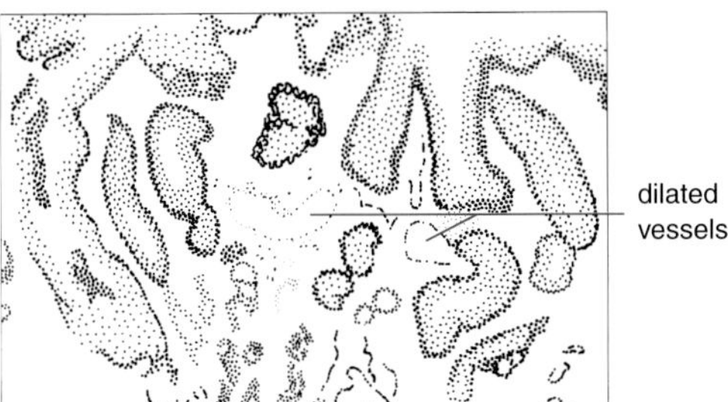

Fig. 12.50 Gastric biopsy in portal hypertension showing dilated mucosal and submucosal vessels. Despite the macroscopic reddened mucosa there is no inflammatory infiltrate. H&E stain.

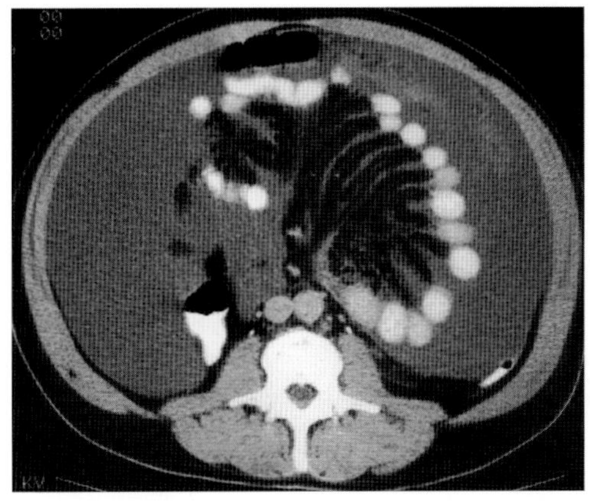

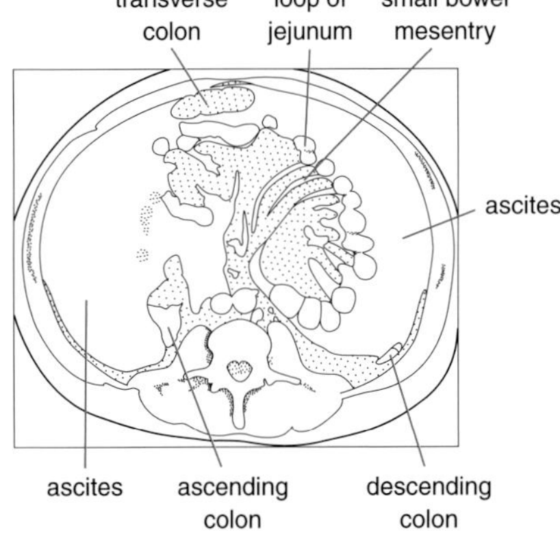

Fig. 12.51 CT demonstrating marked ascites and the leaves of the small bowel mesentery.

left anterior perihepatic space
body of pancreas
stomach
fluid in lesser sac
splenic flexure of colon
spleen
splenic vein
tail of pancreas

Fig. 12.52 CT demonstrating ascites in the left anterior perihepatic space and in the lesser sac (lesser omental bursa).

merely reflects cholestasis (Fig. 12.65). Mallory's hyaline is occasionally found in primary biliary cirrhosis.

CONGENITAL HEPATIC FIBROSIS AND CYSTS

In congenital fibrosis the liver is usually enlarged, firm and has a fine reticular pattern of fibrosis. Cysts are unusual but they can be associated with bile duct abnormalities. Histology shows diffuse periportal and perilobular fibrous bands (Fig. 12.66). The isolated parenchyma maintains a normal architecture, and there is little inflammation. Bile duct proliferation is present in the fibrous tracts, with mild ductular dilatation. Congenital hepatic fibrosis is occasionally associated with abnormalities of the renal tract, including medullary sponge kidney and polycystic disease.

Cysts of the liver can be solitary or multiple. When solitary cysts of the liver occur, 95% are unilocular and 5% multilocular. They are lined by a single layer of columnar epithelium. Polycystic disease of the liver is divided into adult or childhood varieties. In the childhood type, small cysts are usually visible macroscopically (Fig. 12.67). Histologically the cysts are derived from branches of

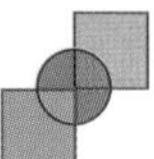

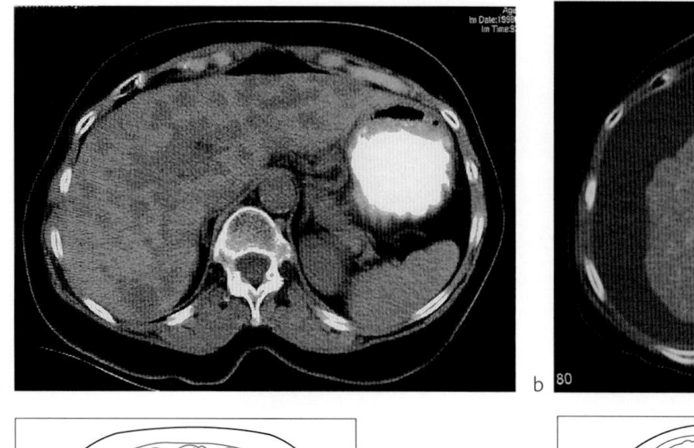

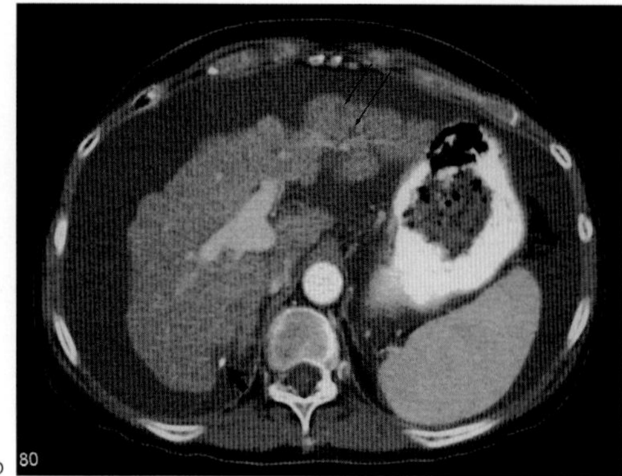

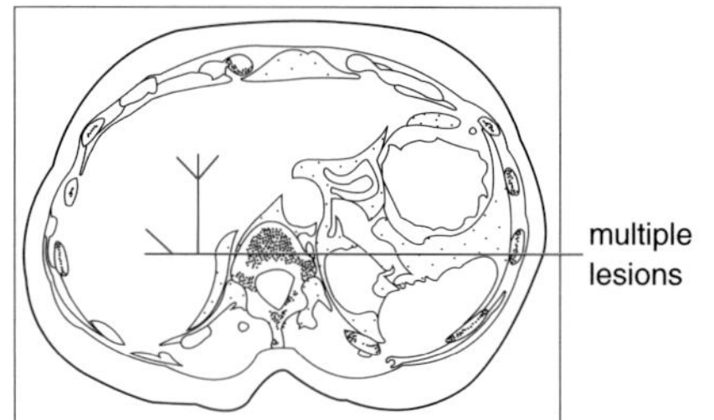

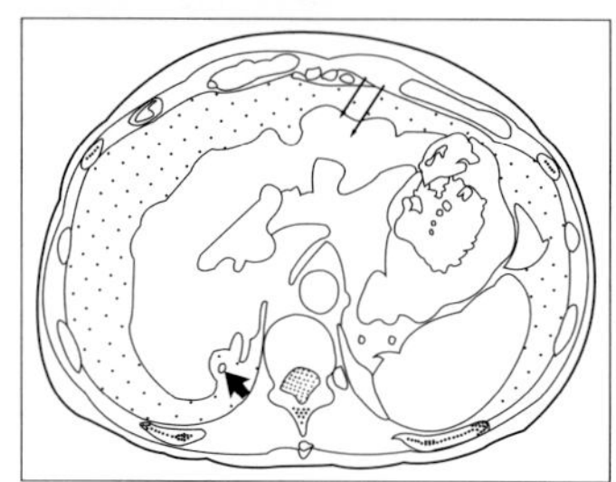

Fig. 12.53 CT demonstrating 'pseudocirrhosis' due to treated breast cancer. (a) Unenhanced CT of liver shows numerous 0.5–2.0 cm low-attenuation masses throughout the liver. (b) Several years after chemotherapy, an enhanced CT of the liver shows marked regression of metastatic disease. A few tiny low-attenuation lesions (thin arrows) are seen. One is focally calcified (thick arrow). The liver is now shrunken with a coarsely lobulated contour. Ascites is present.

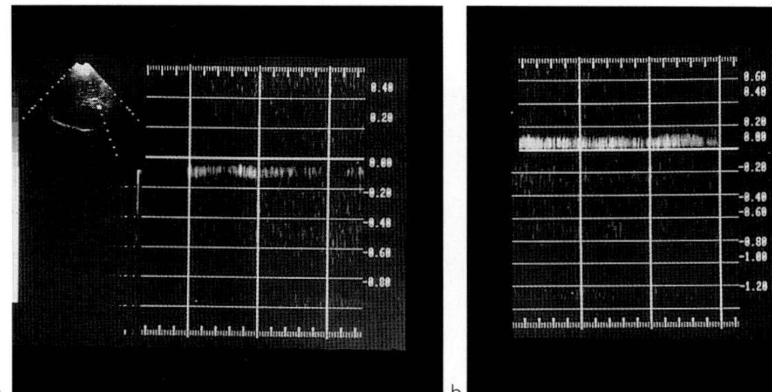

Fig. 12.54 Doppler ultrasound showing direction of blood flow in the portal vein. The cursor to the extreme left indicates the plane of measurement. (a) shows hepatofugal (retrograde) flow in contrast to the normal hepatopedal flow (b). Courtesy of Dr M.C. Collins.

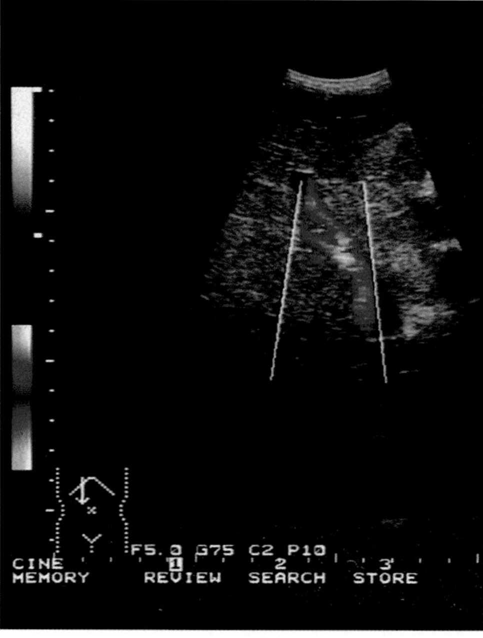

Fig. 12.55 Color Doppler ultrasound showing normal portal vein blood flow. The color signal indicates the rate/direction of flow, red being normal forward flow. Courtesy of Dr M.C. Collins.

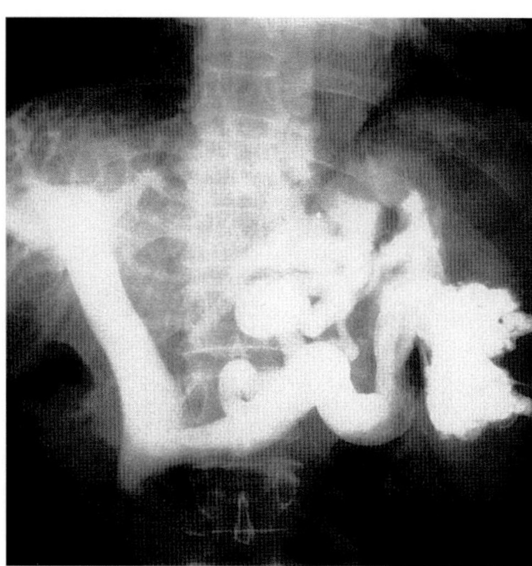

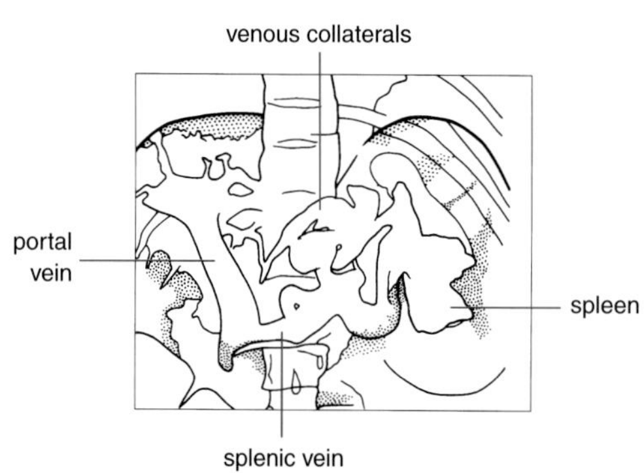

Fig. 12.56 Dilated portal vein and venous collaterals demonstrated by splenoportography. Courtesy of Prof A.P. Hemingway.

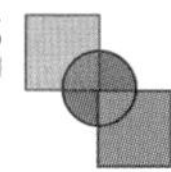

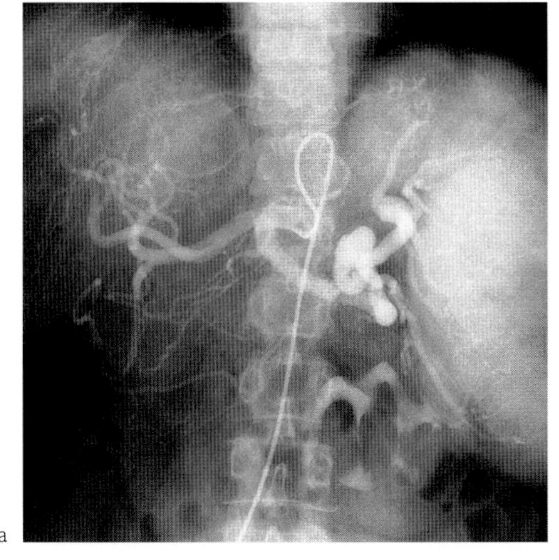

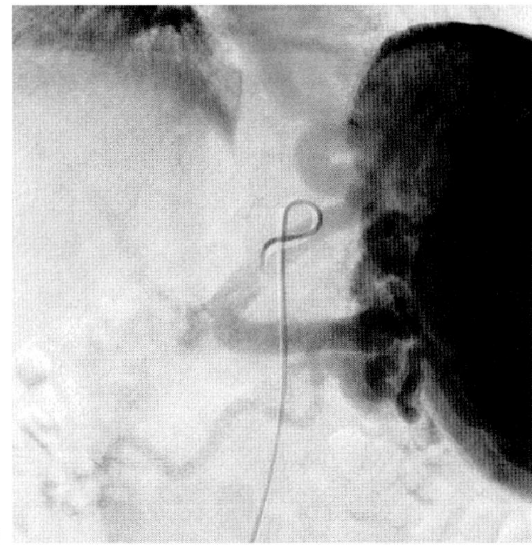

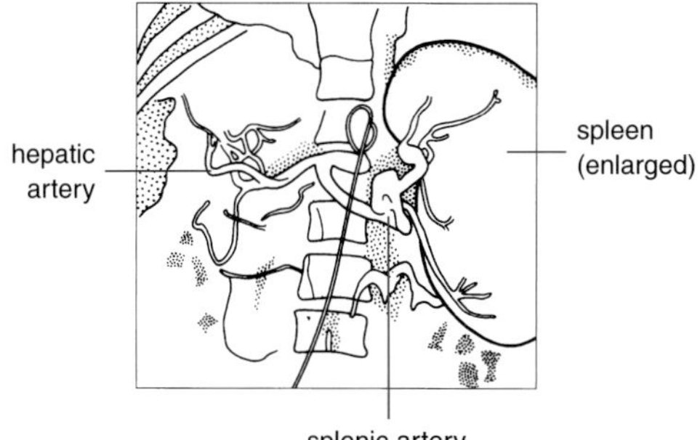

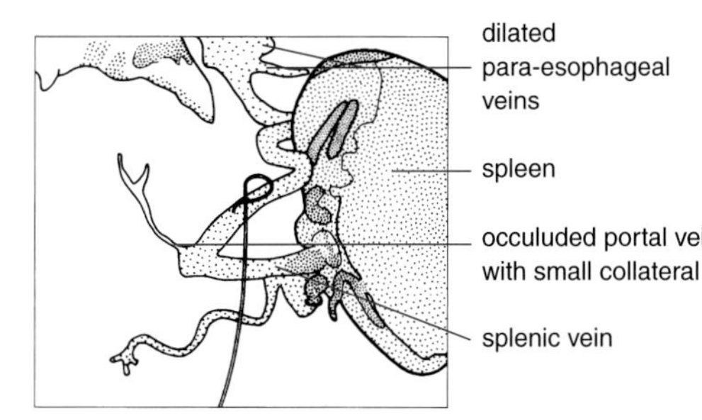

Fig. 12.57 Celiac angiography of a patient with cirrhosis, portal venous occlusion, and portal hypertension. Note the abnormal intrahepatic vessels and enlarged spleen following arterial injection (a). The venous phase (b) shows portal vein obstruction together with dilated para-esophageal veins. Courtesy of Prof A.P. Hemingway.

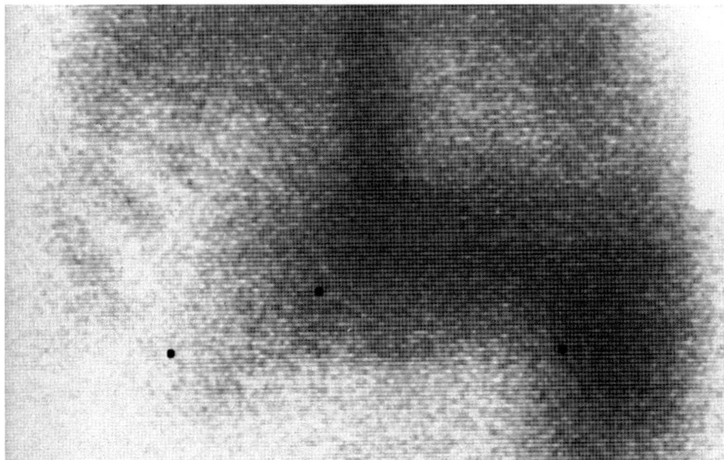

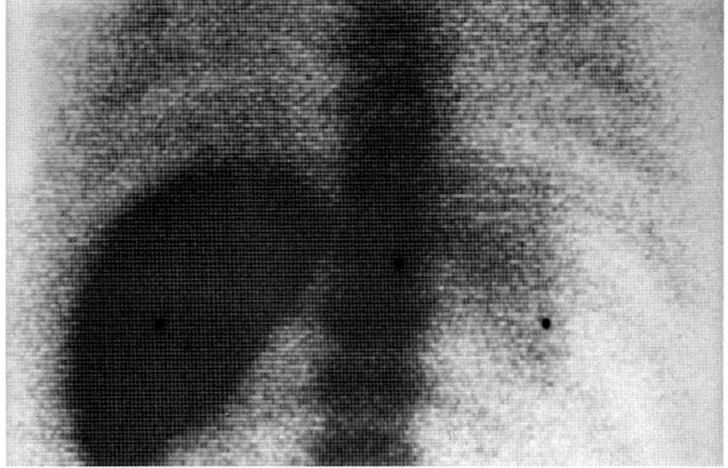

Fig. 12.58 Technetium sulfur colloid scan showing anterior (a) and posterior (b) views in a patient with severe alcoholic hepatitis and cirrhosis. There is virtually no uptake of isotope by the liver, with consequent diversion to the vertebrae and ribs and enlarged spleen.

dilated bile ducts. The disease occurs in association with renal polycystic disease (Fig. 12.68), which is a different variety from that seen in association with congenital hepatic fibrosis. Multiple congenital cysts in the liver may be found by chance during surgery, or can produce huge enlargement of the liver with larger cysts and filling defects on scintigraphy (Fig. 12.69a). The topographical limitations of ultrasonography make it difficult to encompass all of these lesions in other than composite scans (Fig. 12.69b), and CT may prove the most suitable specific technique for confirming the diagnosis (Fig 12.70, 12.71). The liver is diffusely cystic and cysts may measure up to 10–12 cm in diameter; the cysts have a flat epithelial lining. Microhamartomata (Von Meyenberg complexes), are tiny periportal collections of dilated ducts which are often found incidentally in biopsy or autopsy specimens, representing one end of the spectrum of cystic disease.

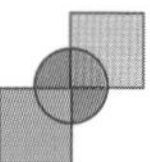

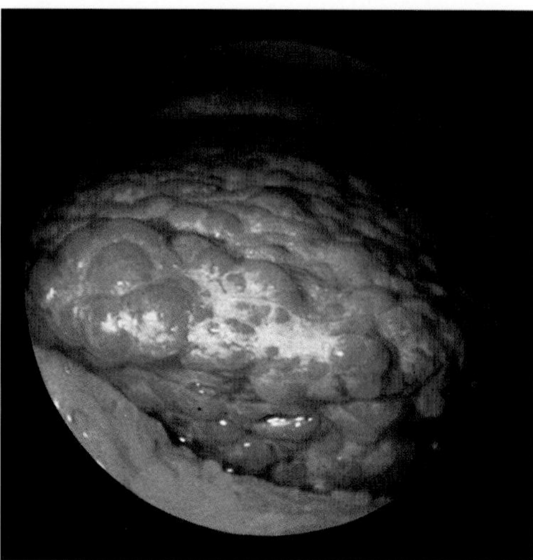

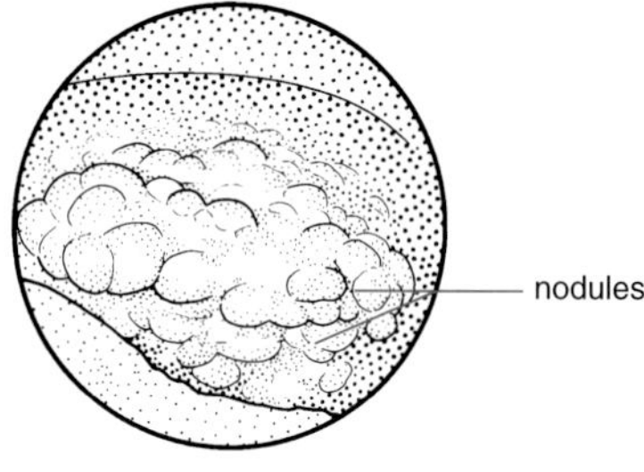

■ **Fig. 12.59** Laparoscopic view of the surface of a nodular cirrhotic liver.

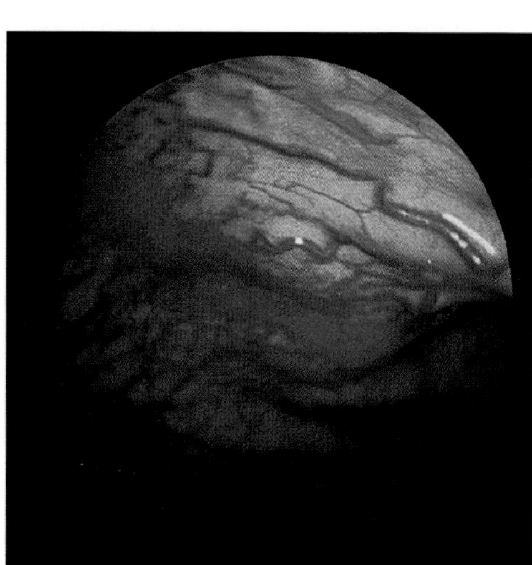

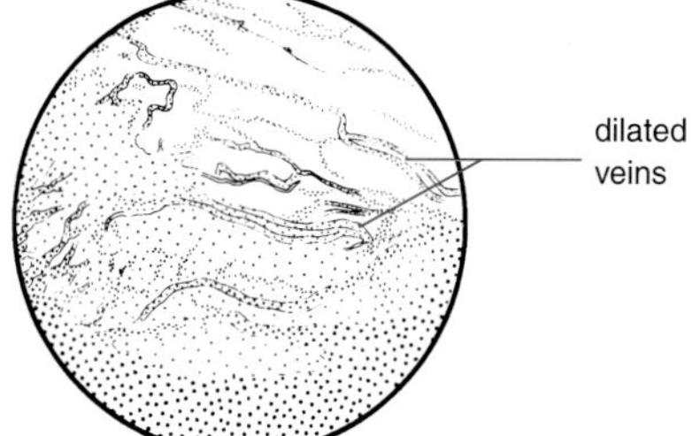

■ **Fig. 12.60** Laparoscopic view of dilated peritoneal veins in portal hypertension.

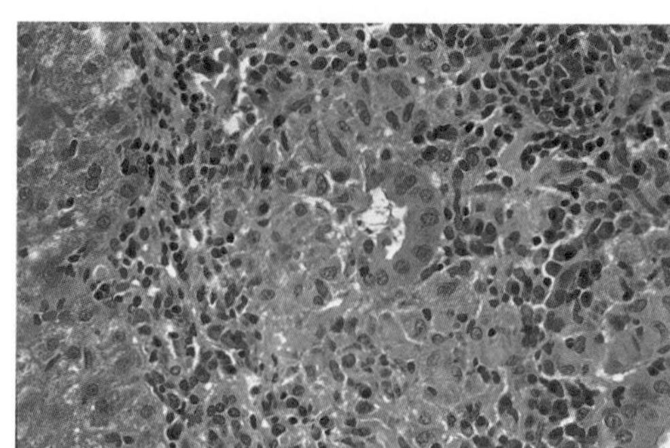

■ **Fig. 12.61** Primary biliary cirrhosis, stage 1. Microscopic view of the first stage of primary biliary cirrhosis showing a duct-destructive lesion with a granulomatous histiocytic reaction associated with the injured, disrupted biliary epithelium.

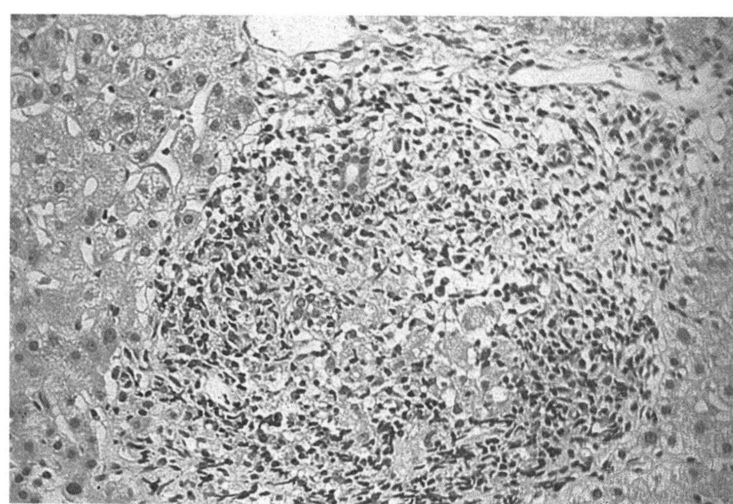

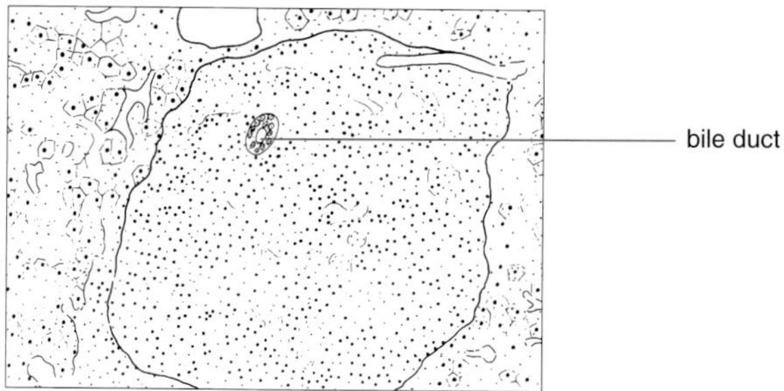

■ **Fig. 12.62** Primary biliary cirrhosis, stage 2. Microscopic view of the second stage of primary biliary cirrhosis showing an irregular portal tract that is markedly expanded by a dense lymphoplasmacytic infiltrate, and lacks a bile duct, but contains a proliferation of small ductules, many of which are immature and lack lumens, at the periphery. H&E stain (x 180). Courtesy of Prof I. Talbot.

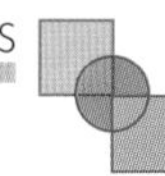

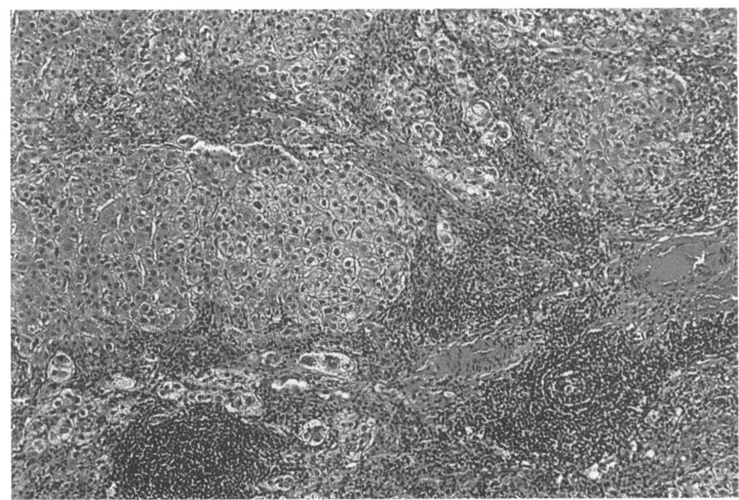

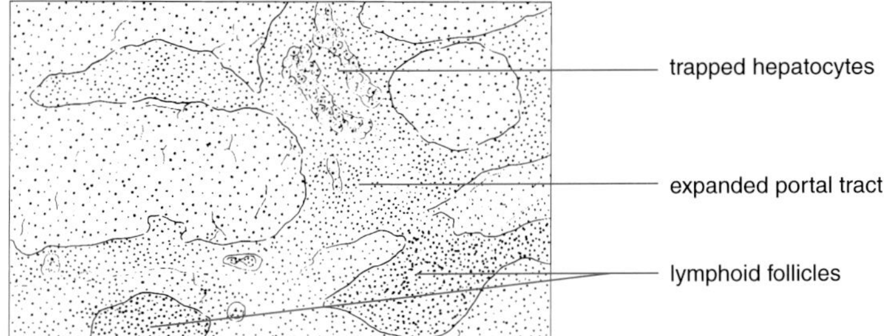

■ **Fig. 12.63** Liver histology showing the second stage of primary biliary cirrhosis. Lymphoid follicles mark the site of destroyed bile ducts, and piecemeal necrosis has trapped hepatocytes. H&E stain (x 75).

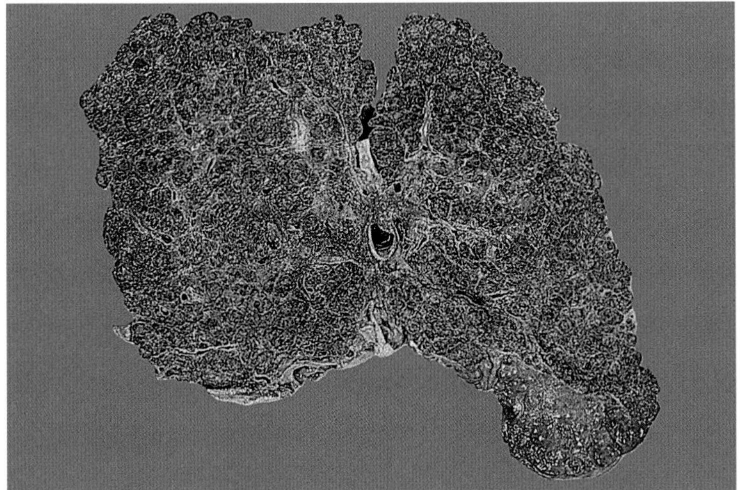

■ **Fig. 12.64** A cirrhotic liver in primary biliary cirrhosis. Courtesy of Prof I. Talbot.

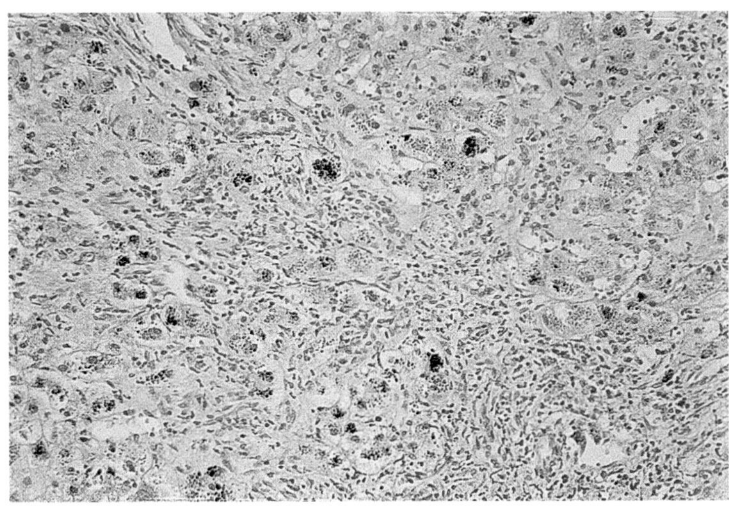

■ **Fig. 12.65** Liver biopsy in primary biliary cirrhosis stained specifically for copper. Rubeanic acid stain.

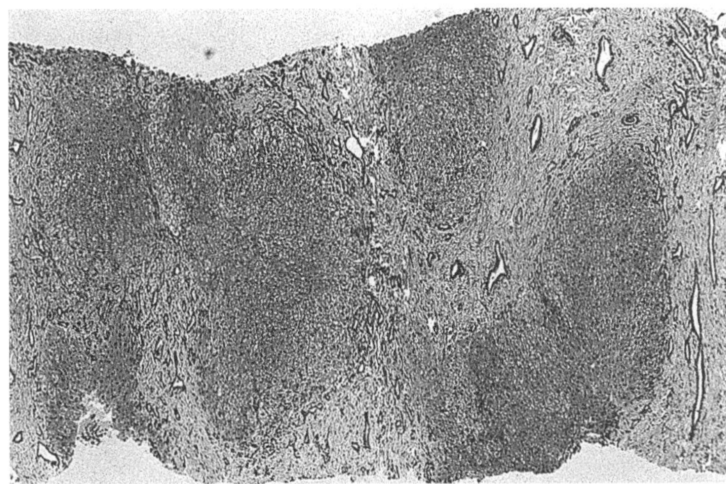

■ **Fig. 12.66** Histology in congenital hepatic fibrosis. H&E stain (x 30). Courtesy of Prof I. Talbot.

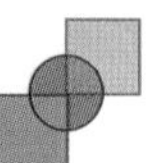

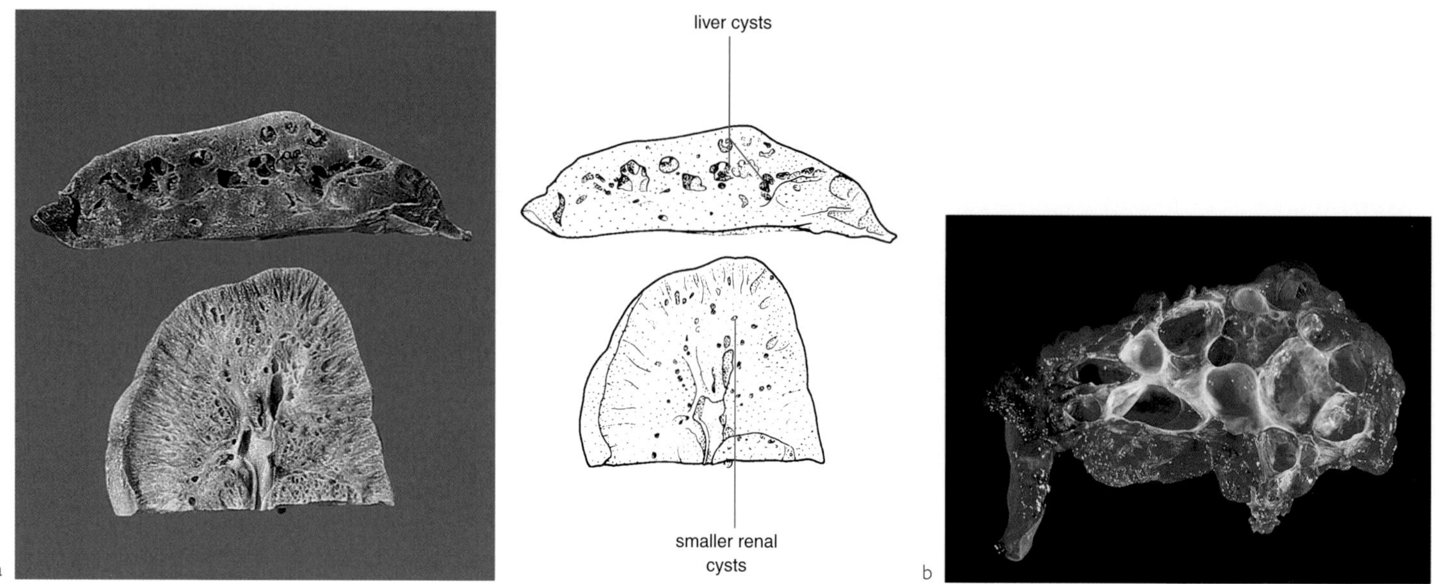

■ **Fig. 12.67** (a) Liver and kidney slices from a child who died with childhood polycystic disease. (b) Adult polycystic liver disease. Hepatic lobectomy specimen from a patient with adult polycystic kidney disease showing a cluster of simple cysts with smooth linings derived from biliary epithelium.

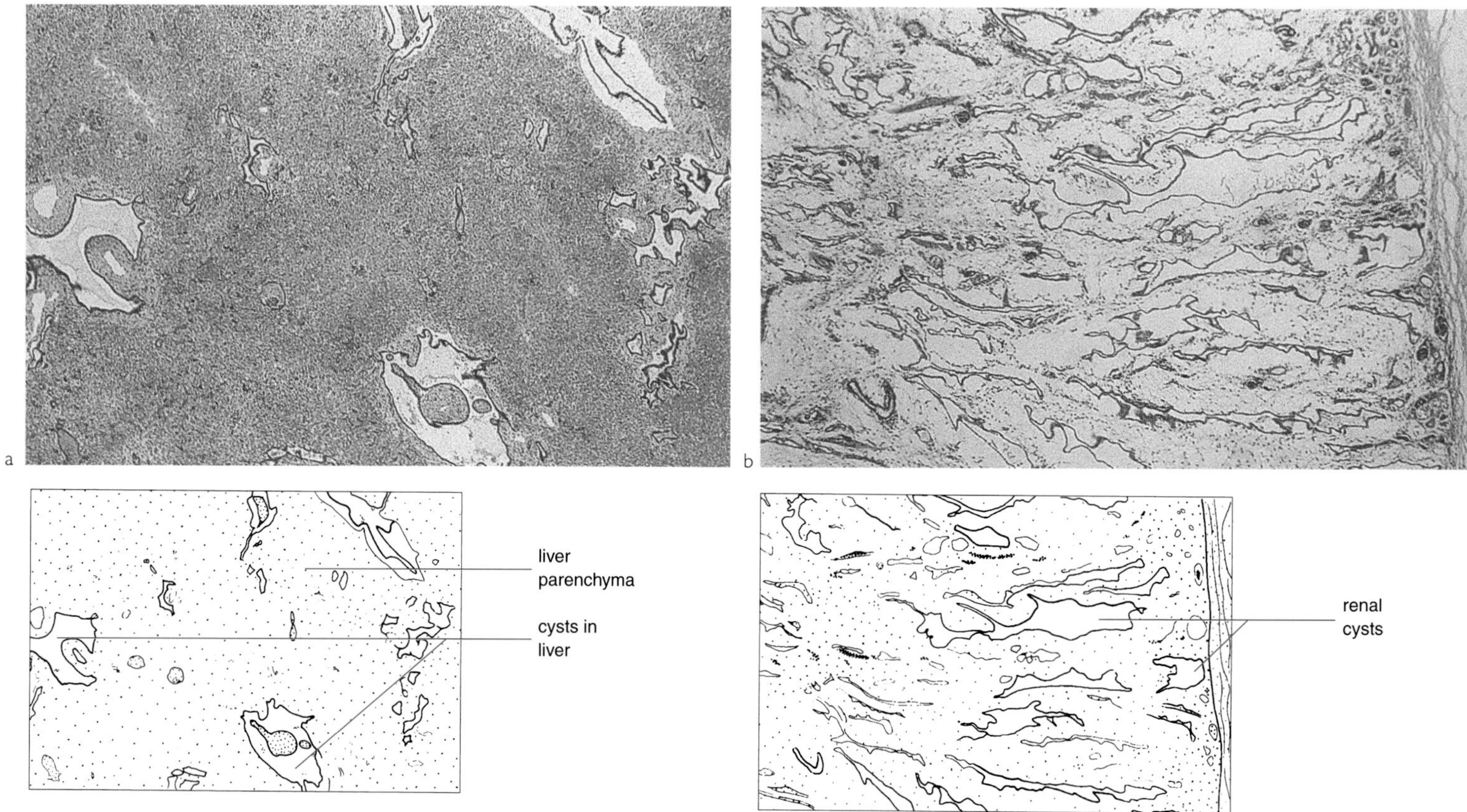

■ **Fig. 12.68** Histological appearances of the liver (a) and kidney (b) showing extensive cyst formation in a case of childhood polycystic disease. H&E stain (x 30).

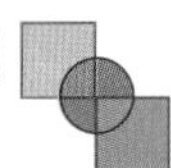

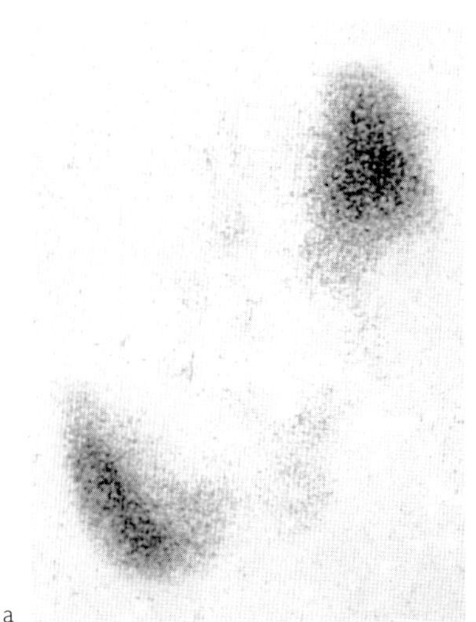
a

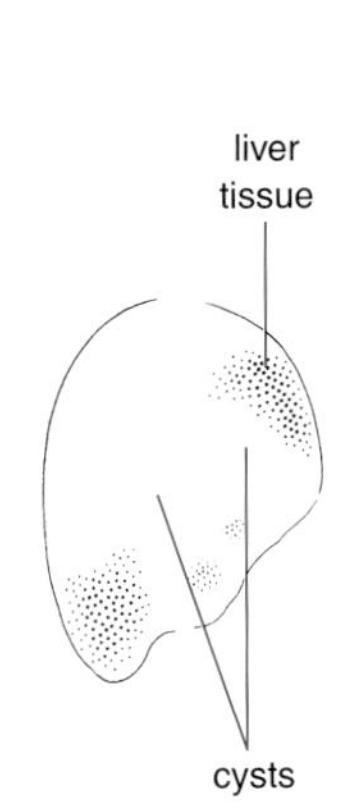

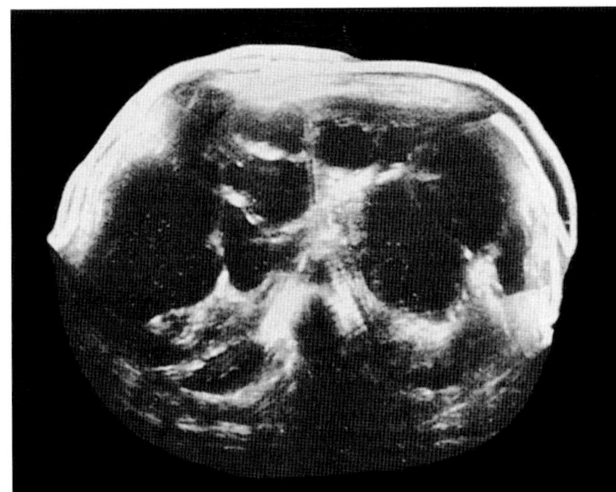
b

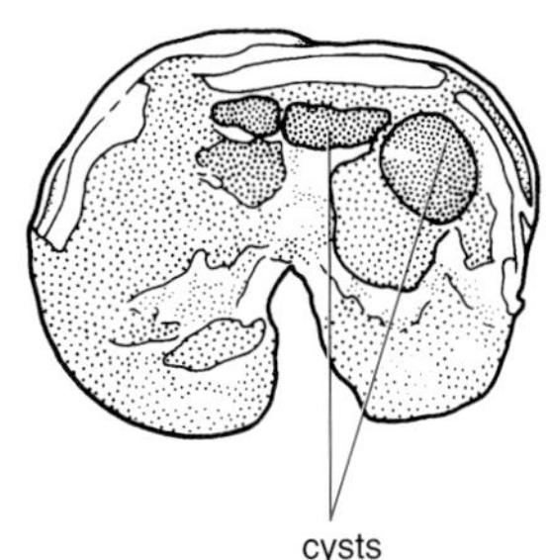

Fig. 12.69 Polycystic liver showing large filling defects on the scintiscan (a), and the ultrasound (b).

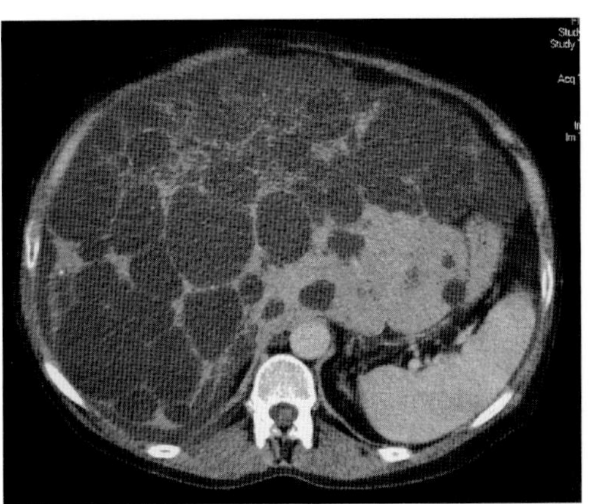

Fig. 12.70 CT demonstrating polycystic liver disease. Numerous fluid-attenuation masses (cysts) are seen throughout a markedly enlarged liver. The patient had autosomal dominant polycystic kidney disease and a renal transplant.

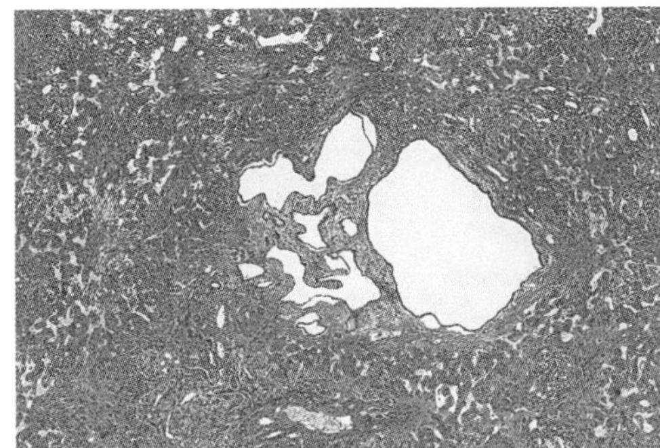

Fig. 12.71 Von Meyenburg complex. Microscopic appearance of the von Meyenburg complex showing the small collection of cystically dilated ductal structures in the portal tract of an asymptomatic patient.

METABOLIC AND VASCULAR DISORDERS OF THE LIVER AND HEPATIC TUMORS

13

METABOLIC DISORDERS OF THE LIVER

Many metabolic disorders affect the liver. Although most present during childhood the age of presentation is very variable, and the commonest, hemochromatosis, is essentially a disease of adults.

Hemochromatosis

Liver disease due to iron overload may be either primary or secondary. Primary (idiopathic) hemochromatosis is an inherited disorder of excessive iron absorption presenting in adult life with chronic liver disease associated with excess iron deposition in the liver and pancreas, and more obvious distinction in radiographic characteristics of these organs from the spleen (Figs 13.1–13.3). Iron is deposited in the hepatocytes, Kupffer cells and portal tract septae (Figs 13.4–13.6).

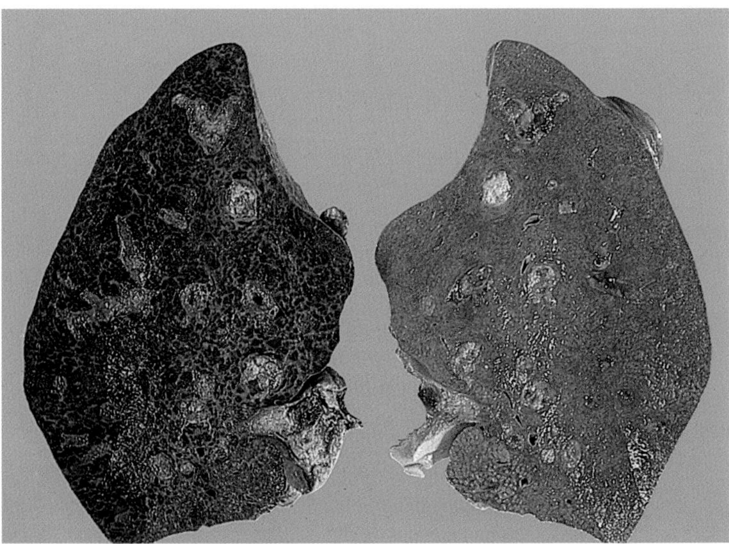

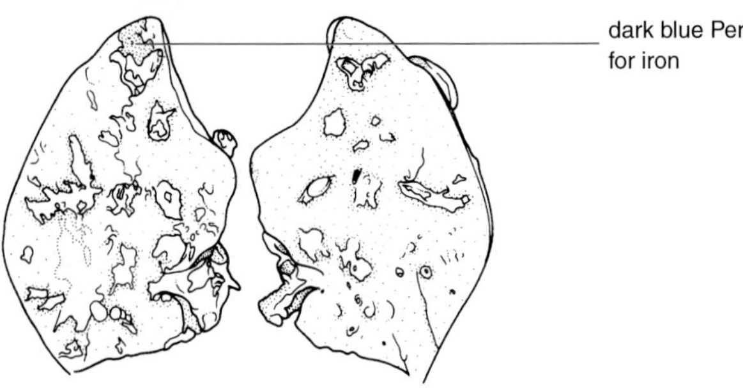

■ **Fig. 13.1** A cirrhotic liver in hemochromatosis staining blue with Perls' stain. Courtesy of Prof I. Talbot.

Once cirrhosis is established, it is initially micronodular but subsequently becomes macronodular and is associated with a high incidence of hepatocellular carcinoma (Figs 13.3, 13.7).

Secondary hemochromatosis arises as a consequence of multiple blood transfusions, chronic iron administration and hemolytic anemia in which the iron deposition is primarily in the Kupffer cells and leads to hemosiderosis. Iron accumulation may also occur as a secondary complication of alcoholic liver disease, and in this case distinction from primary hemochromatosis may be difficult.

Wilson's disease

The cirrhosis of Wilson's disease is due to abnormal absorption of copper and accumulation of the metal in hepatocytes (Figs 13.8–13.10). Fatty change and progressive cholangiolar proliferation are precirrhotic features of the condition which may be reversed in the early stages with chelating drugs.

Indian childhood cirrhosis

This condition is marked by fibrous hepatocellular degeneration, Mallory's hyaline and copper deposition preceding the development of cirrhosis and liver failure (Fig. 13.11). The etiology of the disorder is poorly understood, but the excess deposition of copper is considered by many to be a primary, rather than a secondary, feature.

Galactosemia

Congenital absence of the enzyme galactose-1-phosphate uridyl transferase leads to the accumulation of toxic amounts of galactose and other metabolites in the liver. This autosomal recessive disease starts in infancy with vomiting, malnutrition and hepatosplenomegaly. Cataracts, brain damage, and macronodular cirrhosis develop later. Fatty change in the liver is the earliest histological feature (Fig. 13.12). Subsequently the hepatocytes show a striking pseudoglandular arrangement, which diminishes as cirrhosis develops.

Glycogen storage diseases

In von Gierke's disease there is a defect in glucose-6-phosphatase production. This leads to hepatomegaly due to excessive deposition of glycogen. Feeding difficulties and hypoglycemia are the major symptoms in infancy, followed by impaired growth and gross hepatic enlargement. Liver biopsy shows a characteristic appearance of hepatocytes with pale cytoplasm (Fig. 13.13). Special processing measures have to be undertaken in order to permit histochemical distinction between fat and glycogen deposition.

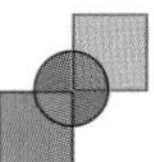

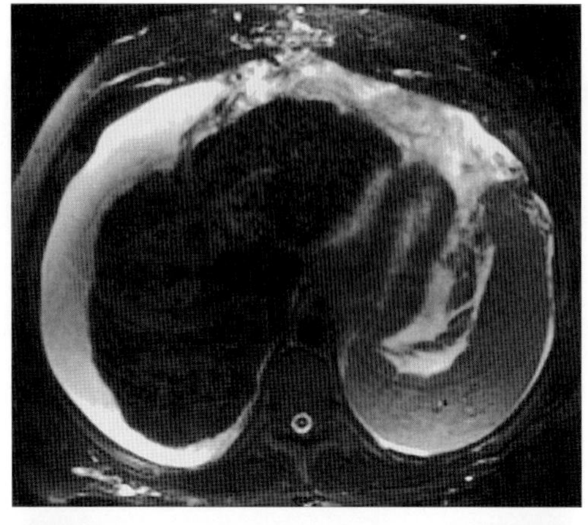

a

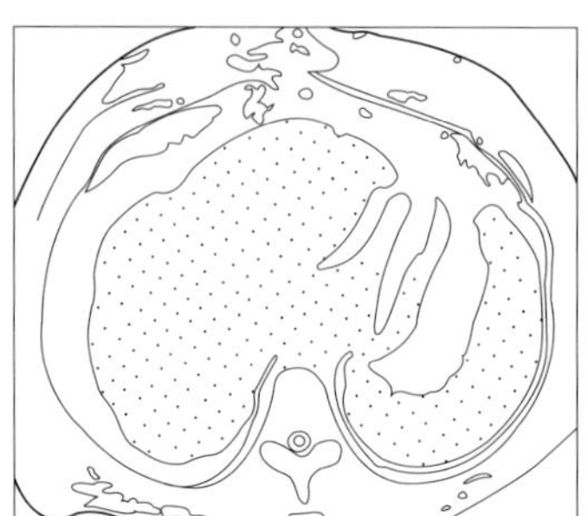

■ **Fig. 13.2** MRI demonstrating liver and pancreas in a patient with hemochromatosis. (a) T_2-weighted, fat-suppressed MRI shows that the liver is of much diminished intensity ('darker') due to increased iron. (b) T_2-weighted, fat-suppressed MRI shows the pancreas is of very low intensity related to iron deposition. Courtesy of Drew Torigian, MD, Philadelphia.

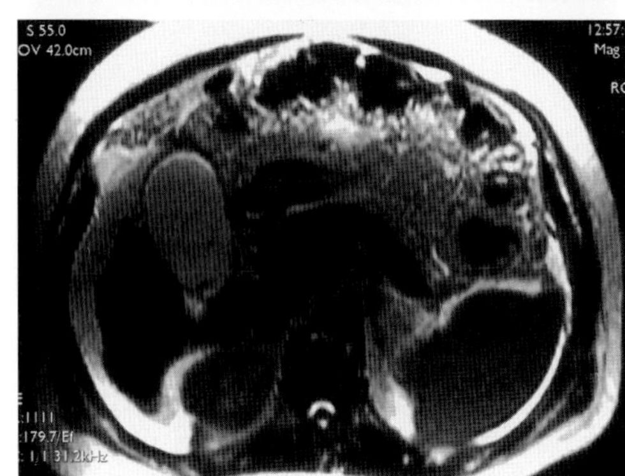

b

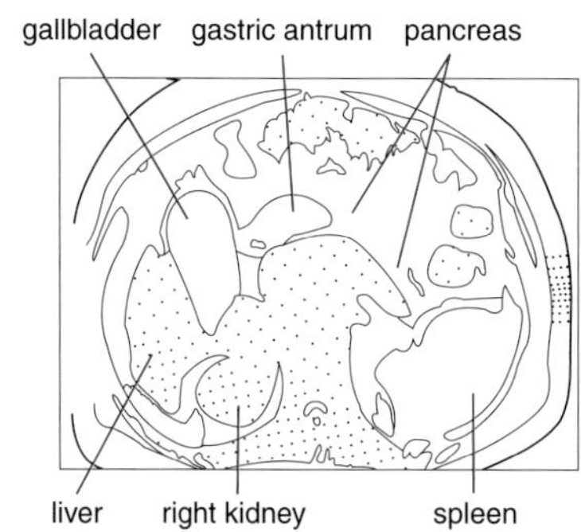

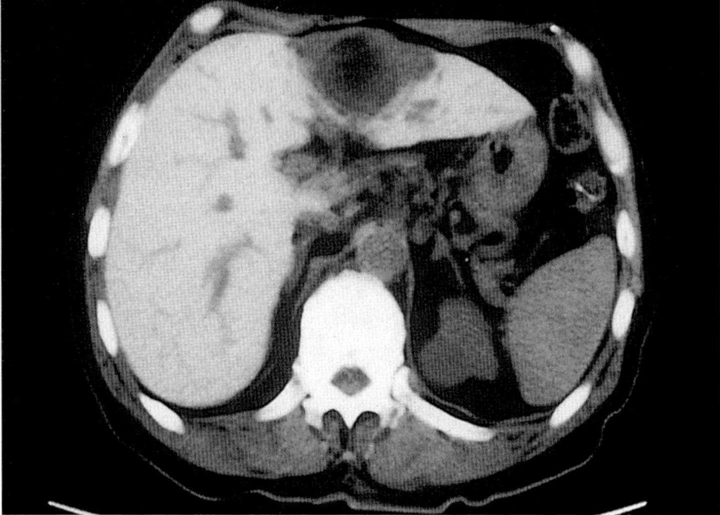

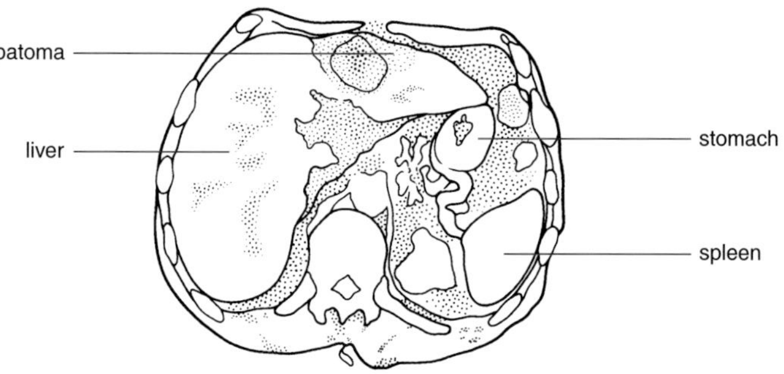

■ **Fig. 13.3** CT scan of the liver in hemochromatosis with an associated hepatoma. The excess iron deposition is reflected by the increased density of the liver image compared with the spleen. Courtesy of Dr R.A. Nakielny.

Niemann–Pick disease

This is a rare disease that chiefly affects Jewish children. Sphingomyelin accumulates in the reticuloendothelial system throughout the body. The changes in the liver include hypertrophy of the Kupffer cells and vacuolation of their cytoplasm. As a consequence of the Kupffer cell hypertrophy, the hepatocytes tend to atrophy. The foamy Kupffer cells are autofluorescent, and birefringent with polarized light and weakly PAS-positive (Fig 13.14).

Gaucher's disease

As in Niemann–Pick disease the major hepatic involvement of Gaucher's concerns the Kupffer cells, which are distended by glucocerebroside. The cells are lightly eosinophilic and the cytoplasm has a faintly crinkled or striated appearance. Their pyknotic nuclei and cytoplasm are best visualized with periodic acid-Schiff reagent (Figs 13.15–13.17).

Alpha-1-antitrypsin deficiency

In children serum deficiency of alpha-1-antitrypsin is associated with neonatal jaundice and progressive liver damage; in teenagers and adults it is associated with chronic liver disease and/or pulmonary emphysema. The characteristic histological feature is the presence of brown, lightly stained acidophilic bodies within hepatocytes (Figs 13.18, 13.19). These are strongly PAS-positive (Fig. 13.20), and

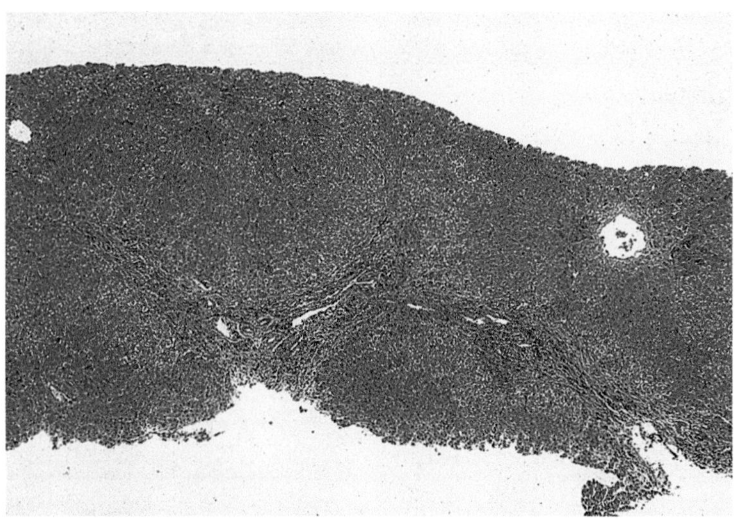

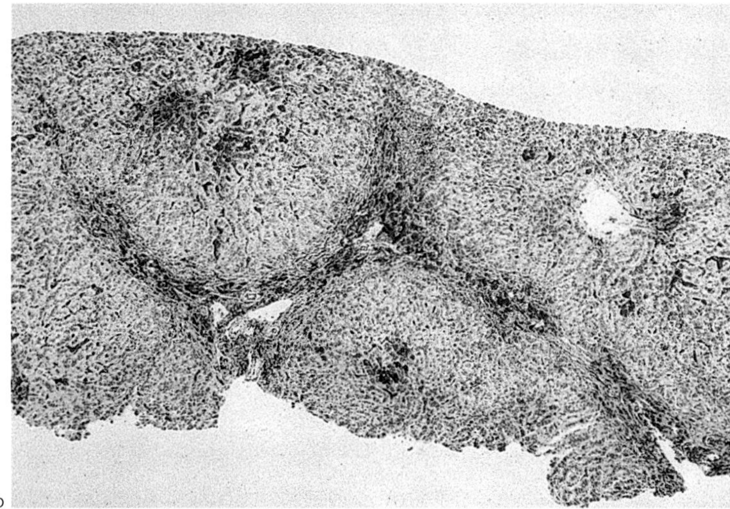

■ **Fig. 13.4** Histological appearance of the liver in hemochromatosis showing brown hemosiderin granules. (a) H&E stain (x 30) and (b) Perls' stain (x 35). Courtesy of Prof I. Talbot.

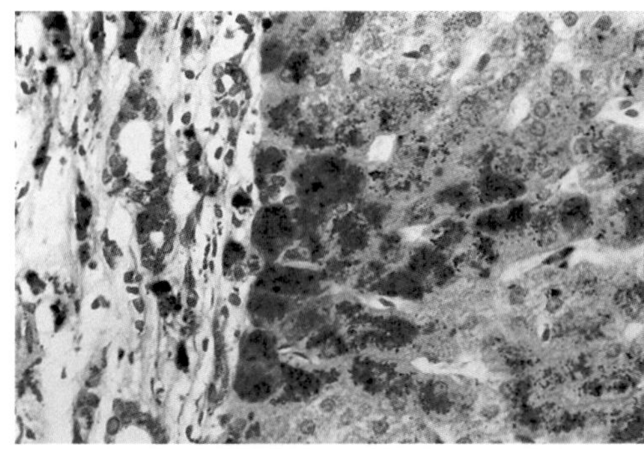

■ **Fig. 13.5** Hereditary hemochromatosis. High-magnification view of a Prussian blue iron stain of the liver showing the dense deposits of iron in both the periportal hepatocytes and the biliary ductal epithelium (seen at left); iron deposition is, to a lesser degree, also seen in non-epithelial cells such as Kupffer cells and portal stromal cells.

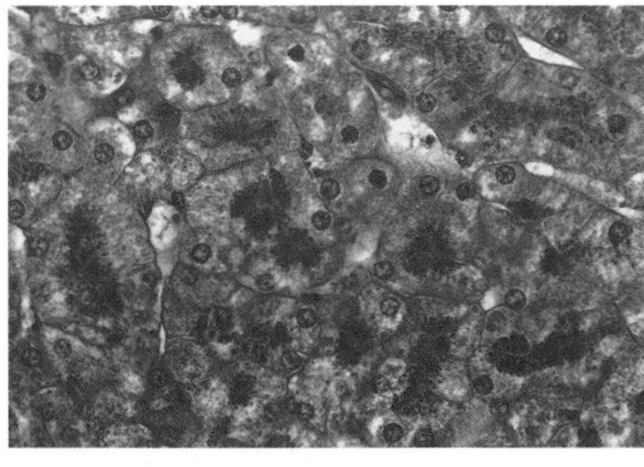

■ **Fig. 13.6** Hereditary hemochromatosis. High-magnification microscopic appearance of hepatocytes showing the typical pericanalicular location of the intracellular iron.

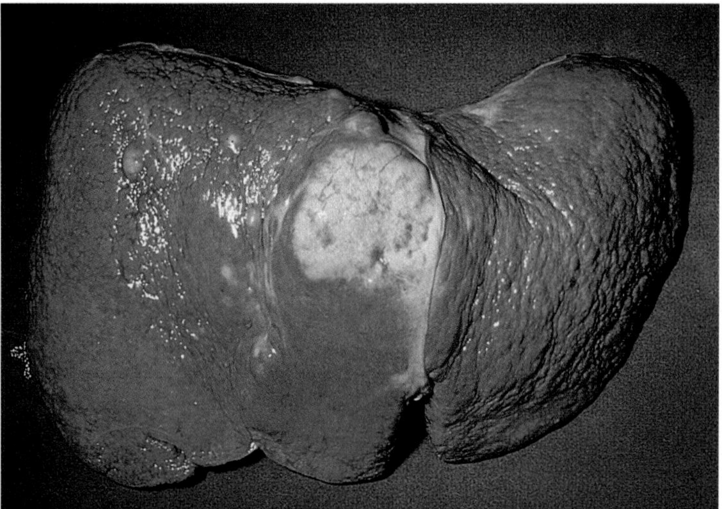

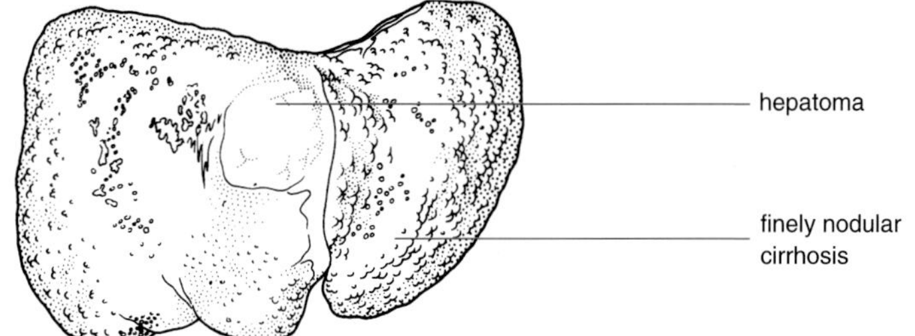

■ **Fig. 13.7** Macroscopic appearance of a cirrhotic liver and hepatoma secondary to hemochromatosis.

this can be shown by immunocytochemical means to be due to the enzyme itself (Fig. 13.21).

Amyloidosis

Hepatic involvement is common in all types of amyloid disease, but liver function is impaired only rarely. Amyloid is deposited in a perisinusoidal position in the space of Disse. The adjacent hepatocytes are often compressed, and the portal tract vessels may

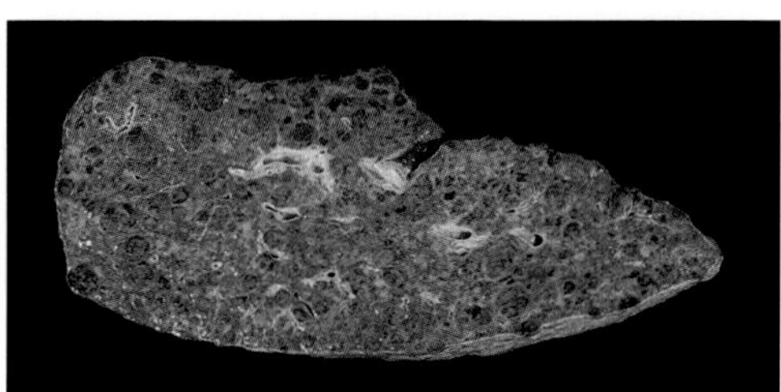

■ **Fig. 13.8** Wilson's disease. Hepatectomy (explant) specimen showing macronodular cirrhosis.

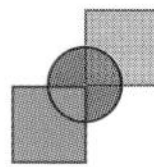

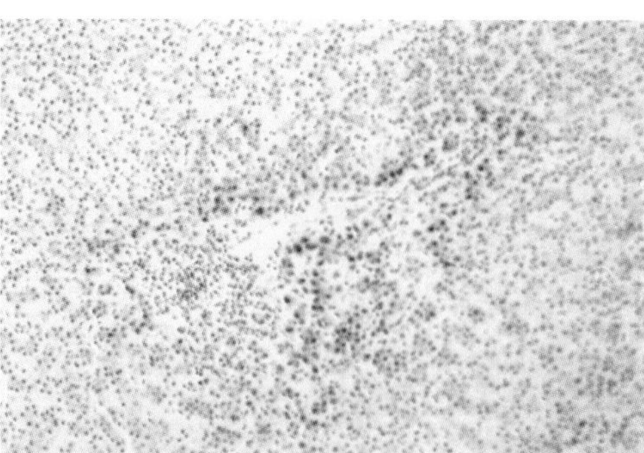

■ **Fig. 13.9** Microscopic view of copper stain in Wilson's disease showing red-brown stained copper accumulation in periportal hepatocytes.

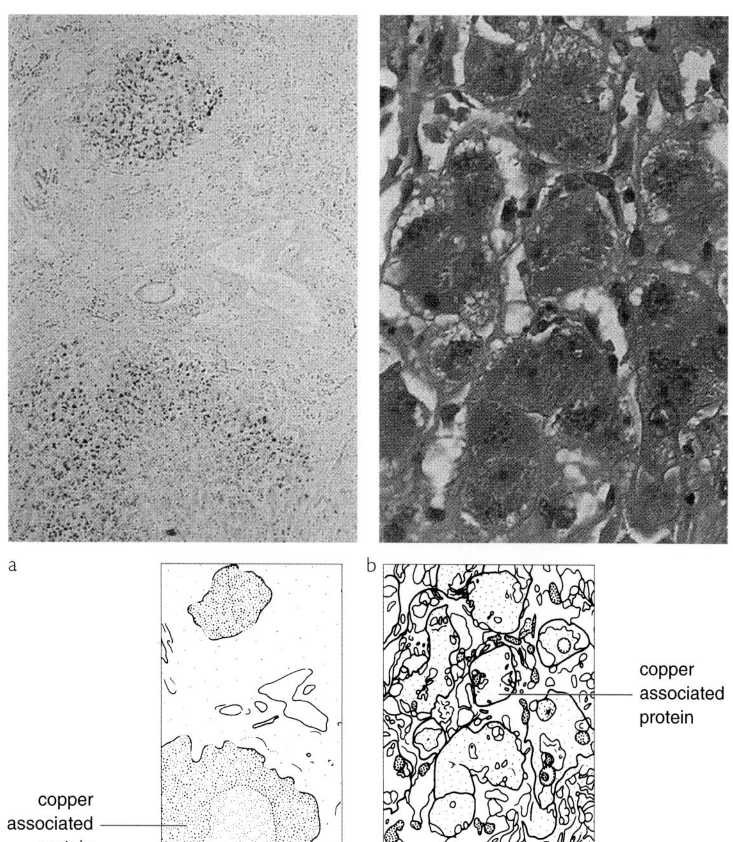

■ **Fig. 13.10** Histological appearance of the liver in Wilson's disease showing copper associated protein deposits. (a) Rubeanic acid stain (x 20) and (b) H&E stain (x 320). Courtesy of Prof I. Talbot.

also be involved (Fig. 13.22). Amyloid material shows a characteristic stain with Congo red and also gives typical apple-green birefringence when examined under polarized light (Fig. 13.23). Myeloma-related amyloid has different characteristics (Fig. 13.24).

Cystic fibrosis (mucoviscidosis) (see also Chapter 9)

Liver abnormalities are being seen with increasing frequency in patients with cystic fibrosis, especially as such individuals survive longer following improved treatment of the pulmonary and pancreatic disease. Fatty change is the most frequent histological abnormality in the liver, and this may be related to problems with malabsorption. Focal biliary fibrosis is often seen in which portal tracts are expanded with ductular proliferation and periportal fibrosis. The bile ducts are distended by inspissated bile (Fig.13.25). Ultimately the fibrosis may progress to macronodular cirrhosis.

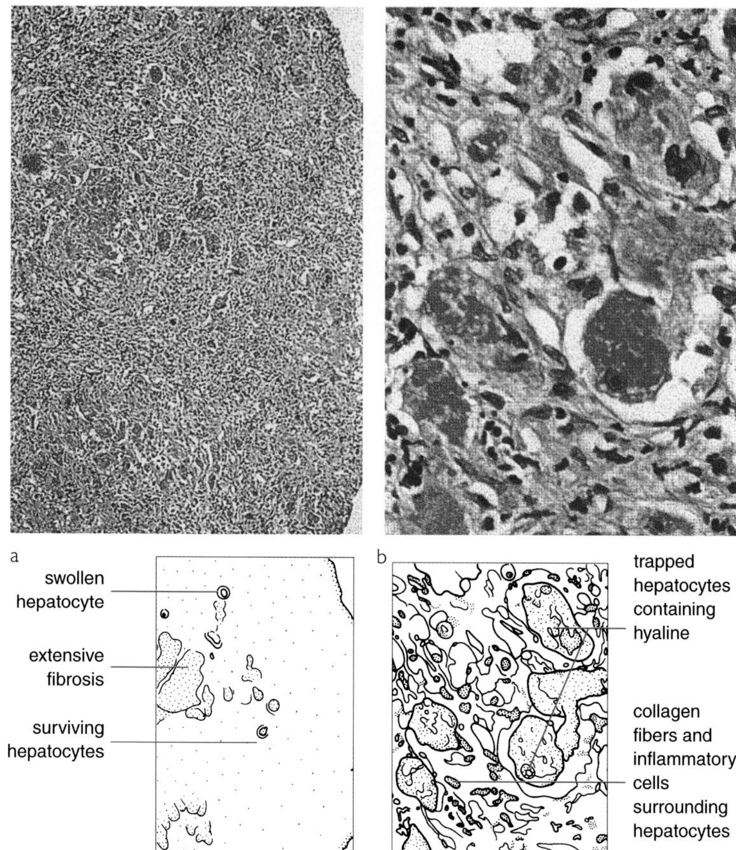

■ **Fig. 13.11** Liver histology in Indian childhood cirrhosis showing 'creeping fibrosis' isolating hepatocytes; (a) H&E stain (x 120) and enlarged hepatocytes containing hyaline material; (b) H&E stain (x 320). Courtesy of Prof I. Talbot.

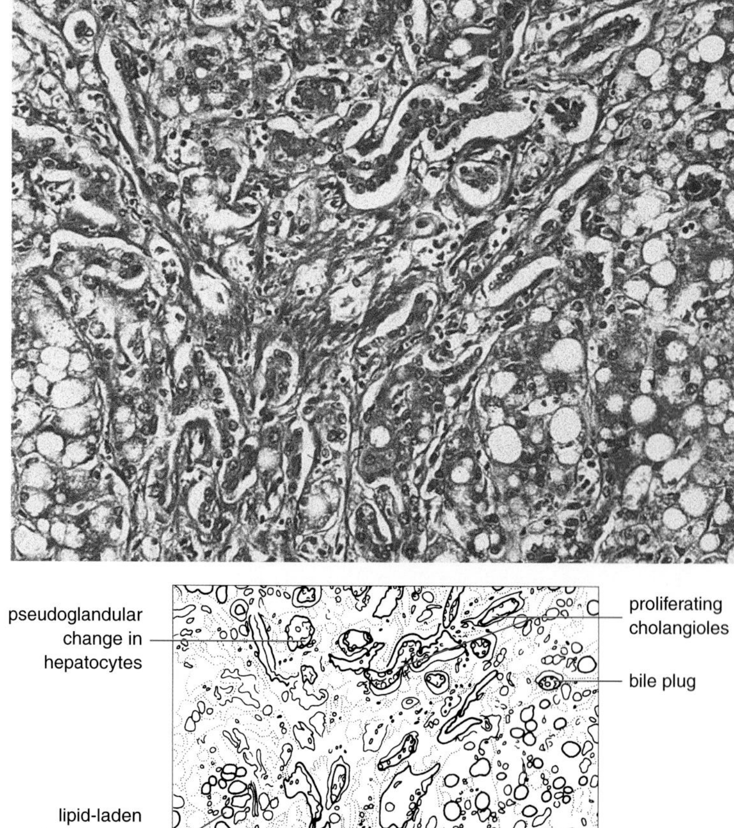

■ **Fig. 13.12** Histology of fatty infiltration, pseudoglandular alteration in hepatocytes, and bile duct proliferation in galactosemia. H&E stain (x 120). Courtesy of Prof B. Portmann.

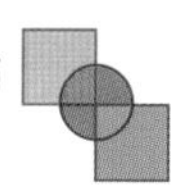

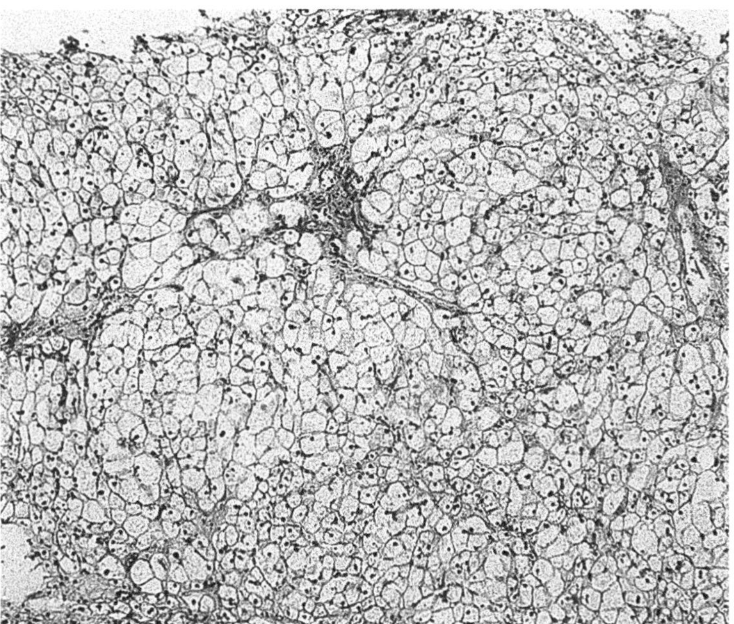

■ **Fig. 13.13** Histology in glycogen-storage disease, showing swollen hepatocytes with pale or rarefied cytoplasm where glycogen has dissolved out during the processing. H&E stain (x 75). Courtesy of Prof I. Talbot.

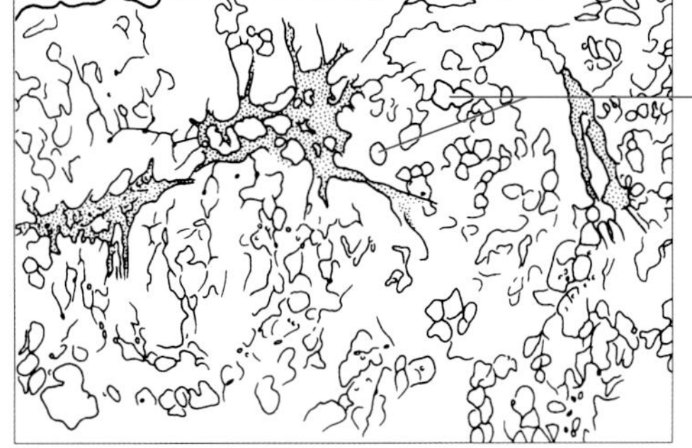

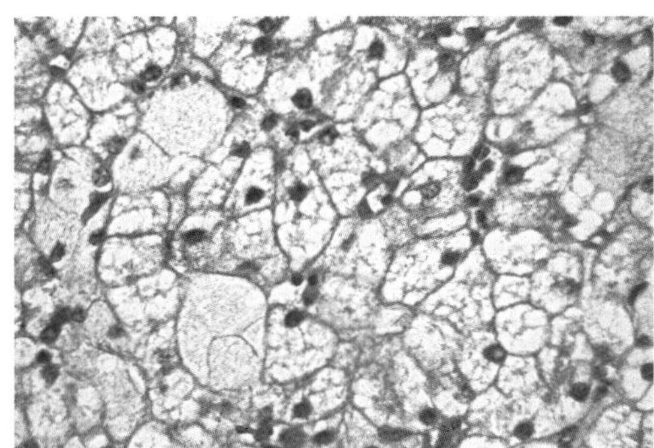

■ **Fig. 13.14** Niemann–Pick disease (sphingomyelin-cholesterol lipidosis). High-magnification micrograph of sheets of enlarged, foamy Kupffer cells filled with sphingomyelin-cholesterol.

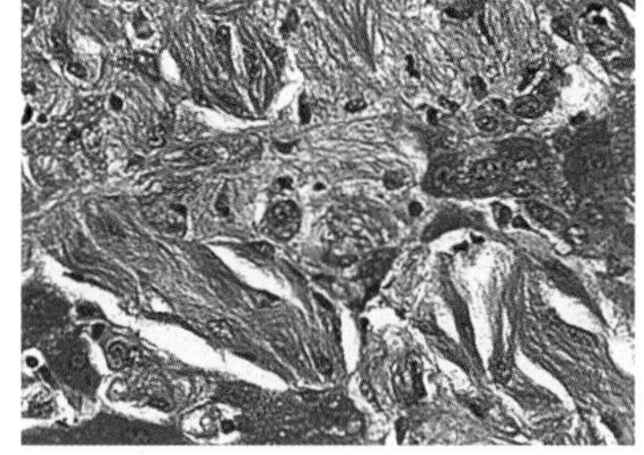

■ **Fig. 13.17** Gaucher's disease. High magnification of Gaucher's cells showing the characteristic delicate striations of the cytoplasm.

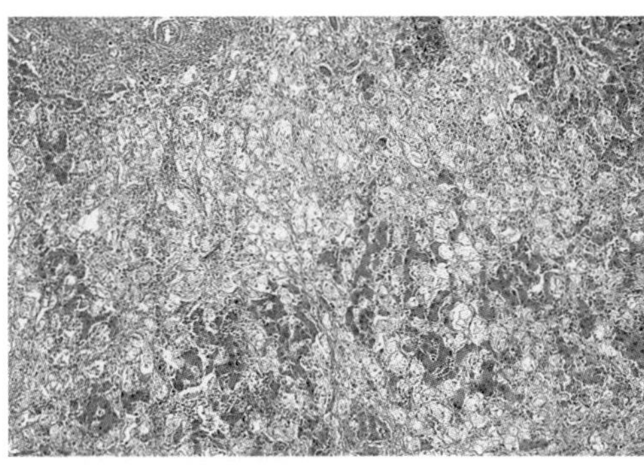

■ **Fig. 13.15** Gaucher's disease (glycosyl ceramide lipidosis). Microscopic view showing masses of pale-staining Gaucher's cells replacing large areas of the hepatic parenchyma (upper left) and disrupting and distorting remaining hepatic cords (lower right).

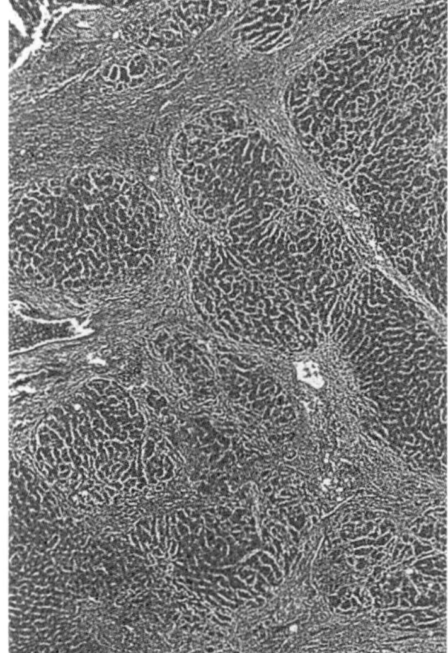

■ **Fig. 13.18** Alpha-1-antitrypsin deficiency. Established cirrhosis in alpha-1-antitrypsin deficiency showing a micronodular pattern.

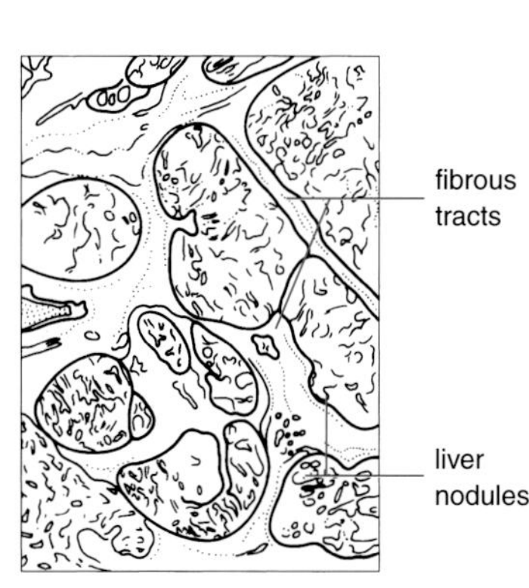

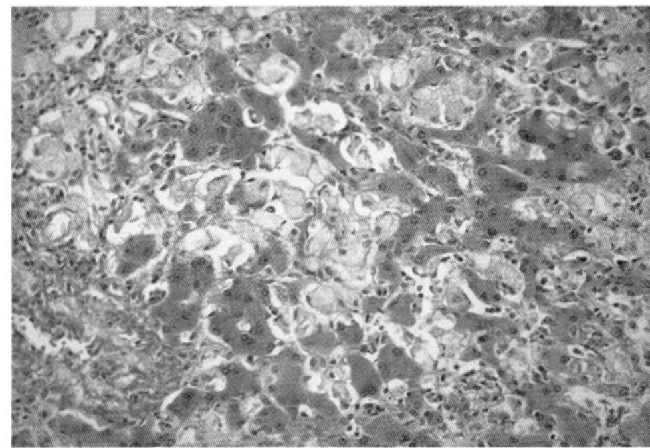

■ **Fig. 13.16** Gaucher's disease. High-magnification appearance of pale-staining Kupffer cells filled with glycocerebroside filling and expanding sinusoids and compressing atrophic-appearing pink-staining hepatocytes in adjacent cords.

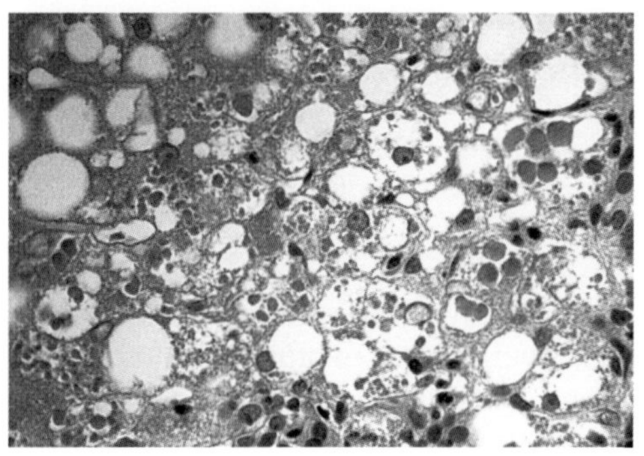

■ **Fig. 13.19** Alpha-1-antitrypsin deficiency. Microscopic view of parenchyma showing lymphocytic inflammatory infiltrates among periportal hepatocytes that display steatotic and ballooning changes indicative of injury and contain numerous eosinophilic cytoplasmic globules of alpha-1-antitrypsin.

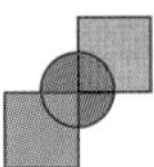

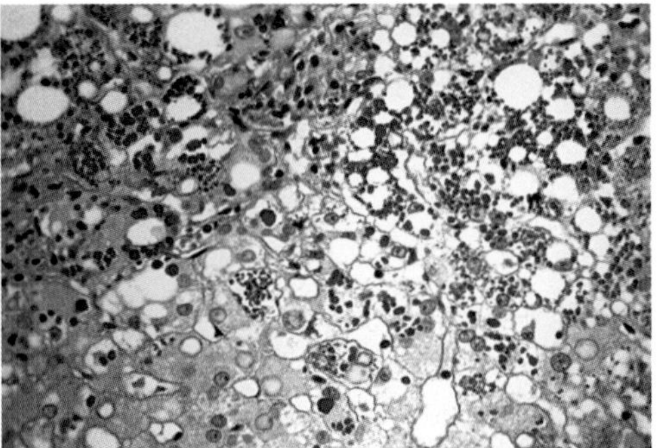

■ **Fig. 13.20** Alpha-1-antitrypsin deficiency. PAS stain showing intense magenta staining of the cytoplasmic globules of alpha-1-antitrypsin.

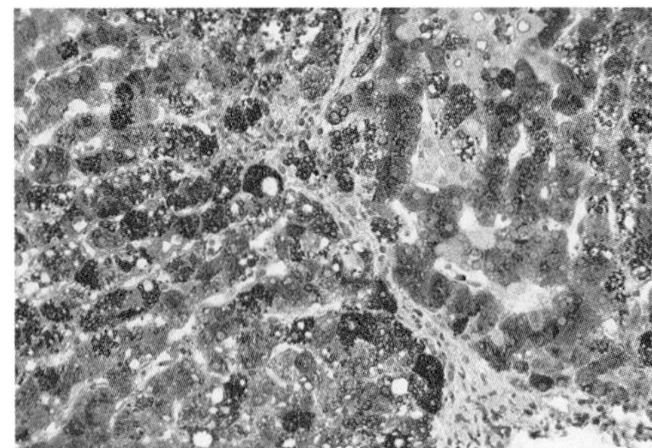

■ **Fig. 13.21** Alpha-1-antitrypsin deficiency. Immunohistochemical stain for alpha-1-antitrypsin showing the intense positive staining of the cytoplasmic globules and the paler staining of the entire hepatocyte cytoplasm.

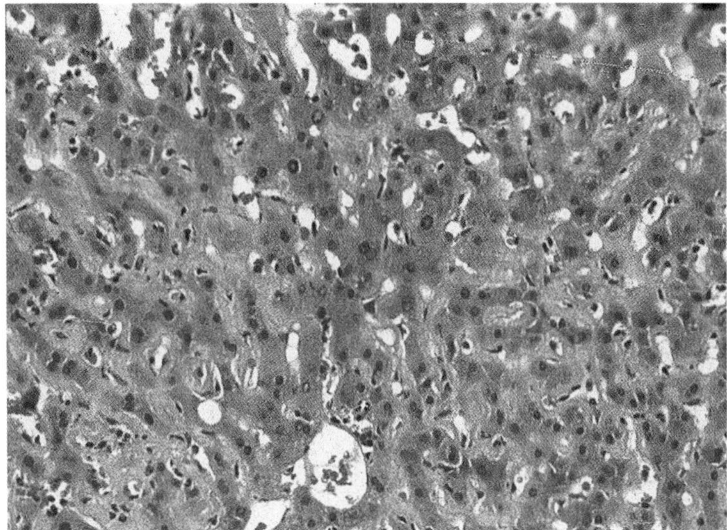

■ **Fig. 13.22** Amyloid deposition in hepatic sinusoids is seen as amorphous pink-staining material with H&E (x 180).

Hepatic porphyria

Two varieties of porphyria are associated with liver abnormalities.

Porphyria cutanea tarda

This condition is characterized by photosensitive blistering of the face and hands (Fig.13.26). It is particularly associated with alcohol abuse and Hepatitis C (HCV) (see Chapter 11). Electron microscopy reveals needle-shaped cytoplasmic inclusions in some cases.

Protoporphyria

This rare form of porphyria may lead to progressive jaundice and liver failure (Fig. 13.27). Dense brown deposits of protoporphyrin can be seen in bile duct canaliculi and Kupffer cells. The deposits are birefringent and give a bright red color (Fig. 13.28).

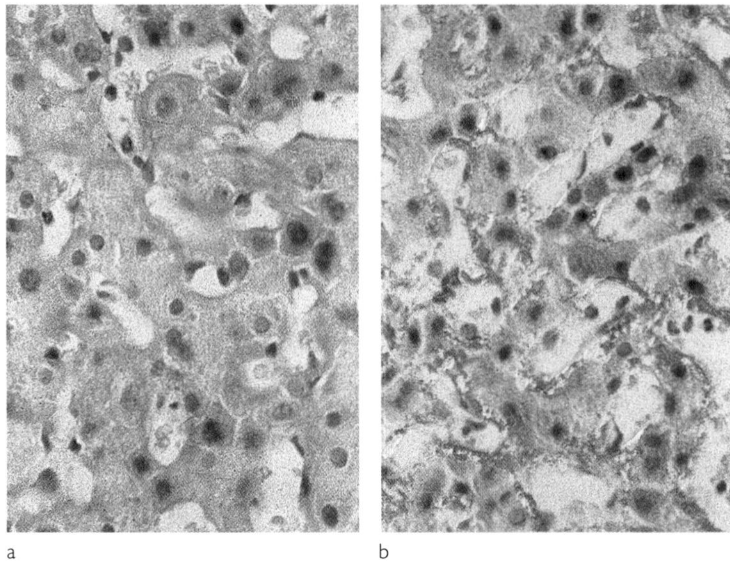

■ **Fig. 13.23** Amyloid in the sinusoids is clearly shown by staining with Congo red ((a), x 320) and gives a green birefringence with polarized light ((b), x 320).

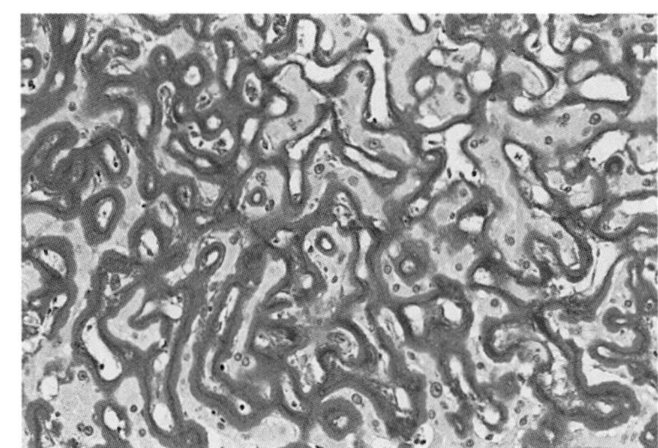

■ **Fig. 13.24** Light chain deposition disease and amyloidosis of the liver. PAS stain showing the PAS-positive, diastase-resistant staining of myeloma-related light chain-related (AL) amyloid (it is Congo red negative) and highlighting a sinusoidal deposition pattern that outlines the hepatic cords.

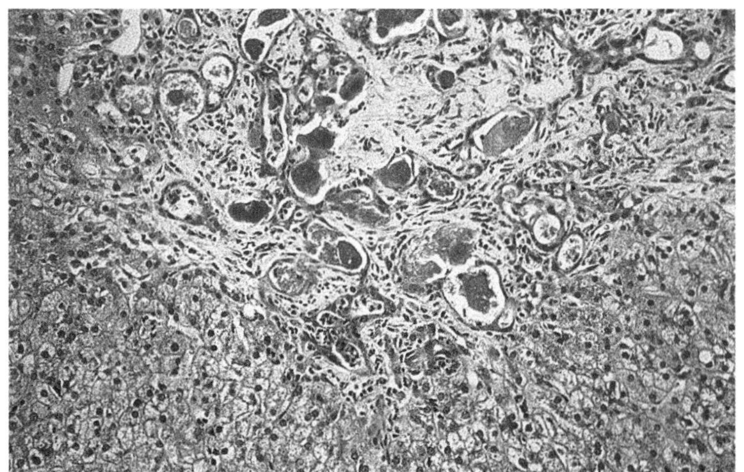

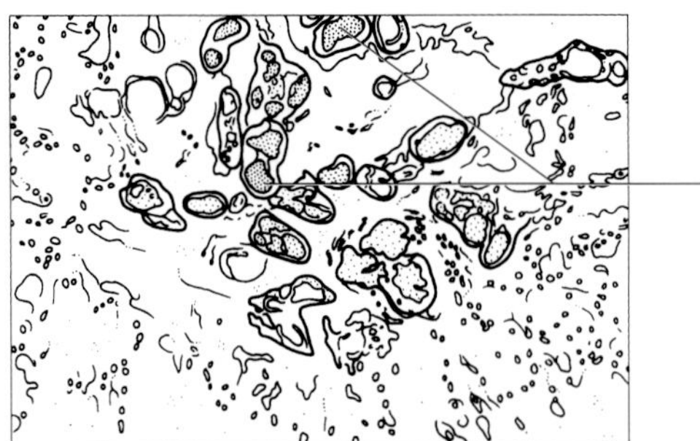

■ **Fig. 13.25** Liver histology in cystic fibrosis. There is mild periportal fibrosis and striking portal tract proliferation of the bile ducts, which contain inspissated secretions and atrophic epithelium. H&E stain (x 180). Courtesy of Prof P. Scheuer.

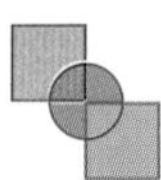

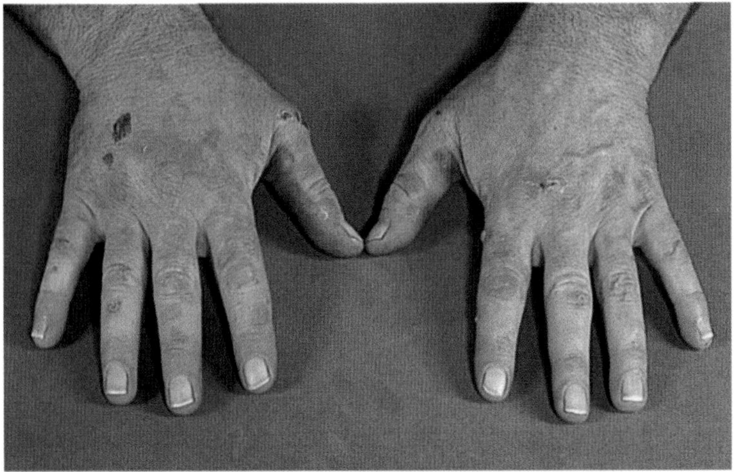

■ **Fig. 13.26** Photosensitive blistering of the skin in porphyria cutanea tarda.

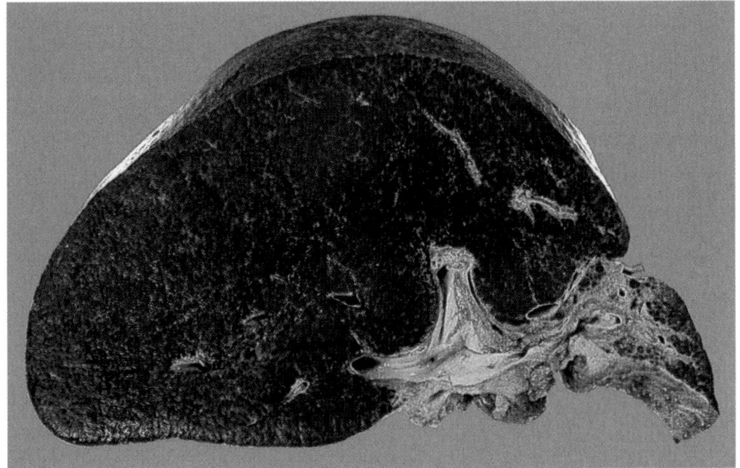

■ **Fig. 13.27** Slice of liver from a patient with erythropoietic protoporphyria, showing pigmentation. Courtesy of Prof I. Talbot.

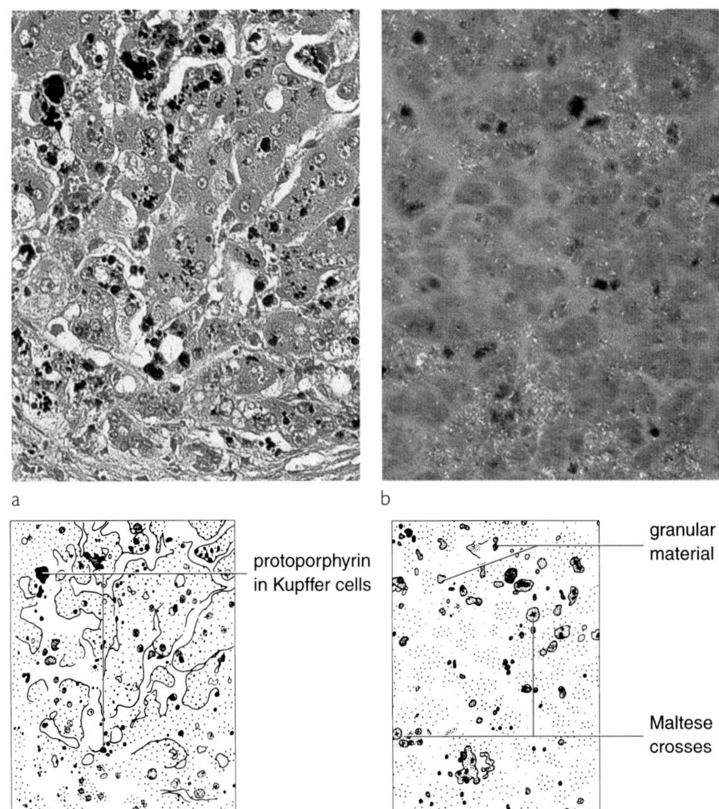

■ **Fig. 13.28** Liver histology in protoporphyria, showing dark-brown deposits of protoporphyrin in Kupffer cells and bile canaliculi ((a), H&E stain (x 140), courtesy of Prof I. Talbot). Under polarized light the classical Maltese crosses of protoporphyrin, and also granular material, are seen ((b), x 160).

Fatty liver of pregnancy

Acute fatty liver is a rare but serious complication of pregnancy. It usually occurs in the last trimester and is associated with a high mortality. It is more common in primigravidae and with twin pregnancies. Histologically the striking feature is the presence of microvesicular steatosis (Fig. 13.29) with little evidence of liver cell necrosis. In patients who survive, the liver returns to normal completely.

Reye's syndrome

This condition is characterized by the development in children of an acute encephalopathy with coma associated with fatty liver. The etiology is unknown, but epidemiological studies have shown a high correlation with aspirin ingestion, and the condition has become much rarer since the widespread withdrawal of junior aspirin. Reye's syndrome is characterized by a diffuse infiltration of hepatocytes with small fatty droplets (Fig. 13.30). These fat globules are particularly obvious if a specific fat stain is used (Fig. 13.31). As with acute fatty liver of pregnancy, necrosis is not a prominent feature, but Reye's syndrome is associated with a significant mortality.

Sarcoidosis

The liver is one of many organs which may be involved in sarcoidosis. Non-caseating granulomas are seen (Fig. 13.32), and these are indistinguishable from those seen in a variety of other conditions. Fibrosis

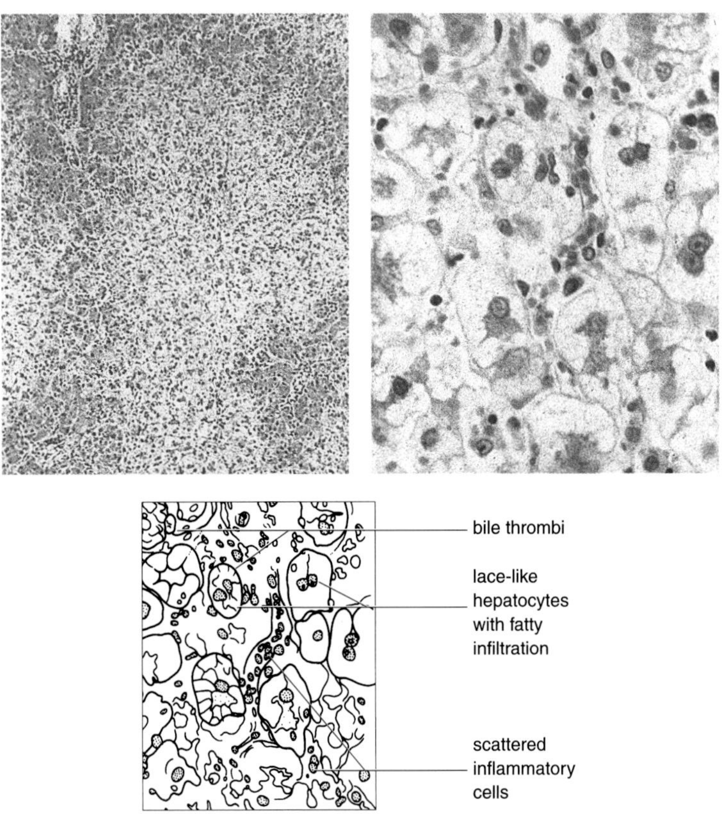

■ **Fig. 13.29** Fatty liver of pregnancy showing the characteristic distribution of pale fat-laden cells ((a), H&E stain, x 50) and the lace-like pattern at higher magnification ((b), H&E stain, x 320).

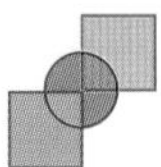

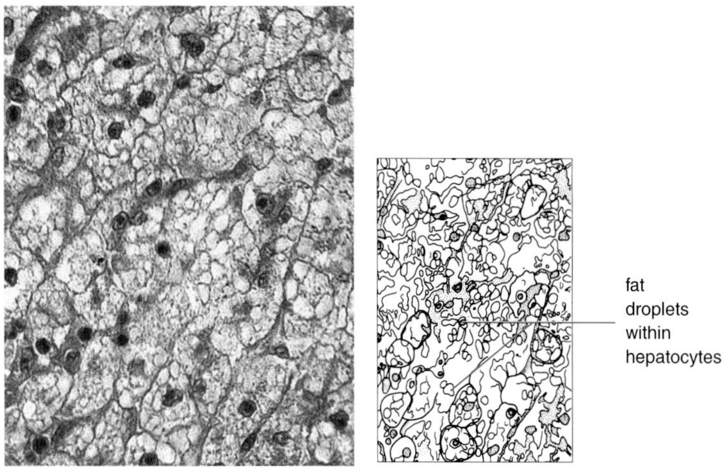

■ **Fig. 13.30** Liver histology in Reye's syndrome showing fat within cytoplasmic microvesicles. H&E stain (x 320). Courtesy of Prof I. Talbot.

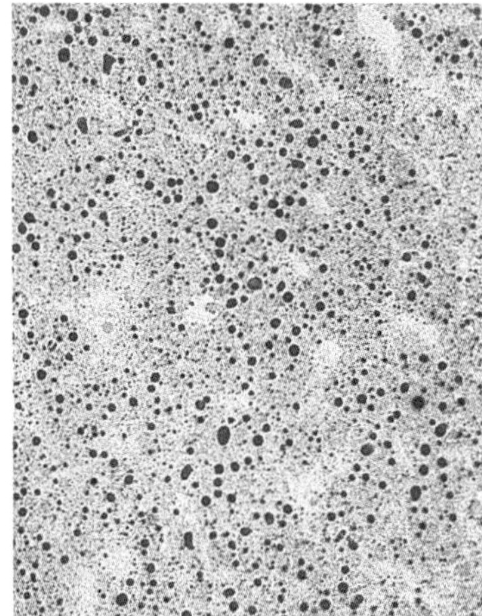

■ **Fig. 13.31** Liver section in Reye's syndrome, with fat globules stained by oil red (x 40). Courtesy of Prof I. Talbot.

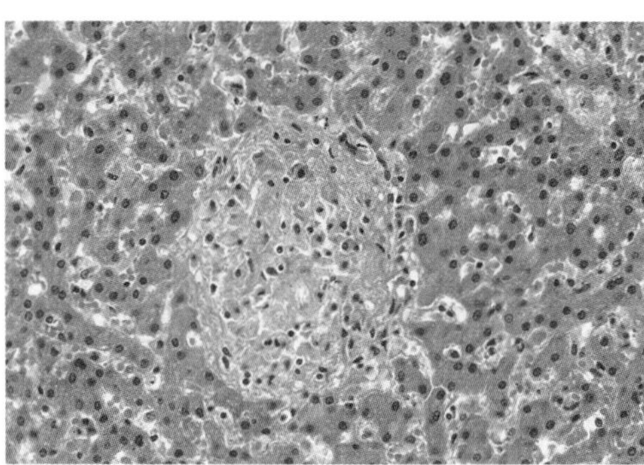

■ **Fig. 13.32** Hepatic granuloma. Microscopic appearance of a discrete, non-caseating granuloma in the liver of a patient with sarcoidosis.

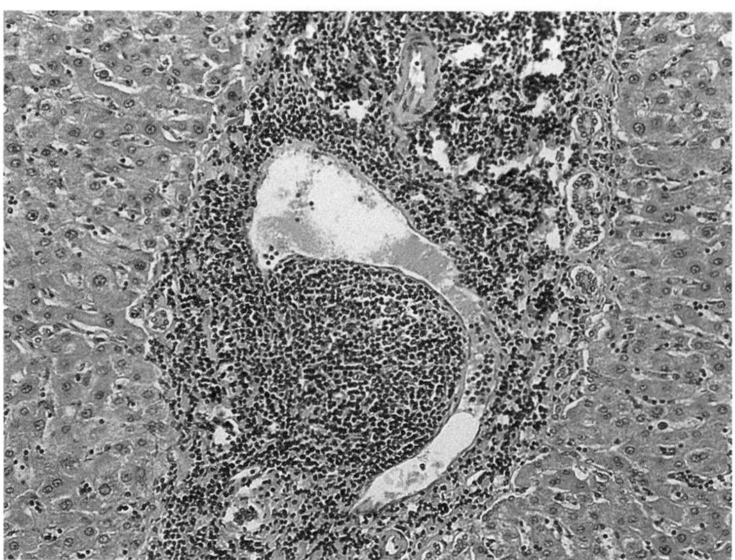

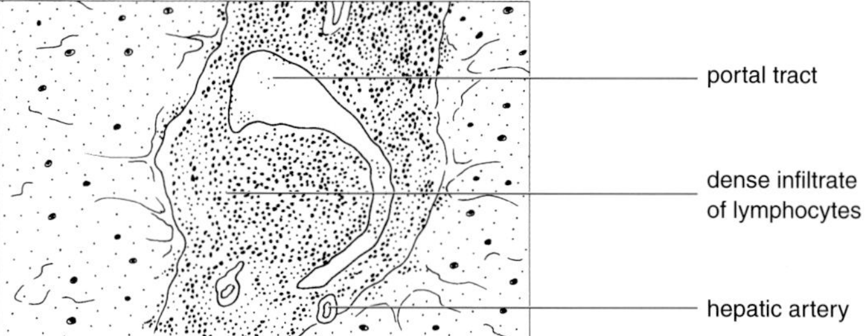

■ **Fig. 13.33** Liver biopsy of chronic lymphatic leukemia showing a portal tract surrounded by a dense infiltrate of mature lymphoid cells. H&E stain. Courtesy of Professor J.C.E. Underwood.

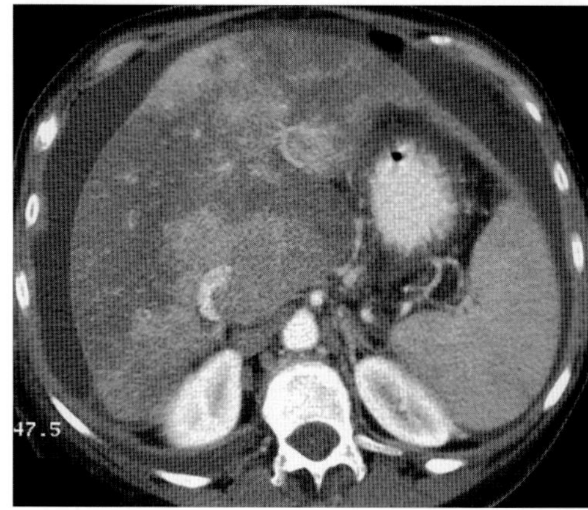

■ **Fig. 13.34** CT scan of Budd–Chiari syndrome. The appearances are not immediately diagnostic for the non-expert and infiltrative disease is sometimes suspected.

leading to portal hypertension is a rare complication of sarcoid liver disease.

Lymphoma/leukemia

Infiltration of the portal tracts and sinusoids is commonly seen in the liver of patients with leukemia or lymphoma (Fig. 13.33), although clinical evidence of liver dysfunction is unusual. Although Reed–Sternberg cells are occasionally found in patients with Hodgkin's disease, the infiltrate is usually non-specific. Very occasionally indeed lymphoma may present with fulminant hepatic failure.

VASCULAR DISORDERS

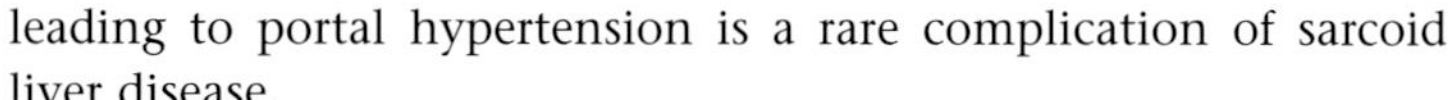

Budd–Chiari syndrome

Obstruction of the hepatic venous blood flow leads to hepatomegaly, jaundice, ascites, and liver failure. When obstruction is complete it is usually fatal unless transplantation is possible, but partial obstruction will result in portal hypertension. By virtue of its separate venous drainage, the caudate lobe is relatively spared; the radioisotope scan is said to be characteristic of this condition, although in practice this is seen in only a minority of cases. Ultrasound and CT scanning are valuable techniques for establishing the diagnosis (Fig. 13.34) although the changes are often subtle and will only be recognized if specifically sought. MR scanning also has an important place now (Fig. 13.35). The hypertrophy of the caudate lobe may result in constriction of the inferior vena cava (IVC) (Fig. 12.36). The diagnosis is ultimately confirmed by hepatic venography (Fig. 13.37). During venography, pressure readings are taken from the supra- and infrahepatic portions of the IVC to help plan the treatment strategy.

Budd–Chiari syndrome is usually secondary to thrombus (Fig. 13.38), but may follow tumor invasion (Fig. 13.39) or, rarely, a congenital web

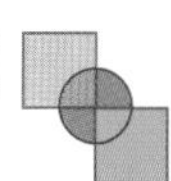

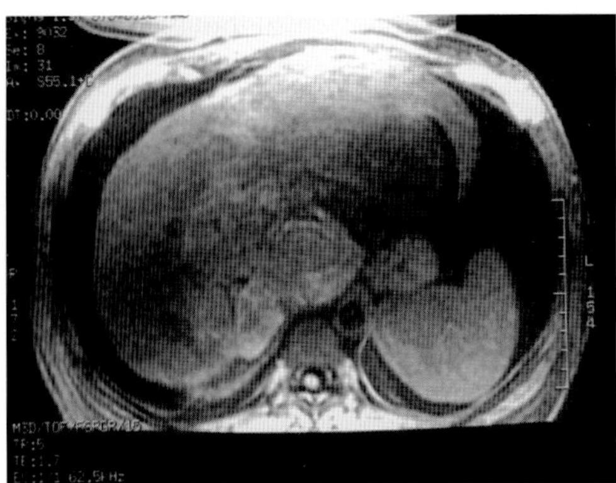

■ **Fig. 13.35** MRI appearances of Budd–Chiari syndrome. As with CT the appearances are not at first clear but the differentiation between the caudate lobe and the rest of the liver can be discerned.

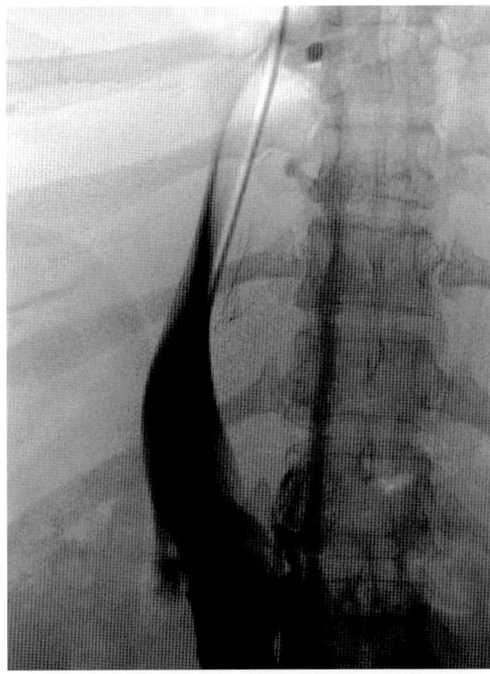

■ **Fig. 13.36** Cavagram showing compression by the enlarged caudate lobe in Budd–Chiari syndrome.

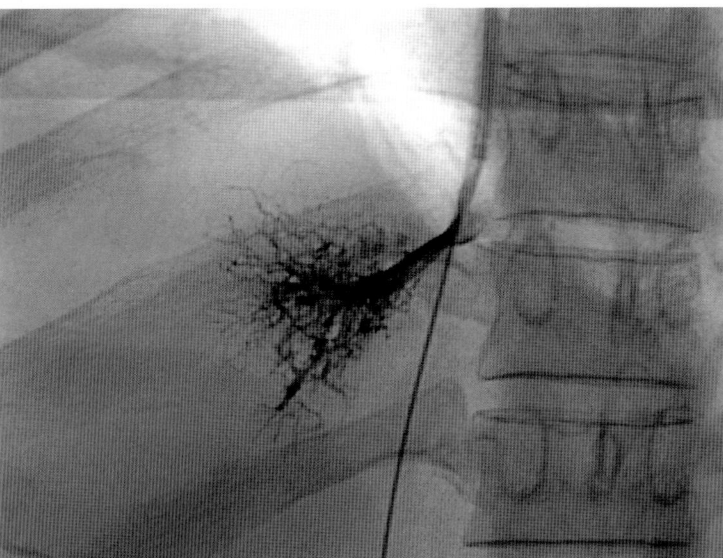

■ **Fig. 13.37** Hepatic venogram in Budd–Chiari syndrome. Contrast fills only some spidery veins in the caudate lobe.

lesion. The major pathological features are centrilobular congestion and sinusoidal dilatation, which lead to atrophy and hepatocyte destruction around the central veins (Figs 13.40–13.43). As fibrosis develops, hepatocyte regeneration is seen near the portal tracts.

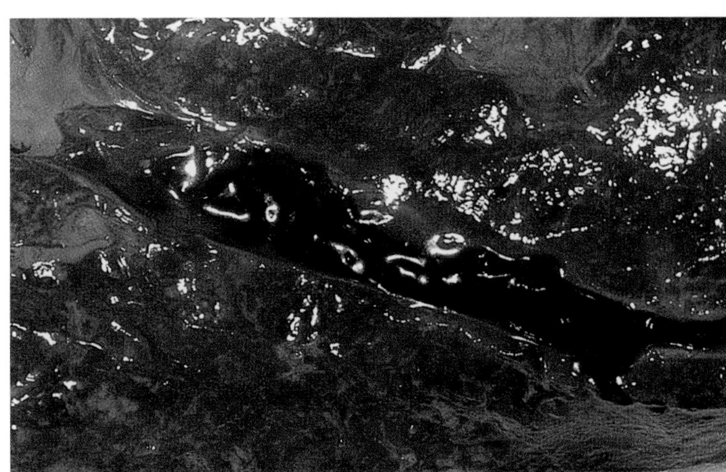

■ **Fig. 13.38** Gross appearance in Budd–Chiari syndrome, showing a thrombus in an hepatic vein. Courtesy of Prof I. Talbot.

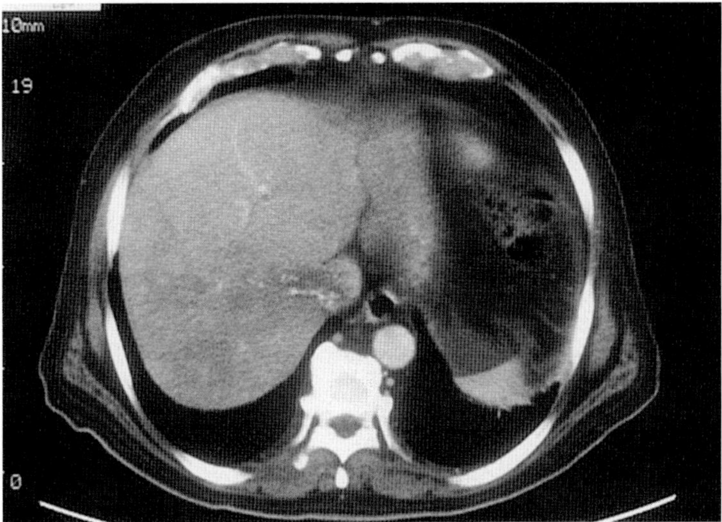

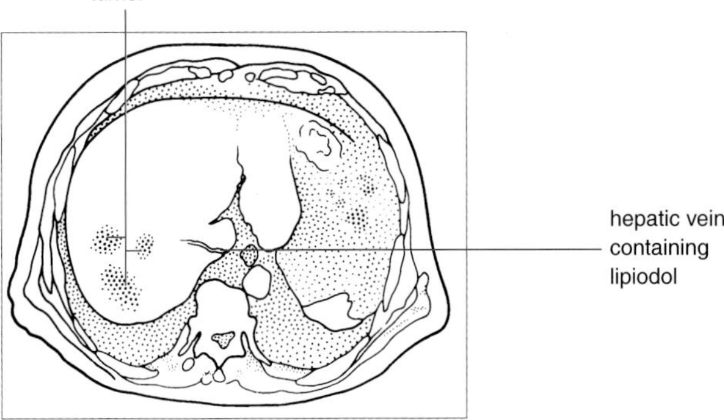

■ **Fig. 13.39** CT scan following injection of intravenous lipiodol. There is a hepatoma in the right lobe of the liver; tumor in the hepatic vein has selectively taken up the oil emulsion. Courtesy of Dr. R.A. Nakielny.

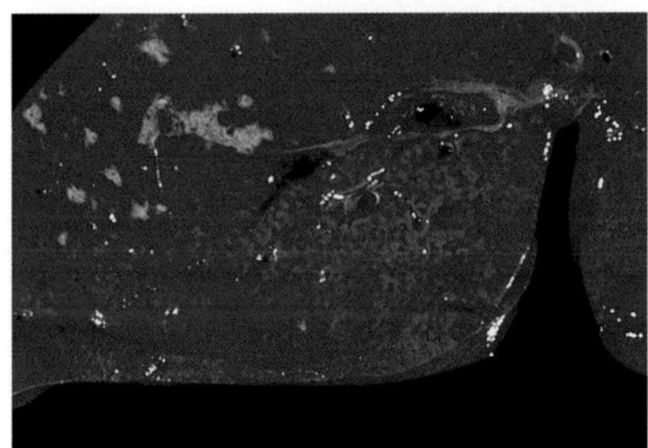

■ **Fig. 13.40** Budd–Chiari syndrome. Cut surface of the liver in the Budd–Chiari syndrome showing the deep red mottled appearance of acute centrilobular congestion and irregular yellow-tan foci of parenchymal infarction.

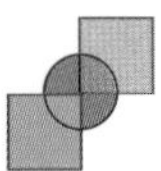

The combination of inferior vena caval thrombosis and hepatic vein thrombosis leading to hepatic infarction also has characteristic radiological features (Fig. 13.44).

Veno-occlusive disease

Obstruction of the small intrahepatic veins occasionally follows ingestion of 'bush teas' which contain senecio alkaloids that damage the intima of small veins. Histology shows centrilobular congestion, necrosis, fibrosis (Figs 13.45–13.48) and, eventually, cirrhosis.

Congestive cardiac failure

Long-standing heart failure due to mitral valve disease or constrictive pericarditis leads to chronic congestion, the so-called nutmeg liver (Figs 13.49, 13.50). Although this is commonly referred to as cardiac

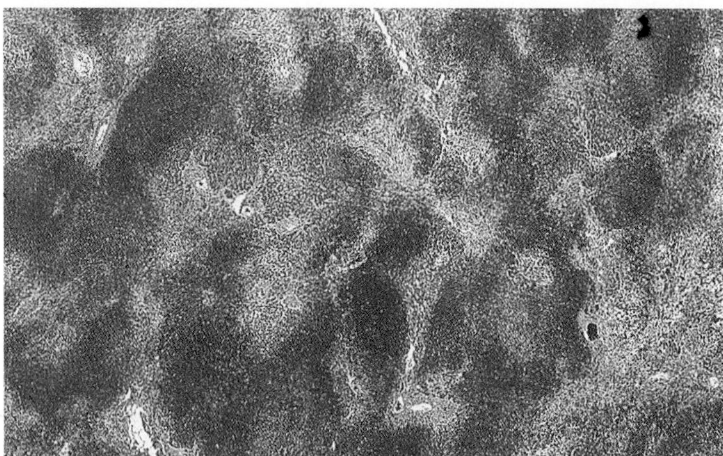

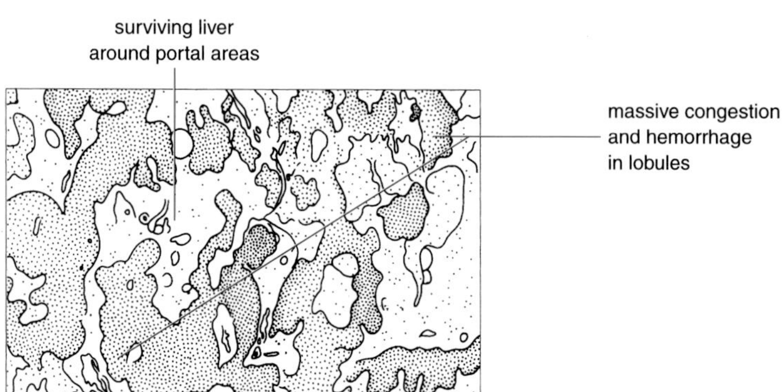

Fig. 13.41 Liver histology in Budd–Chiari syndrome showing greatly congested sinusoids and atrophy of hepatocytes around a central vein. H&E stain (x 35). Courtesy of Prof I. Talbot.

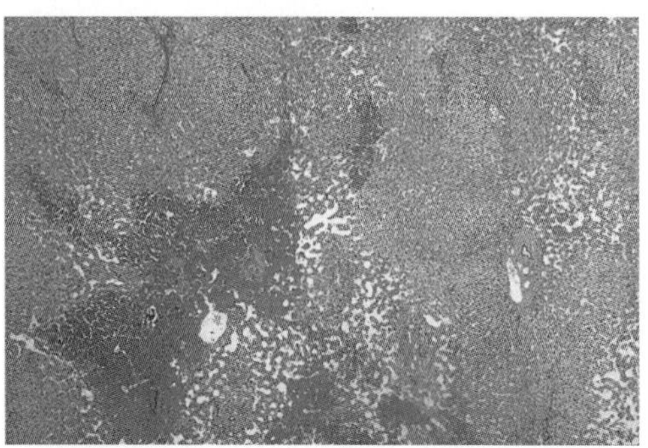

Fig. 13.42 Budd–Chiari syndrome. Microscopic view of the grossly congested and dilated sinusoids in the centrilobular region with hepatic parenchymal replacement by red cells, changes that reflect the rapid onset of venous outflow obstruction in hepatic vein thrombosis.

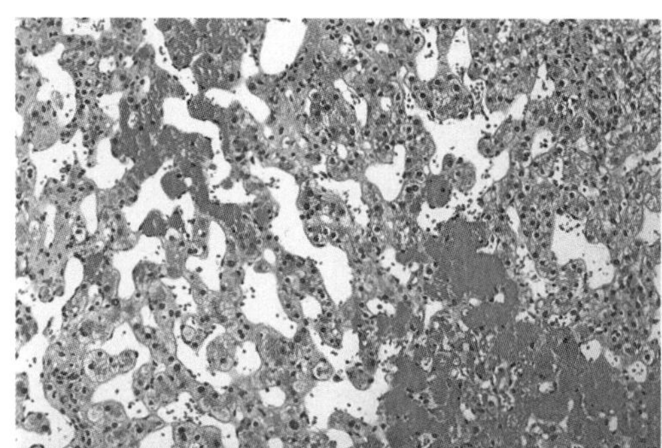

Fig. 13.43 Budd–Chiari syndrome. Higher magnification of the centrilobular region shows the characteristic finding of hemorrhage into the space of Disse and hepatic cords, with red blood cells displacing and replacing hepatocytes, well seen in cords flanked by dilated, but empty sinusoids.

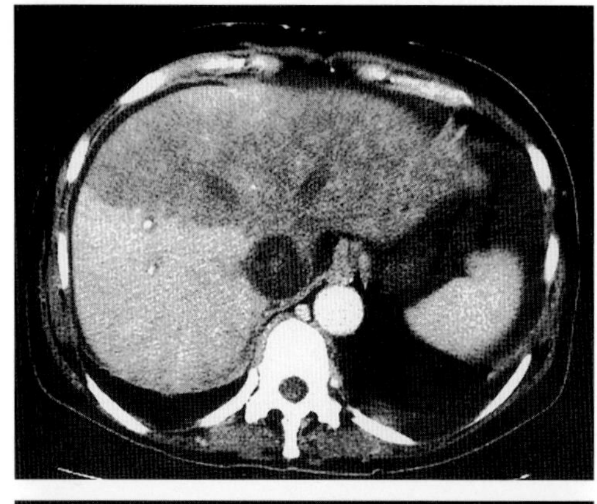

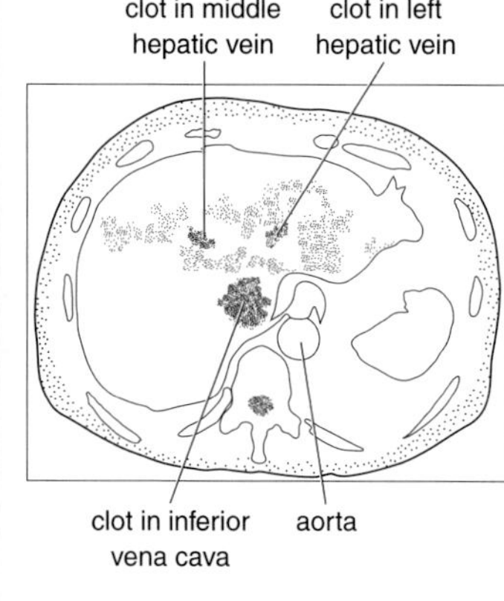

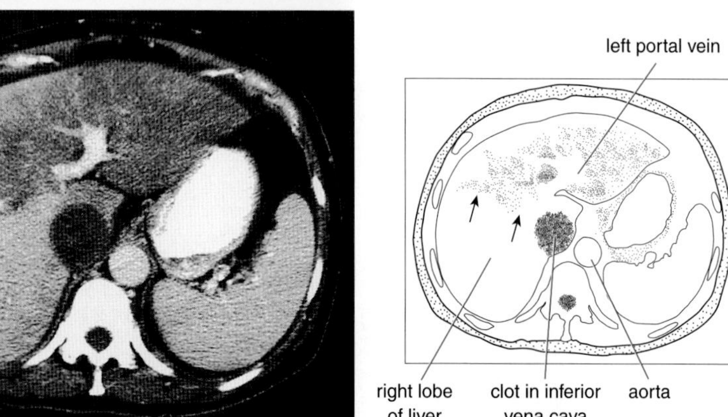

Fig. 13.44 Thrombosis of inferior vena cava and hepatic veins resulting in venous infarction. (a) CT demonstrates low-attenuation clot distending the left and middle hepatic veins and the inferior vena cava. The left lobe of the liver and a small part of the anterior segment of the right lobe are of diffuse low attenuation. (b) CT through level of mid liver shows contrast enhancement of the left portal vein and marked distension of the inferior vena cava with clot.

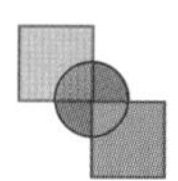

cirrhosis, true cirrhosis rarely occurs. Histologically it is associated with sinusoidal dilatation followed by centrilobular congestion with loss of hepatocytes (Fig. 13.51).

Peliosis hepatitis

This uncommon vascular condition is associated with the use of oral contraceptives and a number of systemic disorders, for example carcinoma and tuberculosis. Blood-filled vascular spaces or lacuna-like holes are present (Fig. 13.52), and these may rupture causing intraperitoneal bleeding.

Shock

In severe shock, areas of centrilobular necrosis may be seen as a terminal lesion due to poor perfusion and hypoxia. In eclampsia or severe toxemia of pregnancy there are often widespread hepatic periportal infarcts and extensive fibrin deposition (Figs 13.53, 13.54).

Arterial infarction

Ligation or occlusion of the hepatic artery causes only temporary hepatic disturbance, due to the dual blood supply of the liver (75% from the portal vein). Nevertheless, localized areas of infarction may occur (Figs 13.55, 13.56). Smaller hepatic arteries may be affected by polyarteritis nodosa (Fig. 13.57).

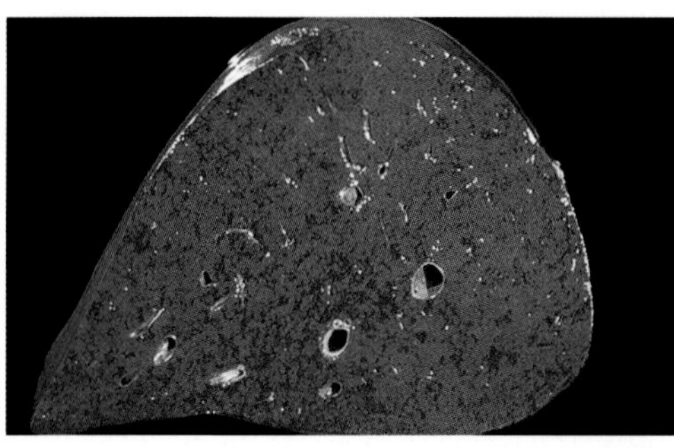

■ **Fig. 13.45** Veno-occlusive disease. Hepatectomy explant specimen in veno-occlusive disease complicating bone marrow transplantation showing an irregular, arborized pattern of congestion with rimming by yellow-tan discoloration indicative of necrosis.

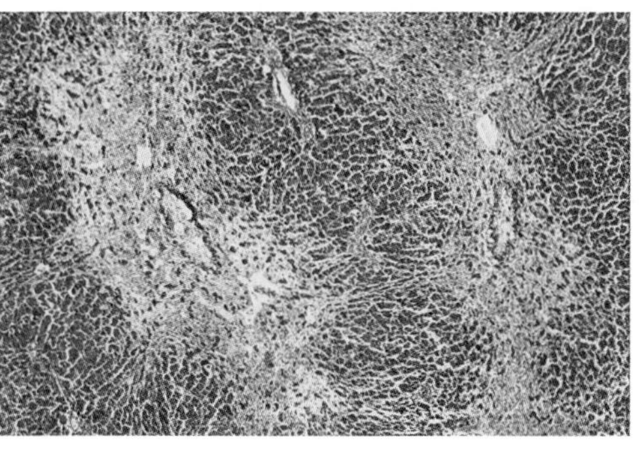

■ **Fig. 13.46** Veno-occlusive disease. Low-magnification view of trichrome stain showing the blue-rimmed central veins (normal perivascular collagen) and the pale zones of perivenular hepatocyte atrophy surrounding them.

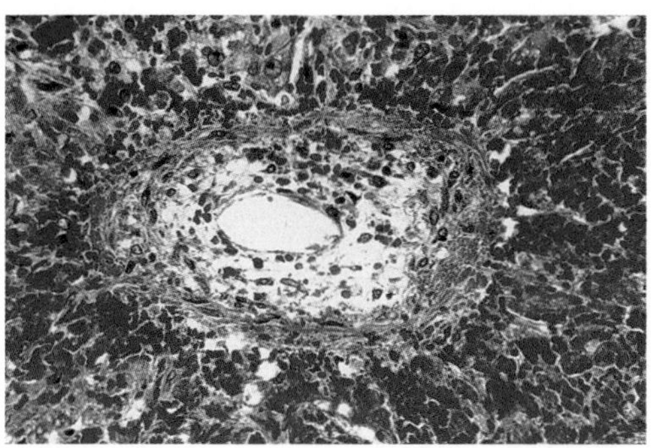

■ **Fig. 13.47** Veno-occlusive disease. Trichrome stain of central vein showing an early lesion of endothelial injury with subendothelial edema, hemorrhage and monocytic infiltrates.

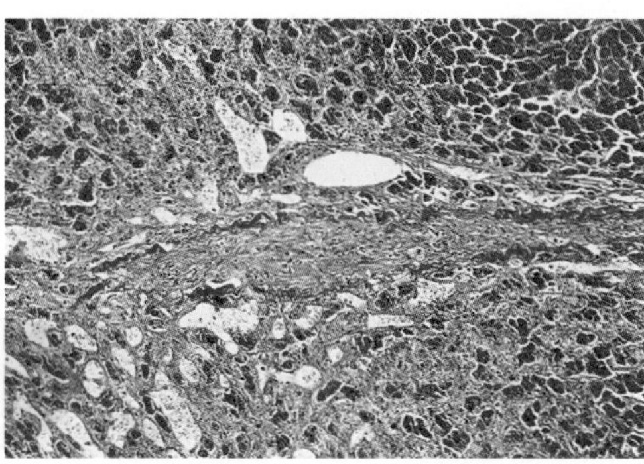

■ **Fig. 13.48** Veno-occlusive disease. Trichrome stain of central vein showing fibrous obliteration of the lumen of a central vein.

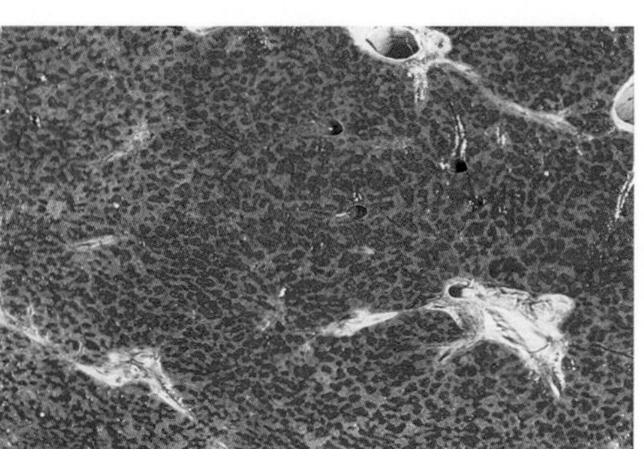

■ **Fig. 13.49** Passive hepatic congestion in heart failure. Cut surface of the liver with passive congestion due to heart failure showing the classic pattern of 'nutmeg liver' characterized by bridging central–central zones of yellow-tan necrosis rimmed by hemorrhage that encircles islands of periportal parenchyma.

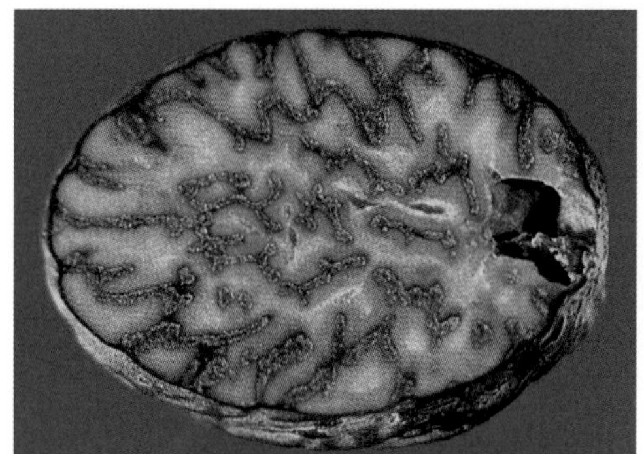

■ **Fig. 13.50** Cut surface of a nutmeg showing the veining pattern to which the gross appearance of the liver parenchyma in passive congestion has been likened.

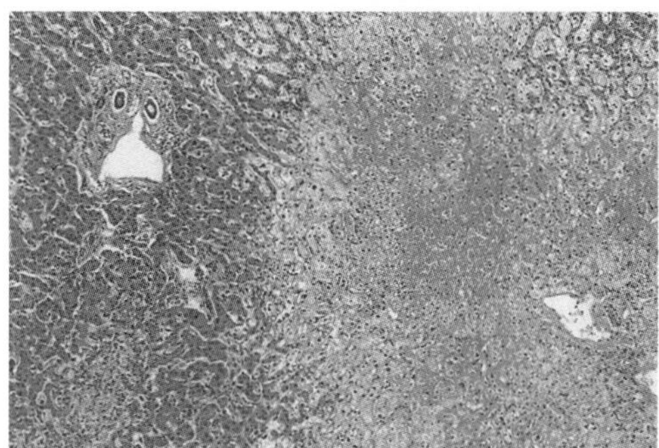

■ **Fig. 13.51** Nutmeg liver: passive hepatic congestion in heart failure. Microscopic view showing a centrilobular zone of necrosis and hemorrhage surrounding a central vein (extreme right) and a portal area (extreme left) surrounded by viable hepatocytes.

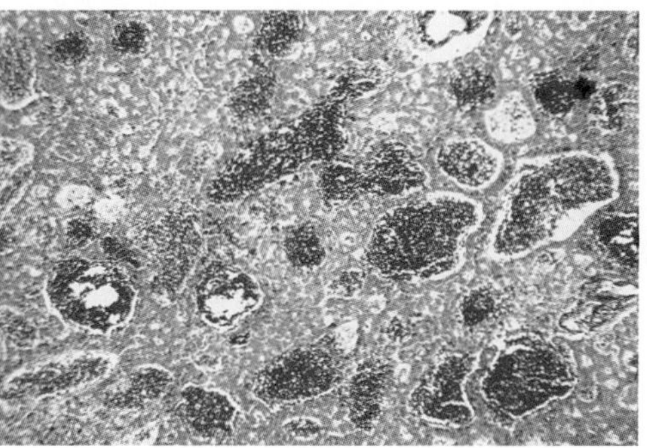

■ **Fig. 13.52** Peliosis hepatis. Microscopic view showing the characteristic cystically dilated blood-filled spaces lacking endothelial linings within the hepatic parenchyma.

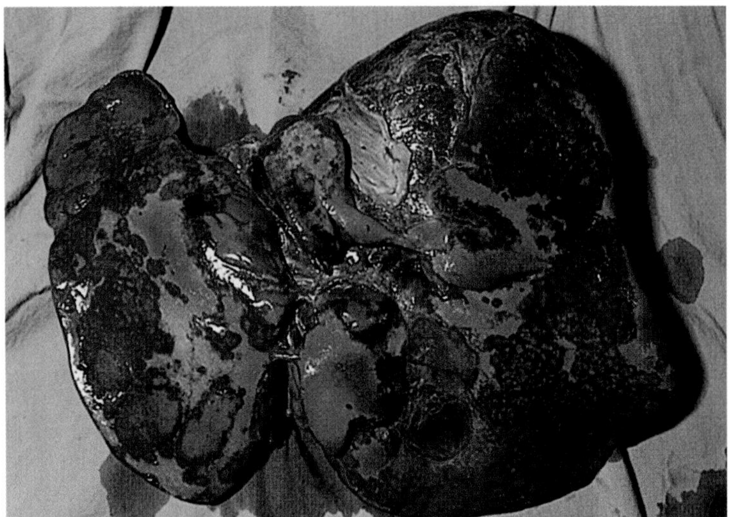

Fig. 13.53 Liver of a patient who died from eclampsia, showing areas of massive infarction.

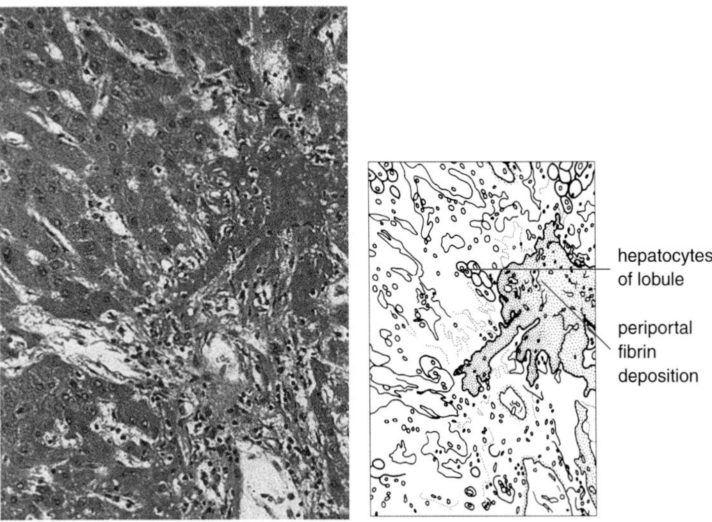

Fig. 13.54 Characteristic periportal fibrin deposition in eclampsia. H&E stain (x 120).

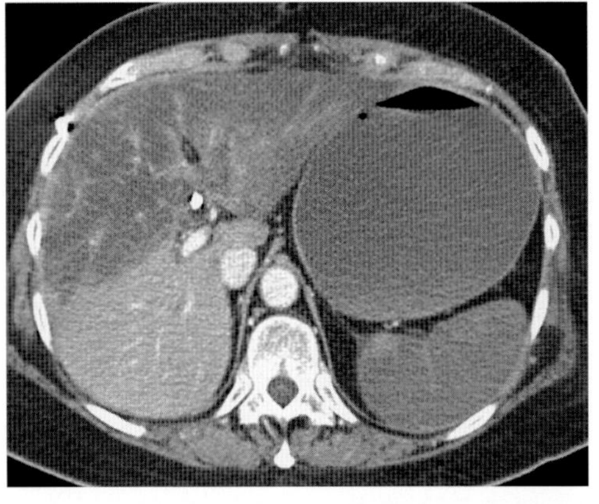

Fig. 13.55 CT scan exhibiting the characteristic appearance of hepatic infarction; this degree of hepatic damage is rare because of the multiple blood supplies of the liver. Surviving normal tissue can also be seen.

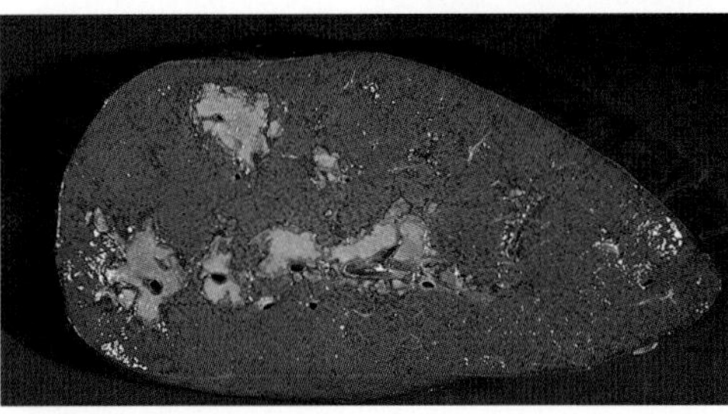

Fig. 13.56 Hepatic infarction. Macroscopic view of liver in arterial thrombosis and infarction showing large irregular foci of yellowed, necrotic parenchyma rimmed by hemorrhage. The intervening liver shows the green discoloration of cholestasis.

Extrahepatic portal venous obstruction

There are many causes of extrahepatic obstruction involving the portal venous system (Fig. 13.58). The site of obstruction may be demonstrated (very rarely these days) by splenic venography following direct percutaneous puncture of the spleen, or indirectly by examining the venous return following splenic arterial injection of contrast (see below). Simple ultrasound is relatively unhelpful in the imaging of portal vein obstruction, but its usefulness can be substantially increased by the addition of Doppler techniques (see Chapter 12). CT scanning (Fig. 13.59) is a useful non-invasive technique for visualizing portal vein occlusion, gradually being superseded by the more sensitive magnetic resonance imaging (Fig. 13.60).

Hereditary hemorrhagic telangiectasia (Osler–Weber–Rendu disease)

Hereditary hemorrhagic telangiectasia (see also Chapters 2, 3, and 4) is associated mainly with hemorrhagic lesions in the mouth and gastrointestinal tract, but some vascular dilatations may be found in the liver (Fig. 13.61). This condition is asymptomatic but the vascular nature of the lesions is such that percutaneous liver biopsy should only be carried out with great caution.

Arteriovenous malformation

Arteriovenous malformation (AVM) within the hepatic vasculature is not common. Although it may be responsible for catastrophic bleeding it may also be an incidental finding. The appearances on scanning may be misleading until the phasic sequence of contrast enhancement is appreciated (Fig. 13.62). Confusion with hemangiomas (see below) should then be avoided.

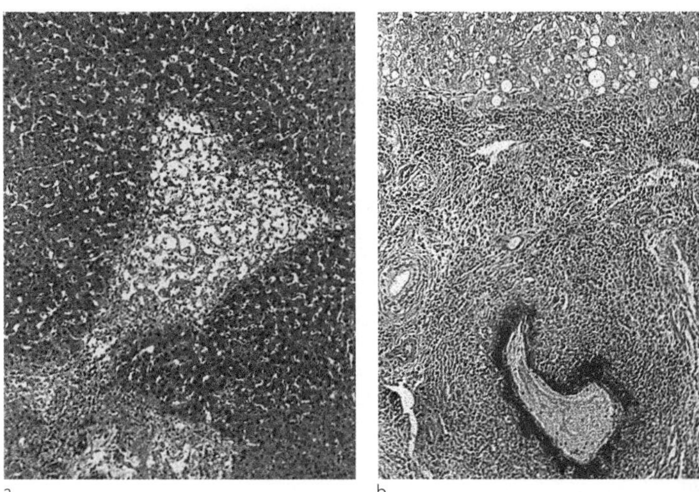

Fig. 13.57 Liver sections in polyarteritis nodosa showing a small triangular zone of liver cell death ((a), H&E stain, x 50) and fibrinoid necrosis of an hepatic artery with heavy surrounding inflammatory infiltrate ((b), H&E stain, x 50).

Etiology of Extrahepatic Portal Venous Obstruction		
Splenic	trauma	neoplasia
	pancreatitis	idiopathhic
Portal	sepsis	thrombotic disorders
	trauma	cirrhosis
	neoplasia	idiopathic

Fig. 13.58 The etiology of extrahepatic portal venous obstruction

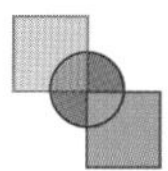

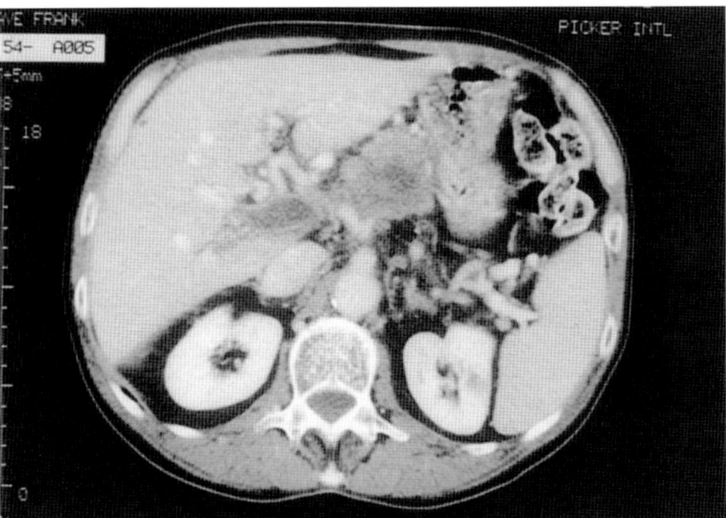

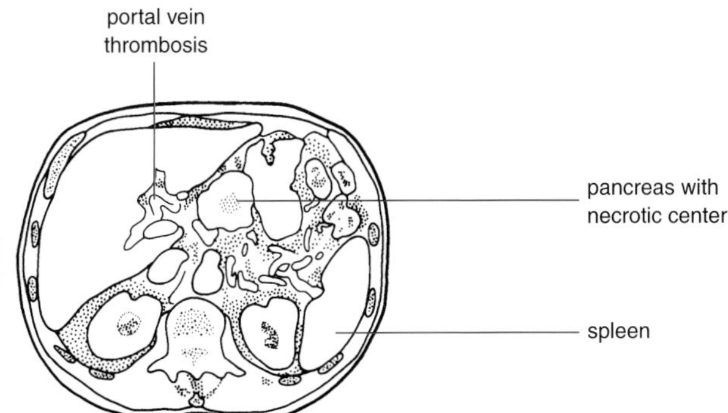

Fig. 13.59 CT scan showing portal vein thrombosis secondary to carcinoma of pancreas. Courtesy of Dr R.A. Nakielny

a

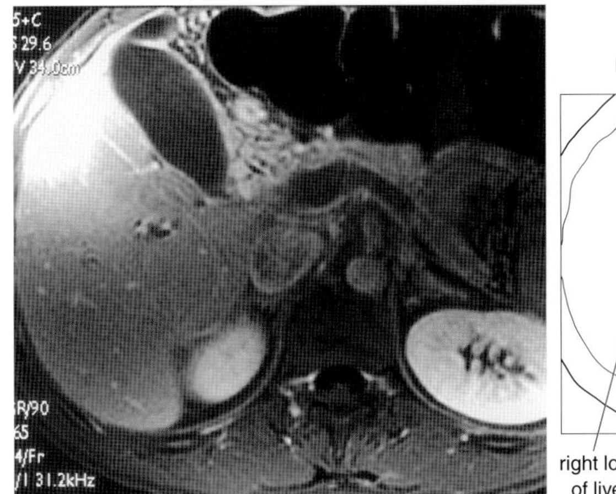

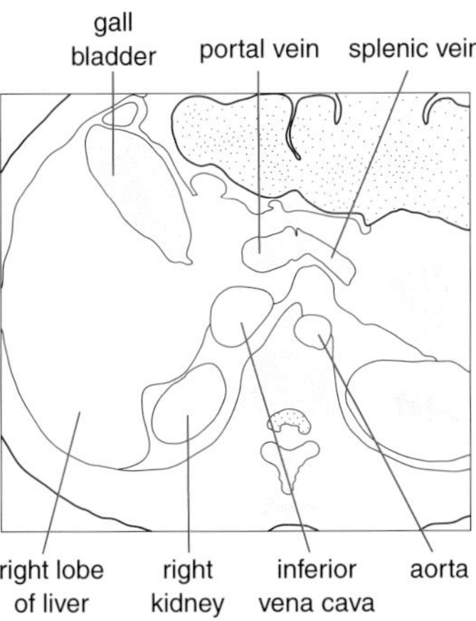

b

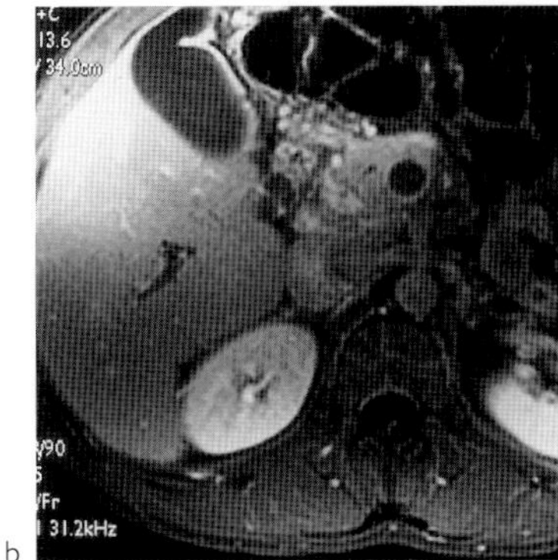

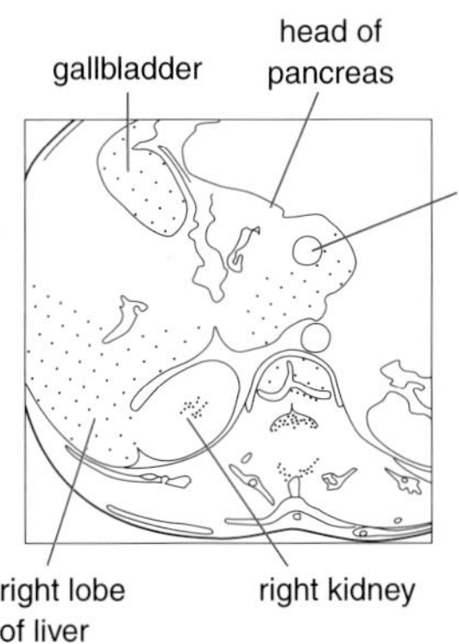

Fig. 13.60 Portal vein thrombus and obstruction in a patient with hypercoagulable state. (a) MR through neck of pancreas shows low-intensity clot distending distal splenic vein and the proximal portal vein. Compare the intensity of the blood in the normal inferior vena cava with that in the splenic and portal veins. (b) MR through the head of the pancreas shows a dilated, clot-filled low-intensity distal superior mesenteric vein.

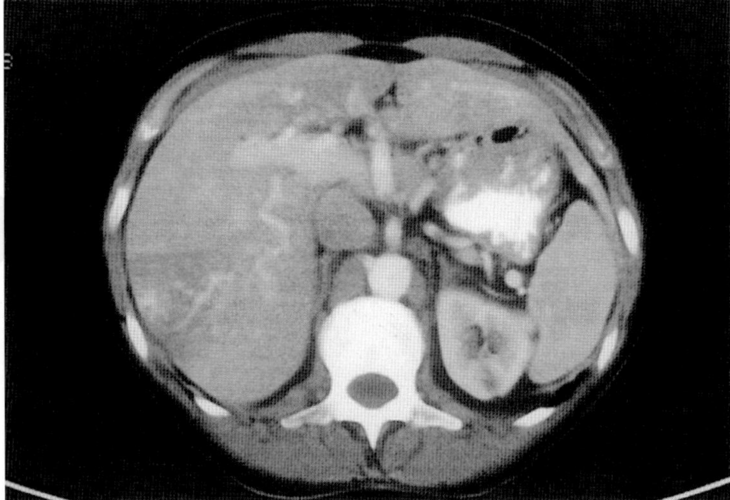

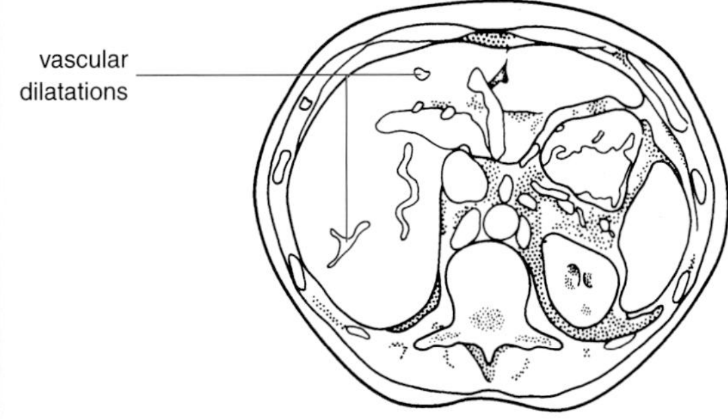

Fig. 13.61 CT scan of hereditary hemorrhagic telangiectasia showing multiple vascular dilatations. Courtesy of Dr R.A. Nakielny.

Trauma

Although the liver is well protected from external trauma by the rib cage, lacerations may occur as a result of road traffic accidents and other major abdominal injuries. Ultrasound (Fig. 13.63) and/or CT scanning (Fig. 13.64) are valuable tools for detecting such injuries, which may be fatal unless diagnosed promptly. Percutaneous liver biopsy resulting in subcapsular hematoma which may rupture into the peritoneum is an important cause of traumatic damage to the organ with its own particular imaging characteristics (Fig. 13.65). On rare occasions malignant infiltration of the peritoneum may cause changes misleadingly suggestive of subcapsular hemorrhage (Fig. 13.66). Hemobilia is a well-recognized consequence of trauma and ERCP may then provide useful additional information (Fig. 13.67 and see Chapter 14).

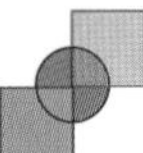

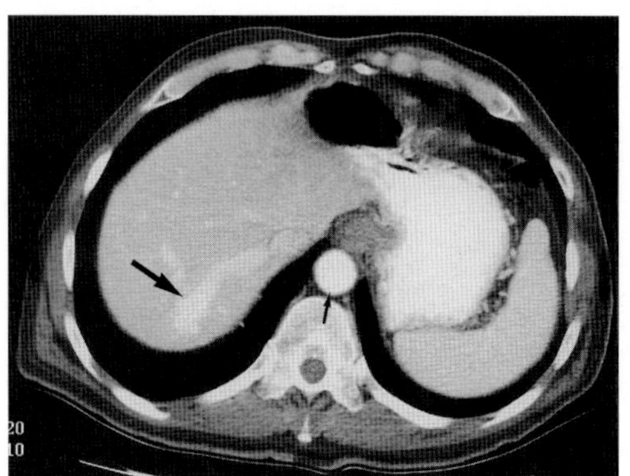

a

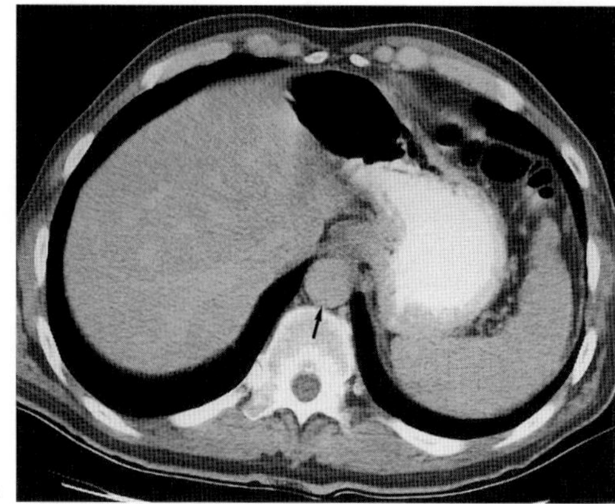

b

■ **Fig. 13.62** CT demonstrating portovenous malformation. (a) Image obtained during the late hepatic arterial phase shows a tubular shaped contrast-enhancing mass (long arrow). Compare its density with the contrast in the aorta (small arrow). The right hepatic vein is enlarged. (b) Image obtained during the late portal venous/near equilibrium phase, shows diminished contrast enhancement. A hemangioma would show increasing enhancement.

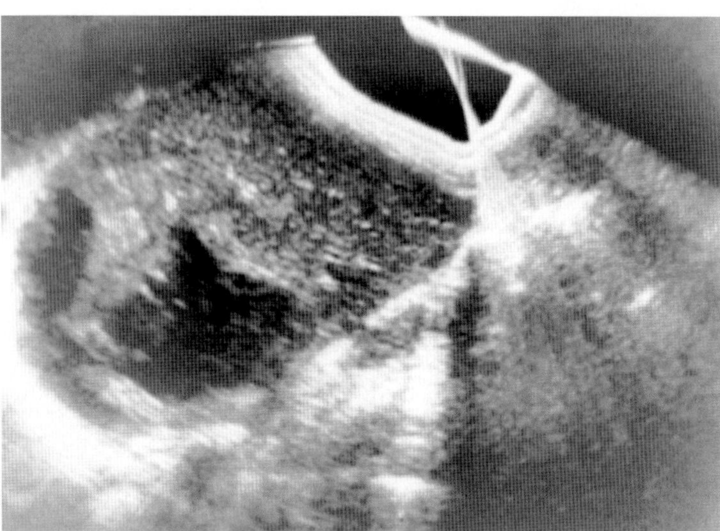

■ **Fig. 13.63** Ultrasonogram showing traumatic liver injury following a road traffic accident. There is an intrahepatic collection of blood and a subcapsular hematoma.

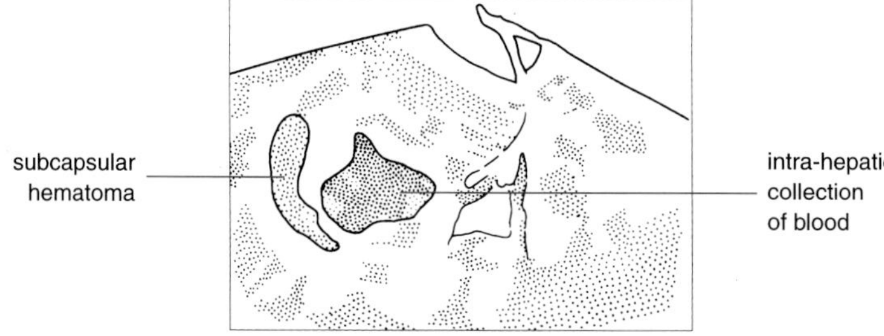

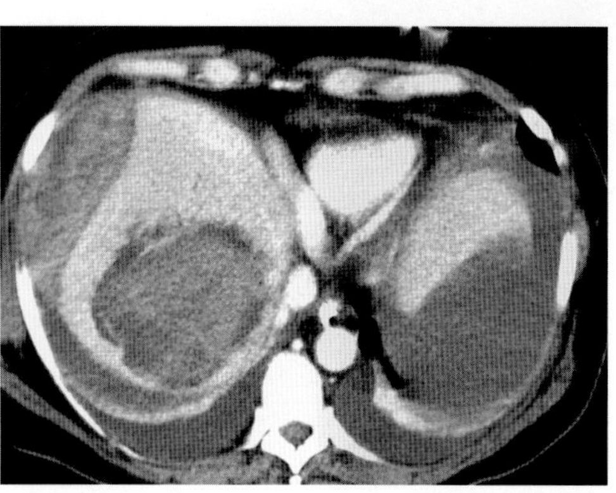

■ **Fig. 13.64** CT from a similar case showing massive intra-abdominal hematoma formation including intrahepatic and subcapsular bleeding.

LIVER CYSTS AND TUMORS

Cysts

Solitary cysts are a common chance finding at ultrasonography, surgery, or postmortem and involve the right lobe of the liver more often than the left (Figs 13.68–13.70). Most cysts are unilocular and are lined by a single layer of cuboidal cells, but multiple cysts are also seen (Fig 13.71). Malignant transformation occurs very rarely. Fortunately CT scanning can usually make a ready distinction between metastases and concomitant incidental cysts (Fig. 13.72).

Multiple hepatic cysts are often seen in association with the polycystic kidney syndrome, but can occur as a heritable form of isolated polycystic liver disease. Diagnosis is obvious on CT (Fig. 13.73)

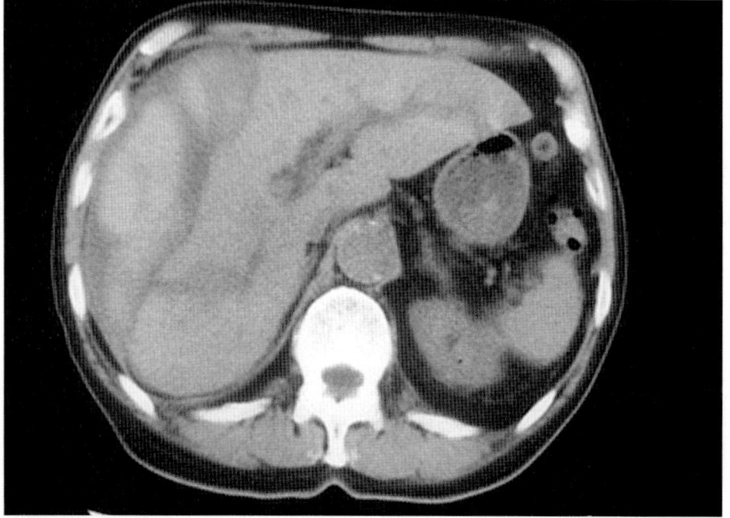

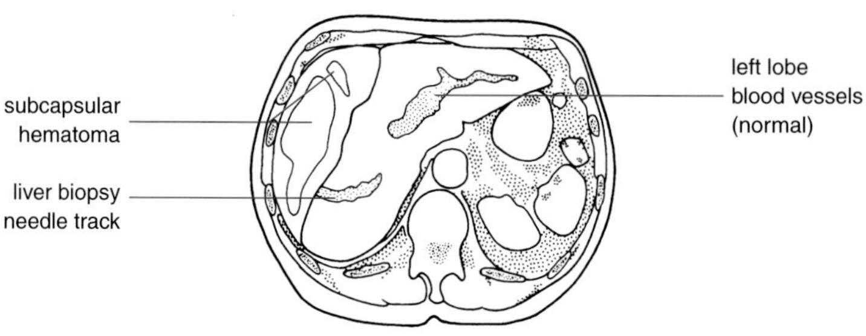

■ **Fig. 13.65** CT scan showing a subcapsular hematoma indenting the liver. The darker shadow is caused by the presence of fresh blood. Bleeding occurred as a result of liver biopsy, and the needle track is clearly visible. Courtesy of Dr R.A. Nakielny.

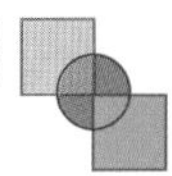

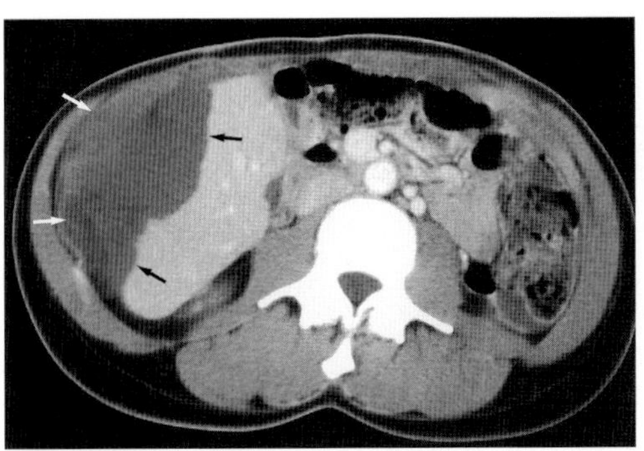

Fig. 13.66 Huge intraperitoneal implant mimicking subcapsular hematoma. A large 8 cm thick non-homogeneous mass (white arrows) indents the contour of the liver (black arrows).

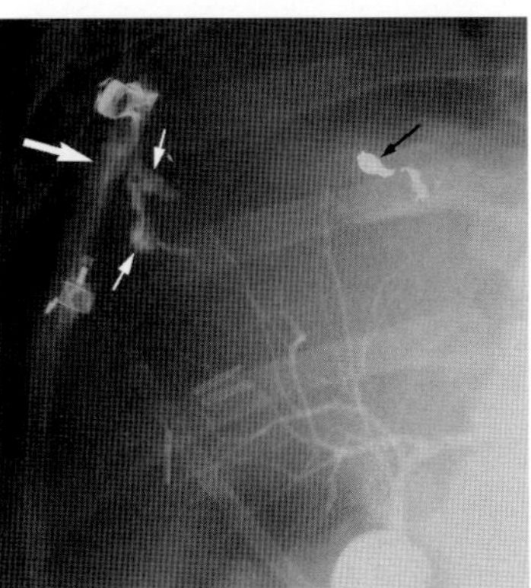

Fig. 13.67 ERCP demonstrating leak from anterior right lobe of liver into right perihepatic space. Many irregular metallic-density bullet fragments (black arrow) lie in the hepatic parenchyma. Contrast leaks (short white arrows) out of peripheral branches and enters a drainage tube (long white arrow) in the right perihepatic space.

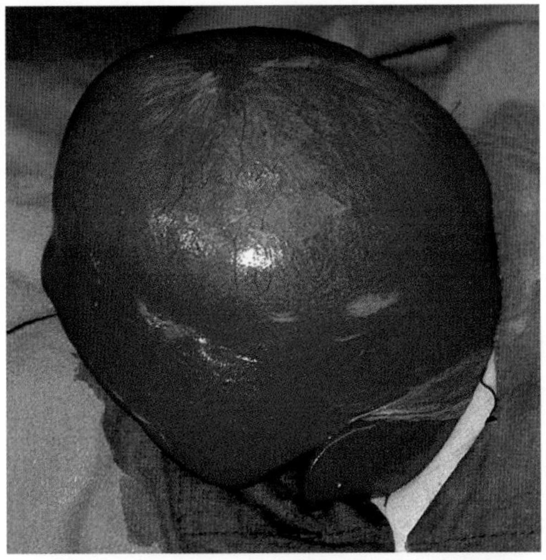

Fig. 13.68 A developmental cyst at surgery. Courtesy of Prof I. Talbot.

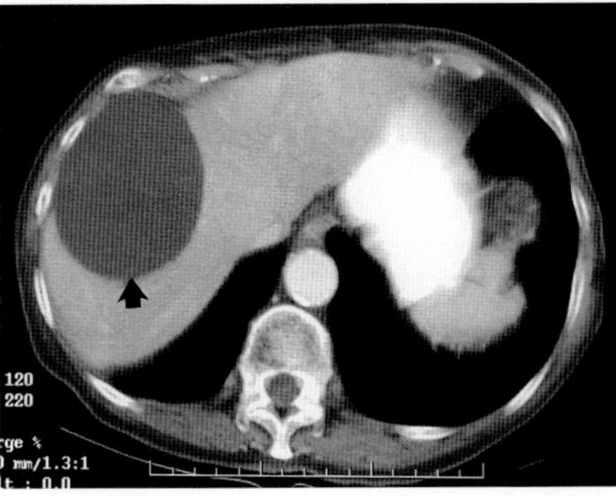

Fig. 13.69 CT showing simple cyst of liver. A fluid-attenuation mass (arrow) is present in the anterior segment of the right lobe of the liver.

or MRI (Fig. 13.74). Symptomatic lesions may require surgical management (Fig. 13.75) and very rarely liver transplantation.

Adenoma and other focal benign lesions

Adenomas are benign tumors of liver cells, typically seen in young women as a well-recognized complication of oral contraceptive use.

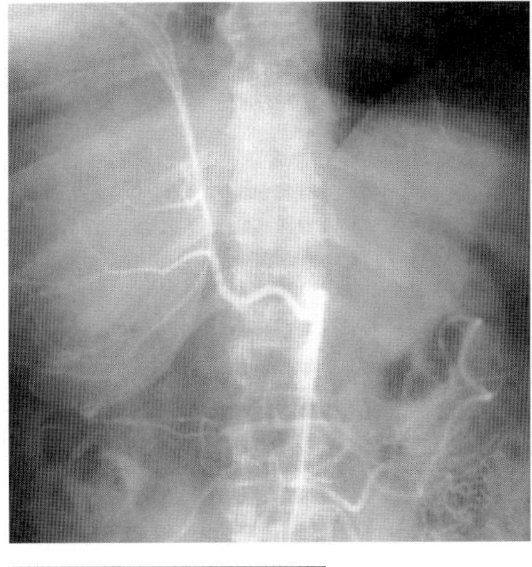

Fig. 13.70 Hepatic arteriogram showing gross displacement of blood vessels by a large avascular cyst.

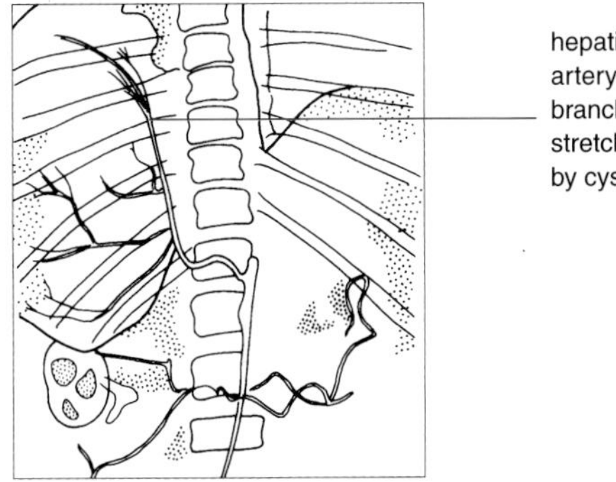

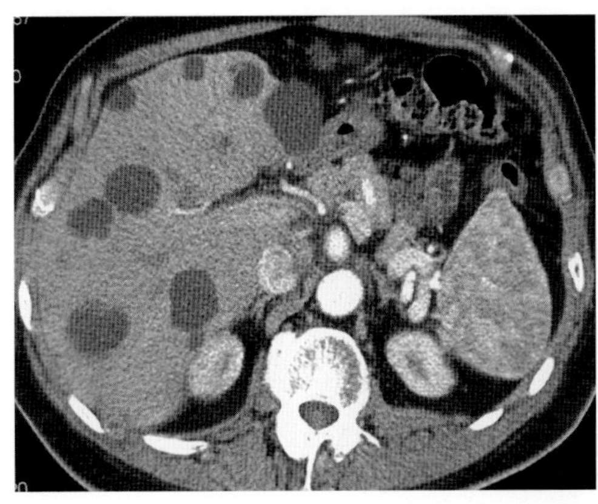

Fig. 13.71 Multiple benign hepatic cysts in a non-syndromic patient.

Hepatic adenomas are also seen in glycogen storage disease (type 1a). Since adenomas may undergo malignant transformation, it is important to make a firm diagnosis of adenoma when it is suspected and to differentiate it from focal nodular hyperplasia (FNH) (see below). The typical adenoma consists of a solitary nodule, which may be up to 15 cm in diameter, in an otherwise normal liver. Adenomas appear hypodense on non-contrast CT, with variable enhancement with contrast (Figs 13.76, 13.77). When the clinical diagnosis is in doubt, technetium-sulfur colloid scintigraphy may differentiate adenoma from FNH as the adenoma does not have Kupffer cells and therefore does not take up the sulfur colloid. Surgical excision may be necessary for larger lesions or where persisting doubt about malignant status exists (Fig. 13.78). The histology comprises trabeculae of slightly enlarged liver cells (Figs 13.79, 13.80). Large, thin-walled vessels may be present which may thrombose, rupture, or bleed. Adenomas of bile duct origin comprising subcapsular nodules of proliferating small ducts may occur, but these are usually incidental findings at operation or autopsy (Fig. 13.81).

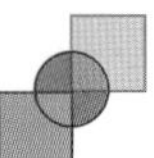

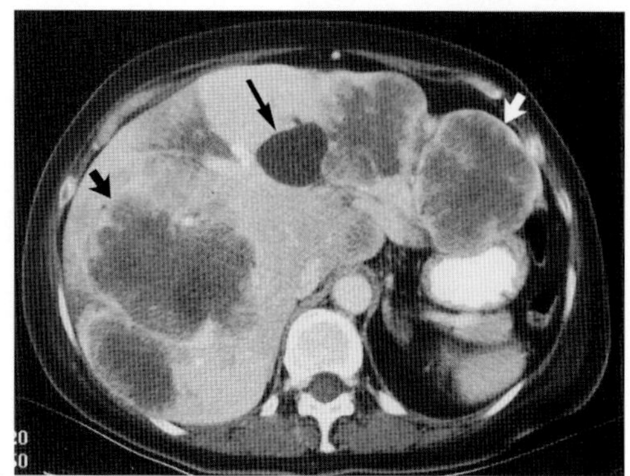

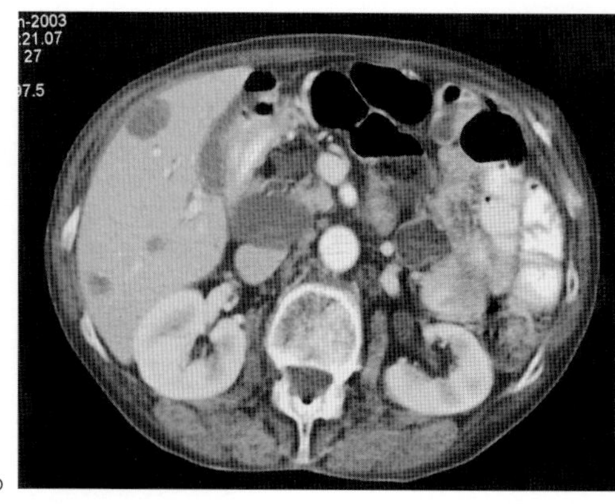

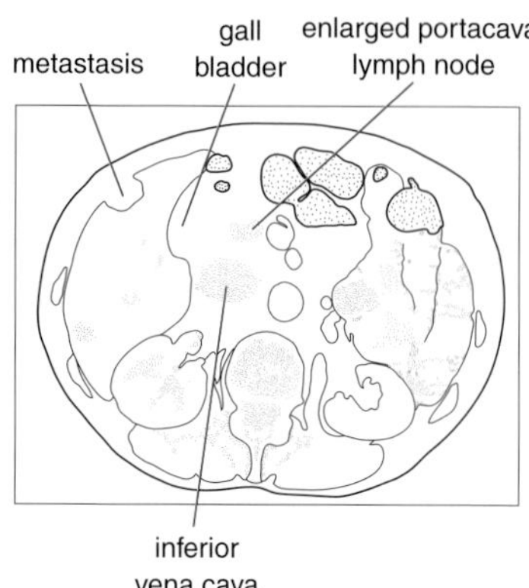

Fig. 13.72 (a) CT comparing simple cyst and multiple low-attenuation metastases. A simple cyst (long arrow) is manifest as a uniform fluid attenuation (less than 20 Hounsfield units) mass in the medial segment of the left lobe of the liver. Many large metastases are manifested as inhomogeneous low-attenuation masses (short arrows) with contrast enhancing rims and central foci. (b) CT demonstrating 'fluid-attenuation' metastases in a patient with colloid carcinoma of the breast. Compare the density of the three liver metastases with the density of the bile in the gallbladder. Not all fluid attenuation lesions in the liver are simple cysts. Metastasis to a lymph node in the portacaval space is also present. Note the very low attenuation of this nodal metastasis.

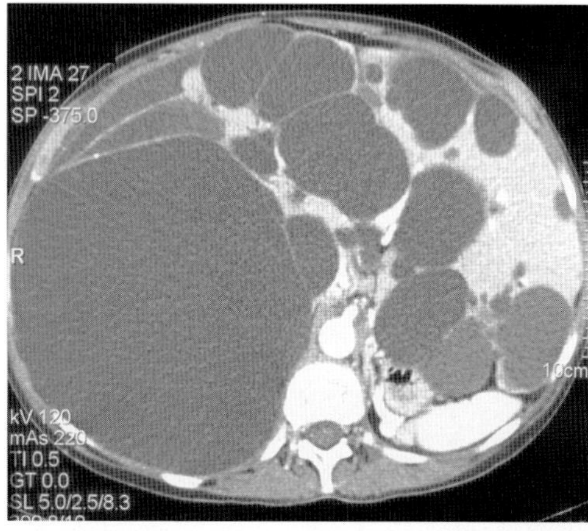

Fig. 13.73 Polycystic liver disease seen at CT scanning. Courtesy of Richard Schulick, MD.

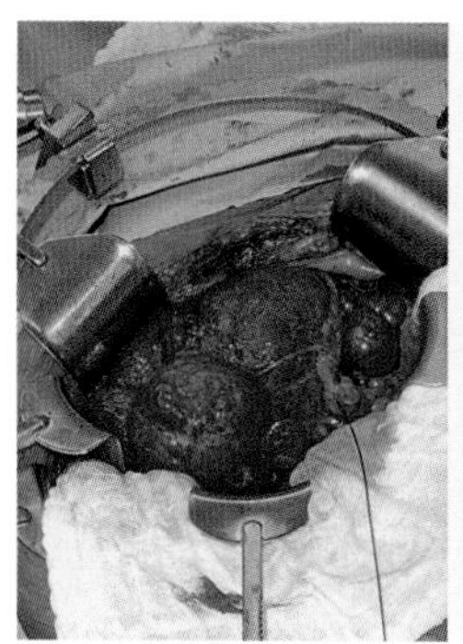

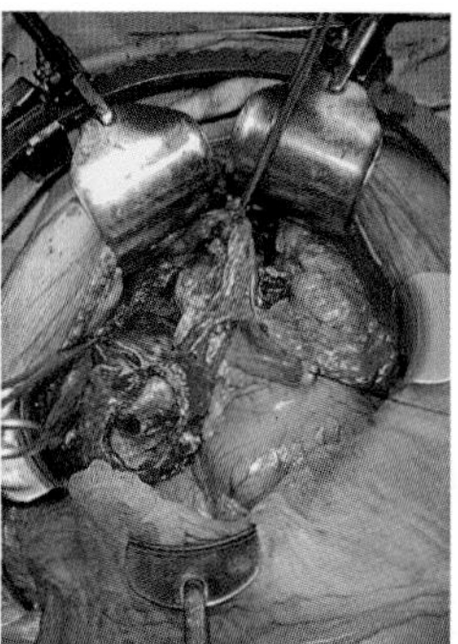

Fig. 13.75 Resection in polycystic liver disease.

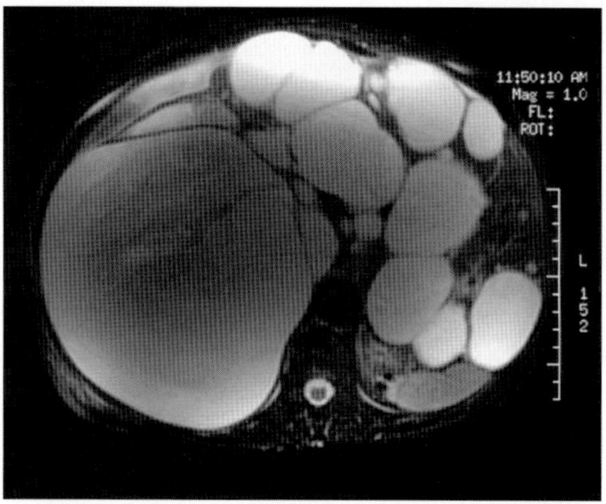

Fig. 13.74 MR appearances of polycystic liver disease. Courtesy of Richard Schulick, MD.

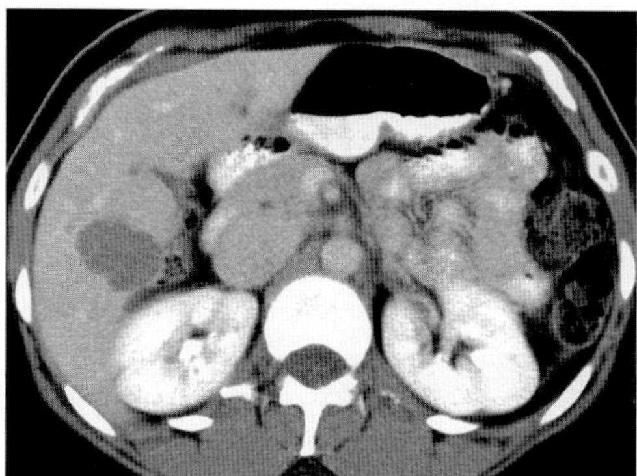

Fig. 13.76 CT scan of hepatic adenoma. A single small lesion.

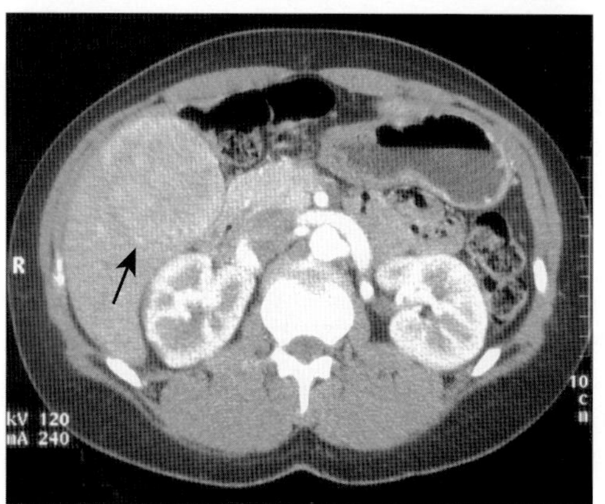

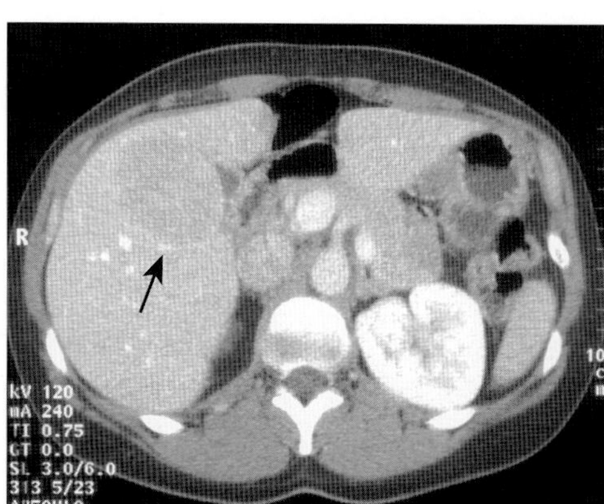

Fig. 13.77 CT scan of hepatic adenoma. (a, b) Images from the arterial and venous phases of contrast scanning in a patient with a larger adenoma.

Other rare benign nodular parenchymal lesions occur in the liver and their cause is unknown. Within this category are focal nodular hyperplasia (Figs 13.82–13.86) and partial nodular transformation; both are normally asymptomatic but may be responsible for abnormal liver function tests. In the former, which is demonstrated well on CT or MR scanning, there is a characteristic central scar with radiating fibrous bands around nodules of hepatocytes without a lobular pattern. In the latter, hilar nodules of hepatocytes grow and compress adjacent liver tissue, and clinical presentation is with symptoms and complications of portal hypertension. This condition is most commonly associated with Felty's syndrome.

Hemangioma

In infancy, these benign vascular tumors may cause transient cardiac failure before regressing spontaneously. In adults hemangiomas are the most common incidental tumors found on liver imaging (~7%). Although small hemangiomas are almost always asymptomatic, their discovery may cause serious concerns of 'cancer' among patients and their relatives. Occasionally, hemangioma may cause abdominal pain, and, most unusually, they may rupture spontaneously (or cause hemorrhage if inadvertently punctured during liver biopsy). A bruit may be audible over larger lesions. The sonographic appearances are usually diagnostic (Fig. 13.87), but the characteristic vascular pattern is also well shown on rapid sequence, contrast-enhanced CT. On unenhanced CT, these lesions appear as relatively hypodense, well-circumscribed masses. After IV contrast, they typically show peripheral enhancement, followed by homogeneous near-complete filling in the case of smaller lesions (Figs 13.88, 13.89); note the distinction from AVM shown above. Even huge tumors may be readily visible only in specific phases of the contrast cycle (Fig. 13.90). The obvious differences between the appearances on different phases of MR scanning can also be diagnostic, and this may be especially helpful in smaller lesions (Fig. 13.91). Arteriography (Fig. 13.92) is not normally necessary, although it may be used in atypical cases as well to define the blood supply if surgical ligation or excision are contemplated because of major symptoms or complications (Fig. 13.93). Histologically the lesions consist of dilatations of proliferating blood vessels (Fig. 13.94).

Hemangiopericytomas are very occasionally seen, and now will usually be managed surgically (Fig. 13.95). Malignant vascular tumors, hemangiosarcomas (Fig. 13.96), are rare. They are often associated with industrial exposure to polyvinyl chloride. The tumors are usually multicentric hemorrhagic nodules. Mostly the endothelial cells use the pre-existing liver trabeculae as a scaffold, but solid cellular masses or cavernous blood spaces may be found (Fig. 13.97).

Hepatoma (primary hepatocellular carcinoma: HCC)

Primary carcinomas of the liver are usually derived from parenchymal cells. Those derived from bile ducts, the cholangiocarcinomas, will be considered in Chapter 14. The majority (>85%) arise in cirrhotic livers, and cirrhosis of any etiology may predispose to primary liver

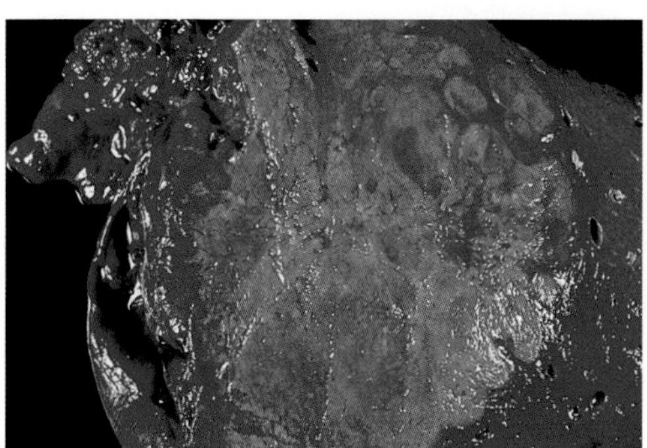

Fig. 13.78 Hepatocellular adenoma. Surgical resection specimen showing slightly irregular borders and a vaguely nodular, fleshy yellow-pink cut surface.

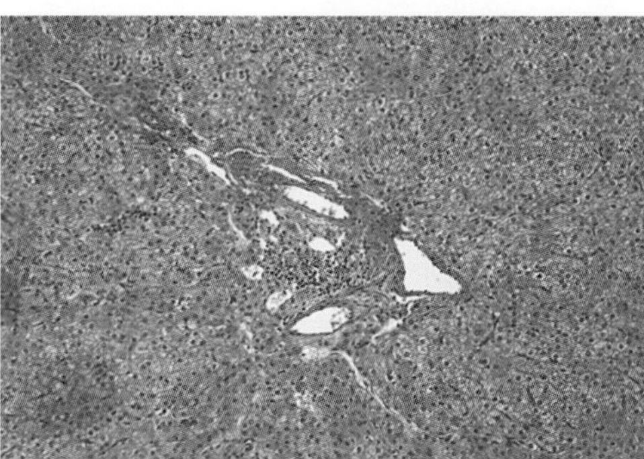

Fig. 13.79 Hepatocellular adenoma. Microscopic section showing the uniform hepatocellular composition, the abnormal vascular pattern, and the absence of portal tracts.

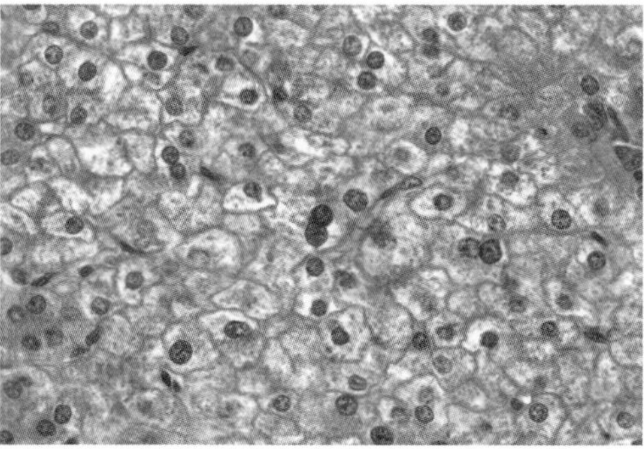

Fig. 13.80 Hepatocellular adenoma. High magnification showing the monomorphous appearance of the hepatocytes, the lack of mitotic activity, and the growth in thick disorganized cords that, like normal liver, contain Kupffer cells and endothelial cells.

a

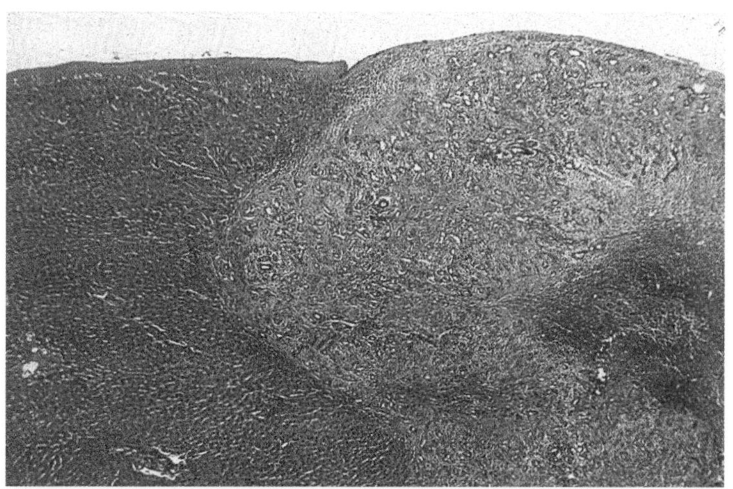

b

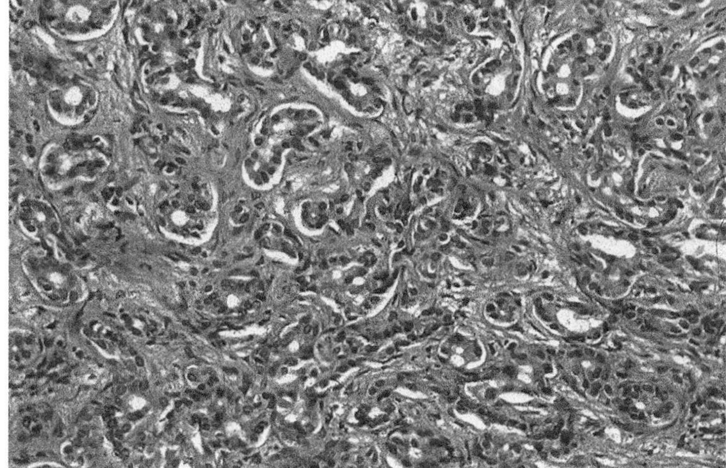

Fig. 13.81 Bile duct adenoma, with a dark patch of inflammation, found incidentally at autopsy ((a), H&E stain, x 30). At higher magnification, the proliferating bile ductules can be seen ((b), x 180).

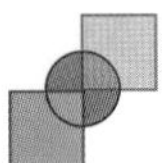

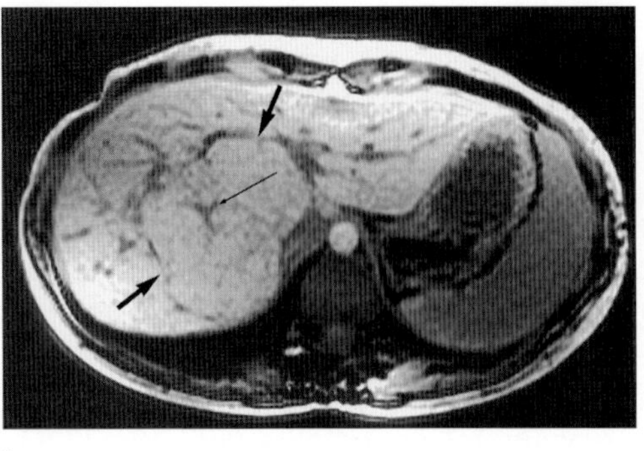

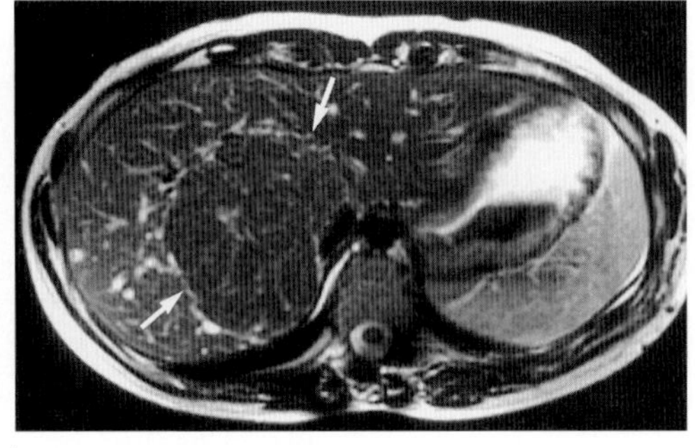

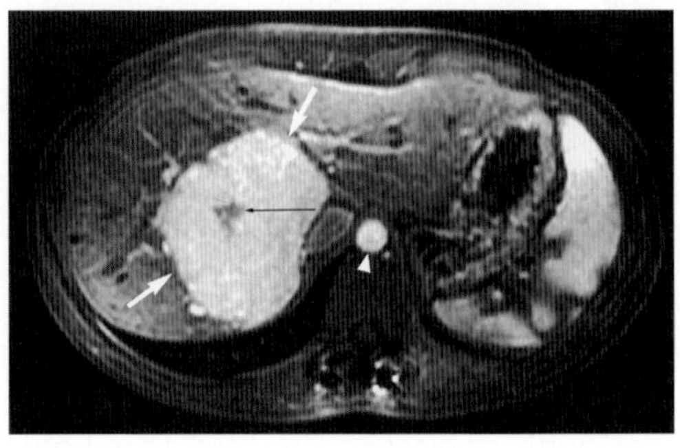

a b c

Fig. 13.82 MRI demonstrating focal nodular hyperplasia. (a) T_1-weighted image demonstrates a subtle mass (thick arrows) that is isointense to the liver parenchyma. A central stellate scar (thin arrow) is seen. (b) T_2-weighted image demonstrates a subtle mass (arrows) that is slightly hypointense to normal parenchyma. (c) Image obtained in the arterial-dominant phase after intravenous injection of gadodiamide (Omniscan, Nycomed, Princeton, NJ) demonstrates a hypervascular mass (white arrows) with a central scar (black arrow). The aorta brightly enhances (arrowhead). Courtesy of Drew Torigian, MD, Philadelphia.

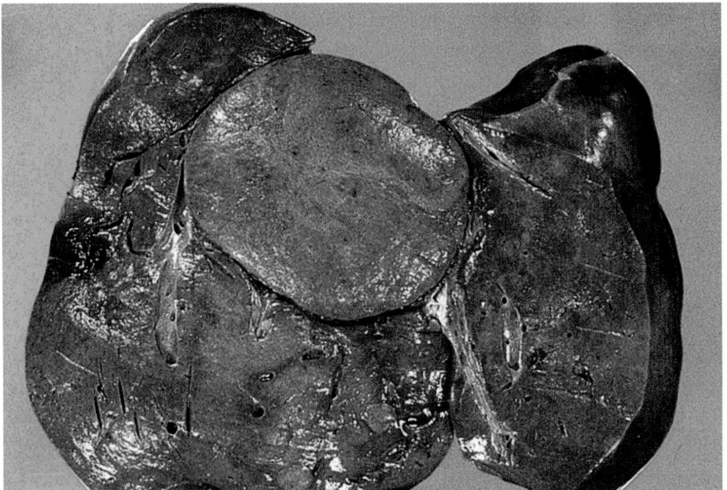

Fig. 13.83 Focal nodular hyperplasia found at autopsy in a case of glycogen-storage disease. Courtesy of Prof I. Talbot.

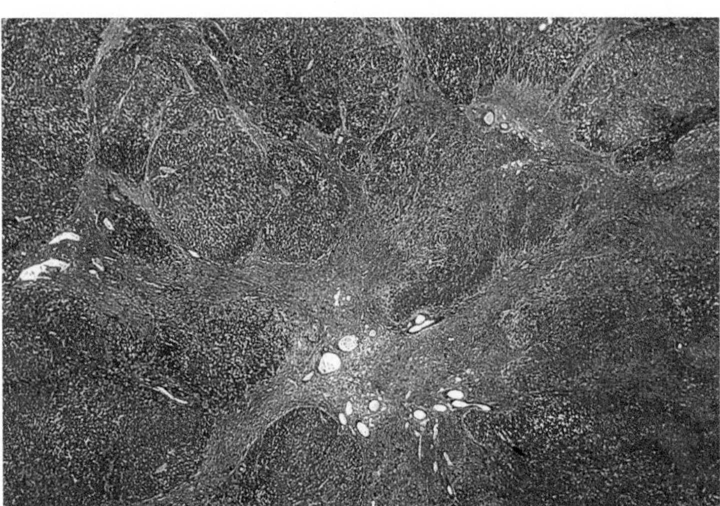

Fig. 13.84 Focal nodular hyperplasia showing central stellate scar. Masson trichrome stain (x 12).

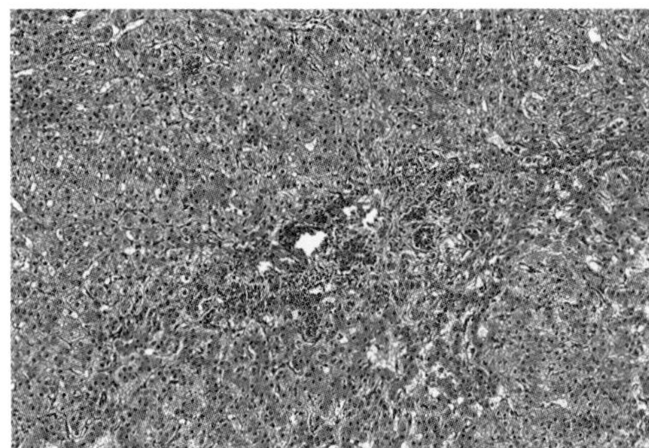

Fig. 13.85 Focal nodular hyperplasia. Microscopic section showing the hamartomatous composition of the lesion, which includes both hepatocytic parenchyma and portal areas that are cytologically normal but architecturally atypical.

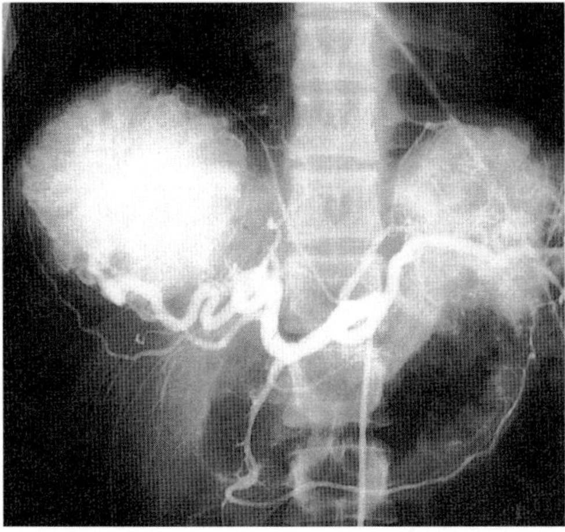

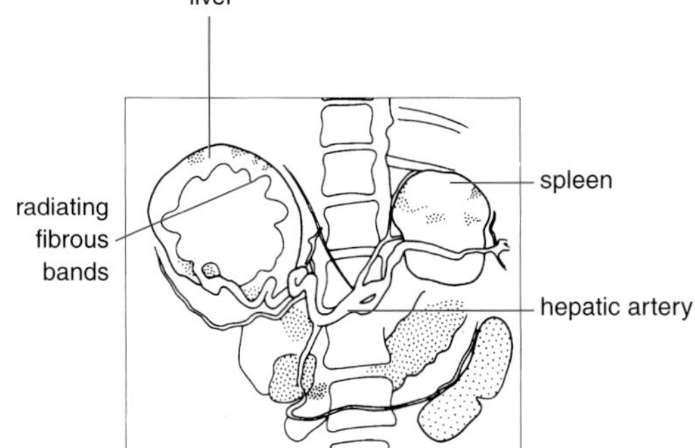

Fig. 13.86 Hepatic arteriogram showing the stellate appearance produced by radiating fibrous bands in a nodule in focal nodular hyperplasia. Courtesy of Professor A.P. Hemingway.

cancer. Hepatitis B has been unquestionably the most important predisposing factor, and there is a close geographical association between the prevalence of this tumor and that of chronic hepatitis B (see Chapter 11); hepatitis C is now becoming more important in this arena. Hepatoma may present initially with features of chronic decompensated liver disease, or it may develop as a terminal complication in patients with long-established cirrhosis. Spontaneous rupture of malignant nodules of the liver may also occur. Less commonly, hepatomas may arise in an otherwise normal liver. Dramatically elevated alpha-feto-protein and positive ultrasound scanning are the least invasive effective routes to diagnosis (Fig. 13.98). The sensitivity of CT scan to diagnose HCC has improved with the use

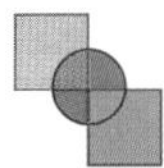

of dual-phase helical scanning (Fig. 13.99). The tumor may appear hypodense without contrast and hyperdense during the arterial phase. About 10% of HCCs are seen only in the arterial phase, some becoming isodense during the portal venous phase. Since necrosis is common in large tumors, the appearances may be non-homogeneous (Fig. 13.100). Smaller lesions may be seen only on MRI (Fig. 13.101), and it is useful to bear in mind that up to 15% of hepatomas are missed with any one imaging technique, and that the overall sensitivity of CT or MRI for small HCCs (<1 cm) is only around 50%. Intravenous injection of the oily contrast medium lipiodol can help to establish the diagnosis since this is selectively taken up by tumor tissue (Fig. 13.102). Arteriography (Fig. 13.103) will demonstrate the blood supply, and is of value in determining the operability of such tumors. Laparoscopy will reveal the tumor (if it occurs on the inferior or anterior surface of the liver) as well as the accompanying cirrhosis (Fig. 13.104). Radioisotope scanning of the liver is now rarely used for diagnosing liver tumors. Macroscopically, liver cell carcinomas often appear as soft hemorrhagic masses which may be nodular or diffuse (Fig. 13.105). Microscopic examination usually shows that the tumor cells resemble normal hepatocytes (Figs 13.106, 13.107). Liver cell dysplasia is a marker of potential malignant change (Fig. 13.108).

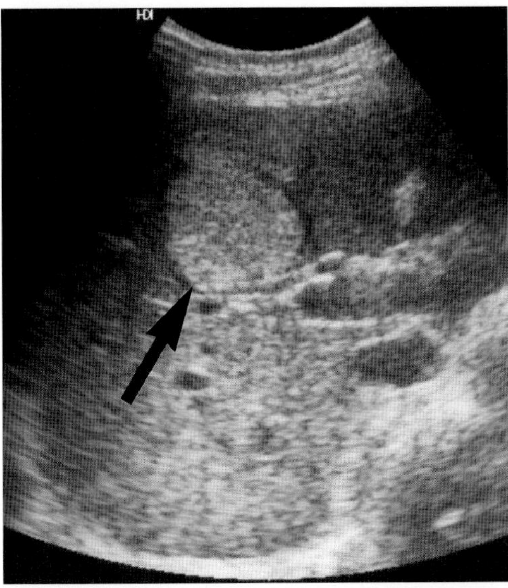

Fig. 13.87 Ultrasound demonstrating hemangioma. A 3 cm hyperechoic mass (arrow) is seen in the left lobe of the liver. Courtesy of Jill Langer, M.D., Philadelphia.

Hepatic metastasis

The liver is a frequent site for metastasis from any primary tumor site (Fig. 13.109). Ultrasound (Fig. 13.110), CT scanning (Figs 13.111, 13.112) and MRI (Fig. 13.113) are all valuable non-invasive techniques for detecting such tumor deposits. Their appearance depends on their vascularity: colorectal metastatic lesions for example typically exhibiting peripheral enhancement. Most lesions require histological confirmation. The newer technique of positron emission tomography combines scintigraphic imaging with some of the computer software of CT and MR to give a 'functional' scan which can permit the characterization of small lesions (Fig. 13.114). The PET scan itself is poor at localization, and future combined scanners that allow simultaneous PET and CT (or MR) scanning could revolutionize our ability to image in difficult situations. Each of these imaging techniques may provide a route-map for biopsy, which can of course also be performed under direct laparoscopic vision (Fig. 13.115).

Deep jaundice is a relatively uncommon complication of metastatic liver disease, but may occur if the tumor distorts and blocks the hepatic ducts (Fig. 13.116). The histological appearances of metastatic

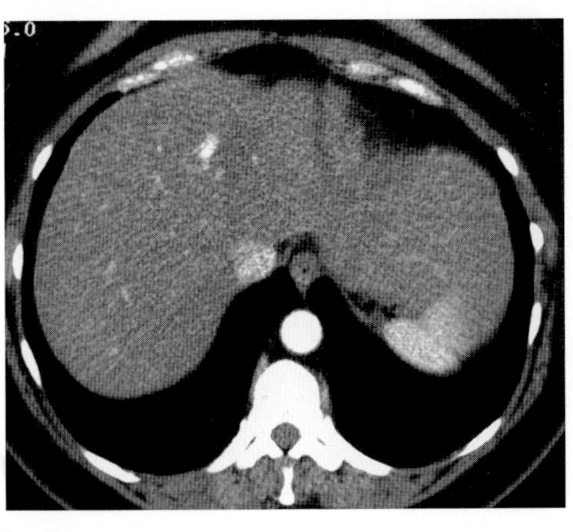

a

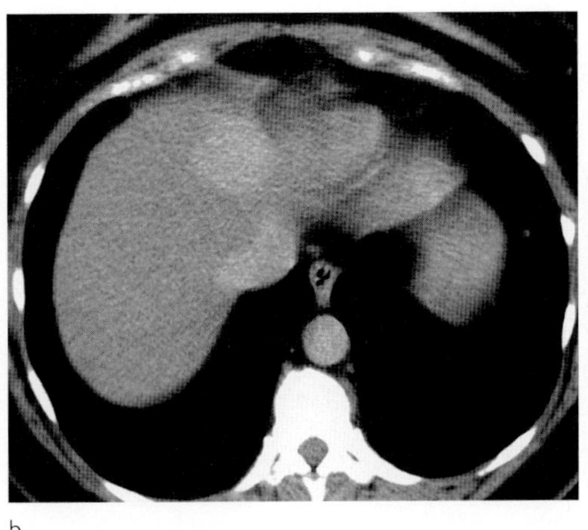

b

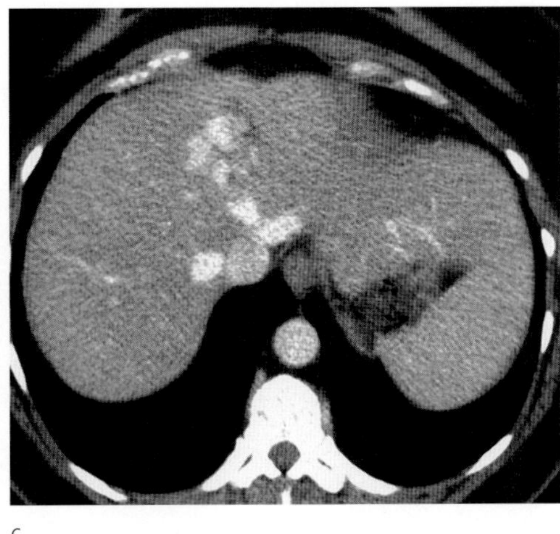

c

Fig. 13.88 A dynamic CT sequence in a patient with a small posterior hemangioma (a: early arterial phase; b: late arterial phase; c: venous phase).

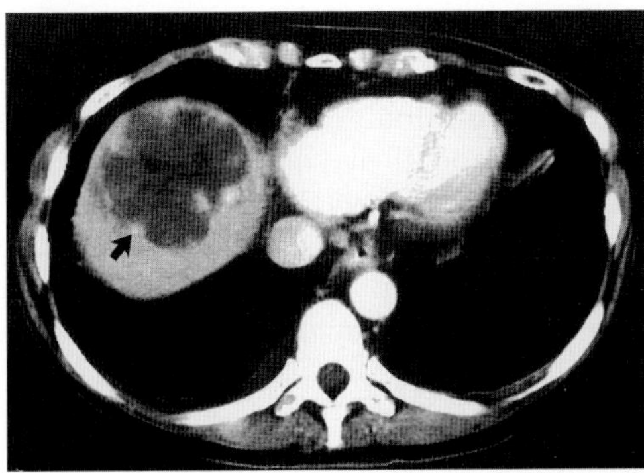

a

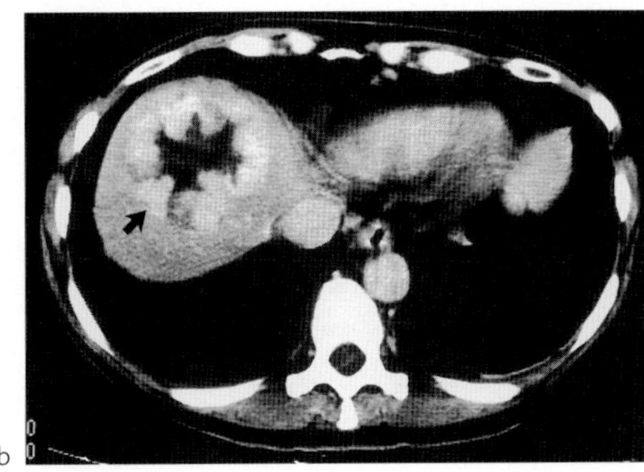

b

Fig. 13.89 CT showing large hemangioma in the dome of the liver. (a) Image obtained during the hepatic arterial phase shows an 8 cm inhomogeneous low-attenuation mass with densely enhancing nodules in its periphery (arrow) ('peripheral nodular enhancement'). (b) Image obtained during the portal venous phase demonstrates progressive but incomplete enhancement ('fill-in') of the outer parenchyma of the tumor (arrow).

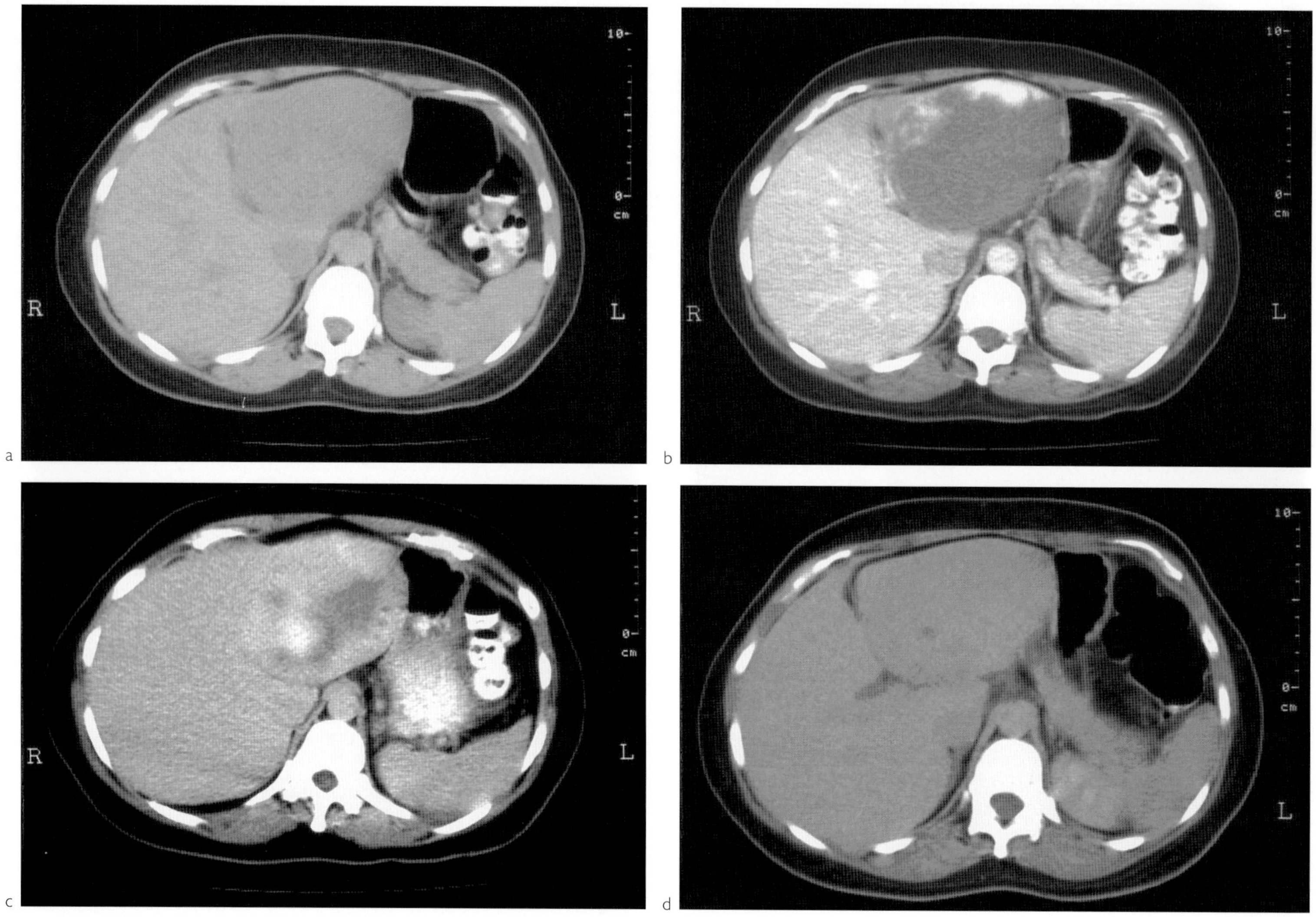

Fig. 13.90 A large left lobe hemangioma is obvious in the early contrast phase but almost invisible, both prior to intravenous contrast, and remarkably shortly afterwards (a: oral contrast has been given and the liver is almost within normal limits; b: the hemangioma is obvious immediately after intravenous contrast; c: within seconds the infilling pattern is seen and the tumor begins to disappear; d: after a few minutes (the contrast is still being excreted by the kidney) the tumor is again almost invisible).

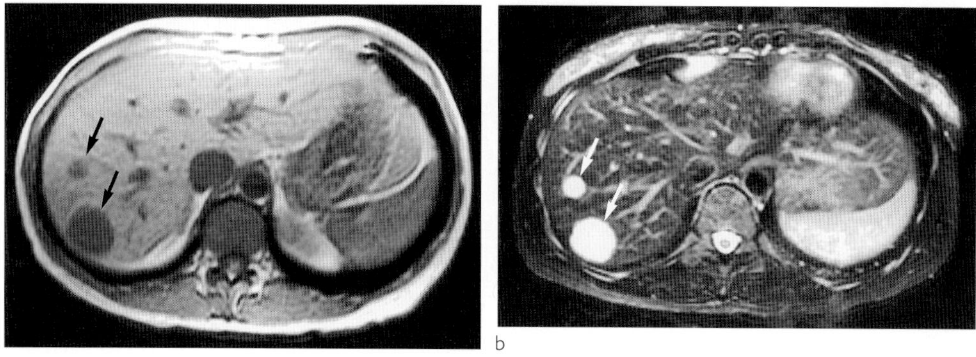

Fig. 13.91 MRI demonstrating two hemangiomas in the right lobe of the liver. (a) T_1-weighted image shows two low-intensity masses (arrows). (b) T_2-weighted image demonstrates two masses of very high intensity (arrows) (the so-called 'light bulb'). Courtesy of Drew Torigian, MD, Philadelphia.

tumors commonly resemble those of the primary neoplasm, and in addition there may be invasion and compression of the normal liver (Fig. 13.117).

Carcinoid and other endocrine tumors

It is important to distinguish metastatic liver disease as a result of the carcinoid syndrome from other types since carcinoid tumors tend to spread slowly and have a much better prognosis than most other malignant tumors with secondary deposits. Macroscopically, carcinoid metastases have a characteristic umbilicated appearance (Fig. 13.118). The histological appearance is of nests of small hyperchromatic cells with characteristic staining properties (Fig. 13.119).

A range of other gastrointestinal endocrine tumors may also metastasize to the liver, and their characterization will be influenced by their function or lack of it (Fig. 13.120). One useful innovation has been the addition of imaging with the somatostatin analog octreotide, illustrated here in a case of (disseminated) Zollinger–Ellison syndrome (see also Chapter 3). These tumors can be difficult to diagnose on CT or MRI. The patient had undergone pancreatic resection 20 years previously. Two lesions were found incidentally on ultrasound; one was thought cystic and the other

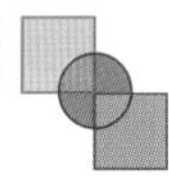

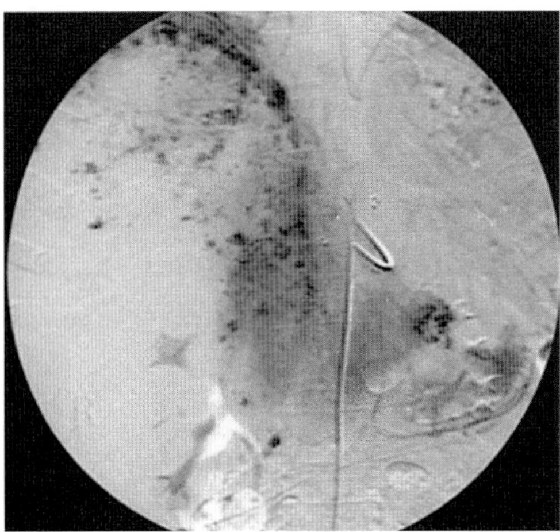

Fig. 13.92 Hepatic arteriogram showing displacement of the right hepatic artery by a large hemangioma. Pooling of blood within dilated vessels is visible. Courtesy of Professor A.P. Hemingway.

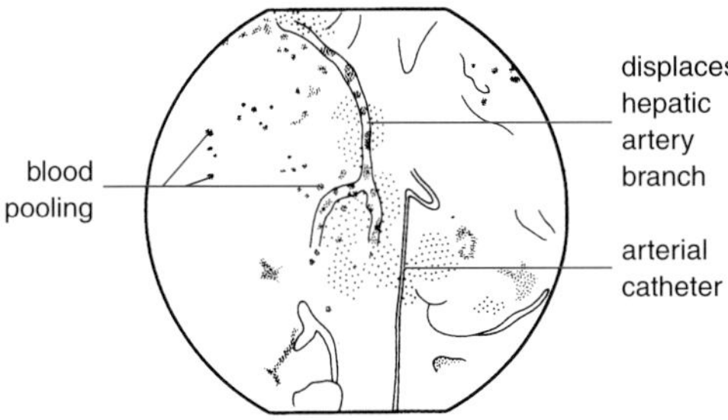

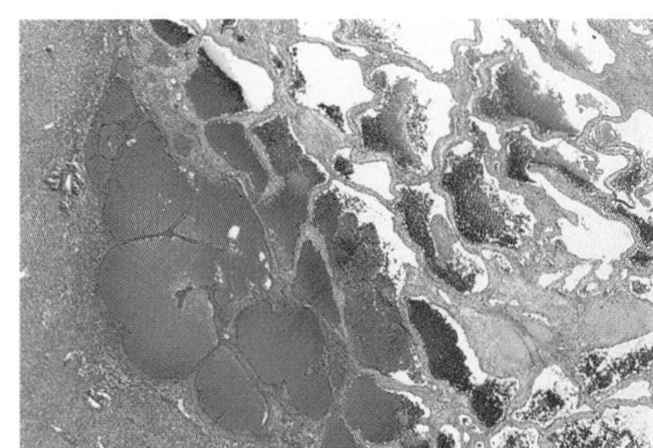

Fig. 13.94 Microscopic view of a cavernous hemangioma of the liver composed of collections of large, blood-filled, thin-walled, endothelial-lined vascular structures

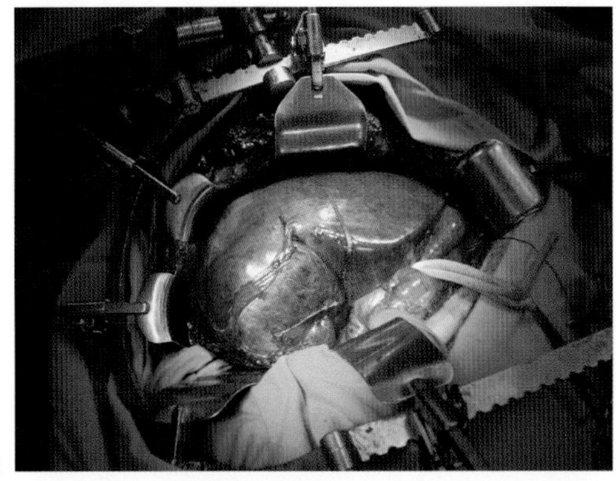

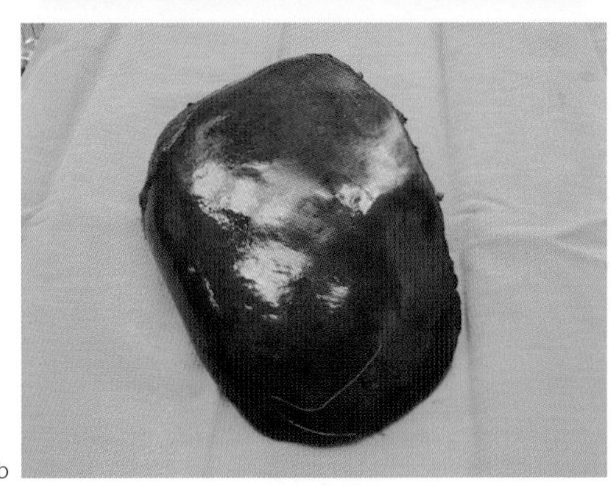

Fig. 13.95 Operative photograph of an hemangiopericytoma (a), and (b) the resected specimen. Courtesy of Richard Schulick, MD.

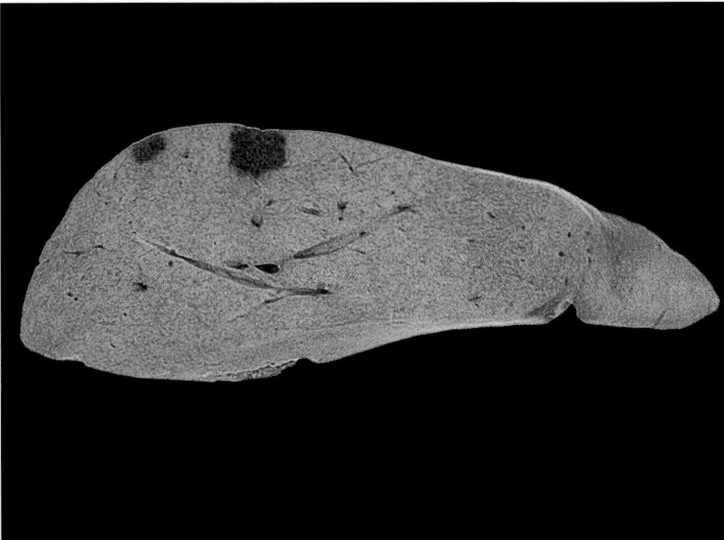

Fig. 13.93 Cut liver surface showing dark patches of hemangiomas. Courtesy of Prof P. Scheuer.

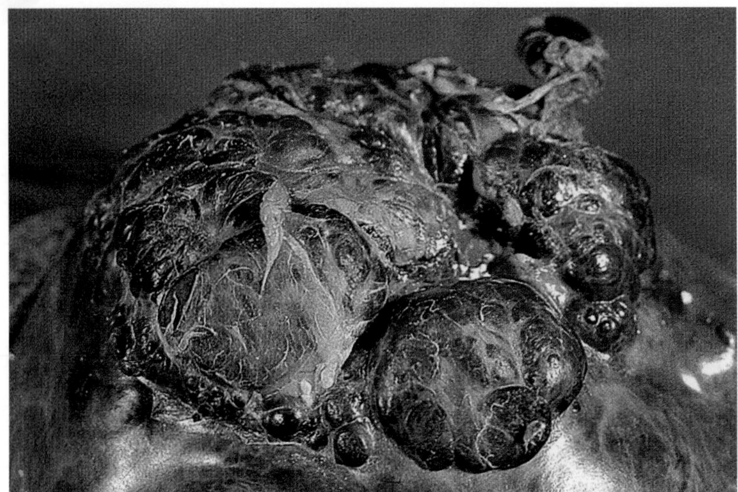

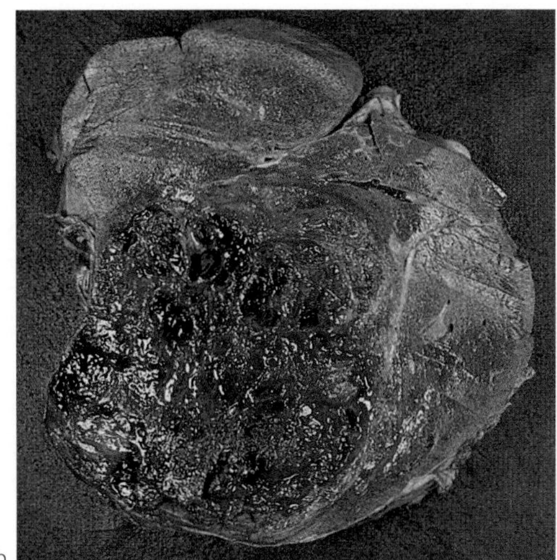

Fig. 13.96 Two typical appearances of hemangiosarcoma: a surface vascular tumor (a) and a hemorrhagic tumor mass (b). Courtesy of Professor K. Weinbren.

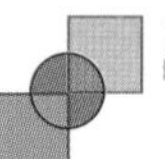

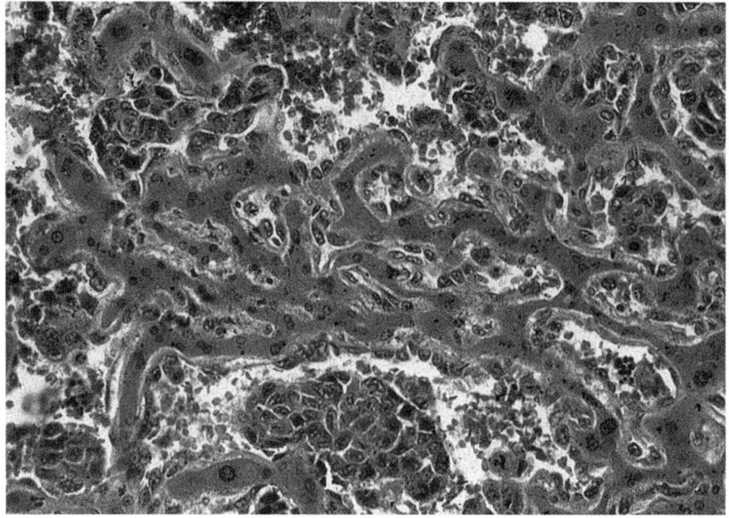

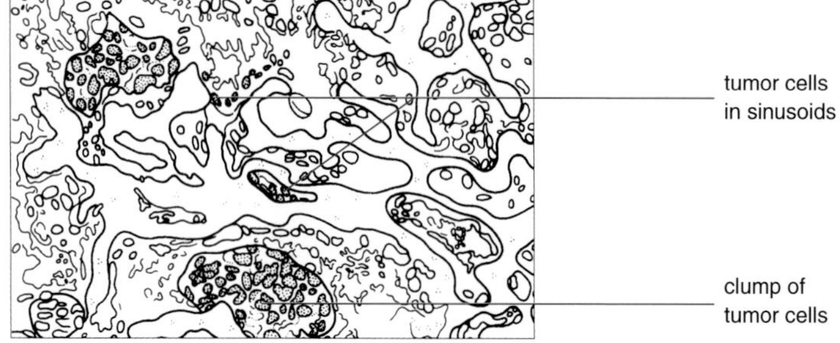

■ **Fig. 13.97** The characteristic growth pattern of an angiosarcoma along the sinusoids can be seen. H&E stain (x 48).

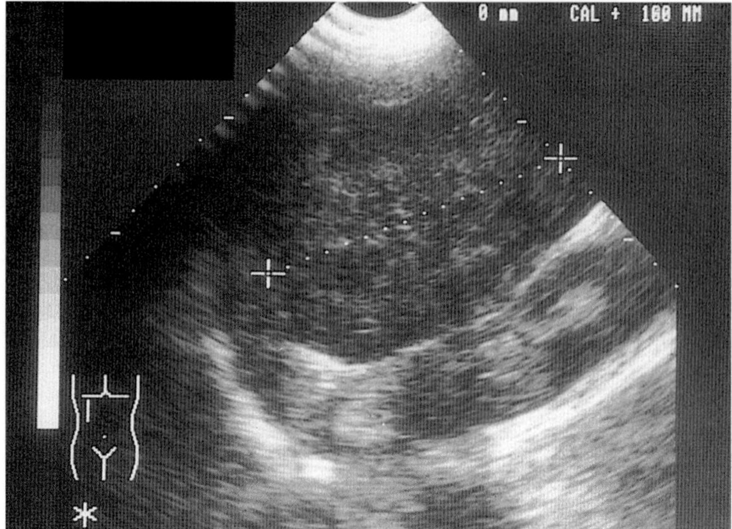

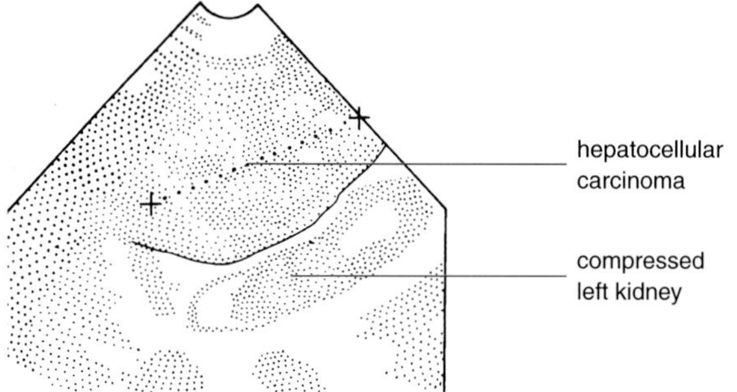

■ **Fig. 13.98** Ultrasonogram showing a large hepatocellular carcinoma (marked by the line joining the crosses) compressing the left kidney. Courtesy of Dr M.C. Collins.

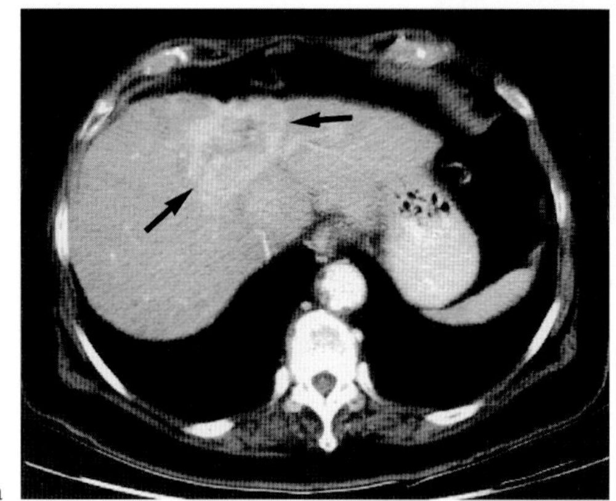

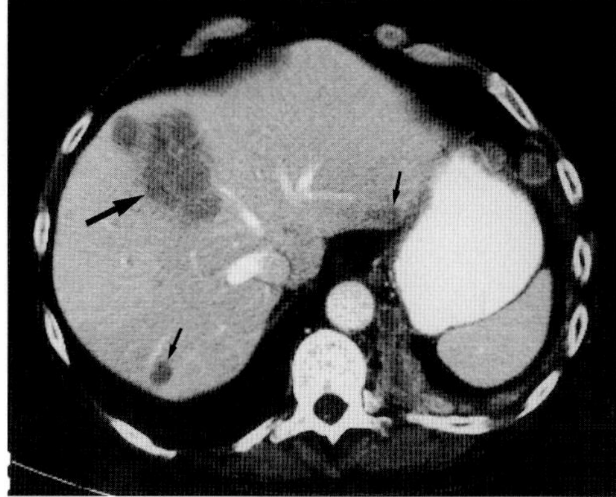

■ **Fig. 13.99** (a) CT demonstrating a hypervascular hepatocellular carcinoma. A contrast enhancing mass (arrows) is seen in the late hepatic arterial phase. (b) CT demonstrating hypovascular hepatocellular carcinoma with satellite metastases. A 4 cm low-attenuation mass (large arrow) spans the anterior segment of the right lobe and the medial segment of the left lobe of the liver. Low-attenuation metastases (small arrows) are seen.

was a solid lesion that was barely visible on T_1-weighted images, but bright on T_2 MRI (Fig. 13.121). The tumor enhanced on arterial images (Fig. 13.122). An atypical hemangioma was suspected, but because of the history, an octreotide scan was performed which showed a metastatic lesion subsequently confirmed at surgery (Fig. 13.123).

Pediatric tumors

Primary tumors of the liver are rare in children; hepatoblastoma accounts for barely 5% of all pediatric malignancies. Progressive abdominal distention due to hepatomegaly is the most common presenting feature, and surgical excision of such tumors may be curative (Fig. 13.124). Histologically, such tumors consist of one of two types of primitive cells, either embryonal (Fig. 13.125), or fetal (Fig. 13.126).

REFERENCE

Dobos N, Rubesin SE. Radiologic imaging modalities in the diagnosis and management of colorectal cancer. Hem Onc Clin North Am 2002; 16: 875–895, Figs 8A–C.

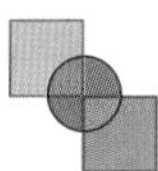

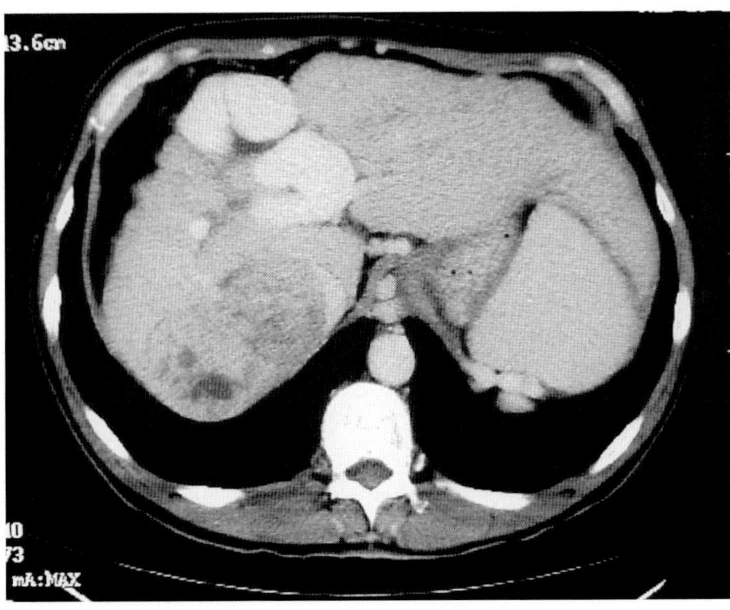

■ **Fig. 13.100** CT of a larger more heterogeneous hepatoma in a patient with portal hypertension and obvious varices.

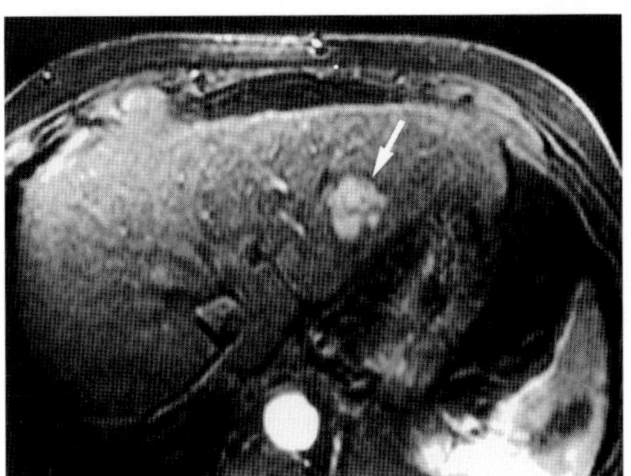

■ **Fig. 13.101** MRI demonstrating hepatocellular carcinoma. T_1-weighted sequence performed after intravenous administration of gadodiamide. A high-intensity mass (arrow) is seen in the left lobe of the liver. Courtesy of Drew Torigian, MD, Philadelphia.

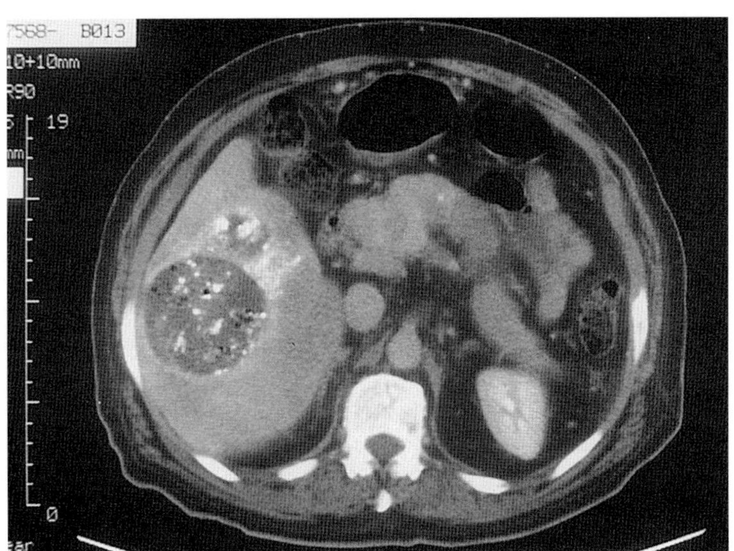

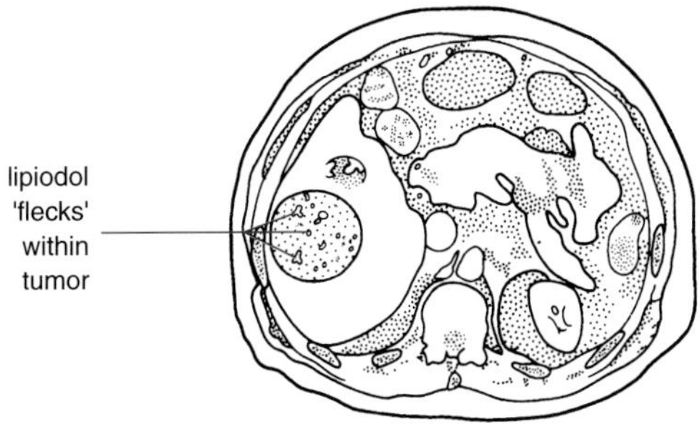

■ **Fig. 13.102** CT scan of a hepatoma following injection of intravenous lipiodol selectively taken up by tumor tissue. Courtesy of Professor A.P. Hemingway.

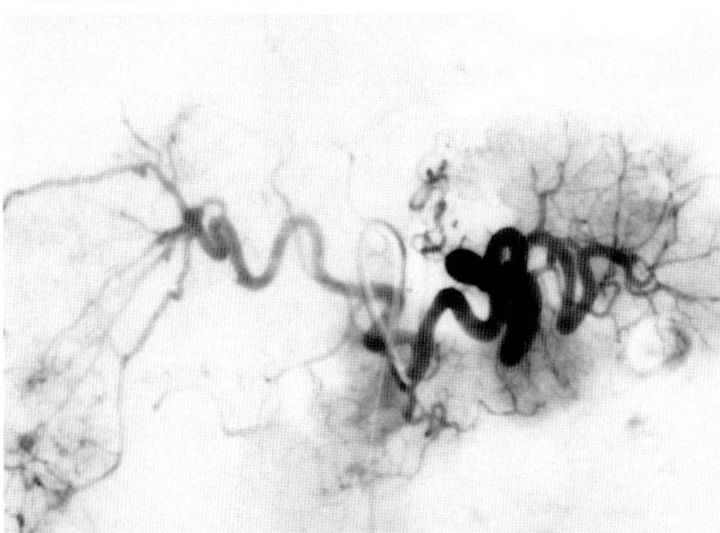

■ **Fig. 13.103** Hepatic arteriogram of the same tumor as Fig. 13.101. Digital subtraction angiography shows pathological blood vessels in addition to the large mass – diagnosing the tumor as being unresectable. Courtesy of Professor A.P. Hemingway.

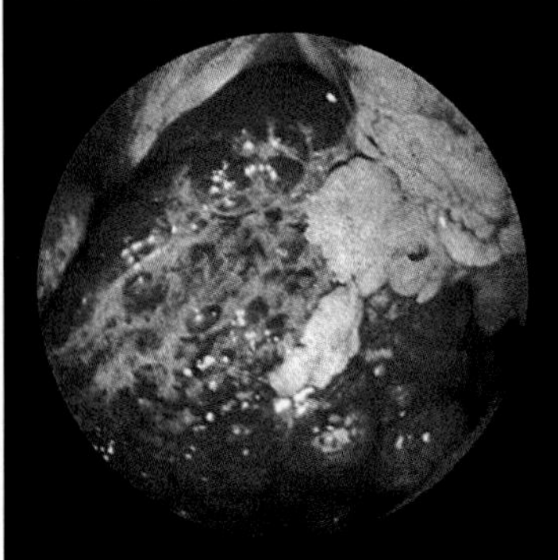

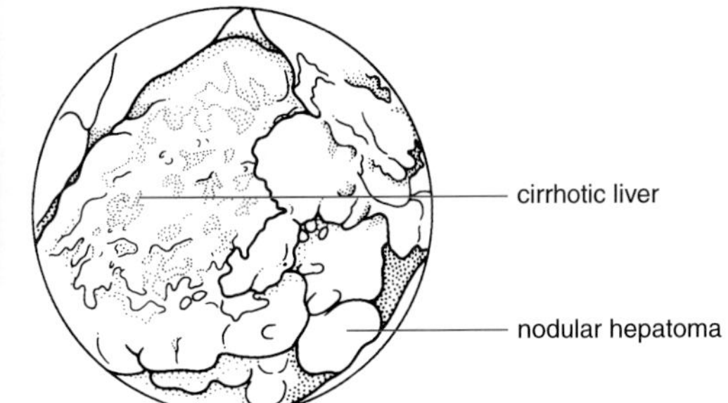

■ **Fig. 13.104** Laparoscopic view of a cirrhotic liver with a nodular hepatoma.

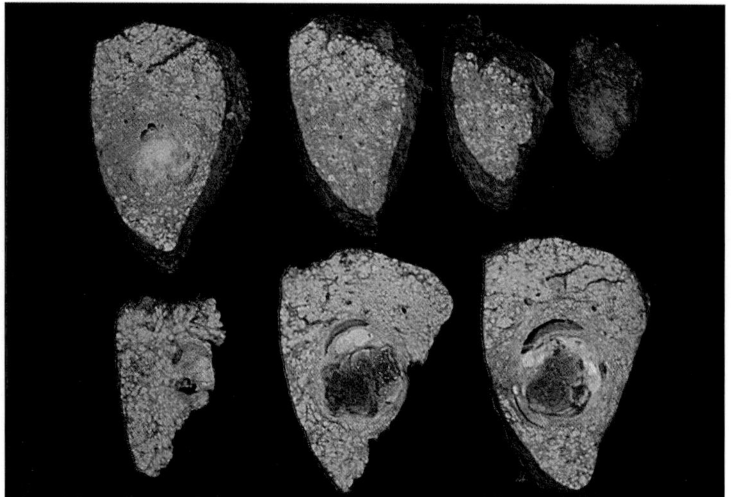
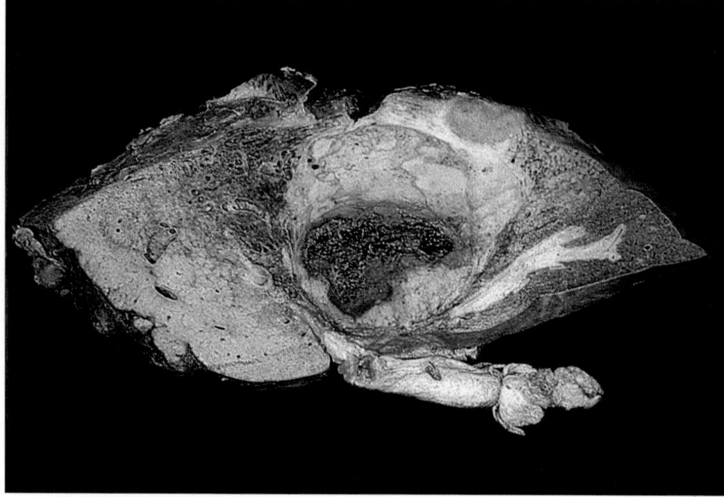

■ **Fig. 13.105** Hepatocellular carcinomas in a cirrhotic (a) and a non-cirrhotic (b) liver. (b) Courtesy of Professor K. Weinbren.

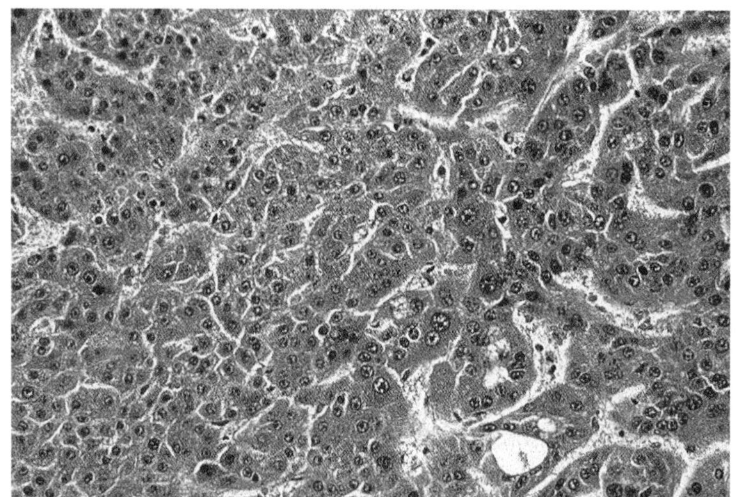
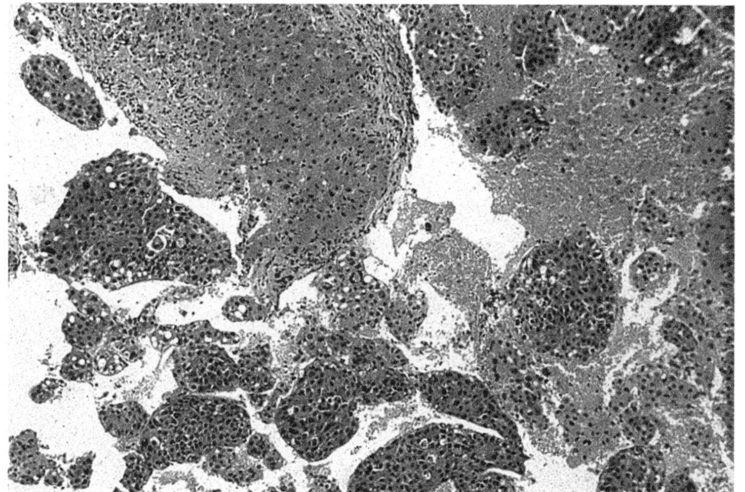

■ **Fig. 13.106** Histology of a typical hepatoma ((a), H&E stain, x 48) and the appearance in a typical, fragmented biopsy ((b), H&E stain, x 180) with nests of tumor cells and a fragment of cirrhotic liver.

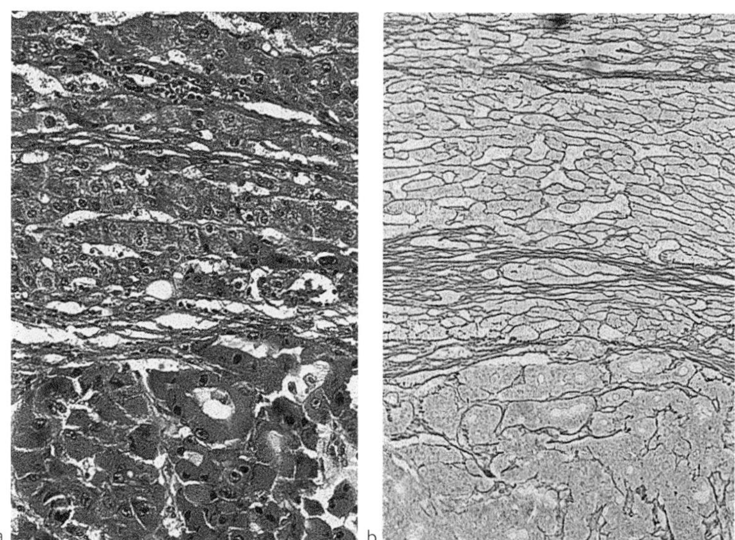

■ **Fig. 13.107** Differing growth patterns but close resemblance of cell types in a hepatoma (lower field) and adjacent normal liver (upper field). (a), H&E stain (x 120); (b), stained for reticulin, (x 120).

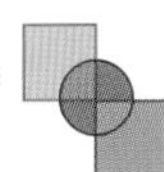

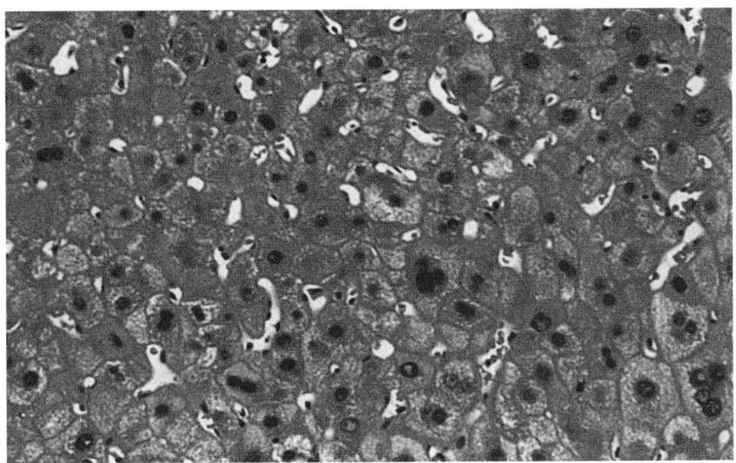

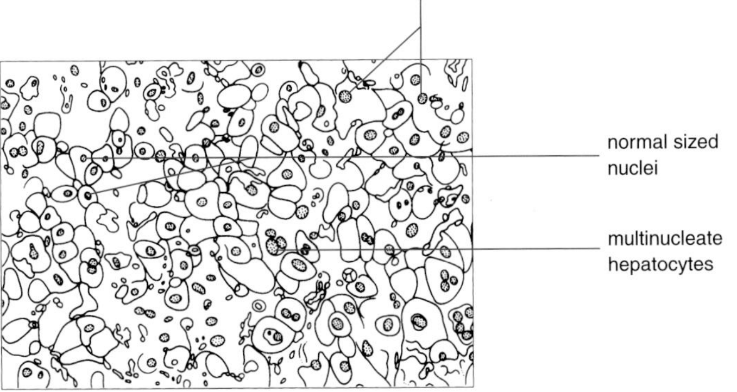

■ **Fig. 13.108** Liver histology showing marked variability in hepatocyte size amounting to dysplasia. H&E stain (x 180).

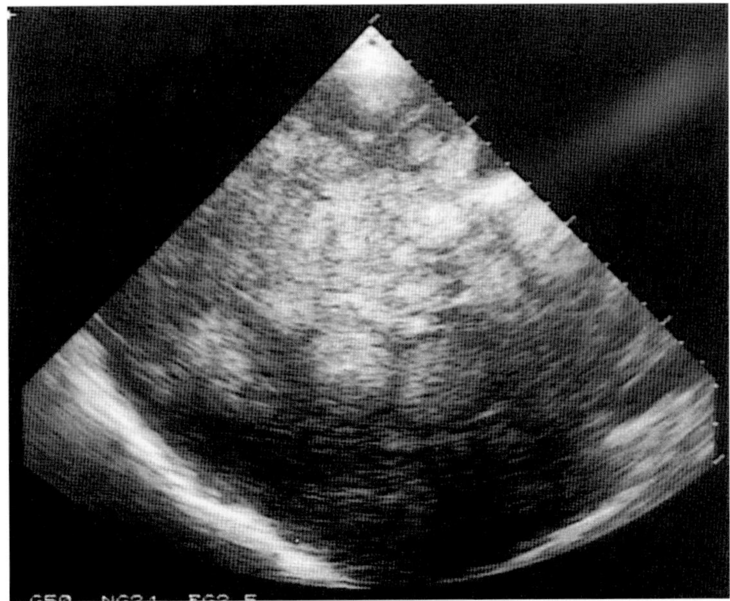

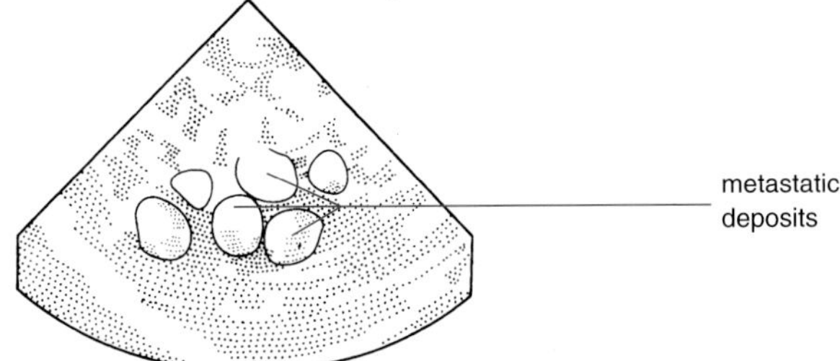

■ **Fig. 13.110** Ultrasonogram showing multiple hepatic metastases. Courtesy of Dr M.C. Collins.

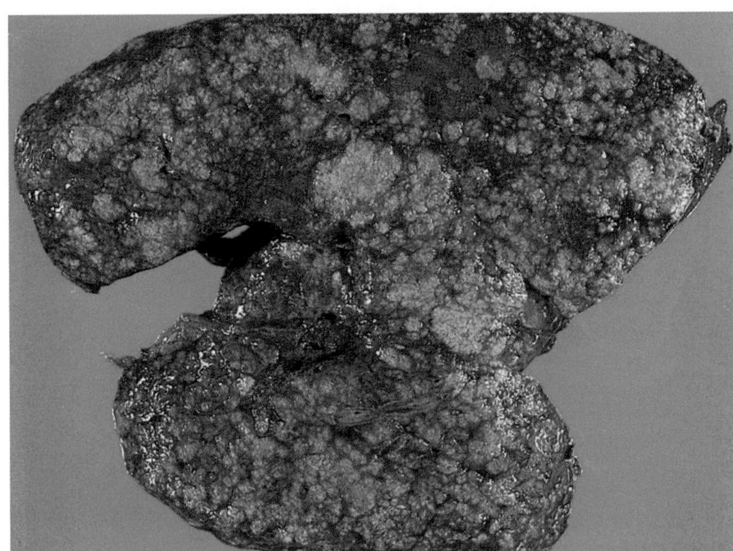

■ **Fig. 13.109** Gross appearance of a liver with numerous metastases. Courtesy of Prof I. Talbot.

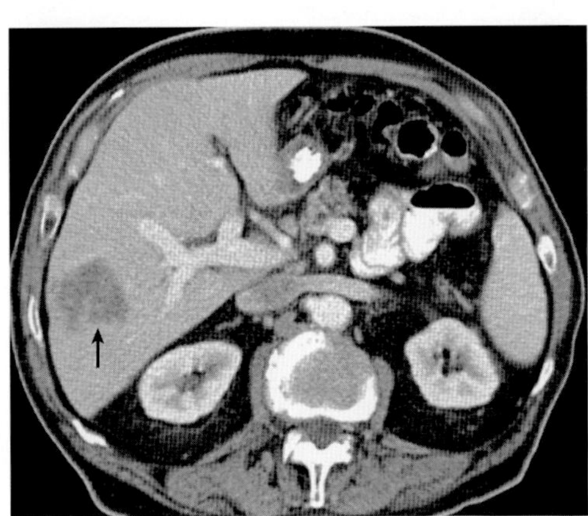

■ **Fig. 13.111** Single well-defined metastasis (arrow) in the right lobe seen here on CT scanning

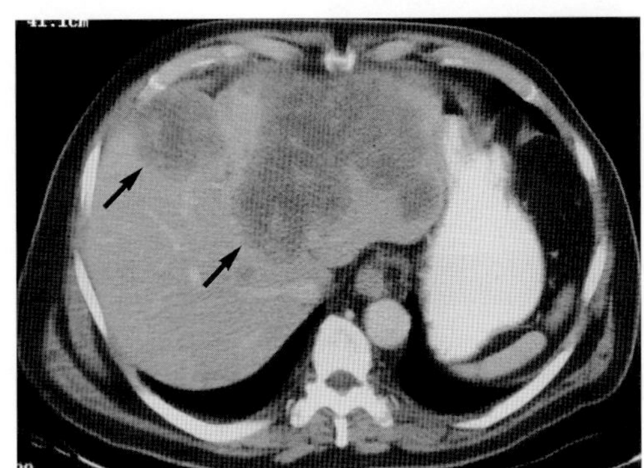

■ **Fig. 13.112** CT demonstrating liver metastases from colonic carcinoma. Large, lobulated, non-homogeneous, low-attenuation masses (arrows) replace most of the left lobe of the liver.

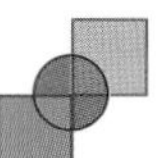

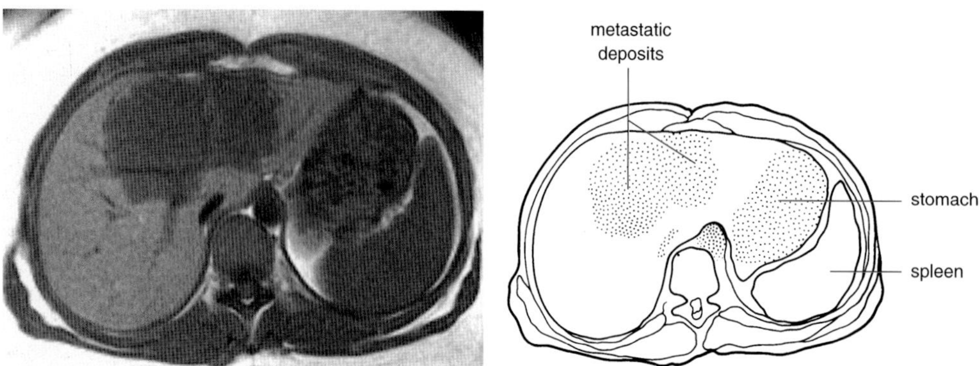

Fig. 13.113 Magnetic resonance image showing a large hepatic mass. This 'turboflash' image was obtained in a single 2-second exposure. Courtesy of Dr L.W. Turnbull.

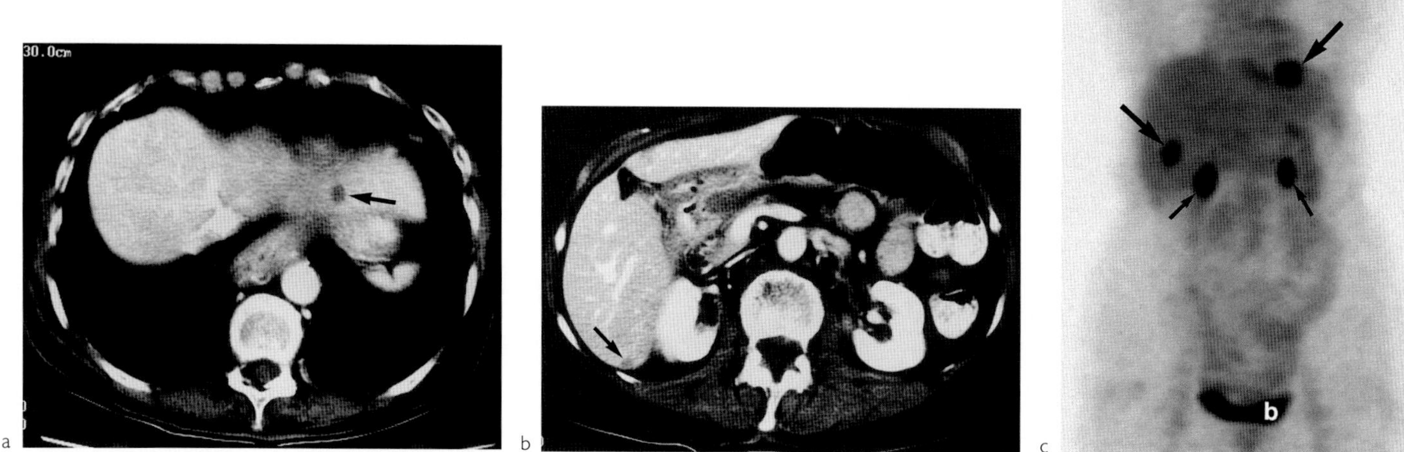

Fig. 13.114 PET characterizing small liver lesions as metastases. CT through the dome of the liver (a) and the posterior segment of the right lobe (b) shows two 9 mm 'too small to characterize' low-attenuation lesions (arrows). (c) Coronal image from positron emission tomography (PET) with FDG-glucose demonstrates intense metabolism in two small liver lesions (large arrows), corresponding to the indeterminate lesions shown on the CT scan. The renal collecting systems (small arrows) and urinary bladder (b) are also seen. (Reproduced with permission from reference 1, Figs 8A–C.)

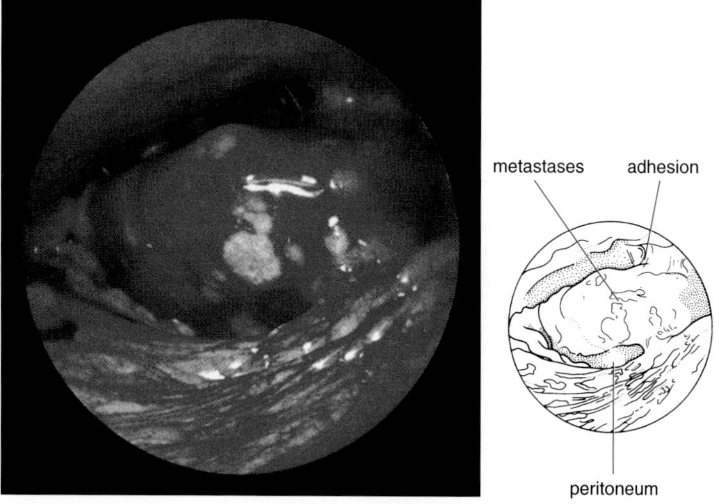

Fig. 13.115 Laparoscopic view of an irregular liver infiltrated by metastases.

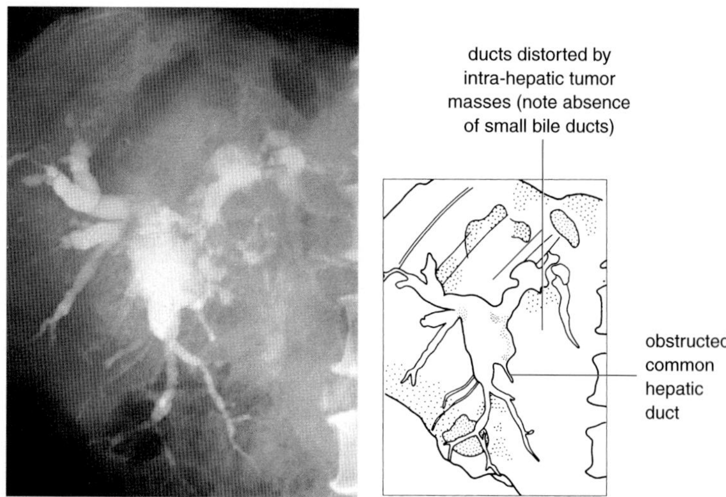

Fig. 13.116 Endoscopic retrograde cholangiogram showing metastatic deposits from a carcinoma of pancreas. In addition to obstruction at the porta hepatis, there is distortion of the intrahepatic duct system by tumor.

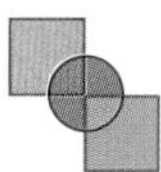

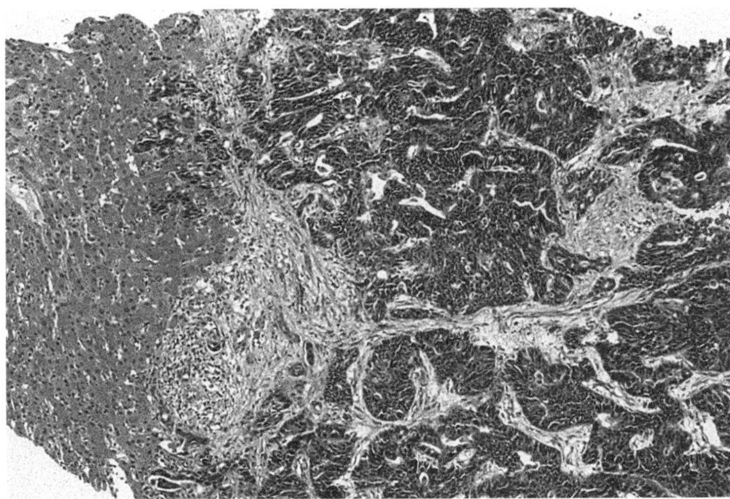

■ **Fig. 13.117** Section of liver showing metastatic adenocarcinoma (right field). H&E stain (x 18).

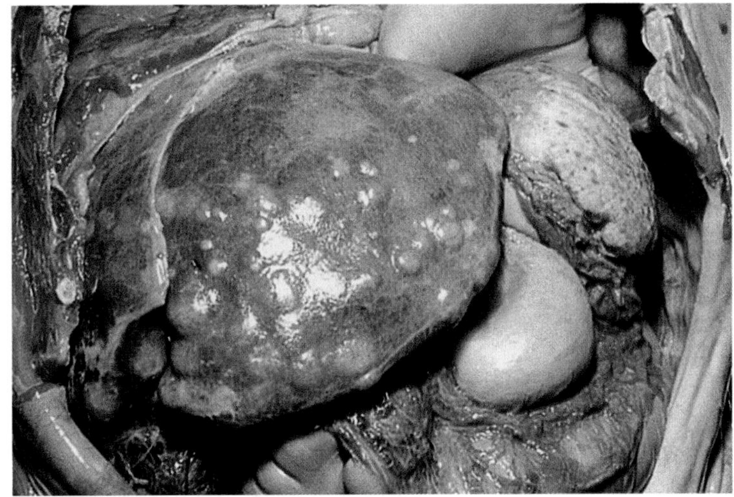

■ **Fig. 13.118** Macroscopic appearance of a liver studded with carcinoid deposits. Courtesy of Dr N.D.S. Bax.

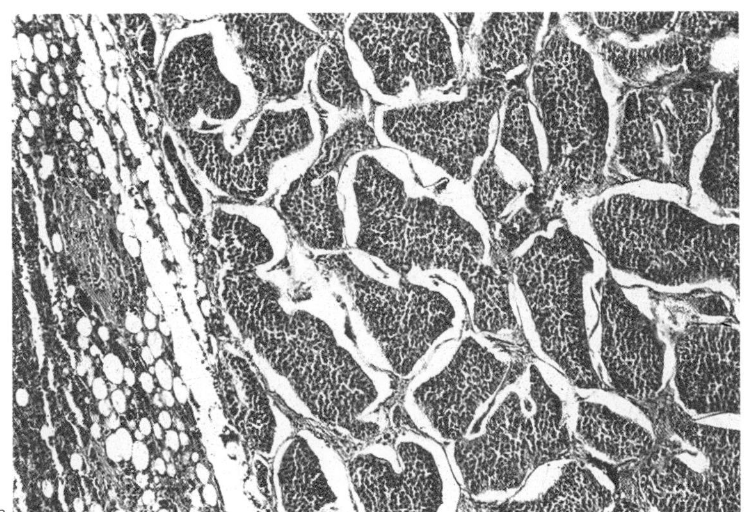

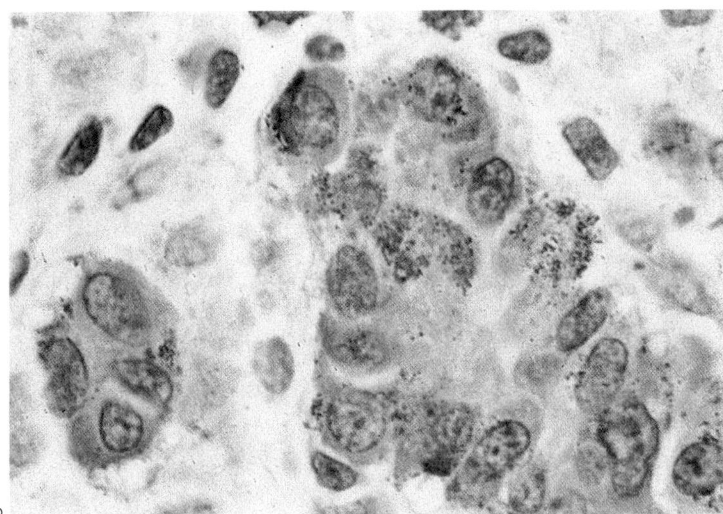

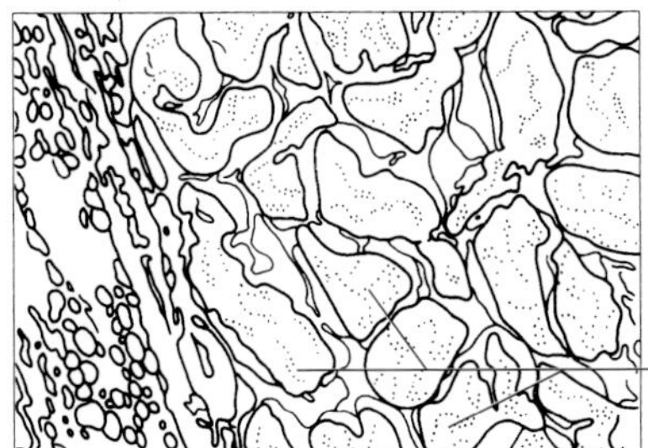

■ **Fig. 13.119** Liver histology showing characteristic regular islands of metastatic carcinoid tumor ((a), H&E stain, x 150). With higher magnification and an alkaline diazo reaction, red-brown neurosecretory granules are seen ((b), x 480).

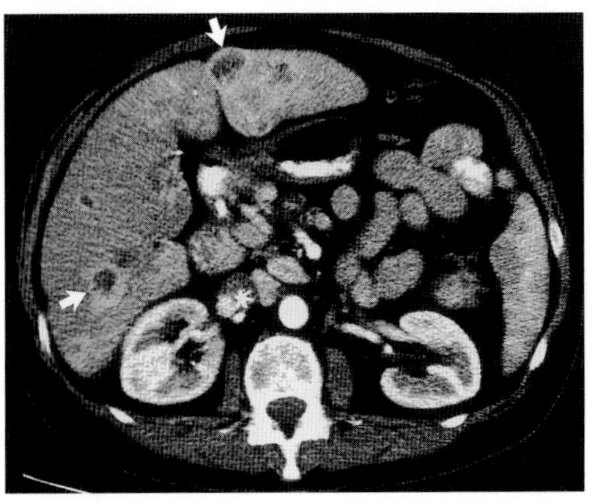

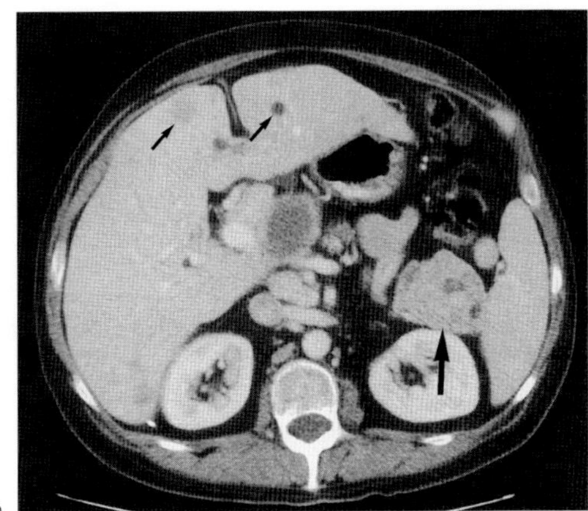

■ **Fig. 13.120** Hypervascular metastases from non-functioning islet tumor of the pancreas. (a) CT obtained during hepatic arterial phase (filmed using a 'liver window') shows numerous metastases (arrows) with contrast-enhancing rims and low-attenuation centers. (b) CT obtained in portal venous phase demonstrates washout of the hypervascular rims (small arrows). A 4 x 6 cm enhancing inhomogeneous mass (large arrow) is seen in the tail of the pancreas.

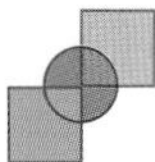

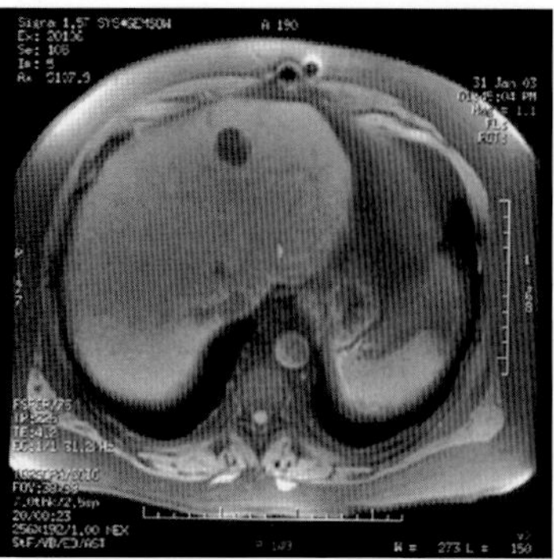

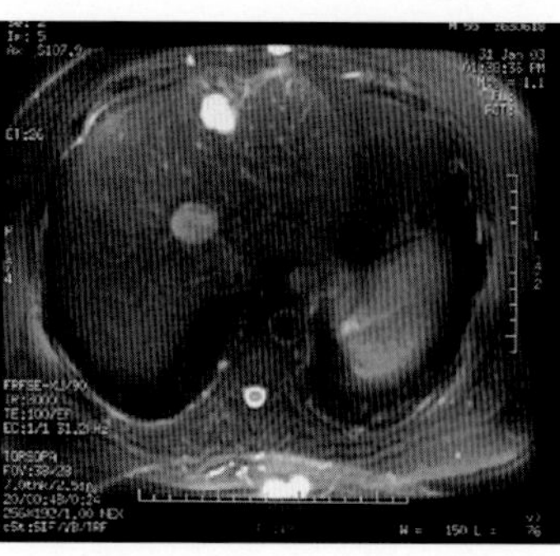

Fig. 13.121 Two incidental ultrasound images were further investigated. The solid lesion was barely visible on T_1-weighted MR images and bright on T_2 MRI.

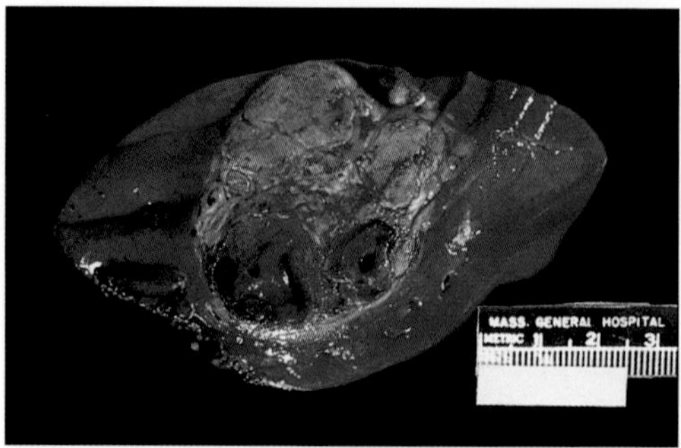

Fig. 13.124 Hepatoblastoma. Macroscopic view of a surgically resected hepatoblastoma treated with neoadjuvant chemotherapy for 4 days prior to resection showing the typically solitary lesion with a solid, well-circumscribed appearance. The cut surface of the viable tumor is yellow-tan; necrotic tumor are hemorrhagic and cavitated.

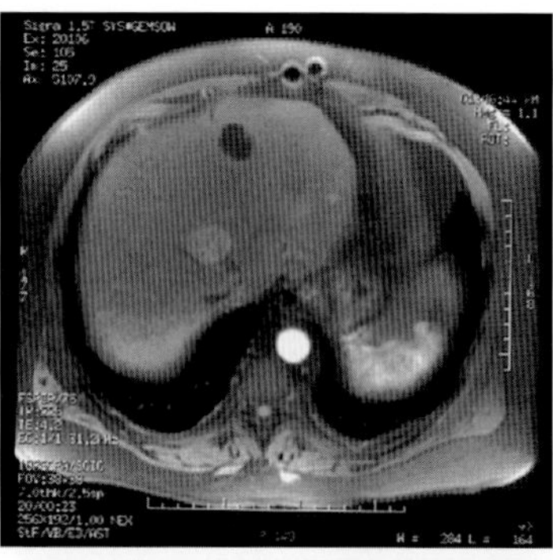

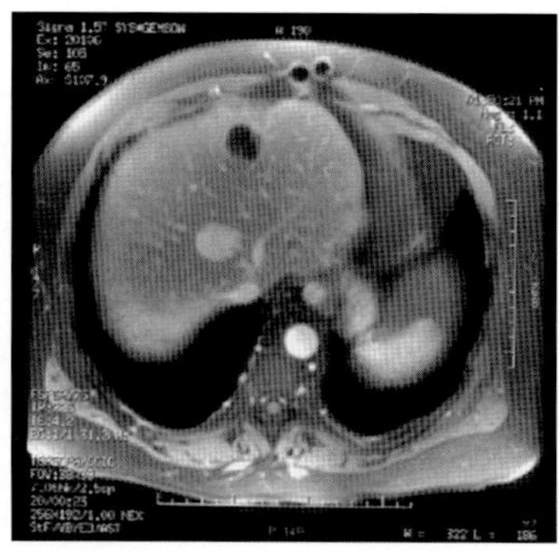

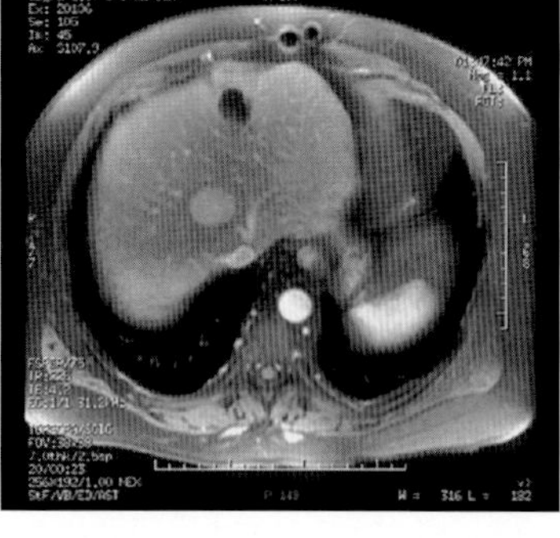

Fig. 13.122 The tumor investigated in Fig 13.120 enhanced in the arterial phase of contrast imaging.

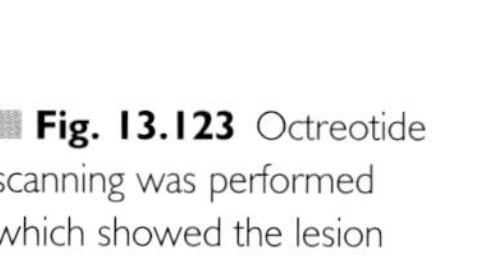

Fig. 13.123 Octreotide scanning was performed which showed the lesion to be metastatic.

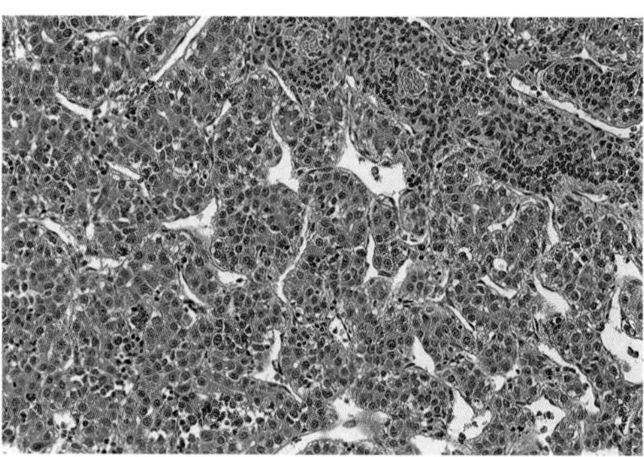

Fig. 13.125 hepatoblastoma. Hepatoblastoma of a pure epithelial type showing tumor cells resembling fetal hepatocytes arranged in irregular cords.

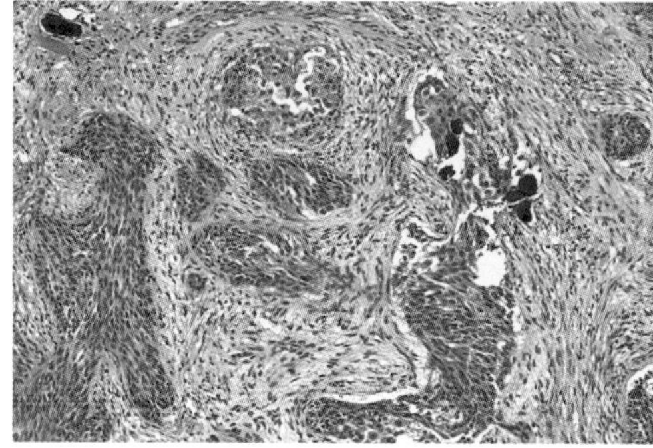

Fig. 13.126 Hepatoblastoma of a mixed type showing solid cords of hepatocytic epithelial cells and spindle cells of embryonic appearance.

DISEASES OF THE GALL BLADDER AND BILE DUCTS

14

INTRODUCTION

The normal biliary tree has been described in Chapter 10 and is illustrated here radiographically and anatomically (Figs 14.1–14.3). The gall bladder is usually a pear-shaped sac that is 8–10 cm long with a capacity of about 50 ml. It is divided into a neck, body and fundus. The mucosa comprises tall columnar epithelium, which is thrown into simple folds. There is no muscularis mucosa distinct from the main muscle coat, which consists of interlacing bundles of fibers lacking a regular pattern. Loose connective tissue separates the muscle from the serosa (Fig. 14.4). In the neck of the gall bladder is a small pouch (Hartmann's pouch), which is particularly marked in pathological states, and it is here that stones commonly impact (Fig. 14.5). The normal gall bladder contracts briskly after fat ingestion. This is most readily demonstrable by ultrasound (Fig. 14.6).

GALLSTONES

Three major types of gallstones are described: pure cholesterol stones; pure pigment stones; and mixed stones, which include calcium salts as well as cholesterol and bile pigment (Figs 14.7–14.10). Pigment stones are associated with hemolysis and biliary infection, whereas cholesterol and mixed stones are more

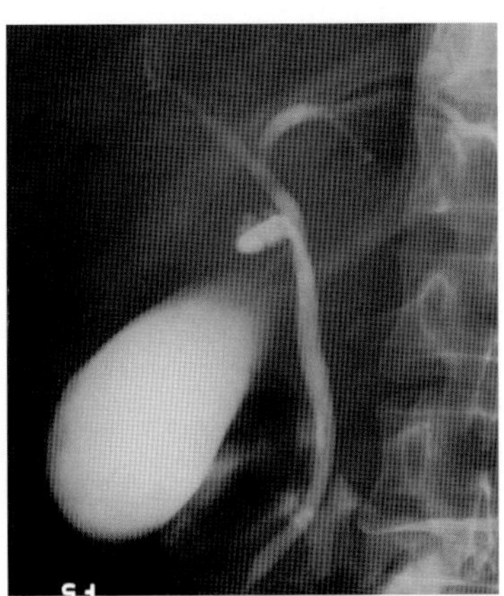

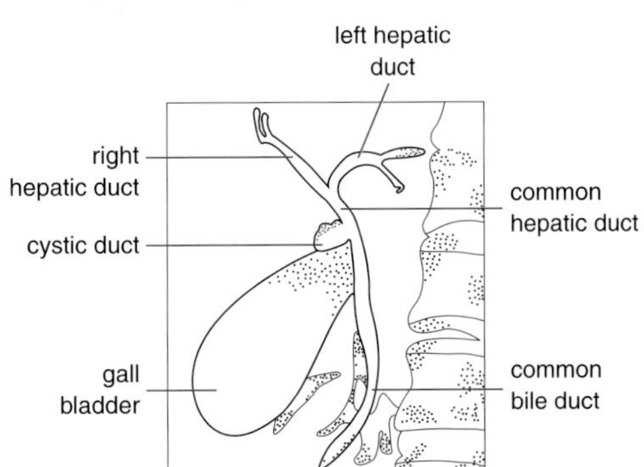

Fig. 14.1 Endoscopic retrograde cholangiogram showing normal biliary tree.

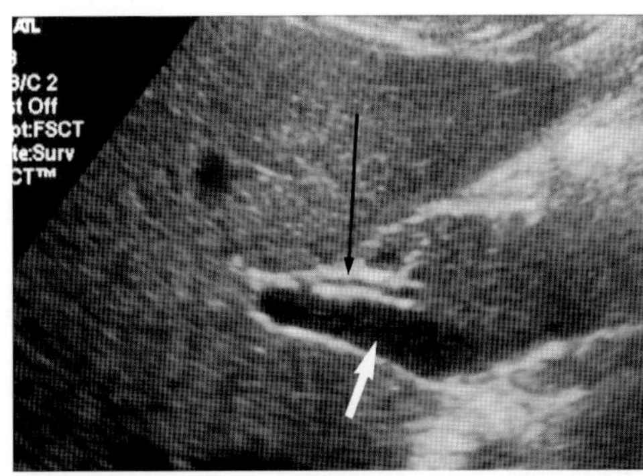

Fig. 14.2 Ultrasound showing normal hepatic duct. The hepatic duct (black arrow) lies superior to the portal vein (white arrow). Courtesy of Jill E. Langer, M.D., Philadelphia.

a

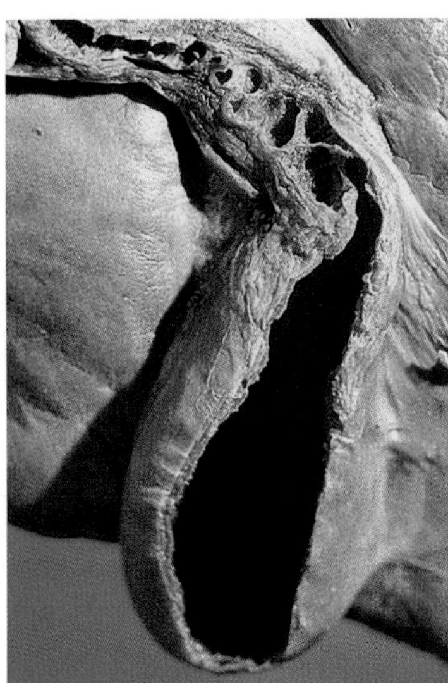

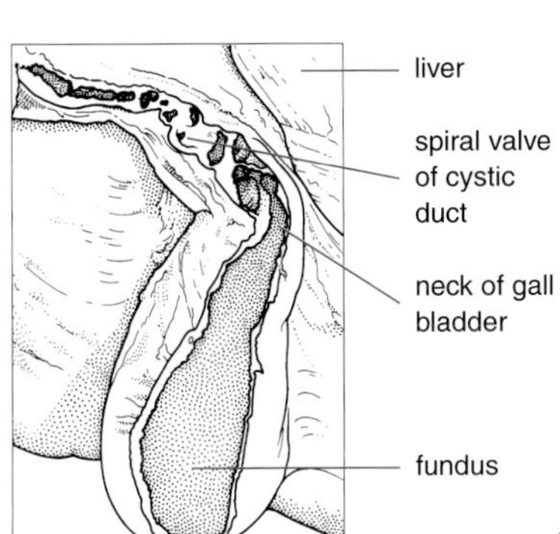

b

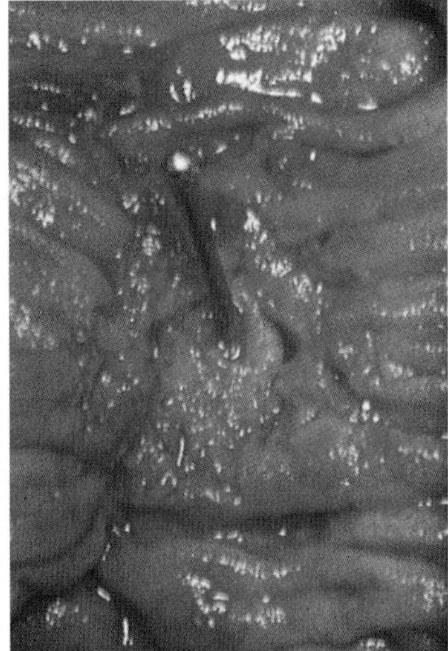

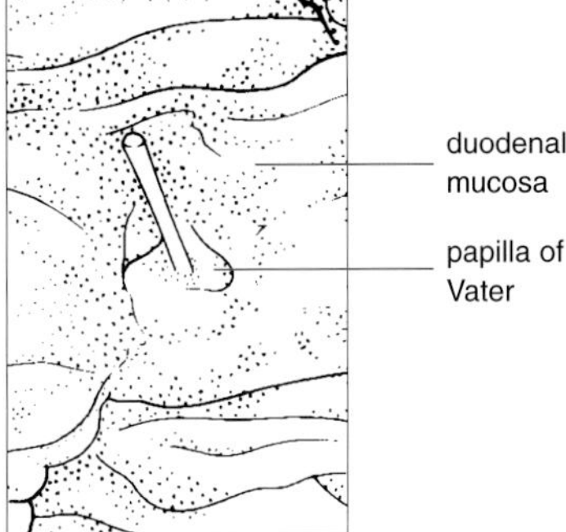

Fig. 14.3 The normal gall bladder (a) and the papilla of Vater (b) at autopsy with a probe passed into the duodenum.

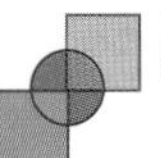

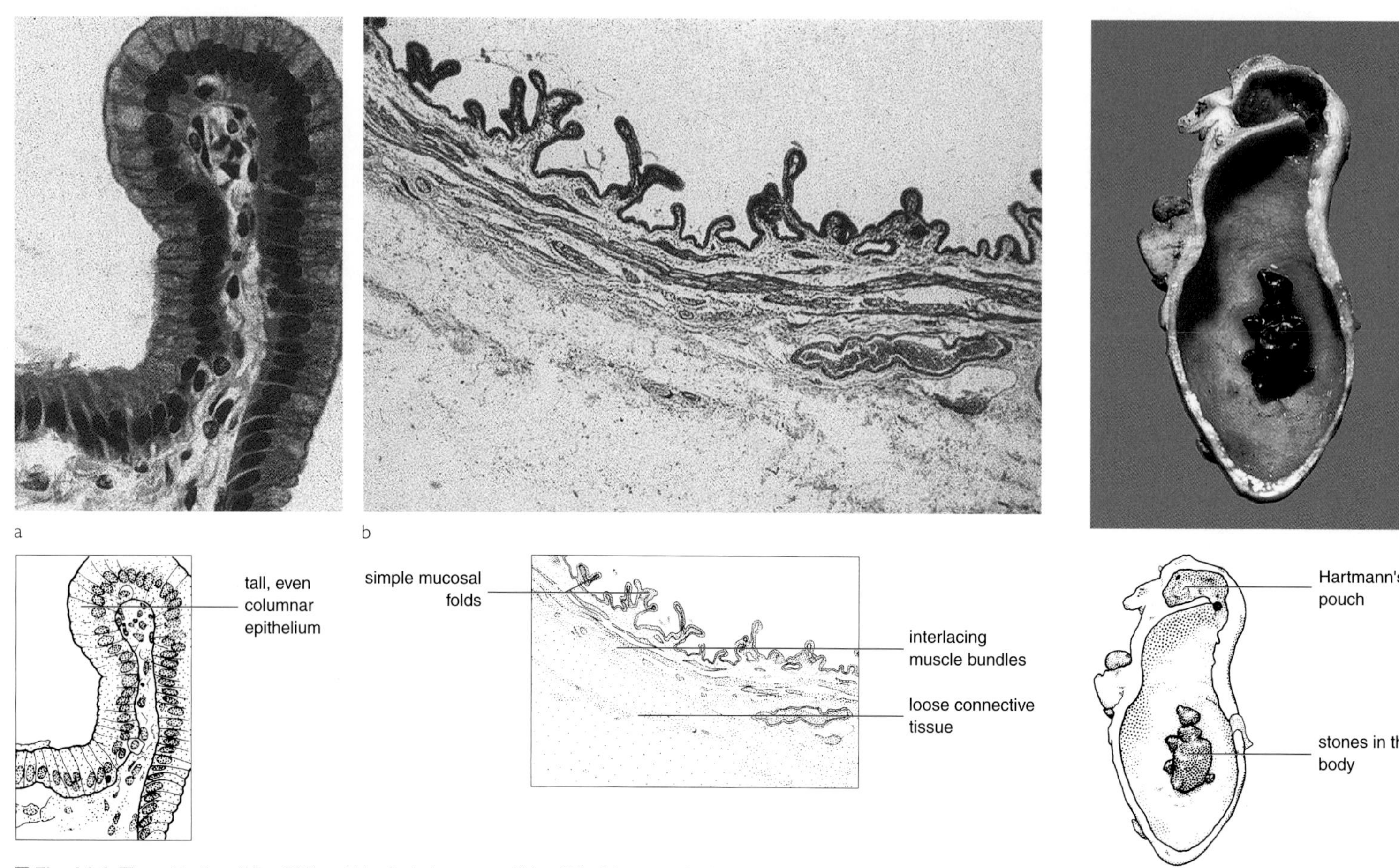

■ **Fig. 14.4** The epithelium ((a), x 320) and histological structure ((b), x 30) of the normal gall bladder. H&E stain.

■ **Fig. 14.5** Gall bladder showing Hartmann's pouch and pigment stones.

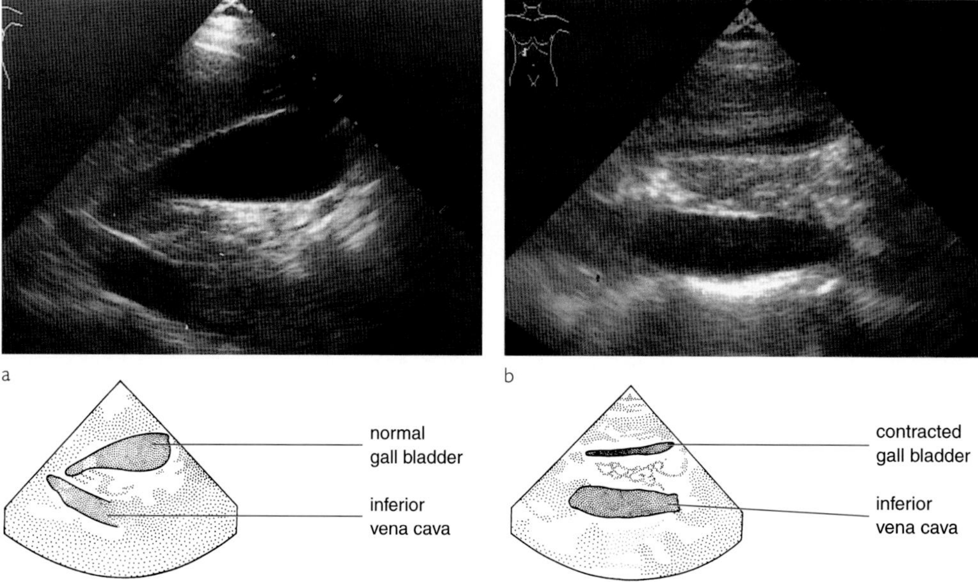

■ **Fig. 14.6** Ultrasound showing a normal gall bladder before (a) and 30 minutes after (b) ingestion of a fatty meal. Courtesy of Dr M.C. Collins.

commonly found in females and the obese; they are also associated with interruption of the enterohepatic circulation of bile acids by surgery or by diseases of the small bowel such as Crohn's disease.

There are marked racial differences in the prevalence of stones. Stones may occur singly or in large numbers (Fig. 14.11).

Calcified stones

A minority of gallstones contains sufficient calcium to be visible on a plain abdominal X-ray (Figs 14.12, 14.13), and rarely they contain gas (Fig. 14.14). Cholecystography may confirm that they are in the biliary system (Fig. 14.15), but ultrasound has now almost completely replaced the oral cholecystogram (Fig 14.16).

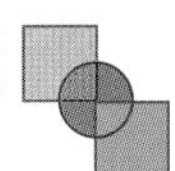

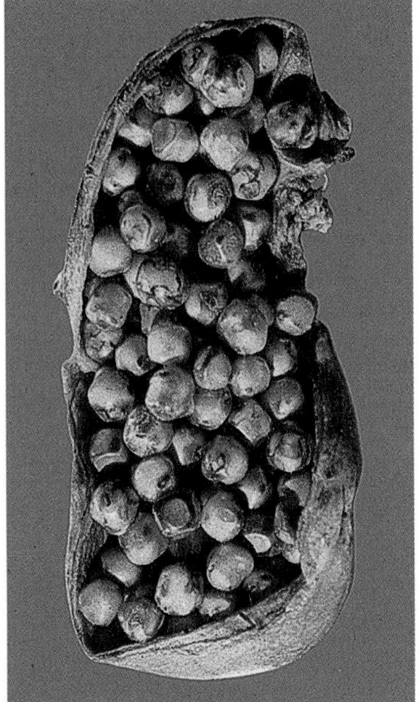

■ **Fig. 14.7** A gall bladder containing at least 50 mixed stones.

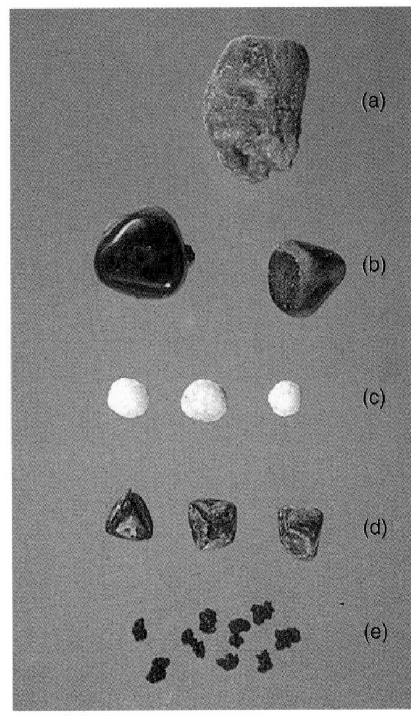

■ **Fig. 14.8** Common varieties of gallstones: a cholesterol stone (a); mixed gallstones (b–d); and pigment stones (e).

Translucent stones

Over 80% of gallstones are radiolucent as they contain too little calcium to render them visible on a plain X-ray. The oral cholecystogram will only confirm their presence if the gall bladder function is good enough to concentrate contrast media. Ultrasound is unquestionably the technique of choice as it is quick, accurate, safe, and non-invasive. Stones are diagnosed by the acoustic shadow that they cast (Fig. 14.16). Smaller stones may be detected by CT scanning (Fig. 14.17). MRI cholangiography (MRC) scanning is proving of some

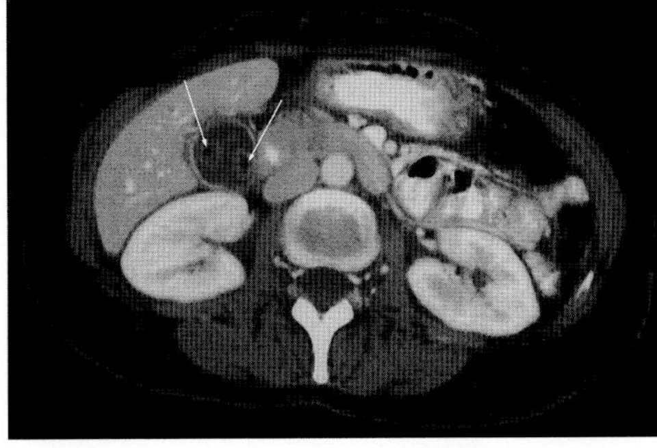

■ **Fig. 14.10** CT demonstrating two non-calcified gallstones. Concentric rings of varying attenuation are seen. Two black dots of gas composed mainly of nitrogen (arrows) are present centrally.

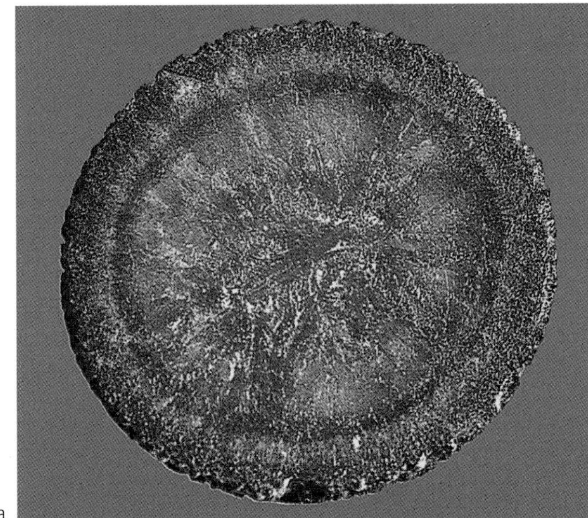

a

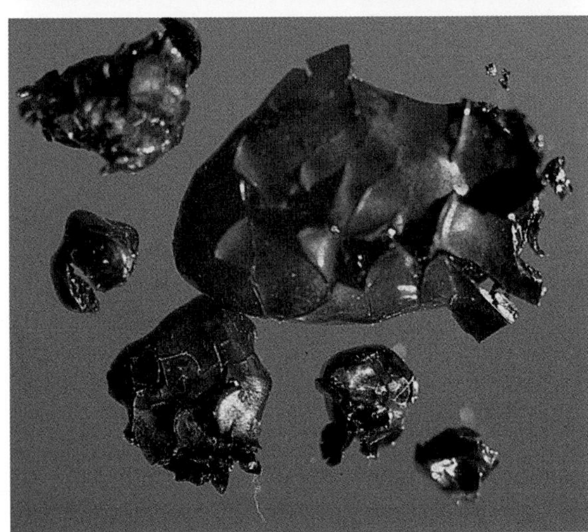

b

■ **Fig. 14.9** A cholesterol stone (a) and pigment stones (b).

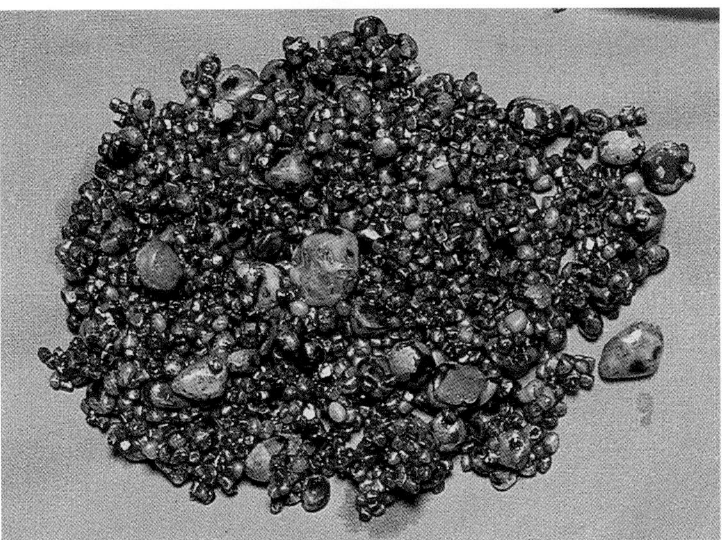

■ **Fig. 14.11** Mixed gallstones that were removed at one cholecystectomy – 2942 in total.

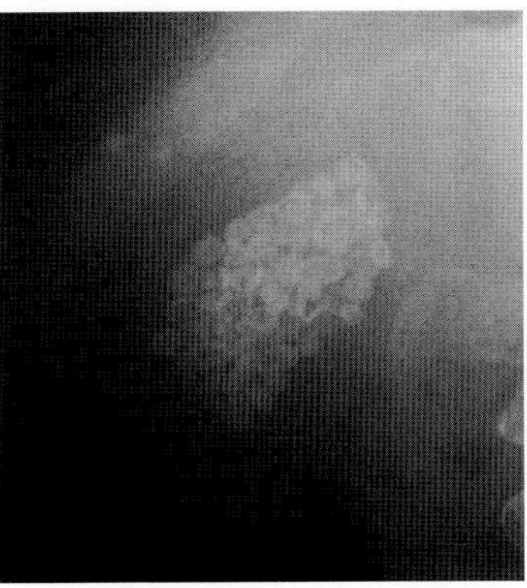

■ **Fig. 14.12** Plain radiograph of the right upper quadrant shows numerous small (2–3 mm) calcified, faceted gallstones.

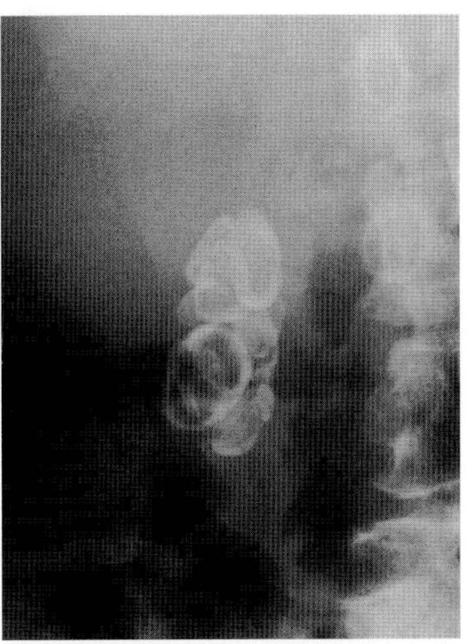

■ **Fig. 14.13** Plain radiograph of the right upper quadrant shows 11 large (5–10 mm) calcified gallstones.

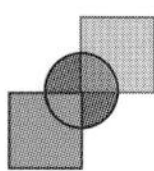

Epidemiology of Pigment and Mixed/Cholesterol Stones	
Pigment stones	**Mixed/cholesterol stones**
increase with age	increase with age
female = male	female > male
increased incidence in:	increased incidence in:
hemolysis	ileal disease
biliary infection	cystic fibrosis
alcoholic cirrhosis	hyperlipoproteinemia (type IV)

Fig. 14.14 Some clinical associations of mixed/cholesterol and pigment stones.

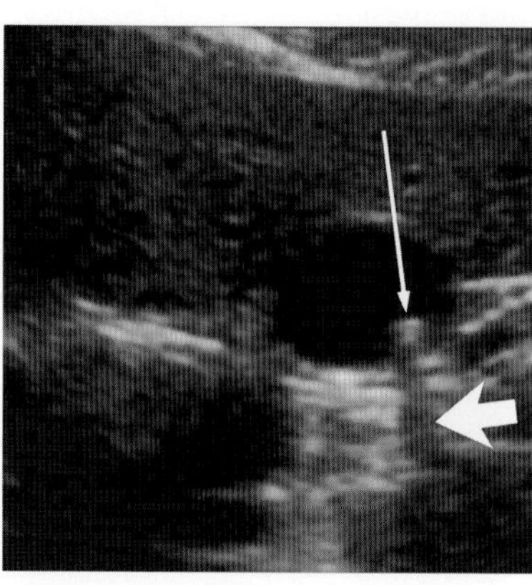

Fig. 14.17 Ultrasound showing a gallstone. A 3 mm round, echogenic structure (thin arrow) is seen in the dependent portion of the gallbladder. Shadowing (thick arrow) is seen below the gallstone. Courtesy of Jill E. Langer, M.D., Philadelphia.

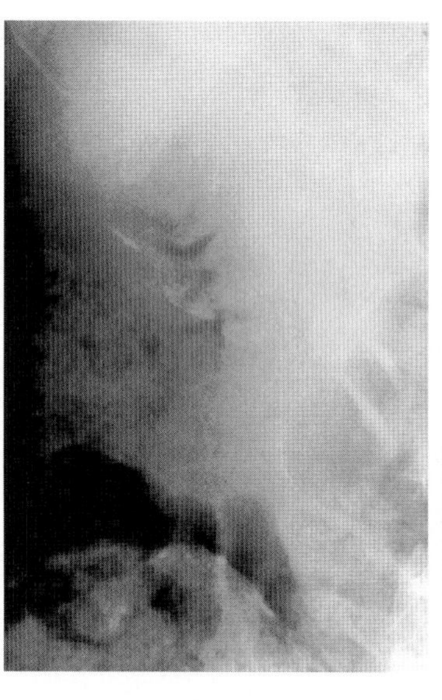

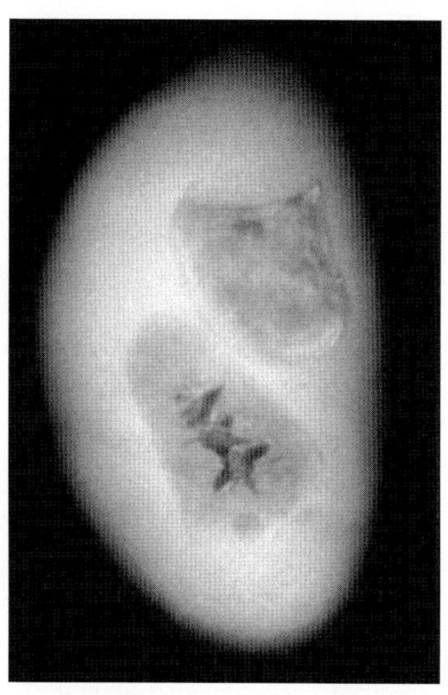

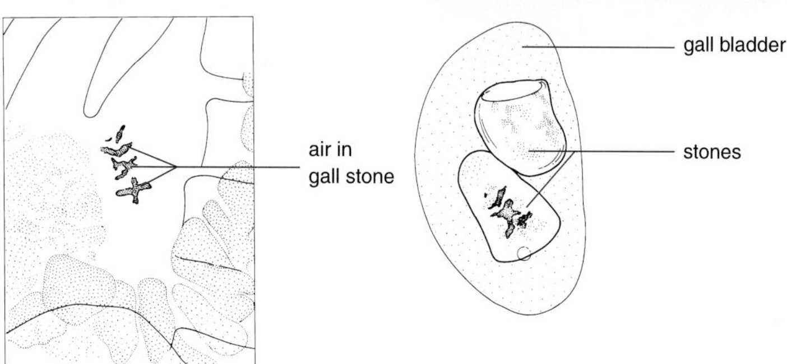

Fig. 14.15 Plain abdominal radiograph of the gall bladder showing air in a gallstone (left), and a radiograph of the same stone after cholecystectomy (right).

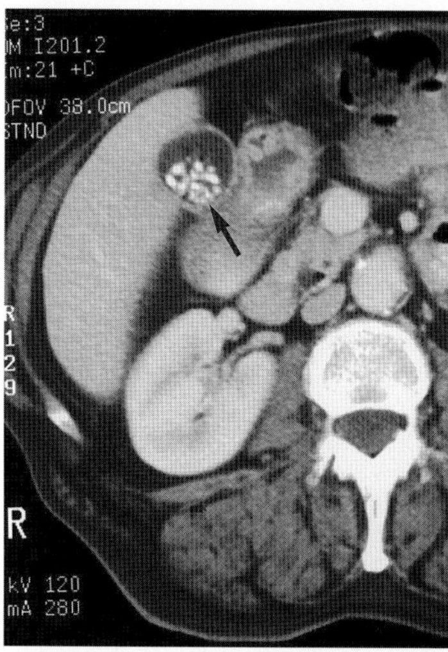

Fig. 14.18 CT demonstrating numerous tiny calcified gallstones (arrow).

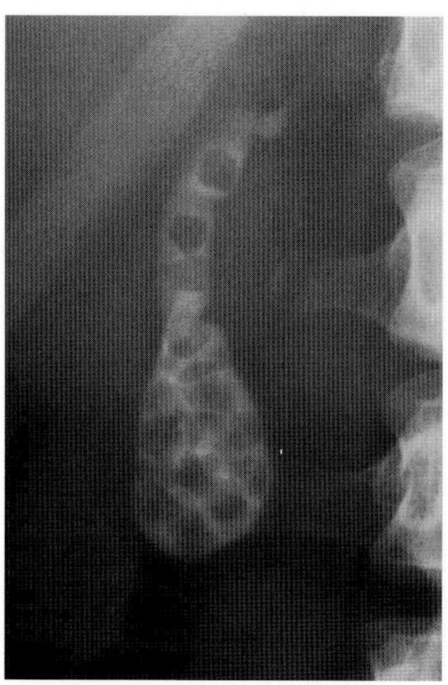

Fig. 14.16 Oral cholecystogram demonstrating about 20 radiolucent, 5–7 mm polygonally shaped gallstones. The gallbladder is contracted about the stones.

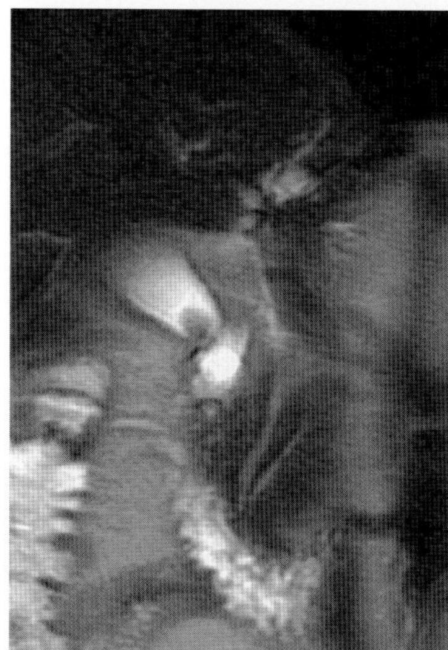

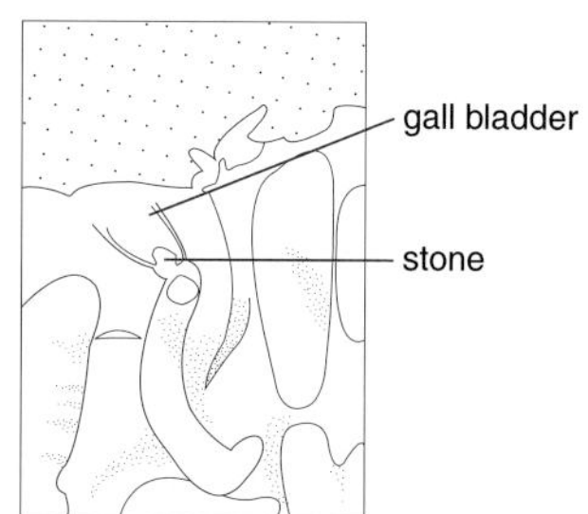

Fig. 14.19 MRI scan showing gallstones in the gall bladder. Courtesy of Ihab Kamel, MD.

help (Fig. 14.18), and although ERCP may also be used to demonstrate gallstones, it should not be employed for simple diagnostic purposes.

CHOLECYSTITIS

Stones in the gall bladder can cause either acute (Figs 14.19, 14.20) or chronic (Figs 14.21, 14.22) cholecystitis. Acute cholecystitis is often a clinical diagnosis that can be confirmed on ultrasound or other imaging modalities such as MRI (Fig 14.23). Occasionally, the cystic duct is blocked by a stone, following which the gall bladder is distended by white mucus and gives rise to a mucocele (Fig. 14.24).

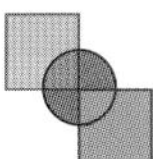

The histological appearances of the gall bladder in acute cholecystitis may range from acute inflammatory changes to widespread hemorrhagic necrosis (Figs 14.25, 14.26). In chronic cholecystitis, the gall bladder is thickened owing to the formation of connective tissue deep to the muscle (Fig. 14.27). The degree of inflammation is variable, and although gallstones are usually present, acalculous cholecystitis may also occur (Fig. 14.28).

Cholesterolosis of the gall bladder is an uncommon condition in which yellow flecks are seen over the mucosal surface, giving an appearance known as the strawberry gall bladder (Fig. 14.29). This is due to large numbers of foamy macrophages in the mucosa (Fig. 14.30) and is a benign asymptomatic abnormality. In contrast, chronic or recurrent inflammation of the gall bladder may be caused by xanthogranulomatous cholecystitis, a condition in which ulceration of the gall bladder wall may occur with or without associated gallstones (Figs 14.31, 14.32).

Conditions associated with cholecystitis

Unless cholecystographic contrast has been administered, an opaque gall bladder (Fig. 14.33) is a rare finding on plain abdominal radiograph. But this can occur when the cystic duct is blocked and concentrated residual bile containing radio-dense calcium – the so-called limey bile – is formed within the gall bladder. Unusually, the wall calcifies, forming the 'porcelain' gall bladder that appears on the radiograph as an outline of radio-opaque calcium (Figs 14.34–14.36).

DIVERTICULA OF THE GALL BLADDER

Out-pouchings of mucosa between the muscle bundles (Aschoff–Rokitansky sinuses) are common (Fig. 14.37). They increase with age and have many features in common with colonic diverticula.

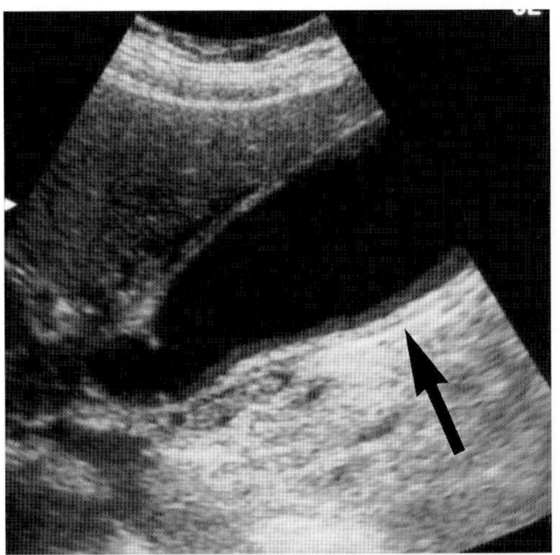

a

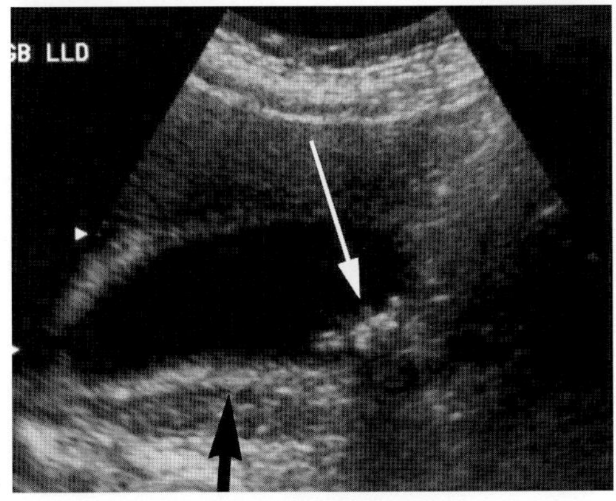

b

Fig. 14.20 Ultrasound demonstrating cholecystitis and gallstones. (a) The wall of the gallbladder (arrow) is thickened. (b) Gallstones (white arrow) are present. Shadowing posterior to the gallstones is present. The wall of the gallbladder is thickened (black arrow). Courtesy of Jill E. Langer, M.D, Philadelphia.

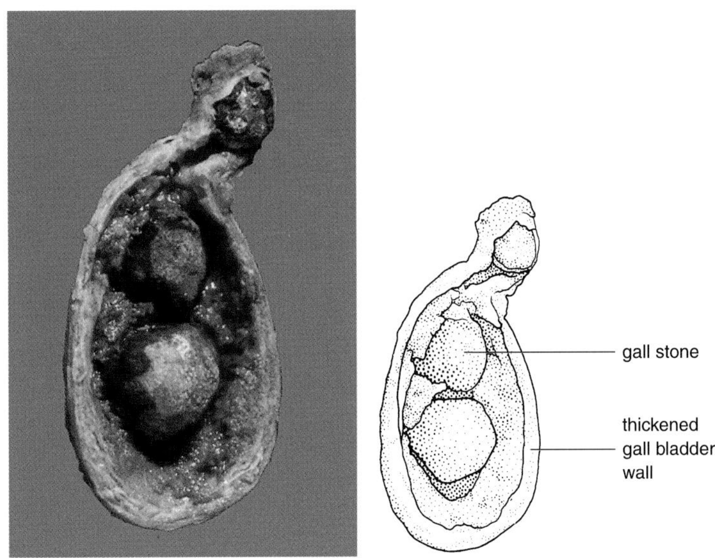

Fig. 14.22 Chronic cholecystitis with the gall bladder contracted around two stones in the body and one in the neck.

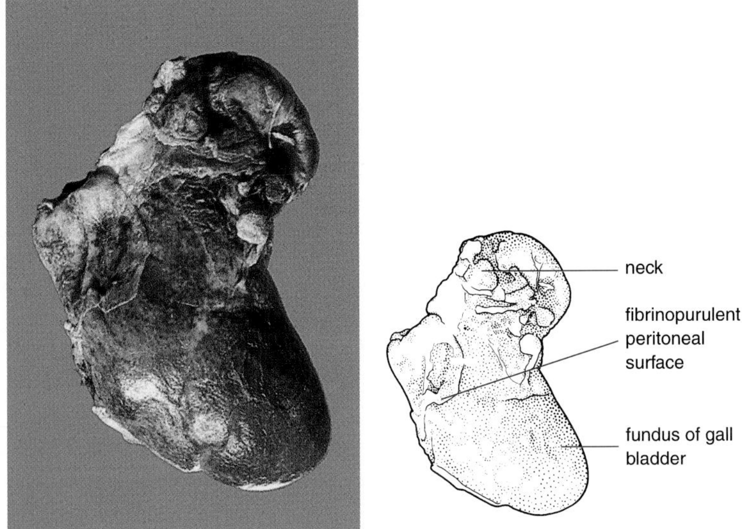

a

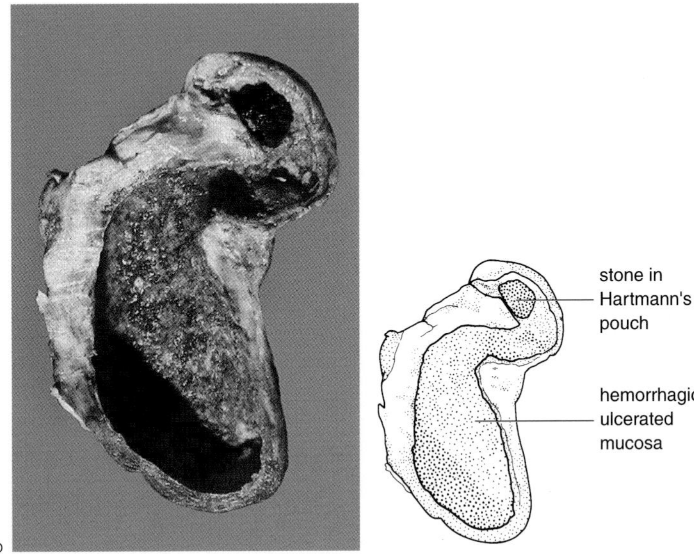

b

Fig. 14.21 The gall bladder in acute cholecystitis showing peritonitis over the surface (a) and mucosal ulceration with a stone in Hartmann's pouch (b).

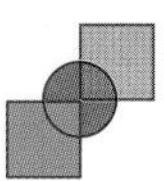

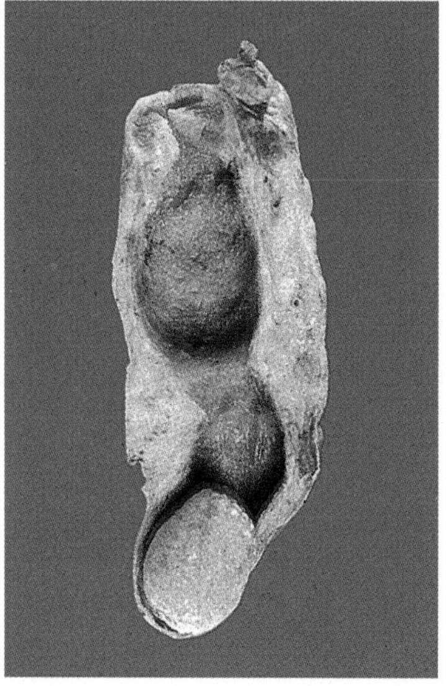

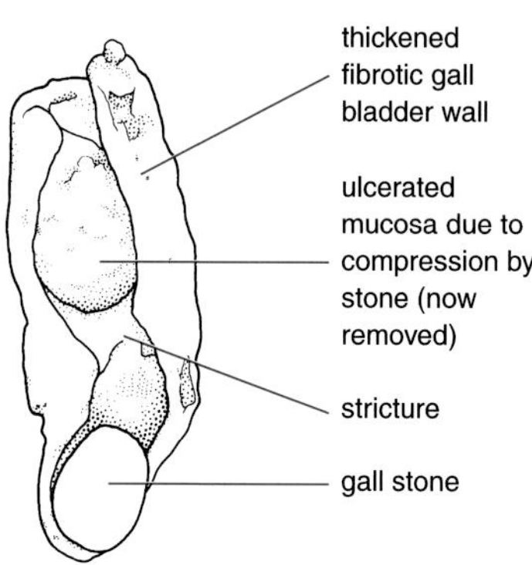

■ **Fig. 14.23** Chronic cholecystitis and cholelithiasis showing a large oval stone in the fundus with a stricture above. The second stone was removed to reveal ulcerated mucosa.

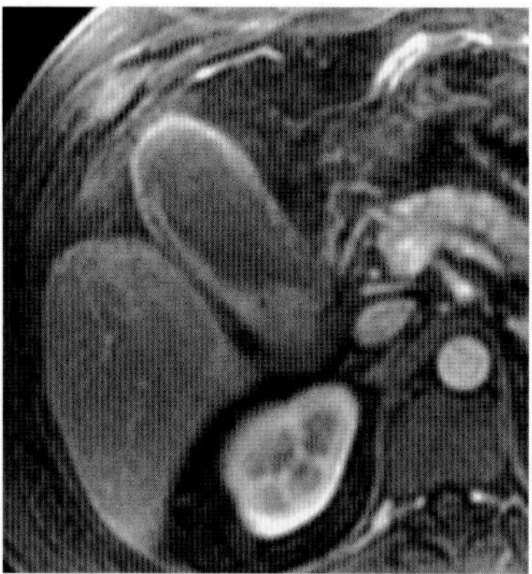

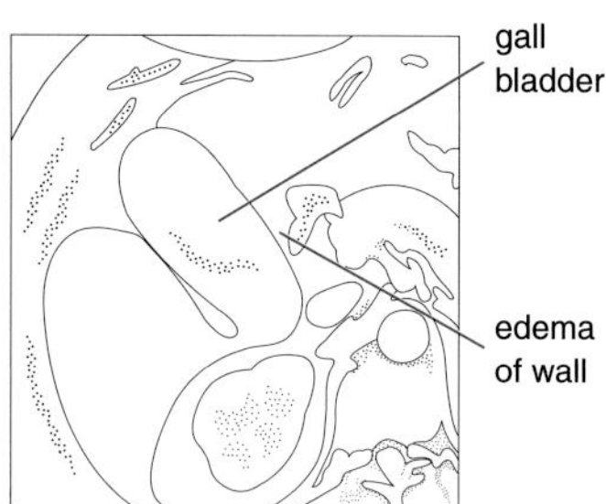

■ **Fig. 14.24** Acute cholecystitis demonstrated by MR. The edema of the gall bladder wall is readily seen. Courtesy of Ihab Kamel, MD.

■ **Fig. 14.25** A mucocele of the gall bladder that is distended, pale, and thin walled.

They are most frequent in the fundus and often become filled with inspissated bile (Fig. 14.38), biliary gravel or cholesterol crystals. Their role in gall bladder disease is not clear. When diverticulae are accompanied by generalized muscle hypertrophy, the term adenomyosis is used (Figs 14.39–14.41), and adenomyoma if localized (Fig. 14.42).

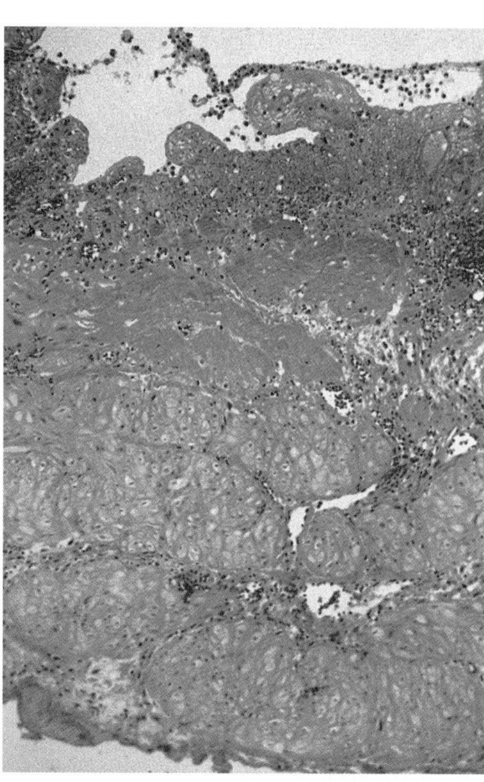

■ **Fig. 14.26** Microscopic appearance of acute cholecystitis showing mucosal ulceration and hemorrhage with fibrinopurulent exudate covering the luminal surface

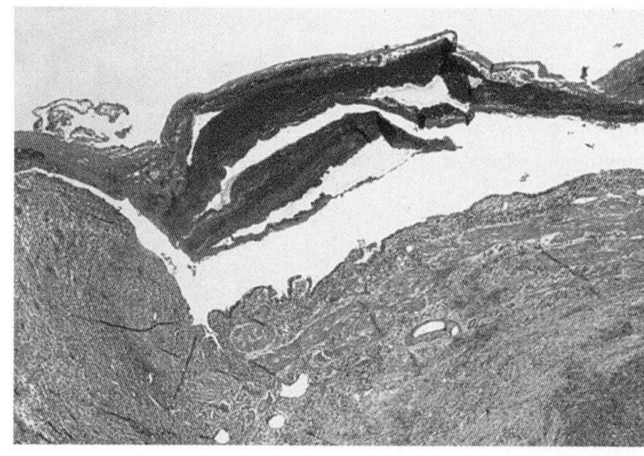

■ **Fig. 14.27** Acute cholecystitis. High magnification view of the edge of a transmural ulcer filled with inflamed granulation tissue (a), hemorrhage in the lumen, and suppurative inflammation involving all layers of the gallbladder wall (b).

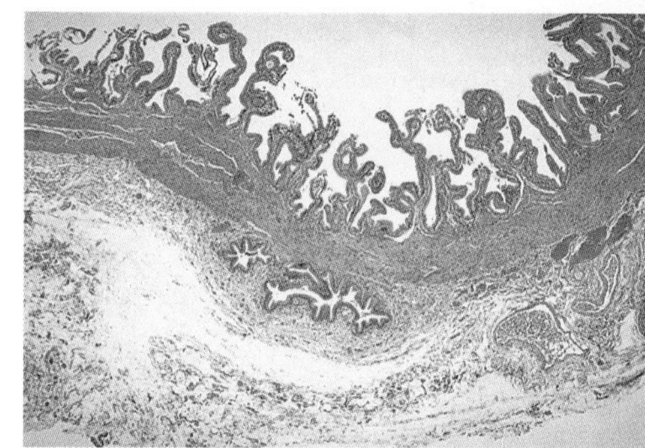

■ **Fig. 14.28** Chronic cholecystitis. Histologic section showing typical features including complex bridging of the mucosal villi, mural thickening, and Rokitansky–Aschoff sinuses extending into the extramural soft tissue.

BILE DUCT STONES

Although valuable as a means of detecting bile duct dilatation, ultrasound is less reliable in identifying calculi within the common bile duct (Figs 14.43, 14.44). Percutaneous transhepatic cholangiography (Fig. 14.45) and endoscopic retrograde cholangiography (Figs 14.46–14.48) which were, in their days, the preferred diagnostic techniques are gradually giving way to CT (Fig. 14.49) and to MRC (Fig. 14.50). Intravenous cholangiography is no longer sanctioned since it is a poor means of visualizing the biliary tree and one which carries a high risk of serious contrast reaction. Endoscopic ultrasound (EUS) is also an excellent way of diagnosing bile duct stones.

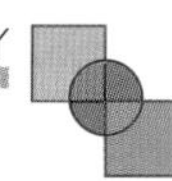

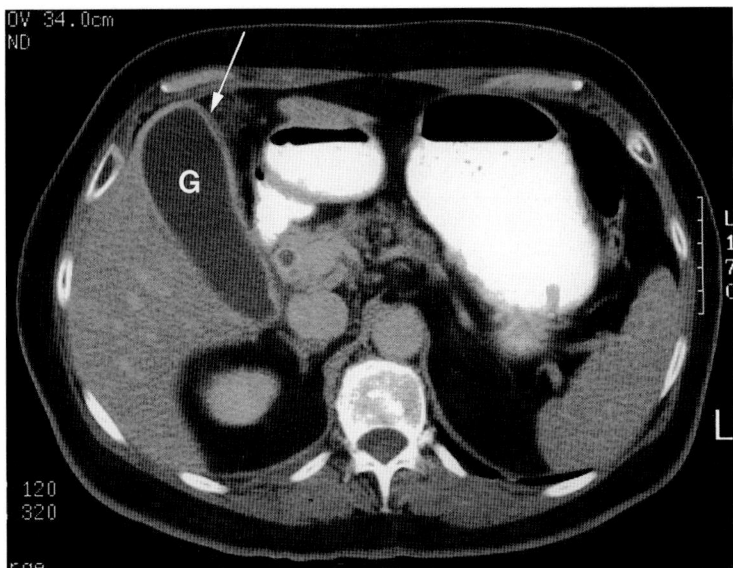

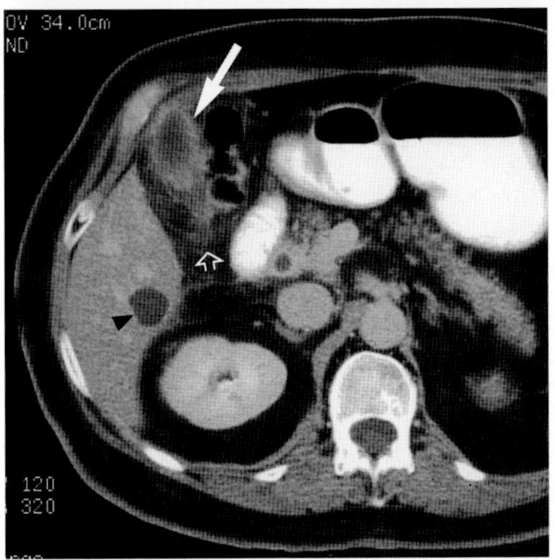

■ **Fig. 14.29** CT demonstrating acute acalculus cholecystitis. (a) Axial image through the level of the pancreatic head shows a dilated gallbladder (G) with a thick wall. A mural stratification pattern is visible in one part of the wall (arrow). (b) CT through the level of the tip of the liver shows that the base of gallbladder has a thickened wall (long arrow). Stranding of the fat (open arrow) adjacent to the gallbladder indicates acute inflammation. A simple cyst (arrowhead) is seen in the liver.

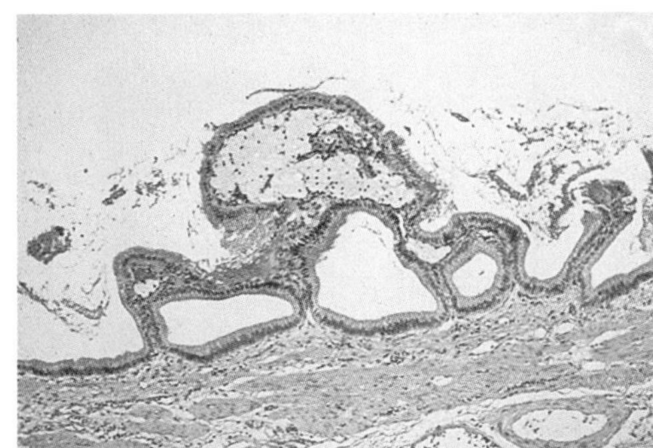

■ **Fig. 14.31** Microscopic view of cholesterolosis showing the characteristic collections of pale, foamy-appearing histiocytes filling the mucosal stroma.

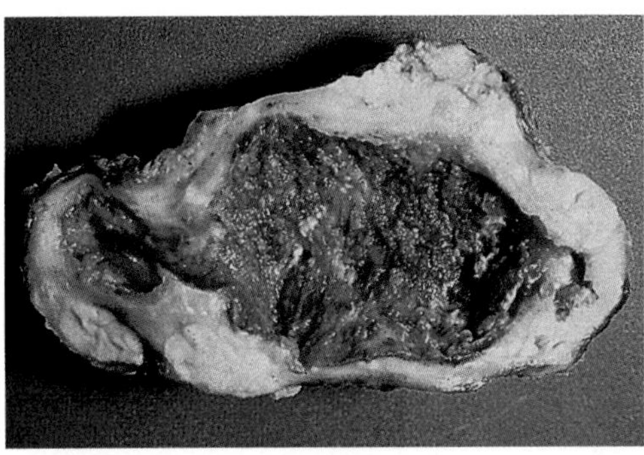

■ **Fig. 14.32** Macroscopic view of gall bladder showing extensive ulceration, with large nodules of xanthogranulomatous material in the wall. Courtesy of Dr M.A. Parsons.

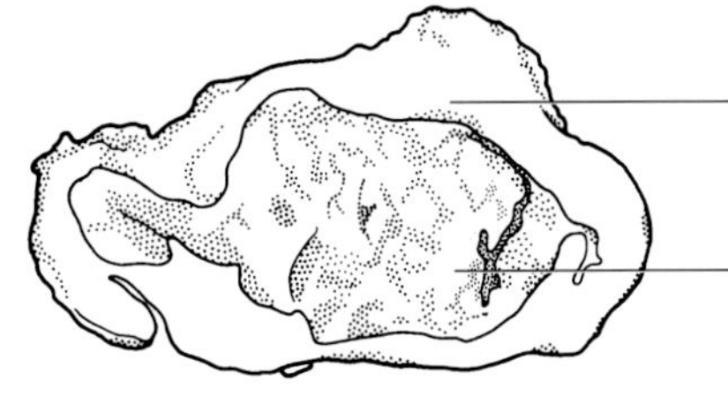

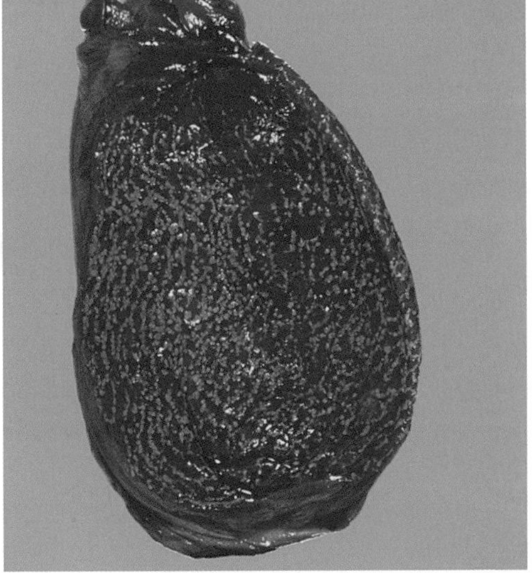

■ **Fig. 14.30** Cholesterolosis (strawberry gallbladder) cholecystectomy specimen showing the reddened mucosa flecked with yellow seed-like deposits of cholesterol that has been likened to the appearance of a strawberry.

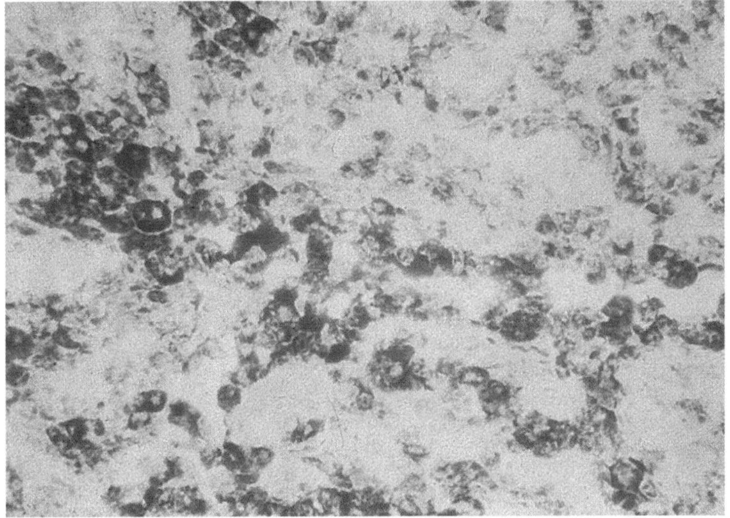

■ **Fig. 14.33** Oil-Red-O stain of a frozen section of xanthogranulomatous tissue. The lipid deposits stain red. Courtesy of Dr M.A. Parsons.

COMPLICATIONS OF BILIARY SURGERY

Calculi may be retained following cholecystectomy or may form *in situ* and this possibility should always be considered in patients presenting with jaundice at any time following cholecystectomy. Bile leaks may occur if operative ligatures slip or if the duct is damaged (Fig. 14.51). Gallstones may also form in the reconstructed biliary tree after liver transplantation (Fig. 14.52).

A plain radiograph will reveal any air present in the biliary tree (Fig. 14.53). This occurs when the ampullary valve is damaged after spontaneous passage of a stone though the ampulla of Vater, and is expected after surgery to the biliary tree or endoscopic sphincterotomy. Rarely, gallstones may spontaneously fistulate from the gall bladder direct into the intestine (Fig. 14.54).

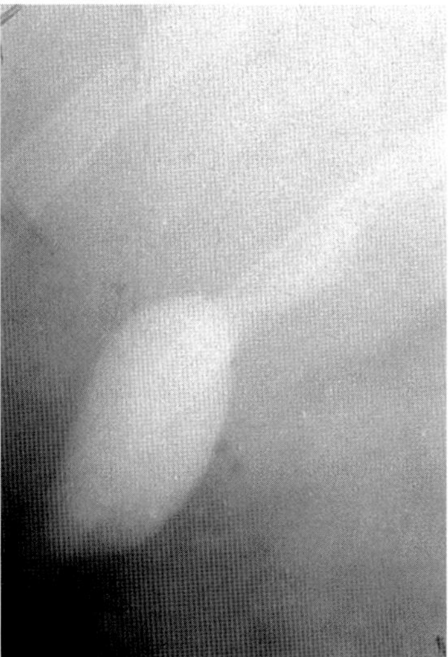

Fig. 14.34 Plain abdominal radiograph showing limey bile without any radio-opaque dye.

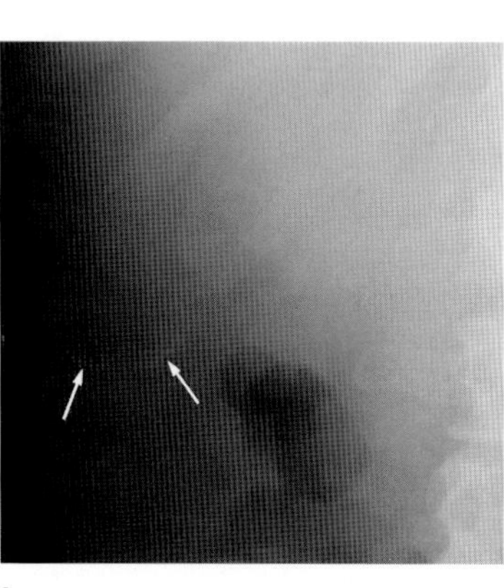

a

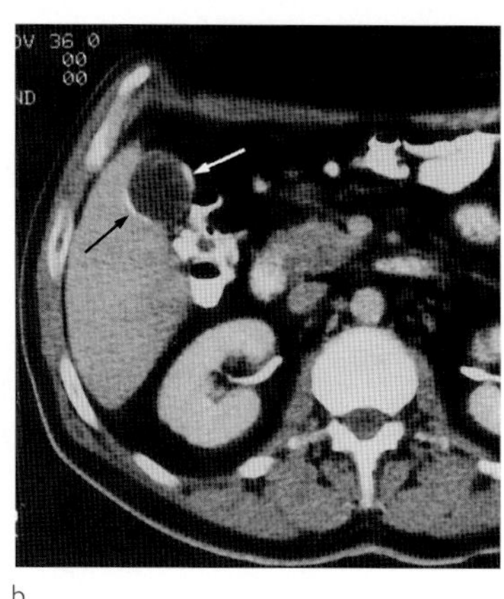

b

Fig. 14.35 Porcelain gallbladder. (a) Plain radiograph of the abdomen shows a curvilinear calcification (arrows) in the right upper quadrant. (b) CT through the tip of the liver shows curvilinear calcifications (arrows) in wall of the gallbladder.

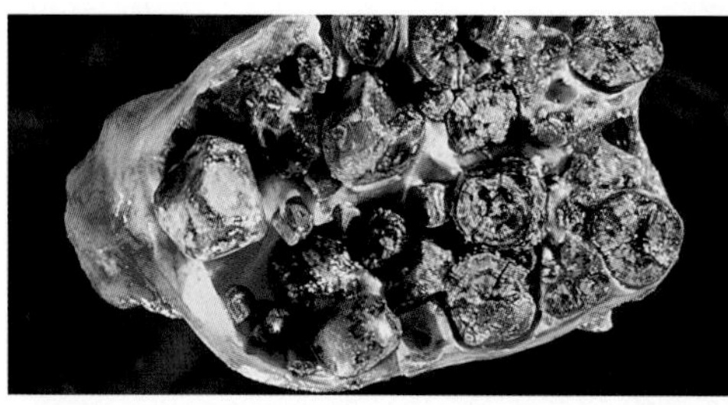

Fig. 14.36 Cholecystectomy specimen of a porcelain gallbladder showing mixed composition stones filling the lumen and irregular white plaques of calcium in the wall (lower left).

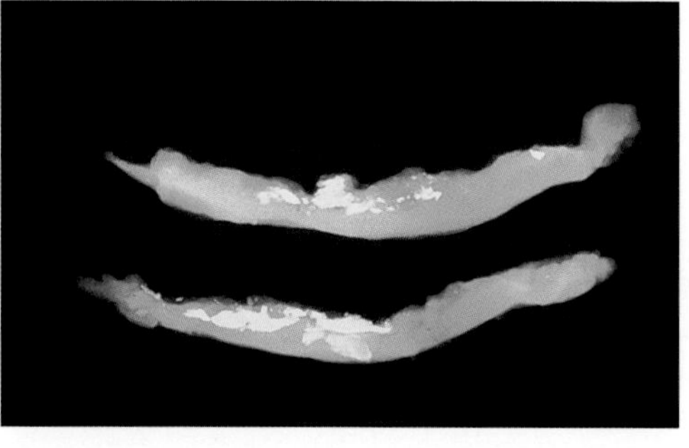

Fig. 14.37 Porcelain gallbladder. Specimen radiograph of full-thickness transverse sections through the gallbladder showing the densely radio-opaque deposits of calcium in the wall.

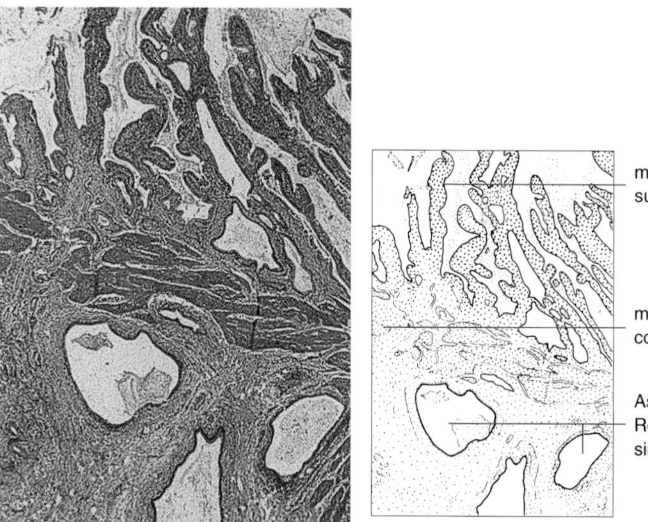

Fig. 14.38 Aschoff–Rokitansky sinuses occurring deep to the muscle of the gall bladder. H&E stain (x 20).

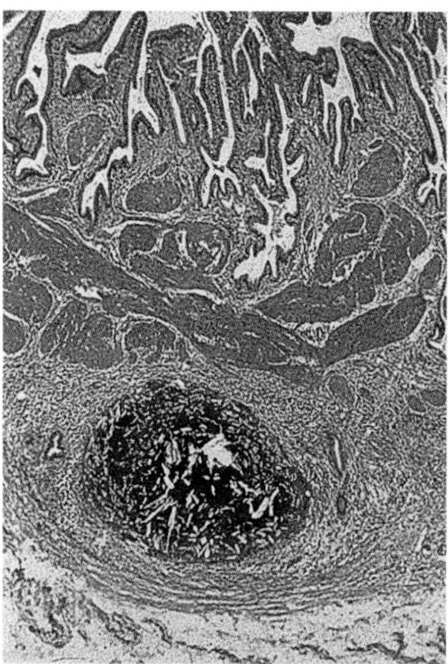

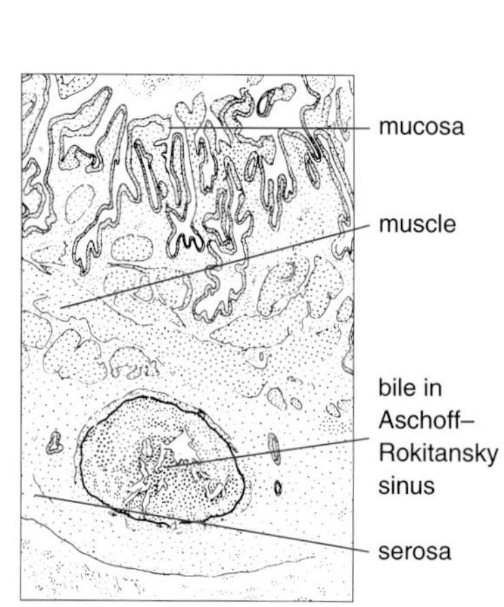

Fig. 14.39 Inspissated bile in a distended Aschoff–Rokitansky sinus penetrating deeply into the muscle. H&E stain (x 16).

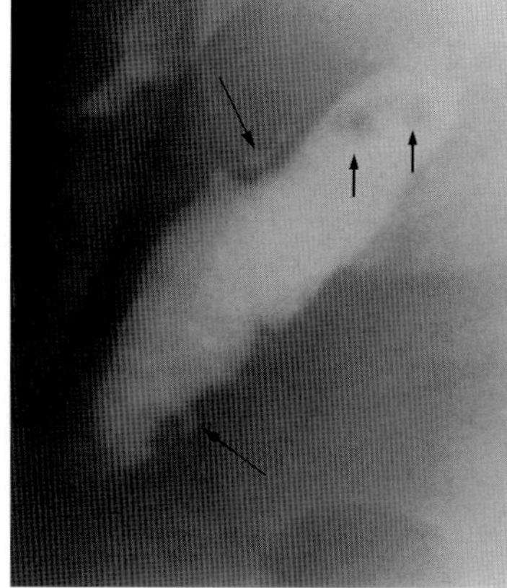

Fig. 14.40 Erect spot radiograph obtained during oral cholecystogram demonstrating adenomyomatosis of the gallbladder. Numerous flask-shaped out-pouchings arise from the wall of the gallbladder, representing dilated Rokitansky–Aschoff sinuses (long arrows). Three radiolucent gallstones (short arrows) are floating in the oral contrast.

Hemobilia

Pain, jaundice and gastrointestinal hemorrhage are the classical presenting symptoms of bleeding into the biliary tree. This may be caused by trauma, an aneurysm, or a hepatic tumor, but it is most commonly associated with liver biopsy. Retrograde cholangiography may reveal clots in the bile duct, but hepatic angiography

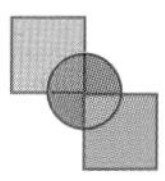

will define the site of hemorrhage (see also Chapter 13). Selective hepatic angiography with embolization of the bleeding vessel is an effective means of treatment which obviates the necessity for laparotomy (Fig. 14.55).

CONGENITAL ABNORMALITIES

Phrygian cap

An unusual but harmless finding on cholecystography is a gall bladder bent upon itself (Fig. 14.56), and so resembling the Phrygian cap taken up by the French revolutionaries. There are many other harmless congenital variations in the shape of the gall bladder.

Choledochal cyst

This rare congenital abnormality is a local dilatation of the common bile duct. It can be huge and may cause biliary obstruction and infection. Although a congenital abnormality, it may present at any stage in life. The lesion is best visualized by percutaneous or retrograde cholangiography (Figs 14.57, 14.58).

Caroli's disease

There are various congenital cystic abnormalities of the bile ducts, some of which are associated with renal disorders. Multiple intrahepatic saccular biliary dilatations are seen in Caroli's disease, often in association with diffuse dilation of the extrahepatic ducts (Figs 14.59–14.61). These patients may also present with cholangitis and jaundice, sometimes with secondary stone formation (Fig. 14.62). The diagnosis can be confirmed on ERC, MRI, or MRCP. The hepatic histology is in line with the dilatation seen macroscopically (Fig. 14.63). The major complication of this condition is cholangiocarcinoma, but progression to liver failure also frequently occurs.

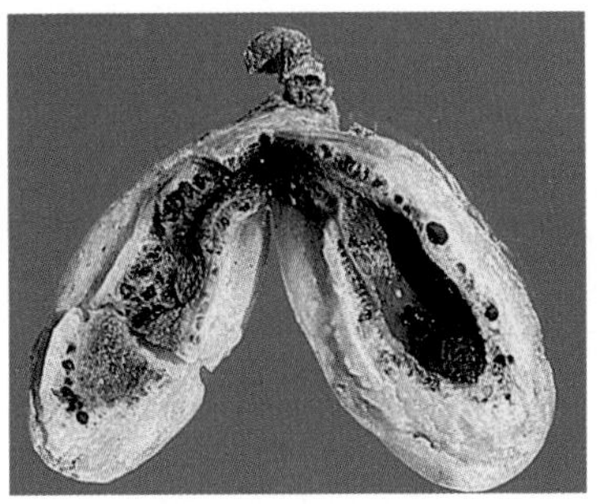

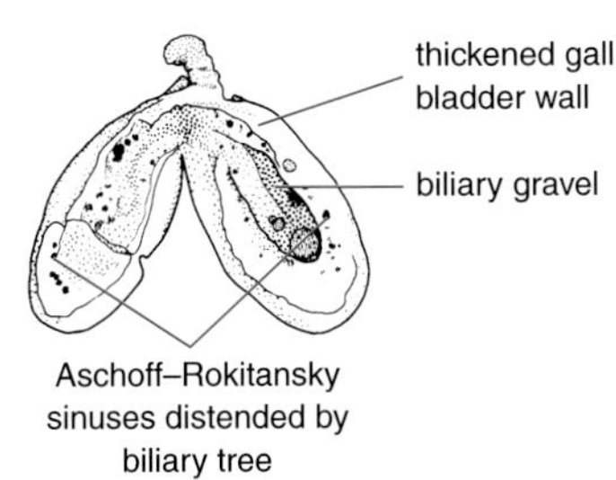

Fig. 14.41 Chronic cholecystitis showing a contracted gall bladder with biliary gravel in the lumen and distended Aschoff–Rokitansky sinuses: the characteristic pattern of diffuse adenomyosis.

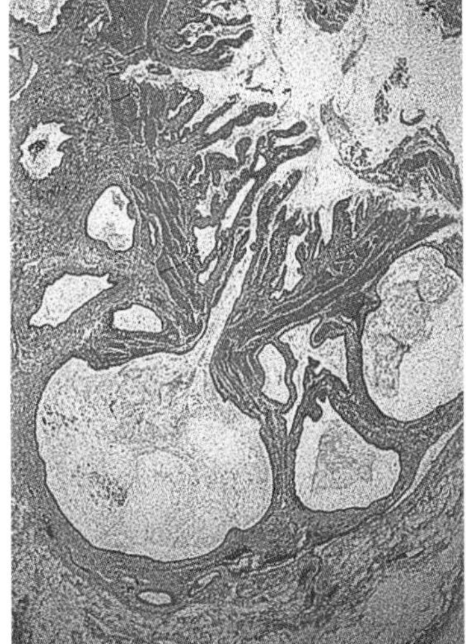

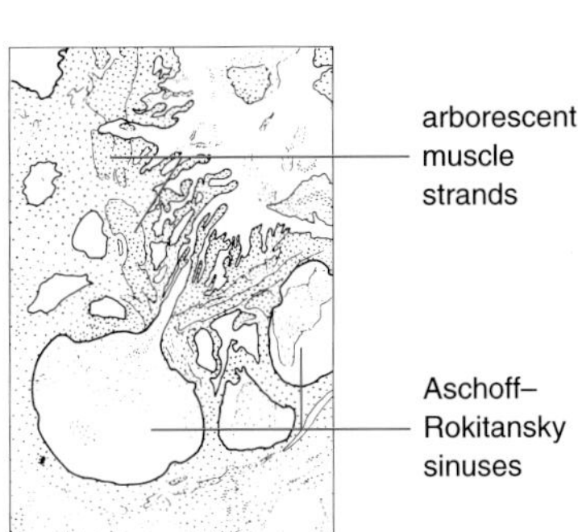

Fig. 14.42 Histological appearance of adenomyosis showing sinuses and arborescent muscle fibres. H&E stain (x 8).

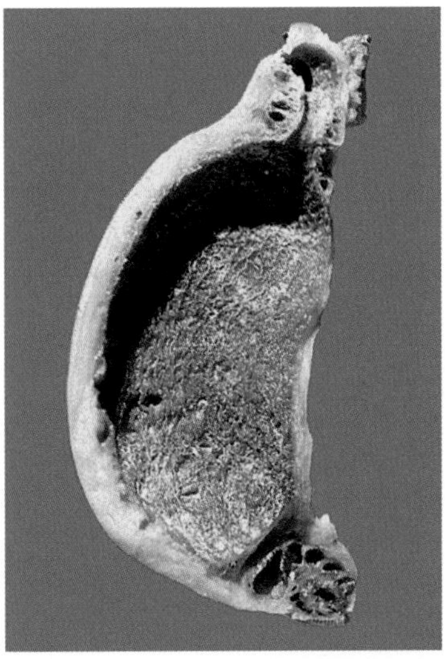

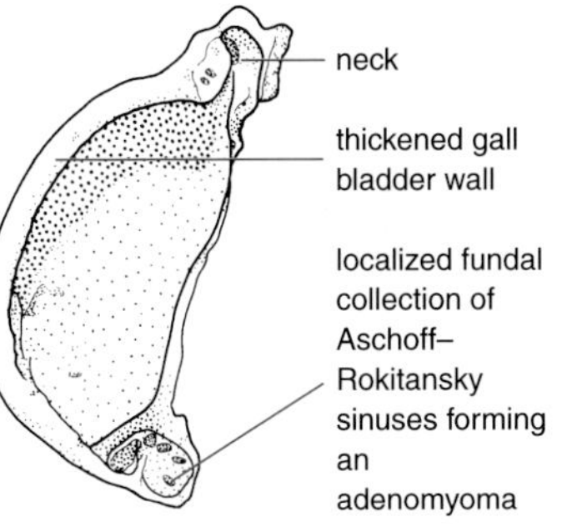

Fig. 14.43 Fundal adenomyoma of the gall bladder.

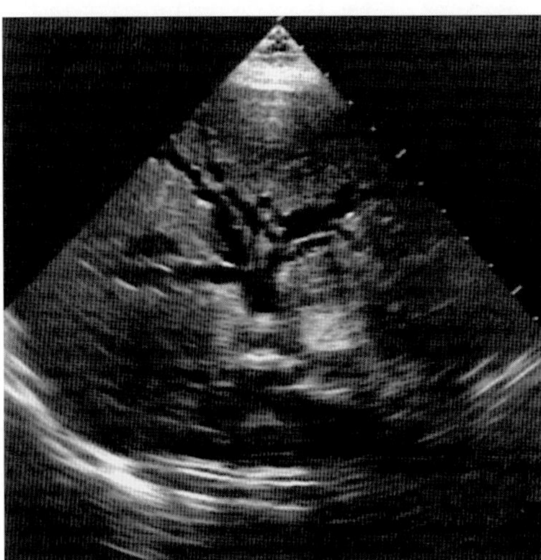

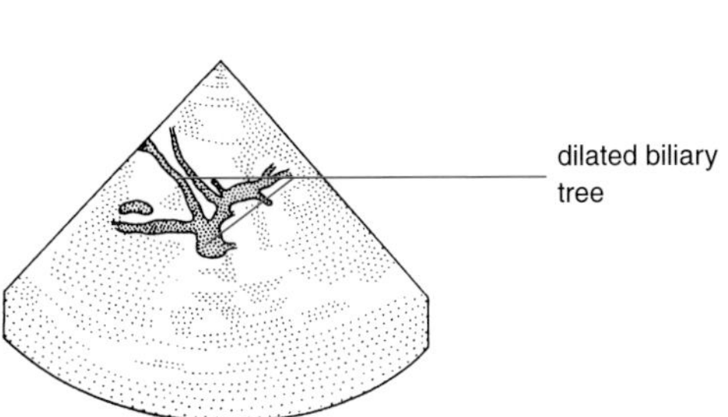

Fig. 14.44 Ultrasound showing dilatation of the intrahepatic biliary tree. Courtesy of Dr M.C. Collins.

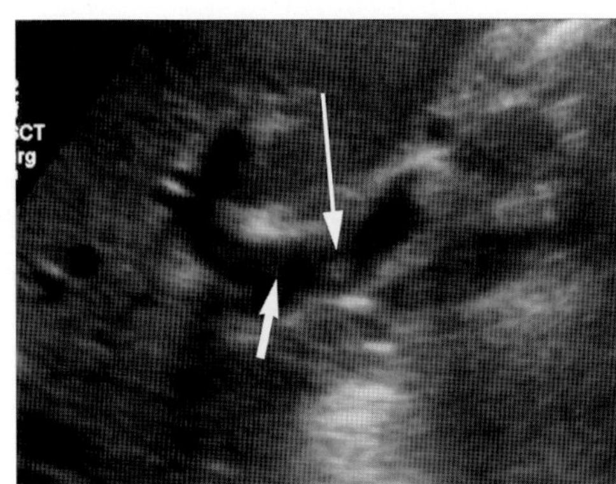

Fig. 14.45 Ultrasound demonstrating common hepatic duct stone. A 4 mm ovoid echogenic structure (long arrow) is seen within the lumen of the common hepatic duct (short arrow). Courtesy of Jill E. Langer, M.D., Philadelphia.

Biliary atresia

Congenital narrowing or absence of the intrahepatic and/or extrahepatic ducts (Fig. 14.64) is an unusual cause of persistent jaundice which starts in infancy and usually continues until death within the first decade of life if untreated. Prolonged cholestasis leads to malabsorption of (lipid soluble) vitamin D and eventually to biliary rickets (Fig. 14.65).

Biliary atresia may be extrahepatic or intrahepatic. In the extrahepatic form the liver is dark green (Fig. 14.66) and extensive fibrosis is seen around the portal areas. This eventually leads to micronodular secondary biliary cirrhosis with proliferation of ductules in fibrous tracts (Fig. 14.67). In intrahepatic biliary atresia, there is usually a paucity of bile ducts in the portal tracts (Fig. 14.68), rather than a complete absence, with progression to cirrhosis. It is associated with neonatal giant cell hepatitis.

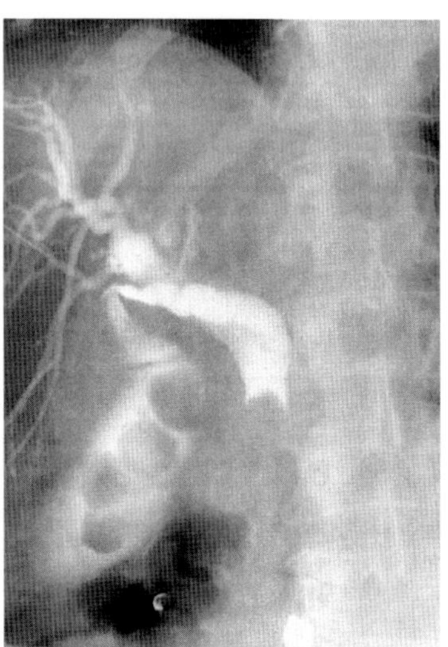

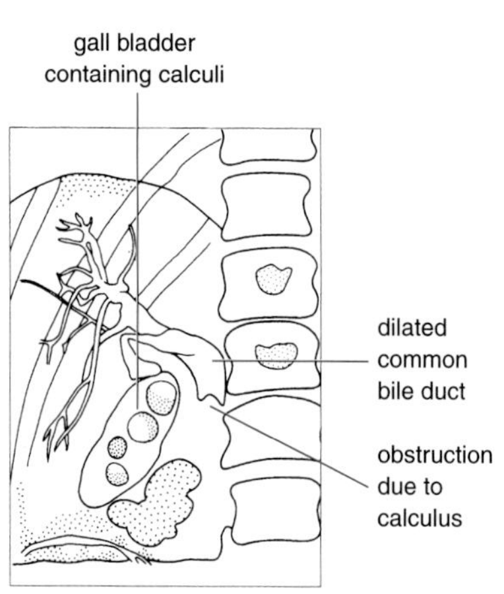

Fig. 14.46 Percutaneous transhepatic cholangiogram showing a dilated biliary tree due to a common bile duct stone. There are several further calculi in the gall bladder.

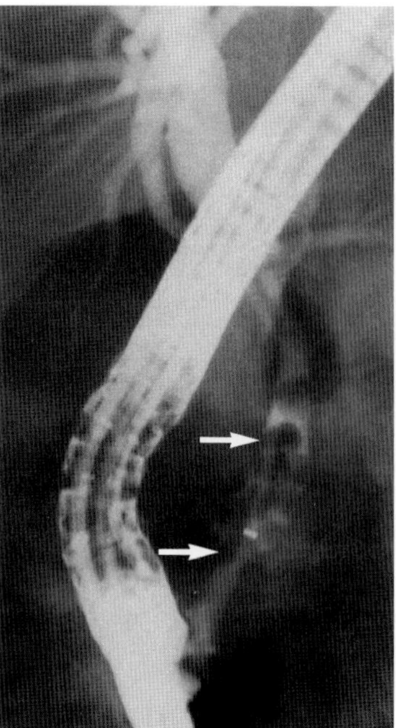

Fig. 14.47 Endoscopic retrograde cholangiogram shows ten 3–4 mm in size, polygonally shaped calculi (arrows) in the common bile duct.

CHOLANGITIS

Biliary worm infestations

In tropical countries, roundworms (*Ascaris*) may invade the biliary tree and cause jaundice, cholangitis, and stones. They are well demonstrated by retrograde cholangiography (Fig. 14.69). In the Far East, the Chinese liver fluke (*Clonorchis*) invades the liver from the blood stream and causes chronic inflammation and fibrosis of the intrahepatic ducts which predisposes to cholangiocarcinoma. In Europe, the sheep liver fluke (*Fasciola*) may be contracted by ingesting its cercaria. It causes cholangitis with fever, hepatic pain and eosinophilia. Histologically, the portal tracts are infiltrated with acute inflammatory cells and eosinophils.

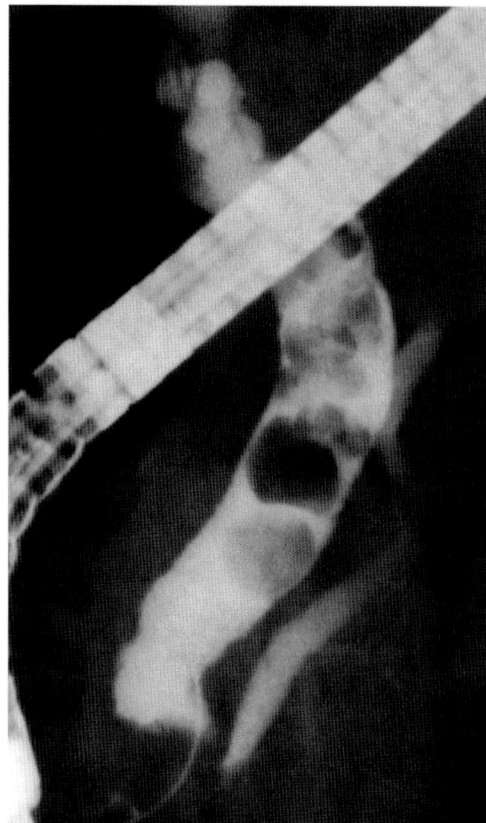

Fig. 14.48 Endoscopic retrograde cholangiogram demonstrates choledocholithiasis with biliary dilatation. Numerous 4–13 mm in size, polygonally shaped, radiolucent filling defects are seen in the common bile and common hepatic duct.

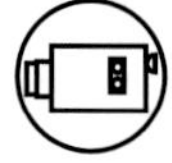

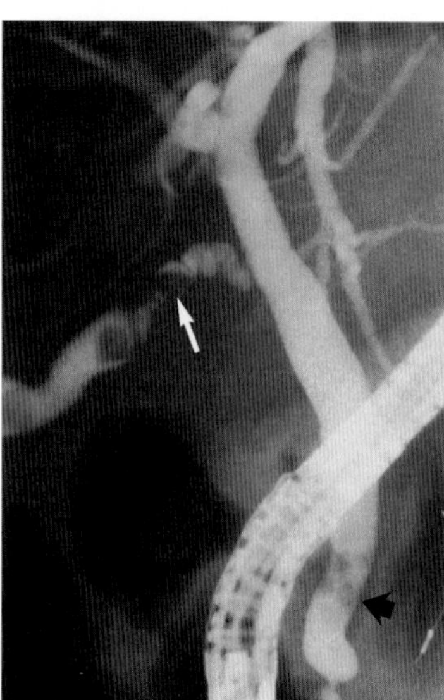

Fig. 14.49 Endoscopic retrograde cholangiogram shows choledocholithiasis and cystic duct lithiasis. Three polygonally shaped radiolucent filling defects (representative calculus – white arrow) are seen in cystic duct and five smaller non-calcified stones (black arrow) are present in the distal common bile duct.

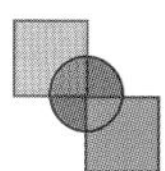

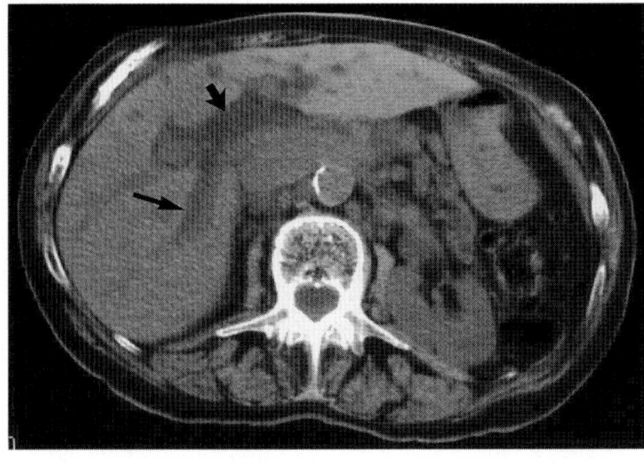

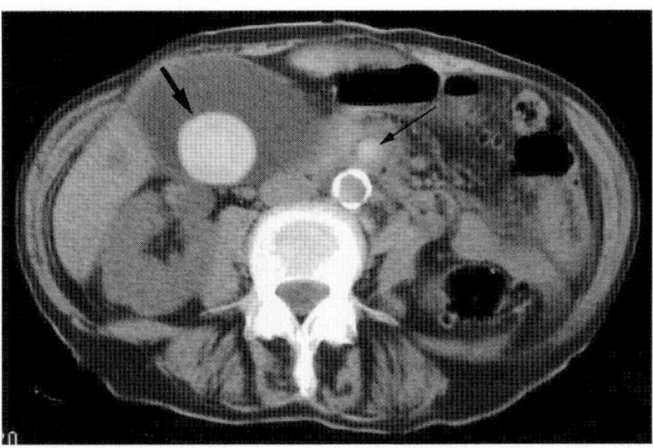

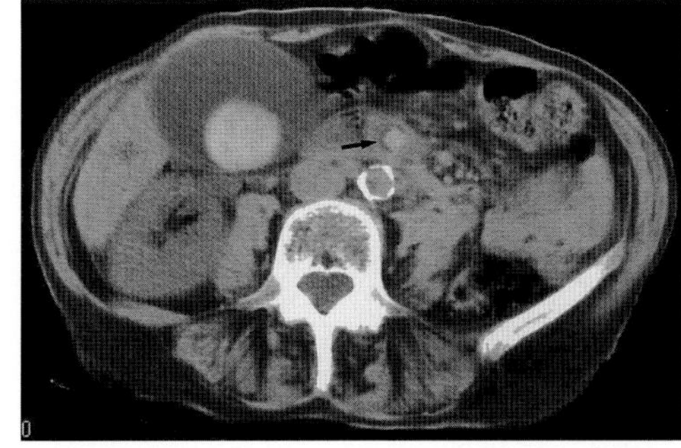

a b c

Fig. 14.50 CT performed without oral, intravenous, or contrast demonstrating cholelithiasis and choledocholithiasis. (a) Image through the mid liver shows intrahepatic bile duct dilatation (long arrow identifies dilated duct to posterior segment right lobe) and a dilated common hepatic duct (short arrow). (b) A large laminated gallstone (thick arrow) is seen in a dilated, thick-walled gall bladder. A faintly calcified calculus (thin arrow) is seen in the region of the head of the pancreas. This patient had previously undergone left nephrectomy accounting for the leftward and inferior deviation of the pancreas and colon, respectively. (c) Shows a crescent-shaped ring of bile (arrow) partially surrounding the common duct calculus.

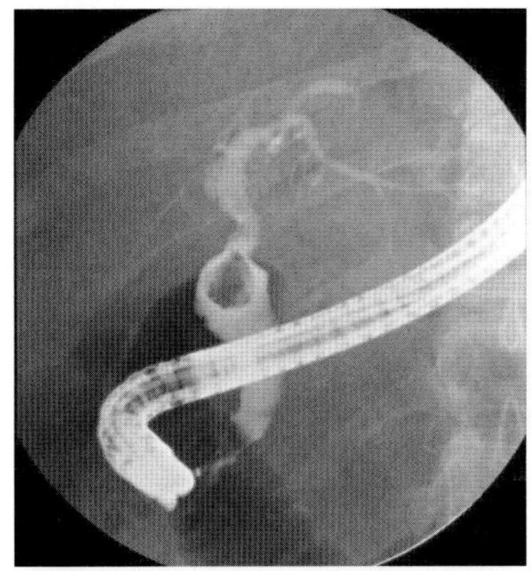

Fig. 14.53 Common bile duct stone in a patient after orthotopic liver transplantation.

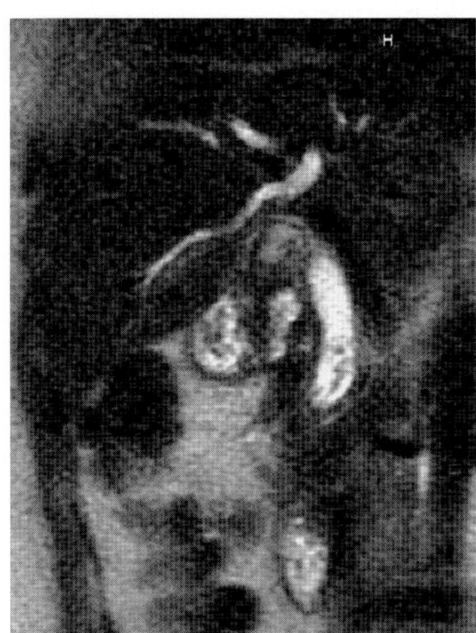

Fig. 14.51 An early MRC clearly showing common bile duct stones despite the very modest overall quality of the scan.

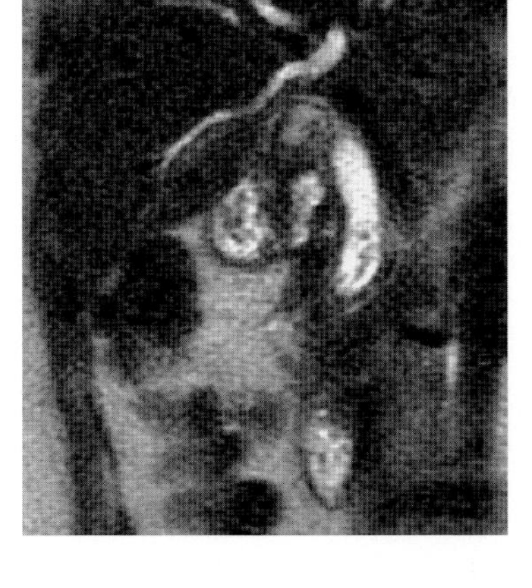

Fig. 14.54 Plain radiograph of abdomen showing air in a dilated biliary tree. The patient had previously undergone sphincterotomy.

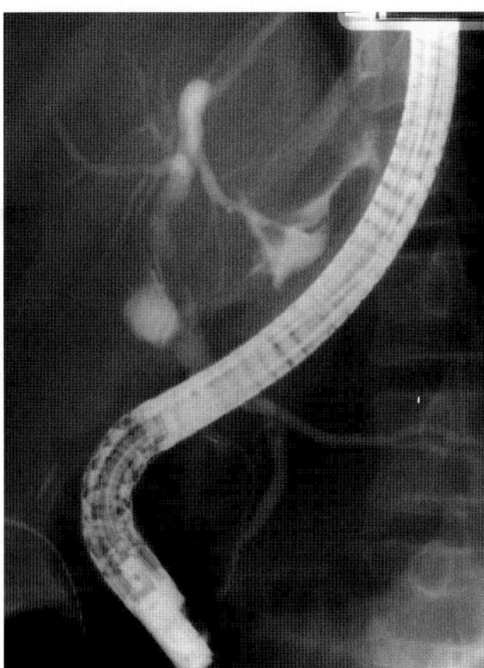

Fig. 14.52 Collection of contrast outside the normal line of the biliary and intestinal lumen in a patient in whom there was a bile leak after cholecystectomy.

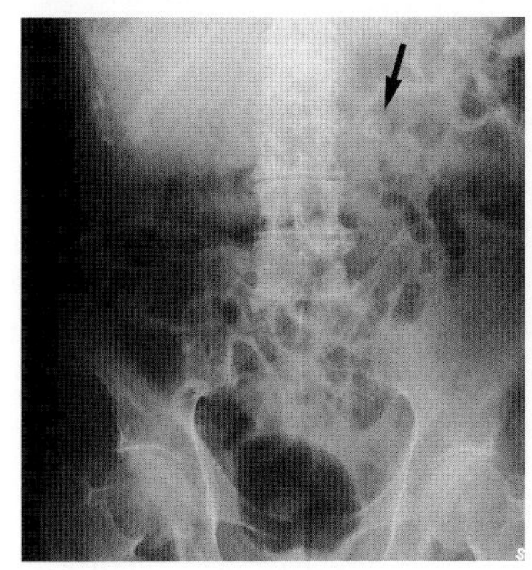

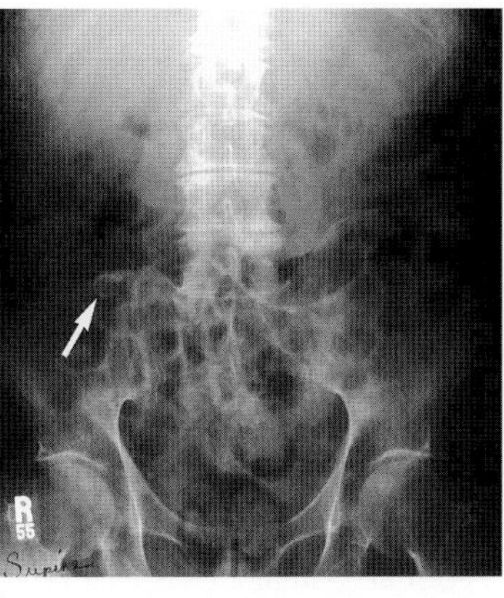

a b

Fig. 14.55 Movement of gallstones through the small intestine. (a) Plain abdominal radiograph shows a 1 cm peripherally calcified polygonally shaped density in the left upper quadrant (arrow). The small intestine is mildly distended but not obstructed. (b) Plain radiograph of the abdomen obtained 2 days later shows that the peripherally calcified calculus (arrow) has moved in the right lower quadrant. No air was seen in the biliary tree.

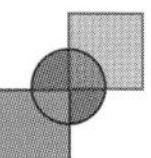

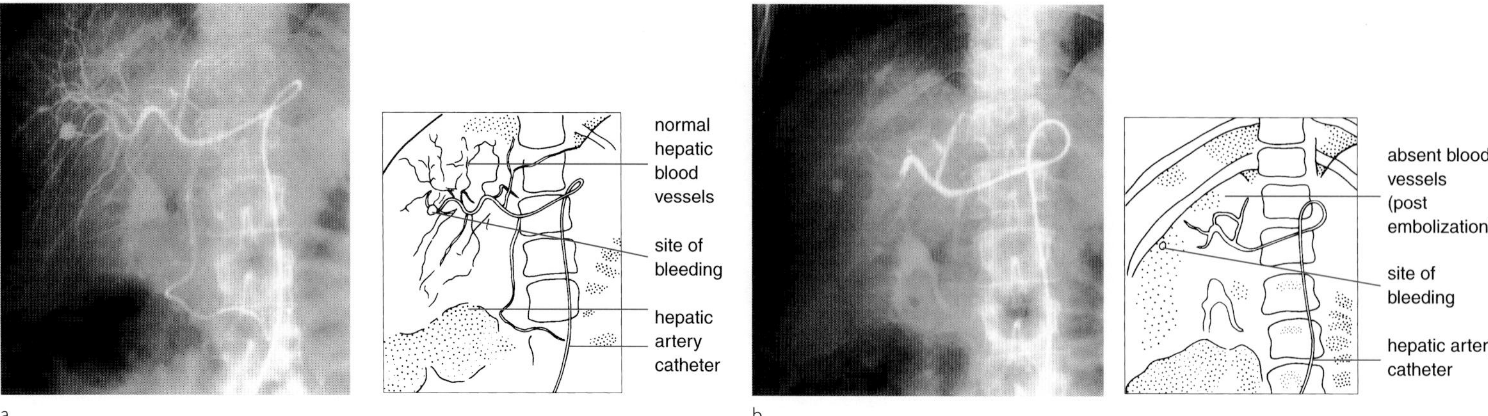

Fig. 14.56 Hepatic angiogram of a patient with hemobilia before (a) and after (b) embolization. The bleeding lesion is readily visible in the right lobe: this part of the liver is completely embolized.

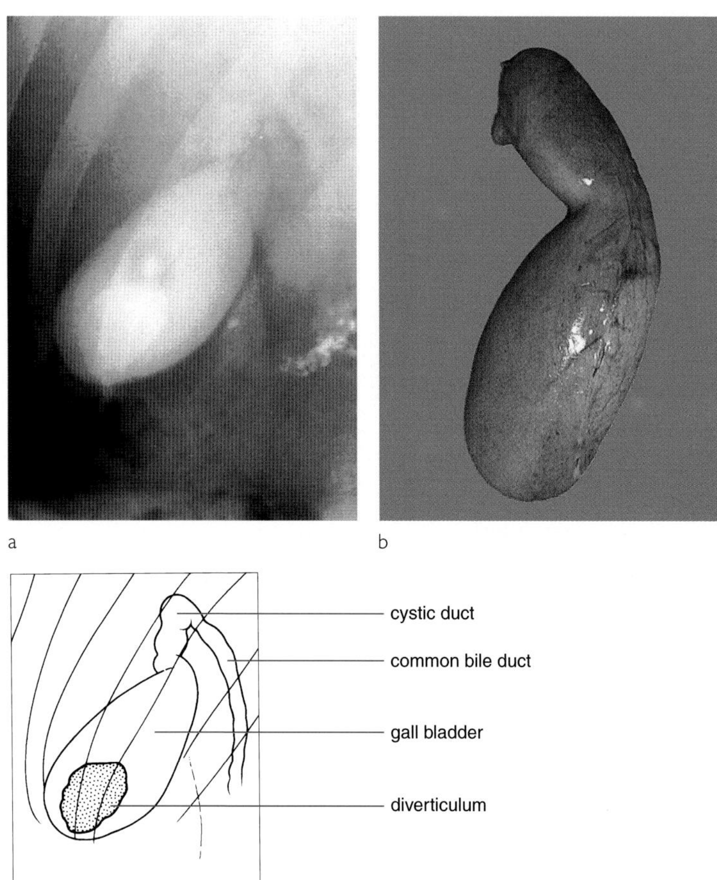

Fig. 14.57 Cholecystogram (a) showing a gall bladder diverticulum (Phrygian cap). The gross specimen (b) shows narrowing of the body of the gall bladder.

Fig. 14.58 Endoscopic retrograde cholangiogram demonstrating choledochal cyst. Fusiform dilatation (large white arrows) of the distal common hepatic duct and proximal and mid common bile duct is present. The distal-most common bile duct (small white arrow) is of normal caliber. No anomalous insertion of the main pancreatic duct (black arrow) is seen in this patient.

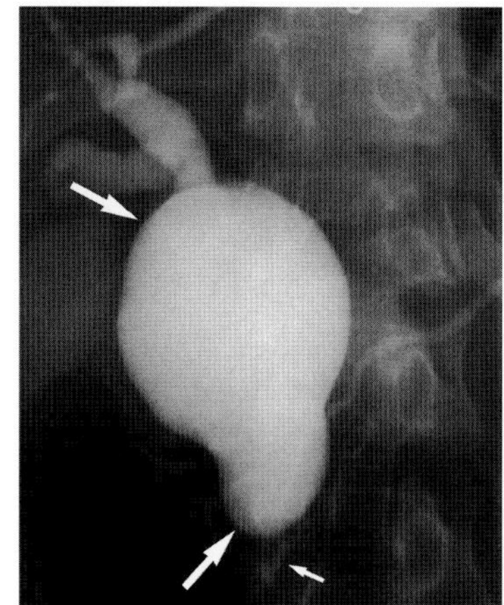

Fig. 14.59 Endoscopic retrograde cholangiogram depicting choledochal cyst. Focal saccular dilatation of the proximal and mid common bile duct (large arrows) is seen. Normal insertion of the main pancreatic duct (small arrow) into normal distal common bile duct is present.

Other infective cholangitis

Cholangitis in the West is associated with gallstones, biliary strictures or any form of intermittent or partial obstruction (Fig. 14.70). The diagnostic histological feature is the presence of neutrophils between the epithelial cells of the bile ductules (Fig. 14.71). Severe and continuing cholangitis may lead to fibrosis and eventually to secondary biliary cirrhosis (Fig. 14.72). In the Far East, recurrent cholangitis is associated with a high incidence of stone formation, particularly within the intrahepatic ducts. In immunosuppressed patients there may be resistant infection with protozoan parasites such as Cryptosporidia, and fungal disease may also be seen (Fig. 14.73).

Sclerosing cholangitis

This may either be a primary phenomenon or occur secondary to gallstones, recurrent infection of the biliary tree or AIDS (see Chapter 11). Primary sclerosing cholangitis may be responsible for intrahepatic cholestasis without much in the way of ascending cholangitis, but as far as the biliary tree is concerned the presentation tends to be associated with the characteristic stricturing that it causes (see below).

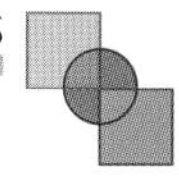

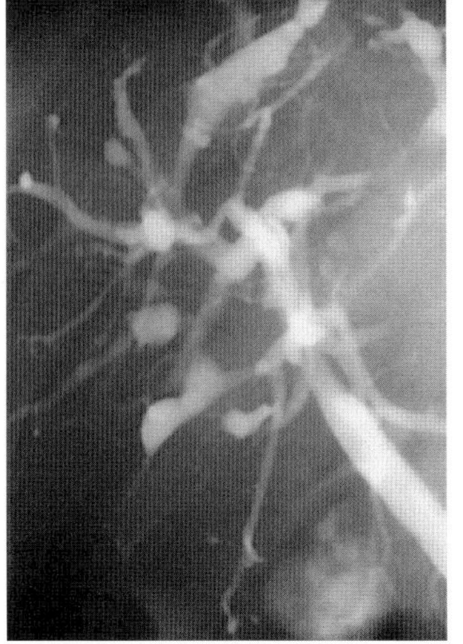

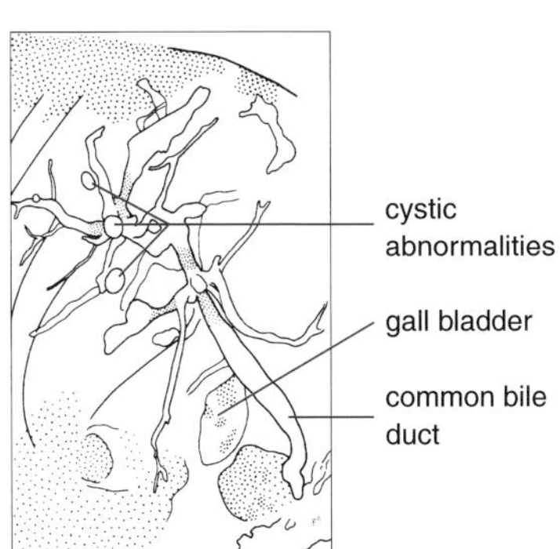

Fig. 14.60 Endoscopic retrograde cholangiogram of Caroli's disease showing multiple cystic abnormalities of the intrahepatic biliary tree.

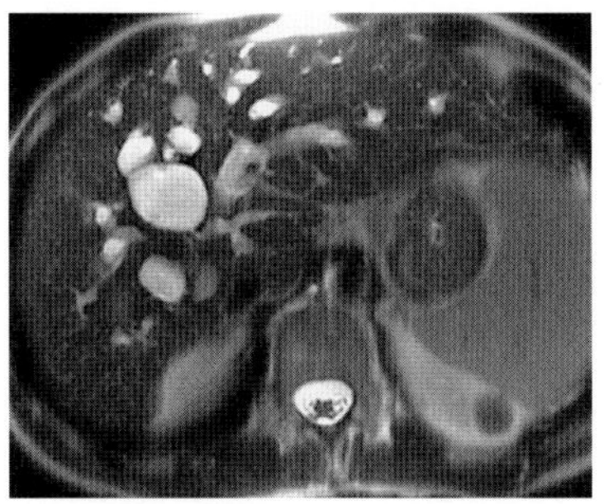

Fig. 14.61 MRI scan showing multiple dilated areas within the intrahepatic biliary system

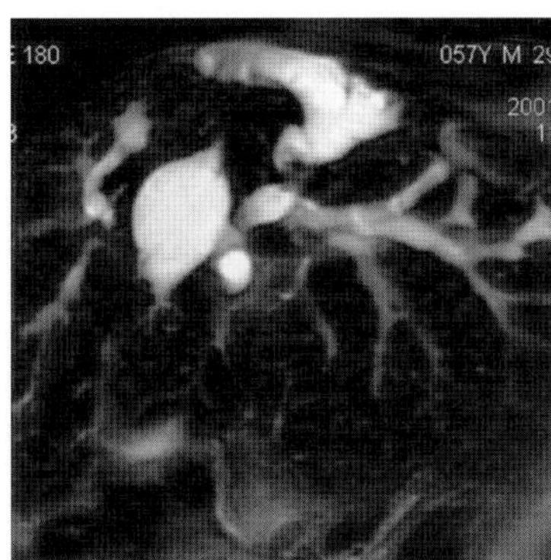

Fig. 14.62 MRC in the same patient as Fig. 16.60 confirms a bizarre pattern of biliary dilatation.

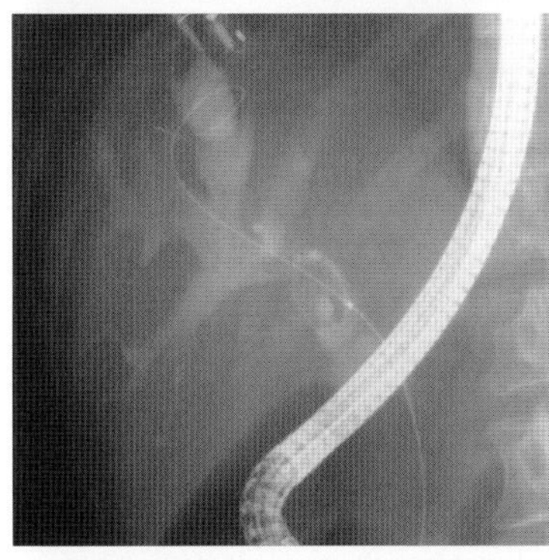

Fig. 14.63 ERCP demonstrating secondary ductal stone in Caroli's syndrome.

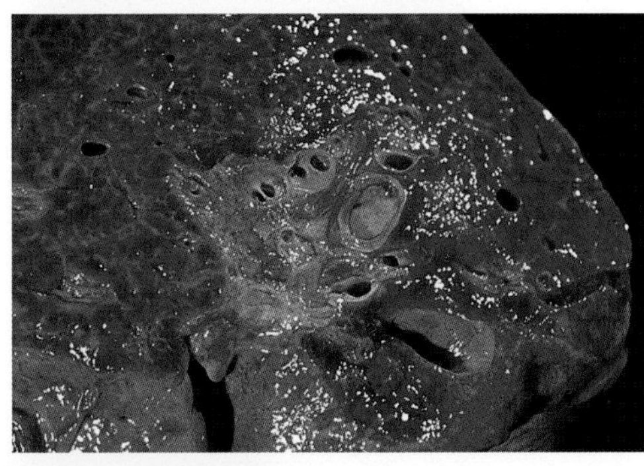

Fig. 14.64 Caroli's disease. Autopsy liver specimen from a patient with Caroli's disease transected through the porta hepatis showing the cystically dilated ductal profiles many of which contain purulent exudate from superimposed suppurative cholangitis.

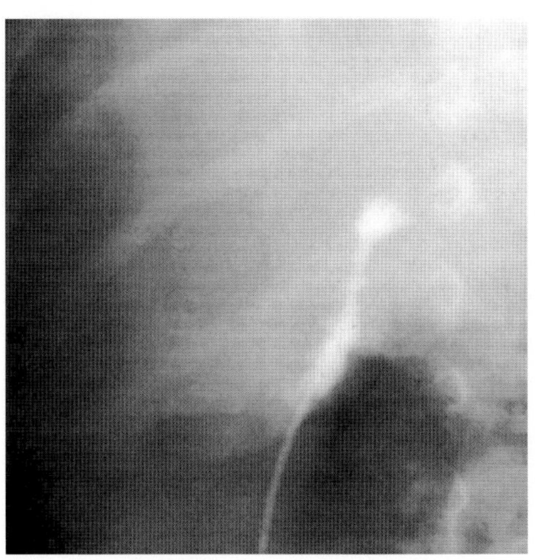

a

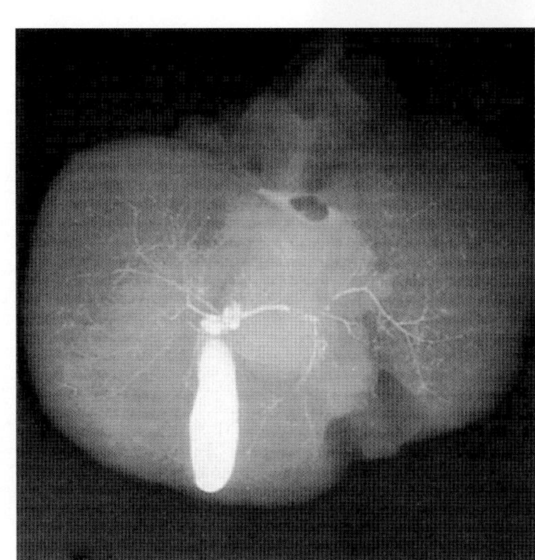

b

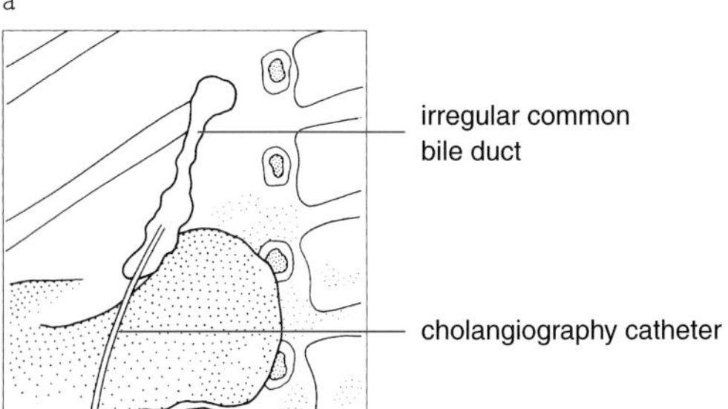

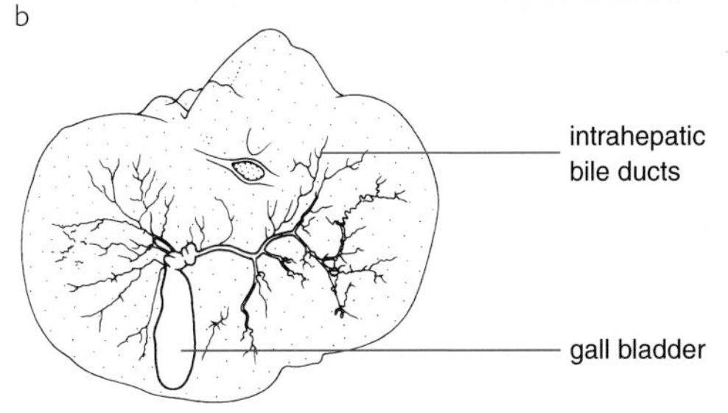

Fig. 14.65 Operative cholangiogram of an infant with intrahepatic biliary atresia (a) and of a normal liver (b). Courtesy of Dr G.M. Steiner.

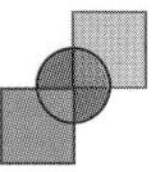

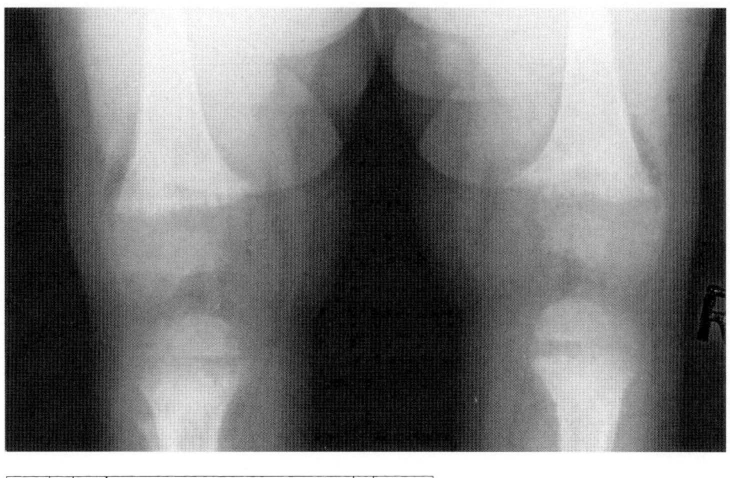

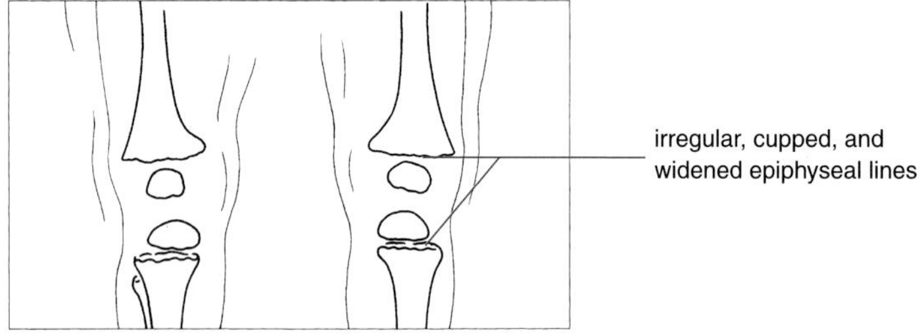

■ **Fig. 14.66** Radiograph of the legs of a child with biliary rickets.

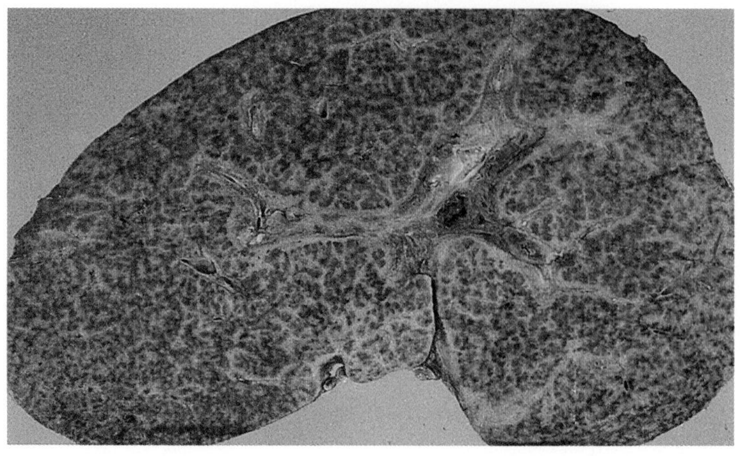

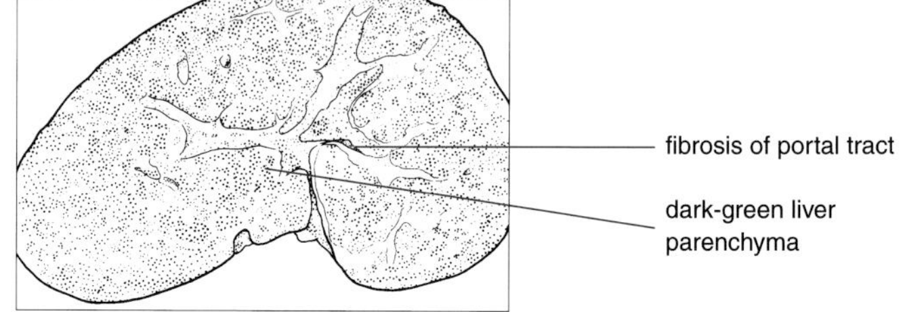

■ **Fig. 14.67** Liver section of extrahepatic biliary atresia showing extensive irregular fibrosis in portal tracts around the dark green hepatic parenchyma. Courtesy of Prof I.Talbot.

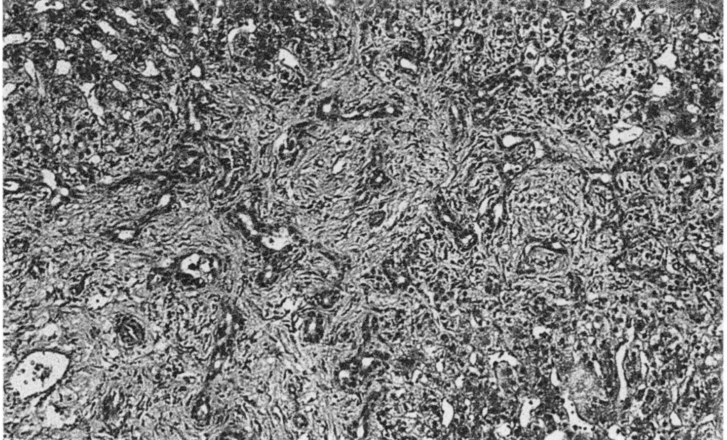

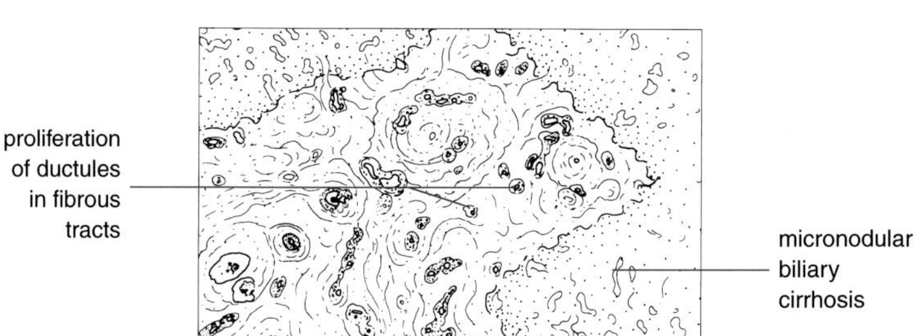

■ **Fig. 14.68** Extrahepatic biliary atresia showing portal fibrosis and proliferation of ductules. H&E stain (x 140). Courtesy of Prof B. Portmann.

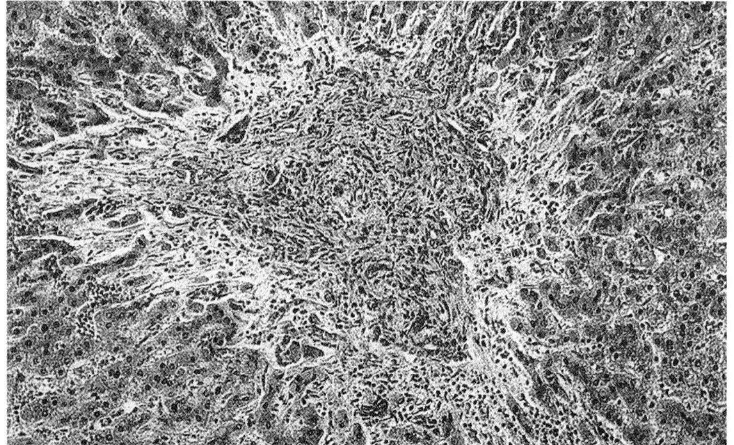

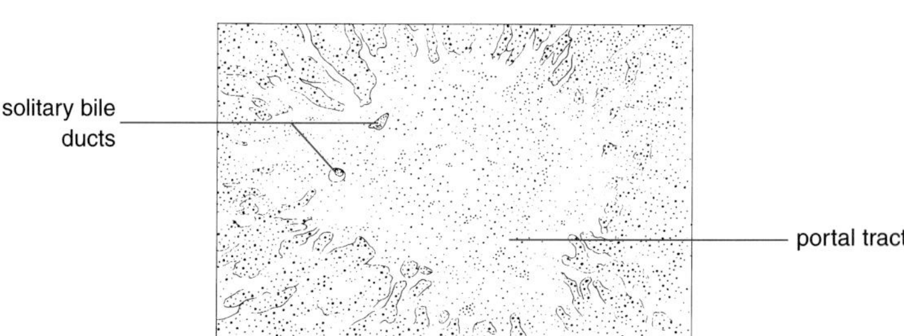

■ **Fig. 14.69** Intrahepatic biliary atresia showing paucity of intrahepatic ducts in the portal areas. H&E stain (x 180). Courtesy of Prof I.Talbot.

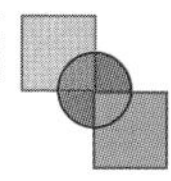

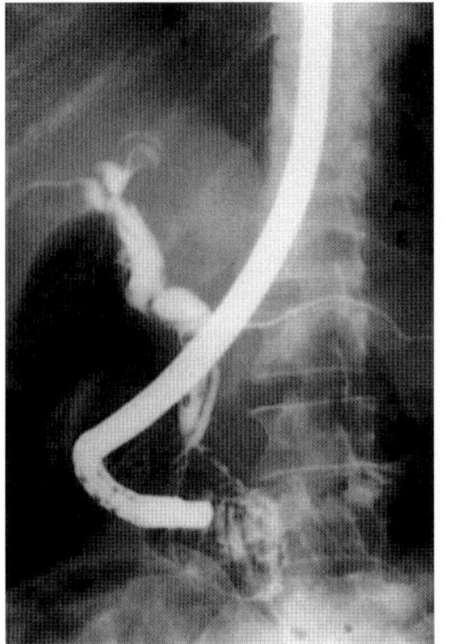

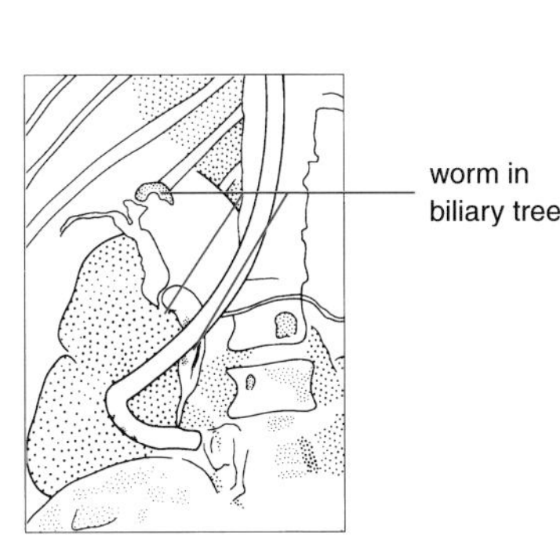

Fig. 14.70 Endoscopic retrograde cholangiogram showing Ascaris in the biliary tree.

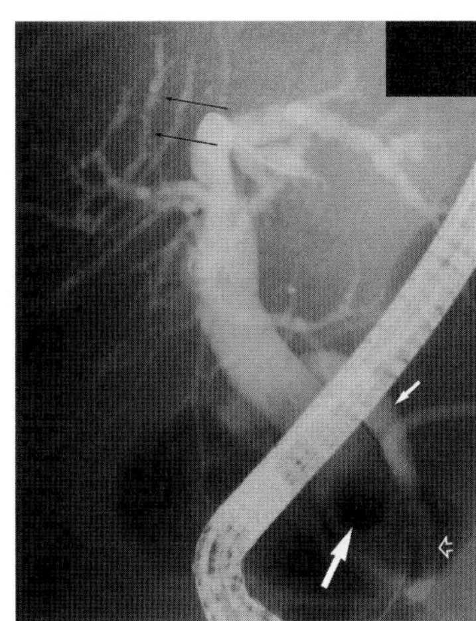

Fig. 14.71 Endoscopic retrograde cholangiogram in patient with bacterial cholangitis associated with common duct stone. A 1.1 cm radiolucent filling defect (large white arrow) is seen in a dilated distal common bile duct. Branches to the anterior segment of the right lobe of the liver have an irregular contour due to cholangitis (black arrows). The cystic duct (with a low entrance into the bile duct) is identified by the small white arrow. The main pancreatic duct is mildly dilated (open arrow) with an irregular contour due to prior pancreatitis.

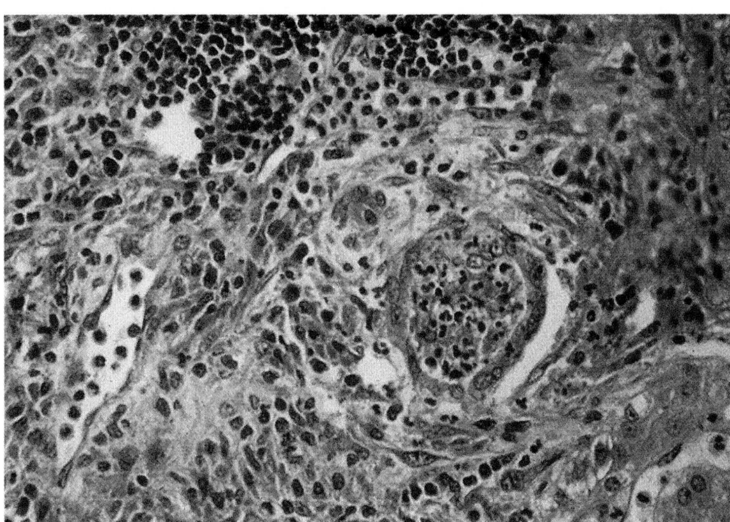

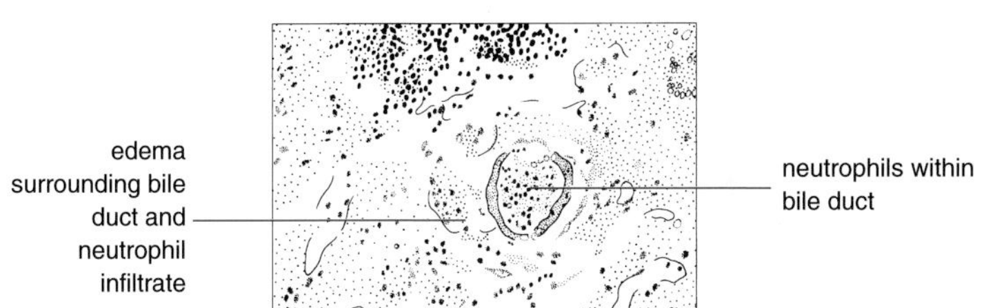

Fig. 14.72 Histology of ascending cholangitis showing an edematous portal tract infiltrated with inflammatory cells. H&E stain. Courtesy of Professor J.C.E. Underwood.

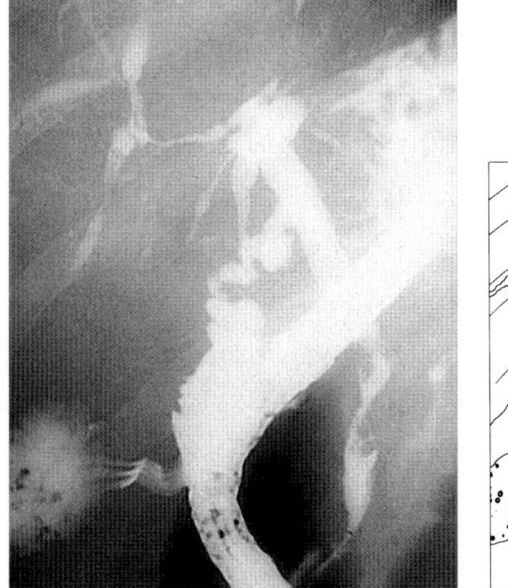

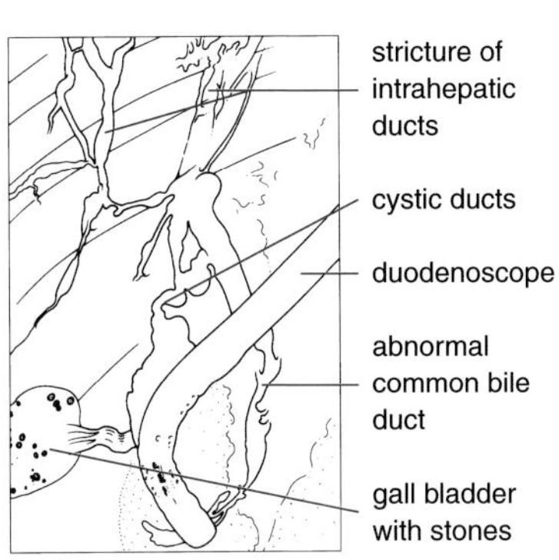

Fig. 14.73 Retrograde cholangiogram showing sclerosing cholangitis secondary to gallstones.

STRICTURING BILIARY DISEASE

Primary sclerosing cholangitis

Primary sclerosing cholangitis (PSC) is now the most common cause of benign stricture of the bile duct. About 5% of patients with inflammatory bowel disease develop PSC, and more than 70% of PSC patients have either UC or Crohn's disease (mostly the former). The disease may involve both intrahepatic and extrahepatic ducts (Figs 14.74, 14.75). ERCP is no longer the diagnostic modality of first choice, but may still be necessary as MRCP misses some early lesions. The sensitivity of the latter continues to improve in experienced hands.

The early histological changes consist of non-specific inflammatory fibrosis in the wall of the bile ducts (Fig. 14.76), but as the disease progresses, the portal tracts are thickened and the bile ducts become progressively obliterated (Fig. 14.77). Unfortunately, PSC is complicated by cholangiocarcinoma in a significant number of patients.

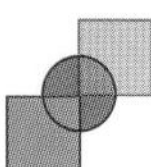

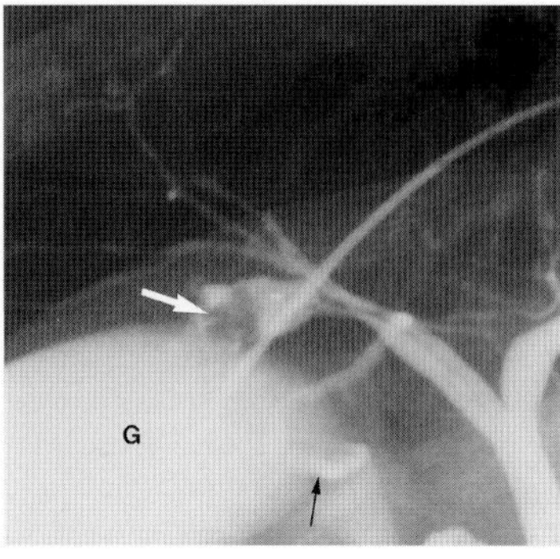

Fig. 14.74 Endoscopic retrograde cholangiogram demonstrating fungus ball in right hepatic duct in diabetic with fever. A 1 cm radiolucent filling defect (white arrow) with contrast in its interstices is seen in a dilated duct in the posterior segment of the right lobe of the liver. The gallbladder (G) and cystic duct (black arrow) are identified.

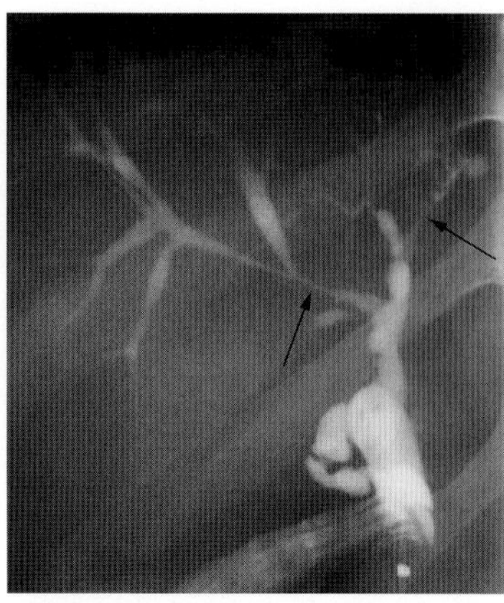

Fig. 14.75 Endoscopic retrograde cholangiogram demonstrating primary sclerosing cholangitis in a patient with ulcerative colitis. Numerous strictures (representative strictures identified by arrows) are seen in the intrahepatic biliary tree. Partial biliary obstruction is implied by the dilated biliary radicles proximal to the strictures.

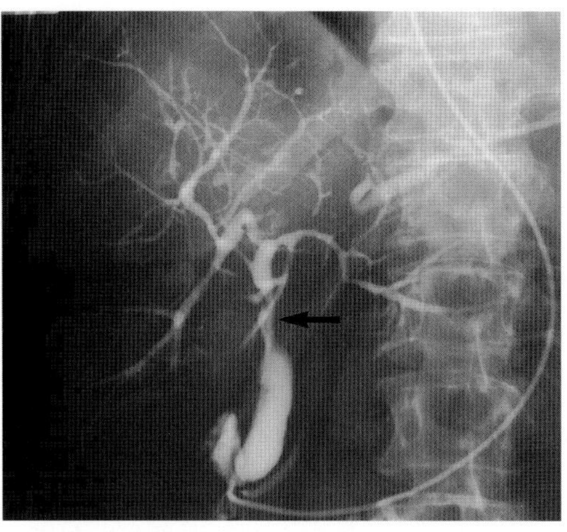

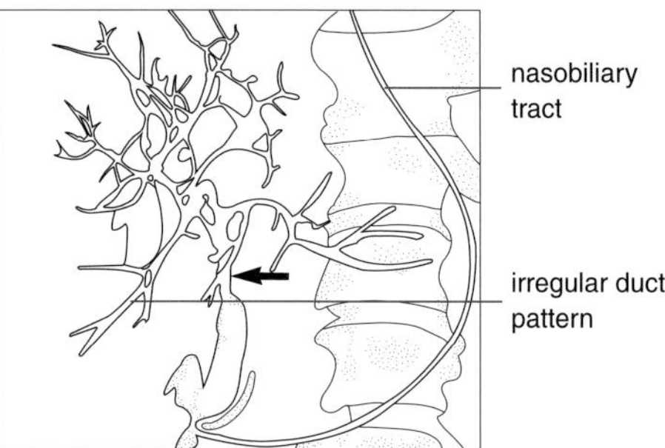

Fig. 14.76 Injection of nasobiliary tube demonstrating primary sclerosing cholangitis. Numerous areas of stricture formation and dilatation are seen in the intrahepatic biliary tree. A long stricture of the common hepatic duct (arrow) is present.

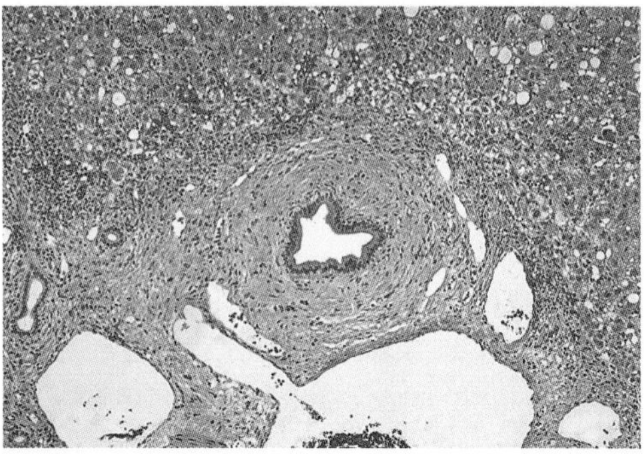

Fig. 14.77 Primary sclerosing cholangitis. Microscopic view of a portal tract showing the concentric periductal fibrosis that results from chronic large duct obstruction.

Other benign biliary strictures

Benign strictures of the extrahepatic biliary system occasionally accompany bile duct stones, owing to complicating cholangitis (Fig. 14.78), and may be seen as a complication of cholecystectomy (Fig. 14.79) and more particularly so after bile duct exploration. These strictures are either secondary to direct trauma, anastomotic narrowing or ischemic in nature. Liver transplantation is, more than most, an operative procedure prone to subsequent stricture formation (Fig. 14.80), but apparent stricturing in the early post-operative phase may be simply the result of a mis-match in duct size between donor and recipient (Fig. 14.81); although technically undesirable it is not necessarily followed by any ill effects (Fig. 14.81). Ischemic strictures can follow apparently uncomplicated biliary tree surgery due, it is assumed, to transient interruption of the blood supply to the bile duct. Rarely there may be dilatation secondary to stones in the cystic duct compressing the main bile duct (Mirizzi syndrome). Benign strictures of whatever cause are often complicated further by proximal stones that can be often challenging for interventional endoscopists. Pancreatitis may lead to compression of the lower end of the common bile duct giving the impression of a biliary stricture, but this is usually transient and resolves once the pan-creatic inflammation subsides (Fig. 14.82). Occasionally strictures are seen without any obvious explanation (Fig. 14.83). Biliary atresia is discussed above.

TUMORS OF THE GALL BLADDER AND BILE DUCTS

Benign tumors and polyps

True neoplastic polyps of the gall bladder and biliary tree are rare (Fig. 14.84) but, like adenomas elsewhere in the gastrointestinal tract, they consist of dysplastic branching acini of columnar epithelium (Fig. 14.85). Tumor-like polyps are commoner (Fig. 14.86). These may be little more than single prominent villi distended into a polypoid excrescence by cholesterol-laden macrophages (Fig. 14.87), but more often they will be adenomyomas (Fig. 14.88). Adenomyomas are more common in the fundus where they produce a filling defect on cholecystography or ultrasound. Microscopically, the adenomyoma is a complex of muscle and out-pouching of the gall bladder mucosa. Papillary lesions may undergo malignant transformation.

Carcinoma of the gall bladder

Carcinoma of the gall bladder is an uncommon cause of jaundice in the elderly, but one which is strongly associated with gallstones (Figs 14.89, 14.90). It is usually first diagnosed at an advanced inoperable stage as the tumor may be very large before symptoms occur (Fig. 14.91). Macroscopically, carcinoma of the gall bladder is usually diffuse but polypoid varieties may be found. Tumors tend to spread by direct invasion into the adjacent liver. Histologically, the majority are adenocarcinomas (Figs 14.92, 14.93).

Carcinoma of the bile duct/cholangiocarcinoma

PSC and cholangiocarcinoma are the two most common causes of obstruction at the hilum of the liver. A typical presentation is with progressive painless cholestatic jaundice. PSC presents a particular diagnostic challenge as it is itself a key premalignant condition with a lifetime risk of secondary cholangiocarcinoma of about 15%. The diagnosis of malignancy is suspected from combinations of imaging techniques including ultrasonography (Fig. 14.94), CT, and cholangiography (Figs 14.95, 14.96). The hilar Klatskin tumor is often difficult to see on CT or MR, but may show peripheral enhancement with IV contrast MRI (Figs 14.97, 14.98).

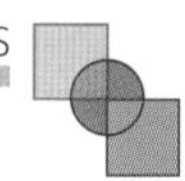

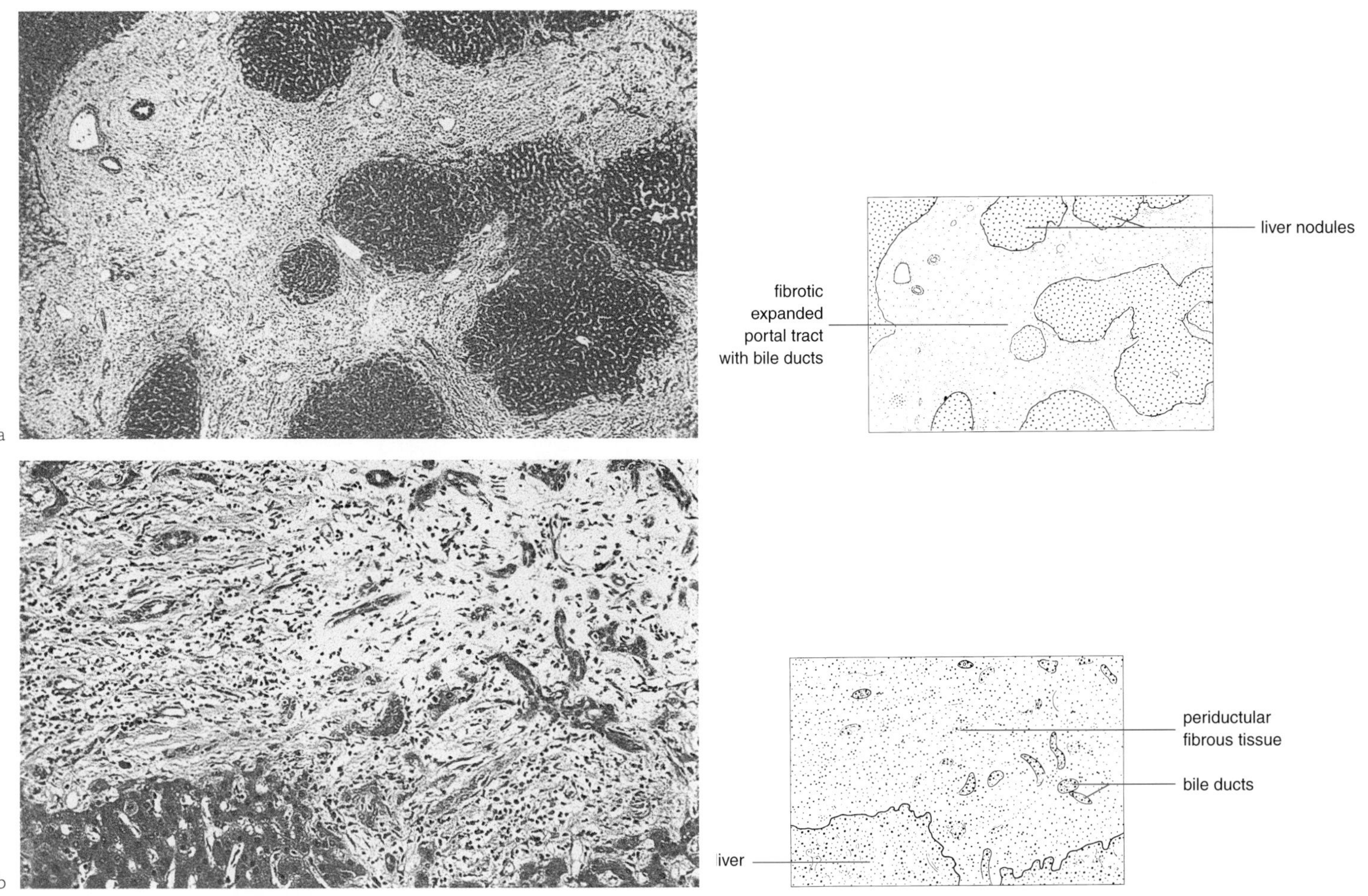

Fig. 14.78 Advanced stage primary sclerosing cholangitis with chronic cholangitis and secondary biliary cirrhosis developing. H&E stain (x 75, upper; x 180, lower).

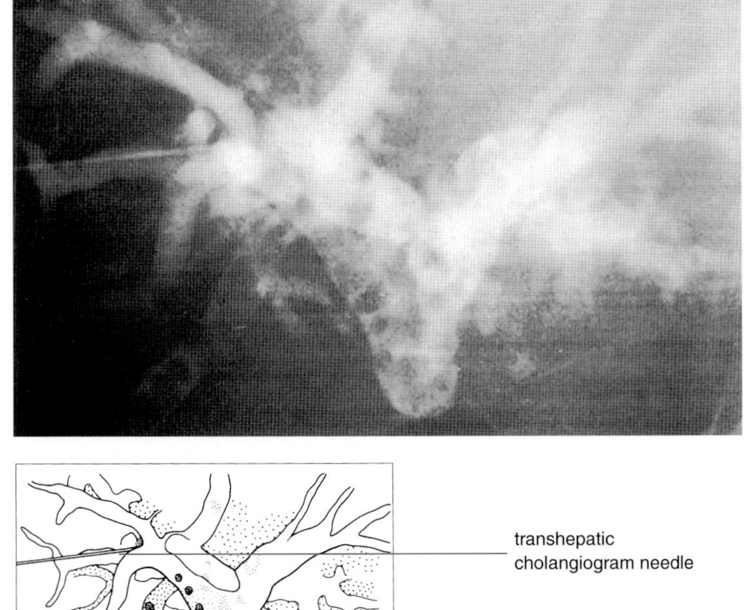

Fig. 14.79 Percutaneous transhepatic cholangiogram showing a stricture of the common hepatic duct associated with gross intrahepatic stone disease. Courtesy of Dr M.C. Collins.

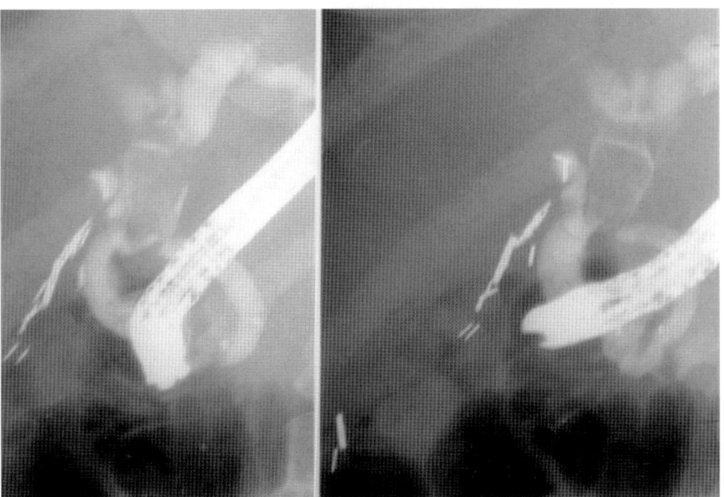

Fig. 14.80 Large bile duct stone above a stricture itself most probably a direct consequence of prior cholecystectomy.

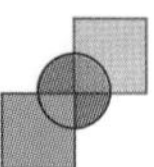

Cancer of the bile duct may also involve peripheral ducts (intrahepatic cholangiocarcinoma), or extrahepatic ducts (Figs 14.99–14.101); the common bile duct is usually implicated to some extent. The tumor may spread in continuity to the ampulla (Figs 14.102, 14.103), but it remains an entity distinct in behavior and prognosis from ampullary carcinoma (see Chapter 3).

Bile duct malignancies are usually adenocarcinomas (Fig. 14.104) and, when intrahepatic, are often indistinguishable from metastatic adenocarcinoma from other sites. The presence of a fibrous stroma distinguishes bile duct cancer (Fig. 14.105) from hepatocellular

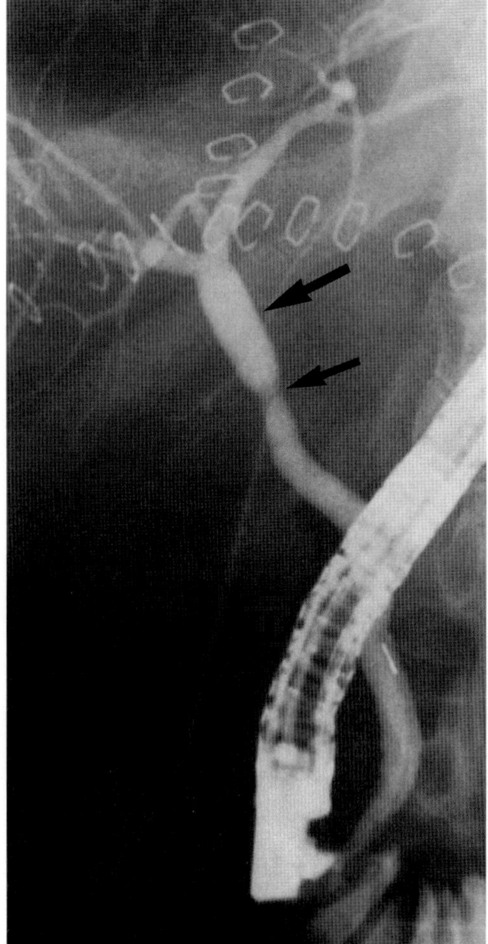

Fig. 14.81 Mild stricture at choledochostomy after liver transplant. A thin, smooth annular narrowing (shorter arrow) is present at the biliary anastomosis. Mild dilatation of the transplant hepatic duct (longer arrow) is seen.

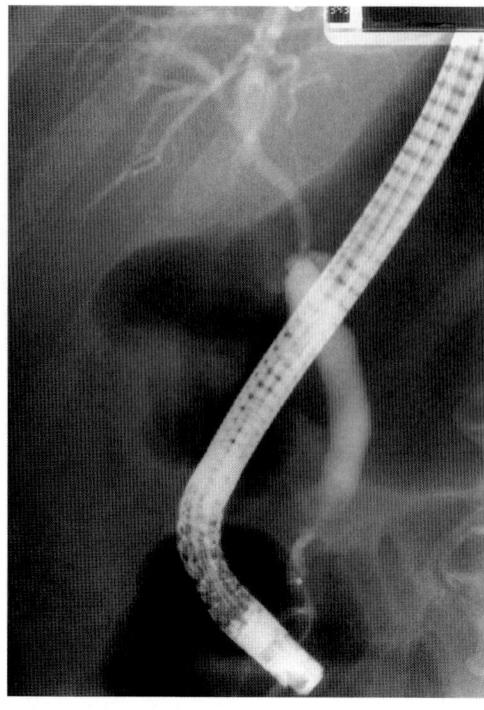

Fig. 14.82 Cholangiogram demonstrating a relatively harmless mismatch in caliber between the donor and recipient biliary trees after liver transplantation.

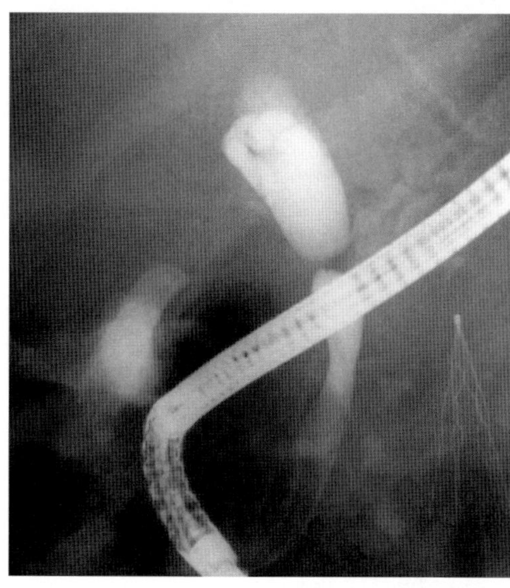

Fig. 14.84 Benign biliary stricture of unknown etiology. A vena caval umbrella is also present,

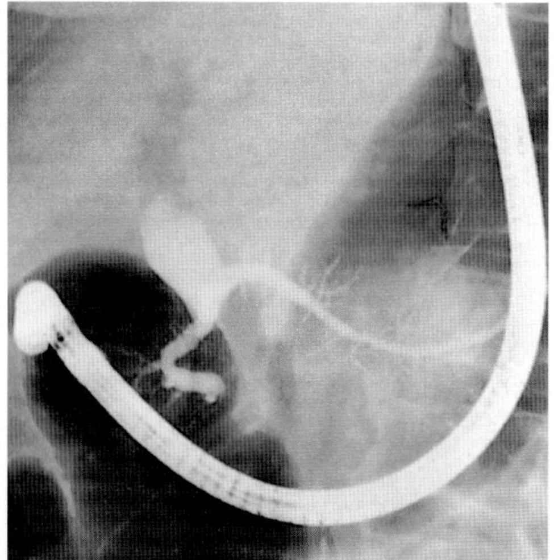

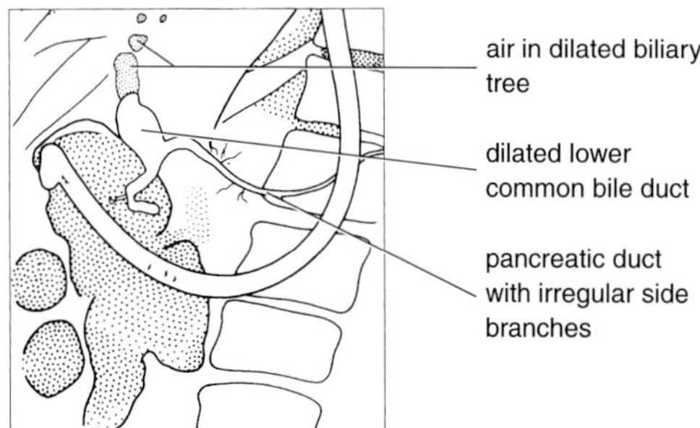

Fig. 14.83 Endoscopic retrograde cholangiopan-creaticogram showing bile duct compression due to pancreatitis. Note the grossly irregular side branches of the pancreatic duct.

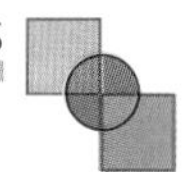

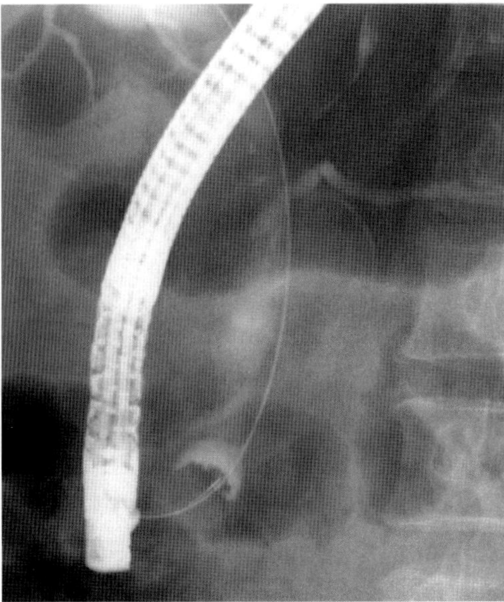

Fig. 14.85 Unusual benign adenoma of the distal common bile duct.

carcinoma, in which a glandular pattern is more commonly seen. This fibrous characteristic may make histological and cytological diagnosis difficult as biopsies may fail, and brushings may include no cellular material.

Other malignancies of the biliary tract

Almost all other neoplastic lesions found in the biliary tree are the result of secondary infiltration, most particularly from the pancreas (see Chapter 9), but occasionally a lymphoma may target the hilar areas and lead to a primary biliary presentation (Figs 14.106–14.108).

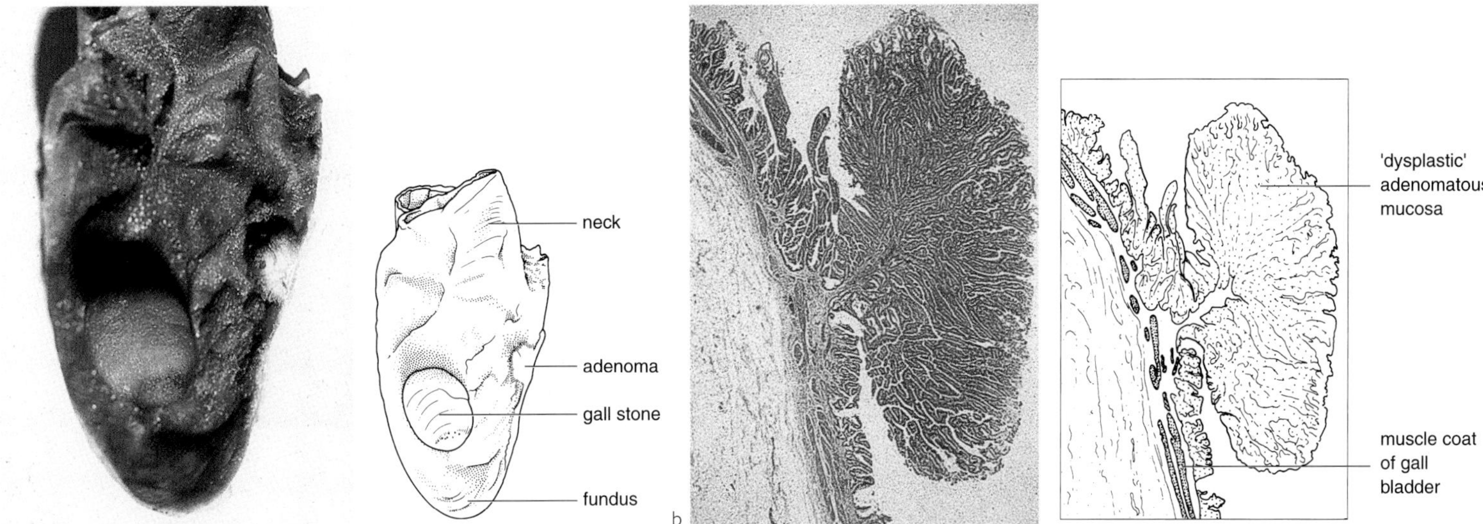

Fig. 14.86 The cut surface of an adenoma is visible in this gall bladder, which also contains a stone (a). The histological appearance is that of dysplastic adenomatous mucosa (b).

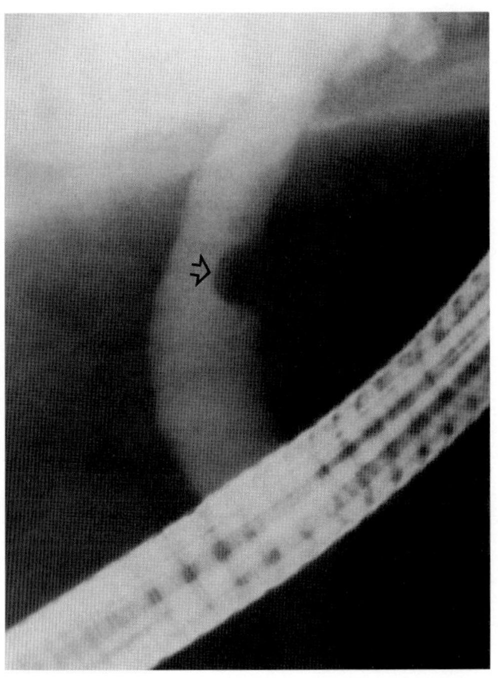

Fig. 14.87 Endoscopic retrograde cholangiogram demonstrating a polyp in the common bile cut. A 5 mm hemispheric protrusion (arrow) into the contrast column is seen. This was an inflammatory polyp.

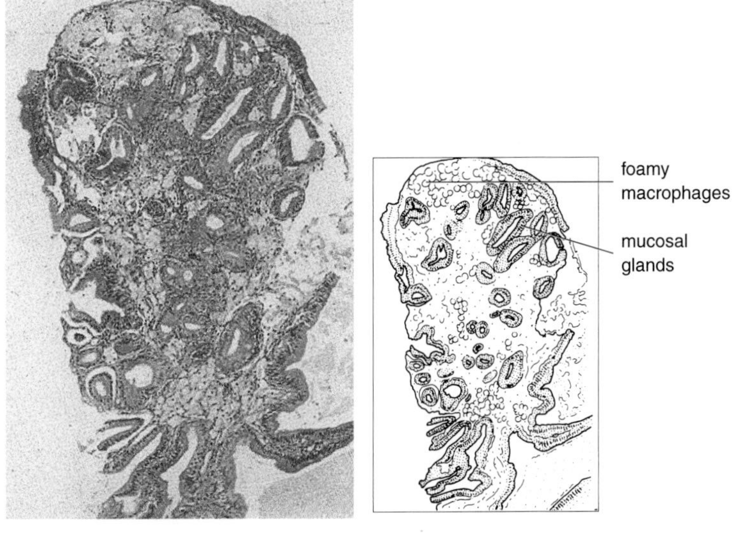

Fig. 14.88 A polyp of the mucosa caused by cholesterolosis. H&E stain (x 50).

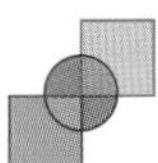

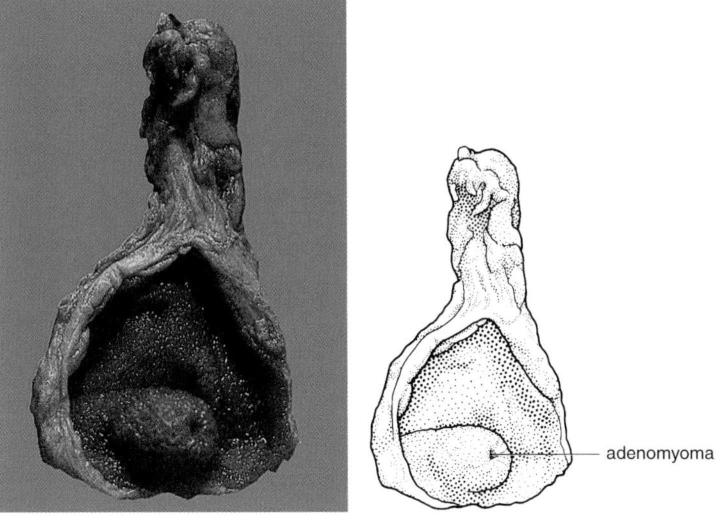

■ **Fig. 14.89** A gall bladder showing a fundal adenomyoma.

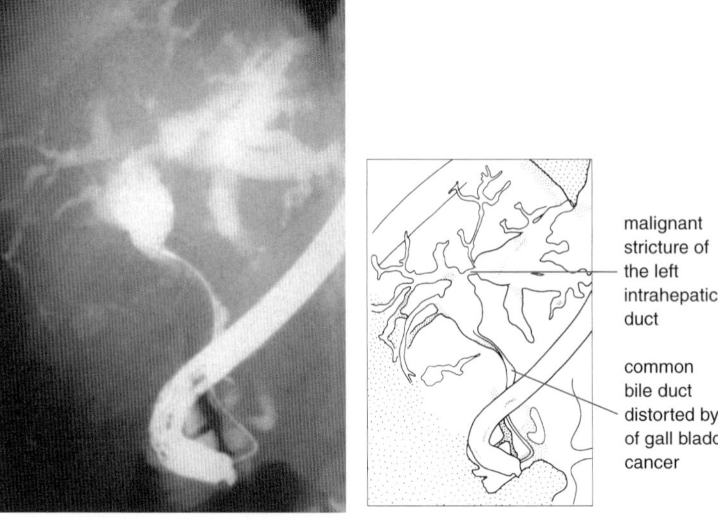

■ **Fig. 14.92** Endoscopic retrograde cholangiogram showing distortion of the bile duct due to carcinoma of the gall bladder. Obstruction of the left intrahepatic duct system caused by tumor is also apparent. Courtesy of Dr M.C. Collins.

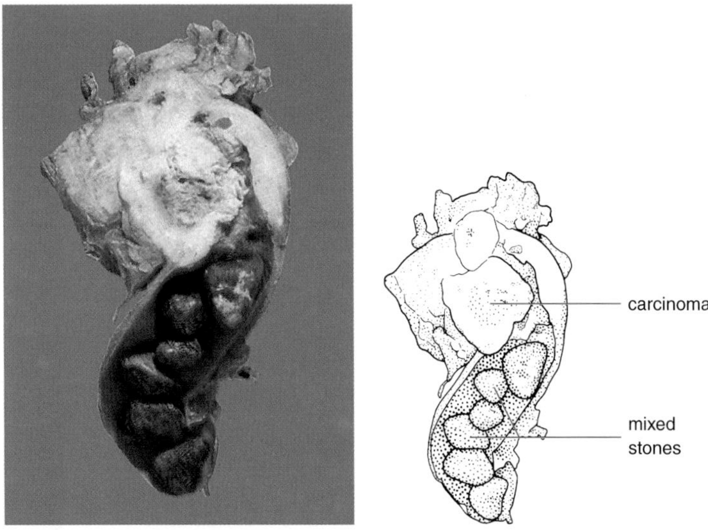

■ **Fig. 14.90** Carcinoma of the neck of the gall bladder.

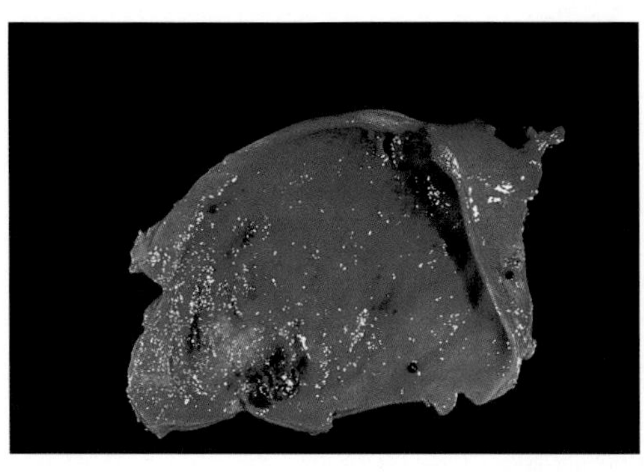

■ **Fig. 14.93** Carcinoma of the gallbladder. Cholecystectomy specimen containing an unsuspected carcinoma seen as an irregular yellow-tan mass with focal hemorrhage in the fundus.

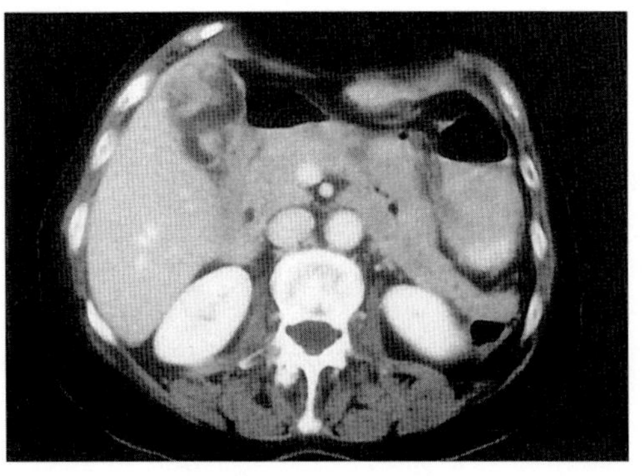

■ **Fig. 14.91** CT scan showing carcinoma of the gall bladder. Gallstone and inspissated bile are readily visible. Courtesy of Dr R.A. Nakielny.

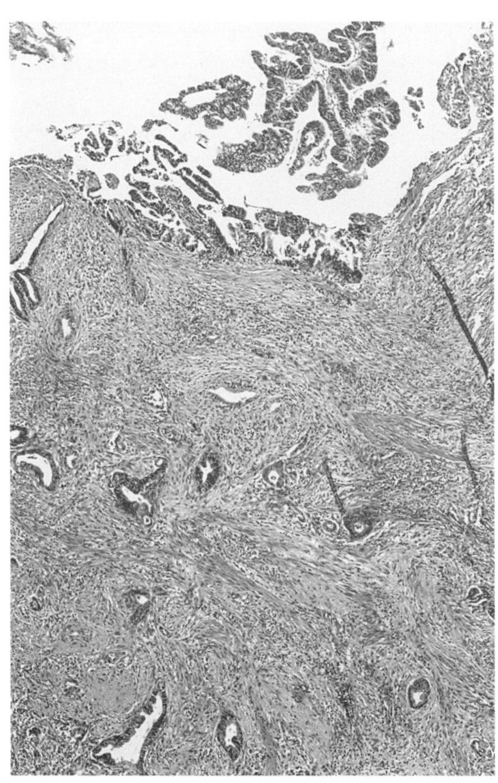

■ **Fig. 14.94** Carcinoma of the gallbladder. Microscopic view of transmurally invasive adenocarcinoma developing from high-grade dysplasia of the overlying mucosa.

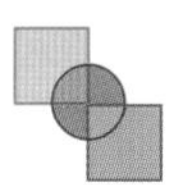

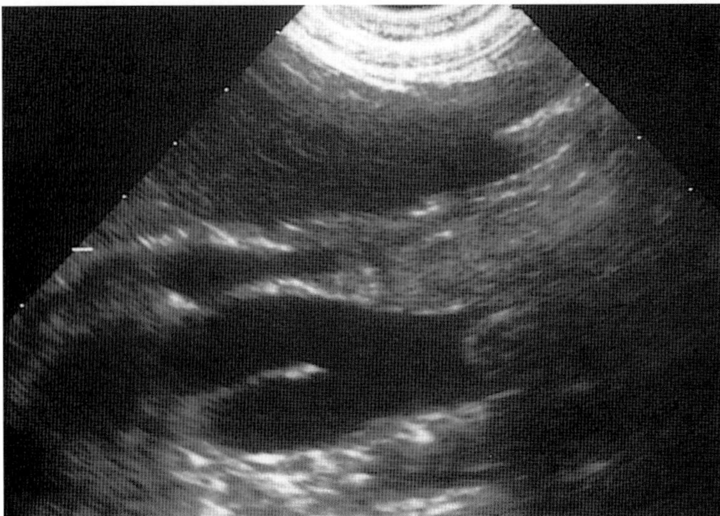

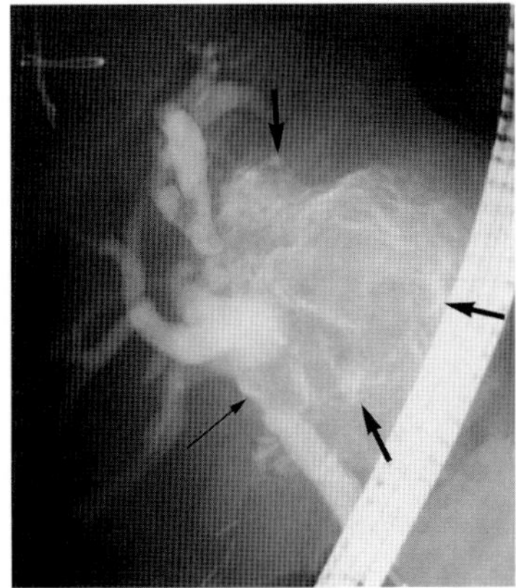

■ **Fig. 14.96** ERCP showing intrahepatic cholangiocarcinoma of the left lobe of the liver invading the proximal common hepatic duct (thin arrow). Contrast fills the interstices of the tumor (thick arrows).

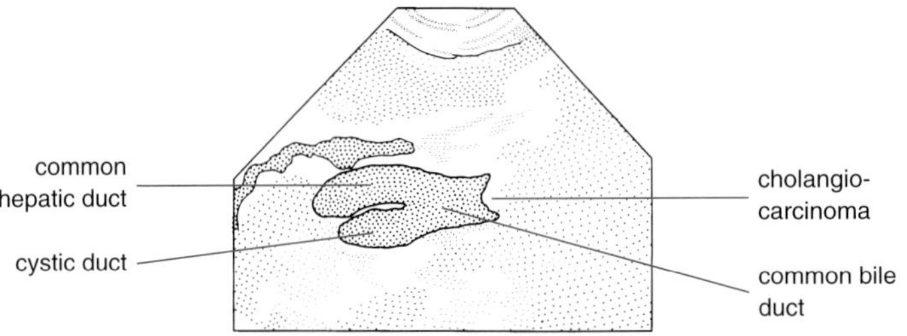

■ **Fig. 14.95** Ultrasonogram showing cholangiocarcinoma of the common bile duct just below the entry of the cystic duct. The smooth rounded appearance of the tumor could be readily mistaken for a stone. Courtesy of Dr M.C. Collins.

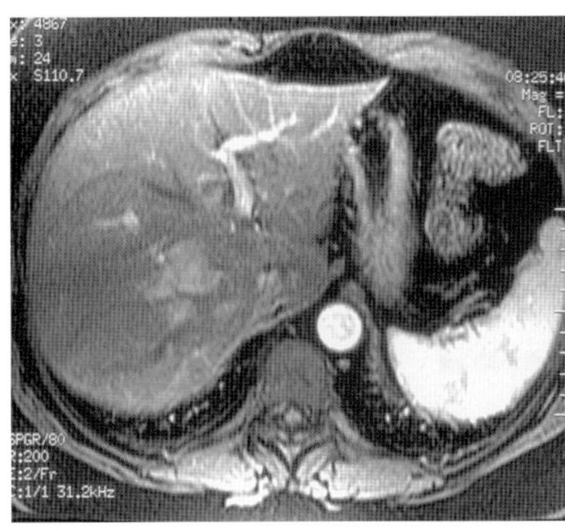

■ **Fig. 14.98** The arterial phase of MRI scanning in a hilar Klatskin tumor.

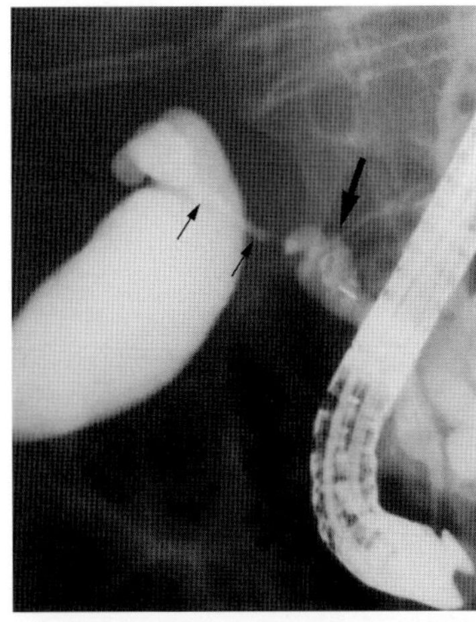

a

■ **Fig. 14.97** ERCP and CT demonstrating cholangiocarcinoma with biliary obstruction. (a) Endoscopic retrograde cholangiogram demonstrating abrupt cut-off of the common hepatic duct (long arrow). A mass in the porta hepatis extrinsically compresses the cystic duct (short arrows). The etiology of this appearance could be to primary cholangiocar-cinoma or extrinsic tumor invading the porta hepatis. (b) Corticomedullary differentiation in the left kidney and dense contrast in the aorta identify this as an image obtained in late arterial/early portal venous phase. Diffuse biliary dilatation is seen (short arrow identifies dilated branch to right lobe). A low-attenuation mass (mid-length arrow) surrounds the hepatic artery (long arrow). Low-attenuation tumor is questionably seen in the left lobe of the liver. (c) Contrast in the renal collecting systems identifies this as a 'delayed' CT image. The hepatic artery (long arrow) is barely visible. Tumor in the porta hepatis (short arrow) demonstrates delayed contrast enhancement. Compare the density of tumor to that of the right portal vein (arrowhead). (d) Tumor in the left lobe of the liver is now clearly identified by its delayed contrast enhancement (arrows).

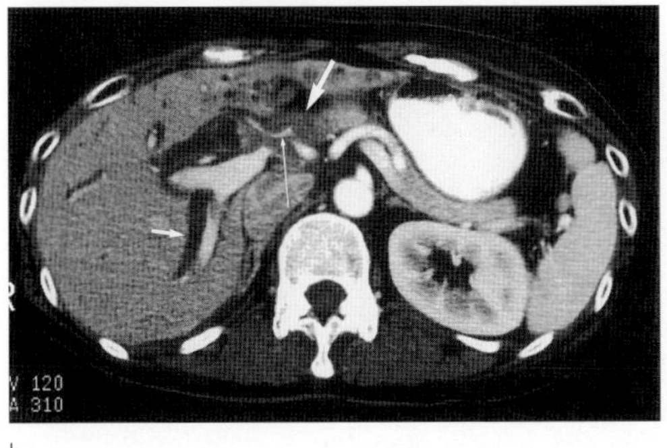

b

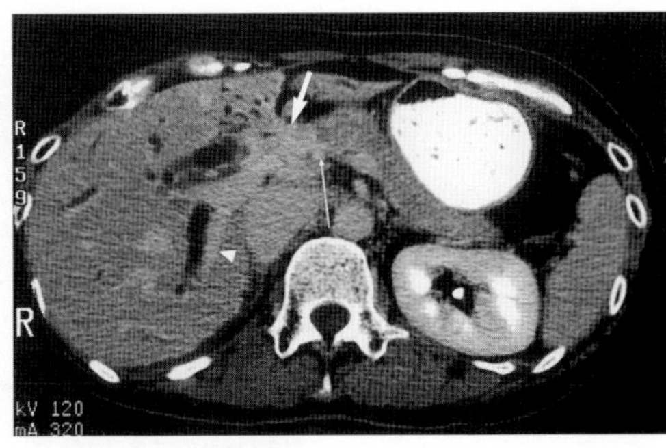

c

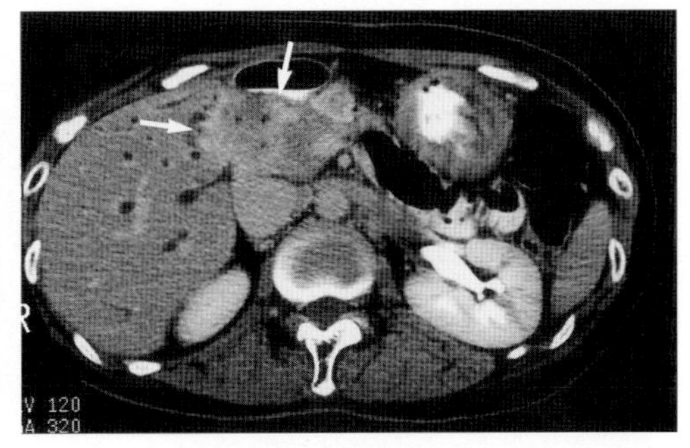

d

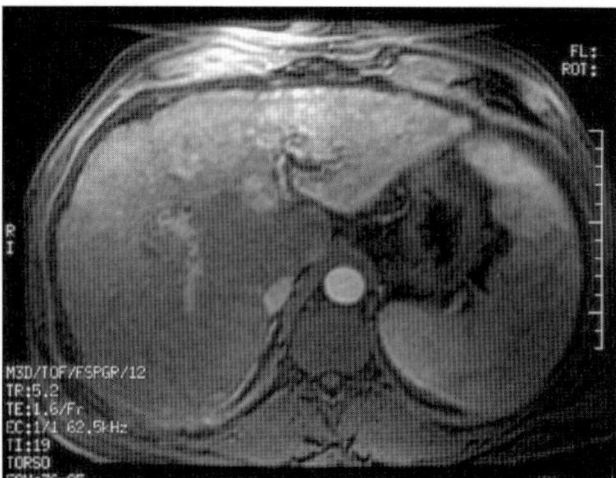

Fig. 14.99 The change in the contrast pattern seen in the venous phase supports the diagnosis.

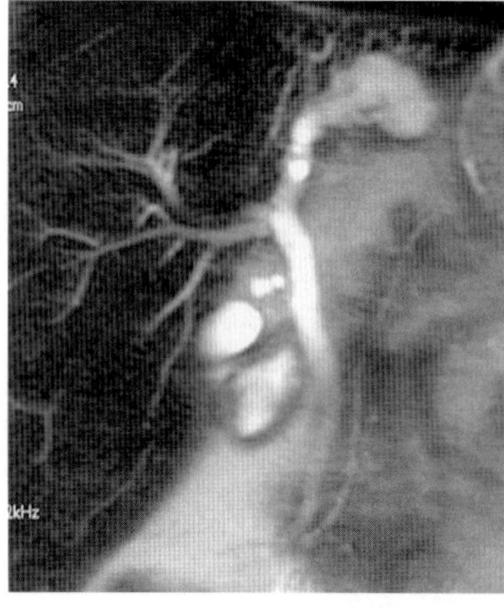

Fig. 14.100 MRC of high left hepatic duct cholangiocarcinoma. Courtesy of Ihab Kamel, MD.

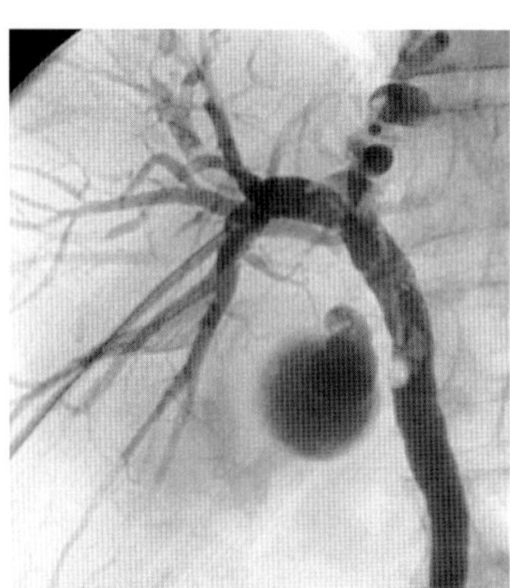

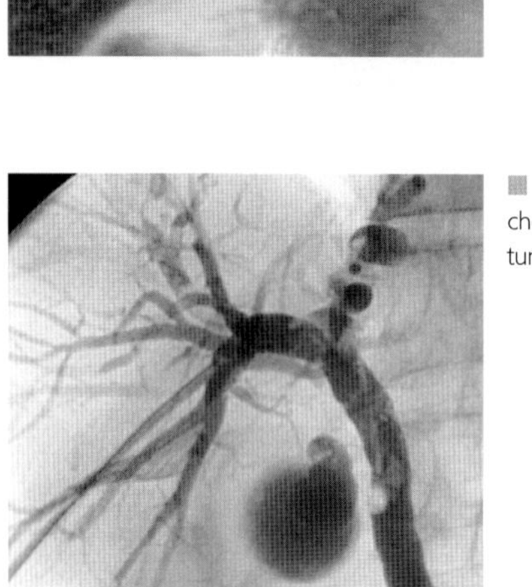

Fig. 14.101 Percutaneous cholangiogram of the same hepatic duct tumor. Courtesy of Ihab Kamel, MD.

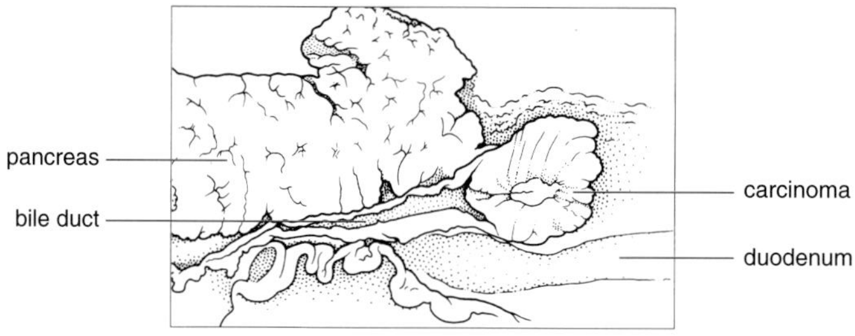

Fig. 14.102 Carcinoma of the bile duct in the middle third. Courtesy of Prof K. Weinbren.

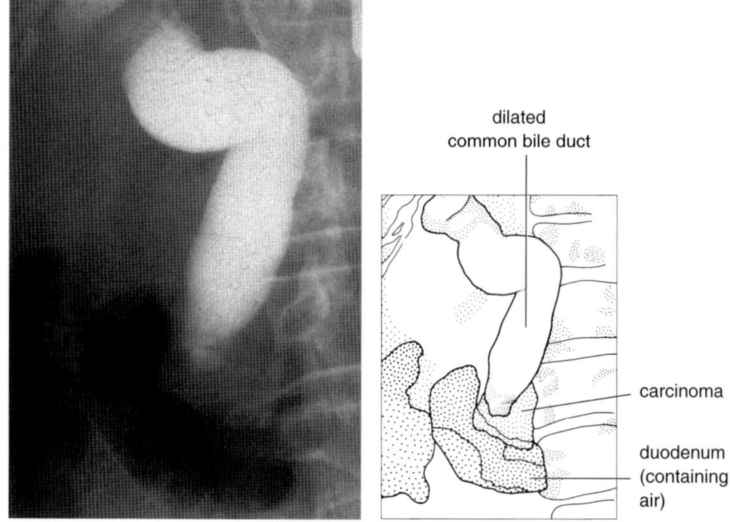

Fig. 14.103 Cholangiogram showing obstruction due to a carcinoma at the lower end of the bile duct which protrudes into the duodenum. Courtesy of Dr M.C. Collins.

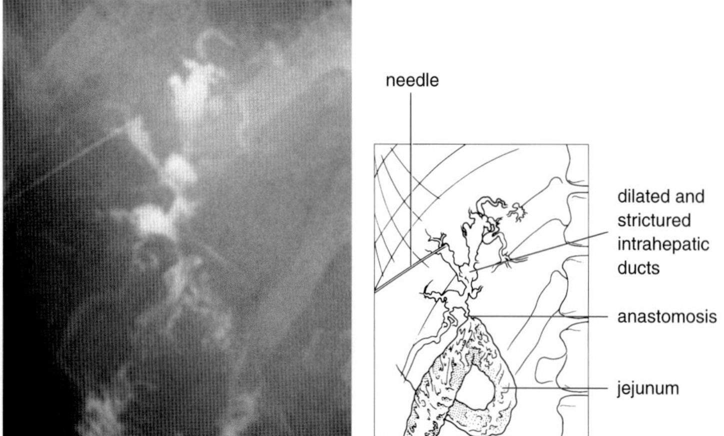

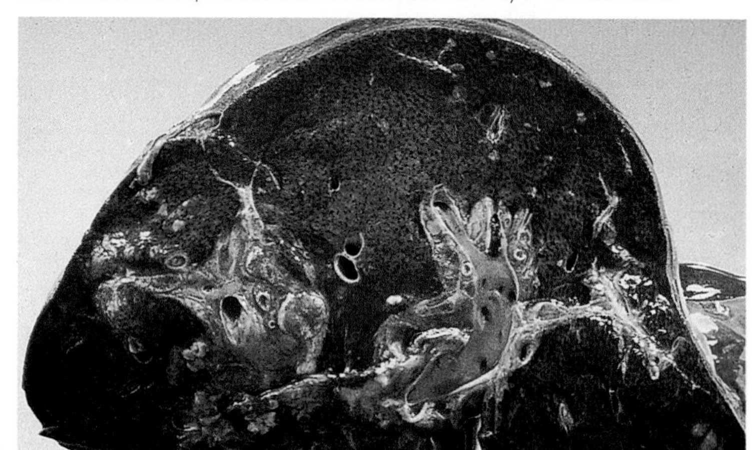

Fig. 14.104 Percutaneous transhepatic cholangiogram (a) showing invasion of the intrahepatic bile ducts by carcinoma of the bile ducts after a choledochojejunostomy. The liver of the same patient removed at post-mortem (b) shows infiltrating carcinoma.

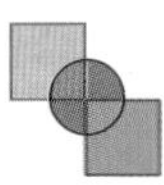

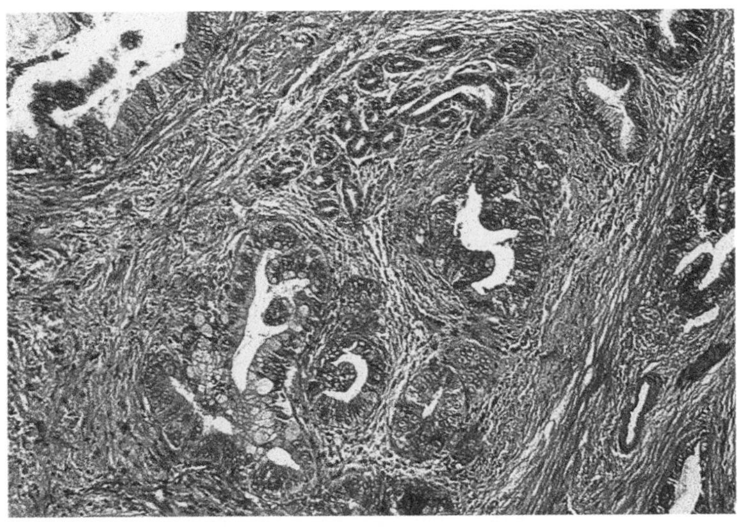

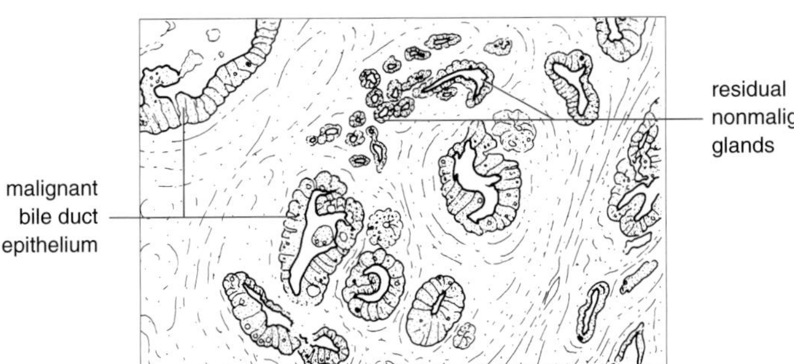

■ **Fig. 14.105** Typical bile duct adenocarcinoma replacing the normal structure. H&E stain (x 160). Courtesy of Prof K. Weinbren.

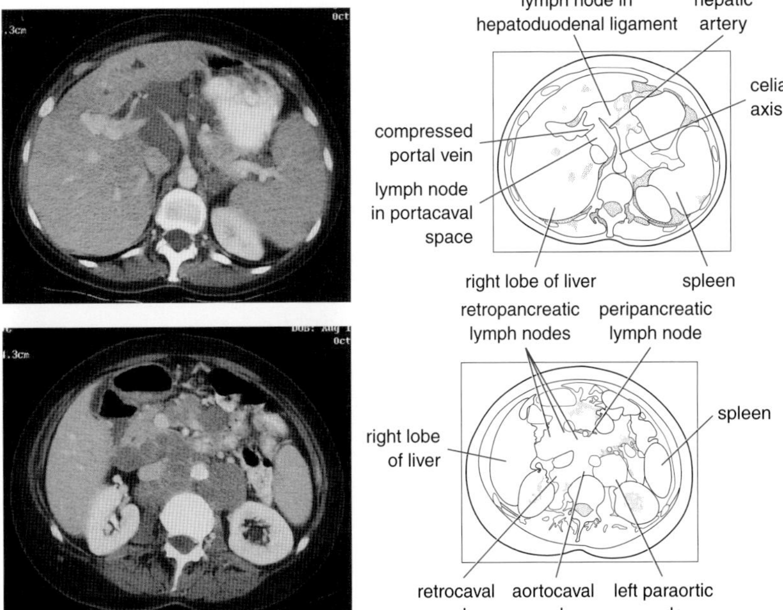

■ **Fig. 14.107** Mantle cell lymphoma invading the porta hepatis. CT through the level of the celiac axis shows enlarged lymph nodes in the hepatoduodenal ligament and in the portacaval space compressing the portal vein. CT through the level of the pancreatic head shows enlarged lymph nodes in the peripancreatic, retrocaval, aortocaval, and left para-aortic regions.

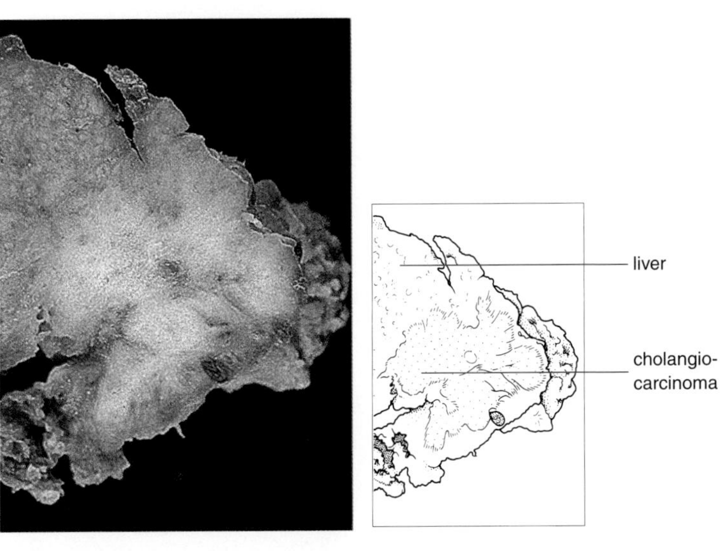

■ **Fig. 14.106** A typical cholangiocarcinoma with its sclerotic outline in contrast to the hepatocellular carcinomas depicted in Chapter 13. Courtesy of Prof K. Weinbren.

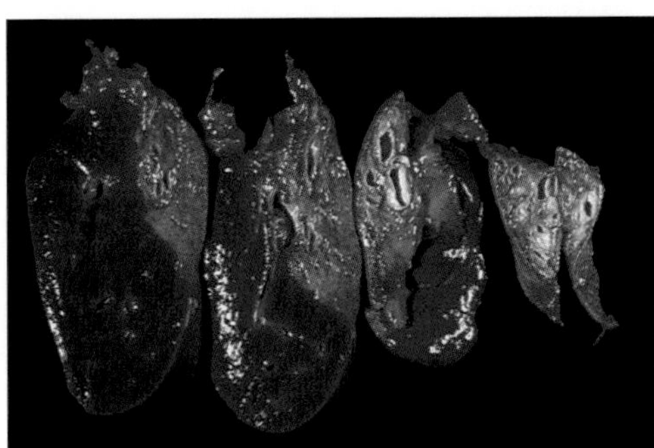

■ **Fig. 14.108** Partial hepatectomy specimen with obstructive cholangiocarcinoma showing dilated bile ducts within an irregular yellow-tan mass that merges with the cholestatic, green-tinged adjacent liver parenchyma.

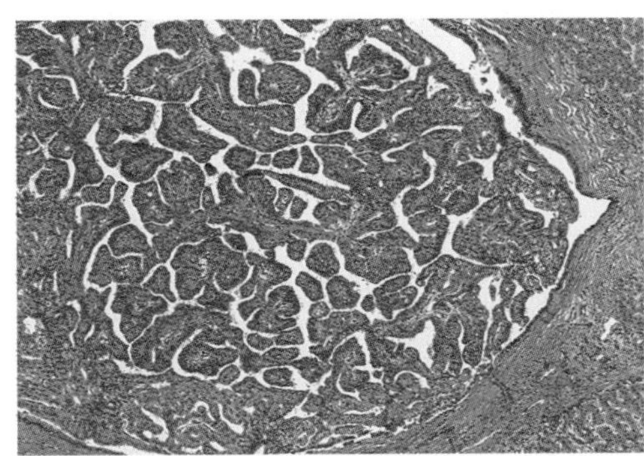

■ **Fig. 14.109** Cholangiocarcinoma. Microscopic section through a bile duct adjacent to an invasive cholangiocarcinoma showing carcinoma *in situ* with a papillary growth pattern filling and expanding the lumen.

INDEX

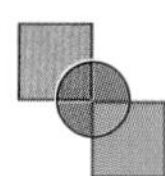